Parkinson's Disease

Diagnosis and Clinical Management

Parkinson's Disease

Diagnosis and Clinical Management

Stewart A. Factor, D.O.
William J. Weiner, M.D.
Editors

DEMOS

New York

Demos Medical Publishing, Inc., 386 Park Avenue South, New York, New York 10016

Library of Congress Cataloging-in-Publication Data
Parkinson's disease : diagnosis and clinical management / Stewart A.
Factor, William J. Weiner, editors.
    p. ; cm.
Included bibliographical references and index.
    ISBN 1-888799-50-1 (hardcover)
1. Parkinson's disease.
    [DNLM: 1. Parkinson Disease—diagnosis. 2. Parkinson Disease—therapy.
WL 359-P24678 2002] I. Factor, Stewart A., 1956– II. Weiner, William J.
    RC382 .P2644 2002
    616.8'33—dc21

                                                              2002002212

Made in the United States of America

Dedication

For my wife, Ann Marie, and my daughters, Katie and Rachel, who provide me with
unconditional love and support.
And for my parents, Mildred and Harry, who taught me well.

S.A.F.

To my friends and colleagues who did so much and left so early.

Harold L. Klawans, M.D.
C. David Marsden, D.Ss., F.R.C.P., F.R.S.
John "Jack" Penny, Jr., M.D.

W.J.W.

CONTENTS

Foreword

With Parkinson's disease research, both basic and clinical, moving at a fast pace, Doctors Factor and Weiner have seized the moment to bring out a comprehensive monograph on this disorder. Research on Parkinson's disease has for decades led the way in pioneering therapeutic advances in the field of neurodegenerative illnesses. Uncovering the biochemical basis of its symptoms and signs made it the first neurodegenerative disease effectively ameliorated by neurotransmitter replacement therapy and subsequently neurotransmitter agonist therapy. Stereotaxic surgery also pioneered with Parkinson's and has resulted in major therapeutic advances, initially with ablations in the thalamus and pallidum and more recently with continuous electrical stimulation in these nuclei and, even more effectively, in the subthalamic nucleus. These therapeutic milestones have not as yet been achieved in any other neurodegenerative disorder.

Beyond symptomatic therapy, though, is protective therapy, restorative therapy, neuronal replacement therapy and gene therapy, and again research on Parkinson's has led the way. Protective therapy is the slowing of the rate of progression or even preventing further progression. There have been and continue to be clinical trials evaluating antioxidants, glutamate antagonists, mitochondrial enhancers and neurotrophic factors as protective therapies. Restorative therapy is the recovery of injured but not-yet-dead neurons, and clinical trials with neuroimmunophyllins are under way. Neuronal replacement therapy is undergoing trials with surgical implantation of fetal cells, and one can anticipate similar attempts in the not distant future with stem cells that have been converted to neurons with the biochemical features of the cells lost in Parkinson's disease. Animal models tested with gene therapy have already shown symptomatic benefit from implantation of cells inserted with genes that form enzymes critical for the synthesis of dopamine.

Parkinson's was also the first neurodegenerative disease to be monitored with positron emission tomography (PET) and single photon emission computed tomography (SPECT). With the radioligand fluorodopa, PET scans show deficient biosynthetic enzyme, dopa decarboxylase, and deficient dopamine transmitter uptake in striatal dopaminergic nerve terminals in the striatum. With ligands that bind to the dopamine transporter, SPECT scans have revealed its deficiency, serving as another indicator for loss of these striatal nerve terminals. Potentially, these PET and SPECT scans can serve as biomarkers for diagnosis and also for the rate of progression of degeneration with serial measurements. The latter function will become most useful for monitoring the effectiveness of protective and restorative therapies; scans have already been successfully used to monitor neuronal replacement therapy.

Although the book's title emphasizes diagnosis and treatment, it includes a number of chapters that deal with the pathology and biochemistry of Parkinson's disease, offering the reader a valuable state-of-the-art overview of this disorder. Despite the effective treatments available today, well described in this voloume, the disease progressively worsens and in its advanced stages remains a difficult burden to patients and their care providers. There is much in this monograph explaining how one can cope with these problems. And there is much to be hopeful for. Research breakthroughs in a disease have always served as a magnet to attract more investigators and clinicians into the field, which in turn leads to more breakthroughs and new therapeutic strategies. The advances achieved in understanding and treating Parkinson's disease in the past three decades reflect this phenomenon, leading one to anticipate even greater progress in the future. The monograph edited by Doctors Factor and Weiner not only provides practical treatment approaches, but also serves as a testament to the state of knowledge about Parkinson's disease at the beginning of the 21st century.

Stanley Fahn, M.D.

Preface

"When, however, the nature of the subject and the circumstances under which it has been taken up, are considered, it is hoped that the offering of the following pages to the attention of the medical public, will not be severely censured. The disease, respecting which the present inquiry is made, is of a nature highly afflictive. Notwithstanding which, it is not yet obtained a place in the classification of nosologists; some have regarded its characteristic symptoms as distinct and different diseases, and others have given its name to diseases differing essentially from it; whilst the unhappy sufferer has considered it as an evil, from the domination of which he had no prospect of escape."

– James Parkinson

Parkinson's disease (PD) is commonly encountered in our practices and is the second most common neurodegenerative disease. As the population of the industrialized world ages, the impact of this disease on clinical neurology will expand. It has been our good fortune to witness the incredible advances that have taken place over the last few decades in the treatment of PD and resultant improvement in the lives of patients with this disorder. The new millennium gives us pause to contemplate those changes and what is yet to come. The growing literature regarding PD reflects this phenomenon. The time is now appropriate for a comprehensive text on PD that provides the reader with an up-to-date review on the multiple aspects of the disease and puts them into perspective. The scholarly contributions from many of the leading researchers in the field have made such a text a reality. We believe that this book will be useful not only to movement disorder specialists and their fellows aspiring to take on this challenging and ever-changing field but also to neurologists, gerontologists, neurosurgeons, neuropsychologists, neuroscience researchers, and neurology residents. The text provides both theoretical and practical approaches to PD, and this book will be an important addition to their libraries.

This book is organized to provide a comprehensive view of PD as we move into the 21st century and takes the reader through nine sections covering clinical presentation, behavioral and psychiatric manifestations, pathology and neurochemistry, diagnosis, etiology and pathogenesis, drugs, treatment issues, surgery and subtypes of parkinsonism as the core of the book. These topics are bracketed in the beginning by a section on history that gives the reader a sense of where we have been with regard to PD starting with James Parkinson's famous essay. This, in turn, gives us an idea of how far we have come. At the end there is a section on social issues that concern PD patients now, at the turn of this century.

In the history section, Louis in Chapter 2 delineates the limited references to the shaking palsy that followed Parkinson's report. As Goetz points out, it was Charcot who was able to separate PD from other diseases with tremor and gait disorders such as multiple sclerosis in a manner similar to the way we now try to separate PD from PSP and MSA. Charcot also expanded the description of PD by adding rigidity to the cardinal features and demonstrating that PD may be diagnosed without the presence of tremor. It was Charcot, because of the inaccuracies associated with the name shaking palsy, who coined the term *Parkinson's disease*. The next chapter is a time line of advances occurring in the 20th century, which serves as a prelude to the core of the text.

The next two sections comprising 15 chapters provide a clinical description of PD. They are organized to emphasize not only the motor aspects but also the nonmotor and behavioral and psychiatric features of the disease which had been ignored in early writings. As patients live longer these latter features are becoming major morbidity issues. Since gait and balance are frequently the primary disabling symptom, Giladi discusses the gait disorder as a separate issue. In this chapter he emphasizes the freezing gait disorder that is so troublesome and, thus far, not amenable to therapy of any kind. Often nonmotor complaints such as sensory symptoms (pain, numbness, tingling, internal tremor), speech dysfunction, gastrointestinal and other autonomic features, or sleep disorders may dominate the discussion with patients at of ce visits. For this reason, we thought that it was important to address them in separate chapters, especially since much has been written about them over the past few decades.

The natural history of PD, including the preclinical period and effect of therapy, has been a matter of discussion in recent years, especially with the examination of putative neuroprotective agents. Feigin and Eidelberg, in Chapter 13, review current knowledge of the progressive nature of PD based on clinical, pathological, and imaging studies showing, for example, that the preclinical period may be less than 10 years. Gancher reviews the clinical rating scales that have revolutionized our ability to quantitate the progressive nature of PD and effects of therapy. He discusses their evolution and validation and provides them for the reader.

Parkinson mistakenly reported that "the senses and intellects being uninjured" in this disorder. As we move into the new millennium, dementia probably represents the greatest unmet need in our patients from a therapeutic standpoint. The definition and concepts concerning the pathogenesis of this phenomenon have changed dramatically in the last decade. Marder presents a very cogent survey of the clinical issues of dementia in PD, while Galasko addresses the relationship of PD to Alzheimer's disease and dementia with Lewy bodies. There is increasing awareness that PD is also associated with a variety of psychiatric disorders. In some patients, these play a significant role in adversely affecting quality of life, and they are discussed in detail in Chapters 17 to 19.

While our grasp of the clinical syndrome has improved, so has our understanding of the pathology and neurochemistry of PD, and these are covered in Section IV, Chapters 20 through 23. Despite our improved understanding of the clinical features, the diagnosis can still be difficult, especially when we attempt to differentiate PD from other degenerative parkinsonian syndromes. In Section V, Lees discusses the problems with diagnosis from a clinical and pathological standpoint, while the following two chapters discuss imaging technology that may have a place as diagnostic tools in the future.

The etiology of PD is still unknown even after 184 years, however, several well-established theories are a key focus in research as we move into the next century. The most commonly held notions are covered in Chapters 28 and 29. Simon and Beal provide a clear, succinct description of the complicated biochemistry surrounding the oxidative processes that may be central to the pathogenesis of PD and their relationship to mitochondrial and excitotoxic mechanisms. Burke introduces the reader to the concept and terminology of apoptosis, which has become prominent in discussions of the pathogenesis of PD in the 1990s and which, no doubt, will continue to be a focus in coming years. The discovery of MPTP has had enormous impact on research related to the etiology, pathogenesis, and treatment of PD in the last 20 years. Langston puts this discovery in perspective as we approach the end of two decades since his initial report with a broad review in Chapter 30.

Parkinson's disease remains the only neurodegenerative disorder that has demonstrated significant responsiveness to therapeutic interventions. Over the last 30 years there has been a revolution in the management of PD patients with the introduction of a wide range of drugs and surgical procedures. Still other treatments that are experimental at this time represent potential for improved care in the future possibly in relation to neuroprotection. With the availability of newer treatments a number of issues have emerged to bring about active discussion and controversy including the approach to treating early disease, motor fluctuations, and psychosis. All these aspects of therapy are extensively treated in this text, being discussed in detail in Chapters 32 to 50 (Sections VII, VIII, and IX). Simuni and Hurtig begin these sections with a detailed discussion of levodopa, including its history, evolution, and the controversies that surround it. Further discussions of newer drug therapy include the dopamine agonists (Chapter 35), COMT inhibitors (Chapter 36), and atypical antipsychotics (Chapter 37). Treatments that have potential for the future, including excitatory amino acid receptor antagonists and gene therapy, are covered separately by Blandini and Greenamyre, and Mouradian. Interest in surgery has been rejuvenated in the 1990s because of improved technology and continued disease morbidity. At the end of the 20th century, ablative techniques, deep brain stimulation, and neural transplants are gaining momentum as important treatments in advanced patients, and these are covered in Section IX, Chapters 47 to 50.

The differential diagnosis of PD is very large. Section X reviews in four chapters those disorders that are most important. A majority of patients with PD have no obvious family history, and a small minority have an autosomal dominant form with some subtle phenotypic differences from the sporadic type. These families and their genetic abnormalities have been a topic of intense discussion in the last decade, especially in relation to the pathogenesis of disease. Are they different diseases? Golbe addresses this question in Chapter 52.

No current text on PD would be complete without a discussion of social issues. Four that have been of greatest importance are quality of life issues for patients, impact of the diseases on the family, driving and PD, and the cost of PD to society. The subjects are covered extremely well in Chapters 55 to 58.

All 58 chapters together form a comprehensive review of the many issues regarding PD that face physicians today. While it was our intent to organize the chapters so that they complement each other and form a very readable and lucent text that can read from beginning to end, we have also provided the reader with extensive cross-referencing of each chapter so that subjects of interest can easily be isolated. Each chapter may also stand on its own as a scholarly review of the individual subject. Each one is concisely written and heavily referenced for this purpose.

As we all move forward in our endeavors to better understand Parkinson's disease, we close in the spirit of James Parkinson:

"The disease had escaped particular notice; and the task of ascertaining its nature and cause by anatomical investigation, did not seem likely to be taken up by those who, from their abilities and opportunities, were most likely to accomplish it. That these friends to humanity and medical science, who have already unveiled to us many of the morbid processes by which health and life is abridged, might be excited to extend their researches to this malady, was much desired; and it is hoped that this might be procured by the publication of these remarks."

Stewart A. Factor
William J. Weiner

Acknowledgements

We would like to thank the contributors to this text. We realize that this is a complicated era in medicine and it is becoming more difficult to find the time to write review articles and book chapters. Despite that, these experts were able to put together timely, cogent and comprehensive reviews of their subject and for that we are grateful. We thank our patients who continually educate and challenge us in this constantly growing field. Our staffs have been invaluable to us as we worked toward the completion of this book. Special thanks, for their editorial and secretarial support, goes to Maria Macias and Faith Wood. Our other staff members are Dinorah Bateman, Maria Gomez, Sharon Evans and, last but not least, Diane Brown. Diane was a co-founder of the Parkinson's Disease and Movement Disorders Center at Albany Medical Center. Her dedication to that program has always been above and beyond the call. During the preparation of this book she was stricken with a serious illness and died on November 13, 2000 at the age of 54. We think of her often. We would like to express our gratitude to the American Parkinson's Disease Association and the National Parkinson's Foundation for the support they provided our programs over the last decade. Finally, we are indebted to Rosalyn Newman, Victor and Marilyn Riley, and Key Bank of New York for their extraordinarily generous support for our programs. They have provided us with the means to continue our work in Parkinson's Disease.

Contributors

Charles H. Adler, *Mayo Clinic, Department of Neurology, Scottsdale, Arizona*

J. Eric Ahlskog, *Mayo Clinic, Rochester, Minnesota*

Patricia G. Archbold, *Oregon Health Sciences University, Portland, Oregon*

Kevin D. Barron, *Albany Medical College, Albany, New York*

M. Flint Beal, *Massachusetts General Hospital, Boston, Massachusetts*

Fabio Blandini, *Neurological Institute "C. Mondino", Pavia, Italy*

Allison Brashear, *Indiana University School of Medicine, Indianapolis, Indiana*

Robert E. Burke, *Columbia University, New York, New York*

Richard Stanley Burns, *Director, Movement Disorders Clinic, Department of Neurology, The Cleveland Clinic Foundation, Cleveland, Ohio*

Donald B. Calne, *Neurodegenerative Disorders Centre, University of British Columbia, Vancouver, British Columbia, Canada*

Julie H. Carter, *Oregon Health Sciences University, Portland, Oregon*

Tiffany W. Chow, *Rancho Los Amigos/USC Alzheimer's Disease Center, Downey, Los Angeles, California*

Cynthia L. Comella, *Rush Medical College, Chicago, Illinois*

Jeffrey L. Cummings, *Rancho Los Amigos/USC Alzheimer's Disease Center, Downey, Los Angeles, California*

David Eidelberg, *North Shore University Hospital, Manhasset, New York*

Stewart A. Factor, *Parkinson's Disease and Movement Disorder Center of Albany Medical Center, Albany, New York*

Andrew Feigin, *North Shore University Hospital, Manhasset, New York*

J. Stephen Fink, *Boston University School of Medicine, Boston, Massachusetts*

Joseph H. Friedman, *Memorial Hospital of Rhode Island, Pawtucket, Rhode Island*

Douglas Galasko, *University of California–San Diego, San Diego, California*

Stephen T. Gancher, *Department of Neurology, Oregon Health Sciences University, Portland, Oregon*

William T. Garrett, *Medical College of Georgia, Augusta, Georgia*

Oscar S. Gershanik, *Centro Neurologico Hospital Francés, Buenos Aires, Argentina*

Nir Giladi, *Movement Disorders Unit, Department of Neurology, Tel-Aviv Sourasky Medical Center, Sackler Faculty of Medicine, Tel-Aviv University, Tel-Aviv, Israel*

Christopher G. Goetz, *Professor of Neurological Sciences, Professor of Pharmacology, Rush Medical College, Rush-Presbyterian–St. Luke's Medical Center, Chicago, Illinois*

Lawrence I. Golbe, *UMDNJ–Robert Wood Johnson Medical School, New Brunswick, New Jersey*

J. Timothy Greenamyre, *Emory University, Atlanta, Georgia*

Mark Guttman, *Department of Medicine (Division of Neurology) and Department of Psychiatry, University of Toronto, Ontario, Canada*

John P. Hammerstadt, *Department of Neurology, Oregon Health Sciences University, Portland, Oregon*

Ruyi Hao, *Senior Scientist, Neuroscience Research, R&D Systems, Minneapolis, Minnesota*

Robert A. Hauser, *University of South Florida, Tampa, Florida*

Robert G. Holloway, *University of Rochester School of Medicine and Dentistry, Rochester, New York*

Jean Pintar Hubble, *Madden/National Parkinson Foundation Center of Excellence, Ohio State University, Columbus, Ohio*

Howard Hurtig, *University of Pennsylvania Health System, Philadelphia, Pennsylvania*

Diane M. Jacobs, *Columbia University College of Physicians and Surgeons, New York, New York*

William C. Koller, *Ph.D. University of Miami, Miami, Florida*

Amos D. Korczyn, *Sackler Faculty of Medicine, Tel-Aviv University Medical School, Ramat-Aviv, Israel*

Roger Kurlan, *University of Rochester Medical School, Rochester, New York*

J. William Langston, *The Parkinson's Institute, Sunnyvale, California*

Anthony E. Lang, *Toronto Western Hospital, Toronto, Ontario, Canada*

Andrew J. Lees, *The National Hospital for Neurology and Neurosurgery, London, United Kingdom*

Peter A. LeWitt, *Clinical Neuroscience Center, Southfield, Michigan*

Elan D. Louis, *Gertrude H. Sergievsky Center, College of Physicians and Surgeons, Columbia University, New York, New York*

Andres M. Lozano, *Toronto Western Hospital, Toronto, Ontario, Canada*

Kelly Lyons, *University of Kansas Medical Center, Kansas City, Kansas*

Karen Marder, *Columbia University College of Physicians and Surgeons, New York, New York*

Kenneth Marek, *Yale University School of Medicine, New Haven, Connecticut*

Deborah C. Mash, *University of Miami School of Medicine, Miami, Florida*

Donna L. Masterman, *Rancho Los Amigos/USC Alzheimer's Disease Center, Downey, Los Angeles, California*

Herbert Y. Meltzer, *Vanderbilt University Medical Center, Nashville, Tennessee*

Eric S. Molho, *The Parkinson's Disease and Movement Disorder Center of Albany Medical Center, Albany, New York*

M. Maral Mouradian, *National Institute of Neurological Disorders and Stroke, National Institutes of Health, Bethesda, Maryland*

Puiu F. Nisipeanu, *Department of Neurology, Hill Yaffe Hospital, Hadera*

John G. Nutt, *Oregon Health Sciences University, Portland, Oregon*

Rajesh Pahwa, *University of Kansas Medical Center, Kansas City, Kansas*

Pramod Kr. Pal, *National Institute of Mental Health and Neurosciences (NIMHANS), Bangalore, Karnataka, India*

Jung Y. Park, *Toronto Western Hospital, Toronto, Ontario, Canada*

Ronald E. Pfeiffer, *Professor and Vice-Chair, Director, Division of Neurodegenerative Diseases, Department of Neurology, University of Tennessee Health Science Center, Memphis, Tennessee*

Eamonn M.M. Quigley, *University of Nebraska Medical Center, Omaha, Nebraska*

Jose Martin Rabey, *Chairman, Department of Neurology, Assaf Harofe Medical Center, Sackler School of Medicine, Tel Aviv University, Israel*

A.H. Rajput, *University of Saskatchewan, Royal University Hospital, Saskatoon, Saskatchewan, Canada*

M.L. Rajput, *University of Saskatchewan, Royal University Hospital, Saskatoon, Saskatchewan, Canada*

Lorraine Olson Ramig, *CCC-SLP, Professor Department of Speech, Language, Hearing Sciences, University of Colorado–Boulder, Research Associate, Wilbur James Gould Voice Research Center, Denver Center for the Performing Arts, Denver, Colorado*

Irene Hegeman Richard, *University of Rochester Medical School, Rochester, New York*

David Riley, *Mount Sinai Medical Center, Cleveland, Ohio*

Jacob I. Sage, *Robert Wood Johnson Medical School, New Brunswick, New Jersey*

Ali Samii, *University of Washington School of Medicine, Harborview Medical Center, Seattle, Washington*

Kapil D. Sethi, *Medical College of Georgia, Augusta, Georgia*

Lisa M. Shulman, *University of Miami School of Medicine, Miami, Florida*

Andrew D. Siderowf, *University of Pennsylvania, Philadelphia, Pennsylvania*

Andrew Siderowf, *University of Pennsylvania School of Medicine, Philadelphia, Pennsylvania*

Eric Siemers, *Lilly Research Laboratories, Indianapolis, Indiana*

David K. Simon, *Beth Israel Deaconess Medical Center, Boston, Massachusetts*

Tanya Simuni, *University of Pennsylvania Health System, Philadelphia, Pennsylvania*

Yoland Smith, *Emory University, Atlanta, Georgia*

Matthew B. Stern, *University of Pennsylvania, Philadelphia, Pennsylvania*

Barbara J. Stewart, *Oregon Health Sciences University, Portland, Oregon*

Caroline M. Tanner, *The Parkinson's Institute, Sunnyvale, California*

Jerrold L. Vitek, *Emory University, Atlanta, Georgia*

Cheryl Waters, *Columbia University, New York, New York*

Carolyn Weeks, *Madden/National Parkinson Foundation Center of Excellence, Ohio State University, Columbus, Ohio*

William J. Weiner, *University of Maryland School of Medicine, Baltimore, Maryland*

Mickie Welsh, *University of Southern California, School of Medicine, Los Angeles, California*

Thomas Wichmann, *Emory University, Atlanta, Georgia*

Steven Wilkinson, *University of Kansas Medical Center, Kansas City, Kansas*

Theresa A. Zesiewicz, *University of South Florida, Tampa, Florida*

Richard M. Zweig, *Department of Neurology, Louisiana State University Medical Center, Shreveport, Louisiana*

1

James Parkinson: The Man and the Essay

Stewart A. Factor, D.O.
Parkinson's Disease and Movement Disorder Center of Albany Medical Center, Albany, New York
and
William J. Weiner, M.D.
Maryland Parkinson's Disease and Movement Disorder Center, University of Maryland, Baltimore, Maryland

INTRODUCTION

Movement disorder specialists utter his name on a daily basis in speaking to patients, talking to colleagues, and giving lectures in medical colleges or to physicians, residents, and students. It was Charcot, in the nineteenth century, who first suggested that the shaking palsy be given the name "Parkinson's disease." Parkinson's disease (PD) has become the subject of intense interest as exemplified by the contents of this text. It is the subject of innumerable scientific papers and is not infrequently mentioned in the lay literature or on the news. Parkinson's disease knows no boundaries with regard to race, nationality, gender, or social class, and we frequently hear about celebrities diagnosed. Who was this man whose fame persists as we move into the twenty-first century? Who was James Parkinson? History portrays him as a Renaissance man who lived at the turn of another century. He was not only a practicing general physician who contributed to the medical literature of his time, but also a man who had interests as wide as politics, chemistry, and paleontology. We thought it would be appropriate to begin this text by discussing James Parkinson, the man, and his famous "An Essay on the Shaking Palsy," which started it all. We do not intend to provide a detailed biography of his life. Others have completed that task, and the reader is referred to two interesting books for additional details (1,2). This chapter is followed by two chapters that discuss how PD was perceived in the nineteenth century. There is an emphasis on Charcot and how he was able to further define the clinical features of the shaking palsy and separate the disorder from other clinical entities. The history section

ends with an outline of important discoveries in the twentieth century.

THE MAN

James Parkinson was born on April 11, 1755, to John and Mary Parkinson (2). They resided at 1 Hoxton Square in the parish of St. Leonard's of Shoreditch, Middlesex County, England, where he lived his entire life. He was the oldest of three children, followed by brother William and sister Mary Sedgewood. His father was a physician and surgeon who practiced in Hoxton. At age 20 James studied at London Hospital Medical College for six months, and that was followed by an apprenticeship with his father that lasted six years. He qualified as a surgeon in 1784 at the age of 29 (3). He later joined his father in a practice referred to as "Parkinson and Son," which was a large lucrative practice that also cared for the poor in the parish. They attended a "private madhouse" for over 30 years. The practice of Parkinson and Son lasted 80 years and four generations.

In 1781 James Parkinson married Mary Dale and they had six children. Two died in infancy or early childhood, their first, James John, and their sixth, Jane Dale. His second son, John William Keys Parkinson, joined him in medical practice and ultimately John's son, James Keys Parkinson, joined the practice as well.

We do not know what James Parkinson looked like except that he was "rather below middle stature" (2). A photograph that was initially identified as James Parkinson was published in *Medical Classics* in 1938 (4) (Figure 1-1), but it turned out that the picture was from a group photo taken in 1872, well after

Parkinson's death, of the membership of the British Dental Association (1). The subject's name was also James Parkinson. James Parkinson died on December 21, 1824, of a dominant hemisphere stroke that initially caused hemiplegia and aphasia. He was buried at the parish of St. Leonard's but his gravestone is not to be found today. A factory occupies the site of his birth on 1 Hoxton Square, and in September 1961 a commemorative blue plaque was placed (2) (Figure 1-2).

James Parkinson had a number of talents that served him well in his career. He was fluent in English, Latin, French, and Greek. He was an expert at shorthand, which he used to take verbatim notes in various lectures he attended. Some of these notes were later used to

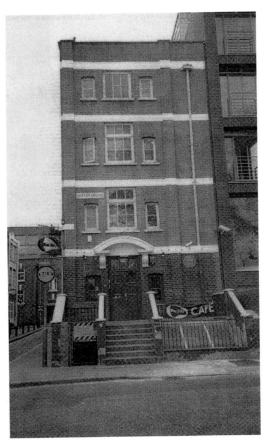

(A)

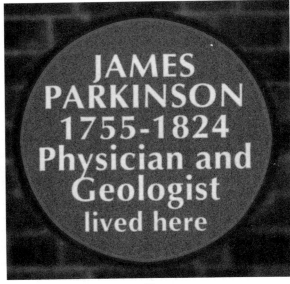

(B)

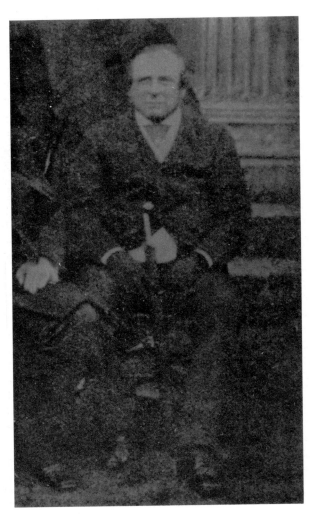

FIGURE 1-1. Photo of a British dentist named James Parkinson. It was taken in 1872 but was misidentified as James Parkinson, author of "An Essay on the Shaking Palsy," who died in 1824. (Reproduced with permission from Robert E. Krieger Publishing Co.).

FIGURE 1-2. A: The building currently located at 1 Hoxton Square, the birthplace of James Parkinson. (Generously provided by Christopher Goetz, MD). B: A closeup of the plaque (actually blue in color) on the building memorializing James Parkinson.

publish the lectures; for example, the surgical lectures of John Hunter were published in 1833 as *Hunterian Reminiscences* (published by Parkinson's son, John William Keys Parkinson). He was also an accomplished artist, a talent that he used in his many writings and emphasized as important to medical students.

James Parkinson was a political activist who found it difficult to remain silent while people suffered. He lived under the monarchy of King George III at a time when the standard of living was declining as the result of war and rising taxes. Representation in parliament for all citizens was nonexistent, and corruption pervaded the government. The French Revolution, which led to the death of Louis XVI, was ongoing, and America had recently gained its freedom from British rule, instigating important discussions by social reformers in Great Britain about democracy, suffrage, and representation for all people, not just the rich. The social reformers were referred to by one conservative political leader, Edmund Burke, as the "swinish multitude." It was also a time when Thomas Paine wrote *The Rights of Man*. James Parkinson was a member of two outspoken societies of that time, The London Corresponding Society, started by Thomas Hardy in 1792, and the Society of Constitutional Information. The monarchy and parliament were exceedingly suspicious about these organizations. There was no freedom of the press or speech, and the right of habeas corpus was suspended to prevent revolution from spilling into Great Britain. Many members of these societies were tried and convicted of treason and received severe punishments. The primary objective of the London Corresponding Society was to bring about reform of the parliamentary representation of the people. While they were put down to some extent by the monarchy, the activities of this group may have ultimately laid the foundation for the change to more representative democracy in Great Britain (2). Parkinson's part was as a writer. In a periodical known as "Politics of the People" he wrote a series of a dozen or so articles under the pseudonym Old Hubert (2,5,6) between 1793 and 1795 (7). These pamphlets were highly critical of the political system and covered a wide range of social topics, while at the same time parrying with Edmund Burke. Some of the titles included *Revolutions without bloodshed or reformation preferable to revolt; Pearls cast before swine by Edmund Burke – scraped together by Old Hubert; A vindication of the London Corresponding Society; and An Address to the Hon. E Burke from the Swinish Multitude*. The writings dealt with such issues as political corruption, poverty, unfairness of taxes and wages, civil disobedience, unfair imprisonment and poor prison conditions, the education of children from poor families, and provisions for the aged and disabled (2,5,7). The proceeds from the sale of the pamphlets were used to support the families of political prisoners (8). He was identified as the author in an advertisement in the *London Times* and during a cross-examination under oath for the Privy Council during an investigation, but he never was accused of wrongdoing. However, the publisher of the periodical was tried and convicted of treason.

Parkinson was also a key character in the "Popgun Plot" to assassinate King George III. Five members of the London Corresponding Society were arrested for high treason in relation to the apparent plan. In fact, a plan never existed except in the mind of one man, Thomas Upton. Three others were falsely accused based on forged letters (forged by Upton), and one was arrested because of his association with Upton. Only one actually went to trial. The plot involved the firing of a poison-tipped arrow from an air gun. No further details were ever devised. Parkinson's role was threefold. He visited one of the prisoners as physician and pleaded for the prisoners' removal from poor prison conditions, and he requested that the prisoner receive regular visits from a physician. He was a spokesperson for the prisoners with regard to bail. Finally, he was a witness for the defense during the Privy Council hearings for the three falsely accused and in the one trial that was held. He did not appear for Upton. He asserted the innocence of the accused. During the Privy Council investigation he initially refused to take the oath unless he received assurances that he would only be asked questions on the topic at hand. This annoyed the attorney general, and he was told he would not be asked questions that might incriminate him (he responded that "there was no question you can produce an answer to criminate me") but he was tricked. He was asked questions on issues regarding society membership and plans and about various writings, including some of his own. He was a formidable witness who disclosed little information but did admit to his memberships and his writings under the pseudonym Old Hubert. When asked if he had seen certain members, he always answered that he had seen them in his own home. None of the accused was found guilty and all were ultimately freed. Parkinson, in his writings and appearances in the Privy Council, took significant risks with regard to his own career and life. He could have been prosecuted for his activities in the societies, for association with others accused, and for writings against the monarchy. But he was a man of principle and honor who believed these issues were too important to remain silent. The Privy Council members respected his forthrightness and as a result he was not prosecuted. He left the London Corresponding

Society shortly after the Popgun trials as more extreme forces took it over. His political writings ended in 1795.

Despite leaving the societies, Parkinson was unwavering in his stance for parliamentary reform. He continued that fight as a trustee of the Vestry for the Liberty of Hoxton (also referred to as parish councilor), to which he was appointed in 1799 (2). He remained at this post for 25 years until his death. While the council was concerned about local affairs such as highway upkeep, illumination of the streets, and support of the church of St. Leonard, they also were active in national affairs. Since there was no parliamentary representation, the council took on that role, using town meetings and petitions as a means of protest. The primary concern was parliamentary reform and improvement of representation. The petition sent to the House of Commons from the parish contained many of the points Parkinson had written about in his earlier political papers, indicating his significant role in its completion.

Through the parish council Parkinson took on other responsibilities, usually with humanitarian goals. He was concerned about the welfare of children who worked as apprentices for mistresses and masters. In the early nineteenth century children of the poor and orphans found second homes when they were taken in to work for those better off. Some of the children were abused in various ways. Parkinson recommended the formation of a team of inspectors who would travel to the various households. In fact, he took on this role himself and discovered some of these abuses. A law that required review and visitation was set into motion based on his findings. His interest in child abuse issues did not start there. He had written about it in 1800 in his article "*The Villagers Friend and Physician*" (9). He also became a trustee for the poor and was appointed surgeon, apothecary, and man-midwife to the poor of the parish in 1813. The later position was salaried and required, among other things, that he make house calls for sick paupers. His accomplishments during this time included the formation of separate fever wards for patients with typhus fever. He emphasized the contagious nature of the disease, a view not universally accepted at that time, and ultimately won support. After four years of discussion a 12-bed ward was completed and the impact was significant. His papers on "Observations on the necessity of Parochial fever wards, with remarks on the present extensive spread of fever" written in 1818 and "*On the treatment of infectious or typhoid fever*" written in 1824 lead to the construction of fever wards in London and the surrounding area and provided for improved treatment with appropriate hospital care and nursing. When

James Parkinson died and his son resigned, it took six physicians to fill their shoes as parish physicians.

James Parkinson made significant contributions to the medical literature beyond the "*Essay on the Shaking Palsy.*" They included books, monographs, and case studies written for physicians and the lay public, some of which are worth mentioning. In 1799 he wrote a two-volume book on domestic medicine entitled "*Medical Admonitions to families, respecting the preservation of health and the treatment of the sick.*" In this 548-page text he examined the symptoms and physical signs of common ailments of the time and emphasized the need for an experienced physician. A table of symptoms, listed alphabetically, was included in the book. This served to point out the difficulty with providing a definite diagnosis early in the course of an illness. He discussed such topics as the problems associated with the improper indulgence of children, epilepsy and pseudoseizures, and resuscitation of the drowned (2,9). He wrote a monograph entitled "*Observations on the nature and cure of Gout*" in 1805. This paper included a clinical description including the presumed experience of his father and himself, both of whom suffered from gout, along with pathology and therapy of the time. He criticized the accepted theories of etiology and treatment practices. In 1802 he wrote "*Hints for the improvement of trusses,*" which included his invention to make their use easier. He complained in the paper about the high price of these devices since they were mostly needed by those of modest means.

Parkinsons first paper was a case report entitled "*Some account of the effects of lightning*" about two men struck by lightning during the same storm. One was outdoors, the other indoors. They both responded to therapy with bleeding, hot brandy and water, and wet flannels. This paper was presented to the Medical Society of London on February 4, 1789. He wrote several papers with his son, John William Keys Parkinson, including "A case of Trismus," which was read to the Medical and Chirurgical Society by John on June 18, 1811. The two also coauthored the earliest reference to appendicitis in the English literature in 1812. The paper entitled "*A case of diseased vermiform appendix*" was read before the Medical and Chirurgical Society on January 21 of that year and included a clinical and pathological discussion of a 5-year-old boy who died from a ruptured appendix and resultant peritonitis. One other interesting publication was "*Cases of hydrophobia,*" which was an account of two cases written from memory because he had either given the notes to another physician *or lost them.* He wrote "*I shall be obliged to rely, in the following account, entirely on my memory, which is however so impressed with the most important facts, that although it has to refer to a rather distant period, it will not, I trust, materially mislead me.*" The case notes, which he had given to another physician, were later published with some discrepancies in a book.

As a physician, Parkinson was concerned about the education and qualifications of physicians in practice and the easy access of untrained "quacks" to medical practice. In 1800 he wrote an article entitled "*The Hospital Pupil: an essay intended to facilitate the study of medicine and surgery,*" in which he addressed qualifications including more than ordinary ability and intelligence and limited levity (5). Although it was a guide for medical students, he used the opportunity to criticize the educational program of the time (2,7,10) and recommended liberal arts education and knowledge of multiple languages for use in reviewing the literature. His proposed curriculum was similar to more modern education (2,10). He also was an active advocate for the Apothecaries Act of 1815, which required licensing examinations for a proper diploma and allowed for prosecution of those who practiced without appropriate qualifications.

James Parkinson had an interest in chemistry that probably started as early as 1780 and ultimately led to the publication of a well-received textbook (2,5). It started with his reading of the works by Dr. Richard Watson and persisted with his attendance at the lectures of Sir Humphrey Davy at the Royal Institution of Great Britain in the early 1800s. Although he never wrote any scientific chemistry articles, in 1800 he wrote "*The Chemistry Pocket Book.*" It was a heavily referenced theoretical text with few experiments included, but it was easy to read and brought chemistry to the level of the "ordinary reader." It was a concise yet comprehensive account of the knowledge in the field and was inexpensive. It sold well, which led to the publication of four editions; the last in 1807 was reissued in 1809. The final edition included chapters on geology, with which he was very familiar, and the biology of bodily fluids.

James Parkinson was also an avid collector of minerals, fossils, and seashells, and he gained notoriety for his knowledge of geology and oryctology (this term was changed to paleontology about 10 years after his death) (2,3,5). He acquired his knowledge by collecting specimens in the field from the gravel and clay pits of Shoreditch, exchanging and trading pieces, and purchasing pieces from dealers and at auctions, and he became a self-educated expert. He apparently became interested in the subject after reading the chemical essays of Richard Watson, the same book that lead to his interest in chemistry. His collection grew to become one of the largest, most valuable collections of fossils in Great Britain, and the collection was displayed in his house at 1 Hoxton Square in his own museum. After his death in 1824, the collection was auctioned off, with many pieces ending up in various museums in Cambridge, Oxford, and Haslemere (2,3).

In the early 1800s he took on the enormous task of writing a three-volume text on oryctology entitled "*Organic remains of a former world.*" It was in these texts that his artistic abilities were of utmost importance as all figures were his drawings of the specimens. Volume I, "*An examination of the mineralized remains of the vegetables and animals of the antediluvian world generally termed extraneous fossils,*" was published in 1804. There were 1,146 pages, 42 plates, and 700 figures. Volume II, "The Fossil Zoophytes," was published in 1808, and Volume III, "Fossil starfish, Echini, Shells, Insects, Amphibia, Mammalia, & c.," was published in 1811. This book was the first systematic examination of oryctology in English and the first comprehensive text to cover both plants and animals including vertebrates (2). It was written for the general public to introduce the public to the study of this subject. He made it a practical guide to help the student who was digging so that he could identify his findings. He did not use the standard chapter format to write this book but instead used a series of letters to an imaginary friend ("with an inquiring mind") to cover the topics. He apparently used this format not only because he thought it would be easier to follow but also because he thought the format would work better with his busy schedule and ability to write only in short time slots. The text included discussion on the history of the science going back to Greek and Roman philosophers. He discussed the effect of Noah's flood and provided a theory of petrification, which differed from the accepted theory of his time. In the second volume he described the muriatic acid test, which he devised to demonstrate the presence of organic matter in the fossilized specimen. He also reported on the structure of pebbles. His classification of fossils was a departure from the standard ones. These volumes solidified his place as a London expert in the field.

The book sold well and was reprinted several times, even after Parkinson's death, and went out of print in the 1840s. The plates were republished in 1850 in Mantell's "*Pictorial Atlas of Fossil Remains.*" Parkinson published a follow-up book in 1822 entitled "*Outlines of Oryctology*" with 343 pages and 220 figures. It was a practical field manual for the oryctology student. It was an easy-to-read introductory book and was reissued in 1830 with corrections that Parkinson had made before his death.

James Parkinson was a founding member of the Geological Society and was present at its inaugural meeting in 1807. He was an active member, serving a two-year term on the society council. In the first issue of the "Transactions of the Geological Society" in 1811 he wrote a paper entitled "*Observations on some of the strata in the neighborhood of London, and on the fossil remains contained in them*," which gave the first detailed description of the strata of the London basin and led to the new field of stratigraphical geology. He made other contributions to the transactions in the following years. He also made contributions to the British encyclopedia and dictionary of the arts and sciences on the subjects of oryctology and conchology. Because of his many important contributions to the field, James Parkinson was made an honorary member of the Wernerian Society of Natural History of Edinburgh and the Imperial Society of Naturalists of Moscow.

James Parkinson received several honors both in life and posthumously. In 1777, while still an apprentice to his father, he received a silver medal for his part in the rescue of a man who attempted suicide by hanging. This was a case his father ultimately reported. In 1823 he was the first recipient of the Honorary Gold Medal from the Royal College of Surgeons for "his promotion of natural knowledge particularly expressed by his splendid work on Organic Remains ..." (2,3,10). He received the award on April 11 of that year, his sixty-eighth birthday (2,3). In September 1955, to commemorate his two hundredth birthday, a marble tablet with the inscription "*James Parkinson, of Hoxton, Surgeon and Apothecary*" was unveiled and a special service was held (3). Among those present were two of his direct descendents and the president of the History of Medicine Section of the Royal Society of Medicine. In that same year a tribute to Parkinson was held at the Second International Congress of Neuropathologists at the Royal College of Surgeons of England. J.G. Greenfield gave an address on "*Historical Landmarks in the Pathology of Involuntary Movement*" and referred to Parkinson's contribution. Also at that meeting a special exhibit was presented by his biographer, A.D. Morris (medical superintendent of St. Leonards Hospital in Shoreditch), reviewing many aspects of his life (3). Because of his work in paleontology a species of Nautilus, a tropical cephalopod mollusk, was named after him; *Nautilus Parkinsoni* (2). His name is also preserved in geological circles for it has been used for well-known fossils from the interior Oolite; the ammonite *Parkinsonia parkinsoni*, the crinoid *Apiocrinus parkinsoni*, a gastropod *Rostellaria parkinsoni,* and a stemless palm *Nipa parkinsoni* (3,11). And, of course, medically his name is attached to that neurologic disorder that he described so well and is the subject of this book and many other books and articles – *Parkinson's disease.*

Yahr described James Parkinson as a "physician for all seasons" (5). He was not only a humane physician in a busy practice who cared for the poor and mentally ill but also a talented writer who added substantially to the medical literature of his time, publishing a series of important papers and books. These publications were directed not only to the medical community but also to the common people. Over 200 years later he continues to be remembered for some of those contributions. In addition, he was an expert in chemistry, paleontology, and geology, making important strides in these sciences through a number of publications, books, and papers and received due recognition for them. Finally, he was a political activist who used his talent as a writer to spearhead a battle against corruption and inequity. With this book we salute him for all his contributions but especially for his writing of the medical classic "*An Essay on the Shaking Palsy*," which is discussed in the next section.

THE ESSAY

James Parkinson published his medical classic, "An Essay on the Shaking Palsy," in 1817 at the age of 62 (Figure 1-3) (12). This was a comprehensive treatise containing five chapters and 66 pages on the subject (which he also called "paralysis agitans"). The review includes his experience with six patients. He must have contemplated this subject for some time because he indicates that the first time he saw it "was observed in a case which occurred several years back, and which, from the particular symptoms which manifested themselves in its progress: from the little knowledge of its nature, acknowledged to be possessed by the physician who attended: and from the mode of its termination: excited an eager wish to acquire some further knowledge of its nature and cause." It is considered a medical classic because of the eloquent and detailed description of the clinical features of this disease. It is unlikely that any of us, having the benefit of nearly 200 years of literature experience, could provide as eloquent a description as James Parkinson did based solely on six patients. It should be noted that, of the six patients that he reports on, three were "casually met on the street" or "only seen at a distance." Despite that, he accumulated a substantial knowledge of the clinical features and natural history of this disorder. Anyone interested in Parkinson's disease should take the time to read this gem of the neurologic literature.

AN

ESSAY

ON THE

SHAKING PALSY.

BY

JAMES PARKINSON,
MEMBER OF THE ROYAL COLLEGE OF SURGEONS.

LONDON:
PRINTED BY WHITTINGHAM AND ROWLAND,
Goswell Street.

FOR SHERWOOD, NEELY, AND JONES,
PATERNOSTER ROW.
1817.

(a)

CONTENTS.

(b)

AN

ESSAY

ON THE

SHAKING PALSY.

CHAPTER I.

DEFINITION—HISTORY—ILLUSTRATIVE CASES.

SHAKING PALSY. *(Paralysis Agitans.)*
Involuntary tremulous motion, with lessened muscular power, in parts not in action and even when supported ; with a propensity to bend the trunk forward, and to pass from a walking to a running pace : the senses and intellects being uninjured.

(c)

FIGURE 1-3. A: Title page of the monograph "An Essay on the Shaking Palsy." B: Table of Contents. C: First page showing the definition of the disease.

He starts in the preface with an apology (as he did in other works), clearly underestimating his abilities and the respect that they engendered. As a clinician, and not having had the opportunity to examine the pathology of any of his cases, he wrote "some conciliatory explanation should be offered for the present publication: in which, it is acknowledged that mere conjecture takes the place of experiment: and, that analogy is the substitute for anatomic examination, the only sure foundation for pathological knowledge." He claims to have taken on the task of writing the paper because he thought that the disease was unrecognized and/or poorly classified and he wanted more effort focused on it. He indicated that "the disease had escaped particular notice: and the task of ascertaining its nature and cause by anatomic investigation, did not seem likely to be taken up by those who, from their abilities and opportunities, were most likely to accomplish it. That these friends of humanity and medical science, who have already unveiled to us many of the morbid processes by which health and life is abridged, might be excited to extend their researches to this malady, was much desired; and it was hoped, that this might be procured by the publication of these remarks." Not only were these words placed in the preface as an introduction to the paper itself but also he concluded with the same comments. He also described this paper as being a work in progress; "considered it to be a duty to submit his opinions to the examinations of others, even in their present state of immaturity and imperfection" (he refers to himself in the third person in the writing of this paper). Other important issues that he discusses in the preface included, from a clinical standpoint, that he recognized that it is a disease of long duration that progresses to a level of significant disability. He indicates "the disease ... is of a nature highly afflictive." He also indicates that the patients themselves understand the chronicity of the disease and the disability associated with it: "whilst the unhappy sufferer has considered it as an evil, from the domination of which he had no prospect of escape." Parkinson indicates that to understand the natural history of the disease one needs to either observe patients as they evolve or see patients at various stages of the disease and receive a "correct history of its symptoms even for several years." He notes in the preface that, in fact, he came to understand the nature of the illness from all three. He also indicates in the preface that he may not be the first to have seen this disease and there are other publications that support this possibility (12,13). But he suggests that very often the authors thought of the individual features of paralysis agitans as separate disorders: "some have regarded its characteristic symptoms as distinct and different diseases, and others have given its name to diseases distinct from it."

The first two chapters (Chapter 1: Definition – history – illustrative cases; Chapter 2: Pathognomonic symptoms examined – Tremor Coactus – Scelotyrbe Festinana) provide the clinical description of this disease and the portions of the paper that have made it so enduring. It is astounding how much he gleaned from the small number of cases that he saw, especially since half of them were seen only briefly and on one occasion. He notes that the tremor and the gait disorder, the most visually dramatic features,

are the pathognomonic symptoms of the disease: "the tremulous agitation, and the almost invincible propensity to run, when wishing only to walk, each of which has been considered by nosologists as distinct diseases, appear to be pathognomonic symptoms of this malady." He indicates quite succinctly that the resting tremor is the characteristic feature and one that could differentiate paralysis agitans from other forms of tremor. And he indicates that the differentiation of tremor is not really that hard: "a small degree of attention will be sufficient to perceive, that Sauvages, by this just distinction, actually separates this kind of tremulous motion, and which is the kind peculiar to this disease, from the Genus Tremor." He wrestled with the appropriate terminology for the tremor to separate it from other forms of tremor that occurred in action. He suggested that the term *palpitation* would be more appropriately used. He indicates that "the separation of palpitation of the limbs from tremor, is the more necessary to be insisted on, since the distinction may assist in leading to a knowledge of the seat of the disease." He also points out clearly that tremor alone can not lead to the diagnosis: "tremor can, indeed, only be considered as a symptom." He then describes in an eloquent fashion the natural history of disease starting from the very earliest points and its insidious nature: "so slight and nearly imperceptible are the first in roads of malady, and so extremely slow is its progress, that it rarely happens, that the patient can form any recollection of the precise period of commencement." He continues: "The first symptoms perceived are, a slight sense of weakness, with a proneness to tremble in some particular part: ... but most commonly of the hands and arms.... These symptoms gradually increase in the part first afflicted; and at an uncertain period, but seldom in less than 12 months or more, the morbid influence is felt in some other part." He continues later writing "after a few months the patient is found to be less strict than usual in preserving an upright posture: this being most observable whilst walking, but sometimes whilst sitting or standing." He points out the benign nature of the early symptoms, indicating that "hitherto the patient will have experienced but little inconvenience." He then goes on to show how the disabling portions of the disease begin to appear: "But as the disease proceeds similar employment's (writing and other dexterous maneuvers) are accomplished with considerable difficulties, the hand failing to answer the exactness to the dictates of the will. Walking becomes a task which can not be performed without considerable attention. The legs are not raised to that height, or with that promptitude which the will directs, so that utmost care is necessary to prevent frequent falls.

At this period the patient experiences much inconvenience, which unhappily is found daily to increase." The discussion provides even further information on the continued progression as he notes: "as time and the disease proceed, difficulties increase: writing can now be hardly at all accomplished. Whilst at meals the fork not being duly directed frequently fails to raise the morsel from the plate ... at this period the patient seldom experiences a suspension of the agitation of his limbs." He then goes on to provide a detailed description of the gait disorder that characterizes paralysis agitans with particular emphasis on festination: "the propensity to lean forward becomes invincible, and the patient is thereby forced to step on the toes and fore part of the feet, whilst the upper part of the body is thrown so far forward as to render it difficult to avoid falling on the face ... irresistibly impelled to take much quicker and shorter steps, and thereby to adopt unwillingly a running pace."

In the very late stages he indicates "the trunk is almost permanently bowed, muscular power is more decidedly diminished, and the tremulous agitation becomes violent. Patients walk now with great difficulty and unable any longer to support himself with his stick."

It is suggested that he did not discuss bradykinesia as a major feature of the disease (7). He does not mention it as a pathognomonic feature of the disease, but he does discuss it in a variety of ways. Bradykinesia is not infrequently described by the patients as a feeling of weakness, and that is how he discusses it as noted in the previous quote in the later stages. In his definition he indicates "with lessened muscular power" but he also notices a decrease in general motion by indicating his description of Case 5 "the inability for motion." It is frequently noted that he does not mention rigidity as a major feature of the disease, and it is suggested that perhaps he did not actually perform a physical examination on these patients but primarily observed them and took histories from them.

He did recognize a variety of other features of the disease, the emphasis of which was not made until much later. Perhaps he did not recognize their high frequency because of the limited number of patients studied. These features are now considered to be important aspects of the disease as noted by the contents of this book. With regard to sleep disorders he writes "in this stage, the sleep becomes much disturbed." The speech disorder is also well recognized, "the power of articulation is lost," and later he indicates in the later stages of disease "his words are now scarcely intelligible." He vividly describes the features of a masked face and drooling by indicating "the chin is now almost immovably bent down upon the sternum. The slops with which he is attempted to be fed, with the saliva, are continually trickling from the mouth." The inability to swallow is also alluded to by the use of soft foods in that comment. Constipation, a feature that we all know to be present in a large percentage of patients, is well recognized; "the bowels, which had been all along torpid, now, in most cases, demand stimulating medicines of very considerable power."

It is frequently attributed to Charcot (see Chapter 3) that Parkinson's disease may occur without tremor, but, in fact, Parkinson himself may have described such a case. In his Case 5 he mentions nothing of tremor in the description but instead only recognizes the akinesia and gait disorder. However, he only saw this patient from a distance. He also probably first described the freezing phenomenon, although this is also usually not attributed to his description. However, a discussion in Case 6 describes it perfectly: "it being asked, if whilst walking he felt much apprehension from the difficulty of raising his feet, if he saw a rising pebble in his path? He avowed, in a strong manner, his alarm on such occasion; and it was observed by his wife, that she believed, that in walking across the room he would consider as a difficulty the having to step over a pin." It is often noted that Parkinson did not recognize any psychiatric or behavioral changes that might be associated with the disease as indicated by his definition, which states "the senses and intellects being uninjured." It may be that he only believed that to be true for the earlier stages of the disease. Later in his description, when discussing advanced disease, he did note that the patients may suffer "with slight delirium." In addition, there was some discussion about the possibility of depression occurring in these patients. In discussing a case described in the literature that he considers very similar to paralysis agitans, there is a comment indicating "a more melancholy object I never beheld. The patient, naturally a handsome, middle-size, sanguine man, of a cheerful disposition, and an active mind, appeared much emaciated, stooped and dejected." There is no further discussion on whether he considered this a major feature of the disease. Finally, we have come to recognize, in the last two or three decades, that sensory symptoms may, in fact, occur in Parkinson's disease, particularly in relation to pain. Pain of various types has been well described (see Chapter 8). In fact, he does describe pain in a variety of ways in this manuscript, even suggesting that it may be an important early feature. In his description of Case 4 he describes that "his application was on account of considerable degree inflammation over the lower ribs on the left side" and after treating him he indicates that "no change appeared to have taken place and his original complaint." Both authors have had patients complain of similar distribution of pain. In addition, in Chapter 4 (the chapter on Proximate cause – Remote causes – illustrative cases), he discusses pain of the radicular type in the arms, which might represent an early feature of the disease. In fact, one female patient that he discussed complained of radicular pain similar to that described by other patients, which he thought might also represent paralysis agitans and attributed it to the disease. He states "on meeting with these 2 cases, it was thought that it might not be improbable that attacks of this kind, considered at the time merely as rheumatic affections, might lay the foundation of this lamentable disease, which might manifest itself at some distant period, when the circumstance in which it had originated, had, perhaps, almost escaped the memory."

He also recognized the more common occurrence of this disease in older patients, since his six patients all were 50 years of age or older. He also recognized, while discussing the literature and other similar cases, that younger age of onset might suggest the presence of a different disorder.

Chapter 3 provides his differential diagnosis for the shaking palsy and, in fact, he mentions how frequently, and inappropriately, that term is used to describe patients: "that the name by which it is here distinguished has been hitherto vaguely applied to diseases very different from each other, as well as from that to which it is now appropriated." He discusses patients with stroke, seizures, and other forms of tremor.

In Chapter 4, Parkinson ventures a guess on the location of the lesion and the etiology of the disease and indicates quite succinctly that it is a guess: "before making the attempt to point out the nature and cause of this disease, it is necessary to plead, that it is made under very unfavorable circumstances. Unaided by previous inquiries immediately directed to this disease, and not having had the advantage, in a single case, of that light which anatomical examination yields, opinions and not facts can only be offered. Conjecture founded on analogy, and an attentive consideration for the peculiar symptoms of the disease, have been the only guides that could be obtained for this research, the result of which is, as it ought to be, offered with hesitation." As in the classic neurologic teaching, Parkinson takes us through the localization process by showing first that it is a nervous disease by writing "by the nature of the symptoms we are taught, that the disease depends upon some irregularity in the direction of the nervous influence," and then he goes on to indicate more specifically that it is a central nervous system disease, and particularly located in the upper cervical spine, instead of a peripheral nervous system disease. He writes "that the injury is rather in the source of this influence than merely in the nerves of the parts; by the situation of the parts whose actions are impaired, and the order in which they become affected, that the proximate cause of the disease is in the superior part of the medulla spinalis." He also points out that it does not go beyond the brain stem by stating "and by the absence of injury to the senses and to the intellect, that the morbid state does not extend to the encephalon." His primary thoughts on the etiological process relate to neck trauma and inflammation. It is interesting that he notes that none of his patients had had any significant trauma that might have caused the type of damage he was considering. In this chapter he provides discussions of appropriate cases. This is the weakest part of his paper because those patients that he discusses do not clearly have the symptoms of paralysis agitans. However, he uses them as an example in much the same way as we hypothesize on etiology and location of the lesion by the discussion of obvious symptomatic cases. In relation to this he notes "although it may not mark an identity of the disease, serves at least to show that nearly the same parts were the seat of disease in both instances. Thus we attain something like confirmation of the supposed proximate cause and of one of the assumed occasional causes. He further discusses the slowly progressive nature of the pathologic process within the brain leading to the progressive nature of the disease: "but taking all circumstances into due consideration, particularly the very gradual manner in which the disease commences, and proceeds in its attacks; as well as the inability to ascribe its origin to any more obvious cause, we are led to seek for it in some slow morbid change in the structure of the medulla, or its investing membranes, or theca, occasioned by simple inflammation or rheumatic or scrophulous affection." He then discusses the order of spreading as the disease progresses in moving downward and further into the cervical spine or upward into the medulla oblongata.

Finally, in Chapter 5, he addresses possible treatments. He probably was the first person to discuss neuroprotective therapies: "There appears to be sufficient reason for hoping that some remedial process may ere long be discovered, by which, at least, the progress of the disease may be stopped." He also notes "and even, if unfortunately deferred to a later period, they might then arrest the further progression of the disease although the removing of the affects already produced, might be hardly to be expected," which indicates that he did not think much of symptomatic therapies at that time. Parkinson was not impressed by the use of oral therapies: " the employment of internal medicines is scarcely warrantable; unless analogy should point out some remedial trial of which rational hope might authorize." He was concerned, however, that because of the slow progression of the disease and the benign nature in the early stages, patients might delay treatment: "seldom occurring before the age of 50, and frequently yielding but little inconvenience for several months, it is generally considered as the ere remediable diminution of the nervous influence, naturally resulting from declining life; and remedies therefore are seldom sought for." When discussing the treatments of the day, he actually speaks about the need for clinical trials to prove their usefulness: "experiment has not indeed been yet employed to prove, but analogy certainly warrants the hope, that similar advantages might be derived from the use of the means enumerated, in the present disease."

The essay was well received in the medical community (15). As this was the latter part of an illustrious career, the reviews indicate knowledge of his previous work and respect for the man, his modesty, and his contributions. In particular, this report was found to be important and continues to be viewed in the same manner today. Despite this, there was no second printing of the monograph and originals became scarce. In the twentieth century attention was drawn back to it by its being reprinted in several books (1,2,4) and in copies provided by pharmaceutical companies.

If one were to look at Parkinson's initial cry for attention to this disease and then look at the contents of this book, it would be clear that his intent was successful. Parkinson's disease continues to be one that receives substantial research attention as well as publicity in the lay literature. In the preface Parkinson says, "should the necessary information be thus obtained, the writer will repine to no censure which the precipitated publication of mere conjectural suggestions may incur; but shall think himself fully rewarded by having excited the attention of those, who may point out the most appropriate means of relieving a tedious and most distressing malady." Although we have not yet cured Parkinson's disease, if he could see the progress made in the last two centuries, as presented in this text, we think he would be "fully rewarded."

Acknowledgments

This chapter was supported by the National Parkinson Foundation, The Albany Medical College Parkinson Research Fund, and the Riley Family Chair in Parkinson's Disease (SAF).

REFERENCES

1. McMenemey WH. James Parkinson 1755–1824: A biographical essay. In: Critchley M (ed.). *James Parkinson (1755–1824)*. London: Macmillan, 1955: 1–143.
2. Morris AD. James Parkinson: His life and times. In: Clifford Rose F (ed.). *History of Neuroscience*. Boston: Birkhauser, 1989.
3. Kelly EC. James Parkinson. *Med Classics* 1938; 2:957–997.
4. Eyles JM. James Parkinson (1755–1824). *Nature* 1955; 176:580–581.
5. Tyler KL, Tyler HR. The secret life of James Parkinson (1755–1824): The writings of Old Hubert. *Neurology* 1986; 36:222–224.
6. Jelinek JE. Parkinson and the plum tree. *Arch Neurol* 1994; 51:1182–1183.
7. Yahr MD. A physician for all seasons: James Parkinson 1755–1824. *Arch Neurol* 1978; 35:185–188.
8. Currier RD, Currier MM. James Parkinson: On child abuse and other things. *Arch Neurol* 1991; 48:95–97.
9. Gibson W. An Essay on Dr. James Parkinson (1755–1824). From the XIII International Congress on Parkinson's Disease. Vancouver, Canada, July 1999.
10. Gibson W. Dr. James Parkinson (1755–1824). *Neurosci News* 1999; 2:11–14.
11. Pearce JMS. Aspects of the history of Parkinson's disease. *J Neurol Neurosurg Psychiatry* 1989; 52(Suppl):6–10.
12. Parkinson J. *An Essay on the Shaking Palsy*. London: Sherwood, Neely, and Jones, 1817.
13. Calne DB, Dubini A, Stern G. Did Leonardo describe Parkinson's disease. *N Engl J Med* 1989; 320:594.
14. Manyam BV. Paralysis agitans and levodopa in "Ayurveda": Ancient Indian medical treatise. *Mov Disord* 1990; 5:47–48.
15. Hertzberg L. An Essay on the Shaking Palsy: Reviews and notes on the journals in which they appeared. *Mov Disord* 1990; 5:162–166.

2

Paralysis Agitans in the Nineteenth Century

Elan D. Louis, M.D., M.S.

Gertrude H. Sergievsky Center, College of Physicians and Surgeons, Columbia University, New York, New York

INTRODUCTION

James Parkinson, a general practitioner, published the first pamphlet devoted exclusively to paralysis agitans ("An Essay on the Shaking Palsy") in 1817 (1). Despite its wide-renown in the present day, Parkinson's work is said to have received little immediate attention in his native country, England, and when he died in 1824, Parkinson was perhaps better known as a geologist and political pamphleteer (see Chapter 1). As late as 1868, one-half century after Parkinson's seminal publication, Sanders implied that nothing new had been added to the literature on this disorder: "succeeding authors have, in general, simply quoted it [Parkinson's initial publication], or have . . . overlooked the disease altogether" (2). He further added that the original contributions made since his [Parkinson's] time have been few and fragmentary" (2). There are several other indications that, before Charcot's studies beginning in 1861, (3–5) the disease had received little attention. In 1861 Charcot wrote that "paralysis agitans is indisputably a very little known disease" (3), and McHenry wrote in 1958 that "Charcot later named this *hitherto unrecognized* [my italics] entity after Parkinson" (6).

The purpose of this chapter is to examine the medical literature on Parkinson's disease during the 45-year period from 1817 to 1861 in order to provide an account of the number and type of references to the shaking palsy. This chapter serves as a supplement to a partial bibliography that has been published elsewhere (7). The year 1861 was chosen as an endpoint because it represents the beginning of Charcot's landmark publications in this area (see Chapter 3) (3–5). This analysis is restricted to the literature published in Parkinson's native country, England.

BACKGROUND

In 1817 (1) Parkinson elegantly described the clinical features of six cases of what he termed the *shaking palsy* or *paralysis agitans* including the resting tremor, flexed posture, festinating gait, and "lessened muscular power" or "paralysis" (1,6,8). He did not distinguish what he referred to as "paralysis" or "lessened muscular power" from what would be recognized by later physicians as bradykinesia and paucity of movement. His detailed and insightful view of the disease was based on only six cases. Further testament to his ability to astutely observe was the fact that several of these cases (cases 2,3,5) had either been "only seen at a distance," "noticed casually in the street," or "casually met with in the street" (1). In 1865 Sanders suggested alternative names for the shaking palsy, including "Parkinson's disease," "paralysis agitans festinia," "paralysis agitans senilis," and "paralysis agitans Parkinsonii" (9). Later, in 1888, Charcot suggested renaming this entity after James Parkinson (Parkinson's disease) (6).

LITERATURE REVIEW

The British literature on paralysis agitans during this 45-year period included 26 references (10–35), apart from Parkinson's treatise (1). These references were published in either general medical textbooks (*N* = 5), textbooks dealing specifically with disorders of the nervous system (*N* = 3), or journals (*N* = 18). Each of these references was relatively brief. None provided an original and comprehensive analysis of the clinical signs, treatment, etiology, and pathology of this newly described disorder. References may be divided into three categories. The first were those that provided no more than a partial reiteration of Parkinson's initial clinical description, often quoting directly from his 1817 treatise (10–16). The second were those that provided somewhat more than a reiteration of Parkinson's description. These consisted either of passing remarks about paralysis agitans or of brief descriptions of original case reports (17–29). The third were those that described cases that today we would classify as other neurologic disorders (e.g., convulsive disorders) (30–35). Each of these categories is discussed further in the following passages.

A substantial number of the references merely provided a partial reiteration of the detailed clinical descriptions of Parkinson. These references, the majority of them in textbooks, did not provide new clinical observations (10–16). They either quoted or paraphrased large sections from Parkinson's treatise. All of these credited James Parkinson with the initial description (e.g., "A disease has been lately described by Mr. Parkinson, under the title *paralysis agitans* or shaking palsy, which appears to me to be highly deserving of our attention" (10) or "Mr. Parkinson's description of the disease, however, is the best we have hitherto had and is as follows (11).)

Several references provided more than a reiteration of Parkinson's description (17–29). These consisted either of passing remarks about paralysis agitans or of brief original case reports. The majority of these were published in journals rather than in textbooks. Many of these were published by Dr. Elliotson, a practitioner at St. Thomas's Hospital in London. In 1827 Elliotson commented on an individual with paralysis agitans to whom he had attended at St. Thomas's Hospital. The patient was briefly described as having "constant shaking of the legs and arms" (17). Elliotson further wrote: "The intensity of the tremor varies. Till within the last week, the agitation would sometimes cease for a few hours or even a whole day, but for the last week has been constant" (17). In 1830 Elliotson described a 38-year-old schoolmaster with right-sided tremor of 18-months' duration. The patient also exhibited a tongue tremor and tachyphemia. Elliotson wrote: "The affection of the tongue is attended by the following very curious result … and suddenly he brings out his words with extreme rapidity; and such is the effort that he cannot stop himself.… It is a phenomenon analogous to the running which occurs on the attempt to walk (19). In 1831, in a clinical lecture published in *The Lancet*, Dr. Elliotson remarked on paralysis agitans. He distinguished between "organic" forms of paralysis agitans arising later in life and paralysis agitans resulting from fright: "There was a case of

acute rheumatism, and one of *paralysis agitans* from fright. I spoke of this disease before. The patient was a man fifty years of age; and usually, I believe, it arises at such an age from an organic cause, for I have never been able to cure a person of it at or after middle life. I cured one between thirty and forty years of age, but he was the oldest. In this case it came on from fright, and therefore there may be nothing organic …" (20). It would seem that Dr. Elliotson had under his care individuals with several distinct disorders, all of which he labeled "paralysis agitans." Among these were cases of paralysis agitans that started in later life and were difficult to cure. These were probably cases of Parkinson's disease. In 1838 (23) and again in 1841 (24), Hall wrote: "I have long had an interesting case under my care" (24). He briefly described a man, 28 years of age who "is affected by weakness and agitation of the right arm and leg; augmented on any occasion of agitation, and on moving; it is observed as he walks or when he passes his cane from one hand to the other; there is, besides, a peculiar lateral rocking motion of the eyes, and a degree of stammering and defective articulation" (24). Hall referred to this entity as "hemiplegic paralysis agitans" (24). In 1842 Thompson commented in *The Lancet* that treatment with the ergot of rye was beneficial in "… the paralysis agitans or tremens in advanced life, where I have seen it of considerable benefit recently myself …" (25). One of the lengthier accounts of paralysis agitans was published in the *Guy's Hospital Reports* in 1853. Four cases in individuals ranging in age from 34 to 60 years were briefly described. Each case was reported by a different author. Consistently noted were the gradual and asymmetric onset of this disorder, the subsequent involvement of both ipsilateral limbs, the progression to a more severe and generalized disorder, and the predominance, clinically, of resting tremor (27). The following passages are excerpted from this report: "a fair healthy looking man, by trade a hatter, states that in October, two years ago, the weather being cold at the time, he got very wet, and sat for a long time in a coffee room with his wet clothes upon him, and afterwards embarked on board a steam boat, remaining on deck all night. The next morning on disembarking, he could scarcely walk, his limbs feeling stiff and tired. After four days, his right hand began to tremble so much that he could not write, and gradually the whole arm became similarly affected. After eight months, his right leg began to feel heavy and tremble like the arm on the same side" (27). One of the other four cases was described as follows: "a 34-year-old man who was an engine driver of the one of the steam-tugboats on the river … dates his first symptoms from four years ago, when he began to have an aching pain in the left shoulder, soon following by trembling of the muscles, and in the course of a year extending down to the hand. The leg on the same side was similarly affected, and for nine months the disease was hemiplegic. During the last three months the other arm has begun to shake ..." (27). Finally, in 1855, Paget reported a man with a third cranial nerve palsy and a gait abnormality. The man, a 41-year-old brick maker, had been admitted to Addenbrooke's Hospital. Paget wrote that the patient's "tendency to fall is chiefly forwards; he has a tendency to lean forwards, and fall on his face.... Whenever he got out of bed, he likewise fell precipitately forward" (28,29). Paget noted that the gait abnormality was progressive, writing as follows: "During the earlier part of the time, he could make two or three steps forward before falling; afterwards, the propensity to fall forwards showed itself before he could take a single step" (28). Interestingly, the pathology in this case was attributed to a lesion in the region of the midbrain: "The disease of the crura was the only peculiar and uncommon lesion of the brain, and is therefore naturally associated with the peculiar and unique symptom" (28). He further noted that the lesion "was deeply seated, occupying in both crura the position of the locus niger, and encroaching on the nervous fibrils around it" (28).

Those references that did not merely reiterate what Parkinson had written consisted either of passing remarks or of brief comments without extensive clinical detail. When original cases were reported, these were isolated cases by single authors. Only one author of this period described having seen more than one case: Elliotson had seen "four or five cases" by 1833 (13).

Several references described cases that today we would classify as other neurologic disorders (30–35). In 1827 a case of "paralysis agitans" was described with unusual features including the onset of tremor in a leg, which was described as "swollen, dark coloured, and painful" (30). The illness was also accompanied by "giddiness, with some pain in the head" (30). In *The Lancet* in 1831, Gowry described a case of "paralysis agitans intermittens" (31). The patient, a 26-year old woman "of sanguine temperament" (31), experienced convulsive paroxysms for a period of less than one week. The author wrote: "Involuntary tremor of upper and lower extremities, continuing for about five or six minutes, occurring twice or three times every hour, and attended with complete loss of power of limbs; muscles of lips re [sic] rapidly and spasmodically brought into contact during paroxysm, and tongue partially protruded, with a corresponding sound, and inability to articulate; orbicular muscles of eyelids, during some of the paroxysms, are similarly affected; paroxysm terminates in a heavy sigh.... During intermission

is able to raise hands to head, but this is done slowly and with great consequent fatigue" (31). In this particular case, the term *paralysis agitans* was used descriptively to refer to the cessation of voluntary movement (paralysis) accompanied by chronic seizure activity (agitans). An anonymous report, dated 1832, described a case seen at St. Thomas's Hospital (32). The diagnosis was given as "paralysis agitans", although the clinical course was unusual. The report described a 54-year old "china-burner, of a spare habit" (32), who had been admitted to the hospital. He had experienced two episodes that were separated by an 18-month period. Each episode was of six weeks duration, during which "the whole of his extremities were in a continual state of tremor; head and jaw also affected" (32). The patient made a "perfect" recovery each time. In 1839 a case of paralysis agitans was reported in *The Lancet* (33). From the description, it seems more probable that the patient, a 14-year-old girl "of apparently good constitution, though slender make" (33), had transiently experienced either epilepsia partialis continua, chorea, or ballism. The author wrote that the patient "... has a constant and violent involuntary motion or shaking of the right forearm, and slightly of the arm; the motion is so violent that it cannot be stopped, though held down. Was seized with the same complaint months ago, and got relief from some medicine taken inwardly" (33). She recovered almost fully from the reported episode after a brief period of four days, with the author writing that she was "almost quite well; only a very slight tremulous motion indeed, so slight as to be scarcely perceptible; has good motion of the arm, and thinks in a few days more shall be perfectly restored" (33). Green described tremor disorders in three children (34). Reynolds reported a case of a 57-year-old carpenter who had a tremor. However, the tremor seemed to be an action tremor rather than a tremor at rest: "any attempt to move the limb voluntarily at once reproduces the shaking" (35). With the use of galvanic stimulation, the tremor resolved to a great extent. In summary, both "paralysis" and shaking or "agitans" were noted to accompany neurologic disorders other than Parkinson's disease, and the term *paralysis agitans* was often loosely applied to these disorders. The problem was well summarized by Sanders in 1865: "In regard to paralysis agitans, it is necessary to remark that this name is sometimes loosely and inaccurately applied .... It may be questioned, however, whether the term paralysis agitans ought to be confined to the senile form of it, associated with a propensity to fall or move forwards, described by Parkinson. I think, that it would be more useful to reserve for Parkinson's disease the specific name of paralysis agitans festinia, or senilis, or Parkinsonii, and thus leave us free to extend the general name of paralysis agitans to other causes occurring at various ages, and not attended by the irresistible impulse to move forwards. Certainly there are many instances of true paralysis (especially spinal paralysis and paraplegia) which are accompanied by jerking and shaking movements without any tendency to move forward, and which require a designation that shall not confound them with Parkinson's disease" (9).

It was clear to Parkinson and others that the motor system was one of the systems principally affected in paralysis agitans. The early view was that the paucity and slowness of movement were the result of weakness or paralysis, and hence, the nomenclature, paralysis agitans, seemed appropriate (1,10,24). Parkinson (1817) noted that patients with this disorder had "lessened muscular power" (1), and he further added that "the weakened powers of the muscles in the affected parts is so prominent a symptom, as to be very liable to mislead the inattentive, who may regard the disease a mere consequence of constitutional debility" (1). Similarly, Cooke (1820) wrote that "this disease begins with some degree of weakness" (10), and Hall (1841) wrote that "the first symptom of this *insidious* [his italics] disease is weakness and tremor" (24). However, several authors questioned whether paralysis was indeed present. In 1836 Watson wrote that "I refer to what has been badly called the *shaking palsy* [his italics] ... badly ... because there is in truth no paralysis at all" (16). In 1855 Reynolds wrote that "The term paralysis agitans is essentially bad, as paralysis does not necessarily exist in the condition referred to, and when present, as in some cases, is not primary.... The patient can do little with his affected limbs; but it is because of their constant agitation, not because of their paralysis" (15). However, a clear separation between signs of pyramidal dysfunction (weakness and spasticity) and extrapyramidal dysfunction (bradykinesia and rigidity) did not arise until the work of Charcot (See Chapter 3). In 1879 Charcot wrote: "According to that author [Parkinson], decreased muscle strength always accompanies the disease, and it is probably true for a good number of cases. But this is far from being the rule. Many patients, including ours today, maintain, at least for a long time, good muscular strength" (4). In the 1880s Charcot (6) began to call to attention the presence of "slow movements" and "muscular rigidity" in his patients with paralysis agitans, distinguishing rigidity from weakness and bradykinesia: "More commonly, muscular rigidity only comes on or predominates in the most advanced stage of paralysis agitans. Yet, long before rigidity actually develops, patients have significant difficulty performing ordinary activities; this problem relates to another cause. In some of the various patients I showed you can easily recognize how difficult it is for them to do things even though rigidity or tremor is not the limiting feature. Instead, even a cursory exam demonstrates that their problem relates more to slowness in execution of movement rather than to real weakness.... These phenomena have often been interpreted as weakness, but you may be assured that until late in the disease these patients are remarkably strong" (6).

Although Parkinson noted that the intellect was "uninjured" in paralysis agitans (1), the prevalence of dementia in Parkinson's disease has been variably estimated to be on the order of 10 percent to 40 percent (36–40). During the 45-year period in question, clinicians sometimes made passing remarks about cognitive compromise observed in later stages of this illness. For example, Reynolds wrote that "the intelligence is enfeebled" (15). However, it was not until after this period that physicians first began to emphasize the presence of cognitive impairment in some of their patients. In 1865 Sanders noted that in the final stages of the disease, "the memory and intellect are weakened" (9). In 1881 Buzzard wrote the following regarding the mental state of one of his patients, a 64-year-old man who had worked as an upholsterer's foreman and who had had paralysis agitans for two years duration: "As regards his mental state, in reply to inquiry he says that 'he feels lost.' He says 'he wants to give his address,' and gives 139 Bow Road, which is not altogether correct. He seems very obtuse, and scarcely speaks at all, though he is always apparently conscious" (41).

During this time period, there was little new knowledge or understanding of the precise location of the pathology in this disorder. In general, authors reiterated Parkinson's explanation that the pathology lay in the superior part of the medulla spinalis (1). However, as noted previously, in 1855 Paget reported a man with a third cranial nerve palsy and the "involuntary tendency to fall precipitately forwards" (28). On autopsy, a mass "... came close to the surface at the origin of the left oculo-motor nerve; but elsewhere it was deeply seated, occupying in both crura the position of the locus niger, and encroaching on the nervous fibrils around it" (28). Paget then wrote: "But, assuming the immediate cause of the falling forward to have been due to the disease of the crura cerebri, we have still some little ambiguity. The structure of each crus is twofold; in its interior is the locus niger, the vesicular substance constituting a nervous centre. The exterior is composed of nervous fibrils, which form the medium of communication between the cerebral and other parts of the nervous system.... It may, then, the asked, whether the peculiar symptoms were due to the disease of the nervous centre or of the fibers of communication.... The locus niger is, with good reason, regarded as the nervous centre of the oculo-motor nerve; and this seems commonly held to be its function. We have no right to presume that its function is thus limited, although, looking to its moderate dimensions, we may incline to the opinion, that it cannot exercise a very considerable influence over the general movements of the body and so may be justified in concluding that the particular derangement of locomotion was rather caused by disease of the fibres whose function is to keep up a communication between the cerebrum and other parts of the nervous system" (28). For the time being, the central role of the substantia nigra in the pathogenesis of Parkinson's disease remained elusive. Later, in the 1870s and again in 1893, Benedikt, Blocq, and Marinesco reported cases of hemi-parkinsonism in the setting of peduncular tuberculomas, and in 1893 Brissaud speculated that the substantia nigra might be the location of the disease process (42–44).

The primary aim of this analysis was to review the literature published in Parkinson's native country, England. During this period, there were also several references to Parkinson's disease in both the German and the French literature. The most notable were those of Romberg (45,46) and Trousseau (47). These have been discussed elsewhere (48).

CONCLUSION

James Parkinson's work in 1817 on the shaking palsy (1) received little initial attention in his country, and before Charcot's work in this area, which began in the early 1860s (3–5), this disease was the subject of little scholarship (2,3,6). In the 45-year period between 1817 and 1861, there are a small number of references in the British literature to "shaking palsy." References that either (1) merely reiterated word for word what had already been written by Parkinson or quoted directly from his text (2) provided passing remarks about paralysis agitans, (3) provided relatively sparse clinical descriptions of newly-reported cases, and (4) did not separate Parkinson's disease from other disease entities characterized by both "shaking" and "palsy" (e.g., tonic-clonic seizures and ballism). During this period, little new information was added to the original clinical observations made by Parkinson in 1817. The separation of extrapyramidal signs (bradykinesia) from pyramidal signs (weakness) did not become apparent until later work by the French neurologic community.

Acknowledgments

This work was supported by Federal Grant NIH NS01863 and the Paul Beeson Physician Faculty Scholars in Aging Research Award.

REFERENCES

1. Parkinson J. *An Essay on the Shaking Palsy*. London: Whittingham and Rowland, 1817.
2. Sanders WR. Paralysis agitans. In: Reynolds JR (ed.). *System of Medicine*. Vol. 2. Philadelphia: J.B. Lippincott and Co., 1868:184–204.
3. Charcot JM, Vulpian A. De la paralysie agitante. *Gaz Hebdomadaire Med Chirurg* 1861; 8:765–767, 816–820; 9:54–59.
4. Charcot JM. *Lectures on Diseases of the Nervous System*. Philadelphia: H.C. Lea and Co. 1879.
5. Charcot JM. Paralysie Agitante, Tremblement Senile, Sclerose en Plaque. *Gaz Hopit Paris* 1881; 54:98–100.
6. McHenry LC Jr. James Parkinson, Surgeon and Paleontologist. *J Okla Med Assn* 1958; 51:521–523.
7. Reynolds JR. *A System of Medicine*. Philadelphia: J.B. Lippincott and Co., 1868:184–204.
8. McMenemey WH. James Parkinson 1755–1824: A Biographical Essay. In: Critchley M (ed.). *James Parkinson (1755–1824)*. London: Macmillan, 1955:1–143.
9. Sanders WR. Case of an Unusual Form of Nervous Disease, Dystaxia or Pseudo-Paralysis Agitans, with Remarks. *Edinburgh Med J* 1865; 10:987–997.
10. Cooke J. *A Treatise on Nervous Disease*. London: Longman and Co., 1820:207.
11. Good JM. *The Study of Medicine, with a Physiological System of Nosology*. 2nd ed. Philadelphia: Bennett & Walton, 1824:297–300.
12. Good JM. *The Study of Medicine*. Vol IV. 3rd ed. London: Thomas and George Underwood, 1829:486–490.
13. Elliotson J. Lectures on the theory and practice of medicine. Diseases of the head and nervous system. *London Med Gaz* 1833; January 5:433–537.
14. Todd RB. Paralysis. In: Forbes J (ed.). *Cyclopaedia of Practical Medicine*. Vol III. London: Sherwood, Gilbert and Piper, 1833:259–260.
15. Reynolds JR. *The Diagnosis of Diseases of the Brain, Spinal Cord, Nerves and Their Appendages*. London: John Churchill, 1855:163–164.
16. Watson T. *Lectures on the Principles and Practice of Physic Delivered at King's College, London*. Vol. I. 5th ed. Philadelphia: Henry C. Lea, 1872:629–631. [A little-revised edition of lectures initially given in 1836-1837].
17. Elliotson J. On the medical properties of the subcarbonate of iron. *Medico-Chirurgic Transact* 1827; 13:232–353.
18. Elliotson J. On the use of subcarbonate of iron in tetanus. *The Lancet* 1829:557–559.

19. Elliotson J. Clinical lecture on paralysis agitans. *The Lancet* 1830:119–123.

20. Elliotson J. Clinical lecture. *Lancet* 1831; I:289–297.

21. Elliotson J. Clinical lecture. *Lancet* 1831:557.

22. Elliotson J. Clinical lecture. *Lancet* 1831:599.

23. Hall M. Lectures on the theory and practice of medicine. *The Lancet* 1838:41.

24. Hall M. *On the Diseases and Derangements of the Nervous System.* London: H Baillière, 1841:320–321.

25. Thompson JB. "Chorea sancti viti," with cases and observations. *Lancet* 1842; I:616–618.

26. Graves RJ. *A System of Clinical Medicine.* Dublin: Fannin & Co., 1843.

27. Birkett EL. Poland A. *Guy's Hospital Reports.* 2nd ser. London: John Churchill, 1853:134–136.

28. Paget GE. Case of involuntary tendency to fall precipitately forwards, with remarks. *Med Times Gaz* 1855; 10:178–180.

29. Reynolds JR. Dr. Paget's case of disease in the crura cerebri. *Med Times Gaz* 1855; 10:218–219.

30. Case of paralysis agitans, or shaking palsy, treated with carbonate of iron. *Lancet* 1827:766–767.

31. Gowery TC. Case of paralysis agitans intermittens. *Lancet* 1831; II:651.

32. Hospital reports. St. Thomas's Hospital. Paralysis agitans. *London Med Surg J* 1832; 11:605–607.

33. Gibson M. On spinal irritation. *Lancet* 1839; II:567–571.

34. Green H. Cases of nervous tremor in children. *Prov Med J* 1844:178.

35. Reyonolds JR. Report of a case of paralysis agitans removed by continuous galvanic current. *Lancet* 1859; II:558–559.

36. Celesia GG. Wanamaker WM. Psychiatric disturbances in Parkinson's disease. *Dis Nerv Syst* 1972; 33:577–583.

37. Lieberman A, Dziatolowski M, Kupersmith M, et al. Dementia in Parkinson's disease. *Ann Neurol* 1979; 6:355–359.

38. Martilla RJ, Rinne UK. Dementia in Parkinson's disease. *Acta Neurol Scand* 1976; 54:431–441.

39. Mayeux R, Stern Y, Rosenstein R, et al. An estimate of the prevalence of dementia in idiopathic parkinson's disease. *Arch Neurol* 1988; 45:260–263.

40. Mayeux R, Chen J, Mirabello E, et al. An estimate of the incidence of dementia in patients with idiopathic Parkinson's disease. *Neurology* 1990; 40:1513–1517.

41. Buzzard T. A clinical lecture on shaking palsy. *Brain* 1881; 4:473–492.

42. Benedikt M. Tremblement Avec paralysie croisée du moteur oculaire commune. *Bull Méd* 1889; 3:547–548.

43. Marinesco G. Blocq P. Sur un cas de tremblement Parkinsonien hémiplégique d'une tumeur du pédoncule cérébral. *Comp Rend Soc Biol* 1983; 5:105–111.

44. Brissaud E. In: Meige H (ed.). *Leçons Sur Les Maladies Nerveuses.* Paris: Masson, 1895.

45. Romberg M. *Lehrbuch der Nervenkrankheiten des Menschen.* Berlin: A. Duncker, 1840–1846.

46. Romberg M. *A Manual of the Nervous Diseases of Man.* Vol II. London: New Sydenham Society, 1853.

47. Trousseau A. Tremblement senile et paralysie agitante. *Clinique Médicale de l'Hotel-Dieu de Paris.* Paris: Bailliere, 1861.

48. Tyler KL. A history of Parkinson's disease. In: Koller WC (ed.). *Handbook of Parkinson's Disease.* New York: Marcel Dekker, 1987.

3

Charcot and Parkinson's Disease

Christopher G. Goetz

Professor of Neurological Sciences, Professor of Pharmacology, Rush Medical College, Rush-Presbyterian–St. Luke's Medical Center, Chicago, Illinois

INTRODUCTION

During their early years at the Salpêtrière in the 1860s, J-M. Charcot and A. Vulpian collaborated so closely in the study of multiple sclerosis and Parkinson's disease that the exact contribution made by each cannot be determined. As early as 1861, they coauthored a three-part summary article in which they reviewed the past medical literature (primarily foreign), referred to a few reports by French colleagues, and added a case that they had observed themselves (1–3). Charcot recalled in 1868 that his well-documented first article still did not clarify the nature and characteristics of multiple sclerosis that he and Vulpian frequently faced in the large population of Salpêtriére invalids. "In all these descriptions, including our own, there was total confusion between paralysis agitans and multiple sclerosis" (4) (161F, 134E). The separation of Parkinson's disease from other neurologic entities was one of Charcot's major clinical contributions, and in facilitating the proper identification of the disease, these studies set the stage for the eventual anatomic link to midbrain lesions by Brissaud in 1895 (5) and nigral degeneration by Greenfield and Bosanquet in 1953 (6).

Jean-Martin Charcot's focused descriptions of Parkinson's disease, its clinical spectrum, and associated features were amplified throughout his career. His amphitheater teaching sessions at the Salpêtrière provided the needed medical and theatrical setting to compare various movement disorders from the vast patient material at Charcot's disposal. Charcot lectured specifically on Parkinson's disease, both in his formal Friday lectures and in his show-and-tell clinical case presentations, known as the "Tuesday lessons." The formal lectures were by and large read from detailed notes that were compiled by his assistant Bourneville into the multivolume complete works *Oeuvres Complètes* (4). The Tuesday lessons were impromptu teaching exercises and primarily aimed at showing diagnostic strategies through history-taking and clinical examination. These doctor–patient dialogues were hand-transcribed by his students, Blin, Colin, and Jean Charcot, the professor's son. These were reproduced in lithograph form in limited edition and later edited (and often purged of interesting comments and reflections) for a more widely available printed version (7).

TREMOROUS DISEASES

The origin of clinical confusion between multiple sclerosis and Parkinson's disease was the prominent shaking or tremor that occurred in both conditions. Charcot approached the problem of differential diagnosis by examining tremor as a clinical phenomenon. These studies stand among Charcot's most perceptive clinical investigations and showed his ingenious methods of collecting clinical data with the tools available at the time. Although today tremors are best analyzed with special electronic detectors that are lightweight and sensitive to small amplitude changes in movement, Charcot adapted the available tools of the era to his advantage. His first studies were purely observational; he noted that some tremor occurred when the patient moved the involved extremity, but it was absent when the limb was completely relaxed and immobile. In contrast, other tremors persisted during rest and often occurred only at rest. Using an adaptation of the bulky apparatus called a sphygmograph, Charcot was able to record various tremors and demonstrate the difference in frequency and amplitude in groups of patients (Figure 3-1). By comparing groups of patients, Charcot noted that those with rest tremor also had rigidity, balance difficulties, and slowness of movement (Figure 3-2). These features constituted the cluster of signs known as paralysis agitans or Parkinson's disease, a condition previously described in 1817

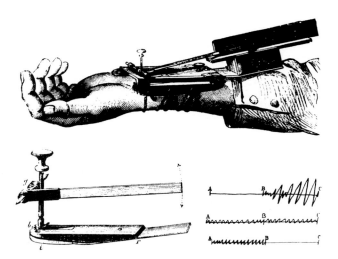

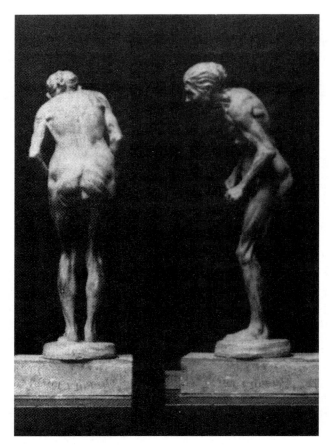

FIGURE 3-1. The sphygmograph was developed originally for recording pulses, but at the Salpêtrière the machine was adapted to allow recording of tremors and movements of the wrist. (From *Dictionnaire Encyclopédique des Sciences Mèdicales*, Ser. 3, Vol. 11, pp. 208–209, 1883). Tremor drawings from Charcot's lesson on tremor classification. AB indicates rest and BC represents action. **Top:** multiple sclerosis; **middle and bottom,** Parkinson's disease.

and well known clinically in spite of its having no identified neuropathologic lesion. In contrast, patients with predominant action tremor had distinctive multifocal sclerotic lesions of the central nervous system that had been termed *sclérose en taches ou en isles* by Cruveilhier (8). Charcot increasingly ascribed this type of tremor clustered with signs of weakness, sensory abnormalities, visual problems, and nystagmus, to multiple sclerosis.

The lectures on comparative features of multiple sclerosis and Parkinson's disease were originally presented in 1868, 1869, and 1871. Thereafter they were repeated in modified form. For many of the studies, Charcot recruited his interns and externs, and the results formed the basis of many medical theses for graduating interns. With his familiar proviso, *"si je ne me trompe pas,"* he remarked on his student's work of 1868: "If I am not mistaken, the line of demarcation between these was determined by me for the first time in the thesis of Dr. Ordenstein" (4) (161F, 134E).

Parkinson's Disease

After a long and frustrating search, Charcot acquired a copy of Parkinson's *"An Essay on the Shaking Palsy"* (1817) through the help of an English librarian, Dr. Windsor. In 1887 there was still no French translation of this work. Speaking in his impromptu Tuesday lessons, he said: "It is a small pamphlet almost impossible to find. . . . As short as the work is, it contains

FIGURE 3-2. Statue by Paul Richer who worked at the Salpêtrière as an artist, physician, and sculptor. This patient shows the flexed posture and joint deformities of Parkinson's disease. The statue today is in the Musée de l'Assistance Publique, Paris.

a number of superb ideas, and I would encourage any one of you to embark on a French translation (7, leçon 9)." He described the features identified by Parkinson, citing the strengths and weaknesses of the original description: "This is a descriptive and vivid definition that is correct for many cases, most in fact, and will always have the advantage over others of having been the first. But it errs by being too general and being inapplicable to the case where tremor is absent. We also do not find here a reference to the element of rigidity that gives to these patients their characteristic appearance. We could go back and improve on this definition as a starting point for more discussion, although we should not stop at Parkinson's definition. Read the entire book, and it will provide you with the satisfaction and knowledge that one always gleans from a direct clinical description made by an honest and careful observer" (7).

Beginning with this essay, Charcot dissected the four cardinal features of Parkinson's disease, and from the definition of archetype cases, he encouraged his students to define and classify clinical variants.

Tremor

On the basis of his early work with Vulpian, Charcot divided tremor by using the same features that modern neurologists employ – the frequency of the movements and the actions associated with the tremor's greatest intensity (1). Charcot placed the tremor of both Parkinson's disease and multiple sclerosis in his first category of slow tremors, that is, 4 to 6 oscillations. He differentiated the two by the observation that multiple sclerosis patients have no tremor at rest and that their tremor becomes evident only with activity and increases with effort. In contrast, Parkinson's disease patients show tremor both at rest and during activity, and the intensity does not increase with action (Figure 3-1). A third type of slow tremor, referred to by others as senile tremor, had the characteristics of Parkinsonian tremor, except that head titubation accompanied the tremor.

Charcot was tenacious in his stand that Parkinson's disease patients had no head tremor and that any shaking of the head that they might show was entirely secondary to trunk or extremity tremor. This stand was contested by other contemporaries and became the source of heated discussion among clinicians in Paris (10). To prove this point, Charcot brought a series of patients to the amphitheater, each wearing a headband to which Charcot had attached a long thin rod with a feather at the end. Charcot instructed the audience to watch the wavering of the feathers from these many patients (Figure 3-3). As those affected with Parkinson's disease sat or stood, the feathers oscillated like those on the heads of patients with other forms of tremor. But if the trunk or arm was suddenly supported or moved, the head tremor promptly ceased. With this famed feather study, Charcot convinced his colleagues that titubation was not an accompanying feature of Parkinson's disease and that any head shaking seen in such patients was mere overflow. However, Charcot clearly recognized jaw and tongue tremors as features of parkinsonism.

The observation that movement or support diminished parkinsonian tremor shows that Charcot realized the importance of movement in the control of Parkinsonian tremor. Early in the disease, movement suspended tremor. Later, however, with disease progression, tremor became continual. Parkinsonian tremor was never exacerbated by patient movement (Figure 3-1).

To contrast with the slow forms of tremor, Charcot identified rapid or vibratory tremors, that is, 8 to 9 oscillations. In this group were tremors associated with alcoholism, Basedow's disease, and general

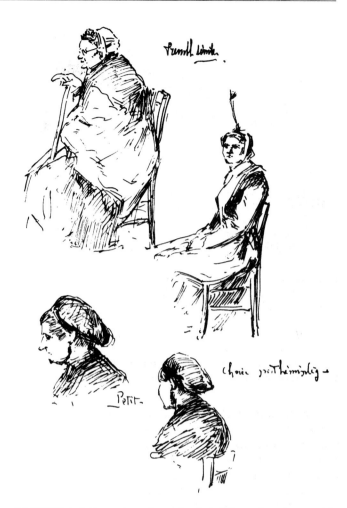

FIGURE 3-3. Drawings from the Salpêtrière of patients with various neurologic conditions. The top two figures are of note for this article: the top figure shows the hunched posture of a patient with Parkinson's disease; the second figure demonstrates Charcot's method of determining titubation and postural head tremor. The patient wore a band around the head with a feather attached to the top, and physicians observed the wavering of the feather when the head was unsupported and supported.

paresis. In his final group of tremor with intermediate oscillatory frequency, he included mainly hysterical tremors and mercurialism. In addition to the frequency, particular characteristics typified the parkinsonian tremor. Charcot described a patient: "The parts of the hand oscillate in almost a pathognomonic manner. The fingers approach the thumb as if to spin wool, and simultaneously the wrist and forearm flex to and fro" (7, Leçon 9).

Although Charcot recognized that tremor was a major manifestation of Parkinson's disease, he was insistent that it was not required for the diagnosis. In this regard he considered the term *paralysis agitans* a misnomer. He recognized that most patients have both rigidity and tremor and divided variants of Parkinsonism into two major categories – cases with tremor and no rigidity and those with rigidity and no tremor. In those patients without marked tremor, he observed that the posture was often less flexed, with the legs and back held in a stiff and even slightly extended attitude.

Bradykinesia

Although Charcot did not speak of akinesia specifically, he clearly recognized it as distinct from rigidity in its clinical significance and often in its independent temporal development. Having spoken of the rare situation in which rigidity may be marked early in the disease, he wrote: "More commonly, muscular rigidity only comes on or predominates in the most advanced stage of paralysis agitans. Yet, long before rigidity actually develops, patients have significant difficulty performing ordinary activities; this problem relates to another cause. In some of the various patients I showed you, you can easily recognize how difficult it is for them to do things even though rigidity or tremor is not the limiting feature. Instead even a cursory exam demonstrates that their problem relates more to slowness in execution of movement rather than to real weakness. In spite of tremor, a patient is still able to do most things, but he performs them with remarkable slowness. I commented on this a few minutes ago in regard to speaking. Between the thought and the action there

is a considerable time lapse. One would think neural activity can only be effected after remarkable effort; in reality, the execution of the slightest movement causes extreme fatigue for the patient. These phenomena have often been interpreted as weakness, but you may be assured that until late in the disease, these patients are remarkably strong" (7, Leçon 21). Commenting on the masked face or blank stare that is so characteristic of the Parkinsonian patient, he continued: "... the muscles of the face are motionless, there is even a remarkable fixity of look, and the features present a permanent expression of mournfulness, sometimes of stolidness or stupidity" (4) (167F, 139E). On masked faces, he continued: "This particular faces was not originally appreciated. It is not in Parkinson's description. I believe I am the first to draw attention to its features that are so arresting and that in fact suffice to establish with ease the proper diagnosis" (4, (168F, 140E).

Stance, Posture, and Gait Abnormalities

Charcot considered drawings, photography, and sculptures to be important medical documents and invested heavily in developing a medical iconography wing of the Salpêtrière service. Charcot himself was an avid sketcher and included his own drawings as part of regular patient notes (*observations*). Although technically crude and rapidly executed, they captured the stature, posture, and gait of Parkinson's disease in its natural evolution (Figure 3-4). Of Charcot's

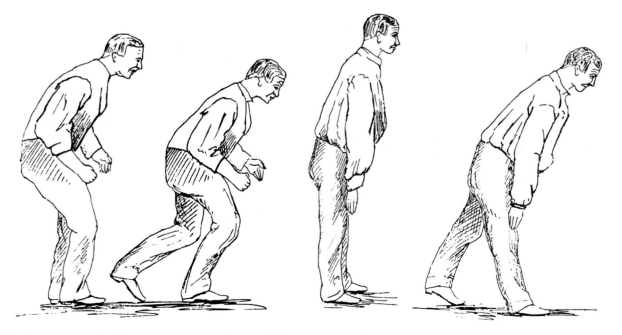

FIGURE 3-4. Drawing by Charcot contrasting the usual flexion posture of Parkinson's disease with one variant of Parkinson's disease with extended posture.

drawings, Henry Meige wrote: "The ability to discern in a country scene or in a human body certain essential contours, to perceive instantly a pattern and to be able to isolate from this pattern the elements necessary for its expression – and to do it exactly in spite of all irrelevant details – this is the faculty that Charcot possessed to a high degree. (11, p. 491)."

In Figure 3-5 Charcot captured the posture, facial expression, and hands of a parkinsonian Jewish merchant seen on one of his voyages to Morocco in 1889. With his junior colleagues he developed *La Nouvelle Iconographie de la Salpêtrière*, a journal that contained an extensive photographic and drawing

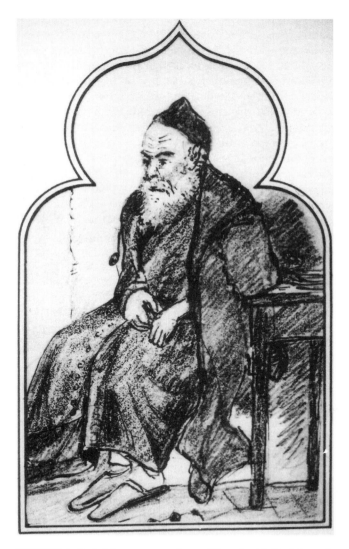

FIGURE 3-5. A Moroccan patient afflicted with Parkinson's disease, drawn by Charcot in 1889 while he was on a voyage As Charcot said to his students, "I have seen such patients everywhere, in Rome, Amsterdam, Spain. They reflect always the same picture. They can be identified from afar. You do not need a medical history" (9, Leçon 21).

collection of the neurologic patients at the Salpêtrière during and after Charcot's tenure until 1918.

Charcot described the slow and hesitant walking of parkinsonian patients and the patient's tendency to retropulse and propulse. "In contrast, if you even tap the second patient, he will propulse forward and his gait will be quite unusual. His head bends forward, he takes a few steps and they become quicker and quicker to the point that he can even bump into the wall and hurt himself. If I pull on his trousers from behind, he will retropulse in the same distinctive way" (7, Leçon 21).

Charcot attempted to analyze propulsion and retropulsion and remained unsatisfied with available theories. "In this regard, I will make a comment on a rather widespread and respected physiologic explanation of propulsion in patients with paralysis agitans. I willingly agree that the tendency to make running steps relates to the thrust-forward posture, so that in walking, these patients will run after their center of gravity. Evidently, however, this explanation will not account for retropulsion, for the body's forward inclination does not change at all as the patient retropulses. In this case, he cannot be said to run after his center of gravity; in fact, he runs away from it" (7) Leçon 21.

Rigidity

Parkinson himself did not speak of rigidity in his description. Charcot, however, identified this important sign and differentiated it from spasticity: "Spasticity, as you know, is of spinal origin and is more or less directly related to a physiologic or structural dysfunction of the descending spinal pyramidal tracts. What is the physiologic explanation for rigidity in Parkinson's disease? As far as I know, nothing is known and it is just this ignorance that I plan to demonstrate to you today. I have two goals, first to stimulate you to study the phenomenon of rigidity and second to impress on you the essential distinction between rigidity and pyramidal or spinal hypertonicity, that is, the absence of reflex accentuation in rigidity" (7, Leçon 22).

The absence of pyramidal weakness in rigid parkinsonian patients was further emphasized by Charcot: "Sooner or later there is an apparent decrease in strength. Movement is slow and seemingly weak, although testing with a dynometer shows that this is not really weakness. Such problems seem rather to relate, as we will see, to muscle rigidity" (7, Leçon 22).

Etiology and Natural Progression

Charcot classified Parkinson's disease as a *névrose*, a term used to designate neurologic conditions, where no identifiable neuroanatomic lesions were present. Although the onset was usually insidious, he believed that two precipitating influences could be identified – prolonged exposure to a damp cold environment, especially a dark first-floor dwelling with poor air ventilation, and a sudden exposure to intensely emotional crisis. In the case report by Romberg of a patient who started his tremor after he was robbed by Cossacks and left in the snow, the two influences could not be easily separated. The disease affected patients in their forties and fifties and was distinctly not a disease that regularly began in the early population. Charcot thought that tremor could cease during the final phase of illness, even when it had been the most prominent feature of the disease in the past (4).

Charcot believed that Parkinson's disease could resolve and be cured in certain cases, but he doubted that such cases related in any way to the various pharmacologic therapies used. He cited several reports of patients who were followed by reputable physicians and whose parkinsonism disappeared. Whether there were toxic or drug-induced forms of reversible parkinsonism in the nineteenth century is not known. After citing the reports of cures coincident with therapy he wrote: "These citations show that the shaking palsy is not incurable, but we must recognize that we know nothing about nature's role in such cases of reversible disability" (7, Leçon 9).

Treatment

"He disdained therapeutic interventions, considering the irregularities of the human body as an astronomer would watch the movements of the stars." (12). These words were written by the writer Léon Daudet, who had known Charcot in several capacities, as the playmate and boyhood friend of Charcot's son, as a medical student under Charcot's watchful eye, and as the son of Charcot's patient, novelist Alphonse Daudet, who suffered from neurosyphilis. The description evokes an image of a scientific purist and a distant, objective, even emotionally cold researcher, an image reinforced by Charcot's silent manner and stern physical bearing. In spite of their drama, however, Daudet's words must be reviewed with circumspection, for throughout the height of his career Charcot was not only a world-renowned scientific researcher but also a prominent and highly sought-after practicing physician. As a clinician, Charcot developed aspects of the modern neurologic examination, introduced diagnostic tools and strategies, and treated numerous neurologic conditions, including Parkinson's disease with traditional and innovative, even controversial, therapies. Although Daudet suggests that Charcot was a therapeutic nihilist, Charcot's lectures, articles, and personal correspondence with patients demonstrated an active interest in therapeutic interventions.

Charcot's attentiveness to treatment, follow-up, and surveillance is evident in a series of 18 unpublished letters located in the archive collection of the Bibliothèque Charcot, Paris (portfolio MA VIII, Parkinson's disease), which concerns a patient with Parkinson's disease. These unnumbered documents, not all dated, cover a period of at least 15 months, from January 1863 through March 1864, and are kept in an envelope with the patient's name and the diagnosis "paralysis agitans" written in Charcot's large script. As a group, these letters reveal how the doctor–patient relationship arose and evolved, as well as the attentiveness offered to the patient by Charcot. Charcot's letters of reply to the patient were based on the patients and his family's assessment of response to treatment. Charcot adopted this system as an efficient form of organization for dealing with outpatients, as shown in an undated letter from the series attached with the prescription: "I would be most obliged, Monsieur, if you would remind me of this prescription the next time you write."

In the first letter, dated January 19, 1863, the patient reminded Charcot that he was originally referred by Brown-Séquard and that Charcot had seen him two months earlier. Charcot had prescribed rest and camphor therapy, which the patient followed, but without respite. Thereafter Charcot embarked on several therapies, and each time he modified his recommendation based on the detailed reports of symptoms and changes. The treatments included hyoscyamine, a centrally active anticholinergic drug that is among the class of agents currently used to treat Parkinson's disease, and ergot products, which are the basis of some modern dopamine agonist drugs. He also used silver nitrate, iron compounds, henbane, pills, and zinc oxide. Charcot was highly specific in his instructions, indicating that quinquina should be diluted with syrup made from orange rind and that pills be made of 0.5 centigrams of silver nitrate impregnated in 9 grams of soft bread to render 100 pills for ingestion.

The documents are particularly revealing of the tone of the doctor–patient relationship. The traditional image, derived from the Tuesday lessons of nearly 25 years later, is Charcot's speaking to the patient, often imperialistically, about his or her symptoms and the patient's generally accepting his recommendations without comment. These earlier letters document instead a lively interchange between doctor and patient, with the patient assertively evaluating Charcot's treatments and, with some audacity, even recommending that he consider others. When the patient was helped,

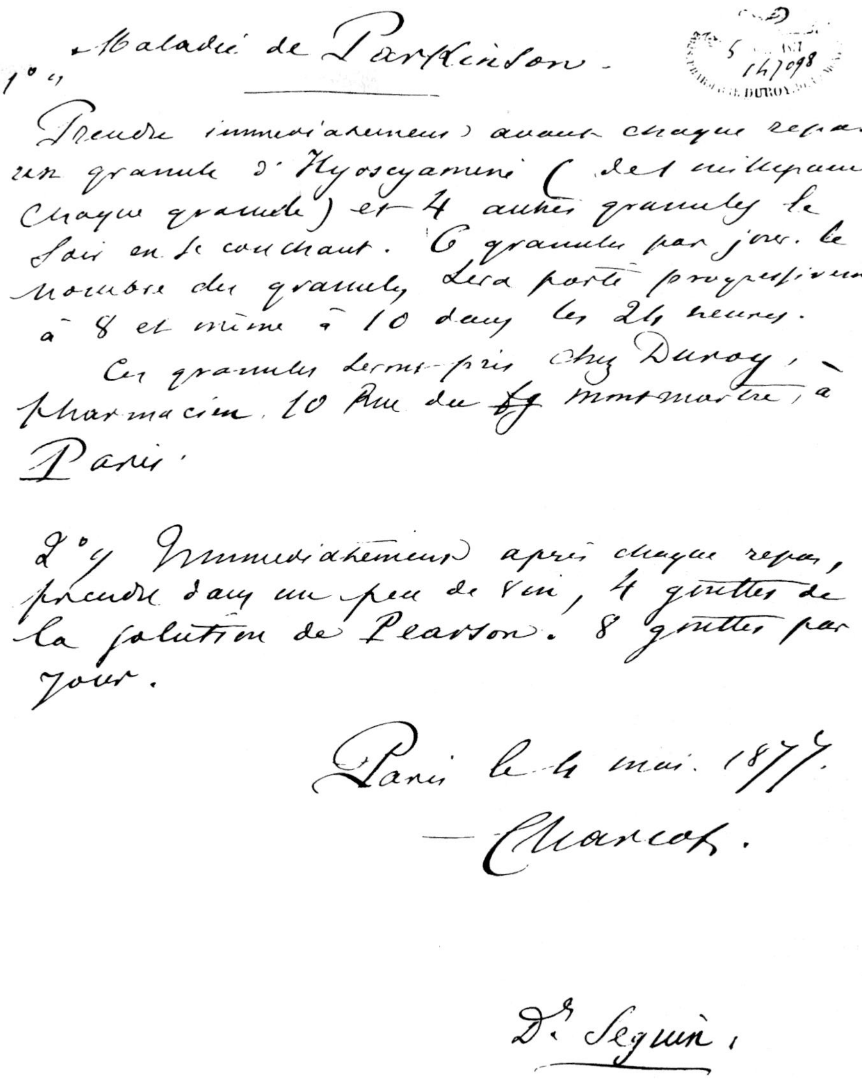

FIGURE 3-6. Prescription written by Charcot for a patient with Parkinson's disease. Translation:
1. Take immediately before each meal, one granule of hyoscyamine (at one milligram per granule) and four additional granules of the same dose at night before retiring. Start with six pills daily and progressively increase to eight and then ten pills daily. These pills may be bought at the Duroy Pharmacy, 10 rue de Faubourg Montmartre in Paris.
2. Immediately following each meal, take in a small glass of wine, 4 drops of Pearson solution, that is 8 drops each day. Paris, May 4, 1877 Charcot.

he openly acknowledged Charcot's contribution, but when he was not, he wrote back promptly asking for better treatments. The tone of Charcot's replies is not known, as his letters are not included, but the dates of the letters demonstrate that he answered the letters quickly and kept them together as a medical dossier. A copy of a prescription written by Charcot for a patient with Parkinson's disease is shown in Figure 3-6.

Drugs that Charcot personally used in treating Parkinson's disease, but without apparent effect, included ergot products from rye and belladonna. Hyoscyamine, an anticholinergic agent, was more useful, but he reminded students of its mere palliative effect. Summarizing his views of the state of therapy for Parkinson's disease in the 1870s, he stated: "Everything, or almost everything, has been tried against this disease. Among the medicinal substances that have been extolled, and which I have myself administered to no avail, I need only enumerate a few." (4)

Charcot's Students and the Salpêtrière

Although Charcot's research focus moved increasingly toward the study of hysteria in the 1880s, he maintained a keen interest in Parkinson's disease throughout his career. Several of his students wrote their medical theses on Parkinson's disease and its variants. After Charcot died, the Salpêtrière remained a focus of Parkinson's disease study, and E. Brissaud, who temporarily assumed Charcot's professorial chair in neurology, reported the cystic brain stem lesions in the midbrain of Parkinson's disease patients in 1895. Several articles on parkinsonian variants were published in the *Nouvelle Iconographie de la Salpêtrière* and other journals that Charcot had established. These reports remain important medical documents on parkinsonian syndromes and their natural evolution and progression, especially because of the accompanying photographs from the Salpêtrière archives.

REFERENCES

1. Charcot J-M, Vulpian A. La paralysie agitante. *Gaz Hebdom Med Chir* 1861; 765–768, 816–823; 1862; 54–64.
2. Charcot J-M, Vulpian A. Sur deux cas de sclérose des cordons postérieurs de la moelle avec atrophie des racines postérieurs (tabes dorsalis, Romberg; ataxie locomotrice progressive, Duchenne de Boulogne). *Comptes-Rendus des Séances et Mémoires de la Société de Biologie* 1862a; 4:155–173.
3. Charcot J-M, Vulpian A. Sur un cas d'atrophie des cordons postérieurs de la moelle épinière et des racines postérieures (ataxie locomotrice progressive). *Gaz Hebdomadaire de Médecine et de chirurgie* 1862b; 9:247–254, 277–283.
4. Charcot J-M. *Oeuvres Complétes*, Vol. 1 (Leçon 5). Paris: Bureaux du Progrés Médical, 1892. In English: Charcot JM. *The Diseases of the Nervous System Delivered at the Salpêtrière* (Translator, G. Sigerson.) London: New Sydenham Society, 1877.
5. Brissaud E. *Leçons sur les maladies nerveuses.* Paris: Masson, 1895.
6. Greenfield JG, Bosanquet FD. The brain stem lesions in parkinsonism. *J Neurol Neurosurg Psychiatry* 1953; 16:213–226.
7. Charcot J-M. *Leçons du Mardi à la Salpêtrière 1887–1888.* Paris: Bureaux du Progrès Mèdical, 1887.
8. Cruveilhier J. (1829–1842). *L'Anatomie Pathologique du Corps Humain.* Paris. Baillière.
9. Parkinson J. *An Essay on the Shaking Palsy.* London: Whittingham and Rowland for Sherwood. Neeley, and Jones, 1817.
10. Charcot J-M. Paralysie agitante, tremblement sénile, sclérose en plaque. *Gaz Hopit Paris* 1881; 54:98–100.
11. Meige H. Charcot Artiste. *Nouvelle Iconographie de la Salpêtrière* 1898; 11:489–516.
12. Daudet L. Devant la douleur. *Nouvelle Librairie Nationale.* Paris, 1944.

4

Twentieth Century – Timeline for PD

William J. Weiner, M.D.

Maryland Parkinson's Disease and Movement Disorder Center, University of Maryland, Baltimore, Maryland

and

Stewart A. Factor, D.O.

Parkinson's Disease and Movement Disorder Center of Albany Medical Center, Albany, New York

1911	First synthesis of D/L dopa	(1)
1912–13	Description of intracytoplasmic eosinophilic inclusions (later referred to as Lewy bodies) in dorsal motor nucleus of vagus and substantia innomita- the substantia nigra was considered unaffected in the original report	(2–3)
1913	Levodopa isolated from broad bean plants at Roche and a simplified manufacturing process described	(4)
1917–26	Encephalitis lethargica- Secondary parkinsonism	(5–6)
1919	Constancy of Nigral Lesions in PD	(7)
1929	Use of large doses of atropine for PD	(8)
1940	First Neurosurgical approach to the basal ganglia for treatment of postencephalitic tremor	(9)
1947	First sterototactic pallidotomy	(10)
1950s	Introduction of synthetic anticholinergics	(11)
1951	Discovery of dopamine ("Encephalin") in the brain and the determination that only levodopa could increase its CNS concentration	(12)
1951	First use of apomorphine in PD	(13)
1952–53	Substantia nigra lesions essential and occurrence of Lewy bodies required as definite criteria in neurologists definition of PD	(14–15)
1955	Introduction of thalamotomy [ventrolateral (VL)] for tremor	(16)
1957	Catechol compounds demonstrated in brains of a variety of animals	(17)
1957	Reserpine demonstrated to reduce brain dopamine; and reserpine-induced bradykinesia in rabbits reversed with levodopa	(18)
1958–59	Dopamine demonstrated to be highly concentrated in the caudate/putamen	(19–20)
1958	Catechol compounds including dopamine demonstrated in human brain	(21)
1960	Description of Shy-Drager syndrome	(22)
1960	Dopamine decreased in the corpus striatum of brain from patients with PD	(23)
1961–62	First reported successful trials of intravenous and oral low dose levodopa.	(24–25)
1964	Description of striatonigral degeneration	(26)
1964	Description of progressive supranuclear palsy (PSP)	(27)
1964–65	Histofluorescence techniques demonstrate that dopamine is concentrated in substantia nigra neurons, and existence of nigrostriatal dopaminergic pathway discovered	(28–29)
1967	First successful oral use of high dose D/L dopa	(30)

1968	Description of corticobasal ganglionic degeneration (CBGD) (31)
1969	First successful use of oral high-dose levodopa (32)
1969	Multiple system atrophy (MSA) – Unifying concept for striatonigral degeneration (SND), Olivoponto–cerebellar degeneration (OPCA) and Shy–Drager syndrome (33)
1969	First successful use of Amantadine (34)
1970	Larodopa (levodopa) approved by Food and Drug Administration for use in PD and levodopa introduced in worldwide distribution for PD (35)
1973	Introduction of decarboxylase inhibitors with levodopa (36)
1973	FDA approval of Sinemet (levodopa/carbidopa)
1973	Concept of dopamine receptor agonists (37)
1974	Identification of striatal dopamine receptors (38)
1974	First clinical use of dopamine receptor agonists in PD (39)
1975	Introduction of levodopa and benserazide (Madopar) (35)
1975	First clinical use of L-deprenyl in PD (35)
1978	Bromocriptine approved for use in the United States
1979	MPTP-induced parkinsonism first reported (40)
1979	Dopamine receptors exist as subtypes (41)
1983	MPTP-induced parkinsonism more fully described (42)
1985	First use of atypical neuroleptics (clozapine) for psychosis in PD (43)
1986	Parkinson Study Group (PSG) formed
1989	Thalamic DBS to treat tremor (44)
1989	Pergolide approved for use in the United States
1989	Selegiline approved for use in the United States
1990	Contursi kindred-large autosomal dominant parkinsonism kindred reported (45)
1990	Description of diffuse Lewy body disease (46–49)
1992	Reintroduction of pallidotomy for PD (50)
1991	Sinemet CR approved for use in the United States
1995	Subthalamic DBS to treat all features of PD (51)
1997	Pramipexole approved for use in the United States
1997	Ropinirole approved for use in the United States
1997	Mutation in Alpha-synuclein gene identified in Contursi and other families with PD (52)
1997	Mutation for juvenile parkinsonism reported (53)
1998	Tolcapone approved for use in the United States
1998	Lewy bodies – stain for alpha-synuclein (54)
1999	Entacapone approved for use in the United States
1999	First double-blind placebo-controlled trial demonstrating efficacy of an atypical neuroleptic (clozapine) in the treatment of psychosis in PD (55)

REFERENCES

1. Funk C. Synthese des d, 1-3-4, Dioxyphenylalanins. *Chem Zentralbl I*, 1911.
2. Lewy FH. Paralysis agitans. I. Pathologische anatomie. In: Lewandowsky M (ed.). *Handbuch der Neurologie.* Berlin: Springer J, 1912: 920–933.
3. Lewy FH. Zue pathologischen Anatomic der Parlysis agitans. *Deutsche Z Nervenheilkunde.* 1913; 50:50–55.
4. Guggenheim M. Dioxyphenylanin, eine neue Aminosaure aus Vicia faba. *Z Physiol Chem* 1913; 88:276–284.
5. Duvoisin RC, Yahr MD. Encephalitis and parkinsonism. *Arch Neurol* 1965; 12:227–239.
6. Von Economo C. Encephalitis lethargica. *Wien Klin Wochenschr.* 1917; 30:581–585.
7. Tretiakoff C. Contribution a l'etude de l'anatomie pathologic du locus niger de soemmering avec quelques deductions relative a la pathogenie des troubles du tunos musculaire et de la maladie de Parkinson. *These*

pour le doctorat en Medicine. Paris: These de Paris, 1919:1–24.
8. Kleemann. Zitiert nach Kapp W, Leickert KH. *Das Parkinson-Syndrom*. Stuttgart: Schattauer, 1971.
9. Meyers R. Surgical procedure for postencephalitic tremor, with notes on the physiology of the premotor ficres. *Arch Neurol Psychiat* 1949; 44:455–459.
10. Spiegel EE, Wycis HT, Marks M, et al. Stereotaxic apparatus for operations on the human brain. *Science* 1947; 106:349–350.
11. Fahn S. The history of parkinsonism. *Mov Disord* 1989; 4(suppl 1): S2–S10.
12. Raab W, Gigee W. Concentration and distribution of "encephalin" in the brain of humans and animals. *Proc Soc Exp Biol Med* 1951; 180:1200.
13. Schwab RS, Amador LV, Lettvin JY. Apomorphine in Parkinson's disease. *Trans Am Neurol Assoc* 1951; 76:251–253.
14. Beheim- Schwarzbach D. Uber-zelleib- veranderungen in nucleus coeruleus bei Parkinson symptomen. *J Nerv Ment Dis* 1952; 116:619–632.
15. Greenfield JG, Bosanquet FD. The brain-stem lesions in Parkinsonism. *J Neurol Neurosurg Psychiatry* 1953; 16:213–226.
16. Hassler R. The pathological and pathophysiological basis of tremor and parkinsonism. *Second Intl Congr Neuropath*. Amsterdam: Excerpta Medical Foundation, 1955:2940.
17. Montagu KA. Catechol compounds in rat disease and in brains of different animals. *Nature* 1957; 180:244–245.
18. Carlsson A, Lindquist M, Magnusson T. 3,4-dihydroxyphenylalaninen and 5-hydroxytryptophan as reserpine antagonists. *Nature* 1957; 180–200.
19. Carlsson A, Lindquist M, Magnusson T, et al. On the presence of 3 hydroxytyramine in brain. *Science* 1958; 127:471–472.
20. Bertler A, Rosengren E. Occurrence and distribution of catecholamines in brain. *Acta Physiol Scand* 1959; 47:350–361.
21. Sano I, et al. Distribution of catechol compounds in human brain. *Biochem Biophys Acta* 1959; 32:586–587.
22. Shy GM, Drager GA. A neurological syndrome associated with orthostatic hypotension. *Arch Neurol* 1960; 2:511–527.
23. Ehringer H, Hornykiewicz O. Verteilung von noradrenalin und dopamin (3-hydroxytyramin) ingerhirn des menschen und ihr verhalten bei erkrankugen des extrapyramidalen systems. *Klin Wochenschr* 1960; 38:1236–1239.
24. Birkmayer W, Hornykiewicz O. Der 1-3,4 Dioxyphenylalanin (= DOPA)- Effekt bei der Parkinson-Akinese. *Wien Jklin Wochenschr* 1961; 73:787–788.
25. Barbeau A, Sourkes TL, Murphy CF. Les catecholamines dans la maladie de Parkinson, In J de Ajuriaguerra (ed). *Monoamines et Systeme Nerveaux Central*. Geneva: Gerog, 1962; 247–262.
26. Adams RD, Van Bogaert L, Van der Eecken H. Striatonigral degeneration. *J Neuropath Exp Neurol* 1964; 23:584–608.
27. Steele JC, Richardson JC, Olszewski J. Progressive supranuclear palsy. *Arch Neurol* 1964; 10:333–359.
28. Anden NE, Carlsson A, Dahlstrom A, Fuxe J\K, Hillarp N-A, Karlsson K. Demonstration and mapping of nigroneostriatal dopamine neurons. *Life Sci* 1964; 3:523–530.
29. Poirier LJ, Sourkes TL. Influence of the substantia nigra on the catecholamine content of the striatum. *Brain* 1965; 88:181–192.
30. Cotzias GC, Van Woert MH, Schiffer LM. Aromatic amino acids and modifications of parkinsonism. *N Eng J Med* 1967; 276:374–379.
31. Rebeiz JJ, Kolodny EH, Richardson EP. Corticodentatonigral degeneration with neuronal achromasia. *Arch Neurol* 1968; 18:20–33.
32. Cotzias GC, Papavasiliou PS, Gellene R. Modification of parkinsonism-chronic treatment with L-dopa. *N Eng J Med* 1969; 280:337–345.
33. Graham JG, Oppenheimer DR. Orthostatic hypotension and nicotine sensitivity in a case of multiple-system atrophy. *J Neurol Neurosurg Psychiatry* 1969; 32:28–34.
34. Schwab RS, England AC, Poskanzer DC, Young RR. Amantadine in the treatment of Parkinson's disease. *JAMA* 1969; 208:1168–1170.
35. Kapp W. The history of drugs for the treatment of Parkinson's disease. *J Neural Transm* 1992; 38:1–6.
36. Rinne UK, Sonninen V, Siirtola T. Treatment of parkinsonism patients with levodopa and extracerebral decarboxylase inbibitor, Ro 4-4062. *Adv Neurol* 1973; 3:59–71.
37. Corrodi H, Fuxe K, Hokfelt T, Lidbrink P, Ungerstedt U. Effect of ergot drugs on central catecholamine neurons. Evidence for a stimulation of central dopamine neurons. *J Pharm Pharmacol* 1973; 25:409.
38. Seeman P. Brain dopamine receptors. *Pharmacologic Rev* 1980; 32:229–313.
39. Calne DB, Teychenne PF, Claveria LE, Eastman R, Greenacre JK, Petrie A. Bromocriptine in parkinsonism. *Br Med J* 1974; 4:442–444.
40. Davis GC, Williams AC, Markey SP, et al. Chronic parkinsonism secondary to intravenous injection of merperidine analogs. Psychiatry Res 1979; Vol 1:249–254.
41. Kebabian JK, Calne DB. Multiple receptors for dopamine. *Nature* 1979; 277:92–96.
42. Langston JW, Ballard P, Tetrud JW, et al. Chronic parkinsonism in humans due to a product or merperidine-analog synthesis. *Science* 1983; 219:979–980.
43. Scholz E, Dichgans J. Treatment of drug-induced exogenous psychosis in parkinsonsim with clozapine and fluperlapine. *Eur Arch Psychiatr Neurol Sci* 1985; 235:60–64.

44. Benabid AL, Pollak P, Hommel M, et al. Treatment of Parkinson tremor by chronic stimulation of the ventral intermediate nucleus of the thalamus. *Rev Neurol (Paris)* 1989; 145:320–323.

45. Golbe LI, Di Iorio G, Bonavita V, Miller DC, Duvoisin RC. A large kindred with autosomal dominant Parkinson's disease. *Am Neurol* 1990; 27:276–282.

46. McKeith IG, Galasko D, Kosaka K, et al. Consensus guidelines for the clinical and pathological diagnosis of dementia with Lewy bodies. (DLB): report of the Consortium on DLB international workshop. *Neurology* 1996; 47:1113–1124.

47. Kosaka K. Diffuse Lewy body disease in Japan. *J Neurol* 1990; 237:197–204.

48. Dickson DW, Ruan D, Crystal H, et al. Hippocampal degeneration differentiates diffuse Lewy body disease (DLBD) from Alzheimer's disease: Light and electron microscopic immunocytochemistry of CA2-3 neurites Lewy body disease. *Archives of Neurol* 1993; 50:140–148.

49. Hansen LA, Masliah E, Terry RD, Mirra SS. A neuropathological subset of Alzheimer's disease with concomitant lewy body disease and spongiform change. *Acta Neuropathologica* 1989; 78:194–201.

50. Latinen LV, Bergenheim AT, Hariz MI. Ventroposterolateral pallidotomy can abolish all parkinsonian symptoms. *Stereotact Funct Neurosurg* 1992; 58:14–21.

51. Limousin O, Pollak P, Benazzouz A, et al. Effect on parkinsonism signs and symptoms of bilateral subthalamic nucleus stimulation. *Lancet* 1995; 345:91–95.

52. Polymeropoulos MH, Lavedan C, Leroy E, et al. Mutation in α-synuclein identified in families with Parkinson's disease. *Science* 1997; 276:2045–2047.

53. Matsumine H. et al. Localisation of a gene for autosomal recessive form of juvenile parkinsonism to chromosome 6q25.2-27. *Am J Hum Genet* 1997; 60:588–596.

54. Spillantini MG, et al. α-synuclein in Lewy bodies. *Nature* 1997; 388:839–840.

55. Parkinson Study Group. Low-dose clozapine for the treatment of drug-induced psychosis in parkinson's disease. *N Engl J Med* 1999; 340: 757–763.

5

Epidemiology of Parkinsonism

M.L. Rajput, MS, and A.H. Rajput, FRCPC

University of Saskatchewan, Royal University Hospital, Saskatoon, Saskatchewan, Canada

The epidemiology of Parkinson's disease (PD) can be divided into three broad categories that cover descriptive, analytic, and experimental or clinical (1). Descriptive epidemiology deals with incidence, mortality, and prevalence rates. Analytic studies identify those factors that influence the frequency of parkinsonism, different variants of parkinsonian syndrome (PS), time trends and their significance. These studies identify association of different events and factors with PD in an effort to determine the cause. Clinical epidemiology includes studies that require repeated careful clinical assessments or autopsy studies, for example, which parkinsonian syndromes respond to which anti-parkinsonian drugs?

Most scientific research occurs in laboratories, where a hypothesis is generated and then tested using controlled experiments. By contrast, epidemiology is the study of nature's experiments that may have been influenced by economic, social, or medical developments. Unlike laboratory experiments, which can be strictly controlled for factors including temperature, dose, and duration to eliminate confounding variables, epidemiologic studies must continuously navigate minefields of biases. Major biases may be introduced during case finding, data collection, data analysis, or interpretation of data. If care is not taken, these biases can render conclusions invalid. Planned laboratory experiments can be verified by others using exactly the same methodology and material. However, no two epidemiologic studies are ever identical because they are conducted using human populations over long periods of time.

Compared to laboratory experiments, epidemiologic studies require considerably more time and effort, and the yield, for example, publications or presentations per unit of effort, is far less. Epidemiologic studies must be planned, conducted, and interpreted carefully – patience truly is a virtue in these studies. The disadvantages are balanced by an important fact. The final objective of biomedical research is the application to human health and disease, and an overwhelming majority of laboratory studies may never reach this goal. In contrast, epidemiologic studies that are done well have direct and immediate application.

Making the connection between an epidemiologic study and daily clinical practice requires interpretation on the part of the clinician. It is important that appropriate significance be given to each aspect of the observations. Any large report may have only a small proportion that is scientifically valid and clinically applicable. A clinician may be faced with having to interpret a one-of-a-kind epidemiologic study. An even more difficult situation is presented when two somewhat similar studies come to different conclusions. In those situations, a rule of thumb is often the best guide – rely on your intuition regardless of who the author is, where the study was conducted, and in which journal the paper is published. If something does not make sense, do not believe it, or at least reserve judgment until further research supports the conclusions. Here we briefly outline some of the issues that are critical for good epidemiologic studies of parkinsonism.

SELECTION OF LOCATION AND POPULATION

There is no community or institution that lends itself to all types of epidemiologic studies. Experimental and clinical studies are conducted in clinic populations. Incidence studies often must focus on physician-diagnosed cases ascertained via health care providers. Prevalence studies can be conducted in any community with appropriate effort. Because there is no biologic marker, the diagnosis of PS cases can only be made by clinical assessment and requires a high level of cooperation on the part of the people being screened. All individuals in the community may not wish to participate. In spite of some limitations, door-to-door survey of a community is the best method to ensure accurate ascertainment of all cases for prevalence studies.

The age distribution of the population being studied must also be considered. Parkinsonism is concentrated in older age, and studies that are restricted to individuals above a certain age would find inflated rates. Unless rates are adjusted for the age distribution of the community residents, these rates are not applicable to the general population. Prevalence studies conducted in community residents often exclude the institutional population. Because a large proportion of advanced parkinsonian patients reside in institutions, these studies provide lower prevalence rates and are therefore not generalizable (2,3).

DIAGNOSIS OF PARKINSONISM AND PARKINSON SYNDROME VARIANTS

Wide variations in the diagnostic criteria utilized in epidemiologic studies make comparisons difficult, if not impossible. While reading the results of a study, it is critical to ascertain the definition used by the researchers to discern exactly which patient population is being described. For the purpose of epidemiologic studies, it should be noted that a de novo emergence of resting tremor in an otherwise healthy elderly individual is a very strong indication of a diagnosis of PD (4). Similarly, resting tremor onset in the lower limbs is usually indicative of PD (5). deRijk and coworkers (6) carefully reviewed the literature on diagnostic criteria of PS used in different epidemiologic studies and concluded that the best criteria are the same as used in clinical studies (6). A patient is diagnosed as having PS if two of the following three symptoms are documented: bradykinesia, rigidity, and tremor (6,7). Of course, an accurate diagnosis of parkinsonism is just the first step as there are several different variants to be distinguished (7) if the objective of the study were to study idiopathic PD alone (8).

The first described anatomic correlation with unilateral parkinsonian features was that by Blocq and Marinesco in 1893, consequent to tuberculoma involving the contralateral substantia nigra (9). The understanding of the anatomical basis of PS however evolved much later. The first description of the disorder was by James Parkinson in 1817 (10). Lewy described Lewy body inclusions in 1912, but their significance to parkinsonism was not established until 1919, more than 100 years after the first clinical description, when Tretiakoff recognized that Lewy body pathology in the substantia nigra was a consistent feature in these patients (11). At that time it was believed that this

disorder represented a single clinicopathologic entity. Following the von Economo encephalitis outbreak in 1916, postencephalitic parkinsonism was first recognized in 1921 (11). Thus it became evident that a focal lesion such as a tuberculoma or an infection such as von Economo encephalitis or an unknown cause such as Lewy body disease can all produce clinical features of parkinsonism. Therefore the terminology was changed to indicate that there are several Parkinson syndromes and the term *Parkinson's disease* was reserved for Lewy body disease (8). There have been no new cases of postencephalitic parkinsonism since the mid-1950s, but other variants have subsequently been recognized. Drug-induced parkinsonism (DIP) was first identified in the late 1950s and is now the second most common variant of parkinsonism in the general population (12–14). Arteriosclerosis, which was once believed to be common pathology in parkinsonism, is now a rare cause of PS (12,13). The rapid drop in diagnoses made of arteriosclerotic parkinsonism from 31 percent of cases in 1965 to 1 percent or less in the same community between 1967 and 1990 indicates better understanding of the etiology of PS rather than a dramatic decline in ischemic parkinsonism (12,13,15). Arteriosclerosis and parkinsonism may coexist in some of these elderly, but the two are not causally linked in most of the cases.

In the early 1960s, progressive supranuclear palsy (PSP) (16), Shy-Drager syndrome (17), and striatonigral degeneration (18) were described as distinct entities. Spinocerebellar ataxias that produce PS as a feature of olivopontocerebellar atrophy were documented in the 1920s. There is some evidence that these disorders are not new entities but that there is simply greater recognition of these variants of PS. For example, Charcot documented a case in the nineteenth century with the clinical picture of PSP (19). Multiple system atrophy (MSA) includes both Shy-Drager syndrome and striatonigral degeneration. In the past many of the MSA patients were probably loosely classified as atypical Parkinson syndrome or arteriosclerotic parkinsonism, or were regarded as postencephalitic parkinsonism because of the younger age at onset.

Most epidemiology studies make no special effort to identify different variants of PS, and this can complicate the interpretation of results and the generalizability of conclusions. There are two North American studies that looked at the entire population and clinically classified the parkinsonian patients into different variants (12,13). In a Rochester study of patients diagnosed between 1967 and 1979, 85.5 percent of the PS cases were PD followed by DIP accounting for 7.2 percent, and there were no new cases of postencephalitic parkinsonism (13). PSP accounted for 1.4 percent and MSA for 2.1 percent of all subjects, whereas vascular parkinsonism was approximately 1% of all cases. The latest Olmsted County study, including Rochester, indicates that 14 percent of the PS cases had dementia as the primary feature and PS was discovered on further neurologic evaluation (12). This category would not be evident without the special project dealing with dementia. That may partly explain the higher incidence of PS in the most recent study (12) compared to the prior incidence study from the same institution, albeit with a somewhat different population base (13). Although Bower and coworkers (12) classified 42 percent of PS cases as PD, Lewy body disease is probably the basis of a much larger proportion of parkinsonism in this community (12), considering that a sizable proportion of the demented cases may have dementia with Lewy bodies (20) and a number of the 20 percent PS cases, who were classified as DIP, may have underlying Lewy body pathology (21). Every recent incidence and prevalence study has noted that the most common parkinsonian variant is PD.

To further complicate matters, the clinical diagnosis of PD is not always accurate (7). In most cases the error involves misdiagnosing other PS variants or essential tremor patients as PD. The other variants such as Jakob-Creutzfeldt disease and PS secondary to toxins or trauma are rare. Epidemiologic studies probably do not accurately reflect the frequency of the uncommon variants. Most such cases are published as single case reports or small case series from specialty clinics that are subject to referral bias. A large proportion with DIP are reported in Rochester/Olmsted county studies (12,22), and in one population study in Italy (14) that noted 8.8% of PS cases as having that diagnosis. Drug-induced parkinsonism patients are concentrated in the chronic care institutions. In our research, parkinsonism was studied in elderly institutionalized individuals and elderly community residents (2,3). Although none of the community residents had DIP (2), one-third of the parkinsonian patients in the institution had DIP (3). Those epidemiologic studies that are all inclusive therefore indicate a larger proportion of DIP (12,13,22). They reflect the PS variants in the entire population and therefore are more meaningful. With the widespread use of newer antipsychotic agents, it is anticipated that DIP will become less common in the future.

In recent years association of dementia and PD has received much attention. There is growing evidence that at any given point nearly one-third of parkinsonian patients have clinically evident dementia (23), and nearly half of Alzheimer's disease patients have some parkinsonian features (24–27).

PROGRESSION OF PARKINSONISM AND STAGING OF DISEASE

The distribution of patients with respect to stage of disease is another important characteristic to know about a study population. Parkinson syndrome progresses through recognizable stages of the disease, but this progression differs in PS variants. The rate of progression of disability is more rapid in MSA and PSP than in idiopathic PD (4,28,29). In the past it has been estimated that the progression from one Hoehn & Yahr stage to the next takes approximately 2 to 2.9 years (30), but our own studies indicate that progression in an optimally treated PD patient is much slower. An average nondemented PD patient with onset at age 62 years treated appropriately progresses by one H & Y stage (31) in approximately six years. The progression rate varies widely from patient to patient.

Despite these variations, in any given individual the disease will advance at a relatively fixed rate (30). With treatment, the disability due to the underlying pathology can be controlled in most patients. In general, severe morbidity is now compressed in the last one to two years of life in most cases.

MANPOWER CONSIDERATION FOR EPIDEMIOLOGIC STUDIES

It goes without saying that the quality of an epidemiologic study depends on the quality of the data collected. Because there is no biologically valid instrument to screen the general population for a diagnosis of PS or PD, it is essential that studies include clinicians with expertise in movement disorders who can make an accurate diagnosis. For example, there is a large body of literature on "family history" based on information obtained from family members and community or church records. These sources may be misleading. In one large family with several autopsy-confirmed PD cases followed in our movement disorder clinic, several family members assured the researchers that a certain deceased family member had PD. It was subsequently discovered that he was a medicolegal case and an autopsy had been done. Careful histologic evaluation of the brain failed to reveal any evidence of PD.

When relatives of PD patients were examined, the concordance of PD in secondary cases with a movement disorder seen in the clinic was 74 percent (32). The second most common diagnosis in secondary cases was essential tremor (21%). Distinction between tremor-dominant parkinsonism and essential tremor can be difficult in some cases (33), and some features of parkinsonism are seen in the majority of normal elderly (34,35). For accurate case finding it is essential therefore that the study team include a qualified neurologist, preferably one specializing in movement disorders, to make the diagnosis. For analytic epidemiology, an expert must see all the patients and, where possible, diagnoses should be verified with autopsy studies. Also, controls used in these studies must be verified to not have PS.

Finally, biostatisticians and epidemiologists are vital team members and should be involved in the study design and data analysis and interpretation. They raise important questions and advise on areas of study in which a clinician may not be qualified. Their involvement throughout the study process can assist in limiting possible biases and enabling accurate conclusions to be drawn from the results of the analyses.

OBJECTIVES OF EPIDEMIOLOGIC STUDIES

Each of the previously mentioned topics must also be evaluated in light of the stated objective for a given study. Each epidemiologic study is conducted with certain primary and secondary objectives designated a priori. If the objective were to identify the number of parkinsonian patients in the general population, it is necessary that all variants of PS be included as each produces disability and needs care. Restricting such studies to PD is not appropriate in this situation. Even after many years of follow-up, up to 24 percent of the patients clinically diagnosed as PD had a different diagnosis (7,36). On the other hand, some DIP patients have subclinical parkinsonian pathology (21). Thus, for the purpose of descriptive epidemiology, all the variants of PS should be included and residents of all ages, in both the community and institutions, be considered.

If the objective were to study etiology of a certain variant of PS, only those patients who suffer from the specific disorder of interest should be included in the study. The most common PS variant is the idiopathic form PD, and therefore most efforts are directed at studying its etiology (8). There is a significant degree of error in predicting the underlying pathology. Although the etiology is not known in several PS variants, it is known that they have different clinical (7), pharmacologic (37), and survival profiles (28,29). Furthermore, it is reasonable to assume that the etiology and pathogenesis of PD is

different from other variants of PS (7,8), and those epidemiologic studies that do not exclude other PS variants are not likely to succeed in identifying the PD cause. Search for an environmental cause of PD should take into consideration that migration and survival both impact prevalence of PD. Thus someone whose disease is consequent to an environmental factor operative at another location would be considered where she or he is currently residing. Therefore prevalent cases are not suitable for assessment of environmental factors; such studies should focus on incident PD cases.

INCIDENCE OF PARKINSONISM

The incidence of a disease is often reported as the number of new cases per year per 100,000 population (38). Reported incidence of PD varies from 4.9 to 25.6 per 100,000 worldwide (12,39). The lowest incidence in Europe is reported from Sardinia at 4.9 per 100,000 (40). Low incidence is also reported from Japan at 10.2 per 100,000 population (41).

Incidence studies are difficult to perform because they require identification of all the new patients in a community. To avoid year-to-year fluctuations, it is necessary that such information be collected over several years and then averaged to determine the annual incidence. The best incidence studies in the world are those based on the population of Olmsted County, Minnesota, and the city of Rochester (12,13,15,42,43). The latest survey revealed PS incidence of 25.6 per 100,000 population (12) in Olmsted County; this is higher than the previous report of 20.5 per 100,000 (13) in the city of Rochester, which accounts for 70 percent of the population in that county. Because of the completeness of case finding and the medical record system in Olmsted County over several decades, most epidemiologists consider these as benchmark incidence figures for the Western countries.

Parkinsonism is concentrated in later age groups and only 4 percent to 10 percent of cases have onset before age 40. In our clinic-based study of 934 patients over 22 years, 6 percent had onset before age 40 (29). The incidence rises with age. For example, in Rochester the annual incidence was 5/100,000 in those between age 40 and 49 years compared with 174 per 100,000 between age 70 and 79 years – a 35-fold increase (15). The most recent Olmsted County study revealed a similar pattern (12). The incidence was 0.8 per 100,000 between age 0 and 29 years and 304.8 per 100,000 in 80 to 99 years (12). If the current survival trends continue, there will be a progressively higher population of elderly in the general population and the overall incidence of parkinsonism will continue to rise. To compare incidence rates in two populations, the rates must be adjusted for age distribution. Other developments that contribute to higher incidence are the increasing recognition that PS may begin at a young age and that a significant proportion of demented patients also have parkinsonian features – this is not a true increase in incidence but an effect of improved case ascertainment.

LIFE EXPECTANCY IN PARKINSONISM

Parkinson syndrome by itself is not fatal; however, it leads to physical disabilities that predispose to deep vein thrombosis, pulmonary embolism, aspiration, falls and resulting complications, and a premature death (44). Life expectancy in Western countries has progressively increased over the last several decades because of improved socioeconomic conditions and better health care. Parkinsonian patients of today would share some of those longevity gains, and hence the life expectancy of contemporary patients would be longer than that of patients diagnosed 30 to 40 years ago. To overcome that bias, patients of past generations should be compared with the general population of that era, and survival in current patients should be compared with the age and sex that matches the contemporary general population. If the survival difference between cases and general population during the period coinciding with modern drug therapy were narrower than in the past, it would indicate that survival gain is due to modern treatment of PS.

The onset of parkinsonism is insidious and difficult to ascertain precisely, and the diagnosis is usually made months or years later. The date of onset of parkinsonism is established retrospectively and is therefore only an approximation rather than an exact date (29,38,43,45,46). Because of the uncertainty of onset date, the life expectancy from the onset of symptoms cannot be measured accurately. Studies that compare survival of patients with that of controls based on a retrospectively identified date of parkinsonism onset erroneously inflate the survival in the patients.

Approximating a time of onset retrospectively for survival analysis artificially inflates the survival in patients compared with that expected in the general population (47). Survival analysis on 934 cases from the date of onset were performed. Indeed, survival in the PS group was longer than expected in the general population. The observation that patients suffering from a chronic, progressively disabling disease such as PS lived longer than the general population of unaffected individuals does not make sense. To overcome this bias, survival must be computed from the date of first contact and controls matched accordingly (29,45). This would allow comparison of survival in patients with the sex and year of birth that match individuals in the general population. By doing so, the benefits of socioeconomic and medical advancements in the general population would be shared by parkinsonian patients equally and would not be a factor in the PS survival gains (48).

The other consideration is that relative frequencies of different parkinsonian variants have changed over the years. For example, postencephalitic parkinsonism (PEP), which had a survival mean of 25.5 years (31) compared with only 9.42 years survival in other variants of parkinsonism, is now extinct. That would influence survival observations in the entire PS population. For assessing survival changes, we must compare the like variety and exclude the previous cases of PEP.

Although expressing survival as a "mean" number of years has value in counseling patients, it does not help to understand any survival changes consequent to current methods of management. As life expectancy in the general population has increased, one would expect some increase in mean life expectancy in parkinsonian patients. Several studies indicate that in the last three decades life expectancy in parkinsonian patients has increased significantly. Uitti et al., using a mathematical model, concluded that levodopa use increased survival considerably (45). Kurtzke et al. (49) observed changes in age at death between 1970 and 1985, and concluded that patients were now living five years longer than prior to access to levodopa. If the five year increase in mean survival in contemporary patients were added to the prelevodopa survival of 9.42 years in the parkinson patients (excluding PEP) (31), the mean survival today would be approximately 15 years (1).

Change in life expectancy with time has implications not only for the individual patient but also for the health care system in order to provide services. If the new cases emerged at the same rate as before but survival was increased, the total number of cases at any given time would be higher than before. If there were indeed an increase in the life expectancy of today's patients compared with the past generations it may reflect the benefits of modern drug therapy. Some observers have concluded that the life expectancy gain is simply an indicator of improved socioeconomic/general medical care leading to increased survival (50). To distinguish between these points of view, case control studies are needed but would be unethical. Levodopa, the most potent drug, or any other symptomatic drug cannot be withheld for a prolonged period of time from any human being with the objective to compare survival in the treated and the untreated patients. By necessity, evaluations of the effect of access to levodopa must be made by other means.

Studies were done on 934 patients seen at the Movement Disorder Clinic in Saskatoon, Saskatchewan, between 1968 and 1990 (29). The severity of disability and the type of parkinsonism in these patients were comparable to that noted in a large prevalence study (51). These 934 patients could be subdivided into prelevodopa and levodopa era cases using two methods: first, visit to the Movement Disorder Clinic and second, the calendar year of onset. Compared with expected rates, survival measured from the first clinic visit in every subgroup was shorter. The most favorable prognosis was noted in 565 cases that had onset after 1973 and had unrestricted levodopa access. In 1975 Saskatchewan prescription drug policy was implemented, whereby cost of levodopa was fully funded by the provincial department of Health for all patients. The observed survival was significantly better in the more recent cases compared with earlier patients when LD was not available or was severely restricted (P < 0.025). This was evident when the grouping was based on first clinic visit or on the PS onset date. Figure 5-1 shows the observed survival in the 565 most recent cases based on first visit compared with the expected survival. Figure 5.2 shows survival comparison of 215 patients who had onset and first clinic visit before 1974 and expected survival in general population. The survival in PS cases was less than expected in both more recent cases and the earlier cases (p-values, P = 0.029 and P<0.0001, respectively). However, the

difference was much greater in cases diagnosed before 1974 with 10-year survival of 46 percent compared with an expected rate of 69 percent. For cases diagnosed in 1974 or later, observed 10-year survival was 78 percent compared with 83 percent expected. It was also identified that the survival benefits were realized only when levodopa was initiated before the patients developed postural instability as indicated by UPDRS stage 2.5 or Hoehn & Yahr stage 3.

Thus the survival in parkinsonian patients has improved remarkably since the widespread use of levodopa, although it remains shortened compared with the general population. It is estimated that the life expectancy of a nondemented patient with onset of idiopathic PD at age 62.4 years will be reduced by approximately two years if treated adequately. The survival is significantly shorter in other variants of parkinsonism and in those who have dementia at first assessment (29). Shortened survival in patients with dementia has also been reported by several other workers (45,52–54).

PREVALENCE OF PARKINSONISM

There is universal agreement that the prevalence of parkinsonism increases with age. One recent study in Holland found prevalence of PS to be 1.4 percent (14 per 1,000 people) over age 55 years and 4.3 percent (43 per 1,000) in the population 85 years and older (55). In two studies restricted to individuals 65 years and

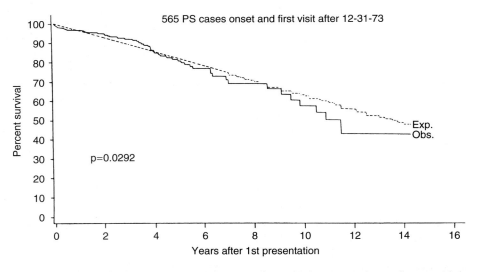

FIGURE 5-1. Obs = Observed survival in patients. Exp = Expected survival in general population. Observed survival in 565 parkinsonian patients who had symptomatic onset after December 31, 1973, compared with the expected survival in the general population matched for age, sex, and the year of birth. Reprinted with permission from: Rajput AH, Uitti RJ, Rajput AH, Offord KP. Timely levodopa (LD) administration prolongs survival in Parkinson's disease. *Parkinsonism and Related Disorders* 1997; 3(3):159–165.

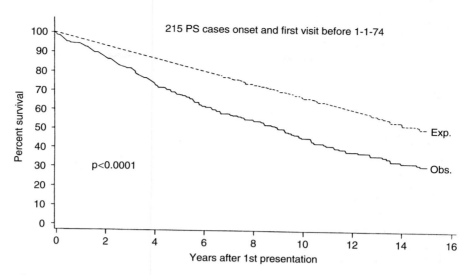

FIGURE 5-2. Obs = Observed survival in patients. Exp = Expected survival in general population. Observed survival in 215 parkinsonian patients who had onset and were first evaluated at Movement Disorder Clinic before 1-1-74 compared with the expected survival in the general population matched for age, sex, and year of birth. Reprinted with permission from Rajput AH, Uitti RJ, Rajput AH, Offord KP. Timely levodopa (LD) administration prolongs survival in Parkinson's disease. *Parkinsonism and Related Disorders* 1997; 3(3):159–165.

older, 3 percent of the community (2) and 9 percent of the institutionalized residents (3) had PS. It is estimated that between 1971 and 1991 the number of individuals over age 85 in Canada and the United States has doubled, thereby markedly enlarging the population at risk of developing parkinsonism.

The best prevalence studies are those in which the entire population of a community is directly surveyed. Most studies are restricted to population 40 years and older, thereby excluding the significant portion of the general population under that age that has lower prevalence. This gives the impression of higher than actual rates in the general population. Worldwide, prevalence rates range from 57/100,000 in China (56) to 371/100,000 in Sicily (14). A prevalence of 347/100,000 was reported in the population over age 40 years in Copiah County, Mississippi (57). As noted earlier, prevalence studies should not rely only upon physician-diagnosed cases. Door-to-door studies have revealed that between 35 percent and 42 percent of the parkinsonian patients were undiagnosed before the survey (14,57).

An indirect method to determine prevalence rate is by multiplying the annual incidence with the mean survival in years. The incidence of 25.6/100,000 population (12) multiplied by an estimated mean survival today of 14.42 years would yield a prevalence rate of 369 per 100,000 in the United States and Canada. In previous reports based on studies in the 1980s, the PS prevalence rate was estimated at 300 per 100,000 (1). This increased prevalence rate is attributable to several factors. The increased

life expectancy in parkinsonian patients since the widespread use of levodopa would translate into higher prevalence rate. Also PS is concentrated in the elderly, a segment of the population that has progressively increased. Diagnosis of PS is now made less reluctantly in those under age 40 or over age 85 and in demented cases than was the case in the past.

There are other means of estimating prevalence but they are not reliable. Death registers as a source of prevalence rate have the lowest yield because, in an overwhelming majority of these patients, the patient dies from a related medical condition and the diagnosis of PS is not noted on the death certificate. The number of antiparkinsonian drug prescriptions in a population is another indicator of prevalence rates. However, as noted earlier, 35 to 42% of cases remain undiagnosed and prevalence estimates based on treatment would be underestimates of the true prevalence. Based on the U.S. population of 1950, the cumulative life time risk of parkinsonism was estimated at 2.4% (43). The recent figures suggest that by age 95 years cumulative risk is nearly 3% (71).

HEALTH SERVICES NEEDS

Although early patients with mild unilateral symptoms can function nearly normally at their usual occupation, those with advanced disease need active intervention. The need for health services in general parallels the severity of disability (31). Those at stage 3 or greater disability, which predisposes them to falling, will need more services. At any given time in the community, it is estimated that between 33% (30) and 37% (29) of PS cases have stage 3 or greater disability. Stage 4 and 5 cases, all of whom need caregiver support, account for 7% (29) to 13% (30) of the prevalent cases.

RACE AND GENDER

Some previous studies based on U.S. private hospital patients indicated that the risk of parkinsonism differed according to skin color, with whites being at increased risk (58,59). One study from Sardinia found a very low prevalence rate and arrived at the same conclusion (40). Assuming that PD may be caused by environmental toxins, it has been suggested that MPTP toxicity is more likely in whites than in blacks (60). On the other hand, studies in Copiah County, Mississippi found no significant differences in PS risk in a mixed race community consisting of nearly equal number of blacks and whites (57). In another mixed race U.S. population survey, the incidence was the highest among black males although there was higher mortality in this group resulting in lower prevalence in blacks (61). The prevalence of parkinsonism in U.S. blacks was fivefold higher than in blacks living in Nigeria, when age of population was taken into account. (62). It should be noted that the studies of blacks and whites in Copiah County, Mississippi (57) and those in Nigeria (62) were conducted using the same methodologic tools by the same principal investigator (B.S.S.) and therefore are not attributable to methodologic bias. Thus the data so far indicate that skin color or race is not related to parkinsonism and that environment plays a large part. The role of environment in the etiology of PS will be covered in later chapters and will therefore not be elaborated upon here.

Several studies have reported higher prevalence in males than in females (43,57,63,64), and large clinical trials often enroll more males than females (65). On the other hand, higher prevalence rates have been reported in women than in men in some carefully conducted door-to-door studies (14,55). The reported difference in prevalence rates between males and females is so small that it can be safely concluded that the risk of disease is not gender-linked.

ANALYTIC AND CLINICAL EPIDEMIOLOGY

This branch of epidemiology analyzes epidemiologic information with the major objective of identifying reasons for changes in disease pattern. The focus of these efforts is the elucidation of the etiology of PD. As the loss of substantia nigra neurons is the hallmark of PD, much work is focused on determining the basis of this selective loss and the formation of Lewy body inclusions. Although the disease is concentrated in older age, the striatal dopamine loss pattern is different and specific for normal aging (66) contrasted to PD (67). Similarly, the subregional patterns of neuronal loss in aging and in PD are different (68). Thus in spite of the concentration of PD in older age, it is neither a manifestation of normal aging nor an acceleration of the aging process.

Clinical epidemiologic studies need a large patient base followed longitudinally using standard measurements. These studies answer many important questions that cannot be answered conclusively by any other types of studies and are performed most appropriatly at special clinics. The Movement Disorder clinics have their own limitations because of the referral bias favoring a larger proportion of unusual cases. However, they are a valuable source of patients to evaluate disease progression (69) and for studies of other illnesses that may be correlated with PD's notably essential tremor (33,70). The evidence, including autopsy studies, thus far indicates that essential tremor neither predisposes nor is a benign variant of PD. Further discussion of the results of both analytical and clinical studies will be covered in later chapters.

REFERENCES

1. Rajput AH, Birdi S. Epidemiology of Parkinson's disease. *Parkinsonism and Related Disorders* 1997; 3(4):175–186.
2. Moghal S, Rajput AH, D'Arey C, et al. Prevalence of movement disorders in elderly community residents. *Neuroepidemiology* 1994; 13:175–178.
3. Moghal S, Rajput AH, Meleth R, et al. Prevalence of movement disorders in institutionalized elderly. *Neuroepidemiology* 1995; 14:297–300.
4. Rajput AH. Clinical features and natural history of Parkinson's disease (special consideration of aging). In: Calne DB (ed.). *Neurodegenerative Diseases*. 1st ed. Philadelphia: W.B. Saunders, 1994:555–571.
5. Rajput AH, Rozdilsky B, Rajput AH. Essential leg tremor. *Neurology* 1990; 40:1909.
6. de Rijk MC, Rocca WA, Anderson DW et al. A population perspective on diagnostic criteria for Parkinson's disease. *Neurology* 1997; 48:1277–1281.
7. Rajput AH, Rozdilsky B, Rajput AH. Accuracy of clinical diagnosis in parkinsonism – A prospective study. *Can J Neurol Sci* 1991; 18:275–278.
8. Duvoisin R, Golbe LI. Toward a definition of Parkinson's disease. *Neurology* 1989; 39:746.

9. Koller WC. Classification of Parkinsonism. In: Koller WC (ed.). *Handbook of Parkinson's Disease.* New York: Marcel Dekker, 1987:51–80.

10. Parkinson J. Critchley M, McMenemey WH, et al. (eds). *A Bicentenary Volume of Papers Dealing with Parkinson's Disease.* London: Macmillan, 1955.

11. Alvord EC, Jr., Forno LS. Pathology. In: Koller WC (ed.). *Handbook of Parkinson's Disease.* New York: Marcel Dekker, 1987:209–236.

12. Bower JH, Maraganore DM, McDonnell SK, et al. Incidence and distribution of parkinsonism in Olmsted County, Minnesota, 1976–1990. *Neurology* 1999; 52:1214–1220.

13. Rajput AH, Offord KP, Beard CM, et al. Epidemiology of parkinsonism: Incidence, classification, and mortality. *Ann Neurol* 1984; 16:278–282.

14. Morgante L, Rocca WA, Di Rosa AE, et al. Prevalence of Parkinson's disease and other types of parkinsonism: A door-to-door survey in three Sicilian municipalities. *Neurology* 1992; 42:1901–1907.

15. Nobrega FT, Glattre E, Kurland LT, et al. Comments on the epidemiology of parkinsonism including prevalence and incidence statistics for Rochester, Minnesota, 1935–1966. In: Barbeau A, Brunette JR (eds.). *Progress in Neurogenetics.* Amsterdam: Excerpta Medica, 1967:474–485.

16. Steele JC, Richardson JC, Olszewski J. Progressive supranuclear palsy. *Arch Neurol* 1964; 10:333–359.

17. Shy GM, Drager GA. A neurological syndrome associated with orthostatic hypotension. *Arch Neurol* 1960; 2:511–527.

18. Adams RD, van Bogaert L, Van der Eecken H. Striato-nigral degeneration. *J Neuropath Exp Neurol* 1964; 23:584–608.

19. Goetz CG. An early photographic case of probable supranuclear palsy. *Mov Disord* 1996; 11(6):617–618.

20. McKeith IG, Galasko D, Kosaka K, et al. Consensus guidelines for the clinical and pathologic diagnosis of dementia with Lewy body (DLB): Report of the Consortium on DLB International Workshop. *Neurology* 1996; 47:1113–1124.

21. Rajput AH, Rozdilsky B, Hornykiewicz O, et al. Reversible drug-induced parkinsonism. Clinicopathologic study of two cases. *Arch Neurol* 1982; 39:644–646.

22. Montgomery EB Jr. Pharmacokinetics and pharmacodynamics of levodopa. *Neurology* 1992; 42(Suppl 1):17–22.

23. Rajput AH, Rozdilsky B. Parkinsonism and dementia: Effects of L-dopa. *Lancet* 1975; 1:1084.

24. Rajput AH. Prevalence of dementia in Parkinson's disease. In: Huber SJ, Cummings JL, (eds.). *Parkinson's Disease. Neurobehavioural Aspects.* New York: Oxford University Press, 1992:119–131.

25. Soininen HL. Extrapyramidal signs in Alzheimer's disease: A 3-year follow-up study. *J Neural Trans Park Dis Dement Sect* 1992; 4(2):107–119.

26. Bennett RG, Greenough WB, Gloth FMI, et al. Extrapyramidal signs in dementia of Alzheimer type. *Lancet* 1989; December 9:1392.

27. Tyrrell PJ, Rosser MN. Extrapyramidal signs in dementia of Alzheimer type. *Lancet* 1989; October 14:920.

28. Rajput AH, Pahwa R, Pahwa P, et al. Prognostic significance of the onset mode in parkinsonism. *Neurology* 1993; 43:829–830.

29. Rajput AH, Uitti RJ, Rajput AH, et al. Timely levodopa (LD) administration prolongs survival in Parkinson's disease. *Parkinsonism and Related Disorders* 1997; 3(3):159–165.

30. Marttila RJ, Rinne UK. Disability and progression of Parkinson's disease. *Acta Neurol Scand* 1977; 56:159–169.

31. Hoehn MM, Yahr MD. Parkinsonism: Onset, progression, and mortality. *Neurology* 1967; 17:427–442.

32. Rajput AH, Fenton ME, George D, et al. Concordance of common movement disorders among familial cases. *Mov Disord* 1997; 12(5):747–751.

33. Rajput AH, Rozdilsky B, Ang L, et al. Significance of parkinsonian manifestations in essential tremor. *Can J Neurol Sci* 1993; 20:114–117.

34. Duncan G, Wilson JA. Normal elderly have some signs of PS. *Lancet* 1989;1392.

35. Jenkyn LR, Reeves AG, Warren T, et al. Neurological signs in senescence. *Arch Neurol* 1985; 42:1154–1157.

36. Hughes AJ, Ben-Shlomo Y, Daniel SE, et al. What features improve the accuracy of clinical diagnosis in Parkinson's disease? A clinicopathologic study. *Neurology* 1992; 42:1142–1146.

37. Rajput AH, Rozdilsky B, Rajput A, et al. Levodopa efficacy and pathological basis of parkinson syndrome. *Clin Neuropharmacol* 1990; 13(6):553–558.

38. Kurland LT, Darrell PH, Darrell RW. Epidemiologic and genetic characteristics of parkinsonism: A review. *International J Neurol* 1961; 2(1):11–24.

39. Marttila RJ. Epidemiology. In: Koller WC (ed.). *Handbook of Parkinson's Disease.* New York: Marcel Dekker, 1987:35–50.

40. Rosati G, Graniere E, Pinna L, et al. The risk of Parkinson's disease in Mediterranean people. *Neurology* 1980; 32:250–255.

41. Harada H, Nishikawa S, Takahashi K. Epidemiology of Parkinson's disease in a Japanese city. *Arch Neurol* 1983; 40:151–154.

42. Kurland LT, Molgaard CA. The patient record in epidemiology. *Sci Am* 1981; 245(4):54–63.

43. Kurland LT. Epidemiology. Incidence, geographic distribution and genetic considerations. In: Fields WS (ed.). *Pathogenesis and Treatment of Parkinsonism.* Springfield, IL: Thomas, 1958:5–43.

44. Mosewich RK, Rajput AH, Shuaib A, et al. Pulmonary embolism: An under-recognized yet frequent cause of death in parkinsonism. *Mov Disord* 1994; 9(3):350–352.

45. Uitti RJ, Ahlskog JE, Maraganore DM, et al. Levodopa therapy and survival in idiopathic Parkinson's

disease: Olmsted County project. *Neurology* 1993; 43:1918–1926.

46. Lees AJ. When did Ray Kennedy's Parkinson's disease begin? *Mov Disord* 1992; 7(2):110–116.

47. Roos RAC, Jongen JCG, Vander Velde EA. Clinical course of patients with idiopathic Parkinson's disease. *Mov Disord* 1996; 11(3):236–242.

48. Lilienfeld DE, Sekkor D, Simpson S, et al. Parkinsonism death rates by race, sex and geography: A 1980's update. *Neuroepidemiology* 1990; 9:243–247.

49. Kurtzke JF, Flaten TP, Murphy FM. Death rates from Parkinson's disease in Norway reflect increased survival. *Neurology* 1991; 41:1665–1667.

50. Lilienfeld DE, Chan E, Ehland J, et al. Two decades of increasing mortality from Parkinson's disease among the US elderly. *Arch Neurol* 1990; 47:731–734.

51. Marttila RJ, Rinne UK. Dementia in Parkinson disease. *Acta Neurol Scand* 1976; 54:431–441.

52. Mindham RHS, Ahmed SWA, Clough CG. A controlled study of dementia in Parkinson's disease. *J Neurol Neurosurg Psychiatry* 1982; 45:969–974.

53. Uitti RJ, Rajput AH, Offord KP. Parkinsonism survival in the levodopa era. *Neurology* 1991; 41(Suppl 1):190.

54. Marder K, Mirabello E, Chen J, et al. Death rates among demented and nondemented patients with Parkinson's disease. *Ann Neurol* 1990; 28(2):295.

55. de Rijk MC, Breteler MMB, Graveland GA, et al. Prevalence of Parkinson's disease in the elderly: The Rotterdam Study. *Neurology* 1995; 45:2143–2146.

56. Li SC, Schoenberg BS, Wang CC, et al. A prevalence survey of Parkinson's disease and other movement disorders in the People's Republic of China. *Arch Neurol* 1985; 42:655–657.

57. Schoenberg BS, Anderson DW, Haerer AF. Prevalence of Parkinson's disease in the biracial population of Copiah County, Mississippi. *Neurology* 1985; 35(6):841–845.

58. Kessler II. Epidemiologic studies of Parkinson's disease, II. A hospital based survey. *Am J Epidemiol* 1972; 95(4):308–318.

59. Kessler II. Epidemiology study of Parkinson's disease. *Am J Epidemiol* 1972; 96:242–254.

60. Lerner MR, Goldman RS. Skin colour, MPTP, and Parkinson's disease. *Lancet* 1987; July:212.

61. Mayeux R, Marder K, Cote LJ, et al. The frequency of idiopathic Parkinson's disease by age, ethnic group, and sex in northern Manhattan, 1988–1993. *Am J Epidemiol* 1995; 142:820–827.

62. Schoenberg BS, Osuntokun BO, Adejua AOG, et al. Comparison of the prevalence of Parkinson's disease in black populations in the rural United States and in rural Nigeria: Door-to-door community studies. *Neurology* 1988; 38:645–646.

63. Bharucha NE, Bharucha EP, Bharucha AE, et al. Prevalence of Parkinson's disease in the Parsi community of Bombay, India. *Arch Neurol* 1988; 45:1321–1323.

64. Mutch WJ, Dingwall-Fordyce I, Downie AW, et al. Parkinson's disease in a Scottish city. *BMJ* 1986; 292:534–536.

65. Parkinson Study Group. Effect of deprenyl on the progression of disability in early Parkinson's disease. *N Engl J Med* 1989; 321:1364–1371.

66. Kish SJ, Shannak K, Rajput A, et al. Aging produces a specific pattern of striatal dopamine loss: Implications for the etiology of idiopathic Parkinson's disease. *J Neurochem* 1992; 58:642–648.

67. Kish SJ, Shannak K, Hornykiewicz O. Uneven pattern of dopamine loss in the striatum of patients with idiopathic Parkinson's disease. *N Engl J Med* 1988; 318:876–880.

68. Fearnley JM, Lees AJ. Aging and Parkinson's disease: Substantia nigra regional selectivity. *Brain* 1991; 114:2283–2301.

69. Lee CS, Schulzer M, Mak E, et al. Patterns of asymmetry do not change over the course of idiopathic parkinsonism: Implications for pathogenesis. *Neurology* 1995; 45:435–439.

70. Rajput AH, Rozdilsky B, Ang L, et al. Clinicopathological observations in essential tremor. Report of 6 cases. *Neurology* 1991; 41:1422–1424.

71. Piccini P, Burn DJ, Ceravolo R, et al. The role of inheritance in sporadic Parkinson's disease: Evidence from a longitudinal study of dopaminergic function in twins. *Ann Neurol* 1999; 45(5):577–582.

6

Cardinal Features of Early Parkinson's Disease

**Pramod Kr. Pal, M.D., D.M., Ali Samii, M.D., F.R.C.P.C., and
Donald B. Calne, D.M., F.R.C.P.C.**

Neurodegenerative Disorders Centre, University of British Columbia, Vancouver, British Columbia, Canada

Pramar Kr. Pal

National Institute of Mental Health and Neurosciences (NIMHANS), Bangalore, Karnataka, India

and

Ali Samii, M.D.

University of Washington School of Medicine, Harborview Medical Center, Seattle, Washington

PARKINSONIAN SYNDROME AND THE DEFINITION OF PARKINSON'S DISEASE

Nearly two centuries ago James Parkinson described a disorder of the elderly under the eponym of "shaking palsy" (1). Over the years the constellation of symptoms and signs of this clinical entity came to be known as "Parkinson's disease." However, the vast clinical experience and emergence of newer diagnostic methods over the past century have forced neurologists to modify their view of this clinical syndrome. It has become evident that the clinical findings described by Parkinson occur in a setting where several different causes can be identified or where the findings are part of other progressive neurodegenerative disorders. Therefore the clinical entity described by Parkinson has been termed *parkinsonism* or the *parkinsonian syndrome* (2) (Table 6-1). Thus it is doubtful whether "Parkinson's disease" is a single entity (2,3) and whether "idiopathic parkinsonism" (IP) may be a suitable name for what is really a syndrome of unknown origin (2). With the advent of modern genetic techniques, a small subgroup of patients who have a familial form of parkinsonism have had their underlying genetic abnormalities identified (4–6).

There is no generally acceptable definition of IP. However, for research purposes, one needs to have a uniform and generally accepted set of inclusion and exclusion criteria. Takahashi and Calne (7) proposed a working definition of IP as a syndrome comprising a combination of the triad – tremor, rigidity, and akinesia, with inclusion and exclusion criteria (Table 6-2).

AGING AND PARKINSON'S DISEASE

Parkinsonian features are seen with normal aging (8–10). Duncan and Wilson (11) noted that almost all elderly people (without any neurologic disorder) attending a day care and nearly one-half of the neurologically "normal" elderly people seen in a community had at least one feature (excluding impaired postural reflex) of parkinsonism. It is difficult to distinguish this apparently "normal" variant of aging from early IP. Old age is the most consistently recognized risk factor for parkinsonism, and its incidence and prevalence increases with age (12). Prevalence has been reported to be 1 percent in patients 60 years or older and 2.6 percent in those over 85 years of age (13).

Like many other, but not all, parts of the central nervous system, there are age-related changes in the nigrostriatal dopaminergic pathways. These are due to (1) age-related, localized neuronal death, and (2) generalized loss of neuronal plasticity (14). There is a decrease in the enzymes involved in dopamine synthesis, especially during the first 20 years of life

Table 6-1   Classification of Parkinsonism

Idiopathic Parkinsonism (commonly known as Parkinson's Disease)
Late-onset (>40 years; generally sporadic)
Early-onset (<40 years; often familial)
  Young-onset (>21 years)
  Juvenile (<21 years)
Parkinsonism due to identifiable cause
Virus (e.g., encephalitis lethargica)
Toxins (e.g., carbon monoxide, manganese, methylphenyltetrahydropyridine)
Drugs (e.g., phenothiazines, reserpine, butyrophenones, metoclopramide)
Vascular (multi-infarct)
Tumors of basal ganglia
Normal pressure hydrocephalus
Hemiparkinsonism-hemiatrophy
Metabolic
  Wilson's disease
  Hepatocerebral degeneration
  Hallervoden-Spatz disease
  Hypoparathyroidism
Parkinsonism in other neurodegenerative disorders
Progressive supranuclear palsy
Cortical-basal ganglionic degeneration
Disorders with cerebellar/autonomic/pyramidal manifestation:
  Multiple system atrophy
    Striatonigral degeneration
    Shy-Drager syndrome
    Olivopontocerebellar atrophy
  Machado-Joseph disease
Disorders with prominent and often early dementia:
  Diffuse cortical Lewy body disease
  Alzheimer's disease with parkinsonism
Parkinsonism-dementia-ALS complex of Guam
Pallidopontonigral degeneration/disinhibition-dementia-parkinsonism-amyotrophy complex

(15,16), a decrease in the dopamine concentration (17,18) most profound from age 60 to 90 years (18), and a fall in the dopamine receptors as documented from postmortem (19) and positron emission tomographic (PET) studies (20). Fearnley and Lees (21) reported a linear fallout of neurons in the substantia nigra with advancing age at a rate of 4.7 percent of the initial number per decade. Idiopathic parkinsonism is clearly not simply a consequence of aging or accelerated aging, as both the extent and pattern of cell loss in the substantia nigra are different in the two conditions. Neuronal loss in IP is curvilinear in contrast to aging, where it is linear, and a 45 percent neuronal loss occurs in the first decade of disease, which is 10-fold greater than that could be accounted for by normal aging (21–23). Neuronal loss in aging is selective and is greatest in the dorsal tier of the substantia nigra followed by the medioventral tier and least in the lateroventral tier, which is reverse of that seen in IP (21). The age-related attrition of dopaminergic nigral neurons is independent of the pathology of IP,

so that these two causes of neuronal death are additive rather than multiplicative (22). Aging must contribute to the appearance and progression of the symptoms of IP (14). The early progression of IP is more rapid in elderly subjects because of a lower "neuronal reserve" (22). The pattern of clinical features is also influenced by the age of onset of IP: young patients often present with dystonic features, whereas those with a later onset have more postural imbalance and difficulty in walking (24–26). This is probably due to the difference in the topography of pathologic changes within the nigrostriatal system seen in aging and IP.

CLINICAL FEATURES

Onset of Symptoms

It is a matter of speculation as to when IP begins. As is the case with other diseases, there is a delay between the onset of the pathologic changes in the nigrostriatal

Table 6-2 Definition of Idiopathic Parkinsonism*

A syndrome comprising a combination of the triad – tremor, rigidity, and akinesia, with inclusion and exclusion criteria:

   (i)   No detectable cause
  (ii)   Therapeutic response to dopaminomimetics
 (iii)   No cerebellar deficits
 (iv)   Pyramidal features limited to possible hyperreflexia and an extensor plantar response
  (v)   No evidence of lower motorneuron dysfunction
 (vi)   Gaze deficits limited to limitation of upward gaze
(vii)   Autonomic deficits limited to minor dysfunction and insufficient to cause repeated syncope: In this context drug-induced autonomic failure must be excluded.

*Takahashi and Calne (7)

pathways and the onset of clinical manifestations. The cause for most patients may be a transient event rather than a prolonged process (27,28). The average age of onset of IP is 55 years (29), although a subset of patients, particularly those with a prominent genetic component to their etiology, may have onset before 40 years (early-onset parkinsonism). The onset is usually insidious and the course is slowly progressive. Initially, symptoms are often intermittent and may be present only during stress. Repeated traumatic events can cause parkinsonism (30). Asymmetry of symptoms is common, and the initial pattern of asymmetry persists, although the deficit on each side progresses (28). The asymmetry is not related to handedness.

Extrapyramidal motor symptoms are usually taken to mark the onset of this disease. However, it is well known that many patients, on retrospective analysis, realize that they had several nonmotor symptoms, before the diagnosis of IP could be made (31).

Early Nonspecific Features

The early symptoms of IP are usually nonspecific and may be seen in many other neurologic syndromes or even normal aging. The symptoms are often related to the occupation and lifestyle of the patients. Loss of energy, easy fatigability, myalgia, arthralgia, stiffness and tightness of muscles, cramps or vague sensory disturbances – dysesthesias and paraesthesias – may suggest a neuromuscular disorder. The latter suspicion is often strengthened by symptoms such as inability to get out of a low chair, dragging of feet or tripping after walking a distance, and clumsiness of hands. The patient or his relatives may notice that a longer time is needed by the patient to do his daily activities such as taking a shower, shaving, dressing, cooking, or eating. Before the emergence of classical rest tremor, there may be a feeling of internal tremulousness and transient appearance of postural tremor in one or both hands, especially in stressful situations. Deterioration in handwriting, in the form of a gradual decrease in the size of letters (micrographia) may be noticed. Inability to achieve high notes can be an early complaint of singers; others may complain of hypophonia after speaking for a while. There are reports of sleep disturbances and bad dreams preceding emergence of IP (32). Further early manifestations that have been reported include dizziness, constipation, seborrheic dermatitis, decreased perception of smell, sudden transient weakness of limbs, dystonic posturing of a limb or hemidystonia, sweating disturbances, and bladder dysfunction. Change in personality, difficulty in concentrating, slowed thinking (bradyphrenia), mood changes especially depression, and impaired cognition may be mistaken for a primary psychiatric disorder or early dementia.

Cardinal Features

Tremor at rest, rigidity, bradykinesia, and abnormalities of posture, gait, and balance are the cardinal manifestations of IP. In the early stages, any combination of tremor, rigidity, or bradykinesia may be present and a neurologic examination may be required to elicit these signs.

Tremor

Approximately 70% of patients notice tremor as the first symptom (33). Tremor is classically described to be present at rest. Characteristically, the tremor is 3–5 Hz rhythmic "pill-rolling" movements of the thumb and forefinger (biplanar) and has varying amplitude. There is abduction and adduction of the thumb and flexion and extension of the metacarpophalyngeal and interphalyngeal joints. At a later stage the tremor may spread to the proximal joints of the limb causing pronation–supination movements of the forearm and to and fro movement of the arm. Onset of tremor is usually in one of the hands (34) and it progresses to involve the other upper limb or ipsilateral lower limb. Rarely, onset is in one or both lower limbs. Onset of tremor in the upper limbs is nearly 10 times more common than in the lower limbs (12). Tremor may be confined to one limb or one side for many years, and in some patients it may be even confined to a single finger for years before the appearance of other signs (35). The jaw, tongue, head, or trunk may be affected by tremor, although trunkal or head tremor is unusual in early IP unless it is a part of postural tremor. Tremor confined to the head or predominating there probably is not parkinsonism (36).

During early disease, tremor is often intermittent for many years (37) and is evident only under stress. Tremor is worsened by nervousness, fatigue, and stress, and it diminishes with voluntary activity or sleep and may have diurnal fluctuations. Tremor in the legs may be seen only when the patient is supine or keeps the legs in a certain posture and it usually disappears when walking. Tremor often increases in the arms while walking. Placing the patient under simultaneous physical and mental stress, such as requesting serial seven subtractions and contralateral tight hand gripping, can bring out tremor even in apparently noninvolved limbs.

It is common for the early tremor of IP to be seen when the hands are held in a posture against gravity or when the hands are being employed to execute voluntary movements (33,34,38).

Rigidity

Rigidity is an increased resistance to passive movement. The resistance is fairly regular and equal in both agonist and antagonist groups of muscles. It may be sustained (plastic or lead pipe) or intermittent and rachetty (cogwheel). Although the latter is usually thought to be parkinsonian rigidity complicated by parkinsonian tremor, it may occur in the absence of tremor and its frequency is often higher (6–12 Hz) (36). Rigidity is differentiated from (a) spasticity, which is classically velocity-dependent (clasp-knife phenomenon) and is associated with hyperreflexia, Babinski's sign, and a pyramidal distribution weakness; (b) geganhalten or paratonic rigidity, seen in dementia, and a variety of encephalopathic conditions, which are characterized by an opposition to passive movement that adjusts to the force applied (9,39); and (c) cogwheeling phenomenon, which may be seen in some cases of advanced essential tremor (40) as a result of coarse tremor interrupting passive movement, without an increase in tone.

Rigidity is often asymmetrical in the early stages of IP. It is commonly present at one or both wrists and in the neck. Like tremor, it may vary during the course of the day and with stress. As disease progresses the characteristic "flexed posture" evolves.

Assessment of rigidity is often difficult because the patient is unable to relax and cooperate; repeated examinations may be needed in both sitting and lying postures. Moreover, arthritic conditions, which are common in the elderly, can also cause local muscle spasm. Rigidity can be elicited by asking the patient to perform voluntary repetitive movements of the contralateral limb.

Bradykinesia

Akinesia (absence of movements) and hypokinesia (reduced amplitude of movement) are characteristics of IP (41). Bradykinesia, a general term used to describe the overall slowness of voluntary movements and poverty of normal associated movements, will be used in this chapter.

Bradykinesia is the most disabling component of IP and of all the clinical signs, its severity has the best correlation with dopaminergic dysfunction and cell loss as revealed by autopsy and PET scan studies. Moreover, it has the best symptomatic response to dopaminomimetic therapy. However, in early stages of IP, bradykinesia may manifest only as minimal slowness.

Bradykinesia and rigidity usually occur together and in most cases are comparable in severity (12). In the early stages, the signs may be confined to the distal muscles, but later in the disease the proximal muscles are involved. Before assessing bradykinesia, special care should be taken to exclude local painful lesions, corticospinal tract involvement, impaired cardiopulmonary reserve, dizziness, and visual impairment that may affect performance of the tests (12). Due consideration should also be given to the handedness of the patient during assessment of dexterity of the limbs. The following observations and tests are part of the Unified Parkinson's Disease Rating Scale (UPDRS) and are often useful for assessing bradykinesia involving different parts of the body:

1. REDUCTION OF NORMAL ASSOCIATED MOVEMENTS
   These include arm swing while walking, spontaneous facial expressions, gestures associated with conversation, and the frequency of blinking. Loss of arm swing is usually asymmetric in early IP, unlike that seen in normal aging.

2. SPEECH
   The patient is asked to speak loudly and clearly, for example, to repeat the names of the months. In early IP the voice may lack the normal fluctuations of volume and pitch and may fatigue quickly. In later stages there is slow initiation of speech, which is weak and monotonous.

3. DECREASED SPEED, AMPLITUDE AND RHYTHM OF REPETITIVE OR SEQUENTIAL SIMPLE MOVEMENTS ON ONE SIDE OF BODY
   Movements often tested include repeated opposition of the forefinger and the thumb, alternating pronation–supination of the hand held vertically and then horizontally, opening and closing fists, quick repetitive hand, and heel

or toe tapping. Initially there is slowing and fatigue, then diminution in amplitude, and subsequently the movements becomes arrhythmic with frequent hesitations and arrests.

4. IMPAIRED DEXTERITY IN COMPLEX MOTOR TASKS THAT NEED FREQUENT CHANGES IN DIRECTION
   Tasks include asking the patient to button a coat, write a long sentence, write 'm' and 'n' alternately for a minute, and copy a horizontal or Archimedes spiral. A progressive decrease in the size of the letters or the spiral (micrographia) is useful, and serial documentation on follow-up helps to follow progression.

5. DIFFICULTY IN PERFORMING SIMULTANEOUS REPETITIVE MOTOR TASKS INVOLVING BOTH SIDES
   Typically, the patient is asked to do alternate pronation and supination of both hands simultaneously. During this task the asymmetry often becomes more pronounced.

6. MOTOR TASKS INVOLVING PROXIMAL AND TRUNKAL MUSCULATURE
   Bradykinesia related to these tasks are obvious in the later stages of IP. There may be difficulty in arising from a low chair without using the hands that are folded across the chest. In advanced stages, walking becomes slow and eventually impossible.

7. OBJECTIVE METHODS OF ASSESSING BRADYKINESIA
   Different methods have been devised to quantify bradykinesia objectively and these are helpful in documenting the effects of therapy. These methods are less affected by inter-rater variabilities. One of the most accurate tests is performance on the Purdue Peg Board (42). The patient is asked to insert pegs in the holes on the Purdue Peg Board, first with each hand separately and then simultaneously, over a specified period of time (usually 30 seconds). The Purdue Peg Board score has been shown to correlate strongly with nigral dysfunction observed in PET scans (43). Rapid alternate tapping of forefinger and index finger on two separate keys of a computerized electronic drum with simultaneous contralateral hand activation has also been found to be a reliable test of bradykinesia with good correlation with fluorodopa PET scans (44). Of course, the severity of rigidity and tremor also influence the performance on all these tests.

Postural Instability and Gait Disorder

Impairment of postural reflexes and abnormality of gait (P.I.G.D.) usually occur about 5 years after the onset of IP (45), although sometimes earlier (26,46,47). Very early impairment of balance warrants a search for other causes of parkinsonism such as progressive supranuclear palsy.

There may be subtle changes in the posture and gait in early stages of IP. The posture may show a slight flexion of the neck or trunk or a lean to one side. Abnormalities of gait may include: (a) loss of arm swing on one or both sides; (b) slowing, especially after walking for a long time; (c) shortened stride length and intermittent shuffle; (d) tripping over objects; (e) difficulty in negotiating narrow lanes; (f) difficulty in walking on toes, heels, tandem or backwards; and (g) inability to turn quickly. As the disease progresses, gait initiation becomes a problem, the steps become more uncertain, and there is festination. Short term arrests of ongoing movements, also known as freezing, usually occur in advanced disease (48) (see Chapter 7).

Postural reflexes are preserved in early IP and the "pull" test is usually negative. The patient is asked to stand with eyes open and feet comfortably apart. He is instructed to resist falling by taking one step using either foot when necessary. A sudden modest pull is applied on the shoulders, initially from the front and then from the back. Patients with impaired righting reflexes will take more than two steps to prevent themselves from falling (49,50).

DIFFERENTIAL DIAGNOSIS

In the early stages of IP, the following conditions often need to be differentiated from it (See Chapters 53 and 54). Table 6-3 summarizes the most important features of some parkinsonian syndromes.

Normal Aging

Normal elderly persons can have some bradykinesia and slowed motor performance (11,51), loss of postural reflexes (50,52,53), slow and short-stepped gait (51,52), and an increased prevalence of essential tremor (54–56). These findings may lead to an erroneous diagnosis of IP. Although muscle tone is normal in the elderly, assessment of tone may be difficult in those with cognitive decline because of gegenhalten (52) or arthritis or there may be increased tone due to spondylotic myelopathy or vascular disease. In normal aging (a) disabilities tend to be symmetric; (b) heel strike and arm swings are normal while walking and the gait is slightly wide-based unlike that seen in IP; (c) alternating

Table 6-3   Differential Diagnosis of Idiopathic Parkinsonism

	IP	SND	OPCA	SDS	CBGD	PSP	NPH	DLBD	ADP	PDCG
Asymmetry at onset	++	−	−	−	++	−	−	−	±	−
Rigidity	++	++	+	+	++	++	+	++	++	+
Resting tremor	++	±	−	−	±	−	±	+	−	±
Bradykinesia	++	+	±	+	++	++	+	++	±	+
Dystonia	±	−	−	−	++	±	−	−	−	−
Myoclonus	±	−	−	−	++	−	−	−	±	−
Abnormal ocular motility	−	−	++	±	+	++	−	±	±	+
Eyelid apraxia	−	±	−	−	±	+	−	−	−	−
Limb apraxia	−	−	−	−	++	−	−	++	±	−
Speech apraxia	−	−	−	−	−	−	−	++	±	±
Dysarthria/hypophonia/ Dysphagia	++	++	++	±	++	++	±	−	±	−
Cerebellar signs	−	+	++	±	−	−	−	−	−	−
Pyramidal signs	−	+	+	±	+	+	++	±	±	++
Perpheral neuropathy	−	−	+	±	−	−	−	−	−	−
Motor neuron disease	−	±	−	±	−	−	−	−	−	++
Autonomic dysfunction	±	+	+	++	±	±	−	−	−	−
Cognitive decline	± (L)	±	±	±	+	++	++ (E)	++ (E)	++ (E)	++ (E)
Sleep abnormalities	±	+	±	+	−	±	−	−	−	−
Gait disturbance/ Postural imbalance	++ (L)	++	++	++	++	++ (E) FF	++ (E)	+	+	++
L-Dopa responsiveness	++	±	±	±	−	±	−	±	−	−

Key: IP – Idiopathic parkinsonism; SND-Striatonigral degeneration; OPCA-Olivopontocerebellar atrophy; SDS-Shy–Drager syndrome; CBGD-Cortical basal ganglionic degeneration; PSP-Progressive supranuclear palsy; NPH-Normal pressure hydrocephalus; DLBD-Diffuse Lewy body disease; ADP-Alzheimer's disease with parkinsonism; PDCG-Parkinsonism-dementia complex of Guam.
− Absent; ± Inconsistent/Variable/Mild; +, Common/Moderate; ++, Frequent/Severe; (E)-Early, (L)-Late, FF-Frequent falls

movements are normal or only slightly slowed; and (*d*) there is no improvement of functions with levodopa.

Essential Tremor (ET)

Essential Tremor is the most common movement disorder and there is a dramatic increase in its prevalence with age (54,57,58). Essential Tremor is typically postural, may be accentuated with goal-directed movements of limbs, and is only occassionally present at rest (58–61). Moreover, with advancing age ET involves other body parts and there is increase in the amplitude and decrease in the frequency of the tremor (60,62–64). A diagnosis of ET is favored by (*a*) tremor of faster frequency (6–9 Hz); (*b*) tremor primarily on sustained posture or action; (*c*) bilateral involvement; (*d*) involvement of other parts of body such as head, voice, trunk; (*e*) absence of micrographia; (*f*) minimal or no signs of rigidity or bradykinesia; (*g*) family history of ET in some 50 percent of cases; (*h*) early age of onset; and (*i*) no response to levodopa.

Drug-Induced Parkinsonism (DIP)

Elderly subjects are especially prone to the development of drug-induced parkinsonism, perhaps because of underlying age-related striatal dopamine deficiency (65–67). The drugs responsible may be dopamine receptor antagonists, such as haloperidol or metoclopramide or dopamine depletors, such as reserpine or tetrabenazine. A history of such medications and improvement on discontinuation of the offending drug may help to distinguish DIP from IP. When parkinsonism continues or worsens slowly, even after discontinuation of the drug, there may be a preexisting preclinical nigrostriatal dopamine deficiency (preclinical parkinsonism) (68,69).

Vascular Parkinsonism (VP)

Multiple basal ganglionic infarcts can lead to parkinsonism that mainly affects the legs (lower body parkinsonism) (70,71). Characteristic features that help to differentiate VP from IP include (*a*) more symmetric signs; (*b*) short-stepped, wide-based, shuffling gait (*marche à petits pas*) with or without freezing, and without festination; (*c*) gegenhalten but no cogwheeling and no tremor; (*d*) pyramidal, cerebellar, and pseudobulbar signs, mild hemiparesis, dysarthria (prominent), dementia, urinary incontinence; (*e*) documented vascular risk factors (such as hypertension, diabetes mellitus, previous strokes and heart disease); (*f*) acute or subacute onset and stepwise progression; (*g*) improvement of clinical signs without the use of levodopa; (*h*) imaging studies showing basal-ganglionic infarcts or frontal and periventricular white matter lesions (72,73).

Progressive Supranuclear Palsy (PSP)

A diagnosis of PSP needs to be considered in patients with progressive parkinsonism and disturbances of gaze. Clinical features favoring a diagnosis of PSP include (*a*) symmetric onset; (*b*) lack of tremor; (*c*) early falls, especially backwards, because of postural imbalance; (*d*) prominent axial (especially neck) rigidity; (*e*) extended knee and trunk with stiff and broad-based gait; (*f*) pseudobulbar features such as early dysarthria, dysphagia, and emotional lability; (*g*) "astonished" facial expression caused by overaction of the frontalis muscles; (*h*) supranuclear ophthalmoparesis typically manifested by paralysis of vertical gaze (especially downgaze); (*i*) defective ocular fixation; (*j*) blepharospasm and apraxia of eyelid opening, eyelid closure, or both; (*k*) early cognitive dysfunction; and (*l*) lack of significant response to levodopa (74–81).

Cortical-Basal Ganglionic Degeneration (CBGD)

Cortical-Basal Ganglionic Degeneration is a rare disorder characterized by asymmetric motor impairment and both cerebrocortical and basal ganglionic dysfunction. Features that distinguish it from IP include (*a*) presence of ideational and ideomotor apraxias; (*b*) rapid (6–8 Hz), irregular, jerky, action/and postural tremor, usually starting in one upper limb; (*c*) limb dystonia; (*d*) cortical sensory loss with accompanying complaints of numbness and paraesthesia in the fingers; (*e*) alien limb phenomenon; (*f*) cortical myoclonus; (*g*) pyramidal signs; (*h*) oculomotor and eyelid abnormalities; (*i*) dysarthria and dysphagia; and (*j*) lack of response to levodopa (82–84).

Parkinsonism with Cerebellar and Autonomic Dysfunction: The Multiple System Atrophies (MSA)

MSA is a group of disorders clinically characterized by any permutations of the designated clinical syndromes of extrapyramidal, pyramidal, cerebellar, or autonomic dysfunctions (85). Nearly 89% of the patients have parkinsonism at some point in the course of their illness (86), yet they seldom respond well to levodopa. Striatonigral degeneration (SND), Shy–Drager syndrome (SDS), and olivopontocerebellar atrophy (OPCA) are the three best characterized subtypes of MSA

Striatonigral Degeneration (SND)

Striatonigral Degeneration is difficult to differentiate from IP. Autopsy-proven cases of SND have been misdiagnosed to have IP largely because of occasional good response to levodopa (87). Differentiating features from IP include (*a*) symmetric onset; (*b*) minimal or no resting tremor, but may have a fast jerky *postural tremor*; (*c*) early-onset falling; (*d*) severe dysarthria, and dysphonia; (*e*) excessive snoring, respiratory stridor, and sleep apnoea; (*f*) cerebellar or pyramidal signs; (*g*) rapid progress; and (*h*) poor or transient response to levodopa (87–89).

Shy-Drager Syndrome (SDS)

Shy-Drager Syndrome (90–92) is characterized by an akinetic-rigid parkinsonism with early onset of severe postural hypotension not related to drugs. Other typical findings include (*a*) bowel and bladder dysfunction, impotence, upper airway obstruction, cardiac arrhythmia, disturbances of sweating and temperature regulation, and pupillary changes (a progressive pandysautonomia); and (*b*) symmetrical manifestations. Sometimes patients have cerebellar signs, corticospinal signs , corticobulbar signs, peripheral neuropathy, and muscle wasting. Patients seldom respond to levodopa, which may worsen postural hypotension.

Olivopontocerebellar Atrophy (OPCA)

Progressive cerebellar ataxia (appendicular and gait) with or without parkinsonism characterize this disorder (93,94) and some of these patients may have parkinsonism as the initial manifestation. Parkinsonian features are usually symmetric and do not respond to levodopa. Other manifestations of OPCA include (*a*) oculomotor abnormalities such as horizontal nystagmus, gaze paresis, impaired convergence, jerky pursuit, and slow saccades; (*b*) dysarthria and dysphagia; (*c*) upper and lower motor neuron signs; (*d*) peripheral neuropathy; (*e*) retinal degeneration; (*f*) cognitive dysfunction; and (*g*) autonomic dysfunction.

Disorders with Dementia as an Important and Often Early Manifestation

Diffuse Lewy Body Disease (DLBD)

DLBD is a chronic progressive disorder of parkinsonian symptoms accompanied by dementia (95–98). DLBD patients usually have an earlier age of onset and multiple psychiatric features (depression, auditory and visual hallucinations, and paranoid ideations), cognitive dysfunction (especially fluctuating features), and are prone to levodopa-induced psychosis. Parkinsonian features are initially mild and patients more frequently have bradykinesia rather than tremor. However, these differences may not be reliable to distinguish DLBD presenting with parkinsonism as the initial manifestation from IP, especially because some patients with DLBD may have partial benefit from levodopa (see Chapters 15 & 16).

Alzheimer's Disease with Parkinsonism (ADP)

Parkinsonism is significantly more common in Alzheimer's disease (AD) than expected in a matched general population (99). Some causes can be identified such as: neuroleptic usage (100), concomitant IP (101), and DLBD (102,103). In addition, advanced AD may lead to degeneration extending to the pyramidal pathways. When parkinsonian features are early in evolution of deficits, ADP may be clinically indistinguishable from IP (101).

Parkinsonism-Dementia Complex of Guam (PDCG)

PDCG, also known as Lytico-Bodig, was first observed in Guam and is characterized by parkinsonian features and dementia (104,105). Other features that may be seen are those of motor neuron disease (106) and supranuclear ocular motility disorder (107).

Normal Pressure Hydrocephalus (NPH)

NPH is characterized by a triad of symptoms: gait abnormality, urinary incontinence, and dementia (108–110). The gait is slow and short-stepped but is reputed to differ from the gait of IP in that it is wide-based, apractic, and irregular, and patients find it difficult to lift the feet from the floor. The leg function improves in a recumbent position. Other differentiating features from IP include: (a) symmetric signs; (b) brisk tendon reflexes in the legs; (c) minimal or absent tremor; (d) history of head trauma, meningitis, or subarachnoid haemorrhage; (e) lack of response to levodopa; (f) computerized tomography scanning or magnetic resonance imaging of brain showing dilatation of all ventricles.

Creutzfeldt–Jakob Disease (CJD)

Although the majority of patients with CJD may have extrapyramidal symptomatology during the course of their illness, only few (9 percent) have them on their first examination (111). The main features that distinguish CJD from IP are rapidly progressive dementia, personality changes, cerebellar ataxia, and myoclonus.

Pallidopontonigral Degeneration (PPND) and Disinhibition-Dementia-Parkinsonism-Amyotrophy Complex (DDPAC)

These are different phenotypic expressions of the same genotype. Distinguishing features from IP include an autosomal dominant disorder characterized by a typical onset in the fourth decade and rapid progression (112). There may be early personality changes, psychiatric symptoms, profound memory loss, and a frontal lobe type of dementia. In addition, gaze paresis, levodopa unresponsive parkinsonism progressing to akinetic mutism, and clinical features resembling motor neuron disease may also be seen (113). A gene for this disorder has been identified on chromosome 17 (113).

Early-Onset Parkinsonism (EOP)

Although IP is a disorder of the elderly, symptoms may begin at a younger age. According to the age of onset, EOP has been classified as (a) "young-onset" (IP beginning between 21 and 40 years of age), or (b) "juvenile-onset" (symptom onset ≤21 years of age) (114). A positive family history is common in both (115), and clinical features are similar to late onset IP, except for more prominent dystonia in the younger patients, and an initial brisk improvement with a low dose of levodopa, followed by an earlier onset of motor fluctuations. EOP needs to be distinguished from other parkinsonian syndromes in adolescence and young adults.

Dopa-Responsive Dystonia (DRD)

Dopa-Responsive Dystonia is an autosomal dominant disorder usually presenting at 4 to 8 years of age with dystonic gait that worsens as the day progresses and improves with sleep. Tremor is uncommon. There may be hyperreflexia in the legs and extensor plantars. Diurnal variation of symptoms, a dramatic response to low doses of levodopa (50–200 mg per day with a decarboxylase inhibitor), and maintenance of the excellent response without development of motor fluctuations all distinguish DRD from juvenile IP (116,117). DRD can present at an older age and then it resembles IP more closely.

Hemiparkinsonism-Hemiatrophy-Syndrome (HPHA)

HPHA is a rare condition in which parkinsonian features, often with dystonia, are confined to one side of the body with hemiatrophy, probably as a result of brain injury at an early stage of brain development (118,119). Younger age of onset, persistent unilateral localization, slow progression, hemiatrophy, lack of a good response to levodopa, and neuroradiologic abnormalities (120) all help to differentiate this condition from IP.

Toxin-Induced Parkinsonism

Methylphenyltetrahydropyridine (MPTP) can cause levodopa-responsive extrapyramidal features indistinguishable from IP (121,122). A history of intravenous drug use, sudden onset of symptoms (not always) and early complications of levodopa therapy (such as dyskinesias, motor fluctuations, psychiatric symptoms) may help to distinguish MPTP-induced parkinsonism from IP.

Chronic manganese intoxication can result in a progressive parkinsonian syndrome. However, these patients must be differentiated from early IP by a confirmed history of exposure to manganese, disturbances of gait ("cock-walk") and balance (tendency to fall backwards), prominent dystonia, infrequent tremor, lack of response to levodopa (123), and a normal fluorodopa PET scan (124).

Hereditary/Metabolic Parkinsonism

Wilson's Disease (WD)

Wilson's Disease, a treatable condition, needs to be ruled out in all patients with early onset parkinsonism. WD can be of pseudoparkinsonian type (125) with asymmetric tremor (resting, postural, or kinetic), akinesia, dystonia, dysarthria, and gait abnormalities as the presenting symptoms. Distinguishing features from IP include a coarse proximal component of the tremor (wing-beating), early psychiatric symptoms, cerebellar signs, diagnostic Kayser–Fleischer rings as determined by slit-lamp examination in the eyes, nonneurologic manifestations (such as hepatic and renal disturbances) and diagnostic laboratory tests for copper and ceruloplasmin.

Juvenile Huntington's Disease

Juvenile Huntington's disease can present with rigidity, dystonia, and bradykinesia as the predominant manifestations (126,127). Chorea, subcortical dementia, and abnormal ocular motility are the important manifestations that differentiate it from IP. Dopaminomimetics may alleviate bradykinesia and rigidity (128) but can cause exacerbation of chorea and dementia. Genetic testing is the most accurate diagnostic tool.

Machado-Joseph Disease

Type I Machado-Joseph disease can lead to prominent extrapyramidal manifestations such as dystonia and rigidity (129). Additional features of progressive cerebellar ataxia and external ophthalmoplegia help to distinguish Machado-Joseph disease from early onset IP.

Hallervorden-Spatz Disease

Hallervorden-Spatz disease is an autosomal recessive disorder with onset of neurologic dysfunction mainly in childhood. The cardinal symptoms are an extrapyramidal movement disorder (mainly rigidity and dystonia), intellectual impairment, and pyramidal tract signs. Nonneurologic symptoms may include foot deformities, skin pigmentation, and tapetoretinal degeneration. Magnetic resonance imaging and bone-marrow studies are helpful for diagnosis (130).

DIAGNOSIS OF EARLY IDIOPATHIC PARKINSONISM

Screening Questionnaire – Validity, Sensitivity, and Specificity

Epidemiologic studies for early detection of IP (131–135) have addressed the validity, specificity, and sensitivity of different screening questionnaires. A set of nine questions (Table 6.4) was originally devised by Tanner and coworkers (135). Duarte and coworkers (131) applied specific weights to each of these questions. A cutoff point of 42 on this weighted questionnaire achieved both 100 percent sensitivity and 100 percent specificity when tested on 50 IP patients and 100 ophthalmological patients, respectively. However, this questionnaire needs further validation on a larger population.

Criteria for Diagnosis of Idiopathic Parkinsonism

Clinicopathologic studies have shown a false-positive rate of about 20 to 25 percent (89,136) and a false-negative rate of 5 to 10 percent, depending on patient selection (136,137). The use of strict exclusion and inclusion criteria may increase the specifity at the cost of reducing the sensitivity. For epidemiologic and screening purposes it is important to have criteria with higher sensitivity as achieved by a screening questionnaire. Subsequently, the positive cases may be categorized as (a) clinically possible, (b) clinically probable, and (c) clinically definite, according to the criteria proposed by Calne and coworkers (138) (Table 6.5). To each of these levels may be added a designation "with" or "without" laboratory support.

Table 6-4   Screening Questionnaire for Detection of Parkinson's Disease*

No.	Question	Score
1	Do you have trouble arising from a chair?	6
2	Is your handwriting smaller than it once was?	7
3	Do people tell you that your voice is softer than it once was?	8
4	Is your balance, when walking, poor?	9
5	Do your feet suddenly seem to freeze in door-ways?	6
6	Does your face seem less expressive than it used to?	6
7	Do your arms and legs shake?	9
8	Do you have trouble buttoning buttons?	8
9	Do you shuffle your feet and take tiny steps when you walk?	8

*Duarate et al. (131)

Table 6-5   Categories of Idiopathic Parkinsonism*

1. **Clinically possible IP:**
   The presence of *any one* of the salient features: tremor, rigidity, or bradykinesia. Impairment of postural reflexes is not included because it is too nonspecific. The tremor must be of recent onset, but may be postural or resting.
2. **Clinically probable IP:**
   A combination of *any two* of the cardinal features: resting tremor, rigidity, bradykinesia, or impaired postural reflexes. Alternatively, asymmetrical resting tremor, asymmetrical rigidity, or asymmetrical bradykinesia are sufficient.
3. **Clinically definite IP:**
   Any combination of *three* of the features: resting tremor, rigidity, bradykinesia, or impaired postural reflexes. Alternatively, two of these features are sufficient, with one of the first three displaying asymmetry.

*Calne et al. (138)

Laboratory Features

There are no absolute diagnostic laboratory tests for the premortem diagnosis of IP and even the pathologic criteria are unclear. High-resolution magnetic resonance imaging and computerized tomography scanning of the brain may be helpful to exclude secondary causes of parkinsonism such as normal pressure hydrocephalus, cerebrovascular disease, progressive supranuclear palsy, Huntington's disease, and olivopontocerebellar atrophy. PET scanning and [123I]ßCIT single photon emission tomography (SPECT) are useful to detect nigrostriatal changes. (See Chapters 25 and 26) [123I]ßCIT SPECT (139) and [123I]FP-CIT SPECT (140) are useful in demonstrating loss of striatal dopamine transporter content in early IP. Functional imaging with PET scanning has provided many insights into the pathophysiology of neurodegenerative disorders including IP. [18F]6-fluoro-L-dopa ([18F]FD) has been used to quantitate presynaptic nigrostriatal function and its reproducibility in normal human subjects has been well established (141). It has been shown that [18F]FD uptake rate constant (Ki) has significant correlations with the dopamine levels in the striatum and with the dopaminergic cell densities in the substantia nigra (142). Similar conclusions have been reached from experimental studies of the nigrostriatal pathways in animals (143). Age-related neuronal loss or impaired function in the nigrostriatal pathways result in a linear decrease in the striatal Ki (144). Nigrostriatal dopaminergic neurons have a high degree of plasticity (145) and a prolonged clinically silent stage of nigral neuronal loss exists before the early symptoms of IP appear. The clinical signs do not appear until 50% of nigral neurons and 80 percent of striatal dopamine is lost (21,145).

Preclinical detection of parkinsonism has been reported (146,147) where asymptomatic subjects had reduced striatal FD uptake and had developed parkinsonism within months. Striatal dopamine deficiency has also been observed in subjects at risk of developing parkinsonism, for example, after exposure to MPTP (148), in Guamanians from regions with Lytico-Bodig (149,150), in co-twins of patients with IP (151–153), in first-degree relatives in a family with dominantly inherited parkinsonism (154), and in individuals who have recovered from drug-induced parkinsonism (68). In early IP symptom onset has been estimated at a putamen Ki of between 57 percent and 80 percent of normal (155). These findings are consistent with the observation by Fearnley and Lees [21] of a curvilinear decline in the nigral cell count with increasing symptom duration in IP and a short presymptomatic period of 4.7 years at the age of 60. Moreover, in a mathematical model, the presymptomatic period was calculated to be 5 to 14 years for patients aged 65 years, depending on the severity of impact of the initial result (23). The rate of progression of the nigrostriatal lesion in IP has been estimated to be 2.5 times that of normal aging (156), but since progression is faster initially, this figure only gives a crude estimate.

Of the four cardinal signs of IP (rigidity, tremor, bradykinesia, and postural imbalance) only bradykinesia, as measured by the UPDRS/Modified Columbia Scale (MCS) or Purdue pegboard, has been found to have the best correlation with the striatal Ki of FD scans (22,43,157). A less robust correlation has been observed with the axial (posture, stability, and gait) and rigidity subscales of MCS, but not with the tremor subscale (43). The methods of assessment of bradykinesia by the MCS and by pegboard are complementary and a combination of these methods improved the correlation with PET (43). Bradykinesia measurements showed the highest correlation with the contralateral but not ipsilateral Ki, implying lateralization of the dopaminergic deficit (43). Bradykinesia has also been shown to have significant correlation with the degree of postmortem striatal dopamine deficiency (158), with nigral cell count (159), and with the decreased concentration of homovanillic acid in cerebrospinal fluid (160). Thus bradykinesia has the best correlation with the nigrostriatal dopaminergic deficit in IP, and therefore the pegboard value and bradykinesia score should be the primary outcome variables for studies addressing the natural evolution of the disorder (22,23).

Response to Dopaminomimetics

Virtually all patients with IP benefit from dopaminomimetic therapy provided they are able to tolerate a reasonable intake of these drugs (up to 1,500 mg of levodopa per day with a peripheral decarboxylase inhibitor (138,161). When in doubt about the response of IP, a sudden cessation of the dopaminomimetic treatment should help answer the question, particularly if the dose is high (138). Injection of a dopaminomimetic agonist such as lisuride or apomorphine (after prior treatment with domperidone) is an alternative and quicker method of detecting a response, although not always practical. Though unresponsiveness to dopaminomometics strongly argues against a diagnosis of IP, responsiveness is not a diagnostic criterion because some other forms of Parkinsonism such as progressive supranuclear palsy (78,162) and multiple system atrophies (86,163) may show a transient or partial response to dopaminomimetics and some pathologically proven cases of IP have been found to be unresponsive (164).

CONCLUSION

Tremor at rest, rigidity, and bradykinesia are the early manifestations of Idiopathic Parkinsonism. The average age of onset of symptoms is the middle of the sixth decade. These symptoms are usually asymmetric and in the initial stages may be intermittent and only worsened by stress. In the early stages of the disease, patients may have nonspecific symptoms such as fatigability, arthralgia, cramps, internal tremulousness, and vague sensory disturbances that may be mistaken for aging, neuromuscular diseases, or other systemic disorders. Initially symptoms are often related to specific tasks. A therapeutic response to an adequate dose of levodopa is seen in virtually all patients. Early impairment of postural reflexes, significant abnormalities of gait, disturbances in ocular motility, autonomic dysfunction unrelated to drugs, progressive dementia, cerebellar signs, focal neurolologic deficits, and unresponsiveness to levodopa warrant a search for other causes of parkinsonism. There are no absolute diagnostic tests for the premortem diagnosis of idiopathic parkinsonism. Functional imaging with [^{18}F]6-fluoro-l-dopa positron emission tomography is useful to quantitate the presynaptic nigrostriatal dysfunction and it correlates well with the clinical manifestation of bradykinesia.

Acknowledgments

The authors thank Susan Calne for editorial assistance. This work was supported by the Pacific Parkinson Research Institute, Vancouver, Canada; The National Parkinson Foundation, Inc, Miami, USA; The Medical Research Council of Canada.

REFERENCES

1. Parkinson J. *An Essay on the Shaking Palsy*. London: Sherwood, Neely, and Jones, 1817.

2. Calne DB. Is "Parkinson's disease" One disease? *J Neurol Neurosurg Psychiatry* 1989; 18–21.

3. Calne DB. Parkinson's disease is not one disease. *Parkinsonism* and real disord 2000; 7:1, 3–9.

4. Kitada T, Asakawa S, Hattori N, et al. Mutations in the *parkin* gene cause autosomal recessive juvenile parkinsonism. *Nature* 1998; 392:605–608.

5. Polymeropoulos MH, Lavedan C, Leroy E, et al. Mutation in the alpha-synuclein gene identified in families with Parkinson's disease. *Science* 1997; 276:2045–2047.

6. Polymeropoulos MH, Higgins JJ, Golbe LI, et al. Mapping of a gene for Parkinson's disease to chromosome 4q21–q23. *Science* 1996; 274:1197–1199.

7. Takahasi H, Calne DB. What is Parkinson's disease? In: Agnoli A, Fabbrini G, Stochii F (eds.). *Parkinson's Disease and Extrapyramidal Disorders: Pathophysiology and Treatment*. London: John Libbey, 1991:25–32.

8. Galasko D, Kwo-on-Yuen P, Klauber MR, et al. Neurological findings in Alzheimer's disease and normal aging. *Arch Neurol* 1990; 47:625–627.

9. Jenkyn LR, Reeves AG, Warren T, et al. Neurological signs in senescence. *Arch Neurol* 1985; 42:1154–1157.

10. Teräväinen H, Calne DB. Motor system in normal aging and Parkinson's disease. In: Katzman R, Terry R (eds.). *The Neurology of Aging*. Philadelphia: F.A. Davis, 1983:85–109.

11. Duncan G, Wilson JA. Normal elderly have some signs of PS. *Lancet* 1989; 2:1392.

12. Rajput AH. Clinical features and natural history of Parkinson's disease (special consideration of aging). In: Calne DB (ed.). *Neurodegenerative Diseases*. Philadelphia: W.B. Saunders, 1994:555–571.

13. Kurland LT. Incidence, geographic distribution and genetic considerations. In: Fields WS (ed.). *Pathogenesis and Treatment of Parkinsonism*. Springfield, IL: Charles C Thomas, 1958:5–43.

14. Wolters EC, Calne DB. Is Parkinson's disease related to aging? In: Calne DB, et al. (eds.). *Parkinsonism and Aging*. New York: Raven Press, 1989:125–132.

15. Côtè LJ, Kremzner LT. Biochemical changes in normal aging in human brain. In: Mayeux R, Rosen WG (eds.). *The dementis, Advances in Neurology*. Vol 38 New York: Raven Press, 1983:19–30.

16. Calne DB., McGeer E., Eiaon A., and Spencer P. Alzheimer's disease, Parkinson's disease, and Motoneuron disease: Abiotrophic interaction between aging and environment? *Lancer* 1067–1070, 1986.

17. Carlsson A, Nyberg P, Winblad B. The influence of age and other factors on concentration of monoamines in the human brain. In: Nyberg P (ed.). *Brain monoamines in normal aging and dementia*. Sweden: Umea University Medical Dissertations, 1984:53–84.

18. Carlsson A, Winblad B. Influence of age and time interval between death and autopsy on dopamine and 3-methoxytyramine levels in human basal ganglia. *J Neural Transm* 1976; 38:271–276.

19. Severson JA, Marcusson J, Winblad B, et al. Age-correlated loss of dopaminergic binding sites in human basal ganglia. *J Neurochem* 1982; 39:1623–1631.

20. Wong DF, Wagner HNJ, Dannals RF, et al. Effects of age on dopamine and serotonin receptors measured by positron tomography in the living human brain. *Science* 1984; 226:1393–1396.

21. Fearnley JM, Lees AJ. Ageing and Parkinson's disease: Substantia nigra regional selectivity. *Brain* 1991; 114:2283–2301.

22. Lee CS, Schulzer M, Mak EK, et al. Clinical observations on the rate of progression of idiopathic parkinsonism. *Brain* 1994; 117:501–507.

23. Schulzer M, Lee CS, Mak EK, Vingerhoets FJG, and Calne DB. A mathematical model of pathogenesis in idiopathic parkinsonism. *Brain* 117:509–516, 1994.

24. Gibb WRG, Lees AJ. The relevance of the Lewy body to the pathogenesis of idiopathic Parkinson's disease. *J Neurol Neurosurg Psychiat* 1988; 51:745–752.

25. Golbe LI. Young-onset Parkinson's disease: a clinical review [Review]. *Neurology* 1991; 41:168–173.

26. Zetusky WJ, Jankovic J, Pirozzolo FJ. The heterogeneity of Parkinson's disease: Clinical and prognostic implications. *Neurology* 1985; 35:522–526.

27. Calne DB. Is idiopathic parkinsonism a consequence of an event or a process? *Neurology* 1994; 44:5–10.

28. Lee CS, Schulzer M, Mak E, et al. Patterns of asymmetry do not change over the course of idiopathic parkinsonism: Implications for pathogenesis. *Neurology* 1995; 45:435–439.

29. Hoehn MM, Yahr MD. Parkinsonism: Onset, progression, and mortality. *Neurology* 1967; 17:427–442.

30. Koller WC, Wong GF, Lang A. Post-traumatic movement disorders: a review. *Mov Disord* 1989; 4:20–36.

31. Koller WC. When does Parkinson's disease begin? *Neurology* 1992; 42:27–31.

32. Schenck CH, Bundlie SR, Mahowald MW. Delayed emergence of a parkinsonian disorder in 38% of 29 older men initially diagnosed with idiopathic rapid eye movement sleep behavior disorder. *Neurology* 1996; 46:388–393.

33. Calne DB, Stoessl AJ. Early Parkinsonism. *Clin Neuropharmacol* 1986; 9:S3–S8.

34. Findley LJ, Gresty MA. Tremor. *Br J Hosp Med* 1981; 26:16–32.

35. Paulson HL, Stern MB. Clinical manifestations of Parkinson's disease. In: Koller WC, Watts RL, (eds.). *Move Disord*. New York: McGraw-Hill, Health Professions Division, 1997:183–199.

36. Calne DB. Parkinsonism. *Med. Int.* 1992; 4177–4183.

37. Hallett M. Differential diagnosis of tremor. In: Vinken PJ, Bruyn GW, Klawans HL (eds.). *Handbook of Clinical Neurology: Extrapyramidal Disorders*. New York: Elsevier Science, 1986:583–595.

38. Findley LJ, Gresty MA. Tremor and rhythmical involuntary movements in Parkinson's disease. In: Findley LJ, Capildeo R (eds.). *Movement Disorders: Tremor*. London and Basingstoke: Macmillan, 1984:295–304.

39. Klawans HL. Abnormal movements in the elderly. *Sandorama* 1981; 15–18.

40. Findley LJ, Gresty MA, Halmagyi GM. Tremor and cogwheel phenomena and clonus in Parkinson's disease. *J Neurol Neurosurg Psychiat* 1981; 44: 534–546.

41. Marsden CD. Slowness of movement in Parkinson's disease. *Mov Disord* 1989; 4:S26–S37.

42. Hietanen M, Teräväinen H, Tsui JK, et al. The pegboard as a measurement of parkinsonian deficit. *Neurology* 1987; 37:266(Abstract).

43. Vingerhoets FJG, Schulzer M, Calne DB, et al. Which clinical sign of Parkinson's disease best reflects the nigrostriatal lesion? *Ann Neurol* 1997; 41: 58–64.

44. Pal P, Lee CS, Tsui JKC, et al. Rapid alternating two-finger tapping test is an age-independent, objective measurement of parkinsonism, and correlates well with Ki of [18F]-DOPA PET scan. Parkinsonism, Rel. Disord. In press.

45. Marttila RJ, Rinne UK. Disability and progression of Parkinson's disease. *Acta Neurol Scand* 1977; 56:159–169.

46. Gibb WR, Lees AJ. A comparison of clinical and pathological features of young- and old-onset Parkinson's disease. *Neurology* 1988; 38:1402–1406.

47. Jankovic J, McDermott M, Carter J, et al. Variable expression of Parkinson's disease: A base-line analysis of DATATOP cohort. *Neurology* 1990; 40:1529–1534.

48. Giladi N, McMahon D, Przedborski S. Motor blocks in Parkinson's disease. *Neurology* 1992; 42:333–339.

49. Sudarsky L. Gait disorders in the elderly. *N Engl J Med* 1990; 322:1441–1446.

50. Weiner WJ, Nora LM, Glantz RH. Elderly inpatients: Postural reflex impairment. *Neurology* 1984; 34:945–947.

51. Drachman DA, Long RR, Swearer JM. Neurological evaluation of the elderly patient. In: Albert ML, Knoefel JE (eds.). *Clinical Neurology of Aging*. New York: Oxford University Press, 1994:159–180.

52. Rajput AH. Parkinsonism, aging and gait apraxia. In: Stern MB, Koller WC (eds.). *Parkinsonian syndromes*. New York: Marcel Dekker, 1993:511–532.

53. Tinetti ME, Speechley M, Ginter SF. Risk factors for falls among elderly persons living in the community. *N Engl J Med* 1988; 319:1701–1707.

54. Rajput AH, Offord KP, Beard CM, et al. Essential tremor in Rochester, Minnesota: A 45-year study. *J Neurol Neurosurg Psychiat* 1984; 47:466–470.

55. Rautakorpi I, Takala J, Marttila RJ, et al. Essential tremor in a Finnish population. *Acta Neurol Scand* 1982; 66:58–67.

56. Salemi G, Savettieri G, Rocca WA, et al. Prevalence of essential tremor: A door-to-door survey in Terrasini, Sicily. *Neurology* 1994; 44:61–64.

57. Findley LJ, Koller WC. Essential tremor: A review. *Neurology* 1987; 37:1194–1197.

58. Larsen TA, Calne DB. Essential tremor. *Clin Neuropharmacol* 1983; 6:185–206.

59. Critchley M. Observations on essential (heredofamilial) tremor. *Brain* 1949; 72:113–139.

60. Elbe RJ. Physiologic and essential tremor. *Neurology* 1986; 36:225–231.

61. Koller WC. Diagnosis and treatment of tremor. *Neurol Clin* 1984; 2:499–514.

62. Calzetti S, Baratti M, Findley LJ. Frequency/amplitude characteristics of postural tremor of the hands in a population of patients with bilateral tremor: Implications for the classification and mechanism of essential tremor. *J Neurol Neurosurg Psychiatry* 1987; 50:561–567.

63. Koller WC, Hubble JP, Busenbark KL. Essential tremor. In: Calne DB (ed.). *Neurodegenerative diseases*. Philadelphia: WB Saunders, 1994:717–742.

64. Rajput AH, Rozdilsky B, Ang L, et al. Significance of Parkinsonian manifestations in essential tremor. *Can J Neurol Sci* 1993; 20:114–117.

65. Friedman JH. Drug-induced parkinsonism. In: Lang AE, Weiner WJ (eds.). *Drug-Induced Movement Disorders*. Mount Kisco, NY: Futura Publishing Co., 1992:41–83.

66. Kish SJ, Shannak K, Rajput A, et al. Aging produces a specific pattern of striatal dopamine loss: Implications for the etiology of idiopathic Parkinson's disease. *J Neurochem* 1992; 58:642–648.

67. Rajput AH, Rozdilsky B, Hornykiewicz O, et al. Reversible drug-induced parkinsonism: Clinicopathological study of two cases. *Arch Neurol* 1982; 39:644–646.

68. Calne DB, Langston JW, Martin WRW, et al. Positron emission tomography after MPTP: observations relating to the Parkinson's Disease. *Nature* 1983; 317:246–248.

69. Hardie RJ, Lees AJ. Neuroleptic-induced Parkinson's syndrome: Clinical features and results of treatment with L-dopa. *J Neurol Neurosurg Psychiat* 1988; 51:850–854.

70. Fitzgerald PM, Jankovic J. Lower body parkinsonism: Evidence for a vascular etiology. *Mov Disord* 1989; 4:249–260.

71. Thomson PD, Marsden CD. Gait disorder of subcortical arteriosclerotic encephalopathy: Binswanger's disease. *Mov Disord* 1987; 2:1–8.

72. Critchley M. Arteriosclerotic parkinsonism. *Brain* 1929; 52:23–83.

73. Hurtig HI. Vascular parkinsonism. In: Stern MB, Koller WC (eds.). *Parkinsonian syndromes*. New York: Marcel Dekker, 1993:81–93.

74. Duvoisin RC, Golbe LI, Lepore FE. Progressive supranuclear palsy. *Can J Neurol Sci* 1987; 14:547–554.

75. Golbe LI, Davis PH, Schoenberg, BS, et al. Prevalence and natural history of progressive supranuclear palsy. *Neurology* 1988; 38:1031–1034.

76. Jankovic J, Friedman DI, Pirozollo FJ, et al. Progressive supranuclear palsy: Motor, neurobehavioral, and neuroophthalmic findings. In: Streifler MB, et al. (eds.). *Parkinson's disease: Anatomy, Pathology, and Therapy.* New York: Raven Press, 1990:293–303.

77. Jankovic J. Apraxia of eyelid opening in progressive supranuclear palsy. *Ann Neurol* 1984; 15:115–116.

78. Jankovic J. Progressive supranuclear palsy: Clinical and pharmacologic update. *Neurol Clin* 1984; 2:473–486.

79. Maher ER, Lees AJ. The clinical features and natural history of Steele–Richardson–Olszewski syndrome (progressive supranuclear palsy). *Neurology* 1986; 36:1005–1008.

80. Steele JC. Progressive supranuclear palsy. *Brain* 1972; 95:693–704.

81. Steele JC, Richardson JC, Olszewski J. Progressive supranuclear palsy: A heterogeneous degeneration involving the brainstem, basal ganglia and cerebellum with vertical gaze and pseudobulbar palsy, nuchal dystonia and dementia. *Arch Neurol* 1964; 2: 473–486.

82. Doody RS, Jankovic J. The alien hand and related signs. *J Neurol Neurosurg Psychiat* 1992; 55:806–810.

83. Rebeiz JJ, Kolodny EH, Richardson EP. Corticodentatonigral degeneration with neuronal achromasia. *Arch Neurol* 1968; 18:20–33.

84. Riley DE, Lang AE, Lewis A. Cortical-basal ganglionic degeneration. *Neurology* 1990; 40:1203–1212.

85. Quinn N. Multiple system atrophy-the nature of the beast. *J Neurol Neurosurg Psychiat* 1989; 89.

86. Quinn NP. Multiple system atrophy. In: Marsden CD, Fahn S (eds.). *Movement Disorders 3.* Oxford: Butterworth-Heinemann, 1994:262–281.

87. Fearnley JM, Lees AJ. Striatonigral degeneration: A clinicopathological study. *Brain* 1990; 113:1823–1842.

88. Gouider-Khouja N, Vidailhet M, Bonnet AM, et al. "Pure" striatonigral degeneration and Parkinson's disease: A comparitive clinical study. *Mov Disord* 1995; 10:288–294.

89. Rajput AH, Rozdilsky B, Rajput AA. Accuracy of clinical diagnosis in Parkinsonism: A prospective study. *Can J Neurol Sci* 1991; 18:275–278.

90. Mathias CJ, Williams AC. The Shy–Drager syndrome (and multiple system atrophy). In: Calne DB (ed.). *Neurodegenerative Disorders.* Philadelphia: WB Saunders, 1994:743–767.

91. Munschauer FE, Loh L, Bannister R, et al. Abnormal respiration and sudden death during sleep in multiple system atrophy with autonomic failure. *Neurology* 1990; 40:677.

92. Shy GM, Drager GA. A neurological syndrome associated with orthostatic hypotension. *Arch Neurol* 1960; 2:511–527.

93. Berciano J. Olivopontocerebellar atrophy. In: Jankovic J, Tolosa E (eds.). *Parkinson's Disease and Movement Disorders.* Baltimore: Williams & Wilkins, 1993:163–189.

94. Duvoisin RC. The olivopontocerebellar atrophies. In: Marsden CD, Fahn S (eds.). *Movement Disorders 2.* London: Butterworth, 1987:249–271.

95. Byrne EJ, Lennox G, Lowe J, et al. Diffuse Lewy body disease: Clinical features in 15 cases. *J Neurol Neurosurg Psychiat* 1989; 52:709–717.

96. Kosaka K. Dementia and neuropathology in Lewy body disease. In: Narabayashi H, et al. (eds.). *Parkinson's Disease: From basic research to treatment. Advances in Neurology.* Vol 60 New York: Raven Press, 1993:456–463.

97. Kosaka K. Diffuse Lewy body disease in Japan. *J Neurol* 1990; 237:197–204.

98. Louis ED, Goldman JE, Powers JM, et al. Parkinsonian features of eight pathologically diagnosed cases of diffuse Lewy body disease. *Mov Disord* 1995; 10:188–194.

99. Rajput AH. Movement disorders and aging. In: Watts RL, Koller WC (eds.). *Movement disorders: Neurologic principles and practice.* New York: McGraw-Hill, 1997:673–686.

100. Morris JC, Drazner M, Fulling K, et al. Clinical and pathological aspects of parkinsonism in Alzheimer's disease: A role for extranigral factors? *Arch Neurol* 1989; 46:651–657.

101. Rajput AH, Rozdilsky B, Rajput A. Alzheimer's disease and idiopathic Parkinson's disease coexistence. *J Geriat Psychiat Neurol* 1993; 6:170–176.

102. Crystal HA, Dickson DW, Lizardi JE, et al. Antemortem diagnosis of diffuse Lewy body disease. *Neurology* 1990; 40:1523–1528.

103. Dickson DW, Ruan D, Crystal H, et al. Hippocampal degeneration differentiates diffuse Lewy body disease (DLBD) from Alzheimer's disease: Light and electron microscopic immunocytochemistry of CA2-3 neurites specific to DLBD. *Neurology* 1991; 41:1402–1409.

104. Hirano A, Kurland LT, Krooth RS, et al. Parkinsonism-dementia complex, an endemic disease on the island of Guam. I. Clinical features. *Brain* 1961; 84: 642–661.

105. Mulder DW, Kurland AT, Iriarte LLG. Neurological disease on the island of Guam. *US Armed Forces Med J* 1954; 5:1724–1739.

106. Lavine L, Steele JC, Wolfe N, et al. Amyotrophic lateral sclerosis/parkinsonism-dementia complex in Southern Guam: Is it disappearing? In: Rowland LP (ed.). *Amyotrophic Lateral Sclerosis and Other Motor Neuron Diseases: Advances in Neurology, vol. 56.* New York: Raven Press, 1991:271–285.

107. Lepore FE, Steele JC, Cox TA, et al. Supranuclear disturbances of ocular motility in Lytico-Bodig. *Neurology* 1988; 38:1849–1853.

108. Hakim S, Adams RD. The special clinical problem of symptomatic hydrocephalus with normal cerebrospinal fluid pressure: Observations on cerebrospinal fluid hydrodynamics. *J Neurol Sci* 1965; 2:307–327.

109. Knutsen E, Lying-Tunnel V. Gait apraxia in normal-pressure hydrocephalus: Patterns of movement and muscle activation. *Neurology* 1985; 9:155–160.

110. Shannon KM. Hydrocephalus and parkinsonism. In: Stern MB, Koller WC (eds.). *Parkinsonian Syndromes*. New York: Marcel Dekker, 1993:123–136.

111. Brown P, Gibbs CJ, Jr, Rodgers-Johnson P, et al. Human spongiform encephalopathy: The NIH series of 300 cases of experimentally transmitted disease. *Ann Neurol* 1994; 35:513

112. Wszolek ZK, Pfeiffer RF, Bhatt MH, et al. Rapidly progressive autosomal dominant parkinsonism and dementia with pallido-ponto-nigral degeneration. *Ann Neurol* 1992; 32:312–320.

113. Lynch T, Sano M, Marder KS, et al. Clinical characteristics of a family with chromosome 17-linked disinhibition-dementia-parkinsonism-amyotrophy complex. *Neurology* 1994; 44:1878–1884.

114. Quinn N, Critchley P, Marsden CD. Young onset Parkinson's disease. *Mov Disord* 1987; 2:73–91.

115. Muthane UD, Swamy HS, Satishchandra P, et al. Early onset Parkinson's disease: Are juvenile- and young-onset different? *Mov Disord* 1994; 9:539–544.

116. Nygaard TG, Marsden CD, Fahn S. Dopa-responsive dystonia: Long-term treatment response and prognosis. *Neurology* 1991; 41:174–181.

117. Nygaard TG, Marsden CD, Duvoisin RC. Dopa-responsive dystonia. In: Fahn S, Marsden CD, Calne DB (eds.). *Dystonia 2, Advances in Neurology*. Vol. 50 New York: Raven Press, 1988:377–384.

118. Buchman AS, Christopher CG, Goetz MD, et al. Hemiparkinsonism with hemiatrophy. *Neurology* 1988; 38:527–530.

119. Klawans HL. Hemiparkinsonism as a late complication of hemiatrophy: A new syndrome. *Neurology* 1981; 31:625–628.

120. Giladi N, Burke RE, Kostic V. Hemiparkinsonism-hemiatrophy syndrome: Clinical and radiologic features. *Neurology* 1990; 40:1731–1734.

121. Ballard PA, Tetrud JW, Langston JW. Permanent parkinsonism in humans due to 1-methyl-4-phenyl-1,2,3,6-tetrahydropyridine (MPTP): Seven cases. *Neurology* 1985; 35:949–956.

122. Langston JW, Ballard PA. Parkinsonism induced by 1-methyl-4-phenyl-1,2,3,6-tetrahydropyridine (MPTP): Implications for treatment and the pathogenesis of Parkinson's disease. *Can J Neurol Sci* 1984; 11:160–165.

123. Lu CS, Huang CC, Chu NS, et al. L-dopa failure in chronic manganism. *Neurology* 1994; 44:1600–1602.

124. Wolters EC, Huang C, Clark C, et al. Positron emission tomography in manganese intoxication. *Ann Neurol* 1989; 26:647–651.

125. Oder W, Prayer L, Grimm G, et al. Wilson's disease: Evidence of subgroups derived from clinical findings and brain lesions. *Neurology* 1993; 43:120–124.

126. Adams P, Falek A, Arnold J. Huntington's disease in Georgia: Age at onset. *Am J Hum Genet* 1988; 43:695–704.

127. Oliver JE. Huntington's chorea in Northhamptonshire. *Br J Psychiat* 1970; 116:241–253.

128. Jongen PJ, Reiner WO, Gabreels FJ. Seven cases of Huntington's disease in childhood and L-dopa-induced improvement in the hypokinetic rigid form. *Clin Neurol Neurosurg* 1980; 82:251–261.

129. Barbeau A, Roy M, Cunha L, et al. The natural history of Machado-Joseph disease. An analysis of 138 personally examined cases. *Can J Neurol Sci* 1984; 11:510–525.

130. Swaiman KF. Hallervorden–Spatz syndrome and brain iron metabolism. *Arch Neurol* 1991; 48:1285–1293.

131. Duarte J, Claveria LE, Pedro-Cuesta JD, et al. Screening Parkinson's disease: A validated questionnaire of high specificity and sensitivity. *Mov Disord* 1995; 10:643–649.

132. Gutierrez MC, Schoenberg BS, Portera A. Prevalence of neurological diseases in Madrid, Spain. *Neuroepidemiology* 1989; 8:43–47.

133. Meneghini F, Rocca WA, Anderson DW, et al. Validating screening instruments for neuroepidemiologic surveys: Experience in Sicily. *J Clin Epidemiol* 1992; 45:319–331.

134. Mutch WJ, Smith WC, Scott RF. A screening and alerting questionnaire for parkinsonism. *Neuroepidemiology* 1991; 10:150–156.

135. Tanner CM, Gilley DW, Goetz CG. A brief screening questionnaire for parkinsonism. *Ann Neurol* 1990; 28:267–268.

136. Hughes AJ, Daniel SE, Kilford L, et al. The accuracy of the clinical diagnosis of Parkinson's disease: a clinicopathological study of 100 cases. *J Neurol Neurosurg Psychiat* 1992; 55:181–184.

137. Joachim CL, Morris JH, Selkoe DJ. Clinically diagnosed Alzheimer's disease: autopsy results in 150 cases. *Ann Neurol* 1988; 24:50–56.

138. Calne DB, Snow BJ, Lee C. Criteria for Diagnosing Parkinson's Disease. *Ann Neurol* 1992; 32:S125–S127.

139. Marek KL, Seibyl JP, Zoghbi SS, et al. [123I] beta-CIT/SPECT imaging demonstrates bilateral loss of dopamine transporters in hemi-Parkinson's disease. *Neurology* 1996; 46:231–237.

140. Booji J, Tissingh G, Boer GJ, et al. [123I] FP-CIT SPECT shows a pronounced decline of striatal dopamine transporter labelling in early and advanced Parkinson's disease. *J Neurol Neurosurg Psychiat* 1997; 62:133–140.

141. Vingerhoets FJG, Snow BJ, Schulzer M, et al. Reproducibility of fluorine-18-6-fluorodopa positron emission tomography in normal human subjects. *J Nucl Med* 1994; 35:18–24.

142. Snow BJ, Tooyama I, McGeer EG, et al. Human positron emission tomographic [^{18}f]fluorodopa studies correlate with dopamine cell counts and levels. *Ann Neurol* 1993; 34:324–330.

143. Pate BD, Kawamata T, Yamada T, et al. Correlation of striatal fluorodopa uptake in the MPTP monkey with dopaminergic indices. *Ann Neurol* 1993; 34:331–338.

144. Martin WRW, Palmer MR, Patlak CS, et al. Nigrostriatal function in humans studied with positron emission tomography. *Ann Neurol* 1989; 26:535–542.

145. Hornykiewicz O, Kish SJ. Biochemical pathophysiology of Parkinson's disease. In: Yahr MD, Bergman KJ (eds.). *Parkinson's disease*. New York: Raven Press, 1986:19–34.

146. Sawle GV, Wroe SJ, Lees AJ. The identification of presymptomatic parkinsonism: clinical and [^{13}F]dopa positron emission tomography studies in an Irish kindred. *Ann Neurol* 1992; 32:609–617.

147. Snow BJ, Martin WRW, Calne DB. A case of subclinical idiopathic parkinsonism detected with fluorodopa PET. *Abstract of the 10th International Symposium on Parkinson's Disease, Tokyo*, 1991:p 222.

148. Guttman M, Calne DB. In vivo characterization of cerebral dopamine systems in human parkinsonism. In: Jankovic J, Tolosa E (eds.). *Parkinson's disease and movement disorders*. Baltimore: Urgan and Schwarzenberg, 1988:49–58.

149. Snow BJ, Peppard RF, Guttman M, et al. Positron emission tomographic scanning demonstrates a presynaptic dopaminergic lesion in Lytico-Bodig: the amyotrophic lateral sclerosis parkinsonism dementia complex of Guam. *Arch Neurol* 1990; 47:870–874.

150. Burn DJ, Mark MH, Playford ED, et al. Parkinson's disease in twins studied with 18F-dopa and positron emission tomography. *Neurology* 1992; 42:1894–1900.

151. Holthoff VA, Vieregge P, Kessler J, et al. Discordant twins with Parkinson's disease: Positron emission tomography and early signs of impaired cognitive circuits. *Ann Neurol* 1994; 36:176–182.

152. Takahashi H, Bhatt M, Snow BJ, et al. Fluorodopa PET studies of twins in idiopathic parkinsonism. *Abstract of the 10th International Symposium on Parkinson's Disease, Tokyo*, 1991; p. 176.

153. Kishore A, Wszolek ZK, Snow BJ, et al. Presynaptic nigrostriatal function in genetically asymptomatic relatives from the pallido-ponto-nigral degeneration family. *Neurology* 1996; 47:1588–1590.

154. Morrish PK, Sawle GV, Brooks DJ. Clinical and [^{18}F] dopa PET findings in early Parkinson's disease. *J Neurol Neurosurg Psychiat* 1995; 59:597–600.

155. Vingerhoets FJG, Snow BJ, Lee CS, et al. Longitudinal fluorodopa positron emission tomographic studies of the evolution of idiopathic Parkinsonism. *Ann Neurol* 1994; 36:759–764.

156. Eidelberg D, Moeller JR, Dhawan V, et al. The metabolic anatomy of Parkinson's disease : Complementary [^{18}F]fluorodeoxyglucose and [^{18}F]fluorodopa positron emission tomographic studies. *Mov Disord* 1990; 5:203–213.

157. Bernheimer H, Birkmayer W, Hornykiewicz, O, et al. Brain dopamine and the syndromes of Parkinson and Huntington. *J Neurol Sci* 1973; 20:415–455.

158. Rinne JO, Rummukainen J, Paljarvi L, et al. Dementia in Parkinson's disease is related to neuronal loss in the medial substantia nigra. *Ann Neurol* 1989; 26:47–50.

159. Rinne UK, Sonninen V. Acid monoamine metabolites in the cerebrospinal fluid of patients with Parkinson's disease. *Neurology* 1972; 22:62–67.

160. Calne DB. The Nature of Parkinson's Disease. *Neurochem Int* 1992; 20:1S–3S.

161. Neiforth KA, Golbe LI. Retrospective study of drug response in 87 patients with progressive supranuclear palsy. *Clin Neuropharmacol* 1993; 16:338–346.

162. Rajput AH, Rodzilsky B, Rajput A, et al. L-dopa efficacy and pathological basis of Parkinson syndromes. *Clin Neuropharmacol* 1990; 13:553–558.

163. Murh MH, Sage JI, Dichson DW, et al. Levodopa-Nonresponsive Lewy Body Parkinsonism: Clinicopathologic study of two cases. *Neurology* 1992; 42:1315–1322.

7

Gait Disturbances

Nir Giladi, MD

Movement Disorders Unit, Department of Neurology, Tel-Aviv Sourasky Medical Center, Sackler Faculty of Medicine, Tel-Aviv University, Tel-Aviv, Israel

INTRODUCTION

It was James Parkinson who first described gait disturbances in the disorder later named after him in his original "An Essay on the Shaking Palsy" (1): "The propensity to lean forward becomes invincible, and the patient is thereby forced to step on the toes and fore part of the feet, whilst the upper part of the body is thrown so far forward as to render it difficult to avoid falling on the face. In some cases, when this state of the malady is attained, the patient can no longer exercise himself by walking in his usual manner, but is thrown on the toes and forepart of the feet; being, at the same time, irresistibly impelled to make much quicker and short steps, and thereby to adopt unwillingly a running pace. In some cases it is found necessary entirely to substitute running for walking; since otherwise the patient, on proceeding only a very few paces, would inevitably fall."

Gait disturbances such as festination, described by Parkinson, are characteristic integral elements of the classical picture of Parkinson's disease (PD). However, it was not until recently that abnormal gait has been recognized as a major parkinsonian feature when it was added as the fifth cardinal sign of parkinsonism together with rest tremor, rigidity, bradykinesia, and abnormal postural reflexes (2).

Parkinsonian gait is considered as one of the middle level gait disorders according to the classification of Nutt and coworkers (3) (Table 7-1). However, the underlying mechanism of gait disturbances in PD is heterogeneous and complex. It is affected by muscle rigidity, hypokinesia, bradykinesia, and abnormal preparation and execution of motor sets. A patient with PD develops increasing dependence on attention and external cueing or visual triggers to maintain normal gait. In addition, the ability to initiate and maintain locomotion is heavily dependent on postural reflexes, which are frequently disturbed in PD. The contribution of each one of the aforementioned disturbances to the final parkinsonian gait abnormalities differs from one patient to another and in the same individual at different stages of the disease.

The purpose of this chapter is to characterize the different subtypes of gait disturbances in PD, to correlate them with the clinical syndrome, and to discuss the effects of different therapeutic modalities.

GAIT DISTURBANCES AS PART OF THE CLINICAL SYNDROME

Gait disturbances are the presenting symptom in only 3.5% to 18% of patients clinically diagnosed as having PD (4,6). Gomez and coworkers (7) compared PD patients with symptom onset before the age of 40 years with those with symptom onset after age 60 and found that gait disturbances were the presenting symptom in 39 percent of the late-onset patients compared with only 3 percent of the early-onset subgroup. Others contended that gait disturbances are more frequent in older PD patients (8) and in patients with older age of symptom onset (8,9). However, a significant number of patients who present with gait disturbance as the initial motor symptom of parkinsonism (frequently in association with postural reflex abnormalities) are eventually diagnosed as having other parkinsonian syndromes, such as progressive supranuclear palsy (PSP), normal pressure hydrocephalus (NPH), or vascular parkinsonism, and not idiopathic PD. In a retrospective analysis of patients with pathologically confirmed diagnosis of Lewy body PD, none had gait disturbances as the presenting symptom, whereas 100 percent of patients with pathologically observed significant vascular changes at the level of the basal ganglia and parkinsonism

Table 7-1 Classification of Gait Syndromes

Lowest level gait disorders
  Peripheral skeletomuscle problems
    Arthritic gait
    Myopathic gait
    Peripheral neuropathic gait

  Peripheral sensory problems
    Sensory ataxic gait
    Vestibular ataxic gait
    Visual ataxic gait

Middle-level disorders
  Hemiplegic gait
  Paraplegic gait
  Cerebellar ataxic gait
  Parkinsonian gait
  Choreic gait
  Dystonic gait

Highest-level gait disorders
  Cautious gait
  Subcortical disequilibrium
  Frontal disequilibrium
  Isolated gait ignition failure
  Frontal gait disorder
  Psychogenic gait disorder

Adapted from Nutt et al., 1993

presented with gait disturbances (10). In other clinical-pathologic studies 13 percent to 33 percent of patients presented with postural instability or gait disturbances (PIGD) as the initial motor symptom (11,13). In agreement with the clinical observation, those who presented with PIGD as initial motor symptom were significantly older (11). These observations raise the question of whether a significant part of PIGD symptoms in PD is related to nondopaminergic or extrastriatal brain dysfunction, possibly related to aging and not purely to the nigrostriatal dopaminergic degeneration (9).

It is more common for gait disturbance to be a feature of advanced PD. As the disease progresses, all patients lose their ability to walk independently because of a combination of severe rigidity, akinesia, and postural instability. Hoehn and Yahr (4) based their clinical scale for PD progression on this observation, defining the most advanced stages (stages 4 and 5) according to the individual's ability to stand and walk.

Since the introduction of levodopa 30 years ago (14), the relationship between disease progression and deterioration of gait has become more complex. Because of recent therapeutic advances, patients often can walk in the "on" state even in the advanced stages of the disease, whereas akinesia can be seen at earlier stages as part of the "off" state. Furthermore, the beneficial effect of levodopa treatment has created new types of gait disturbances, such as choreic or dystonic gait and "on" freezing. Moreover, the use of levodopa has delayed patients' becoming wheelchair-bound. Consequently, disturbed postural reflexes, orthostatism, or severely distorted posture have become major contributory factors in gait disturbances in advanced stages of PD.

ASSESSMENT OF GAIT

Gait should be assessed in every patient as part of the basic neurologic examination. A patient is asked to stand up and walk forward 10 meters, turn around, and return back to his chair, the "Get-Up-and-Go Test" (15,16). It is important to be explicit about the speed with which this should be accomplished: the patient should be asked to walk first at his most comfortable pace and then to perform the task as fast as he can or, alternatively, to walk in one direction at a comfortable pace and return to his chair at the fastest pace he can manage. While the patient is performing the task, the examiner should assess the patient's ability to initiate gait, keep an upright position, walk toward a destination, perform a turn in place, and locate himself correctly back in the chair. Other features that should be observed are body posture, speed and fluency of stepping, and stride length and the distance between the feet (base). While looking carefully at a single step, one should note the height to which the swinging leg is raised above the ground and how this foot meets the floor (heel-toes) and rolls forward. In addition, attention should be paid to the degree of arm swinging and other axial movement. Such an examination should be performed in an open space free of obstacles to allow the patient to perform at his best. There are several clinical scales in use to evaluate gait. The most widely used is the Tinetti Scale, which assesses balance and mobility in two different measurements that yield a maximum of 28 points, 16 for balance and 12 for gait (17). There is no universally accepted scale that specifically assesses parkinsonian gait. However, almost all clinical scales in use for evaluation of parkinsonism include several items to rate gait.

The clinical assessment of gait is ultimately based on the examiner's observational impression. For more detailed and precise evaluation of gait, however, the assessment takes place in a highly sophisticated computerized gait laboratory, where cadence, stride length, velocity, and double limb support are measured while obtaining information on muscle activation, joint movement, and analysis of limb movement in space (18).

Gait Initiation

Initiation of gait can be subdivided into a movement preparation period and a movement execution phase. Movement preparation represents the *"motor planning"* phase, in which an overall strategy is taken "where, when, and how" to initiate gait (19). In PD patients the preparation time was found to be significantly prolonged, with a tendency to be longer as the disease progressed (20). Execution time was prolonged as well, but to a lesser degree (20). Normally the Bereitschafts potential (BP) (the preparatory cortical potential proceeding a motor act) is larger in amplitude when executing complex sequences of movements such as stepping than when simple motor tasks are performed (21). Vidailhet and coworkers (22) found that the BP did not increase in amplitude in PD patients when foot tapping was compared with step initiation. Such abnormal response of BP in step initiation in PD was interpreted as an indirect neurophysiological sign for abnormality in the central preparatory phase of gait initiation in PD (22).

During gait initiation, posture is adjusted by first shifting the center of gravity (COG) laterally and rotating the body before weight is taken on the stance foot to allow the leading leg to swing forward while the COG is shifted anteriorly to create the forward momentum (23). This shift in the COG anteriorly is accomplished by bending the ankle and trunk (24). The anterior shift of the trunk was found to be slow in advanced PD patients (20). In addition to slowness in anterior shift of COG, there is reduced lateral shift of the body mass over the stance limb, decreased propulsive forces, and prolonged anticipatory postural adjustments (25,26). Alteration in postural stability might interfere with the performance of an otherwise intact motor program and movement sequencing and create specific difficulties in gait initiation (27). Interestingly, submovement sequence and timing associated with gait initiation were similar in PD patients and age-matched controls (20).

All of these motor deficits reported in PD patients are most pronounced in self-initiated gait, whereas external cues and sensory stimulation as well as levodopa treatment can improve these parameters significantly (25). One can conclude from these observations that disturbances in gait initiation frequently reported in PD are directly related to dysfunction of the basal ganglia to control internal cued movement sequences and not to slowness in execution of all

subcomponents of gait initiation that are better preserved (20,25).

Start hesitation is the classic parkinsonian disturbance experienced at gait initiation. It has been described as the most common type of freezing of gait (FOG), having been documented in 275 of 318 (86%) patients with PD (Table 7-2). Start hesitation is best described by the patients as a feeling that their feet are "stuck or glued to the ground." It is frequently seen at initiation of gait, but it also occurs while changing from one mode of movement to another, for example, while completing a turn and trying to move forward. Although most episodes of start hesitation last a few seconds, such an episode can sometimes last long enough to make gait impossible. At those times, the patients are actively trying to overcome the block either by making small and ineffective movements with their legs or by using motor, sensory, or cognitive tricks (28).

The mechanism responsible for start hesitation is not clear, but Burleigh-Jacobs and coworkers (25) have shown that it was associated with no anticipatory postural adjustment at all, suggesting that it is related to lack of initiation of postural adjustments. Andrews (29) recorded leg muscle activation of PD patients during freezing episodes and demonstrated coactivation of agonist and antagonist muscles without the temporal activation pattern seen in normal gait initiation. Such synchronization disturbance of muscles activation can explain the inability to initiate a step in spite of a real effort.

The gait initiation pattern of PD patients is difficult to assess objectively both in gait laboratories and during the office visit because it is highly variable and influenced by many sensory and cognitive factors. Several studies that have tried to assess start hesitation or other FOG episodes failed to analyze them scientifically (25,30). As a result, we have recently proposed a freezing of gait self-report questionnaire, which is a

Table 7-2 Type of Motor Blocks Reported in 318 PD Patients with Freezing of Gait

Start hesitation	275 (86%)
On turning	145 (45%)
At doorway	79 (25%)
On open runway	72 (23%)
At destination	56 (18%)
Other nongait	36 (11%)
When "on"	69 (22%)

*Some patients had more than one type of motor block.
Adapted from Giladi et al., 1992.

highly validated scale for evaluating freezing episodes and the frequency of start hesitation (31).

Locomotion

Abnormal locomotion is characteristic of parkinsonism. The parkinsonian gait is described as slow with reduced stride length, decreased cadence (steps per minute), and increase in the proportion of gait cycle spent in the double limb support phase of stance (9,32,36). Shuffling and festinating gait, freezing episodes, abnormal arm swing, and abnormal posture are additional features that contribute to the typical parkinsonian gait. Taking into account that gait velocity, step length, and cadence are parameters that interact, Morris and coworkers (37,38) demonstrated in a series of experiments that patients with PD have a fundamental disturbance in stride length regulation, whereas their cadence control remains intact. Interestingly, the second step is shorter only in the first stride, and this phenomenon is directly associated with progression of the disease (20). In addition, there is higher step-to-step variability of stride length (35,39) and increased variability of leg muscles activation during stepping in PD (40,41). Stride length can become normal by use of visual cues or strategies that increase attention to gait performance. In contrast, a task that competes for the individual's attention while he attempts to walk (distraction) can worsen gait performance (38). Attention is also playing a major role in the ability of parkinsonian patients to modulate gait patterns according to circumstances, for example, walking on a slippery floor, around a corner, at doorways, as well as over obstacles.

Shorter stride length and increased step-to-step variability are indirect signs of a disturbance at the level of the basal ganglia and the supplementary motor area (SMA)–associated loops, which are important structures for the internal control of automatic gait pattern. In other words, the primary disturbance in parkinsonian gait is in motor set or motor programming (38), both of which affect gait as an automatic task. Attention and other motor or sensory tricks help to overcome the disturbance in automatic motor program by shifting to a more controlled gait.

Freezing of Gait

Freezing episodes while in motion (motor blocks) represent a special form of locomotive disturbance seen only in parkinsonism. This phenomenon refers to transient episodes, usually lasting seconds, in which continuation of walking is halted. It is a negative symptom of parkinsonism even though the block is due to unsynchronized overactivation of leg muscles.

Freezing episodes are unrelated to weakness, flaccidity, or decreased muscle tone, and once freezing has dissipated, the patient is free to move or perform the task at the usual pace (42).

The pathophysiology of freezing of gait is poorly understood. It seems to be part of bradykinesia or, more precisely, related to abnormal execution of complex motor tasks such as repetitive, simultaneous, or sequential motor acts (19,43). Freezing of gait can be subclassified into two general types according to its relation with dopaminergic treatment: (1) as a symptom of a hypodopaminergic state that will improve with dopaminergic treatment, and (2) as an event that occurs during relatively normal gait ("on" freezing), does not improve with apomorphine injections and can worsen with dopaminergic treatment (44).

Freezing of gait is associated with decreased concentrations of norepinephrine (45) and serotonin (46) in the cerebrospinal fluid (CSF) of patients with parkinsonism. Andrews (29) recorded electromyographic activity with surface electrodes in five PD patients who suffered from frequent gait freezing episodes. All five patients had similar electromyographic activity during the FOG episode, which was initial activity of the gastrocnemius-soleus muscles, followed approximately 7 millisecond later by simultaneous activity of the tibialis posterior muscle. This activity of flexors and, shortly later, the coactivation of flexors and extensors was observed during freezing episodes in the muscles of the knee as well. Ueno and coworkers (47) confirmed Andrews's original observation that frozen gait was associated with reciprocal or concomitant activation of antagonistic leg muscles.

Freezing phenomenon is common in PD (5,48) and has been reported in most other hypokinetic movement disorders (48). It is part of parkinsonian akinesia (29,43,49,50) reported in about 7 percent of early untreated parkinsonian patients (5,51), whereas later when levodopa became necessary, 26 percent of the patients ultimately experienced FOG (51,53). This increment in the percentage of "freezers" before levodopa was given demonstrates the relationships between FOG and the progression of PD, unrelated to treatment.

Barbeau (54,55) and Ambani and Van Woert (56) were the first to notice a significant increase in freezing, starting about one year after the introduction of high-dose levodopa treatment. In advanced PD it is difficult to differentiate between the contribution of the underlying pathologic process, disease progression, and the possible effect of levodopa treatment on the development of freezing. Several reports have demonstrated an association between FOG and duration of levodopa treatment (5,52,54), although Lamberti and coworkers (53) found no such association. An association between freezing and dopamine agonist therapy has also been alluded to (76). The answer to this controversy will come from a prospective study that will assess the question directly.

Several reports showed that there was an increased risk of FOG in PD when initial symptoms began on the left side in association with speech or balance problems (5,51,53). In contrast, the risk of developing freezing significantly decreased if the initial motor symptom was tremor (51).

Freezing episodes usually can be overcome by increased attention to the motor task and by the use of external cues and a variety of behavioral and motor tricks (28). Stressful situations, especially time-limited ones such as entering an elevator or crossing the street when the light is green, exacerbate FOG. Curiously, a visit to the doctor's office or the gait laboratory improves FOG severity (30), a phenomenon that frequently amazes the caregiver and probably is related to attention and stress. Freezing can be a very disabling symptom of parkinsonism. It is especially difficult when it occurs on every attempt to move. At these times it might be difficult to differentiate it from akinesia during the "off" state.

The clinical evaluation and quantification of motor blocks during motion is difficult because of the highly variable and transitory nature of this motor disturbance. This feature is partly related to the important influence of external cueing or attention on the expression or severity of freezing episodes (28,42).

Festinating Gait

Festinating gait is another very typical disturbance of locomotion seen in parkinsonian patients. Its frequency is undetermined, but it is known to be more common in older patients or in more advanced stages of PD (57). Festinating gait is seen commonly in idiopathic PD and rarely in symptomatic parkinsonism (58). It is described as rapid small steps done in an attempt to keep the COG between the feet while the trunk leans forward involuntarily and shifts the COG forward. It is considered a sign of hypokinesia that effects locomotion. In an attempt to correct balance in response to an external perturbation or excessive body sway, the parkinsonian patient takes steps that are not large enough to place the COG in front of his feet. To compensate and in an attempt to prevent falling, the patient increases stepping velocity and further shortens the stride (59).

Arm Swing

One of the clinical features associated with parkinsonian gait is decreased arm swing. It is frequently a very early sign of parkinsonism. Decreased arm swing was reported as the most bothersome presenting symptom in 2.5 percent of 800 recently diagnosed unmedicated patients enrolled in the Deprenyl and Tocopherol Antioxidative Therapy of Parkinsonism (DATATOP) study (6). The reduction in associated upper limb movements in PD patients was shown to be associated with significant delayed onset of arm swing, reduced length of arm cycle, and reduced velocity of arm swing in the gait cycle (20). All these parameters were further disturbed as the disease progressed (20).

TREATMENT OF PARKINSONIAN GAIT

Levodopa, the most effective and commonly used antiparkinsonian drug, has significant and long-lasting effects on parkinsonian gait. Shortly after levodopa was introduced for the treatment of parkinsonism in the late 1960s, its effect on gait velocity became clear (60,61). Its use led to significant improvement of stride length, velocity and synchronization of movements, double support time, and control of foot landing (8,9,62,65). Levodopa improved stride length and decreased double support time with a ceiling effect, that is, there was no further improvement above a certain dose (62), even though the addition of motivational or arousal processes and external cueing could yield further improvement of stride length (38,66). The effect of levodopa on locomotion occurs through mechanisms involved in control of force and amplitude rather than rhythmicity or automaticity (62). For example, improvement of muscle tone at the knee extensors can improve the angular excursion of the knee joint, which could provide better utilization of energy during propulsive phase and thus increase stride length (32).

Levodopa treatment did not effect stride-to-stride variation and had little effect on the ability to produce rhythmic stepping in response to an external cue or on the amplitude of associated arm movements (9,67). The symptomatic benefit of levodopa is better in younger onset (<40 years) patients, suggesting again that gait disturbances in the older PD population are related to nondopaminergic mechanisms.

The motor complications of long-term treatment with levodopa, especially dyskinesia (dystonia and chorea), have serious implications with regard to gait. Severe painful foot or leg dystonia as well as violent generalized or crural chorea/ballism, frequently aggravated by walking, have become a major problem of advanced PD patients. Patients often have to choose between akinetic "off" state with freezing or "on" with disabling dyskinesias.

These hyperkinetic complications of levodopa treatment are much more common in younger patients (68), and they appear initially in the legs, affecting walking.

Dopamine agonists are frequently used as monotherapy in the symptomatic treatment of the younger population and as add-on therapy to improve levodopa benefit or to spare levodopa dosage in all patients. Agonist clinical benefit on gait, as measured by the Unified Parkinson's Disease Rating Scale (UPDRS) (69) and by other clinical assessment tools, has been shown by numerous studies. Amantadine, selegiline, and the new COMT inhibitors are all known for their symptomatic benefit on almost all parkinsonian parameters, including gait disturbances. However, there has been no systematic physiologic study that assessed the effect of any of these drugs on parkinsonian gait.

In addition to medications, it is generally agreed that nonpharmacologic treatment can improve parkinsonian gait disturbances (70). The use of sensory cues to facilitate locomotor activity has been reported (50,71). Of special interest are the reports by several groups regarding the benefit of rhythmic auditory stimulation with a metronome (66,72).

Treatment of Freezing of Gait

Freezing is considered to be one of the more resistant symptoms in PD. "Off" freezing might respond to dopaminergic treatment, whereas "on" freezing sometimes improves by lowering the dosage of dopaminergic medications.

One of the most characteristic features of freezing is its response to tricks. Stern et al. (28) were the first to report such tricks in detail, dividing them into (1) gait modification by the patient alone or with the assistance of another person, and (2) assistance by auditory (nonverbal), verbal, or visual stimuli. The use of motor tricks is highly recommended because of their effectiveness, safety, and availability. Metronome rhythmic auditory stimulation can also be effective in abolishing freezing episodes and increasing stride length in PD (66,73,74).

Selegiline was shown to decrease the frequency of FOG in the early PD in a prospective double-blind study (51). The mechanism of selegiline's action on freezing is poorly understood. Theoretically, it might act either by its inhibitory effect on monoamine oxidase type B (MAO-B) to increase dopaminergic activity or through the amphetaminergic activity of its metabolites or through another undefined mechanism. A recent study, which demonstrated a significant effect of selegiline on a higher level of movement control and directional control of arm movement (75),

raised the possibility that it has a specific effect on motor programming. Whether selegiline has the same symptomatic effect on FOG in more advanced cases, when taken concomitantly with levodopa, remains to be determined.

The direct effect of levodopa on FOG has never been assessed. However, it is a common experience that when freezing episodes are directly related to a hypodopaminergic state, any dopaminomimetic treatment that will decrease the "off" severity or duration will decrease the number of freezing episodes as well. The effect of dopamine agonist drugs on FOG is not clear. Two small studies have suggested that treatment with dopamine agonist drugs can exacerbate freezing episodes (76,77), but these observations have never been confirmed in a large-scale prospective study. In contrast, apomorphine injections have been reported to produce good symptomatic effect on severe freezing episodes where other antiparkinsonian agents failed (44,78).

L-threo 3,4-dihydroxyphenylserine (DOPS) (a chemical precursor of norepinephrine) has been reported to have a moderate symptomatic effect on FOG, mainly in patients with "pure freezing syndrome" (45). A similar study (79) reported a complete disappearance of freezing in two patients with PD that lasted three weeks, after which the freezing returned and showed no additional response even when higher doses of L-threo-DOPS was given. Two additional patients had transient subjective improvement for four weeks. Another report described only transient benefit from L-threo-DOPS in a patient with pure akinesia (80). Two small double-blind studies found no benefit from L-threo-DOPS treatment for freezing in advanced PD (Fahn, personal communication) (81). Although the role of L-threo-DOPS in FOG in parkinsonian patients is limited, it seems to have mild and temporary benefit only for patients with "pure freezing syndrome," an entity that is currently believed to be a subtype of PSP (82).

FUNCTIONAL NEUROSURGERY FOR GAIT DISTURBANCES

Stereotactic neurosurgery has become an increasingly common approach for treating patients with advanced PD. Unilateral pallidotomy has been shown to have significant beneficial effect in decreasing "off" duration and severity as well as dyskinesia severity (83–91). The effect of such an intervention on neurophysiologic parameters of parkinsonian gait is not known. However, some studies reported significant improvement of gait disturbances that were associated with the "off" state (85,89). Bilateral, high-frequency, deep brain stimulation (DBS) of the globus pallidum interna (Gpi) have shown that gait can be significantly improved when the dorsal Gpi was stimulated, whereas stimulation of the posteroventral Gpi caused significant worsening of parkinsonian gait (92). Gait has also improved significantly with bilateral subthalamic nucleus stimulation (93). Fetal cell graft transplantation is a procedure under investigation, and it is too early to reach any conclusions on its selective effect on gait other than that some patients experienced functional improvement and were able to decrease the amount of antiparkinsonian medications. Freezing of gait seems to be resistant to these treatment approaches thus far.

Acknowledgments

I would like to thank Dr. Shabtai, Dr. Gurevitch, Dr. Anka, and Dr. Simon for their help in the preparation of this chapter and Mrs. Ungar for her continuous technical support.

REFERENCES

1. Parkinson J. *An Essay on the Shaking Palsy.* London, Sherwood: Neely and Jones, 1817.

2. Fahn S. Parkinsonism. In: Rowland L, ed. *Merritt's Textbook of Neurology.* Philadelphia: Lea & Febiger, 1994.

3. Nutt JG, Marsden CD, Thompson PD. Human walking and higher-level gait disorders, particularly in the elderly. *Neurology* 1993; 43:268–279.

4. Hoehn MM, Yahr MD. Parkinsonism: Onset, progression, and mortality. *Neurology* 1967; 50:318.

5. Giladi N, McMahon D, Przedborski S, et al. Motor blocks in Parkinson's disease. *Neurology* 1992; 42:333–339.

6. Parkinson Study Group. Effect of deprenyl on the progression of disability in early Parkinson's disease. *N Engl J Med* 1989; 321:1364–1371.

7. Gomez AG, Jorge R, Garcia S, et al. Clinical and pharmacological differences in early- versus late-onset Parkinson's disease. *Mov Disord* 1997; 12:277–284.

8. Bowes SG, Charlet A, Dobbs RJ, et al. Gait in relation to ageing and idiopathic parkinsonism. *Scand J Rehabil Med* 1992; 24:181–186.

9. Blin O, Ferrandez AM, Pailhous J, et al. Dopa-sensitive and dopa-resistant gait parameters in Parkinson's disease. *J Neurol Sci* 1991; 103:51–54.

10. Yamanouchi H, Nagura H. Neurological signs and frontal white matter lesions in vascular parkinsonism. A clinicopathologic study. *Stroke* 1997; 28:965–969.

11. Gibb WR, Lees AJ. A comparison of clinical and pathological features of young- and old-onset Parkinson's disease. *Neurology* 1988; 38:1402–1406.

12. Rajput AH, Pahwa P, Pahwa P, et al. Prognostic significance of the onset mode in parkinsonism. *Neurology* 1993; 43:829–830.

13. Hughes AJ, Daniel SE, Blankson S, et al. A clinicopathologic study of 100 cases of Parkinson's disease. *Arch Neurol* 1993; 50:140–148.

14. Cotzias GC, Van WM, Schiffer LM. Aromatic amino acids and modification of parkinsonism. *N Engl J Med* 1967; 276:374–379.

15. Podsiadlo D, Richardson S. The timed "Up & Go:" A test of basic functional mobility for frail elderly persons. *J Am Geriatr Soc* 1991; 39:142–148.

16. Mathias S, Nayak U, Isaacs B. Balance in the elderly patient: The "get-up and go" test. *Arch Phys Med Rehabil* 1986; 67:387–389.

17. Tinetti ME. Performance-oriented assessment of mobility problems in elderly patients. *J Am Geriatr Soc* 1986; 34:119–126.

18. Elble J. Clinical and research methodology for study of gait. In: Masdeu J et al. (eds.). *Gait Disorders of Aging.* Philadelphia, New York: Lippincott-Raven, 1997:123–134.

19. Marsden CD. What do the basal ganglia tell premotor cortical areas? *Ciba Found Symp* 1987; 132:282–300.

20. Rosin R, Topka H, Dichgans J. Gait initiation in Parkinson's disease. *Mov Disord* 1997; 12:682–690.

21. Simonetta M, Clanet M, Rascol O. Bereitschaftspotential in a simple movement or in a motor sequence starting with the same simple movement. *Electroencephalogr Clin Neurophysiol* 1991; 81:129–134.

22. Vidailhet M, Stocchi F, Rothwell JC, et al. The Bereitschaftspotential preceding simple foot movement and initiation of gait in Parkinson's disease. *Neurology* 1993; 43:1784–1788.

23. Elble J, Moody C, Leffler K, et al. The initiation of normal walking. *Mov Disord* 1994; 9:139–146.

24. Breniere Y, Cuong Do M. Control of gait initiation. *J Mot Behav* 1991; 23:235–240.

25. Burleigh JA, Horak FB, Nutt JG, et al. Step initiation in Parkinson's disease: Influence of levodopa and external sensory triggers. *Mov Disord* 1997; 12:206–215.

26. Crenna P, Frigo C. A motor programme for the initiation of forward-oriented movements in humans. *J Physiol (Lond)* 1991; 437:635–653.

27. Horak F. Postural inflexibility in parkinsonian subjects. *J Neurol Sci* 1992; 111:46–58.

28. Stern GM, Lander CM, Lees AJ. Akinetic freezing and trick movements in Parkinson's disease. *J Neural Transm Suppl* 1980; 16:137–141.

29. Andrews CJ. Influence of dystonia on the response to long-term L-dopa therapy in Parkinson's disease. *J Neurol Neurosurg Psychiatry* 1973; 36:630–636.

30. Nieuwboer A, de Weerdt W, Dom R, et al. A frequency and correlation analysis of motor deficits in Parkinson's disease. *Disabil Rehabil* 1998; 20:142–150.

31. Giladi N, Shabtai H, Simon ES, et al. Construction of freezing of gait questionnaire for patients with Parkinsonism. *Parkinsonism and Related Disorders* 2000; 6:165–170.

32. Knutsson E, Martensson A. Quantitative effects of L-dopa on different types of movements and muscle tone in Parkinsonian patients. *Scand J Rehabil Med* 1971; 3:121–130.

33. Murray MP, Sepic SB Gardner GM, et al. Walking patterns of men with parkinsonism. *Am J Phys Med* 1978; 57:278–294.

34. Stern GM, Franklyn SE, Imms FJ, et al. Quantitative assessments of gait and mobility in Parkinson's disease. *J Neural Transm Suppl* 1983; 19:201–214.

35. Blin O, Ferrandez AM, Serratrice G. Quantitative analysis of gait in Parkinson patients: Increased variability of stride length. *J Neurol Sci* 1990; 98:91–97.

36. Bowes SG, Clark PK, Leeman AL, et al. Determinants of gait in the elderly parkinsonian on maintenance levodopa/carbidopa therapy. *Br J Clin Pharmacol* 1990; 30:13–24.

37. Morris ME, Lansek R, Matyas TA, et al. The pathogenesis of gait hypokinesia in Parkinson's disease. *Brain* 1994; 117:1169–1181.

38. Morris ME, Lansek R, Matyas TA, et al. Stride length regulation in Parkinson's disease. Normalization strategies and underlying mechanisms. *Brain* 1996; 119:551–568.

39. Vieregge P, Stolze H, Klein C, et al. Gait quantitation in Parkinson's disease – locomotor disability and correlation to clinical rating scales. *J Neural Transm* 1997; 104:237–248.

40. Miller RA, Thaut MH, McIntosh GC, et al. Components of EMG symmetry and variability in parkinsonian and healthy elderly gait. *Electroencephalogr Clin Neurophysiol* 1996; 101:1–7.

41. Cioni M, Richards CL, Malouin F, et al. Characteristics of the electromyographic patterns of lower limb muscles during gait in patients with Parkinson's disease when OFF and ON L-dopa treatment. *Ital J Neurol Sci* 1997; 18:195–208.

42. Giladi N, Fahn S. Freezing phenomenon, the fifth cardinal sign of parkinsonism. In: Fisher A et al. (eds.). *Progress in Alzheimer's and Parkinson's Diseases*. New York and London: Plenum Press, 1998:329–335.

43. Schwab R, England A, Peterson E. Akinesia in Parkinson's disease. *Neurology* 1959; 9:65–72.

44. Linazasoro G. The apomorphine test in gait disorders associated with parkinsonism. *Clin Neuropharmacol* 1996; 19:171–176.

45. Narabayashi H, Kondo T, Nagatsu T, et al. DL Threo-3,4-Dihydoxyphenylserine for freezing symptom in parkinsonism. In: Hassler R, et al. (eds.). *Advances in Neurology*. New York: Raven Press, 1984: 497–552.

46. Tohgi H, Abe T, Takahashi S, et al. Concentrations of serotonin and its related substances in the cerebrospinal fluid of parkinsonian patients and their relations to the severity of symptoms. *Neurosci Lett* 1993; 150:71–74.

47. Ueno E, Yanagisawa N, Takami M. Gait disorders in parkinsonism. A study with floor reaction forces and EMG. *Adv Neurol* 1993; 60:414–418.

48. Giladi N, Kao R, Fahn S. Freezing phenomenon in patients with parkinsonian syndromes. *Mov Disord* 1997; 12:302–305.

49. Luria A. The nature of human conflicts. *Liverghite* 1932; 153.

50. Martin J. Disorder of locomotion associated with disease of the basal ganglia. In: *The Basal Ganglia and Posture*. Philadelphia: J.B. Lippincott, 1967:24–35.

51. Giladi N, McDermott M, Fahn S, et al. and the Parkinson Study Group. Freezing of gait in Parkinson's disease. *Neurology* 1996; 46:A377(Abstract).

52. Kizkin S, Ozer F, Ufacik M, et al. Motor blocks in Parkinson's disease. *Mov Disord* 1997; 12:101(P378).

53. Lamberti P, Armenise S, Castaldo V, et al. Freezing gait in Parkinson's disease. *Eur Neurol* 1997; 38:297–301.

54. Barbeau A. Long term appraisal of levodopa therapy. *Neurology* 1972; 22:22–24.

55. Barbeau A. Six years of high level levodopa therapy in severely akinetic parkinosnian patients. *Arch Neurol* 1976; 33:333–338.

56. Ambani L, Van Woert M. Start hesitation – a side effect of long-term levodopa therapy. *N Engl J Med* 1973:1113–1115.

57. Imai H. [Festination and freezing]. *Rinsho Shinkeigaku* 1993; 33:1307–1309.

58. Thompson P, Marsden CD. Clinical neurological assessment of balance and gait disorders. In: Bronstein A et al. (eds.). *Clinical Disorders of Balance Posture and Gait*. London: Arnold, 1996:79–84.

59. Brown P, Steiger M. Basal ganglia gait disorders. In: Bronstein A et al. (eds.). *Balance Posture and Gait*. New York: Arnold with co-publishers Oxford University Press, 1996:156–167.

60. Mones RJ. An evaluation of L-dopa in Parkinson patients. *Trans Am Neurol Assoc* 1969; 94:307–309.

61. Boshes B, Blonsky ER, Arbit J, et al. Effect of L-dopa on individual symptoms of parkinsonism. *Trans Am Neurol Assoc* 1969; 94:229–231.

62. Ferrandez AM, Blin O. A comparison between the effect of intentional modulations and the action of L-dopa on gait in Parkinson's disease. *Behav Brain Res* 1991; 45:177–183.

63. Pedersen SW, Eriksson T, Oberg B. Effects of withdrawal of antiparkinson medication on gait and clinical score in the Parkinson patient. *Acta Neurol Scand* 1991; 84:7–13.

64. Azulay JP, van-Den BC, Mestre D, et al. Automatic motion analysis of gait in patients with Parkinson disease: Effects of levodopa and visual stimulations. *Rev Neurol (Paris)* 1996; 152:128–134.

65. Pederson S, Oberg B, Larsson L, et al. Gait analysis, isokinetic muscle strength measurement in patients with Parkinson's disease. *Scand J Rehab Med* 1997; 29:67–74.

66. Thaut MH, McIntosh GC, Rice RR, et al. Rhythmic auditory stimulation in gait training for Parkinson's disease patients. *Mov Disord* 1996; 11:193–200.

67. Hausdorff JM, Cudkowicz ME, Firtion R, et al. Gait variability and basal ganglia disorders: Stride-to-stride variations of gait cycle timing in Parkinson's disease and Huntington's disease. *Mov Disord* 1998; 13:428–437.

68. Kostic V, Przedborski S, Flaster E, et al. Early development of levodopa-induced dyskinesias and response fluctuations in young-onset Parkinson's disease. *Neurology* 1991; 41:202–205.

69. Fahn S, Elton R. Members of the UPDRS development committee. Unified Parkinson's Disease Rating Scale. In: Fahn S et al. (eds.). *Recent Developments in Parkinson's Disease.* Florham Park, NJ: Macmillan Health Care Information, 1987:153–163.

70. Weiner WJ, Singer C. Parkinson's disease and nonpharmacologic treatment programs. *J Am Geriatr Soc* 1989; 37:359–363.

71. Iansek RT, Morris M. Rehabilitation of gait in Parkinson's disease [letter]. *J Neurol Neurosurg Psychiatry* 1997; 63:556–557.

72. McIntosh GC, Brown SH, Rice RR, et al. Rhythmic auditory-motor facilitation of gait patterns in patients with Parkinson's disease. *J Neurol Neurosurg Psychiatry* 1997; 62:22–26.

73. Enzensberger W, Oberlander U, Stecker K. [Metronome therapy in patients with Parkinson disease]. *Nervenarzt* 1997; 68:972–977.

74. Enzensberger W, Fischer PA. Metronome in Parkinson's disease [letter]. *Lancet* 1996; 347:1337.

75. Giladi N, Honigman S, Hocherman S. The effect of deprenyl treatment on directional and velocity control of arm movement in patients with early stages of Parkinson's disease. *Clin Neuropharmacol* 1999; 22:54–59.

76. Weiner WJ, Factor SA, Sanchez RJ, et al. Early combination therapy (bromocriptine and levodopa) does not prevent motor fluctuations in Parkinson's disease. *Neurology* 1993; 43:21–27.

77. Ahlskog J, Muenter M, Bailey P, et al. Dopamine agonist treatment of fluctuating parkinsonism: D-2 (controlled release MK-458) vs. combined D-1 and D-2 (pergolide). *Arch Neurol* 1992; 49:560–568.

78. Corboy DL, Wagner ML, Sage JI. Apomorphine for motor fluctuations and freezing in Parkinson's disease. *Ann Pharmacother* 1995; 29:282–288.

79. Oribe E, Kaufman H, Yahr M. Freezing phenomena in Parkinson's disease: Clinical features and effect of treatment with L-threo-DOPS. In: Narabayashi H, et al. (eds.). *Norepinephrine Deficiency and Its Treatment with L-threo DOPS in Parkinson's Disease and the Related Disorders.* New York: Parthenon Publishing Group, 1993:89–96.

80. Yamamoto M, Fujii S, Hatanaka Y. Result of long-term administration of L-threo-3,4-dihydroxyphenyl-serine in patients with pure akinesia as an early symptom of progressive supranuclear palsy. *Clin Neuropharmacol* 1997; 20:371–373.

81. Quinn N, Perlmutter J, Marsden CD. Acute administration of DL-threo DOPS does not affect the freezing phenomenon in parkinsonian patients. *Neurology* 1984; 34:149.

82. Imai H, Narabayashi H, Sakata E. "Pure akinesia" and the later added supranuclear ophthalmoplegia. *Adv Neurol* 1987; 45:207–212.

83. Meyer CH. Unilateral pallidotomy for Parkinson's disease promptly improves a wide range of voluntary activities – especially gait and trunk movements. *Acta Neurochir Suppl Wien* 1997; 68:37–41.

84. Kumar R, Lozano AM, Montgomery E, et al. Pallidotomy and deep brain stimulation of the pallidum and subthalamic nucleus in advanced Parkinson's disease. *Mov Disord* 1998; 13:73–82.

85. Baron MS, Vitek JL, Bakay RA, et al. Treatment of advanced Parkinson's disease by posterior GPi pallidotomy: 1-year results of a pilot study. *Ann Neurol* 1996; 40:355–366.

86. Dogali M, Fazzini E, Kolodny E, et al. Stereotactic ventral pallidotomy for Parkinson's disease. *Neurology* 1995; 45:753–761.

87. Iacono RP, Shima F, Lonser RR, et al. The results, indications, and physiology of posteroventral pallidotomy for patients with Parkinson's disease. *Neurosurgery* 1995; 36:1118–1125.

88. Laitinen LV, Bergenheim AT, Hariz MI. Leksell's posteroventral pallidotomy in the treatment of Parkinson's disease. *J Neurosurg* 1992; 76:53–61.

89. Lang AE, Lozano AM, Montgomery E, et al. Posteroventral medial pallidotomy in advanced Parkinson's disease. *N Engl J Med* 1997; 337:1036–1042.

90. Lozano AM, Lang AE. Pallidotomy for Parkinson's disease. *Neurosurg Clin N Am* 1998; 9:325–336.

91. Ondo WG, Jankovic J, Lai EC, et al. Assessment of motor function after stereotactic pallidotomy. *Neurology* 1998; 50:266–270.

92. Bejjani B, Damier P, Arnulf I, et al. Pallidal stimulation for Parkinson's disease. Two targets? *Neurology* 1997; 49:1564–1569.

93. Krack P, Pollak P, Limousin P, et al. Subthalamic nucleus or internal pallidal stimulation in young onset Parkinson's disease. *Brain* 1998; 121:451–457.

8

Sensory Symptoms

Richard M. Zweig, M.D.

Department of Neurology, Louisiana State University Medical Center, Shreveport, Louisiana

INTRODUCTION

Parkinson's disease (PD) provides opportunities, arguably unparalleled among neurologic disorders, for the study of various aspects of central nervous system function and pathophysiology. However, answering even a simple question, such as why certain patients have tremor whereas others do not, requires an understanding of: (*1*) tremor-generating neuronal pathways, (*2*) how these pathways are suppressed by the normally functioning brain, (*3*) whether lack of tremor in patients reflects this normal brain function and/or additional pathology within tremor-generating pathways (or at sites influencing these pathways), and (*4*) the factors that underlie this phenotypic variability. Sensory symptoms broadly defined are perhaps as common as tremor in PD, and the question of why they occur is anything but simple.

In discussions of PD, "sensory symptoms" usually refer to painful or nonpainful somatosensory symptoms. Like tremor, these are usually "positive" symptoms. Whether described as burning, stabbing, aching, paresthesia-like, cramplike, an inner tremor, or an inner restlessness (akathisia) (Table 8-1), somatosensory symptoms share with another common sensory symptom, visual hallucinations (or a predisposition toward drug-induced visual hallucinations), an interesting paradox. Hallucinations and other psychotic symptoms, whether in schizophrenics or in patients with PD (or dementia with Lewy bodies), are best suppressed by blocking dopamine receptors. Neuroleptics are not commonly used as analgesics but are fairly effective in treating migraine (1). Typical neuroleptics greatly worsen motor symptoms of patients with PD. Why should a disease characterized by loss of dopaminergic neurons have symptoms that can be treated by blocking dopamine receptors? Do sensory symptoms occur because of, or despite, dopaminergic neuronal loss? The chapter begins with an illustrative case

report followed by a discussion of reported somatosensory symptoms in patients with PD and a review of pathophysiologic processes. Finally, a brief discussion of the evaluation and treatment of somatosensory symptoms is included.

CASE REPORT

A 76-year-old man, with a 13-year history of PD, had a four-year history of pain in his left lower extremity. This was described as an electric-like, stabbing pain that traveled from the left thigh and groin to his ankle. Before the onset of pain, symptoms consisted primarily of levodopa-responsive hypophonic dysarthria, hypomimia, tremor of his lower lip, and mild generalized bradykinesia. Although gait and posture were mildly affected, he was golfing regularly. The pain became severe, was unresponsive to conservative therapy, and did not appear to be associated with or affected by levodopa treatment. Spondylitic changes and lumbar disc herniation (L5–S1) were seen on imaging studies. Despite a decompressive laminectomy, pain persisted. Pain was aggravated by standing and walking, but relieved by bending forward. No sensory changes were found on examination, but weakness of the left extensor hallucis longus was noted, as was pain with extension of his lumbar spine and with straight leg raising. Repeat imaging and EMG were consistent with L5 radiculopathy and a second surgical procedure was performed – without success. Following a third unsuccessful procedure, less than two years after onset of pain, placement of a temporary spinal cord–stimulating electrode was undertaken. Although paresthesias elicited by stimulation corresponded to the distribution of his usual pain, there was no relief from pain. Initially change in posture and reluctance to walk were attributed to pain resulting from his spinal

Table 8-1   Somatosensory Symptoms in Parkinson's Disease

Symptom	Localization	Levodopa Response	Other Therapy	Refs.
Paresthesia-like: numbness tingling coldness	Extremities, esp. side of greatest motor signs	Variable	Possibly anxiolytics	2,3,4,9,11
Aching pain	Extremities, joints	Variable		2,3,4,5, 6,11
Burning	Extremities > head or body	May worsen		2,3,4,9
Radicular	Extremities	Variable		5,6
Cramps, tightness	Neck, calf, paraspinal	Often responsive		5
Painful dystonias	Usually feet	Often responsive	Possibly lithium	5,6
Genitalia (in women)		Often responsive		4,8
Unilateral oral (esp. burning)		Usually none	Clozapine, possibly other analgesics	8
Sensory dyspnea		May be responsive		9
Internal tremor	Axial +/− limb	Usually none	Anxiolytics	10
Akathisia		Occasional	Clozapine	11,12
Headache	Esp. nuchal	Occasional	Amitriptyline	15,16,17
Back pain	Mid/lower back	May be responsive		18

disease. However, a severe parkinsonian gait disorder, with propulsion and frequent freezing, evolved.

FREQUENCY, LOCATION, AND QUALITY OF SOMATOSENSORY SYMPTOMS

Although sensory symptoms have been reported to occur in approximately 40 percent of PD patients, they probably are present in a large majority of patients. The 40 percent figure derives from surveys of 101 and 50 ambulatory patients. The larger series includes patients with postencephalitic parkinsonism (2,3). Patients with diabetes, arthritis, musculoskeletal diseases, or other medical illnesses were excluded. Pain, tingling, numbness, coldness, or burning were primarily localized to one or more limbs, typically ipsilateral to the side of the body with the greater motor deficit. Aching or cramplike sensations were included. However, in the larger series (3), patients with pain or other sensory symptoms thought to be associated with increased muscle contraction (painful dystonic spasms, cramps) or otherwise caused by the motor disorder (heaviness, stiffness) were excluded. Both studies emphasized the paresthesia-like quality of most of the symptoms, and in several patients, sensory symptoms preceded the onset of motor symptoms (4). In the smaller series, nerve conduction and somatosensory evoked potential studies were within normal limits

and did not distinguish patients with and without somatosensory symptoms (2). Response to levodopa was not emphasized but was variable, with increased pain (especially a burning sensation) occurring more often than pain relief in the larger series (3).

In contradistinction to these studies, other authors have emphasized sensory and other nonmotor symptomatology that specifically parallel levodopa-related fluctuations in motor signs. In a series of 95 patients with Parkinson's disease, 46 percent reported pain that, in two-thirds of the patients, was related to motor fluctuations (5). The majority of these patients had cramps or muscle tightness (neck, paraspinal, calf). Painful foot and other dystonias were also common, while radicular-like pain, joint pain, or akathitic-related sensations occurred less commonly. Quinn and coworkers (6) proposed a classification of pain in Parkinson's disease primarily based on timing of (and response to) levodopa. In these patients, with or without associated dystonic spasms, pain would occur in the early morning, with "beginning of dose," "end of dose," or with "wearing-off." They also recognized levodopa-responsive pain preceding the diagnosis of Parkinson's disease and peak-dose pain associated with "on-period" dyskinesias. Pains were quite variable from case to case in location and description (7).

Ford and coworkers (8) reported a series of eight patients with Parkinson's disease (one case of atypical parkinsonism) with severe oral or genital pains of unknown etiology. The genital pain (in three women) was generally responsive to levodopa and was associated with motor fluctuations or wearing-off. Oral pains, which were unilateral and burning in quality in three of the patients, were less responsive to levodopa. In all cases the pain syndromes were described as having "a relentless and distressing quality that overshadowed the other features of the parkinsonism (8)." Psychiatric disturbances were noted in six patients, including depression and anxiety. Other nonmotor "off" symptoms described by Hillen and Sage (9) included sensory dyspnea and autonomic disturbances such as limb edema, drenching sweats, urinary frequency, facial flushing, cough, abdominal bloating or pains, and hunger (see Chapter 41).

An apparently common sensory syndrome in patients with Parkinson's disease, typically associated with other sensory symptoms (aching, tingling, or burning) but only recently studied in some detail, is "internal tremor." In a series of 100 consecutive patients, internal tremor was reported as a sensory symptom in 44 percent (10). Overall, 69 percent of the patients had internal tremor, other sensory symptoms, or both. Internal tremor was most often localized axially (chest, abdomen, and neck), with or without limb involvement. There was no statistical association of internal tremor with presence or severity of resting tremor. This symptom was typically not associated with motor fluctuations and was not relieved by antiparkinsonian medications. There was an association of internal tremor with symptoms of anxiety and use of (and response to) anxiolytics. The authors recognized the similarity of internal tremor and paresthesia-like sensory symptoms of Parkinson's patients and somatic symptoms associated with primary anxiety disorders. They distinguished internal tremor from another common symptom in Parkinson's patients that can arguably be considered "sensory," akathisia.

In a series of 100 patients with Parkinson's disease, 68 percent acknowledged feelings of inner restlessness resulting in a need to move (11). In the majority of patients, this was attributed to parkinsonian motor disturbances or various sensory complaints. However, "pure" akathisia, that is, not attributable to other features of the disease, was reported by 26 percent of the total group. This symptom, typically found in patients with more advanced disease, usually was not responsive to antiparkinsonian medications and was not associated with motor fluctuations. The authors distinguished akathisia from the restless leg syndrome; for example, only two of the patients with pure akathisia had symptoms primarily in the evening or at night.

In another study, clozapine-responsive nocturnal akathisia was reported in nine patients with Parkinson's disease (12). Five of the patients had stereotyped repetitive lower extremity movements that were thought to be associated with the akathisia. Because of the lack of lower extremity paresthesias in these patients, the authors differentiated this syndrome from restless leg syndrome (with periodic limb movements). However, typical levodopa-responsive restless leg syndrome has been described in Parkinson's disease (13).

Five of the patients from the nocturnal akathisia group also had a confusional state associated with the akathisia (12). Although not discussed by the authors, it is possible that at least some of these patients had a REM behavior disorder. This disorder is characterized by vivid dreaming associated with vigorous and sometimes injurious motor activity. This phenomenon has been described in patients with Parkinson's disease associated with fluctuating or episodic confusion. REM behavior disorder, often resulting from or exacerbated by antiparkinsonian medications can occur before the onset of parkinsonism (14).

Frequency and characteristics of headache and back pain have been studied individually in patients with Parkinson's disease. Headache, more commonly nuchal than occipital, temporal or frontal but not associated with nuchal (or extremity) rigidity, was present in 35 percent of a series of 71 patients (15). Although early morning headache responsive to levodopa has been described (16), larger studies report tension-like headaches responsive to amitriptyline (15,17). Middle or lower back pain was reported to be present at some stage of the illness in 68 percent of a series of 60 patients with Parkinson's disease without "conditions well known to cause back pain (18)." Back pain preceded the onset of recognized parkinsonism in almost half of these patients. In several patients back pain was responsive to levodopa.

None of the studies reporting frequency of headache, back pain, or akathisia included control groups without PD. Tension-like headaches and low back pain must be among the most common symptoms reported to the general neurologist or primary care physician. Thus the relationship between Parkinson's disease–specific pathology and these symptoms must be considered to be unclear. Yet, as a practical matter, movement disorder specialists certainly see many Parkinson's disease patients with these symptoms in their practice.

PATHOPHYSIOLOGY

The basal ganglia are thought to participate in motivationally or behaviorally relevant sensorimotor integration (19,20). However, current models of basal ganglia physiology emphasize somatotopically and functionally segregated parallel circuits (21,22);

less attention has been directed toward defining sensorimotor integrative properties. Basal ganglia output from the traditionally recognized output nuclei, that is, the globus pallidus interna and substantia nigra pars reticulata, is inhibitory (21,22). Output directed toward regions of thalamus that project to the frontal lobe is highly segregated somatotopically. In PD, increased globus pallidus interna and substantia nigra reticulata activity, due to a shift in balance between so-called "direct" and "indirect" basal ganglia pathways, results in excessive inhibition of thalamocortical activity (23). Frontal hypometabolism, which has been demonstrated in patients with PD using [^{18}F] fluorodeoxyglucose positron emission tomography (PET) scanning (24), is thought to underlie "hypokinetic" features of PD. However, positive symptomatology, and in particular somatosensory disturbances, are not well accounted for by the "direct/indirect" model of basal ganglia function. [see Figure 8-1].

The striatum receives sensory input from numerous sources (19,22). As the entire neocortex projects to the striatum, any cortical area involved in sensory processing could theoretically utilize basal

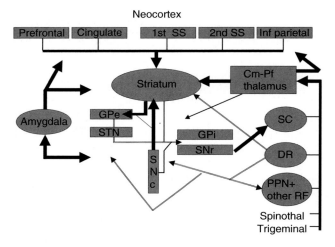

FIGURE 8-1. Possible basal ganglia–related pathways involved in nociceptive and nonnociceptive somatosensory processing. Most of these pathways are described in the text. Thicker arrows reflect relatively larger or better-studied pathways. Excitatory versus inhibitory aspects are not indicated in this figure.
Abbreviations: Cm-Pf = centre median and parafascicular nuclei; DR = dorsal raphe; GPe = globus pallidus externa; GPe = globus pallidus interna; Inf = inferior; PPN = pedunculopontine nucleus; RF = reticular formation; SC = superior colliculus; Spinothal = spinothalamic; SS = somatosensory; SNc = substantia nigra pars compacta; SNr = substantia nigra pars reticulata; STN = subthalamic nucleus.

ganglia connectivity. Projections to the striatum from cortical areas involved in somatosensory function include somatotopically organized input from the first somatosensory cortex (19). This input to the putamen parallels input from the primary motor cortex. Dense topographic projections also arise from the second somatosensory cortex and inferior parietal area 7b (25), which contains somatosensory, multisensory, and task-related neurons. All of these regions contain neurons selectively responsive to painful stimuli (nociceptive). Regions of prefrontal and cingulate cortex that contain nociceptive neurons also project to the striatum (19). The principal thalamic input to the striatum arises from the intralaminar nuclei, including the centre median and parafascicular nuclei (22,26). The specific function of this thalamic input is not known, but in experimental animals the majority of neurons within these structures (or at least major areas within these structures) respond to somatosensory, and in particular nociceptive, stimuli (26).

With the exception of the first somatosensory cortex, somatosensory-responsive (and in particular nociceptive) neurons within the other cortical areas noted earlier and in the intralaminar thalamic nuclei often have large, bilateral receptive fields or have no somatotopic organization (19,25). This parallels striatal (and pallidal) somatosensory-responsive neurons, which also tend to have large cutaneous receptive fields (19). Nociception-related inputs to the intralaminar thalamic nuclei arise from (or are modulated by inputs from) numerous sites, including spinothalamic and spinoreticulothalamic tracts and their trigeminal equivalents, the superior colliculus (27), the pedunculopontine nucleus (cholinergic and noncholinergic neurons located within the mesopontine reticular formation) (28), the dorsal raphe, and the substantia nigra reticulata (29). Of course, many of these sites connect with each other or to other basal ganglia–related structures (19), possibly relaying somatosensory information (e.g., substantia nigra reticulata projections to the superior colliculus, pedunculopontine connections to the substantia nigra, globus pallidus, and subthalamic nucleus (28)).

The majority of dopaminergic substantia nigra neurons are also responsive to somatosensory input, but only if the input is of specific behavioral significance. For example, in a monkey study (30), over 85 percent of 171 dopaminergic neurons evaluated in the awake animal increased firing rates that followed the spontaneous touch of food, but not of nonfood objects, hidden behind a box. In anesthetized monkeys, 68 percent of 140 dopaminergic neurons responded to painful stimulation by decreasing firing rates in the majority of neurons. There was no response in this setting to nonpainful somatosensory stimulation (even if intense). Responses in both paradigms (awake and anesthetized) were nonsomatotopic and bilateral. However, evidence has been provided that dopaminergic substantia nigra neurons can encode stimulus intensity (31).

Dopaminergic nigrostriatal projections appear to significantly influence sensory responsiveness of striatal neurons, although the effect may be indirect (19,32). Striatal neurons normally are highly responsive to external sensory stimulation. Responsiveness in the caudate nucleus is decreased and altered qualitatively (less selective, larger receptive fields) in cats treated with the dopamine-selective neurotoxin MPTP (32). The onset of this effect is coincident with the onset of parkinsonian motor deficits. With recovery of motor function, striatal neuronal responses return to baseline. Decreased responsiveness of striatal neurons to sensory input may contribute to the contralateral sensory neglect that results from the intrastriatal administration of the dopamine depleting agent 6-hydroxydopamine (19).

Paradoxically, dopamine depletion appears to increase nociception (as discussed by Chudler and Dong (19); see also (33,34)). Although both basal ganglia–related and spinal-mediated dopaminergic responses have been implicated, the effect appears to be predominantly supraspinal (19,29,35). For example, in a mouse study demonstrating hyperalgesia following systemic administration of MPTP (33), the effect attenuated after about two weeks, coincident with a marked increase in serotonin activity (despite low dopamine concentrations). Dopamine (and serotonin) mediation of nociception may involve interactions with opiate activity.

Best known for their analgesic properties, opiates are found in high concentrations in the basal ganglia, and co-localize with GABA in both "direct" and "indirect" striatopallidal projections (22): "direct" pathway projections to the globus pallidus interna and substantia nigra reticulata co-localize dynorphin (and substance P), whereas indirect pathway projections to the globus pallidus externa co-localize enkephalin. Kurumaji and coworkers (36) provided indirect evidence favoring a role of basal ganglia met-enkephalin in pain responsiveness by finding a close relationship in the rat between circadian fluctuations in pain responsiveness and met-enkephalin–like immunoreactivity in selective brain regions, including the striatum and "mesolimbic" area, but not within the thalamus or amygdala.

Although early studies emphasized the role of the periaqueductal gray and the serotonergic nucleus raphe magnus in morphine-induced analgesia, morphine injected into various regions of rat pallidum or substantia nigra reticulata also produces a dose-dependent analgesia (inhibited by naloxone) (37,38). This effect appears to be specific, as responses on nonnociceptive sensorimotor tasks are generally unaffected. At least within the substantia nigra, this effect appears to be mediated by the mu receptor (37). Similarly, intravenous morphine significantly depresses nociception-related responses in various brain regions including, in a rat study (39), the ventral globus pallidus and the central nucleus of the amygdala. Putative nociception-related pathways between this region of amygdala and basal ganglia (including globus pallidus and substantia nigra) have also been reported (19).

Dopamine agonists, both in experimental animals and in humans, appear to potentiate the analgesic effect of morphine, whereas depletion of dopamine, for example, by 6-hydroxydopamine lesions of the substantia nigra compacta and adjacent ventral tegmental area, attenuates morphine analgesia, at least in certain pain models (19,40–43). In humans dextroamphetamine has been added to morphine to enhance analgesia, for example, postoperatively (40). In the rat model, an analgesic effect of dextroamphetamine is blocked by 6-hydroxydopamine lesions (42).

Interestingly, certain pain syndromes similar to those described in patients with Parkinson's disease have also been described in psychiatric patients following neuroleptic use. In a series of 107 psychiatric inpatients (44), 23 percent of 60 patients being treated with neuroleptics experienced pain, as compared with only 1 of 47 patients been treated with other psychotropic drugs. In general, the pain described was a poorly localized aching in the extremities. Sensory complaints of heaviness, stiffness, or those associated with acute dystonic reactions were excluded. Pain occurred more frequently in patients with parkinsonism, akathisia, or both, and tended to correlate with severity of parkinsonism. Ford and coworkers (45) described 11 patients with tardive oral (9 patients) and genital (2 patients) pains. These were similar in character to that which the same authors described in patients with Parkinson's disease, for example, severe, relentless, and overshadowing other neurologic symptoms (8). All of the patients also had typical orolingual dyskinesia, and most had tardive dystonia or akathisia as well.

Nondopaminergic mechanisms may also be responsible for some of the sensory symptoms in patients with Parkinson's disease. There is moderate to severe loss of cholinergic pedunculopontine nucleus neurons in Parkinson's disease (46–48). In addition to projecting to intralaminar thalamic nuclei, projections to other sites may contribute to a role of this nucleus in nonopiate analgesic systems (49,50). These cholinergic neurons have also been implicated in an experimental model of morphine addiction (51,52), possibly via projections to the dopaminergic mesolimbic system.

At least two studies have reported an association of pain with depression in PD (53,54). In one study of 95 patients, 46 percent had pain thought to be associated with the disease. Severe depression was noted in 34 percent of those with pain but in only 13 percent of those without pain. Although, as suggested by the authors (53), depression may color "the interpretation of pain" or "pain can exacerbate an already present depression," it is also possible that underlying serotonergic pathology could predispose to both pain and depression. The latter possibility was supported by a study of cerebrospinal fluid from 10 PD patients with pain, 14 Parkinson's patients without pain, and 8 non-Parkinson's patients with post-stroke thalamic pain syndrome (54). In addition to having the highest scores on a self-depression scale, the Parkinson's patients with pain had significantly lower spinal fluid levels of the serotonin metabolite 5-HIAA than the other groups. Low spinal fluid 5-HIAA had previously been associated with depression in PD without reference to pain (55).

EVALUATION AND TREATMENT OF SOMATOSENSORY SYMPTOMS

As we enter a new era of "evidence-" or "outcome-" based medical practice, the evaluation and treatment of sensory symptoms in patients with Parkinson's disease still requires the nuanced, subjective, qualitative approach (i.e., the "art of medicine") practiced by many of the best physicians of past eras. Parkinson's is primarily a disease of the elderly, who often have (or develop) multiple medical problems. The treating physician must obviously look for "flags" that suggest other disease processes, such as weakness (focal or out of proportion to that due to deconditioning), axial sensory level, hyperreflexia or reflex loss, astereognosia, or joint deformity. Although a certain restraint in ordering diagnostic studies to evaluate each sensory symptom is often warranted, where to "draw the line" can be difficult to determine. For example, a normal EMG/NCV study can be reassuring in certain situations. However, patients often have several normal or otherwise unhelpful studies. For example, cervical or lumbar MRI scans are rarely normal in the elderly, yet they are often not helpful.

In evaluating sensory complaints, the physician should always try to determine if there is a relationship to levodopa-related fluctuations in motor symptoms or to other aspects of the motor disturbance. Although certain somatosensory symptoms would be more likely to respond to levodopa than other symptoms (Table 8-1), increasing the dosage of levodopa (or dopamine agonist) might be remarkably effective in the individual patient. In other patients, levodopa can aggravate or cause pains (e.g., burning). In some patients "on" period pain does not respond to manipulation of oral dopaminergic medications, and the only course is to stop levodopa and sacrifice mobility for comfort (6). Transient drug holidays may stop pain, but they do not provide a long-term solution. Two papers have reported on the usefulness of subcutaneous apomorphine injections for off period pain refractory to levodopa (55a,55b). In this situation the apomorphine injection acts to abort a painful episode early on with its rapid action. The effects have been shown to last several years (55b). Apomorphine can be effective in patients who are refractory to treatment with other dopamine agonists. Leg edema, a common side effect of amantadine and dopamine agonists, can be associated with sensory symptoms. Long-acting benzodiazepines (e.g., clonazepam) may be useful for patients with internal tremor and in patients with nocturnal akathisia (10,56), particularly if they also have symptoms suggestive of a REM behavior disorder. The atypical neuroleptic clozapine has also been reported to be effective in patients with nocturnal akathisia (12), whereas inconsistent benefits from this medication have been reported in small series of patients with pelvic, back, or lower extremity pains (56,57). Unfortunately, the efficacy of narcotics, aspirin, acetaminophen, nonsteroidal anti-inflammatory drugs, anticonvulsants, or other agents with analgesic actions have not been systematically evaluated for the treatment of sensory symptoms in PD. From practical experience, they often do not appear to be very useful.

REFERENCES

1. Silberstein SD, Lipton RB. Overview of diagnosis and treatment of migraine. *Neurology* 1994; 44:S6–S16.
2. Koller WC. Primary sensory symptoms in Parkinson's disease. *Neurology* 1984; 34:957–959.
3. Snider SR, Fahn S, Isgreen WP, et al. Primary sensory symptoms in parkinsonism. *Neurology* 1976; 26:423–429.
4. Schott GD. Pain in Parkinson's disease. *Pain* 1985; 22:407–411.

5. Goetz CG, Tanner CM, Levy M, et al. Pain in Parkinson's disease. *Mov Disord* 1986; 1:45–49.

6. Quinn NP, Koller WC, Lang AE, et al. Painful Parkinson's disease. *Lancet* 1986; 1:1366–1369.

7. Nutt JG, Carter JH. Sensory symptoms in parkinsonism related to central dopaminergic function. *Lancet* 1984; 2:456–457.

8. Ford B, Louis ED, Greene P, et al. Oral and genital pain syndromes in Parkinson's disease. *Mov Disord* 1996; 11:421–426.

9. Hillen ME, Sage JI. Nonmotor fluctuations in patients with Parkinson's disease. *Neurology* 1996; 47:1180–1183.

10. Shulman LM, Singer C, Bean JA, et al. Internal tremor in patients with Parkinson's disease. *Mov Disord* 1996; 11:3–7.

11. Lang AE, Johnson K. Akathisia in idiopathic Parkinson's disease. *Neurology* 1987; 37:477–481.

12. Linazasoro G, Marti Masso JF, Suarez JA. Nocturnal akathisia in Parkinson's disease: Treatment with clozapine. *Mov Disord* 1993; 8:171–174.

13. Riley DE, Lang AE. The spectrum of levodopa-related fluctuations in Parkinson's disease. *Neurology* 1993; 43:1459–1464.

14. Schenck CH, Bundie SR, Mahowald MW. Delayed emergence of a parkinsonian disorder in 38% of 29 older men initially diagnosed with idiopathic rapid eye movement sleep behavior disorder. *Neurology* 1996; 46:388–393.

15. Indo T, Naito A, Sobue I. Clinical characteristics of headache in Parkinson's disease. *Headache* 1983; 23:211–212.

16. Indo T, Takahashi A. Early morning headache of Parkinson's disease: A hitherto unrecognized symptom? *Headache* 1987; 27:151–154.

17. Indaco A, Carrieri PB. Amitriptyline in the treatment of headache in patients with Parkinson's disease: A double-blind placebo-controlled study. *Neurology* 1988; 38:1720–1722.

18. Sandyk R. Back pain as an early symptom of Parkinson's disease. *SA Med J* 1982; 2:3.

19. Chudler EH, Dong WK. The role of the basal ganglia in nociception and pain. *Pain* 1995; 60:3–38.

20. Marsden CD. The mysterious motor function of the basal ganglia: The Robert Wartenberg Lecture. *Neurology* 1982; 32:514–539.

21. Alexander GE, Crutcher MD. Functional architecture of basal ganglia circuits: Neural substrates of parallel processing. *Trends Neurosci* 1990; 13:266–271.

22. Flaherty AW, Graybiel AM. Anatomy of the basal ganglia. In: Marsden CD, Fahn S (eds.). *Movement Disorders 3*. Oxford, U.K.: Butterworth-Heinemann, 1994: 3–27.

23. DeLong MR. Primate models of movement disorders of basal ganglia origin. *Trends Neurosci* 1990; 13:281–285.

24. Eidelberg D, Moeller JR, Dhawan V, et al. The metabolic topography of parkinsonism. *J Cereb Blood Flow Metab* 1994; 14:783–801.

25. Dong WK, Chudler EH, Sugiyama K, et al. Somatosensory, multisensory, and task-related neurons in cortical area 7b (PF) of unanesthetized monkeys. *J Neurophysiol* 1994; 72:542–564.

26. Dong WK, Ryu H, Wagman IH. Nociceptive responses of neurons in medial thalamus and their relationship to spinothalamic pathways. *J Neurophysiol* 1978; 41:1592–1613.

27. Krauthamer GM, Krol JG, Grunwerg BS. Effect of superior colliculus lesions on sensory unit responses in the intralaminar thalamus of the rat. *Brain Res* 1992; 576:277–286.

28. Manaye KF, Zweig R, Wu D, et al. Quantification of cholinergic and select non-cholinergic mesopontine neuronal populations in the human brain. *Neuroscience* 1999; 89:759–770.

29. Li J, Ji YP, Qiao JT, et al. Suppression of nociceptive responses in parafascicular neurons by stimulation of substantial nigra: An analysis of related inhibitory pathways. *Brain Res* 1992; 591:109–115.

30. Romo R, Schmaltz W. Somatosensory input to dopamine neurones of the monkey midbrain: Responses to pain pinch under anaesthesia and to active touch in behavioural context. *Prog Brain Res* 1989; 80:473–478.

31. Gao DM, Jeaugey L, Pollak P, et al. Intensity-dependent nociceptive responses from presumed dopaminergic neurons of the substantia nigra, pars compacta in the rat and their modification by lateral habenula inputs. *Brain Res* 1990; 529:315–319.

32. Rothblat DS, Schneider JS. Response of caudate neurons to stimulation of intrinsic and peripheral afferents in normal, symptomatic, and recovered MPTP-treated cats. *J Neurosci* 1993; 13:4372–4378.

33. Rosland JH, Humskaar S, Broch OJ, et al. Acute and long term effects of 1-methyl-4-phenyl-1,2,3,6-tetrahydropyridine (MPTP) in tests of nociception in mice. *Pharmacol Toxicol* 1992; 70:31–37.

34. Lin MT, Wu JJ, Chandra A, et al. Activation of striatal dopamine receptors induces pain inhibition in rats. *J Neural Transm* 1981; 51:213–222.

35. Sage JI, Kortis HI, Sommer W. Evidence for the role of spinal cord systems in Parkinson's disease-associated pain. *Clin Neuropharmacol* 1990; 13:171–174.

36. Kurumaji A, Takashima M, Ohi K, et al. Circadian fluctuations in pain responsiveness and brain met-enkephalin-like immunoreactivity in the rat. *Pharmacol Biochem Behav* 1988; 29:595–599.

37. Baumeister AA. The effects of bilateral intranigral microinjection of selective opioid agonists on behavioral responses to noxious thermal stimuli. *Brain Res* 1981; 557:136–145.

38. Anagnostakis Y, Zis V, Spyraki C. Analgesia induced by morphine injected into the pallidum. *Behav Brain Res* 1992; 48:135–143.

39. Huang G-F, Besson J-M, Bernard J-F. Intravenous morphine depresses the transmission of noxious messages to the nucleus centralis of the amygdala. *Eur J Pharmacol* 1993; 236:449–456.

40. Forrest Jr. WH, Brown BW, Brown CR, et al. Dextroamphetamine with morphine for the treatment of postoperative pain. *N Engl J Med* 1977; 296:712–715.

41. Price MTC, Fibiger HC. Ascending catecholamine systems and morphine analgesia. *Brain Res* 1975; 99:189–193.

42. Morgan MJ, Franklin KBJ. 6-Hydroxydopamine lesions of the ventral tegmentum abolish D-amphetamine and morphine analgesia in the formalin test but not in the tail flick test. *Brain Res* 1990; 519:144–149.

43. Gupta YK, Chugh A, Seth SD. Opposing effect of apomorphine on antinociceptive activity of morphine: A dose-dependent phenomenon. *Pain* 1989; 36:263–269.

44. Decina P, Mukherjee S, Caracci G, et al. Painful sensory symptoms in neuroleptic-induced extrapyramidal syndromes. *Am J Psychiatry* 1989; 149:1075–1080.

45. Ford B, Greene P, Fahn S. Oral and genital tardive pain syndromes. *Neurology* 1994; 44:2115–2119.

46. Hirsch EC, Graybiel AM, Duyckaert C, et al. Neuronal loss in the pedunculopontine tegmental nucleus in Parkinson's disease and progressive supranuclear palsy. *Proc Nat Acad Sci USA* 1987; 84:5976–5980.

47. Jellinger K. The pedunculopontine nucleus in Parkinson's disease, progressive supranuclear palsy and Alzheimer's disease. *J Neurol Neurosurg Psychiatry* 1988; 51:540–543.

48. Zweig RM, Jankel WR, Hedreen JC, et al. The pedunculopontine nucleus in Parkinson's disease. *Ann Neurol* 1989; 26:41–46.

49. Iwamoto ET. Characterization of the antinociception induced by nicotine in the pedunculopontine tegmental nucleus and the nucleus raphe magnus. *J Pharmacol Exp Ther* 1991; 257:120–133.

50. Katayama Y, De Witt DS, Beeker DP, et al. Behavioral evidence for a cholinoceptive pontine inhibitory area: Descending control of spinal motor output and sensory input. *Brain Res* 1984; 296:241–262.

51. Becara A, van der Kooy D. The tegmental pedunculopontine nucleus: A brainstem output of the limbic system critical for the conditioned place preferences produced by morphine and amphetamine. *J Neurosci* 1989; 9:3400–3409.

52. Klitinick MA, Kalivas P. Behavioral and neurochemical studies of opioid effects in the pedunculopontine nucleus and mediodorsal thalamus. *J Pharmacol Exp Ther* 1994; 269:437–478.

53. Goetz CG, Wilson RS, Tanner CM, et al. Relationships among pain, depression, and sleep alterations in Parkinson's disease. *Adv Neurol* 1986; 45:345–347.

54. Urakami K, Takahashi K, Matsushima E, et al. The threshold of pain and neurotransmitter's change on pain in Parkinson's disease. *Jpn J Psychiatr Neurol* 1990; 44:589–593.

55. Mayeux R, Stern Y, Williams J, et al. Clinical and biochemical features of depression in Parkinson's diseases. *Am J Psychiatry* 1986; 143:756–759.

55a. Frankel JP, Lees AJ, Kempster PA, et al. Subcutaneous apomorphine in the treatment of Parkinson's disease. *J Neurol Neurosurg Psychiatry* 1990; 53:96–101.

55b. Factor SA, Brown DL, Molho ES. Subcutaneous apomorphine injections as treatment for intractable pain in Parkinson's disease. *Mov Disord* 2000; 15:167–169.

56. Trosch RM, Friedman JH, Lannon MC, et al. Clozapine use in Parkinson's disease: A retrospective analysis of a large multicentered clinical experience. *Mov Disord* 1998; 13:37–38.

57. Juncos JL. Clozapine treatment of parkinsonian pain syndromes. *Mov Disord* 1996; 11:603–604.

9

Speech, Voice, and Swallowing Disorders

Lorraine Olson Ramig, Ph.D., CCC-SLP, Professor

Department of Speech, Language, Hearing Sciences, University of Colorado–Boulder, Research Associate, Wilbur James Gould Voice Research Center, Denver Center for the Performing Arts, Denver, Colorado

Stefanie Countryman, M.A., CCC-SLP, Speech-Language Pathologist

Wilbur James Gould Voice Research Center, Denver Center for the Performing Arts, Denver, Colorado

Cynthia Fox, M.A., CCC-SLP, Speech-Language Pathologist

National Center for Neurogenic Communication Disorders, Department of Speech and Hearing Sciences, University of Arizona–Tucson

and

Shimon Sapir, Ph.D., CCC-SLP

Wilbur James Gould Voice Research Center, Denver Center for the Performing Arts, Denver, Colorada

INTRODUCTION

Speech and voice disorders have been reported in 75 to 89 percent of individuals with Parkinson's disease (PD). The most common of these characteristics include reduced loudness, monotone and hoarse voice, and imprecise articulation (1–12). These disorders can be among the first signs of PD (13) and may limit the quality of life in these individuals. Speech and voice disorders may reduce the ability to socialize, convey important medical information, interact with family, and maintain employment (8,14).

Swallowing disorders (dysphagia) occur in as many as 95 percent of individuals with PD (15) and occasionally have been reported as one of the first signs of the disease (16). Symptoms of swallowing problems in this population include difficulty with lingual motility, reduced initiation of swallow, difficulty with bolus formation, delayed pharyngeal response, and decreased pharyngeal contraction (15,17,18). In addition, individuals with PD often report weight loss and lack of enjoyment in eating following recognition of swallowing difficulties. Aspiration pneumonia in the later stages of the disease is common and is sometimes the cause of death (19).

While neuropharmacologic (20,21) and neurosurgical (22,23) approaches may be effective in improving limb symptoms in individuals with PD, their impact on speech production and swallowing remains unclear (24,25). Speech treatment has traditionally focused on rate, articulation, and prosody (26,27). Swallowing treatment has focused on behavioral changes and diet modifications (18). A recently developed approach, the Lee Silverman Voice Treatment (LSVT®), has generated the first short- and long-term efficacy data (28,29) for successfully treating disordered speech in this population. In addition, recent research indicates the LSVT® may also improve swallowing ability in this population (17).

SPEECH AND VOICE CHARACTERISTICS IN PARKINSON'S DISEASE

Speech and voice characteristics have been associated with the primary physical features of PD (rigidity, bradykinesia, hypokinesia, and tremor), although the exact pathophysiologic cause remains unclear (30–33). Perceptual, acoustic, aerodynamic, kinematic, videostroboscopic, electroglottographic, and electromyographic data document disorders of laryngeal, respiratory, articulatory, and velopharyngeal function in individuals with PD (34–37).

Laryngeal and Respiratory Disorders

Darley and coworkers reported one of the first systematic descriptions of perceptual characteristics of speech and voice in individuals with PD (38–40). They identified reduced loudness; monopitch; monoloudness; reduced stress; breathy, hoarse voice quality; imprecise articulation; and short rushes of speech as classic features of speech and voice in these individuals. The vocal characteristics were further described by Logemann, Boshes, and Fisher (6,41), who reported voice quality problems such as hoarseness, roughness, breathiness, and tremor in 89 percent of 200 patients they studied. Similarly, Ludlow and Bassich (42) reported that 83 percent of the individuals they studied a had harsh voice and 17 percent of them had a breathy voice. They suggested that harsh voice quality may be associated with drug-related dyskinesias. Furthermore, Aronson (13) and Stewart and coworkers (43) are among those who observed that voice disorders may occur very early in the disease process.

Acoustic data have been used to describe the speech and voice characteristics of individuals with PD and seem to parallel perceptual descriptions. These acoustic measures include sound pressure level (SPL), fundamental frequency and its variability, and phonatory stability.

Early studies (3,4,42–46) did not confirm a reduction in SPL consistent with perceptual reports of *reduced loudness* in these individuals. However, a recent report by Fox and Ramig (47) documented SPL that was 2 to 4 decibels (at 30 cm) lower across a number of speech tasks when comparing 29 individuals with PD and an age- and gender-matched control group. A 2 to 4 decibel change is equal to a 40 percent perceptible change in loudness (47).

Fundamental frequency variability in speech has been reported to be consistently lower in individuals with PD when compared with a nondisordered control group (3,4,42). These findings support the perceptual characteristics (38–40) of *monopitch* or *monotonous speech*, typically observed in these individuals. A reduction in maximum fundamental frequency range has also been observed in PD when compared with nondisordered speakers (3,42,48).

Measures of short-term phonatory stability (e.g., jitter, shimmer, harmonics-to-noise ratio) are consistent with various perceptual characteristics of *disordered voice quality* (e.g., *hoarse, breathy, harsh*) (49,50). Long-term phonatory instability, reflecting vocal tremor in the range of 3 to 7 Hz during sustained vowel phonation, has been documented in individuals with PD (50–54).

Disordered laryngeal function has been documented through a number of videoendoscopic studies. Hansen and coworkers (34) reported vocal fold bowing (lack of medial vocal fold closure) together with greater amplitude of vibration and laryngeal asymmetry in 30 of 32 individuals with PD. Smith and coworkers (55) made videostroboscopic observations of individuals with PD and reported that 12 of 21 patients had a form of glottal incompetence (bowing, anterior or posterior chink) on *nasal* fiberoptic views. In a more recent study, Perez and coworkers (56) observed laryngeal tremor in 55 percent of the 29 individuals with PD they studied. The primary site of tremor was vertical laryngeal motion. However, the most striking stroboscopic findings in this study were abnormal phase closure and phase asymmetry.

Additional data to support laryngeal closure problems come from analysis of the electroglottographic (EGG) signal. Uziel (11) reported EGG waveforms with reduced amplitude in individuals with PD relative to nondisordered speakers. Gerratt and coworkers (57) reported abnormally large speed quotient and poorly defined closing period in this population. These observations were consistent with slow vocal fold opening relative to the rate of closure and incomplete closure of the vocal folds.

Hirose and Joshita (58) studied data derived from the thyroarytenoid (TA) muscles in an individual with PD who had limited vocal fold movement. They observed no reduction in the number of motor unit discharges and no pathologic discharge patterns (such as polyphasic or high-amplitude voltages). They reported loss of reciprocal suppression of the TA during inspiration and interpreted this as evidence of deterioration in the reciprocal adjustment of the antagonist muscles associated with PD rigidity. Luschei and coworkers (59) studied single motor unit activity in the TA muscle in individuals with PD and suggested that the firing rate of the TA motor units was decreased in male subjects. The authors report that these findings and past reports suggest that PD affects rate and variability in motor unit firing in the laryngeal musculature. A study completed by Baker and coworkers (33) found that absolute TA amplitudes during a known loudness level task in individuals with PD were the lowest when compared with young normals and normal aging controls. Relative TA amplitudes were also decreased in both the aging and PD groups when compared with the young normals. The authors concluded that reduced levels of TA muscle activity may contribute to the reduced vocal fold adduction and vocal loudness that is observed in PD and aging populations.

A number of studies have documented evidence of disordered respiratory function in individuals with PD through various aerodynamic measurements. Reduced vital capacity, a reduction in the total amount of air expended during maximum phonation tasks (63), has been reported (60–62). Reduced intraoral air pressure during consonant or vowel productions and abnormal airflow patterns (66,67) have been reported (63–65). It has been suggested that the origin of these airflow abnormalities may be variations in airflow resistance. This may be caused by abnormal movements of the vocal folds and supraglottic area (67) or abnormal chest wall movements and respiratory muscle activation patterns (35,65,68).

Articulatory and Velopharyngeal Disorders

Imprecise consonants have been observed in individuals with PD (6,41,60). Logemann and coworkers (6,41) reported articulation problems in 45 percent of 200 individuals studied. They suggested that inadequate narrowing of the vocal tract may underlie problems with stops /p/, /b/, affricates /sh/, /ch/, and fricatives /s/, /f/.

Disordered rate has also been reported in some individuals with PD. Although rapid rate has been reported in 6 to 13 percent of individuals (3,4,69–71), Canter (44) reported slower than normal rates. Palilalia or stuttering has been observed in a small percentage of patients (38,72).

Acoustic correlates of disordered articulation have been studied and include problems with timing of vocal onsets and offsets (voicing during normally voiceless closure intervals of voiceless stops) (11,36,73) and spirantization (presence of fricative-like, aperiodic noise during stop closures). In addition, Forrest and coworkers (74) reported that speakers with PD demonstrated longer voice onset times (VOT) and suggested that this observation was consistent with a movement initiation problem at the level of the larynx.

Disordered articulatory movements have been documented in PD through kinematic analysis of jaw movements (74–82). It has been consistently reported that individuals with PD show a significant reduction in the size and peak velocity of jaw movements during speech when compared with nondisordered speakers (74,79). In fact, on average, jaw movements of individuals with PD have been reported to be approximately half the size of the jaw movements observed in nondisordered subjects. However, duration of movements in PD and nondisordered individuals have been reported to be similar (74).

Electromyographic characteristics of speech mechanism musculature have provided evidence of rigidity in lip and jaw muscles. Some reports include evidence of increased levels of tonic resting and background activity (30–32,83,84). Others observe loss of reciprocity with increased EMG coactivation patterns in functionally antagonistic muscle groups (30,31,80,81,83).

Although nasality and nasal emission have not been significant or consistent perceptual problems in the speech of individuals with PD, aerodynamic and kinematic studies suggest that velopharyngeal movements may be reduced in some of these individuals (37,80,85). In addition, symptoms of hypernasality may signal other neurologic symptoms besides those caused by PD.

Sensory Observations

Whereas the speech and voice symptoms associated with PD are generally considered in relation to motor output problems, sensory abnormalities in these individuals have been recognized for years (20,86,87). Albin and coworkers (88) and Penny and Young (89) suggest that basal ganglia excitatory circuits inadequately activate cortical motor centers, and as a result, motor neuron pools are not provided with adequate facilitation; thus movements are small and weak. Berardelli (90) suggested that the defect in motor cortex activation is due to a perceptual failure to select the muscle commands to match the external force and speed requirements. Hallet (91) and Demirci and coworkers (92) have suggested that this is a problem with as kinesthesia and have stated that when individuals with PD match their effort to their kinesthetic feedback, they will constantly underscale their movement.

Sensory problems have been studied in relation to speech output in individuals with PD (93–95) and may play an important role in motor speech disorders (96). Recently, problems in sensory perception of effort have been identified as an important focus of successful voice treatment for individuals with PD (97). Consistent with suggestions by Hallet and colleagues, it has been observed that when individuals with PD are asked to produce "loud" speech (i.e., attempt large movements), they increase their otherwise underscaled "soft" speech to a level within normal limits. However, when they produce this "upscaled" speech that is within normal limits to a listener, these patients will complain that they are talking "too loud." Furthermore, individuals with PD often report people around them "must need hearing aids" rather than recognize that their speech has become "too soft." Thus it appears that sensory processing deficits may be a factor in speech and voice characteristics observed in individuals with PD. Research on the role of sensory problems in the speech and voice characteristics will probably further enhance our understanding of this relationship (96).

Swallowing Disorders

Swallowing disorders (see Chapter 10) occur in as many as 95 percent of individuals with PD (98) and may be among the first signs of the disease (18).

Identification of swallowing disorders is extremely important in this population, given the ramifications on nutrition and the ability to take oral medication appropriately. Silent aspiration may be observed, and pneumonia is sometimes the cause of death in individuals in the later stages of the disease (98).

Swallowing abnormalities have been reported in all stages of the disease (98), and many individuals with PD have more than one type of swallowing dysfunction (15). Disorders in both oral and pharyngeal stages of swallowing have been observed (15,98,99). A recent study by El Sharkawi and coworkers (17) found dysfunctions during the oral phase of swallowing to be the most predominant and included reduced tongue control and strength and reduced oral transit times. Others have reported a "rockinglike" motion of the tongue during the oral phase (18). This motion seemed to occur when the patients were unable to lower the posterior portion of the tongue to propel the bolus into the pharynx. Inability or delayed ability to trigger the swallowing reflex has also been observed in this population (18). These disorders may limit the ability of the individual with PD to control the food or liquid bolus while in the oral cavity. This may lead to choking or aspiration of food or liquid. Reduced nutritional intake, lack of enjoyment in eating, and difficulty in taking medications also result from oral phase swallowing dysfunction.

Pharyngeal stage dysfunction includes residue in the valleculae due to reduced tongue base retraction. El Sharkawi and coworkers (17) reported that this was the most common problem in the pharyngeal stage of swallowing. Aspiration may occur in these patients as a result of the residue left in the pharynx after the swallow is complete (18). Leopold and Kagel (15) found several disorders of laryngeal movement during swallowing. These included slow closure, incomplete closure, absent closure, and slowed or delayed laryngeal excursion (15). Increased pharyngeal transit time has also been reported. Silent aspiration has been observed in the later stages of the disease and can be a contributory cause of death (19). Dysfunction in the pharyngeal stage of swallowing may also lead to a feeling that food is stuck in the throat, choking, penetration, aspiration, reduced nutritional intake, or reduced ability to self-medicate.

Swallowing dysfunction occurs in this population even when the individual is considered optimally medicated for motor symptoms (98). Referral for swallowing evaluation is extremely important at the first sign of problems. The need for this referral may occur during the early stages of the disease.

TREATMENT

Medical Treatments

Neuropharmacologic and neurosurgical approaches for the treatment of PD have had positive outcomes on motor function. However, the impact of these treatments on speech, voice production, and swallowing is less compelling. Although some studies have reported on the positive effects of levodopa on limb function (100–106), the magnitude and consistency of improvement in speech tends to be much less (104,105). More recent studies (24,65) reported little consistent variation in speech, voice and respiratory characteristics at different points in the *drug* treatment cycle. Few systematic studies exist on the effect of various *surgical* treatments on speech and voice. Baker and coworkers (25) observed limited effects of fetal dopamine transplant on speech in patients with documented limb function improvement. In addition, significant negative effects on speech, voice, and swallowing have been reported following *bilateral* thalamotomy (107) and pallidotomy (108). Schultz and coworkers (109) analyzed acoustic measures following unilateral pallidotomy in six individuals with PD. At three months post surgery, the authors found that all patients demonstrated positive changes in at least one acoustic measure; however, not all of the six patients consistently demonstrated those changes. It appears that neuropharmacologic and neurosurgical approaches alone do not consistently and significantly improve speech and voice. Therefore, behavioral speech treatment is warranted even for individuals who have optimum medical treatment.

Behavioral Speech, Voice, and Swallowing Treatment

Although there is a high incidence of disordered speech and voice in PD, reports suggest that only 3 to 4 percent of these individuals receive speech therapy (7,12). One explanation for this discrepancy may be that carryover and long-term treatment outcomes have been disappointing. In fact, "conventional wisdom" has been that "changes that occur in the treatment room disappear on the way to the parking lot" (110–113). This challenge of carryover and long-term treatment outcomes has been observed consistently over a wide range of speech treatments that have been applied to this population (71). These approaches have included a combination of training in rate control, prosody, loudness, articulation, and respiration (26). In addition, some forms of treatment have included devices such as delayed auditory feedback (DAF), amplification devices, and pacing boards (27,45,71,114).

In general, when individuals with PD are in the treatment room and receiving direct stimulation or feedback from the speech clinician or an instrument (external cue) (71,115,116), they are able to improve speech and voice production. However, maintaining these improvements (training the ability to internally cue) has been a challenge. This consistent observation provides potential insight into the underlying basis for the problems in carryover. One explanation relates to the sensory processing and internal cueing problems frequently experienced by these individuals (20,90,94). Recognition of these problems may improve treatment of motor speech output. Support for these ideas come from the work of Ramig and coworkers (28,29), who documented that training sensory perception of effort appears to be a key element in successful speech treatment in PD. In addition, neuropsychological problems, such as deficits in procedural learning (117,118) may underlie the challenges that individuals with PD have in maintaining long-term treatment effects and in learning new habits.

Intensive Voice Treatment

Ramig and colleagues developed an approach to the treatment of speech in PD patients. Unlike approaches that focus on rate or articulation, the Lee Silverman Voice Treatment (LSVT®) focuses on the speech problem observed most often in individuals with PD: *disordered voice.*

It was hypothesized by Ramig and coworkers that there are at least three features underlying the voice disorder of PD. These features include (*1*) an overall amplitude scale down (20,88,89) to the speech mechanism (reduced amplitude of neural drive to the muscles of the speech mechanism) that may result in a "soft voice that is monotone," (*2*) problem in sensory perception of effort (20,90) that prevents the individual with PD from accurately monitoring his/her vocal output and results in (*3*) the individual's difficulty in independently generating (internal cueing/scaling) the right amount of effort (91,92,119) to produce adequate loudness. It is hypothesized that the combination of these three features is a significant factor that underlies the speech and voice problems in individuals with PD and makes them particularly resistant to successful treatment. The LSVT® has been designed to address these issues. The LSVT® has five essential concepts: (*1*) increasing the vocal loudness (2) improving sensory perception of effort, that is, "calibration," (*3*) the treatment is administered in a high-effort style and, (*4*) treatment is administered intensively (four times a week for 16 sessions in one month), and (*5*) all speech and voice output is quantified. Every element of treatment is delivered consistently with these five

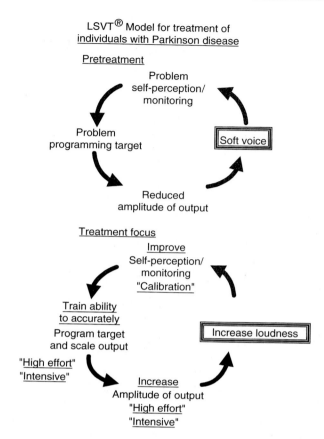

FIGURE 9-1. This figure graphically summarizes the hypothesized neural basis for the LSVT® approach to treating individuals with PD. Pretreatment (top circle) the "soft" voice of the patient may be a result of reduced amplitude of output to the speech mechanism. The "soft" voice is maintained because patients have reduced self-perception or self-monitoring and fail to realize that the voice is "too" soft. Therefore, when they program output for another utterance, they downscale the output and continue to produce a "soft voice."

The LSVT® focus (bottom circle) addresses the "soft" voice at three levels. High effort, intensive treatment is designed to train increased amplitude of output to the respiratory phonatory system to generate increased loudness. Patients are then trained to improve self-perception or self-monitoring of effort so that they understand the relationship between increased effort and successful communication. In this way, when they generate an utterance on their own, they are able to "carry over" adequate effort and loudness for communication success outside the treatment room.

concepts. Treatment techniques are designed to scale-up amplitude to the respiratory and phonatory system and train sensory perception of effort and internal cueing and scaling of adequate output. This approach is graphically represented in Figure 9-1. Administration of treatment four times a week for one month is consistent with principles of motor learning and skill

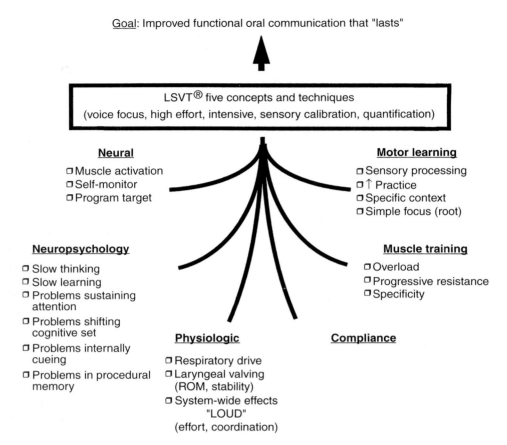

Goal: Improved functional oral communication that "lasts"

LSVT® five concepts and techniques
(voice focus, high effort, intensive, sensory calibration, quantification)

Neural
- ☐ Muscle activation
- ☐ Self-monitor
- ☐ Program target

Motor learning
- ☐ Sensory processing
- ☐ ↑ Practice
- ☐ Specific context
- ☐ Simple focus (root)

Neuropsychology
- ☐ Slow thinking
- ☐ Slow learning
- ☐ Problems sustaining attention
- ☐ Problems shifting cognitive set
- ☐ Problems internally cueing
- ☐ Problems in procedural memory

Muscle training
- ☐ Overload
- ☐ Progressive resistance
- ☐ Specificity

Physiologic
- ☐ Respiratory drive
- ☐ Laryngeal valving (ROM, stability)
- ☐ System-wide effects "LOUD" (effort, coordination)

Compliance

FIGURE 9-2. This figure graphically summarizes the rationale underlying the five essential concepts and techniques of the LSVT® from a neural, speech mechanism physiology, motor learning, muscle training, and neuropsychological compliance perspective. The *neural bases* are the reduction in muscle activation and self-monitoring and consequent problem in programming an output target with adequate amplitude. The *physiologic basis* is the focus on respiratory drive and laryngeal valving to generate a maximally efficient vocal source. "Loud" is used as the system trigger for improving effort and coordination across the speech mechanism. The LSVT® is administered in a manner consistent with *principles of motor learning* in order to maximize treatment effectiveness. Emphasis on sensory processing, increased practice, practice within specific context, and a simple "root" focus (e.g., "loud") are key elements of treatment. The LSVT® is also administered in a way consistent with *principles of muscle training*. Treatment technique overload the muscles using progressive resistance in specific activities. The *neuropsychological aspects* of Parkinson's diseases that may make learning challenging include slow thinking, slow learning, problems sustaining attention, problems shifting cognitive set, problems internally cueing, and problems in procedural memory. These aspects are also considered in the LSVT® through the simplicity and redundancy of treatment. The LSVT® is designed to maximize patient *compliance*. From day 1 of treatment, activities are designed to maximize impact on daily functional communication.

acquisition (120,121) and muscle training (122). In addition, the LSVT® is administered in a manner to maximize patient compliance by assigning treatment activities that make an *immediate* impact on daily functional communication. The rationale for the five concepts of the LSVT® is graphically represented in Figure 9-2.

Treatment Effectiveness Data for the LSVT®

The LSVT® was initially developed during the late 1980s, and initial Phase 1 type studies (e.g.,

case studies, single subject, designs, nonrandomized studies) were published based on that early work (123,124). These studies documented the first evidence of successful treatment outcomes and suggested that intensive treatment (four times a week for one month) focusing on increasing phonatory effort could improve communication in individuals with PD.

Based on those findings, a number of Phase 2 experimental studies (e.g., randomized, blinded) were carried out. In one study 45 individuals with PD were randomly assigned to one of two forms of treatment: respiratory treatment or respiratory and voice treatment (LSVT®). Short- (28) and long-term (29,125,126) outcome data have been reported from these studies. Significant pretreatment to posttreatment improvements were observed for more variables and were of greater magnitude for the subjects who received the voice and respiratory treatment (LSVT®) than for the subjects who received the respiratory treatment alone. Only subjects who received the LSVT® rated a significant posttreatment decrease on the impact of PD on their communication. Corresponding perceptual ratings by "blind" raters (127) revealed that listeners' perception of articulation and hoarseness pre- to posttreatment improved for males in *both* treatment groups. However, *only* the male subjects who had the LSVT® improved in ratings of breathiness and intonation. These findings were supported in studies at one-year (29,128) and two-year follow-up (126). Only those subjects in the LSVT® group improved or maintained vocal intensity above pretreatment levels. In addition, perceptual reports by patients and family members supported the positive impact of treatment on functional daily communication.

In another study (129), 29 individuals with PD were evaluated over six months. Half the group received the LSVT® and half of the group served as an untreated control group. In addition, an age-matched, nondisordered, nontreated control group was studied over this time period. Only subjects who received the LSVT® demonstrated significant increases in variables such as sound pressure level (related to loudness) and semitone standard deviation (related to intonation) at pre-, post-, and six-month follow-up.

An important aspect of this work was to evaluate the underlying speech mechanism changes accompanying treatment. A study by Smith and coworkers (55) documented increases in vocal fold closure following treatment in individuals who received the LSVT® but not in individuals who received respiratory treatment only. These data were collected outside of the treatment clinic by clinicians not directly involved in the study and therefore support *generalization* of treatment effects. Consistent with these findings, Ramig and Dromey (130) reported increased subglottal air pressure and maximum flow declination rate accompanying increased vocal SPL following the LSVT®. These findings were interpreted to be consistent with increased respiratory drive and vocal fold adduction accompanying successful treatment.

To evaluate application of the LSVT® to individuals with other neurologic disorders or conditions, a number of case studies were carried out during this time as well. In one case study, the LSVT® was applied to an individual with PD who had had thalamotomy (bilaterally) (107). In another study, the

LSVT® was applied to three individuals who had Parkinson plus syndromes of multisystem atrophy and progressive supranuclear palsy (131). Although improvements were documented in speech and voice characteristics in these individuals following treatment, the magnitude was not as great as in the subjects with PD. It was recommended that application of the LSVT® to individuals such as these be done on a case-by-case basis and that these patients be referred for treatment *early* in the course of their disease.

A finding of interest following the LSVT® has been the apparent generalization of effects starting with phonatory effort, from a focus on phonation, to additional changes throughout the vocal tract. Not only does increased phonatory effort apparently improve vocal characteristics (loudness, pitch variability, vocal quality), but also it appears to trigger effort and coordination across the speech mechanism. The observation of apparently larger movements in the upper articulatory system following the LSVT® is consistent with reports of Schulman (132) that as a speaker talks "louder" there are accompanying vocal tract and articulatory changes. Ramig and coworkers first reported documentation of this observation in individuals with PD pretreatment, to posttreatment (133). These generalized effects have since been reported in a pre-, post-, six-, and 12-month follow-up by Dromey and coworkers (125) and compared in subjects who received the LSVT® and respiratory treatment by Johnson and coworkers (134). These findings are graphically illustrated in Figure 9-3 and may be extremely useful observations in the attempt to improve efficiency and simplify speech treatment for individuals who may have

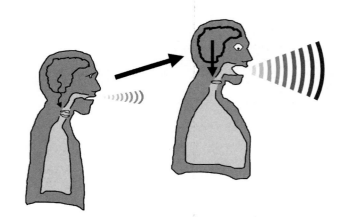

FIGURE 9-3. The LSVT® is designed to improve the phonatory source and scale-up amplitude across the speech mechanism with the global variable "LOUD." Increases in loudness can trigger increases in respiratory volumes, vocal fold adduction, articulatory valving, and vocal tract opening. These factors may all contribute to improved speech intelligibility with the simple target of "LOUD."

multiple speech mechanism problems and cognitive limitations, as is common in motor speech disorders.

PET scan data (135) found functional reorganization of speech motor areas within the brain following the LSVT®. Treatment-related changes were found in the right globus pallidus (GP) and in the supplementary motor area (SMA). In the GP resting state rCBF was significantly reduced posttreatment when compared with pretreatment and significantly increased during sustained phonation when compared with rest. The authors concluded that the LSVT® reduced baseline GP overactivity resembling the effect of pallidotomy. In addition, LSVT® increased GP activity during vocalization. These findings are important because they document the potential neural basis for behavioral changes following the LSVT®.

The goal of the LSVT® is to improve functional communication that lasts for at least six to 12 months without additional treatment. After the 16 sessions of individual treatment in one month, most patients will be able to maintain speech and voice changes for at least six months and sometimes for up to two years (29,126) without additional speech therapy. Within the 16 initial sessions of treatment, patients are encouraged to establish a daily homework routine that they maintain on their own once treatment is over. All patients are encouraged to return for a reassessment at six months, at which time some patients may benefit from a few "tune-up" sessions. Details of the LSVT® have been described elsewhere (97).

Treatment data suggest that individuals with mild to moderate PD have the most positive treatment outcomes following the LSVT®. Patients with co-occurring mild to moderate depression and dementia have succeeded in treatment as well (28). Because treatment focuses on voice, all patients must have a laryngeal examination before treatment to rule out any contraindications (vocal nodules, gastric reflux, laryngeal cancer). It is important to clarify that the goal of the LSVT® is to maximize phonatory efficiency. It is never the goal to teach "tight or pressed" voice but rather to improve vocal fold adduction for optimum loudness and quality.

Swallowing Treatment for Individuals with Parkinson's Disease

Treatment of the swallowing disorders that occur in PD has not been extensively studied. Conventional treatment techniques have included oral motor exercises to improve muscle strength, range of motion and coordination, and behavioral modifications such as the Mendelsohn maneuver, effortful breath-hold, swallow-cough, chin positioning, double swallow, effortful swallow, and diet and liquid modifications (18,136).

Effectiveness of these techniques varies and can be dependent on patient motivation and cooperation, family support, and the timeliness of the referral for a swallowing evaluation. A recent report studied the effects of the LSVT® on swallowing disorders that occur in individuals with PD (17). This study was conducted because of anecdotal reports from patients that their swallowing improved during or after the therapy course was finished. El Sharkawi and coworkers (17) found that the LSVT® reduced the swallowing motility disorders in the group studied by 51 percent. Some temporal measures of swallowing were also reduced, as was the amount of residue. This is the first study of its kind to find positive changes in *both* voice *and* swallowing function following intensive voice therapy alone without a therapy focus on swallowing. More research in this area is needed.

CONCLUSION

Speech, voice, and swallowing problems occur in most individuals with PD and may limit quality of life. Although all aspects of speech production may be affected, disordered voice is one of the most common problems. Previous forms of treatment for the disorder of speech and voice in individuals with PD have had modest effectiveness. The LSVT®, which addresses increased vocal effort and improved sensory perception of effort and is administered in 16 high-effort sessions in one month, has been extensively documented to be a successful approach in the short and long terms.

A wide variety of swallowing disorders in both the oral and pharyngeal stages of swallowing may occur in these patients as well. There are limited efficacy data on the treatment of these disorders, but behavioral and diet modification and the LSVT® may help minimize these difficulties. Although the degenerative course of PD cannot be altered at this time, improving oral communication and swallowing function are important components in developing the highest levels of functioning and independence for these individuals.

Acknowledgment

NIH-NIDCD RO1-DC01150 and P60 DC-00976

REFERENCES

1. Scott S, Caird FI, Williams BO. *Communication in Parkinson's Disease*. Rockville, MD: Aspen, 1985.
2. Atarashi J, Uchida E. A clinical study of parkinsonism. *Rec Adv Res Nerv Syst* 1959; 3:871–882.

3. Canter GJ. Speech characteristics of patients with Parkinson's disease: III. Articulation, diadochokinesis and overall speech adequacy. *J Speech Hearing Disord* 1965a; 30:217–224.

4. Canter GJ. Speech characteristics of patients with Parkinson's disease: II. Physiological support for speech. *J Speech Hearing Disord* 1965b; 30:44–49.

5. Hoberman SG. Speech techniques in aphasia and parkinsonism. *J Michigan State Med Soc* 1958; 57:1720–1723.

6. Logemann J, Fisher H, Boshes B, et al. Frequency and concurrence of vocal tract dysfunctions in the speech of a large sample of parkinson patients. *J Speech Hearing Disord* 1978; 43:47–57.

7. Mutch R, Strucwick A, Roy S, et al. Parkinson's disease: Disability review and management. *Br Med J* 1986; 293:675–677.

8. Oxtoby M. *Parkinson's Disease Patients and Their Social Needs*. London: Parkinson's Disease Society, 1982.

9. Selby G. Parkinson's disease. In: Vinken PJ, Bruyn GW (eds.). *Handbook of Clinical Neurology*. Amsterdam: North Holland, 1968.

10. Streifler M, Hofman S. Disorders of verbal expression in parkinsonism. In: Hassler RG, Christ JF (eds.). *Advances in Neurology*. New York: Raven Press, 1984.

11. Uziel A, Bohe M, Cadilhac J, et al. Les troubles de la voix et de la parole dans les syndromes Parkinson'siens. *Folia Phoniatrica* 1975; 27(3):166–176.

12. Hartelius L, Svensson P. Speech and swallowing symptoms associated with Parkinson's disease and multiple sclerosis: A survey. *Folia Phoniatrica Logopedica*. 1994; 46:9–17.

13. Aronson AE. *Clinical Voice Disorders*. New York: Thieme-Stratton, 1990.

14. King J, Ramig LO, Lemke J. Communication ability in Parkinson's disease in relation to employment satisfaction: A survey. Unpublished manuscript. 1996.

15. Leopold NA, Kagel MA. Laryngeal deglutition movement in Parkinson's disease. *Neurology* 1997; 48:373–375.

16. Croxson SC, Pye I. Dysphagia as the presenting symptom of Parkinson's disease. *Geriatr Med* 1988.

17. El Sharkawi A, Ramig LO, Logemann JA, et al. Swallowing and voice effects of of Lee Silverman Voice Treatment (LSVT®): A pilot study. In submission.

18. Logemann JA. *Evaluation and Treatment of Swallowing Disorders*. Texas: Pro-Ed, 1998.

19. Robbins J, Logemann JA, Kirshner H. Swallowing and speech production in Parkinson's disease. *Ann Neurol* 1986; 11:283–287.

20. Barbeau A, Sourkes TL, Murphy CF. Les catecholamines de la maladie de Parkinson's. In: Ajuriaguerra J (eds.). *Monoamines et Systeme Nerveux Central*. Geneve: George, 1962.

21. Birkmayer W, Kiewicz GH. Oder l-dioxyphenyalanin (l-dopa) effekt deim Parkinson-syndrom des menschen. *Arch Psychiatr Nervenkr* 1962; 203:560–574.

22. Svennilson E, et al. Treatment of parkinsonism by stereotactic thermolesions in the pallidal region: A clinical evaluation of 81 cases. *Acta Psych Neurol Scand* 1960; 35:358–377.

23. Freed CR, Breeze RE, Rosenberg NL, et al. Survival of implanted fetal dopamine cells and neurologic improvement 12 to 46 months after transplantation for Parkinson's disease. *N Engl J Med* 1992; 327(22):1549–1555.

24. Larson K, Ramig LO, Scherer RC. Acoustic and glottographic voice analysis during drug-related fluctuations in Parkinson's disease. *J Med Speech-Language Pathol* 1994; 2:211–226.

25. Baker K, Ramig LO, Johnson A, et al. Preliminary speech and voice analysis following fetal dopamine transplants in 5 individuals with Parkinson disease. *J Speech Hearing Res* 1997; 40(3):615–626.

26. Yorkston KM. Treatment Efficacy: Dysarthria. *J Speech Hearing Res* 1996; 39:S46–S57.

27. Helm N. Management of palilalia with a pacing board. *J Speech Hearing Disord* 1979; 44:350–353.

28. Ramig L, Countryman S, Thompson L, et al. Comparison of two forms of intensive speech treatment for Parkinson disease. *J Speech Hearing Res* 1995; 38:1232–1251.

29. Ramig LO, Countryman S, O'Brien C, et al. Intensive speech treatment for patients with Parkinson's disease: Short and long term comparison of two techniques. *Neurology* 1996; 47:1496–1504.

30. Leanderson R, Meyerson BA, Persson A. Lip muscle function in parkinsonian dysarthria. *Acta Otolaryngol* 1972; 74:350–357.

31. Leanderson R, Meyerson BA, Persson A. Effect of L-dopa on speech in parkinsonism: An EMG study of labial articulatory function. *J Neurol Neurosurg Psychiatry* 1971; 43:679–681.

32. Moore CA, Scudder RR. Coordination of jaw muscle activity in parkinsonian movement: Description and response to traditional treatment. In: Yorkston KM, Beukelman DR (eds.). *Recent Advances in Clinical Dysarthria*. Boston: College-Hill Press, 1989.

33. Baker K, Ramig LO, Luschei E, et al. Thyroarytenoid muscle activity associated with hypophonia in Parkinson disease and aging. *Neurology* 1998; 51(6):1592–1598.

34. Hansen DG, Gerratt BR, Ward PH. Cinegraphic observations of laryngeal function in Parkinson's disease. *Laryngoscope* 1984; 94:348–353.

35. Estenne M, Hubert M, Troyer AD. Respiratory-muscle involvement in Parkinson's disease. *N Engl J Med* 1984; 311:1516.

36. Ackermann H, Ziegler W. Articulatory deficits in parkinsonian dysarthria. *J Neurol Neurosurg Psychiatry* 1991; 54:1093–1098.

37. Hoodin RB, Gilbert HR. Nasal airflows in Parkinsonian speakers. *J Comm Disord* 1989a; 22:169–180.

38. Darley FL, Aronson AE, Brown JR. Clusters of deviant speech dimensions in the dysarthrias. *J Speech Hearing Res* 1969a; 12:462–469.

39. Darley FL, Aronson A, Brown J. Differential diagnostic patterns of dysarthria. *J Speech Hearing Res* 1969b; 12:246–269.

40. Darley FL, Aronson AE, Brown JR. *Motor Speech Disorders*. Philadelphia: W.B. Saunders, 1975.

41. Logemann J, Boshes B, Fisher H. The steps in the degeneration of speech and voice control in Parkinson's disease. In: J. Siegfried (eds.). *Parkinson's Diseases: Rigidity, Akinesia, Behavior*. Vienna: Hans Huber, 1973.

42. Ludlow CL, Bassich CJ. Relationships between perceptual ratings and acoustic measures of hypokinetic speech. In: McNeil MR, Rosenbek JC, Aronson AE (eds.). *The Dysarthrias: Physiology, Acoustics, Perception, Management*. San Diego: College-Hill Press, 1984.

43. Stewart C, Winfield L, Hunt A, et al. Speech dysfunction in early Parkinson's disease. *Mov Disord* 1995; 10(5):562–565.

44. Canter GJ. Speech characteristics of patients with Parkinson's disease: I. Intensity, pitch and duration. *J Speech Hearing Disord* 1963; 28:221–229.

45. Ludlow CL, Bassich CJ. Relationships between perceptual ratings and acoustic measures of hypokinetic speech. In: McNeil MR, Rosenbek JC, Aronson AE (eds.). *Dysarthria of Speech: Physiology-Acoustics-Linguistics-Management*. San Diego: College-Hill Press, 1983.

46. Metter EJ, Hanson WR. Clinical and acoustical variability in hypokinetic dysarthria. *J Comm Disord.* 1986; 19:

47. Fox C, Ramig L. Sound pressure level and self-perception of speech and voice in men and women who have idiopathic Parkinson disease. *Am J Speech Language Pathol* 1997.

48. King J, et al. Parkinson's disease: Longitudinal changes in acoustic parameters of phonation. *J Med Speech-Language Pathol* 1994; 2:29–42.

49. Zwirner P, Murry T, Woodson GE. Phonatory function of neurologically impaired patients. *J Comm Disord* 1991; 24:287–300.

50. Ramig LA, Titze OR, Scherer R, et al. Acoustic analysis of voices of patients with neurologic disease: Rationale and preliminary data. *Ann Otolaryngol Rhinol Laryngol* 1988; 97:164–172.

51. Ramig LA, Shipp T. Comparative measures of vocal tremor and vocal vibrato. *J Voice* 1987; 1:162–167.

52. Ludlow CL, et al. Phonatory characteristics of vocal fold tremor. *J Phonet* 1986; 14: 509–515.

53. Philippbar SA, Robin DA, Luschei ES. Limb, jaw and vocal tremor in Parkinson's patients. In: Yorkston KM, Beukelman DR (eds.). *Recent Advances in Clinical Dysarthria*. Boston: College-Hill Press, 1989.

54. Winholtz WS, Ramig LO. Vocal tremor analysis with the vocal demodulator. *NCVS Status Prog Rep* 1992; 2:119–137.

55. Smith M, Ramig LO, Dromey C, et al. Intensive voice treatment in Parkinson's disease: Laryngostroboscopic findings. *J Voice* 1995; 9:453–459.

56. Perez K, Ramig LO, Smith M, et al. The Parkinson larynx: Tremor and videostroboscopic findings. *J Voice* 1996; 10:354–361.

57. Gerratt BR, Hansen DG, Berke GS. Glottographic measures of laryngeal function in individuals with abnormal motor control. In: Baer T, Sasaki C, Harris K (eds.). *Laryngeal Function in Phonation and Respiration*. Boston: College-Hill Press, 1987.

58. Hirose H, Joshita Y. Laryngeal behavior in patients with disorders of the central nervous system. In: Hirano M, Kirchner JA, Bless DM (eds.). *Neurolaryngology: Recent Advances*. Boston: Little, Brown, 1987.

59. Luschei ES, Ramig LO, Baker KL, et al. Discharge characteristics of laryngeal single motor units during phonation in young and older adults and in persons with Parkinson disease. *J Neurophysiol* 1999; 81:2131–2139.

60. Cramer W. De spaak bij patienten met Parkinsonisme. *Logop Phoniatr.* 1940; 22: 17–23.

61. De la Torre R, Mier M, Boshes B. Evaluation of respiratory function: Preliminary observations. *Quart Bull Northwestern Univ Med School* 1960; 34:332–336.

62. Laszewski Z. Role of the department of rehabilitation in preoperative evaluation of parkinsonian patients. *J Am Geriatr Soc* 1956; 4:1280–1284.

63. Mueller PB. Parkinson's disease: Motor-speech behavior in a selected group of patients. *Folia Phoniatr* 1971; 23:333–346.

64. Marquardt TP. *Characteristics of Speech in Parkinson's Disease: Electromyographic, Structural Movement and Aerodynamic Measurements*. Seattle: University of Washington, 1973.

65. Solomon NP, Hixon TJ. Speech breathing in Parkinson's disease. *J Speech Hearing Res* 1993; 36:294–310.

66. Schiffman PL. A "saw-tooth" pattern in Parkinson's disease. *Chest* 1985; 87:124–126.

67. Vincken WG, Gauthier SG, Dollfuss RE, et al. Involvement of upper-airway muscles in extrapyramidal disorders, a cause of airflow limitation. *N Engl J Med* 1984; 311(7):438–442.

68. Murdoch BE, Chenery HJ, Bowler S, et al. Respiratory function in Parkinson's subjects exhibiting a perceptible speech deficit: A kinematic and spirometric analysis. *J Speech Hearing Disord* 1989; 54:610–626.

69. Hammen VL, Yorkston KM, Beukelman DR. Pausal and speech duration characteristics as a function of speaking rate in normal and parkinsonian dysarthric individuals. In: Yorkston KM, Beukelman DR (ed.). *Recent Advances in Clinical Dysarthria*. Boston: College-Hill Press, 1989.

70. Hanson WR, Metter EJ. DAF speech rate modification in Parkinson's disease: A report of two cases. In: Berry WR (eds.). *Clinical Dysarthria*. San Diego: College-Hill Press, 1983.

71. Adams SG. Hypokinetic dysarthria in Parkinson's disease. In: McNeil MR (ed.). *Clinical Management of*

Sensorimotor Speech Disorders. New York: Thieme, 1997.

72. Sapir S, Pawlas AA, Ramig O, et al. Speech and voice abnormalities in Parkinson disease: Relation to severity of motor impairment, duration of disease, medication, depression, gender, and age. In submission.

73. Weismer G. Articulatory characteristics of parkinsonian dysarthria: Segmental and phrase-level timing, spirantization and glottal-supraglottal coordination. In: McNeil M, Rosenbek J, Aronson A (eds.). *The Dysarthrias: Physiology, Acoustics, Perception and Management.* San Diego: College Hill Press, 1984.

74. Forrest K, Weismer G, Turner G. Kinematic, acoustic and perceptual analysis of connected speech produced by parkinsonian and normal geriatric adults. *J Acoustic Soc Am* 1989; 85:2608–2622.

75. Caliguri MP. Labial kinematics during speech in patients with parkinsonian rigidity. *Brain* 1987; 110:1033–1044.

76. Caliguri MP. The influence of speaking rate on articulatory hypokinesia in parkinsonian dysarthria. *Brain Language* 1989a; 36:493–502.

77. Caliguri MP. Short-term fluctuations in orofacial motor control in Parkinson's disease. In: Yorkson KM, Beukelman DR (eds.). *Recent Advances in Clinical Dysarthria.* Boston: College Hill Press, 1989b.

78. Conner NP, Abbs JH. Task-dependent variations in parkinsonian motor impairments. *Brain* 1991; 114:321–332.

79. Conner NP, Abbs JH, Cole KJ, et al. Parkinsonian deficits in serial mulitarticulate movements for speech. *Brain* 1989; 112(pt. 4):997–1009.

80. Hirose H, Kiritani S, Ushijima T, et al. Patterns of dysarthric movements in patients with parkinsonism. *Folia Phoniatr* 1981; 33(4):204–215.

81. Hirose H. Pathophysiology of motor speech disorders (dysarthria). *Folia Phoniatr (Basel)* 1986; 38:61–88.

82. Hunker CJ, Abbs JH, Barlow SM. The relationship between parkinsonian rigidity and hypokinesia in the orofacial system: A quantitative analysis. *Neurology* 1982; 32:749–754.

83. Hunker CJ, Abbs JH. Physiological analyses of parkinsonian tremors in the orofacial system. In: McNeil MR, Rosenbek JC, Aronson AE (eds.). *The Dysarthrias: Physiology, Acoustics, Perception, Management.* San Diego: College-Hill Press, 1984.

84. Netsell R, Daniel B, Celesia GG. Acceleration and weakness in parkinsonian dysarthria. *J Speech Hearing Disord* 1975; 40:170–178.

85. Hoodin RB, Gilbert HR. Parkinsonian dysarthria: An aerodynamic and perceptual description of velopharyngeal closure for speech. *Folia Phoniatr* 1989b; 41:249–258.

86. Koller WC. Sensory symptoms in PD. *Neurology* 1984; 34:957–959.

87. Tatton WG, Eastman, MJ, Bedingham W, et al. Defective utilization of sensory input as the basis for bradykinesia, rigidity and decreased movement repertoire in Parkinson's disease: A hypothesis. *Can J Neurosci* 1984; 11:136–143.

88. Albin RL, Young AB, Penny JB. The functional anatomy of basal ganglia disorders. *Trends Neurosci* 1989; 12:366–375.

89. Penny JB, Young AB. Speculations on the functional anatomy of basal ganglia disorders. *Annu Rev Neurosci* 1983; 6:73–94.

90. Berardelli A, Dick JP, Rothwell JC, et al. Scaling of the size of the first agonist EMG burst during rapid wrist movements in patients with Parkinson's disease. *J Neurol Neurosurg Psychiatry* 1986; 49(11):1273–1279.

91. Hallet M, (ed.). Sensorimotor integration and mysterious sensory phenomena in movement disorders. *Motor Control.* American Academy of Neurology, 1997.

92. Demirci M, Grill McShane, Hallet M. Impairment of kinesthesia in Parkinson's disease. *Neurology* 1995; 45:A218.

93. Schneider JS, Lidsky TI. *Basal Ganglia and Behavior: Sensory Aspects of Motor Functioning.* Toronto: Hans Huber, 1987.

94. Schneider JS, Diamond SG, Markham CH. Deficits in orofacial sensorimotor function in Parkinson's disease. *Ann Neurol* 1986; 19:275–282.

95. Solomon NP, et al. Tongue function testing in Parkinson's disease: Indicators of fatigue. In: Till JA, Yorkston KM, Beukelman DR (eds.). *Motor Speech Disorders: Advances in Assessment and Treatment.* Baltimore: Paul H. Brookes, 1994.

96. Ramig LO, Fox C, Morrison. Motor, sensory, and neuropsychological bases for successful speech treatment in individuals with Parkinson disease: Why has the LSVT® been successful? Unpublished manuscript.

97. Ramig LO, Pawlas A, Countryman S. *The Lee Silverman Voice Treatment (LSVT): A Practical Guide to Treating the Voice and Speech Disorders in Parkinson Disease.* Iowa City, IA: National Center for Voice and Speech and LSVT Foundation (1-888-606-5788), 1995b.

98. Nilsson H. *Quantitative Aspects of Swallowing.* Department of Neurology, Sweden, 1998.

99. Stroudley J, Walsh M. Radiographic assessment of dysphagia in Parkinson's disease. *Br J Radiol* 1991; 64:890–893.

100. Critchley EMR. Speech disorders of parkinsonism: A review. *J Neurol Neurosurg Psychiatry* 1981; 44:751–758.

101. Mawdsley C, Gamsu CV. Periodicity of speech in parkinsonism. *Nature* 1971; 231:315–316.

102. Mawdsley C. Speech and levodopa. *Adv Neurol* 1973; 3:33–47.

103. Nakano KK, Zubick H, Tyley HR. Speech defects of parkinsonian patients. *Neurology* 1973;

104. Rigrodsky S, Morrison EB. Speech changes in parkinsonism during L-dopa therapy: Preliminary findings. *J Am Geriatr Soc* 1970; 18:142–151.

105. Wolfe VI, et al. Speech changes in Parkinson's disease during treatment with L-dopa. *J Comm Disord* 1975; 8(3):271–279.

106. Yaryura-Tobias JA, Diamond B, Merlis S. Verbal communication with L-dopa treatment. *Nature* 1971; 234:224–225.

107. Countryman S, Ramig LO. Effects of intensive voice therapy on speech deficits associated with bilateral thalamotomy in Parkinson's disease: A case study. *J Med Speech-Language Pathol* 1993; 1(4):233–249.

108. Ghika J, Ghika Schmid F, Fankhauser H, et al. Bilateral contemporaneous posteroventral pallidotomy for the treatment of Parkinson's disease: Neuropsychological and neurological side effects. Report of four cases and review of the literature. *J Neurosurg* 1999; 91(2):313–321.

109. Schultz GM, Peterson T, Sapienza CM, et al. Voice and speech characteristics of persons with Parkinson's disease pre- and post-pallidotomy surgery: Preliminary findings. *J Speech Hearing Res* 1999.

110. Weiner WJ, Lang AE. *Movement Disorders; A Comprehensive Survey.* Mount Kisco, NY: Futura, 1989.

111. Sarno MT. Speech impairment in Parkinson's disease. *Arch Phys Med Rehabil* 1968:269–275.

112. Allan CM. Treatment of non-fluent speech resulting from neurological disease: Treatment of dysarthria. *Br J Disord Comm* 1970; 5:3–5.

113. Greene HCL. *The Voice and Its Disorders.* London: Pitman Medical, 1980.

114. Downie AW, Low JM, Lindsay DD. Speech disorders in parkinsonism: Usefulness of delayed auditory feedback in selected cases. *Br J Disord Comm* 1981a; 16:135–139.

115. Scott S, Caird FL. Speech therapy for Parkinson's disease. *J Neurology Neurosurg Psychiatry* 1983; 46:140–144.

116. Rubow RT, Swift E. A microcomputer-based wearable biofeedback device to improve transfer of treatment in parkinsonian dysarthria. *J Speech Hearing Disord* 1985; 50:178–185.

117. McNamara P, Obler LK, Au R, et al. Speech monitoring skills in Alzheimer's disease, Parkinson's disease and normal aging. *Brain Language* 1992; 42:38–51.

118. Saint-Cyr JA, Taylor AE, Lang AE. Procedural learning and neostriatial dysfunction in man. *Brain* 1988; 111.

119. Stelmach GE. Basal ganglia impairment and force control. In: Requin J, Stelmach GE (eds.). *Tutorial in Motor Neuroscience.* Netherlands: Kluwer Academic Publishers, 1991.

120. Schmidt RA. *Motor Control and Learning.* Champaign, Ill.: Human Kinetic Publishers, 1988.

121. Schmidt RA. A schema theory of discrete motor skill learning. *Psychol Rev* 1975; 82:225–260.

122. Astrand PO, Rodahl K. *Textbook of Work Physiology.* New York: McGraw-Hill, 1970.

123. Ramig LO, Bonitati C, Lemke J, et al. Voice treatment for patients with Parkinson disease: Development of an approach and preliminary efficacy data. *J Med Speech-Language Pathol* 1994; 2:191–209.

124. Ramig LO. The role of phonation in speech intelligibility: A review and preliminary data from patients with Parkinson's disease. In: Kent RD (ed.). *Intelligibility in Speech Disorders: Theory, Measurement and Management.* Amsterdam: John Benjamin, 1992.

125. Dromey C, Ramig LO, Johnson A. Phonatory and articulatory changes associated with increased vocal intensity in Parkinson disease: A case study. *J Speech Hearing Res* 1995; 38:751–763.

126. Ramig LO, Sapir S, Countryman S, et al. Intensive voice treatment (LSVT®) for individuals with Parkinson's disease: A 2 year follow-up. In review.

127. Baumgartner C, Sapir S, Ramig L. Voice quality changes following Phonatory-Respiratory Effort treatment (LSVT®) versus Respiratory Effort Treatment for Individuals with Parkinson Disease. *J. Voice* in press.

128. Sapir S, Ramig LO, Hoyt P, et al. *Phonatory-respiratory effort (LSVT®) vs. respiratory effort treatment for hypokinetic dysarthria: Comparing speech loudness and quality before and 12 months after treatment.* A paper presented to the International Congress on Parkinson Disease. July, 1999, Vancouver.

129. Ramig LO, Sapir S, Fox C, et al. Changes in SPL following intensive voice treatment (LSVT®) in individuals with Parkinson disease: Comparison with untreated patients and with age-matched normal controls. In press.

130. Ramig LO, Dromey C. Aerodynamic mechanisms underlying treatment-related changes in SPL in patients with Parkinson disease. *J Speech Hearing Res* 1996; 39:798–807.

131. Countryman S, Ramig LO, Pawlas AA. Speech and voice deficits in parkinsonian plus syndromes: Can they be treated? *J Med Speech-Language Pathol* 1994; 2:211–225.

132. Schulman R. Articulatory dynamics of loud and normal speech. *J Acoustic Soc Am* 1989; 85: 295–312.

133. Ramig LO, et al. *The Effects of Phonatory, Respiratory and Articulatory Treatment on Speech and Voice in Parkinson's Disease.* Sedona, AZ: 1994

134. Johnson A, Strand E, Ramig L. The effect of intensive respiratory and laryngeal treatment on single word speech intelligibility and select articulatory acoustics in patients with Parkinson's disease. *J Med Speech-Language Pathol.* In preparation.

135. Liotti M, Vogel D, New P, et al. *A PET study of functional reorganization of premotor regions in Parkinson's disease following intensive speech and voice treatment (LSVT®).* A paper presented to the Academy of Neurology, November, 1998.

136. Yorkston KM, Miller RM, Strand EA. *Management of Speech and Swallowig in Degenerative Diseases.* Communication Skill Builders, 1997.

10

Gastrointestinal Features

Eamonn M.M. Quigley, MD, FRCP, FACP, FACG
University of Nebraska Medical Center, Omaha, Nebraska

INTRODUCTION AND BACKGROUND

Although it has been recognized for some time that gastrointestinal problems are common among patients with Parkinson's disease (PD) and are frequently distressing, their pathophysiology, evaluation, and management has until recently received relatively little attention. This chapter reviews the current status of our understanding of gastrointestinal function in PD, outlines an approach to the evaluation and management of these symptoms, and speculates on some future prospects in this area.

AN OVERVIEW OF GASTROINTESTINAL MOTOR FUNCTION

Although in theory several gastrointestinal functions could be disturbed in PD, in relation either to the disease process itself or to its therapy, this chapter focuses on the gastrointestinal function that has received the greatest attention in this context, namely, gastrointestinal motility. Before specific abnormalities in gastrointestinal motor function in PD are discussed, a brief overview of gastrointestinal motor function is appropriate.

Given its essential role in digestion, absorption, secretion, and excretion, the gastrointestinal tract and its associated organs play an essential role in homeostasis. The various physiologic processes of the gastrointestinal tract serve these functions. Thus motility propels food, chyme, and stool and promotes mixing to increase contact time and, thereby, digestion. Gut muscle and nerve are integrated into a "mini-brain" and are adapted to subserve these homeostatic functions. Throughout most of the gastrointestinal

tract gut, smooth muscle is arranged in two layers, an outer longitudinal layer and an inner circular layer. At the beginning and end of the gut, striated muscle is found in the oropharynx, upper esophageal sphincter, and proximal part of the esophagus, and in the external anal sphincter and pelvic floor muscles, respectively. In these locations, somatic innervation plays a crucial role in the regulation of swallowing and defecation; these functions are, not surprisingly, particularly prone to disruption in neurologic disease. Throughout the remainder of the gut, several levels of control are evident. Myogenic regulation of motility refers to the intrinsic properties of gut muscle cells and their interactions with one another. Next comes the enteric nervous system, which is now recognized as a distinct and independent division of the autonomic nervous system (1). The enteric nervous system may represent the most important level of neuronal control of motility and is capable of generating and modulating many functions within the gastrointestinal tract without input from the more traditional divisions of the autonomic and central nervous systems. Through variations in neuronal morphology and in the electrophysiologic properties of individual neurons, as well as through the presence of a wide variety of neurotransmitters and neuromodulatory peptides, the enteric nervous system demonstrates striking plasticity. Of relevance to any discussion of the gut in central nervous system disorders, it is now recognized that the enteric and central nervous systems share many similarities, both morphologic and functional. For example, almost all neurotransmitters identified within the central nervous system are also found in enteric neurons – the concept of enteric nervous system involvement in neurologic disease should not come as a great surprise. Although the enteric nervous system is primarily responsible for the generation and modulation of most motor activities within the gut, input from autonomic nerves and the central nervous system also modulates motor activity – autonomic input in now recognized to be exerted primarily through the modulation of enteric nervous system activity. It has also been recognized recently that the gut has important sensory functions, which are perceived within the central nervous system and play a fundamental role in several reflex events in the gut (2). Indeed, sensory dysfunction is now also believed to play an important role in the pathogenesis of a variety of functional gastrointestinal disorders (2).

The following is a brief overview of the motor functions of the principal organs of the gastrointestinal tract. Swallowing is a complex and highly organized act, traditionally divided into two phases: oropharyngeal and esophageal. The oropharyngeal phase includes the transfer of the food bolus to the pharynx, pharyngeal peristalsis, and propulsion through the upper esophageal sphincter into the esophageal body. This is accomplished through the precisely coordinated action of several muscle groups, including those of the tongue, pharynx, and upper esophageal sphincter. Cranial nerves V, VII, IX, X, and XII convey the afferent and efferent signals involved in this phase of swallowing, which is coordinated in a swallowing center in the reticular formation in the brain stem (3). The esophageal phase of swallowing is primarily a function of the smooth muscle esophagus and is regulated centrally via vagal afferents and peripherally by the intrinsic properties of esophageal smooth muscle (4). Transport of the bolus from the esophagus to the stomach involves the simultaneous generation of a peristaltic sequence in the esophageal body and complete relaxation of the lower esophageal sphincter; the latter is mediated by a prominent inhibitory innervation at the sphincter.

The main functions of gastric motility are to accommodate and store the ingested meal, grind down or triturate the solid particles, and then empty the homogenized meal in a regulated fashion into the duodenum (5,6). Small intestinal motility should serve to mix the meal with intestinal secretions and propel chyme and undigested material in an aboral direction as appropriate (6). The lower esophageal, pyloric, and ileocecal sphincters regulate transit between adjacent organs and prevent oral reflux.

Colonic motility is less well characterized in humans. Mixing and retropulsion appear to dominate in the right colon, whereas storage and intermittent aboral propulsion are the dominant functions on the left side (7,8). Finally, the anal canal and distal rectum play a crucial role in the regulation of defecation and the maintenance of continence.

GASTROINTESTINAL DYSFUNCTION IN PARKINSON'S DISEASE – HISTORICAL BACKGROUND AND PRINCIPAL FEATURES

The cardinal gastrointestinal manifestations of PD were clearly and vividly described in Parkinson's original monograph in 1817 (9). Referring to swallowing difficulties, he stated "food is with difficulty retained in the mouth until swallowed; and then is difficultly swallowed – the saliva fails of being directed to the back part of the fauces, and hence is continually draining from the mouth." He also recognized problems with constipation and defecation: "the bowels, which all along had been torpid, now in most cases, demand stimulating medicines of very considerable power: the expulsion of the feces from the rectum sometimes requiring mechanical aid." Thereafter, gastrointestinal manifestations of PD received relatively little attention until the latter half of the twentieth century. A number of surveys then described a high frequency of drooling, dysphagia, gastroesophageal reflux, delayed gastric emptying, and constipation among patients (10,15). A number of factors were invoked to explain the pathophysiology of these symptoms, including alterations in diet, reduced activity, side effects of antiparkinsonian medications, and associated autonomic dysfunction (16). The true prevalence of gastrointestinal symptoms in PD and their relationship to the disease process itself were not defined until the past decade. In a series of studies that (1) included age- and gender- matched controls, (2) employed validated study instruments, and (3) provided follow-up, Edwards and colleagues confirmed a high prevalence of esophageal and colo-rectal symptoms among patients with PD, regardless of therapy (17,19). Among 98 patients, disordered salivation (70%), dysphagia (52%), nausea (24%), constipation (29%), and defecatory dysfunction (66%) emerged as the gastrointestinal symptoms that were truly more common in PD (17). Only PD severity and the duration of disease correlated with gastrointestinal symptoms; patient age, gender, level of activity, dietary fiber intake, and antiparkinsonian therapy did not (17). These findings appeared to support Parkinson's original hypothesis, namely, that gastrointestinal symptoms are a component of the disease process itself.

DYSPHAGIA IN PARKINSON'S DISEASE

Swallowing difficulty is one of the most common, distressing, and challenging gastrointestinal problems in PD. Because of the risk of aspiration and its impact on nutrition, disordered swallowing function is indeed potentially life-threatening. The primary symptoms are drooling and dysphagia, the latter usually described as a sensation of food sticking at the level of the thyroid cartilage. It is crucial to understand that in PD drooling and difficulty with saliva are manifestations of disordered swallowing and not of abnormal salivation. Patients with PD do not secrete excess saliva; indeed, salivary output in PD is either normal or decreased (10,16). Drooling reflects a difficulty in transporting saliva to the posterior pharynx. Up to 30 percent of patients with PD describe respiratory symptoms such as coughing, choking, or nocturnal dyspnea in association with dysphagia (17). The recent, carefully performed study of Ali and colleagues has considerably clarified the pathogenesis of dysphagia in PD. Among the many components of swallowing studied, lingual tremor, impaired pharyngeal peristalsis, and restricted opening of the upper esophageal sphincter were those that predicted dysphagia in patients (20). Given the important role of tongue pulsion in generating the force that propels the bolus through the upper esophageal sphincter, the central role of lingual tremor in the pathogenesis of dysphagia among these patients can be readily understood. Impaired opening of the upper esophageal sphincter may lead to the appearance of cricopharyngeal "bars" on radiologic studies and to the development of Zenker's diverticula (20).

The clinician needs to be aware of one potential trap in the clinical assessment of the parkinsonian patient with dysphagia, namely, the false localization of dysphagia to the region of the upper esophageal sphincter by PD patients whose disease process lies in the distal esophagus (22). Although the true prevalence of gastroesophageal reflux in PD remains to be determined, it is certainly clear that PD patients are not immune from reflux disease or of such complications such as peptic esophageal strictures. For reasons that remain poorly understood, these patients frequently present with dysphagia, which is indistinguishable from that associated with the PD process itself – a failure to recognize this and to fully investigate all PD patients with dysphagia will lead to inappropriate therapy. If recognized, appropriate therapy of gastroesophageal reflux disease may lead to significant improvement in dysphagia. The true prevalence of disturbed motor function in the esophageal body and lower esophageal sphincter in PD remain to be determined.

NAUSEA, VOMITING, DYSPEPSIA, AND GASTRIC FUNCTION IN PARKINSON'S DISEASE

Nausea and vomiting are common symptoms among patients with PD and are the symptoms that may clearly be directly related to the central effects of dopaminergic medications. However, the survey performed by Edwards and colleagues indicated that nausea may be a feature of PD (17) per se, and some studies suggest a high prevalence of gastroparesis in PD (23,24). Gastric emptying may play a crucial role in the management of patients with PD, especially in those with prominent "on"–"off" fluctuations. These individuals are dependent on an accurately timed delivery of dopaminergic medications from the stomach to their site of absorption in the small intestine (25). In such individuals, relatively minor fluctuations in gastric emptying rate could significantly disrupt PD control. There is some evidence that prokinetic medications may help to smooth control in these patients (23,26). It is surprising that the true status of gastric motility in PD remains unclear and that there have been few, if any, appropriately performed studies of any parameter of gastric motor function in this patient population. Those that have been performed have either not employed appropriate controls or have failed to correct the possible influence of dopaminergic medications. A recent study using the noninvasive technique of electrogastrography also indicated that gastric motility may indeed be disturbed in PD, irrespective of dopaminergic therapy (27). Further studies are clearly needed.

Although severe disruption of small intestinal motility resulting in pseudo-obstruction and ileus has been reported in PD, we know very little regarding small bowel motility in this disease.

CONSTIPATION, DIFFICULT DEFECATION, AND COLONIC AND ANORECTAL FUNCTION

Constipation and difficult defecation are the most common gastrointestinal symptoms among patients with established PD (17). Symptom assessments and formal tests of colonic and anorectal function suggest that both delayed colonic transit (i.e., abnormal motility of the colon) and defecatory dysfunction (i.e., dys-coordinate activity in the pelvic floor and sphincter muscles) contribute to symptom development (17). Furthermore, many patients exhibit features of both abnormalities. Slow transit constipation may progress to megacolon and even fatal perforation.

Formal studies of the defecatory mechanism in these patients suggest that an inability to relax the puborectalis muscle on straining, and thereby "straighten out" the anal canal to facilitate defecation, is a common and important contributing feature (19,28). Direct electromyographic recordings from the sphincter muscles in affected patients have demonstrated that, while the function of the internal anal sphincter is preserved, the external sphincter, puborectalis, and levator ani muscles are stimulated and may "paradoxically" contract as the patient attempts to defecate (29–31). These abnormalities appear similar to those described in the urinary tract in PD.

THE PATHOPHYSIOLOGY OF GASTROINTESTINAL DYSFUNCTION IN PARKINSON'S DISEASE – AVAILABLE EVIDENCE AND FUTURE PROSPECTS

In the past, gastrointestinal symptoms in PD were largely ascribed to side effects of antiparkinsonian medications, inactivity, and dietary changes. It now appears unlikely that, apart from inducing nausea and vomiting, dopaminergic medications have a central role in the pathogenesis of gastrointestinal dysfunction in PD. The balance of evidence now suggests that most gastrointestinal symptoms reflect the direct involvement of parts of the gastrointestinal tract by the primary disease process. Dysphagia, resulting from lingual tremor or impaired opening of the upper oesophageal sphincter, and obstructive defecation, consequent upon an impaired puborectalis response to straining, appear to be based on disturbances in skeletal muscle function analogous to other, better recognized manifestations of this disease process. Although the prevalence and severity of these symptoms have been shown to correlate with the severity and duration of disease (17) and to parallel disease activity in those with prominent "on"–"off" fluctuations, the response of these symptoms to dopaminergic therapy in general has been either disappointing or entirely absent (20). The basis for this paradox remains unexplained.

Skeletal muscle involvement cannot explain gastrointestinal symptoms originating from most of the gastrointestinal tract, lined as it is by smooth muscle and controlled by the enteric and autonomic nervous systems. Autonomic dysfunction could certainly play a role, given its prevalence in PD and its prominence in some PD-related syndromes such as the Shy-Drager syndrome. Relationships between autonomic dysfunction and gastrointestinal dysfunction in PD have not been examined directly.

Evidence has accumulated to suggest a more direct involvement of the gastrointestinal tract in PD. Lewy bodies have been identified in autonomic neurons supplying the gastrointestinal tract (32) as well as in the enteric nervous system of the esophagus and colon (33,34). Furthermore, Singaram and colleagues have documented severe depletion of dopaminergic neurons in the colon in a small number of patients with PD and severe constipation (35). Further studies are needed to delineate the extent of dopamine depletion in the enteric nervous system and to define its relationship to symptoms and motor dysfunction in affected PD patients. It is tempting to speculate that further studies of the enteric nervous system may provide valuable insights into the basic mechanisms of disease initiation and progression in PD. The enteric nervous system could serve as a window to the central nervous system (36).

MANAGEMENT OF GASTROINTESTINAL COMPLICATIONS IN PARKINSON'S DISEASE

Few studies have directly addressed the therapy of gastrointestinal symptoms in PD. Those studies that have examined the symptomatic response to dopaminergic therapy among PD patients with dysphagia have provided disappointing results. For patients with dysphagia, emphasis must be placed, in the first instance, on its early recognition and, second, on the institution of counseling, nutritional modifications, and swallowing maneuvers designed to promote efficient deglutition and to minimize the risk of aspiration. If aspiration has occurred and is likely to recur, alternate routes of nutrition may need to be considered. For most patients a percutaneous, endoscopically placed gastrostomy (PEG) provides an acceptable and safe alternative and avoids the need for intravenous access and total parenteral nutrition.

Nausea and vomiting may present a formidable therapeutic challenge in PD. Metoclopramide and phenothiazines should not be used because of their propensity to cause or exacerbate parkinsonian symptoms. Cisapride, a prokinetic devoid of a central antiemetic action, may accelerate gastric emptying but has not been shown to alleviate nausea and vomiting in this patient population. The peripheral dopamine antagonist domperidone would appear the ideal alternative, given that it does not cross the blood–brain barrier, yet is both an antiemetic and a prokinetic. Limited studies suggest its efficacy, not only as an antiemetic but also as a useful adjunct to dopaminergic therapy in those who may be experiencing impaired delivery of dopaminergic medications from the stomach (37). In patients experiencing nausea and vomiting from levodopa, the use of additional carbidopa (Lodosyn) can be very helpful. Tablets contain 25 mg of carbidopa, and one tablet with each levodopa dose may be sufficient to alleviate these adverse symptoms.

The management of constipation and difficult defecation begins with the exclusion of other causes of these symptoms, particularly depression. Given the increased prevalence of depression among patients with PD and the frequency with which elderly patients with depression present with lower gastrointestinal symptoms, this disorder needs to be considered and sought for in this patient population. The management of constipation can often prove difficult. Although simple measures such as increasing fluid intake and advocating ingestion of dietary fiber (38) may prove helpful in some patients, many continue to be symptomatic; some, and especially those with difficult defecation, are poorly tolerant of conventional laxative approaches. A few therapeutic strategies had been subjected to formal clinical trials in the PD patient with constipation. There are limited data to suggest efficacy for psyllium (39) and cisapride (40,41) in those with slow transit constipation. Short-term studies in a small number of patients provide some evidence to indicate that the potent dopaminergic agent apomorphine may improve anorectal and pelvic floor coordination and promote evacuation (42). A similar approach has been adopted among PD patients with problems with micturition. One approach that we have found helpful is the use of polyethylene glycol–based solutions as laxatives. These agents, commonly used in large volume for bowel cleansing prior to barium enema studies and colonoscopy, are administered on a daily basis in much smaller volumes and increased until a regular soft stool is obtained (43). This approach is generally well tolerated and is usually not complicated by the distension and bloating associated with many osmotic agents. It is important to emphasize that in the patient with severe constipation considerable emphasis must be placed on achieving regular evacuation by whatever means. In this way silent progression to megacolon and perforation may be avoided (44,47).

In non-PD patients with disturbed defecation and similar abnormalities in anal sphincter/pelvic floor coordination, biofeedback has proved effective. This strategy has not been assessed in PD and may be difficult to achieve given the prevalence of cognitive dysfunction and significant physical impairment associated with this disease process.

CONCLUSION

Gastrointestinal symptoms are common in patients with established PD and may represent a major challenge to the patient, their family, and their health care providers. The nature of the gastrointestinal symptoms truly associated with PD has been considerably clarified, and the prominence of disturbed swallowing and difficult defecation has become ever more evident. The pathogenesis of these symptoms has been considerably elucidated, and the balance of evidence now supports the direct involvement of the gastrointestinal tract by the PD process as the primary cause of gastrointestinal symptoms. Recent studies suggesting the direct involvement of the enteric nervous system by the PD process are particularly intriguing, and we look forward to considerable progress in this area. In the meantime, the clinician should remain alert to the importance of gastrointestinal dysfunction in this common degenerative neurologic disease and should be aware of relatively simple management strategies that may serve to avoid complications and significantly alleviate distress.

REFERENCES

1. Goyal RK, Hirano I. Mechanisms of disease: The enteric system. *N Engl J Med* 1996; 334:1106–1115.
2. Mayer EA, Gebhart GF. Basic and clinical aspects of visceral hyperalgesia. *Gastroenterology* 1994; 107:271–293.
3. Morrell RM. The neurology of swallowing, In: Groher ME (ed.). *Dysphagia and Management*. City: Butterworths, 1984; 12–18.
4. Diamant N. Firing up the swallowing. *Mech Mature Med* 1996; 2:1190–1191.
5. Malagelada J-R, Azpiroz F. Determinants of gastric emptying and transit in the small intestine. *Handbook of Physiology*. 2nd ed. *The Gastrointestinal System*, Vol. 1, Part 2, 1989: 909–938.
6. Quigley EMM. Gastric and small intestinal motility in health and disease. *Gastro Clin North Am* 1996; 25:113–145.
7. Sarna SK. Physiology and pathophysiology of colonic motor activity (part one of two). *Dig Dis Sci* 1991; 36:827–862.
8. Sarna SK. Physiology and pathophysiology of colonic motor activity (part two of two). *Dig Dis Sci* 1991; 36:998–1018.

9. Parkinson J. *An Essay on the Shaking Palsy*. London: Whittingham and Rowland, 1817.

10. Eadie MJ, Tyrer JH. Alimentary disorder in parkinsonism. *Aust Ann Med* 1965; 14:13–22.

11. Logemann JA, Blonsky ER, Boshes B. Dysphagia in parkinsonism. *JAMA* 1975; 231:69–70.

12. Bushman M, Dobmeyer SM, Leeker L, et al. Swallowing abnormalities and their response to treatment in Parkinson's disease. *Neurology* 1989; 39:1309–1314.

13. Logemann J, Blonsky ER, Boshes B. Lingual control in Parkinson's disease. *Trans Am Neurol Assoc* 1973; 98:276–278.

14. Calne DB, Shaw DG, Spiers ASD, et al. Swallowing in parkinsonism. *Br J Radiol* 1970; 43:456–457.

15. Palmer ED. Dysphagia in parkinsonism. *JAMA* 1974; 229–1349.

16. Edwards LL, Quigley EMM, Pfeiffer RF. Gastrointestinal dysfunction in Parkinson's disease: Frequency and pathophysiology. *Neurology* 1992; 42:726–732.

17. Edwards LL, Pfeiffer RF, Quigley EMM, et al. Gastrointestinal symptoms in Parkinson's disease. *Mov Disord* 1991; 6:151–156.

18. Edwards LL, Quigley EMM, Hofman R, et al. Gastrointestinal symptoms in Parkinson disease: 18-month follow-up study. *Mov Disord* 1993; 8:83–86.

19. Edwards LL, Quigley EMM, Harned RK, et al. Characterization of swallowing and defecation in Parkinson's disease. *Am Gastroenterol* 1994; 89:15–25.

20. Ali GN, Wallace Kl, Schwartz R, et al. Mechanisms of oral-pharyngeal dysphagia in patients with Parkinson's disease. *Gastroenterology* 1996; 110:383–392.

21. Born LJ, Harned RH, Rikkers LF, et al. Cricopharyngeal dysfunction in Parkinson's disease: Role in dysphagia and response to myotomy. *Mov Disord* 1996; 11:53–58.

22. Byrne KG, Pfeiffer RF, Quigley EMM. Gastrointestinal dysfunction in Parkinson's disease. A report of clinical experience at a single center. *J Clin Gastroenterol* 1994; 19:11–16.

23. Soykan I, Sarosiek I, Schifflet J, et al. The effect of chronic oral domperidone therapy on gastrointestinal symptoms and gastric emptying in patients with Parkinson's disease. *Mov Disord*. 1997; 12:952–957

24. Evans MA, Broe GA, Triggs EJ, et al. Gastric emptying rate and the systemic availability of levodopa in the elderly parkinsonian patient. *Neurology* 1981; 31:1288–1294.

25. Kurlan R, Rothfield KP, Woodward WR, et al. Erratic gastric emptying of levodopa may cause "random" fluctuations of parkinsonian mobility. *Neurology* 1988; 38:419–421.

26. Djaldetti R, Koren M, Ziv I, et al. Effect of cisapride on response fluctuations in Parkinson's disease. *Mov Disord* 1995; 10:81–84.

27. Soykan I, Lin Z, Bennett JP, et al. Gastric myoelectrical activity in patients with Parkinson's disease: Evidence of a primary gastric abnormality. *Dig Dis Sci* 1999 (in press).

28. Ashraf W, Pfeiffer RF, Quigley EMM. Anorectal manometry in the assessment of anorectal function in Parkinson's disease: A comparison with chronic idiopathic constipation. *Mov Disord* 1994; 9:655–663.

29. Ashraf W, Wszolek ZK, Pfeiffer RF, et al. Anorectal function in fluctuating (on-off) Parkinson's disease: Evaluation by combined anorectal manometry and electromyography. *Mov Disord* 1995; 10:650–657.

30. Mathers SE, Kempster PA, Swash M, et al. Constipation and paradoxical puborectalis contraction in anismus and Parkinson's disease: A dystonic phenomenon? *J Neurol Neurosurg Psychiatry* 1988; 51:1503–1507.

31. Mathers SE, Kempster PA, Law PJ, et al. Anal sphincter dysfunction in Parkinson's disease. *Arch Neurol* 1989; 46:1061–1064.

32. Wakabayashi K, Takahashi H, Ohama E, et al. Lewy bodies in the visceral autonomic nervous system in Parkinson's disease. In: Narabayashi H, Yanagisawa N, Mizuno Y (eds.). *Parkinson's Disease. From Basic Research to Treatment (Advances in Neurology, Vol 60)*. New York: Raven Press 1993:609–612.

33. Kupsky WJ, Grimes MM, Sweeting J, et al. Parkinson's disease and megacolon: Concentric hyaline inclusions (Lewy bodies) in enteric ganglion cells. *Neurology* 1987; 37:1253–1255.

34. Wakabayashi K, Takahashi K, Ohama E, et al. Parkinson's disease: An immunohistochemical study of Lewy-body containing neurons in the enteric nervous system. *Acta Neuropathol* 1990; 79:581–583.

35. Singaram C, Ashraf W, Gaumnitz EA, et al. Dopaminergic defect of enteric nervous system in Parkinson's disease patients with chronic constipation. *Lancet* 1995; 346:861–864.

36. Quigley EMM. Epidemiology and pathophysiology of gastrointestinal manifestations in Parkinson's disease. In: Corazziari (ed.). *NeuroGastroenterology*. Berlin: deGruyter, 1996:167–178.

37. Quigley EMM. Gastrointestinal dysfunction in Parkinson's disease. *Semin Neurol* 1996; 16:245–250.

38. Astarloa R, Mena MA, Sanchez V, et al. Clinical and pharmacokinetic effects of a diet rich in insoluble fiber on Parkinson's disease. *Clin Neuropharmacol* 1992; 15:375–380.

39. Ashraf W, Pfeiffer RF, Park F, et al. Constipation in Parkinson's disease: Objective assessment and response to psyllium. *Mov Disord* 1997; 12:946–951.

40. Jost WH, Schimrigk K. Cisapride treatment of constipation in Parkinson's disease. *Mov Disord* 1993; 8:339–343.

41. Jost WH, Schimrigk K. Long-term results with cisapride in Parkinson's disease. *Mov Disord* 1997; 12:423–425.

42. Edwards LL, Quigley EMM, Harned RK, et al. Defecatory function in Parkinson's disease: Response to apomorphine. *Ann Neurol* 1993; 33:490–493.

43. Corazziari E, Badiali D, Habib FI, et al. Small volume isomotic polyethylene glycol electrolyte balanced solution (PMF-100) in treatment of chronic nonorganic constipation. *Dig Dis Sci* 1996; 41:1636–1642.

44. Lewitan A, Nathanson L, Slade WR Jr. Megacolon and dilatation of the small bowel in parkinsonism. *Gastroenterology* 1952; 17:367–374.

45. Caplan LH, Jacobson HG, Rubinstein BM, et al. Megacolon and volvulus in Parkinson's disease. *Radiology* 1965; 85:73–78.

46. Rosenthal MJ, Marshall CE. Sigmoid volvus in association with parkinsonism. Report of four cases. *J Am Geriatr Soc* 1987; 35:683–684.

47. Bak MP, Boley SJ. Sigmoid volvulus in elderly patients. *Am J Surg* 1986; 151:71–75.

11

Autonomic Nervous System Dysfunction

Jean Pintar Hubble, M.D., and Carolyn Weeks, B.S.
Madden/National Parkinson Foundation Center of Excellence, Ohio State University, Columbus, Ohio

INTRODUCTION

Parkinson's disease (PD) is a movement disorder diagnosed on the basis of its classic clinical features – rest tremor, muscle rigidity, bradykinesia, and postural instability. These motor features are primarily ascribed to selective dopaminergic neuronal cell loss within the substantia nigra of the midbrain. Virtually all conventional PD pharmacotherapies are aimed at replenishing, mimicking, and enhancing brain dopamine in order to alleviate the motor manifestations. Although quite common and often disabling, the nonmotor features of PD receive much less attention and are poorly understood. Included in the list of nonmotor manifestations are sleep disturbances, cognitive decline, mood disorders, sensory symptoms, and autonomic nervous system dysfunction. Although autonomic dysfunction is common in PD, the nature and intensity of resulting symptoms varies widely from patient to patient. These can take the form of thermoregulatory dysfunction and skin changes, pupillary abnormalities, gastrointestinal problems and weight loss, cardiovascular abnormalities, and urinary and sexual dysfunction.

Parkinsonism coupled with autonomic failure is often indicative of multiple system atrophy (MSA). Parkinson's disease is clinically and pathologically distinct from MSA (1). Autonomic features of MSA are well described in other works (2). Key aspects of autonomic nervous system dysfunction commonly occurring in idiopathic PD are reviewed in this chapter.

NEUROPATHOLOGY OF AUTONOMIC DYSFUNCTION IN PARKINSON'S DISEASE

The pathology of PD has been shown to extend to regions of the nervous system other than dopaminergic centers, including areas involved in the autonomic

nervous system. Rajput and Rozdilsky described cell loss and Lewy bodies within the sympathetic ganglia of PD patients (3). Antibodies to sympathetic neurons have been detected in PD patients (4). The neurodegeneration of PD and Lewy bodies can be seen in other autonomic regulatory regions, including the hypothalamus, sympathetic system (intermediolateral nucleus of the thoracic cord and sympathetic ganglia), and parasysmpathetic system (dorsal, vagal, and sacral parasympathetic nuclei) (5,6). Lewy bodies were also found in the adrenal medulla and in the neural plexi innervating the gut, heart, and pelvis. This work provides convincing neuropathologic evidence that both the central and peripheral autonomic nervous systems can be affected in PD. The pathology of PD is thoroughly reviewed in Chapter 20.

THERMOREGULATORY DYSFUNCTION AND SKIN CHANGES

Over 100 years ago, Gowers described sweating episodes and abnormal sensations of warmth and coldness in PD patients (7). Levodopa and other dopaminergic medications have since been shown to either accentuate or alleviate these symptoms. In particular, individuals who develop a fluctuating motor response pattern to levodopa are likely to have episodic sweating or other thermoregulatory symptoms. Tanner and coworkers found 48 percent of PD patients to have excessive sweating (8). The majority of these subjects had a fluctuating motor response, including chorea (levodopa-induced dyskinesia); nevertheless, the sweats were not easily attributed to these excessive involuntary movements as 68 percent of these patients described sweating while in the bradykinetic (off) state. These same investigators evaluated thermoregulatory responses to an external heat source before and after the administration of dopaminergic medications. In the premedicated state, PD subjects had more sweating than control subjects. In the absence of medication, these subjects appeared to have impaired peripheral vasodilatation, thereby failing to properly dissipate body heat. After taking their usual medications, sweating and heat dissipation in the PD subjects were no different from the normal controls. Turkka and Myllyla reported similar results and found increased upper body sweating correlated to disease severity in PD (9).

The significance of thermoregulatory dysfunction in PD is underscored by reports of patients who develop profuse sweating, hyperthermia, tachypnea, tachycardia, altered mentation, and rhabdomyolysis when antiparkinsonian drug therapy is abruptly withdrawn (10,11,12). Fatalities have resulted. This drug-withdrawal syndrome is akin to the neuroleptic malignant syndrome associated with dopamine-blocking agents. It appears that antiparkinsonian medications such as levodopa directly or indirectly improve thermoregulation and other features of autonomic dysfunction in PD. With the sudden withdrawal of pharmacotherapy, these vital regulatory mechanisms can totally fail.

The pathophysiology of thermoregulatory dysfunction in PD is not established. It is probable that several neural mechanisms are at play. Experimentally, the hypothalamus has been demonstrated to play an important role in the maintenance of normal core body temperature; infusion of a dopamine agonist on the hypothalamic thermoregulatory center causes a dose-dependent decrease in body temperature via changes in peripheral vasomotor tone (13). Other central neural systems important in the regulation of body temperature are found in the cerebral cortex, thalamus, brain stem, and spinal cord (14).

Peripheral sweat gland function is regulated by the sympathetic nervous system. Sympathetic skin responses (SSR) have been studied in PD patients in an effort to evaluate autonomic dysfunction. Braune and colleagues compared electrically evoked SSRs in the hands and feet of PD patients and controls (15). Patients had longer latencies and reduced amplitudes correlating with age, disease duration, and motor asymmetries. In another study, about 15 percent of PD patients had abnormal SSRs that correlated with disease severity, disease duration, and sexual impotence (16). The authors speculate that SSR abnormalities in PD may reflect changes in the intermediolateral columns of the spinal cord that provide the preganglionic efferent innervation to postsynaptic sympathetic neurons.

The addition or adjustment of dopaminergic medications usually constitutes the initial treatment of sweating and thermoregulatory dysfunction in PD. It has been suggested that longer-acting compounds such as the dopamine agonists may be particularly beneficial,

but no controlled comparisons to levodopa have been undertaken. Propranolol has also been reported to be useful in the control of episodic sweating in PD (8).

Seborrhea or seborrheic dermatitis occurs frequently with normal aging and is particularly common in PD. This overexcretion of sebum has been attributed to hyperactivity of the parasympathetic component of the autonomic nervous system. Martignoni and coworkers compared the sebum excretion rates of 70 PD patients with those of 60 normal control subjects (17). There was no correlation between sebum excretion rates and clinical signs of autonomic nervous system dysfunction in the PD subjects. They found that men (both PD and control subjects) had higher excretion rates than women. Male PD subjects had the highest excretion rate, suggesting a possible role for androgens in the genesis of seborrhea in PD. Seborrhea can result in seborrheic dermatitis in the form of oily, chafing, reddened skin over the eyebrows, forehead, and scalp (dandruff). Men are also apt to develop this rash over the beard region. Dandruff shampoos that contain coal tars or selenium can help control scalp flaking and itching. Over-the-counter creams and ointments may help the facial rash. Prescription creams including corticosteroids and ketoconazole are sometimes effective and can be massaged into the scalp if needed. Sometimes the seborreic rash involves the eyelids (blepharitis). The individual with PD is also prone to inflammation of the eyes and eyelids because of changes in tears and tear duct flow. Cleansing the eyelids with a warm, damp washcloth and the use of artificial tears are usually sufficient. However, secondary infections of the outer covering of the eye (conjunctivitis) may occur. Signs of conjunctivitis include reddening of the whites of the eye and thick white or yellow discharge from the eye. Prescription antibiotic eyedrops are usually needed to effectively treat conjunctivitis.

PUPILLARY CHANGES

The size and reactivity of the pupils are controlled by the sympathetic and parasympathetic components of the autonomic nervous system. Constriction of the pupils is mediated via the parasympathetic fibers of the third cranial nerve that arise from the Edinger-Westphal nucleus of the midbrain. Pupillary dilatation is mediated via the more circuitous sympathetic pathways; cortical and hypothalamic fibers synapse with neurons of the intermediolateral column of the thoracic spinal cord. Fibers of these spinal cells synapse onto superior ganglionic cells in the cervical region. Postganglionic sympathetic axons constitute a part of the carotid plexus and ultimately join the fifth cranial nerve, which innervates the pupil.

Martignoni and coworkers found abnormally slow pupillary responses to light and pain in PD patients (18). Similary, Korczyn and coworkers studied pupillary responses in PD and found that resting diameters were normal but the response to changes in light was less (19). The results of instillation of pharmacologic agents to the eye demonstrated the peripheral autonomic nervous system to be intact in these PD subjects. The authors concluded that pupillary abnormalities in PD result from central autonomic dysfunction centered in the parasympathetic Edinger-Westphal nucleus of the midbrain.

Conventional drugs used to treat PD can cause visual disturbances, including blurred vision and photophobia. The most common offenders are drugs possessing anticholinergic properties such as trihexyphenidyl and benztropine. These drugs block parasympathetic activity, resulting in failure of normal pupillary constriction to light and convergence. Virtually all elderly PD patients have an element of presbyopia causing similar problems. Thus anticholinergic drugs can exaggerate the visual difficulties of older patients. Anticholinergic drugs should be avoided in individuals with narrow-angle glaucoma as these agents can cause an abrupt and dangerous rise in intraocular pressure unless coadministered with a peripheral cholinergic ocular agent such as pilocarpine (20,21).

In contrast to the anticholinergic drugs, the effects of levodopa on pupillary function is not well established. Both miosis (pupillary constriction) and mydriasis (dilatation) have been associated with levodopa use (22,23). Clinically significant pupillary changes do not appear to be common.

GASTROINTESTINAL DYSFUNCTION AND WEIGHT LOSS

A detailed review of gastrointestinal dysfunction in PD is provided in Chapter 10. What follows is a brief synopsis of these problems with emphasis on their possible relationship to the autonomic nervous system. Problems related to the gastrointestinal system in PD include sialorrhea, poor motility, changes in appetite, and weight loss. Sialorrhea is a common complaint in PD. It has been attributed to both overproduction and infrequent swallowing of saliva. Salivary secretion is dependent on parasympathetic cholineric innervation to the salivary glands via fibers in the seventh and ninth cranial nerves. Sympathetic fibers reach the glands via the cervical sympathetic trunk and cause contraction of salivary duct myoepithelial cells, resulting in decreased salivation. Anticholinergic drugs can help reduce sialorrhea in PD, and the sudden cessation of anticholinergic drugs can cause transient hypersalivation. Nevertheless, normal saliva production rates have been reported both in PD patients taking no antiparkinsonian medications and those on stable drug doses (24,25). This suggests that sialorrhea in PD is more likely the result of decreased swallowing rather than overproduction referable to autonomic dysfunction.

Slowed passage (motility) of food and waste can effect the gastrointestinal tract in its entirety in PD. Chewing, swallowing, gastric emptying, intestinal motility, and defecation can all be abnormally slowed in this disease process. At least a component of this is likely referable to autonomic dysfunction in PD. For example, degeneration of the parasympathetic neurons of the enteric plexus may contribute to poor motility and constipation (26). However, gastrointestinal symptoms such as constipation may not be solely due to autonomic dysfunction in PD. Factors contributing to constipation can include decreased physical exercise, diminished intake of food and liquid, reduced force of abdominal muscle contractions, and dysfunction of sphincters. Antiparkinsonian medications can also cause or contribute to constipation.

At least 50 percent of PD patients lose weight (27), but the cause of this is not known. Decreased energy (caloric) intake, increased energy expenditure, or both can cause weight loss. Toth and coworkers found that PD patients had lower daily energy expenditure compared with age-matched controls, suggesting that decreased energy intake is a more likely cause of weight loss (28). Gastrointestinal dysfunction on the basis of autonomic nervous system involvement may contribute to reduced energy (caloric) intake in PD because of impaired swallowing, delayed gastric emptying, early satiety, and bloating. Parkinson's disease patients may be at particular risk for poor nutrition, and dietary counseling is appropriate for those with unexplained weight loss (29).

CARDIOVASCULAR FUNCTION

The autonomic nervous system provides the neural regulation for the heart and vasculature. Proper function is fundamental to survival of the organism. There is evidence of pathologic changes within both the central and peripheral sympathetic and parasympathetic pathways in PD. Nevertheless, clinically significant cardiovascular dysfunction in PD is fortunately rare, with orthostatic hypotension serving as the most notable exception. Parkinson's disease patients often have a slightly lower resting blood pressure compared with age-matched controls (30). Orthostatic hypotension is a drop in blood pressure when arising from a sitting or lying position. This is quite common in PD (31,32). Patients may feel light-headed and complain of graying vision, but frank syncope is rare. The drop in blood pressure most often occurs after a change in posture but can also occur following exercise and after eating, when blood is diverted to the splanchnic vasculature (33).

There have been several attempts to identify a single precise anatomic site responsible for orthostatic hypotension in PD. It is not certain whether the dysfunction lies within the afferent or efferent pathways. For example, some PD patients have an intact efferent sympathetic system as evidenced by a normal response with the Valsalva maneuver (30,34); others have an abnormal response to the Valsalva maneuver (33,35). Reported abnormalities of the renin-aldosterone system with intact sodium homeostasis suggest that the peripheral sympathetic system may play a role in orthostatic hypotension in PD (34,36). Both normal and abnormal changes in serum norepinephrine levels have been reported in PD patients (33,37). In contrast to control subjects, PD patients may have an abnormal increase in the pressor response with norepinephrine infusion (38). Andersen and Boesen examined sympathetic vasoconstrictor responses in 12 PD patients using the 133-Xenon washout technique; their results suggest that sympathetic dysfunction in PD is centrally mediated (39). As single central nervous system lesions do not produce orthostatic hypotension in animal models (40), the notion of generalized sympathetic system degeneration in PD as put forward by Langston and Forno seems most plausible (5).

Orthostatic hypotension is rarely of clinical significance in mild, untreated PD patients. Systemic dopamine can cause or exaggerate hypotension. Orally administered levodopa is readily decarboxylated into dopamine. Less common than nausea and vomiting, orthostatic hypotension was found to be a potential systemic side effect of levodopa when it was first introduced to treat PD in the early 1970s (41). Now levodopa is nearly always coadministered with a decarboxylase-inhibiting drug such as carbidopa or benserazide. The coadministration of a decarboxylase inhibitor greatly reduces peripheral metabolism of levodopa into dopamine and diminishes the likelihood of systemic side effects such as nausea and hypotension. The dopamine receptor agonists can also precipitate significant orthostatic hypotension (1). This side effect may be less likely to occur if the drug is introduced cautiously with a small dose and titrated upward over time. The peripheral dopamine agonist domperidone can sometimes be used to treat intolerable systemic dopaminergic side effects of antiparkinsonian medications. Domperidone is not available in the United

Table 11-1   Strategies to Treat Orthostatic Hypotension
Dietary changes: increase fluids, salt, and caffeine intake
Support stockings, elevation of legs, and other mechanical measures
Reduce or discontinue causative drugs (e.g., dopamine agonists)
Pharmacologic agents to raise blood pressure
Fludrocortisone (Florinef)
Ephedrine
Indomethacin (Indocin)
Midodrine (Proamatine)

States. Other strategies to treat orthostatic hypotension in PD are listed in Table 11-1.

URINARY BLADDER DYSFUNCTION

Urinary frequency and urgency are common complaints in PD. This is probably due to involvement of components of the autonomic nervous system. The pathology of PD targets many brain regions normally involved in detrusor control; this includes pathways of the substantia nigra, basal ganglia, hypothalamus, and locus coeruleus (43). Detrusor hyperactivity occurs in the majority of PD patients (44).

It is important to recognize that other factors can contribute to urinary system problems, particularly in the elderly. Urinary symptoms in PD usually take the form of nocturia, urinary frequency during the day, urinary urgency, and urge incontinence. Redistribution of body fluids in the supine position at night probably adds to nighttime urinary frequency. Many men over age 60 years have benign prostatic hypertrophy, which can cause these same symptoms. Similarly, multiparous women may develop urinary control problems with advancing age, which is ascribed to weakness in the muscles of the pelvis. A complete urologic evaluation is essential to the correct diagnosis and treatment of voiding problems in PD. Urine may turn reddish or orange color when taking some medications (e.g., tolcapone, entacapone). This discoloration is harmless, although it may stain clothing. Medications often used to treat urinary frequency, urgency, and stress incontinence are listed in Table 11-2. Most of these drugs should be used cautiously in men with enlarged prostates because of the possibility of bladder outlet obstruction. All of these medicines have anticholinergic side effects and other potential side effects that may not be particularly problematic in PD.

Table 11-2 Drugs Used to Treat Urinary Symptoms
Oxybutynin (Ditropan)
Tricyclic antidepressant compounds (e.g., imipramine)
Tolterodine tartrate (Detrol)
Bethanechol chloride (Urecholine)
Propantheline (Pro-Banthine)
Prazosin (Hytrin)
Desmopressin inhaler (DDAVP)

Table 11-3 Drugs Used to Treat Male Impotence
Yohimbine
Papaverine
Phentolamine
Prostaglandin E
Sildenafil (Viagra)

SEXUAL DYSFUNCTION

Impotence and other forms of sexual dysfunction are probably underreported in PD. Patients, spouses, and physicians rarely discuss these problems with candor. There are many potential causes of sexual dysfunction in individuals over age 60 years. Included among these are vascular insufficiency, prostatic enlargement, depression, and hormonal conditions such as diabetes and thyroid disease. There are many drugs and over-the-counter medications associated with impotence. Drugs that can cause or contribute to impotence include antihistamines, barbiturates, sedatives, tranquilizers, some antidepressants, antihypertensives, and excessive alcohol use. The anticholinergic medications used to treat PD may also cause impotence, but most other antiparkinsonian drugs are only rarely associated with this side effect.

Parkinson's disease itself can cause sexual dysfunction (44a). This usually takes the form of inability to maintain an erection in men and inability to achieve orgasm in women. The reason for impotence in PD is not entirely clear, but it probably is related to involvement of the autonomic nervous system. In a recent survey in the United States, 36 male and 14 female PD patients were interviewed regarding their sexual function (45). Most patients reported less sexual activity following the diagnosis of PD. About 50 percent of men reported difficulties with ejaculation and 75 percent of women had less frequent orgasms following the onset of PD. There was no relationship between sexual dysfunction and depression in this study. In a Danish study, 25 PD patients were surveyed regarding sexual function (46). Approximately 30 to 40 percent of the male patients and 70 to 80 percent of the female patients reported decreased libido and reduced sexual activity. There was an apparent relationship between sexual dysfunction and PD disease duration and severity. Drugs used to treat the primary symptoms of PD (levodopa) do not usually improve sexual function in parkinson-related impotence. A general physical examination and urologic assessment should be undertaken before treatment is initiated for male impotence.

Treatments for impotence are listed in Table 11-3. Female sexual dysfunction in PD is very poorly understood. It had been thought to be less common than in men, but the recent surveys cited earlier argue against this notion. Painful sexual intercourse warrants a full gynecologic assessment in women. It is important to emphasize that both depression and nocturnal Parkinson's symptoms can lessen sexual drive or hinder sexual performance in men and women; these symptom complexes may be treatable with appropriate antidepressant therapy or the addition of antiparkinsonian medications at bedtime.

REFERENCES

1. Quinn N. Multiple system atrophy: The nature of the beast. *J. Neurol Neurosurg Psychiatry* 1989; Suppl:78–79.
2. Polinsky RJ. Multiple system atrophy and Shy-Drager syndrome. In: Robertson D, Low PA Polinsky (eds.). *Premier in the Autonomic Nervous System*. San Diego: Academic Press, 1996:222–226.
3. Rajput AH, Rozdilsky B. Dysautonomia in parkinsonism: A clinicopathological study. *J. Neurol Neurosurg Psychiatry* 1976; 39:1092–1100.
4. Emile J, Pouplard A, Bossu Van Nieuwenhuyse C, et al. Maladie de Parkinson, dysautonomie at autoanticorps dirges contre les neurones sympathiques. *Rev Neurol* (Paris)1980; 136(3):221–233.
5. Langston JW, Forno LS. The hypothalamus in Parkinson's disease. *Ann Neurol* 1978; 129–133.
6. Wakabayashi K, Takahashi H. Neuropathology of autonomic nervous system in Parkinson's disease. *Eur Neurol* 1997; 38(Suppl 2):2–7.
7. Gowers WR. *Disease of the Nervous System*. Philadelphia: Blakiston, 1893.
8. Tanner CM, Goetz CG, Klawans HL. Paroxysmal drenching sweats in idiopathic parkinsonism: Response to propranolol. *Neurology* 1982; 32(2):A162.
9. Turrka JT, Myllyla VV. Sweating dysfunction in Parkinson's disease. *Eur Neurol* 1987; 26:1–7.
10. Toru M, Matsuda O, Makiguchi K, et al. Neuroleptic malignant syndrome-like state a withdrawal of antiparkinsonian drugs. *J Nerv Ment Dis* 1981; 169(5): 324–327.

11. Friedman JH, Feinburg SS, Feldman RG. A neuroleptic malignant-like syndrome due to L-dopa withdrawal. *Ann Neurol* 1984; 16(1):126.

12. Pfeiffer RF, Sucha EL. On-off induced malignant hyperthermia. *Ann Neurol* 1985; 18(1):138.

13. Cox B. Dopamine. In: Lomax P, Schonbaum E (eds.). *Body Temperature*. New York: Marcel Dekker, 1979.

14. Lowey AD. Central automomic pathways. In: Lowey AD, Apyer KM, (eds.). *Central Regulation of Autonomic Functions*. New York: Oxford University Press, 1990:88–103.

15. Braune JH, Korchounov AM, Schipper HI. Autonomic dysfunction in Parkinson's disease by sympathetic skin response: A prospective clinical neurophysiological trial on 50 patients. *Acta Neurol Scand* 1997; 95(5):293–297.

16. Wang SJ, Fuh JO, Shan DE, et al. Sympathetic skin response and R-R interval variation in Parkinson's disease. *Mov Disord* 1993; 8:151–157.

17. Martignoni E, Fodi L, Pacchetti C. Is seborrhea a sign of autonomic impairment in Parkinson's disease? *J Neural Transm* 1997; 104:1295–1304.

18. Martignoni E, Micieli G, Magri M, et al. *Autonomic Failure in Parkinson's Disease*. Presented at the VIIIth International Syposium on Parkinson's Disease, 1985.

19. Korczyn AD, Rubenstein AE, Yahr MD. *The Pupil in Parkinson's Disease*. Presented at the VIIIth International Syposium on Parkinson's Disease, 1985.

20. Weiner N. Atropine, scopolamine, and related antimuscarinic drugs. In: Goodman LS, Gillman A, (eds.). *The Pharmacological Basis of Therapuetics*. 7th ed. New York: Macmillan, 1985:120–137.

21. Taylor P. Cholinergic agonists. In: Goodman LS, Gillman A (eds.). *The Pharmacological Basis of Therapuetics*. 7th ed. New York: Macmillan, 1985:91–99.

22. Spiers ASD, Calne DB, Fayers PM. Miosis during L-dopa therapy. *Br Med J* 1970; 2:639–640.

23. Weintraub MI, Gasstherland D, Van-Woert MH. Pupillary effects of levodopa therapy. *N Engl J Med* 1970; 283:120–123.

24. Cros P, Peryin J, Freidel M, et al. *Rev Stomatol Chir Maxillofac* 1979; 6:319–324.

25. Bateson MC, Gibberd FB, Wilson RSE. Salivary symptoms in Parkinson's disease. *Arch Neurol* 1973; 29:274–275.

26. van Dijk JG, Haan J, Zwinderman K, et al. Autonomic nervous system dysfunction in Parkinson's disease: Relationship with age, medication, duration and severity. *J Neurol Neurosurg Psychiatry* 1993; 56:1090–1095.

27. Abbott RA, Cox M, Markus H, et al. Diet, body and size, and micronutrient status in Parkinson's disease. *Eur J Clin Nutr* 1992; 55:701–707.

28. Toth MJ, Fishman PS, Poehlman ET. Free-living daily energy expenditure in patients with Parkinson's disease. *Neurology* 1997; 48:88–91.

29. Beyer PL, Palarino MY, Michalek D, et al. Weight change and body composition in patients with Parkinson's disease. *J Am Diet Assoc* 1995; 95:979–983.

30. Brevetti G, Bonaduce D, Breglio R, et al. Parkinson's disease and hypotension: 24-hour blood pressure recording in ambulant patients. *Clin Cardiol* 1990; 13:474–478.

31. Gross M, Bannister R, Godwin-Austin R. Orthostatic hypotension in Parkinson's disease. *Lancet* 1972; 1:174–176.

32. Miceli G, Martignoni E, Cavallini A, et al. Postprandial and orthostatic hypotension in Parkinson's disease. *Neurology* 1987; 37:386–393.

33. Turkka J, Tolonen U, Myllyla V. Cardiovascular reflexes in Parkinson's disease. *Eur Neurol* 1987; 26:104–112.

34. Wilcox CS, Aminoff MH. Blood pressure responses to noradrenaline and dopamine infusions in Parkinson's disease and the Shy-Drager syndrome. *Br Med Clin Pharmacol* 1976; 3:207–214.

35. Goetz CG, Lutge W, Tanner CM. Autonomic dysfunction in Parkinson's disease. *Neurology* 1986; 36:73–75.

36. Barbea A, Gillo-Joffroy L, Boucher R, et al. Renin-aldosterone system in Parkinson's disease. *Science* 1969; 18:291–292.

37. Turrka A, Jujarvi KK, Lapinlampi TO, et al. Serum noradrenaline response to standing up in patients with Parkinson's disease. *Eur Neurol* 1986; 25:355–361.

38. Aminoff MJ, Wilcos MJ. Assessment of autonomic function in patients with parkinsonian syndrome. *Br Med J* 1971; 4:80–84.

39. Andersen EB, Boesen F. Sympathic vasoconstrictor reflexes in Parkinson's disease with autonomic dysfunction. *Clin Autonom Res* 1997; 7:5–11.

40. Talman WT. Cardiovascular regulation and lesions of the central nervous system. *Ann Neurol* 1985; 18:1–12.

41. Calne DB, Brennan AS, Spiers D, et al. Hypotension caused by L-dopa. *Br Med J* 1970; 1:474–475.

42. Quinn N, Illas A, Lehermitte F, et al. Bromocriptine in Parkinson's disease: A study of cardiovascular effects. *J Neurol Neurosurg Psychiatry* 1981; 44:426–429.

43. Sotolonga J. Voiding dysfunction in Parkinson's disease. *Semin Neurol* 1988; 8:166–169.

44. Andersen JT. Disturbances of bladder and urethral function in Parkinson's disease. *Int Urol Nephrol* 1985; 17:35–41.

44a. Singer C, Weiner WJ, Sanchez-Ramos J, et al. Sexual dysfunction in men with Parkinson's disease. *J Neurol Rehab* 1989; 3:189–204.

45. Koller WC, Vetere-Overfield B, Williamson A, et al. Sexual dysfunction in Parkinson's disease. *Clin Neurpharm* 1990; 13:461–463.

46. Wermuth L, Stenager E. Sexual problems in young patients with Parkinson's disease. *Acta Neurol Scand* 1995; 91:453–455.

12

Sleep Disorders

Cynthia L. Comella, M.D., A.B.S.M.

Rush Medical College, Chicago, Illinois

Sleep disturbance is a common yet underdiagnosed feature of Parkinson's disease (PD). A survey study in the United Kingdom illustrated just how common it is (1). Of the 220 patients with PD interviewed, 215 reported nocturnal sleep disruption. Seventy-six percent reported that their sleep was disrupted during the night by frequent awakenings. The most frequent disturbance during the night was the need to urinate, with 80 percent reporting at least two nightly visits to the bathroom and 33 percent getting up at least three times per night. The most frequent motor symptom experienced during the night that led to awakenings was the inability to turn over in bed. Painful leg cramps associated with PD occurred during the night in 55 percent of the patients. The nocturnal occurrences of tremor and foot dystonia represent other common complaints. Sleep disturbance related to PD correlates highly with increased distress scores on the Nottingham Health Profile, a scale measuring quality of life, and also contributes to daytime fatigue (2). Other factors contributing to sleep disturbance in PD include not only symptoms of the disease but also effects of PD medications, related primary sleep disorders, and depression.

The common occurrence of PD-associated sleep disturbances is largely unrecognized by physicians, who tend to focus primarily on the motor symptoms. Detailed assessment of sleep and sleep disturbances are often omitted. Similarly, patients and caregivers frequently do not realize the importance of reporting sleep disturbances to their physician unless the disturbance is severe. Without particular attention to sleep and sleep quality, many PD patients may unnecessarily endure treatable sleep disorders for prolonged periods of time. An increased awareness and more aggressive treatment of the nighttime problems of PD patients will promote a better quality of life for both patients and their caregivers. These issues are covered in this chapter.

SLEEP DISTURBANCES RELATED TO SYMPTOMS OF PARKINSON'S DISEASE

Sleep disturbance related to PD can arise from different sources. Some of the frequently occurring causes are listed in Table 12-1. In early mild PD patients, subjective sleep quality does not differ from that of age-matched controls (3). Polysomnography in this group of patients shows that, with the exception of sleep onset delay, there are no major differences between sleep in mild PD and age-matched normal subjects (4). Untreated PD patients are found to have abnormal movements during sleep, including increased blinking, blepharospasm, and tremor. These movements can occur during any sleep stage (5,6) but are more common in the lighter stages of sleep. As the disease progresses, the frequency and severity of associated sleep disturbances increases. Excessive daytime sleepiness (EDS) may occur as a result of nocturnal sleep disturbance. A community-based sample of PD patients showed EDS affected almost four times the percentage of PD patients than patients with diabetes mellitus and was 15 times greater than normal-aged controls. EDS correlated with more advanced disease (7). Polysomnography shows that patients with advanced PD have reductions in total sleep time compared with normal elderly controls, with the most profound decreases in stages 3 and 4 sleep and frequent nocturnal arousals (5,8–10).

During sleep, untreated PD patients demonstrate an increase in muscle tone, which contributes to nocturnal arousals. Treatment with levodopa reduces the muscle tone and lessens sleep fragmentation (9). Fragmented sleep is characterized by frequent nocturnal awakenings and is the most common sleep disturbance in PD patients (11). One study found that 88.5 percent of PD patients had this problem to some degree compared with 74.4 percent of controls, thus indicating that this was also common in the elderly healthy

Table 12-1 Sleep Disturbances in Parkinson's Disease	
Due to parkinsonian symptoms	Fragmentation due to tremor, stiffness, rigidity, pain, difficulty turning over in bed
Due to medications	Sleep fragmentation, nightmares, hallucinations, insomnia, daytime sleepiness
Due to associated conditions	Depression, dementia
May be associated	Sleep apnea, REM sleep behavior disorder

population, although the number of awakenings per night in controls was smaller than in patients (11). If severe, fragmented sleep leads to a reduction in total night sleep time, daytime fatigue, and EDS. Patients will tend to doze during daytime sedentary activities and will complain that although they may fall asleep quickly when going to bed, they awaken frequently during the night for inexplicable reasons. They may report that they are awakened by the need to urinate. These nocturnal awakenings may be prolonged. Direct interview with the patient, however, may suggest that when awakened, they have tremor, stiffness, or difficulty rolling over in bed, leading to feelings of discomfort. Patients may experience feelings of restlessness and a need to physically move, consistent with nocturnal akathisia. These types of sleep complaints are related directly to the symptoms of PD and tend to occur more frequently as the disease progresses.

Urinary symptoms may be associated with prostatic enlargement in men. In both men and women, age-related urologic abnormalities may be responsible for urinary frequency. Autonomic dysfunction secondary to PD may also be the cause. Symptoms related to structural urologic abnormalities including urinary retention with overflow incontinence and spastic bladder with urinary frequency and urgency may mimic each other. Treatment depends on the type of urinary disorder, and consultation with a urologist is pivotal in determining the approach. Several agents are available for treatment of either hypotonic or hypertonic bladder dysfunction. Peripherally acting cholinergic agents, such as urecholine, may alleviate symptoms of the hypotonic bladder. Conversely, peripherally acting anticholinergic agents may improve the urinary symptoms of a hypertonic bladder. Clearly, appropriate diagnosis is paramount in making the correct treatment choice (12).

In PD patients not on medications, symptoms of PD that are tolerable during daytime hours may interrupt

sleep at night. In more advanced treated PD the effect of daytime medications wanes in the evening and during the night, with a consequent increase in muscle rigidity, slowness, stiffness, and tremor. Some patients with wearing-off will awaken every two to four hours at night to take medication because of the recurrence of motor symptoms. The diagnosis of nocturnal symptoms of PD as the cause of the sleep disturbance can often be made through a careful history.

Nighttime PD symptoms may be treated by providing a sustained dopaminergic effect during the night. The controlled-release formulation of carbidopa-levodopa (Sinemet CR 25/100 or 50/200) with a half-life almost double that of the regular preparations of carbidopa-levodopa has been shown to control the nighttime symptoms of PD in some patients, allowing for more consolidated sleep periods and improved early-morning functioning. For patients who awaken only occasionally during the night because of PD symptoms, the regular preparation given at the time of the nighttime awakening is preferred because of its rapid onset of action. Only small doses (1/2 to 1 tablet of immediate-release 25/100 carbidopa-levodopa) are needed. (9). Another technique to prolong levodopa levels that may be effective is the administration of tolcapone or entacapone, catechol-O-methyl transferase (COMT)-inhibiting compounds. These drugs prolong the duration of action of levodopa by preventing enzymatic degradation of levodopa by COMT. COMT inhibitors would only be effective in patients receiving levodopa, as they have no effect on unmedicated patients or those treated with other antiparkinsonian agents. Clinical experience has shown this to be an effective approach, although clinical trials addressing this issue have not yet been implemented.

In contrast to the levodopa preparations, the usefulness of the direct-acting dopaminergic agonists in the treatment of nocturnal PD symptoms has not been adequately evaluated. Some patients report that these agents are more likely to exacerbate insomnia rather than improve it. They may also increase the frequency of nightmares and nocturnal hallucinations. However, their usefulness in the treatment of nocturnal or early-morning dystonia has been demonstrated (13).

DELAYED SLEEP ONSET

Sleep onset insomnia may also be due to PD symptoms but is less characteristic than sleep fragmentation. Other causes, including medications, concurrent existence of restless legs syndrome (RLS), depression, or anxiety, are more likely culprits.

Of the medications used for the treatment of PD, selegiline is the one most likely to result in sleep onset insomnia. Selegiline is metabolized into an amphetamine and, if taken in the late afternoon or evening, may prolong sleep onset. Anticholinergic agents, dopamine agonists, and amantadine may also cause an alerting effect. Withdrawal from benzodiazepines and other hypnosedatives may cause rebound insomnia unless tapered slowly. Certain types of antidepressant medications, especially the serotonin reuptake inhibitors, are also agents to avoid in the evening hours.

RLS is marked by restless feelings or dysesthesias often localized to the legs that occurs at rest in the evening and improves with walking (14). Patients who experience symptoms of RLS find that small doses of pergolide, pramipexole, or ropinirole may provide relief. RLS can occur as an idiopathic disorder or in association with PD. The sensations are often described as unusual feelings of pain or dysesthesia (creepy crawly feelings) in the calf muscles, occurring at rest and relieved by movement. Symptoms occasionally occur in the arms as well. RLS has a circadian occurrence, and the most reporting symptoms occur in the evening hours before bed. There is an association between RLS, dyskinesias while awake (DWA), and periodic limb movement disorder (PLMD). PLMD occurs primarily during non-REM (rapid eye movement) sleep and is marked by an intermittent rhythmic movement of the legs (triple flexion of hip, knee, and ankle) that can result in arousals and awakenings if severe. For RLS, DWA, and PLMD, the direct-acting dopamine receptor agonists appear to be superior to levodopa, with a reduced occurrence of rebound (RLS symptoms occurring at the end of the effect of a single dose of levodopa) and augmentation (RLS symptoms occurring at an earlier time in the evening). Opiates and benzodiazepines may also be effective treatments.

An additional cause of both fragmented and delayed sleep onset is depression. Depression is estimated to affect approximately 40 percent of PD patients (15). In non-PD patients, depression often causes an associated sleep disturbance. An early REM period is one of the characteristic polysomnographic features. Treatment of depression can improve sleep disturbance in non-PD and PD patients alike. The tricyclic antidepressants (e.g., amitriptyline and nortriptyline), with their sedating anticholinergic side effects, when administered in small doses in the evening hours, may be very beneficial. These agents may, however, exacerbate RLS symptoms and increase PLMD, so it is important to differentiate these problems in the office setting. In addition, in patients with hallucinations, these antidepressants may initiate or worsen nighttime hallucinations in susceptible patients.

In PD patients with situational anxiety or acute insomnia with no other contributing factor, the short-term use of zolpidem immediately at bedtime may provide relief, often without causing rebound insomnia after discontinuation. Melatonin in small doses (less than 3 mg) one to two hours before bedtime may be beneficial, although specific deficits in this hormone have not been demonstrated in PD.

SLEEP APNEA

Sleep apnea has been inconsistently associated with PD (16,17). Patients who are excessively sleepy during the day or who have periods of apnea, loud snoring or gasping, and choking during sleep should be evaluated for sleep apnea using polysomnography. Sleep apnea can cause nocturnal hypoxia, cardiac arrhythmias, and sleep fragmentation. Patients with significant sleep apnea may present solely with EDS. Sleep apnea may be central, (airflow ceases due to absence of activation of respiratory muscles), obstructive (airflow reduced or stopped despite respiratory muscle effort), or mixed (containing elements of both). Obstructive sleep apnea is most effectively treated using continuous positive airway pressure (CPAP). Central sleep apnea is more difficult to treat and may require nocturnal oxygen administration or even tracheostomy at night.

Multiple systems atrophy (MSA) is a neurodegenerative disorder marked by parkinsonism, autonomic instability, and cerebellar abnormalities. Patients with MSA may have life-threatening sleep apnea with glottic closure resulting in nocturnal stridor (18). This variant of obstructive sleep apnea responds poorly to CPAP, and use of a tracheostomy at night may be lifesaving. Rapid evaluation is critical as MSA patients, if untreated, may experience sudden death during sleep.

THE EFFECT OF DOPAMINERGIC THERAPY ON SLEEP IN PARKINSON'S DISEASE

A recent study evaluating continuous electronic activity monitoring in 89 PD patients showed that, compared with normal controls, PD patients had higher levels of activity during the night, reflecting more severe sleep disruption. Of the mild to moderate PD patients studied, the use of levodopa or a direct dopamine agonist best predicted increased nocturnal activity (19). Similar findings of increased activity with levodopa were described using a different activity-monitoring technique, although in this study there were fewer movements measured in bed during sleep than seen in the non-PD controls (20).

Other investigators have shown improvements in sleep following levodopa initiation. Polysomnography in five PD patients with and without levodopa treatment showed that levodopa improved sleep efficiency and normalized muscle activity (9). Improved sleep has also been observed with the use of sustained-release levodopa preparations. Controlled-release levodopa has been shown to improve nocturnal akinesia, tremor, and rigidity (21,22) and to increase sleep efficiency, with a reduction in sleep fragmentation. In some patients receiving the long-acting preparations, beneficial effects were still apparent the following morning (23,24).

Although in some PD patients nocturnal use of levodopa may improve sleep, the effect of chronic dopaminergic treatment on sleep architecture may offset this initial benefit. Parenteral infusions of dopaminergic agents have been shown to delay the onset of REM sleep or acutely inhibit an ongoing REM period (25,26). With chronic dopaminergic treatment some investigators observe that there continues to be a suppression of REM sleep and that the discontinuation of dopaminergic therapy resulted in REM rebound lasting up to 10 days in some patients (27). Others report that in the period immediately following the initiation of levodopa, there is a suppression of REM that resolves to baseline levels with chronic treatment (8,28). Yet another group report that REM time actually increases with prolonged therapy (29). In many reports the clinical staging of the patients and their motoric response to dopaminergic agents is not indicated.

SLEEP DISTURBANCE – HALLUCINATIONS SYNDROME IN PARKINSON'S DISEASE PATIENTS ON CHRONIC DOPAMINERGIC THERAPY

As many as 33 percent of PD patients treated chronically with dopaminergic agents develop dopaminergic drug–induced visual hallucinations (30). Factors reported to be associated with the occurrence of hallucinations include age, duration of levodopa therapy, presence of dementia, use of anticholinergic drugs or amantadine, age of PD onset, PD duration, and abnormal MMPI scores (30–38). Nausieda and associates (39) observed that PD patients with dopaminergic-induced hallucinations had preexisting

sleep complaints, in particular awakenings during the night. These investigators postulated that sleep disturbance and hallucinations were on a continuum, with sleep disruption as the initial event (33,39).

A single report of quantitative sleep studies in PD patients with dysphoric dreams demonstrated an absence of K-complexes and sleep spindles with no specific architectural abnormalities. There was a variable suppression of REM (40). In a subsequent study comparing a group of five hallucinating patients with five nonhallucinating PD patients, matched for severity of PD and dosages of antiparkinsonian medications, polysomnographic comparisons revealed that hallucinations were associated with a reduced sleep efficiency and a marked reduction in REM sleep (41).

The treatment of dopaminergic drug–induced hallucinations has been problematic. Discontinuation of drugs with central effects that are not essential to the patient's well-being is the first approach. This would include elimination of anticholinergic agents, anxiolytics, centrally active pain medications, including codeine compounds, antidepressants, and other drugs that can be discontinued safely. Providing a night-light to increase visual stimulation during the night may be useful. A reduction in dopamine drug dose and avoidance of evening doses may be beneficial but also may result in a worsening of motor symptoms. Shifting from the direct dopamine agonists to shorter-acting levodopa preparations may also be helpful. If reduction in the dopaminergic drugs results in an exacerbation of motor symptoms, the atypical antipsychotics can be used (see Chapters 37,42). Clozapine has been shown to be an effective treatment for drug-induced hallucinations in PD without causing a deterioration in motor symptoms. The major adverse effect from clozapine is the development of agranulocytosis. Monitoring of this potentially life-threatening side effect requires weekly blood counts for the first six months of therapy. If stable after six months, blood tests are a continued requirement at biweekly intervals. Other atypical agents, including quetiapine, are currently being assessed. These latter agents do not require blood monitoring.

SLEEP BENEFIT IN PARKINSON'S DISEASE

The preceding sections have dealt with the effect of PD and antiparkinsonian medications on sleep. Conversely, the effect of sleep on PD has been studied. Sleep benefit in PD describes a clinical phenomenon in which, following sleep, symptoms are improved before any medication doses are given. Factor and colleagues (11) found that 43.6 percent of the 78 PD patients interviewed thought that the morning was the "best time of day" for motor performance. In addition, 37.2 percent found that morning was the worse time of day, while 19.2 percent found the morning time to be no different from the rest of the day. The morning same group had shorter duration of PD, had less severe disease, and required fewer dopaminergic medications. The morning better (those experiencing sleep benefit) and morning worse group were similar regarding age, duration of disease, dopaminergic drug requirements, and predominant motor symptoms. In addition, both groups experienced similar sleep problems (fragmentation and initiation). Clark and Feinstein (42) described sleep benefit in six patients, with a follow-up evaluation in one showing a reduction in the duration of morning benefit with progression of PD. Hogl and coworkers (43) examined 10 PD patients with sleep benefit and 10 matching PD patients without it using motor examination measures, levodopa plasma levels, and polysomnography. There were no differences in polysomnographic measures. However, the patients with sleep benefit had more severe interdose "off" periods, suggesting that they had more severe motor fluctuations. We have recently completed a questionnaire study of 117 PD patients and found that 25 percent experience sleep benefit lasting 2 to 3 hours after nocturnal sleep. The duration of sleep benefit correlated with reported duration of improvement following a single dose of levodopa and was more frequent in milder PD taking less antiparkinsonian medication (44). On the other hand, Factor and coworkers (11) found that sleep benefit occurred much less frequently in nonfluctuators. These observations taken together suggest that sleep may improve symptoms of PD. Although the mechanism remains to be elucidated, it is likely that it actually has little to do with sleep directly. It more likely relates to the timing of awakening and the pattern of motor fluctuations (11,42,43).

REM SLEEP BEHAVIOR DISORDER IN PARKINSON'S DISEASE

REM sleep behavior disorder (RBD) has particular relevance to PD and other parkinsonian syndromes. It occurs in association with PD, and RBD may predate, even predict, its onset. Normal REM sleep is marked by cortical desynchronization similar to that seen in the waking state, rapid eye movements, cardiorespiratory irregularities, and skeletal muscle atonia interrupted by phasic muscle twitches. Although dreams may occur during other sleep stages, during REM sleep the dreams are vivid and more internally organized. The anatomic areas involved in the generation and maintenance of REM sleep lie within the brain stem. In animal models, lesions in these REM-related brain stem areas in the pons result in motor behaviors during REM (45–47). The severity of the pontine lesion determines the extent of the behavioral pattern observed. In humans the occurrence of RBD is similarly thought to reflect damage to these same REM-related areas.

RBD was first described in 1986 by Schenck and colleagues (48,49), who observed abnormal behaviors occurring mostly in elderly men. As subsequent cases were reported, the salient clinical features of this syndrome emerged. The minimal diagnostic criteria for RBD as defined by the International Classification of Sleep Disorders (ICSD) includes movement of limbs or body associated with dream mentation and at least one of the following: potentially harmful sleep behaviors; dreams that appear to be "acted out"; or sleep behaviors that disrupt sleep continuity (50). The dreams recalled during episodes of RBD are usually aggressive or violent in nature. Polysomnography, while not required for clinical diagnosis, demonstrates excessive chin muscle tone and limb jerking during REM. Occasionally, complex, vigorous, and sometimes violent behaviors may also occur (51–58).

Episodes of RBD tend to occur sporadically. There may be a flurry of episodes every night followed by a period of quiescence. In a patient with RBD, dreams of being chased, threatened, or trapped lead to behaviors such as punching, choking, kicking, or leaping out of bed. Patients have sustained ecchymosis, lacerations, fractures, and dislocations as a result. Similarly, the bed partners of RBD patients are at risk for injury and are often frightened by the sudden violent outbursts in a person who may be quiet and mild while awake. Usually it is only upon specific questioning by the physician that these nighttime episodes are revealed. The patient seldom remembers the episode, and the caregiver may believe that the episodes are not part of a neurologic syndrome.

RBD is treatable in the vast majority of patients. Small doses of clonazepam may reduce or eliminate the symptoms. A dose as small as 0.25 mg of clonazepam may allow both patient and caregiver peace during the night and prevent additional sleep-related injuries. Atypical antipsychotics such as quetiapine may also have a role. Furthermore, the knowledge that RBD is a neurologic disorder and not secondary to emotional or psychologic derangements is often a relief to both.

The association between RBD and PD at this time remains unexplained. RBD has also been described in MSA (59), a parkinsonian syndrome with more extensive brain stem degeneration than PD (60). In symptomatic RBD, magnetic resonance imaging (MRI) scans show brain stem pathology (61). Similarly, animal experiments implicate specific brain stem nuclei as the anatomic basis for RBD. The occurrence of RBD in PD suggests that in some PD patients there is more widespread brain stem pathology than in others. This may have prognostic implications, perhaps predicting a poorer outcome. Longitudinal studies are necessary to test that hypothesis. Pathologic studies in moderate to severe PD have shown a 40 percent reduction of cholinergic neurons and Lewy body formation in the pedunculopontine tegmental nucleus, (62). Taken together, these observations suggest that certain REM abnormalities may reflect anatomic subcategories of PD.

EXCESSIVE DAYTIME SLEEPINESS IN PARKINSON'S DISEASE

In one community-based study (63), EDS was seen in 15.5 percent of PD patients compared with 4 percent of patients with diabetes mellitus and 1 percent of controls. This problem was associated with a higher stage of PD, greater disability, greater level of cognitive decline, more frequent hallucinations, and longer duration of levodopa therapy. The occurrence of excess daytime napping followed by nocturnal wakefulness is a frequent complaint of patients and their caregivers. In addition to the specific sleep disorders described, other factors may promote this "reversal" of the normal day-night rhythms. Sedentary PD patients who largely remain indoors during the day may doze frequently. The occurrence of these intermittent sleep periods, especially during the afternoon and evening hours, may impede the ability to fall asleep at night. Further, antiparkinsonian medications may cause sleepiness following a dose. This is particularly true for levodopa and the direct dopamine receptor agonists (64–66). Other medications received for medical indications can aggravate daytime sleepiness. Consultation with the patient's family physician may provide adjustments in these concomitant drugs and eliminate overly sedating drugs.

Treatment of day-night reversal relies heavily on the restoration of normal sleep patterns. Good sleep hygiene includes an established bedtime and wake-up time and exposure to adequate light during the day and darkness at night. Indoor lighting does not have sufficient lux to promote a normal circadian rhythm. Exposure to sunlight or its equivalent during the day is needed. This can be accomplished by frequent trips outside, keeping window shades open during the day, or exposure to a light source specifically designed to provide the needed light strength. Physical exercise appropriate to the patient's level of functioning is essential to maintaining flexibility and promotes daytime wakefulness. Strenuous exercise, however, should be avoided for three to four hours before sleep. Structured daytime activities, preferably out of the home, can promote daytime wakefulness. A hot bath about an hour before bedtime may be relaxing and reduce sleep-onset delay by increasing body temperature before bedtime and by allowing the patient to fall asleep during the cooling phase. A light bedtime snack and avoidance of fluid intake in the evening may alleviate nighttime hunger and reduce nocturnal urination. Relaxation techniques may also be useful in reducing nighttime stress and muscle tension.

Sleepiness following antiparkinsonian medications is sometimes difficult to control. A dose reduction may improve postdrug sleepiness but may also lead to an unacceptable increase in parkinsonian symptoms. If the patient is receiving a direct dopamine agonist, changing to another agonist may provide considerable relief. A few patients have reported the sudden onset of an irresistible urge to sleep associated with pramipexole, ropinirole, and pergolide (64,65). This is alleviated by the discontinuation of the drug or switching to another available agonist.

The administration of daytime stimulant medications is reserved for those patients who are unresponsive to other medication adjustments. The amphetamine metabolites of selegiline may increase alertness. Small doses of methylphenidate administered during the day may also be helpful but can also disrupt nighttime sleep.

REFERENCES

1. Lees AJ, Blackburn NA, Campbell VL. The nighttime problems of Parkinson's disease. *Clin Neuropharmacol* 1988; 11:512–519.
2. Karlsen K, Larsen JP, Tandberg E, et al. Fatigue in patients with Parkinson's disease. *Mov Disord* 1999; 14:237–241.
3. Carter J, Carroll S, Lannon MC. Sleep disruption in untreated Parkinson's disease. *Neurology* 1990; 40(Suppl 1):220.
4. Ferini-Strambi L, Franceschi M, Pinto P, et al. Respiration and heart rate variability during sleep in untreated Parkinson patients. *Gerontology* 1992; 38:92–98.
5. Mouret J. Differences in sleep in patients with Parkinson's disease. *Electroenceph Clin Neurophysiol* 1975; 38:653–657.
6. Stern M, Roffwang H, Duvoisin R. The parkinsonian tremor in sleep. *J Nerv Ment Dis* 1968; 147:202–210.
7. Tandberg E, Larsen JP, Karlsen K. A community based study of sleep disorders in patients with Parkinson's disease. *Mov Disord* 1998; 13:895–899.

8. Kales A, Ansel RD, Markham CH, et al. Sleep in patients with Parkinson's disease and in normal subjects prior to and following levodopa administration. *Clin Pharmacol Ther* 1971; 12:397–406.

9. Askenasy JM, Yahr MD. Reversal of sleep disturbance in Parkinson's disease by antiparkinsonian therapy: A preliminary study. *Neurology* 1985; 35:527–532.

10. Friedman A. Sleep pattern in Parkinson's disease. *Acta Med Pol* 1980; 21:193–199.

11. Factor SA, McAlarney T, Sanchez-Ramos JR, et al. Sleep disorders and sleep effect in Parkinson's disease. *Mov Disord* 1990; 5:280–285.

12. Low PA, Polinsky RJ, Kaufmann HC, et al. Autonomic function and dysfunction. Multiple system atrophy (MSA), pure autonomic failure (PAF) and related extrapyramidal disorders. *Continuum* 1998:441–58.

13. Factor SA, Sanchez-Ramos J, Weiner WJ. Parkinson's disease: An open label trial of pergolide in patients failing bromocriptine therapy. *J Neurol Neurosurg Psychiatry* 1988; 51:529–533.

14. Trenkwalder C, Walters AS, Hening W. Periodic limb movements and restless legs syndrome. *Neurol Clin* 1996; 14:629–650.

15. Cummings JL. Depression and Parkinson's disease: A review. *Am J Psychiatry* 1992; 149:443–454.

16. Efthimiou J, Ellis S, Hardie R, et al. Sleep apnea in idiopathic and postencephalitic parkinsonism. *Adv Neurol* 1986; 45:275–276.

17. Apps M, Shaff P, Ingram D, et al. Respiration and sleep in Parkinson's disease. *J Neurol Neurosurg Psychiatry* 1985; 48:1240–1245.

18. Manschauer FE, Loh L, Bannister R, et al. Abnormal respiration and sudden death during sleep in multiple system atrophy with autonomic failure. *Neurology* 1990; 40:677–679.

19. Van Hilten B, Hoff JI, Middelkoop AM, et al. Sleep disruption in Parkinson's disease. *Arch Neurol* 1994; 51:922–928.

20. Laihinen A, Alihanka J, Raitasuo S, et al. Sleep movements and associated autonomic nervous activities in patients with Parkinson's disease. *Acta Neurol Scand* 1987; 76:64–68.

21. Jansen ENH, Meerwaldt JD. Madopar HBS in Parkinson patients with nocturnal akinesia. *Clin Neurol Neurosurg* 1988; 90:35–39.

22. Nausieda PA, Leo GJ, Chesney C. A comparison of conventional and Sinemet CR on the sleep of parkinsonian patients. *Neurology* 1994; 44(Suppl 2):A219.

23. Lees AJ. A sustained-release formulation of L-dopa (Madopar HBS) in the treatment of nocturnal and early-morning disabilities in Parkinson's disease. *Eur Neurol* 1987; 27(Suppl 1):126–134.

24. UK Madopar CR Study Group. A comparison of Madopar CR and standard Madopar in the treatment of nocturnal and early-morning disability in Parkinson's disease. *Clin Neuropharmacol* 1989; 12:498–505.

25. Gillin JC, Post RM, Wyatt R, et al. REM inhibitory effect of L-dopa infusion during human sleep. *Electroenceph Clin Neurophysiol* 1973; 35:181–186.

26. Cianchetti C. Dopamine agonists and sleep in man. In: Wauquier A (ed.). New York: Raven Press, 1985:121–133.

27. Wyatt RJ, Chase TN, Scott J, et al. Effect of L-dopa on the sleep of man. *Nature* 1970; 228:999–1001.

28. Greenburg R, Pearlman CA. L-dopa, parkinsonism, and sleep. *Psychophysiology* 1970; 7:314.

29. Schmidt HS, Knopp W. Sleep in Parkinson's disease: The effect of L-dopa. *Psychophysiology* 1972; 9:88–89.

30. Tanner CM, Vogel C, Goetz CG, et al. Hallucinations in Parkinson's disease: A population study. *Ann Neurol* 1983; 14:136.

31. Celesia GC, Barr AN. Psychosis and other psychiatric manifestations of levodopa therapy. *Arch Neurol* 1970; 23:193–200.

32. Sacks OW, Kohl MS, Messeloff CR, et al. Effects of levodopa in parkinsonian patients with dementia. *Neurology* 1972; 22:516–519.

33. Moskovitz C, Moses K, Klawans HL. Levodopa-induced psychosis: A kindling phenomenon. *Am J Psychiatry* 1978; 135:669–675.

34. Goetz CG, Tanner CM, Klawans HL. Pharmacology of hallucinations induced by long-term drug therapy. *Am J Psychiatry* 1982; 139:494–497.

35. Pederzoli M, Girotti F, Scigliano G, et al. L-dopa long-term treatment in Parkinson's disease: Age related side effects. *Neurology* 1983; 33:1518–1522.

36. Rondot P, De Recondo J, Coignet A, et al. Mental disorders in Parkinson's disease after treatment with L-dopa. *Adv Neurol* 1984; 40:259–269.

37. Glantz R, Bieliauskas L, Paleologos N. Behavioral indicators of hallucinosis in levodopa-treated Parkinson's disease. *Adv Neurol* 1986; 45:417–420.

38. Factor SA, Molho ES, Podskalny GD, et al. Parkinson's disease: Drug-induced psychiatric states. *Adv Neurol* 1995; 65:115–138.

39. Nausieda P, Weiner W, Kaplan L, et al. Sleep disruption in the course of chronic levodopa therapy: An early feature of the levodopa psychosis. *Clin Neuropharmacol* 1982; 5:183–194.

40. Nausieda PA, Glantz R, Weber S, et al. Psychiatric complications of levodopa therapy of Parkinson's disease. *Adv Neurol* 1984; 40:271–277.

41. Comella CL, Tanner CM, Ristanovic RK. Polysomnographic sleep measures in Parkinson's disease patients with treatment-induced hallucinations. *Ann Neurol* 1993; 34:710–714.

42. Clark EC, Feinstein B. The on-off effect in Parkinson's disease treated with levodopa with remarks concerning the effect of sleep. *Adv Exp Med Biol* 1977; 90:175–182.

43. Hogl BE, Gomez-Arevalo G, Garcia S, et al. A clinical, pharmacologic, and polysomnographic study of sleep benefit in Parkinson's disease. *Neurology* 1998; 50:1332–1339.

44. Comella CL, Boehme J, Jaglin J. Sleep benefit in Parkinson's disease (abstract). *Neurology* 1995; 45(Suppl 4):A286.

45. Jones BE. Paradoxical sleep and its chemical structural substrates in the brain. *Neuroscience* 1991; 40:637–656.

46. Shiromani PJ, Siegel JM. Descending projections from the dorsolateral pontine tegmentum to the paramedian reticular nucleus of the caudal medulla in the cat. *Brain Res* 1990; 517:224–228.

47. Hendricks JC, Morrison AR, Mann GL. Different behaviors during paradoxical sleep without atonia depend on pontine lesion site. *Brain Res* 1982; 239:81–105.

48. Schenk CS, Bundie SR, Ettinger MG, et al. Chronic behavioral disorders of human REM sleep: A new category of parasomnia. *Sleep* 1986; 9:293–308.

49. Schenk CS, Bundie SR, Patterson AL, et al. Rapid eye movement sleep behavior disorder. *JAMA* 1987; 257:1786–1789.

50. American Sleep Disorders Association. REM sleep behavior disorder. *The International Classification of Sleep Disorders*. Kansas: Allen Press, 1990:177–180.

51. Lapierre O, Montplaisir J. Polysomnographic features of REM sleep behavior disorder: Development of a scoring method. *Neurology* 1992; 42:1371–1374.

52. Schenck CH, Milner DM, Hurwitz TD, et al. A polysomnographic and clinical report on sleep-related injury in 100 adult patients. *Am J Psychiatry* 1989; 146:1166–1173.

53. Schenk CH, Mahowald MW. Polysomnographic, neurologic, psychiatric, and clinical outcome report on 70 consecutive cases with REM sleep behavior disorder (RBD): Sustained clonazepam efficacy in 89.5% of 57 treated patients. *Cleve Clin J Med* 1990; 57(suppl):S9–S23.

54. Silber CH, Ahlskog JE. REM sleep behavior disorder in parkinsonian syndromes. *Sleep Res* 1992; 21:313.

55. Silber MH, Ahlskog JE. REM sleep behavior disorder and Parkinson's disease (abstract). *Neurology* 1993; 43(Suppl 2):A338.

56. Comella CL, Ristanovic R, Goetz CG. Parkinson disease patients with and without REM behavior disorder

57. Silber MH, Ahlskog JE. REM sleep behavior disorder in parkinsonian syndromes. *Sleep Res* 1992; 21:313.

58. Schenck CH, Bundlie SR, Mahowald MW. Delayed emergence of a parkinsonian disorder in 38% of 29 older men initially diagnosed with idiopathic rapid eye movement sleep behavior disorder. *Neurology* 1996; 46:388–393.

59. Schenck CH, Mahowald MW. Polysomnographic, neurologic, psychiatric, and clinical outcome report on 70 consecutive cases with REM sleep behavior disorder (RBD): Sustained clonazepam efficacy in 89.5% of 57 treated patients. *Cleve Clin J Med* 1990; 57(Suppl):S9–S23.

60. Plazzi G, Corsini R, Peirangeli G, et al. REM sleep behavior disorders in multiple system atrophy. *Neurology* 1997; 48:1094–1097.

61. Ben-Shlomo Y, Wenning GK, Tison F, et al. Survival of patients with pathologically proven multiple system atrophy: A meta-analysis. *Neurology* 1997; 48:384–393.

62. Culebras A, Moore JT. Magnetic resonance findings in REM sleep behavior disorder. *Neurology* 1989; 39:1519–1523.

63. Hirsch E, Graybiel AM, Duyckaerts C, et al. Neuronal loss in the pedunculopontine nucleus in Parkinson disease and in Progressive Supranuclear Palsy. *Proc Natl Acad Sci USA* 1987; 84:5976–5980.

64. Tandberg E, Larsen JP, Karlsen K. Excessive daytime sleepiness and sleep benefit in Parkinson's disease: A community based study. *Mov Disord* 1999; 14:922–927.

65. Frucht S, Rogers JD, Greene P, et al. Falling asleep at the wheel: Motor vehicle mishaps in persons taking pramipexole and ropinirole. *Neurology* 1999; 52:1908–1910.

66. Schapira AHV. Sleep attacks (sleep episodes) with pergolide. *Lancet* 2000; 355:1332–1333.

67. Ferreira JJ, Galitsky M, Montastruc JL, et al. Sleep attacks and Parkinson's disease treatment. *Lancet* 2000; 355:1333–1334.

(RBD): A polysomnographic and clinical comparison. *Neurology* 1993:43.

13

Natural History

Andrew Feigin, M.D., and David Eidelberg, M.D.
North Shore University Hospital, Manhasset, New York

INTRODUCTION

As new therapies for Parkinson's disease (PD) are developed, the need for accurate and comprehensive descriptions of the natural history of the disease is increasingly important. Specifically, knowledge regarding the length of the preclinical period, age of clinical onset, the rate of progression of both early and late-stage PD, and the common causes of death, is critical for designing clinical trials aimed at demonstrating neuroprotection. In addition, studies aimed at improving the symptoms of PD will be strengthened by a thorough understanding of the usual causes of PD disability and the typical manner and time at which these present. Over the past two decades, much has been learned regarding the natural history of PD, and this chapter reviews this information and its implications for the experimental therapeutics of PD.

PRECLINICAL PERIOD

Estimates of the time between the onset of neurophysiologic dysfunction and clinical onset of PD have been derived from both postmortem pathologic studies and in vivo neuroimaging studies. Although many of these studies have utilized different methods and have made varying assumptions regarding the linearity of the progression of PD, many of the results are in agreement and have narrowed estimates for the proposed preclinical period.

Neuropathologic Studies

Initial neuropathologic studies of PD suggested that patients presenting with the earliest signs of the disease have already lost as much as 50 percent of the pigmented dopaminergic neurons in the substantia nigra and 80 percent of striatal dopamine (1). Subsequent studies have modified these findings, suggesting that clinical signs of PD begin to emerge when there has been an approximately 30 percent reduction in total nigral dopaminergic neurons (2), although the most affected portion of the substantia nigra, the ventrolateral region, has lost greater than 60 percent of its neurons at clinical onset. Using cross-sectional neuropathologic data from patients with PD at various stages, and assuming a nonlinear progression of disease, these authors estimated that the neuropathologic process began approximately five years before clinical onset of symptoms. Although an earlier postmortem study utilizing a vesicular monoamine transporter-binding ligand to quantify striatal dopaminergic innervation found similar reductions in dopaminergic activity, this study suggested a longer preclinical period, estimated at 20 to 30 years (3). The difference is likely due to the absence of patients with very early disease in the latter study; that is, the rate of neuronal loss in PD has been consistently found to be more rapid in the early stages of disease (2,4). Therefore, if the rate of neuronal loss in middle and advanced disease is extrapolated back to the preclinical period, the length of the preclinical period will be overestimated.

Neuroimaging Studies

Estimates of the preclinical period in PD based on neuroimaging studies have varied, but much of this variation may be accounted for by methodological differences. Using [^{18}F]fluorodopa positron emission tomography (PET), Vingerhoets and coworkers studied 16 PD patients on two occasions separated by a mean of seven years (5). Linear regression analysis estimated the preclinical period at 40 to 50 years, although a nonlinear fit of the data predicted a preclinical period of 10 to 15 years. In a similar study involving PD patients with a shorter duration of disease, Moorish and coworkers (6) estimated the preclinical period at three years. As with the neuropathologic studies, the differences in these results are likely due to the different population of patients studied. Again, if the progression of PD is nonlinear with a more rapid rate of decline in early disease and a shallower slope of decline in advanced disease, linear extrapolation from data collected from relatively advanced patients will predict a long preclinical period. Therefore, longitudinal studies in early PD patients are more likely to provide accurate estimates of the preclinical period. A single photon emission computed tomography (SPECT) study utilizing the dopamine transporter ligand [^{123}I]βCIT in a cohort of early PD patients estimated the preclinical period at approximately four years (7), supporting the earlier PET findings. In another study involving largely early PD subjects who underwent [^{18}F]fluorodeoxyglucose (FDG) PET, Moeller and Eidelberg (8) demonstrated an abnormal dissociation between a brain network associated with aging and the actual age of PD patients. Extrapolating back to when this dissociation equaled zero gave an estimate of the preclinical period of PD of approximately five years (8). Thus, neuroimaging studies in relatively early PD patients seem to be consistent in estimating the preclinical period at under 10 years, and perhaps under five years.

Clinical Studies

The neuropathologic and neuroimaging estimates of the duration of the preclinical period are supported by clinical evidence as well. Gonera and coworkers (9) compared medical records from 60 PD patients during the decade preceding the diagnosis of PD with those of 58 matched controls. They found several signs and symptoms that occurred more frequently in the PD group than in the control group, including mood changes, pain, paraesthesias, and hypertension, and these differences were identified in the period 4 to 6 years before PD onset. Others have reported depression, malaise, and nonspecific sensory complaints occurring in the years preceding clinical diagnosis of PD (10). Although unproven, these observations suggest that the preclinical neuropathologic changes of PD may be accompanied by subtle clinical symptoms not normally associated with PD.

CLINICAL PRESENTATION

Age of Onset and Symptoms at Onset

The average age of PD onset is approximately 50 to 60 years (11,12), but the range is quite broad, extending on rare occasion from the twenties to any time in old age. Approximately 5 percent of patients present before the age of 40. The factors that determine age of onset are not known. Sixty to 70 percent of patients present with unilateral rest tremor (13,14), but other common

presenting symptoms may include impaired balance or gait disturbance, slowness, and dystonia. Asymmetry of symptom onset is the norm (15). Interestingly, some investigators have noted a preponderance of right-sided onset of symptoms. For example, Poewe and coworkers (13) noted onset on the right side in 61 percent of patients and on the left side in 39 percent of patients in a retrospective study of 253 patients with the clinical diagnosis of PD. (For a detailed review of early PD features, see Chapter 6).

RATE OF PROGRESSION

Rate of Disease Progression

Clinical Studies

Although James Parkinson described aspects of progression in his original description of the disease (16) the first quantitative observations regarding the rate of progression of PD were provided by Hoehn and Yahr (14) in their landmark study of 856 parkinsonian patients. Utilizing the Hoehn and Yahr (HY) scale, the authors evaluated the progression of PD disability in a cohort of 183 untreated patients. They found that the median time to end-stage PD from onset of symptoms was nine years to HY IV and 14 years to HY V. Nonetheless, the progression of PD was observed to be highly variable, so that 16 percent of patients progressed to HY V in under five years, but 34 percent of patients were still in stage I or II 10 or more years after onset. Although some of this variation was likely due to the inclusion of patients with atypical parkinsonism, subsequent studies have confirmed the extensive variability in the rate of progresssion of PD (17). Overall, the average amount of time in each HY stage has been estimated to be approximately 2 to 3 years (17).

Clinical trials aimed at slowing the progression of PD have provided valuable data regarding the natural history of the disease. The study of patients in the placebo arm of prospective, long-term, controlled studies yields detailed and accurate information regarding progression of untreated PD. The Deprenyl and Tocopherol Antioxidative Therapy of Parkinsonism (DATATOP) study enrolled 800 subjects with early (HY I or II) untreated PD and utilized the Unified Parkinson's Disease Rating Scale (UPDRS; 18). Of these, 353 subjects were treated with either placebo or placebo plus tocopherol (found to be ineffective). Overall, the total UPDRS score worsened by 14 percent per year, and the motor portion of the UPDRS score worsened at a rate of approximately 9 percent per year. Similar to earlier longitudinal progression studies, the DATATOP cohort included a group of patients who appeared to have a more slowly progressive course and did not require symptomatic therapy during follow-up. This group, accounting for approximately one-third of the 353 placebo/placebo + tocopherol subjects, progressed at markedly slower rates (total UPDRS 6% per year, motor UPDRS 4% per year) (19). Other clinical trials have found similar rates of change in UPDRS measures in both treated and untreated PD patients (4,20).

The somatotopic progression of PD has recently been described (13). Patients presenting with unilateral upper extremity symptoms typically proceed to ipsilateral lower extremity involvement in 0.8 to 1.4 years and to bilateral involvement in 2.1 to 3.4 years. Despite the progression to bilateral disease, most patients continue to experience more severe symptoms on the initially affected side throughout the course of the disease (21).

Neuroimaging Studies

Neuroimaging studies with PET and SPECT have examined the rate of progression of PD. Although many studies have established that these methods utilizing different ligands provide objective measures that correlate highly with clinical measures of PD severity, there have been very few longitudinal prospective neuroimaging studies in PD.

[^{18}F]fluorodopa (FDOPA) has been the most extensively used radiotracer. FDOPA/PET accurately distinguishes early PD from normal controls, and significant correlations between UPDRS severity ratings and striatal uptake rate constants have been described (22–24). Analogous clinical correlations have been detected with PET imaging of striatal dopamine transporter (DAT) binding (25). Nonetheless, there have only been two longitudinal PET studies in PD (5,6). The first study demonstrated a 1.7 percent per year decline in striatal-to-background ratios of FDOPA uptake in 16 PD subjects with PET scans repeated over a period of seven years. Similarly, the second study found a 2.3 percent per year decline in FDOPA uptake in 17 patients with scans repeated over a mean of 16.5 months. In a recent placebo-controlled trial of fetal cell implantation for the treatment of PD, young subjects (under age 60) initially undergoing sham surgery, with burr hole placement only, were found to have a decline of approximately 3 percent in FDOPA putamenal uptake over one year (26). The older subjects did not have a significant decline, perhaps suggesting that the rate of decline in more advanced patients is slower (the older group had higher baseline mean UPDRS scores, although they were matched with the young cohort for disease duration and baseline striatal FDOPA uptake). Alternatively, the small number of subjects in the older group (n = 9) may

have provided insufficient power to detect a statistically significant change over one year.

SPECT studies utilizing DAT ligands have also examined the rate of progression of PD. The best-studied SPECT ligand has been [^{123}I]β-CIT (27,28). The annualized rate of loss of striatal [^{123}I]β-CIT uptake has been measured at 12 percent in a cohort of early PD patients followed over a mean of 15 months (7). Using another DAT ligand, [^{123}I]IPT, with SPECT, Schwarz and coworkers (29) reported a decline in uptake of 3 percent in a cohort comprised of both early and late-stage PD patients followed over a mean of 12 months. These studies support the idea that the rate of progression of PD may be more rapid in the earlier stages of the disease.

Clinical Predictors of Progression

Given the variability of the rate of progression of PD, the ability to predict the prognosis for a given patient would be very useful both in clinical practice and for clinical trials. Unfortunately, reliable predictors of disease severity have not been identified. Factors that have been associated with a slow rate of progression of disability include tremor predominance and young age at onset (19). Several studies have reported a slower rate of onset of disability in patients presenting with tremor (17,30,31). Furthermore, those presenting with tremor predominance appear to present at an earlier age and are less likely to develop a dementia (30). Early age of PD onset may be an independent factor associated with a relatively good prognosis (32–34).

Effects of Therapy

Dopaminergic therapy has affected the natural history of PD in two ways. First, the course of progression of disability in PD has been altered, and second, complications of long-term exposure to levodopa must now be considered part of the natural history of the disease.

The rate of progression of PD disability appears to be slower since the advent of levodopa therapy. Hoehn (35) reported that PD patients treated with levodopa spent three to five years more in each HY stage compared with subjects followed in the prelevodopa era. Furthermore, for PD patients with disease duration of 10 to 14 years, 38 percent of levodopa-treated patients had reached HY stage IV or V or had died compared with 83 percent of untreated patients. Despite these observations, it remains uncertain whether levodopa actually alters the neuropathologic progression of PD.

Although levodopa has provided dramatic and sustained symptomatic benefits for patients with PD, these benefits appear to occur at the expense of long-term complications such as dyskinesias and motor fluctuations. Several factors appear to affect the likelihood of developing complications of dopaminergic therapy, including duration of exposure to levodopa, levodopa dose, PD severity, and age (36–38). Overall, between 50 and 100 percent of all PD patients taking levodopa for greater than six years will develop peak-dose dyskinesias (13). In an effort to reduce the incidence of dyskinesias, early treatment of PD often focuses on drugs other than levodopa. Specifically, a recent study has found that PD patients initially treated with the dopamine agonist ropinirole showed a significantly lower rate of dyskinesias at five years; in the ropinlrole group 20% developed dyskinesias compared to 48% in the levodopa-treated group (39). However, ropinirole was not as effective as levodopa in controlling motor symptoms of PD.

DISEASE DURATION AND MORTALITY

Although the overall duration of PD from onset until death may not have changed significantly since the advent of levodopa, mortality in early PD has been dramatically reduced (40,41). In the prelevodopa era, Hoehn and Yahr found a mean duration of disease of 9.4 years and a mean age at death of 67 in a cohort of 672 PD patients (14). They found a mortality rate of 2.9 times that expected for an age-matched population. Subsequently, after the introduction of levodopa, Hoehn (35) reported a mortality ration of 1.5, and other studies have found similar mortality rates (42,43). Mean PD duration has been found to be approximately 13 years, and the mean age at death has been reported at 73 years (43). Therefore, levodopa has reduced the mortality of PD and extended life, although patients with PD still have higher mortality rates compared with age-matched populations.

The causes of death in PD patients have not changed since the advent of dopaminergic therapy. Cardiovascular disease is the most common cause of death in PD followed by pneumonia (43). Malignant neoplasms, although the second most common cause of death in the general population over the age of 65, appears to occur less frequently in PD patients (43,44).

CONCLUSION

Over the past four decades the development and validation of clinical scales and neuroimaging methods have permitted more quantitative and rigorous descriptions of PD onset and progression. Advances in the understanding of the pathophysiology of PD over the same period have begun to suggest therapeutic strategies aimed at altering the course of the disease. The challenge for the new millennium will be to identify disease-modifying agents. The ability to achieve this will be based both on the strong groundwork of knowledge of the natural history of PD already accumulated and on the development of new methods of assessing disease severity and progression.

Acknowledgment

Supported by R01 NS35069, R01 NS32368, K08 NS02011, and the National Parkinson Foundation.

REFERENCES

1. Marsden CD. Parkinson's disease. *Lancet* 1990; 335:948–952.
2. Fearnley JM, Lees AJ. Aging and Parkinson's disease: Substantia nigra regional selectivity. *Brain* 1991; 114:2283–2301.
3. Scherman D, Desnos C, Darchen F, et al. Striatal dopamine deficiency in Parkinson's disease: Role of aging. *Ann Neurol* 1989; 26:551–557.
4. Lee CS, Schulzer M, Mak EK, et al. Clinical observations on the rate of progression of idiopathic parkinsonism. *Brain* 1994; 117:501–507.
5. Vingerhoets FJG, Snow BJ, Lee CS, et al. Longitudinal fluorodopa positron emission tomographic studies of the evolution of idiopathic parkinsonism. *Ann Neurol* 1994; 36:759–764.
6. Morrish PK, Sawle GV, Brooks DJ. [^{18}F]dopa-PET and clinical study of the rate of progression in Parkinson's disease. *Brain* 1996; 119:585–591.
7. Marek KL, Seibyl J, Fussell B, et al. ^{123}I-βCIT: Assessment of progression in Parkinson's disease. *Neurology* 1997; 48(Suppl 2):A207.
8. Moeller JR, Eidelberg D. Divergent expression of regional metabolic topographies in Parkinson's disease and normal aging. *Brain* 1997; 120:2197–2206.
9. Gonera EG, van't Hof M, Berger HJC, et al. Symptoms and duration of the prodromal phase in Parkinson's disease. *Mov Disord* 1997; 12:871–876.
10. Koller WC. When does Parkinson's disease begin? *Neurology* 1992; 42(Suppl 4):27–31.
11. Hoehn MM. The natural history of Parkinson's disease in the pre-levodopa and post-levodopa eras. *Neurol Clin* 1992; 10:331–339.
12. Rajput AH, Offord KP, Beard Cm, et al. Epidemiology of parkinsonism. *Ann Neurol* 1984; 16:278–282.
13. Poewe WH, Wenning GK. The natural history of Parkinson's disease. *Ann Neurol* 1998; 44(Suppl 1): S1–S9.

14. Hoehn MM, Yahr. Parkinsonism: Onset, progression, and mortality. *Neurology* 1967; 17:427–442.

15. Hughes AJ, Ben Schlomo Y, Daniel SE, et al. What features improve the accuracy of clinical diagnosis in Parkinson's disease? *Neurology* 1992; 42:1142–1146.

16. Parkinson J. *An Essay on The Shaking Palsy.* London: Sherwood, Neely, and Jones, 1817.

17. Marttila PJ, Rinne UK. Disability and progression in Parkinson's disease. *Acta Neurol Scand* 1977; 56:159–169.

18. The Parkinson Study Group. Effects of tocopherol and deprenyl on the progression of disability in early Parkinson's disease. *N Engl J Med* 1993; 328:176–183.

19. Jankovic J, McDermott M, Carter J, et al. and the Parkinson Study Group. Variable expression of Parkinson's disease: A baseline analysis of the DATATOP cohort. *Neurology* 1990; 40:1529–1534.

20. Olanow CW, Hauser RA, Gauger L. The effect of deprenyl and levodopa on the progression of Parkinson's disease. *Ann Neurol* 1995; 38:771–777.

21. Lee CS, Schulzer M, Mak E, et al. Patterns of asymmetry do not change over the course of idiopathic parkinsonism: Implications for pathogenesis. *Neurology* 1995; 45:435–439.

22. Eidelberg D, Moeller JR, Dhawan V, et al. The metabolic anatomy of Parkinson's disease: Complementary ^{18}F-fluorodeoxyglucoseand ^{18}F-fluorodopa positron emission tomography studies. *Mov Disord* 1990; 5:203–213.

23. Takikawa S, Dhawan V, Chaly T, et al. Input functions for ^{18}F-fluorodopa quantitation in parkinsonism: Comparative studies and clinical correlations. *J Nucl Med* 1994; 35:955–963.

24. Ishikawa T, Dhawan V, Chaly T, et al. Clinical significance of striatal dopa decarboxylase activity in Parkinson's disease. *J Nucl Med* 1996; 37:216–222.

25. Kazumata K, Dhawan V, Chaly T, et al. Dopamine transporter imaging with [^{18}F]FP-CIT and PET. *J Nucl Med* 1998; 39(9):1521–1530.

26. Dhawan V, Nakamura T, Margouleff C, et al. Double-blind controlled trial of human embryonic dopaminergic tissue transplants in advanced Parkinson's disease: Fluorodopa PET imaging. *Neurology* 1999; 52(Suppl 2):A405–A406.

27. Marek KL, Seibyl JP, Zoghbi S. Iodine-βCIT/SPECT imaging demonstrates bilateral loss of dopamine transporters in hemi-Parkinson's disease. *Neurology* 1996; 46:231–237.

28. Seibyl JP, Marek KL, Quinlan D, et al. Decreased single-photon emission computed tomographic [^{123}I]βCIT striatal uptake correlates with symptom severity in Parkinson's disease. *Ann Neurol* 1995; 38:589–598.

29. Schwarz J, Tatsch K, Linke R, et al. Measuring the decline of dopamine transporter binding in patients with Parkinson's disease using ^{123}I-IPT and SPECT. *Neurology* 1997; 48(Suppl 2):A208.

30. Zetusky WJ, Jankovic J, Pirozzolo FJ. The heterogeneity of Parkinson's disease: Clinical and prognostic implications. *Neurology* 1985; 35:522–526.

31. Roos RAC, Jongen CF, Van der Velde EA. Clinical course of patients with idiopathic Parkinson's disease. *Mov Disord* 1996; 3:236–242.

32. Goetz CG, Tanner CM, Stebbins GT, et al. Risk factors for progression in Parkinson's disease. *Neurology* 1988; 38:1841–1844.

33. Blin J, Dubois B, Bonnet AM, et al. Does aging aggravate parkinsonian disability? *J Neurol Neurosurg Psychiatry* 1991; 54:780–782.

34. Diamond SG, Markham CH, Hoehn MM, et al. Effect of age at onset on progression and mortality in Parkinson's disease. *Neurology* 1989; 39:1187–1190.

35. Hoehn MM. Parkinsonism treated with levodopa: Progression and mortality. *J Neurol Transm* 1983; (Suppl 19):253–264.

36. McDowell FH, Sweet R. Ten-year follow-up study of levodopa-treated patients with Parkinson's disease. *Adv Neurol* 1979; 24:475–480.

37. Quinn N, Critchley P, Marsden CD. Young onset Parkinson's disease. *Mov Disord* 1987; 2:73–91.

38. Horstink MWIM, Zijlmans JCM, Pasman JW, et al. Severity of Parkinson's disease is a risk factor for peak dose dyskinesia. *J Neurol Neurosurg Psychiatry* 1990; 53:224–226.

39. Rascol O, Brooks DJ, Korczyn AD, et al. Ropinirole reduces risk of dyskinesia compared to L-dopa when used in early PD. Abstract presentation at the International Congress on Parkinson's Disease, Vancouver, 1999.

40. Curtis L, Lees AJ, Stern GM, et al. Effect of levodopa on course of Parkinson's disease. *Lancet* 1984; 2:211–212.

41. Uitti RJ, Ahlskog JE, Maranganore DM, et al. Levodopa therapy and survival in idiopathic Parkinson's disease: Olmsted County Project. *Neurology* 1993; 43:1918–1926.

42. Shaw KM, Lees AJ, Stern GM. The impact of treatment with levodopa on Parkinson's disease. *Q J Med* 1980; 49:283–293.

43. Di Rocco A, Molinari SP, Kollmeier B, et al. Parkinson's disease: Progression and mortality in the L-dopa era. *Adv Neurol* 1996; 69:3–11.

44. Jansson B, Jankovic J. Low cancer rates among patients with Parkinson's disease. *Ann Neurol* 1985; 17:505–509.

14

Quantitative Measures and Rating Scales

Stephen T. Gancher, M.D.

Department of Neurology, Oregon Health Sciences University, Portland, Oregon

INTRODUCTION

Before the discovery of levodopa, studies that described the efficacy of drug treatment or of surgical therapy largely relied on subjective impressions of disease severity rather than formal assessments. In more recent years, standardized ratings have been developed to compare the effectiveness of a variety of interventions and to allow studies of the natural history of disease progression.

Several different measures of disease severity are commonly employed. In addition to motor signs, which are used in all objective scales, a number of disease symptoms may also be used to measure overall disease severity. These include patient self-reports such as diaries, estimation of functional performance, and measures of impairments of the quality of life.

Another approach is to use biologic markers of disease severity, such as the uptake of radiolabelled levodopa or the binding of other ligands into the striatum. These measures are especially useful in studies of protective or reparative therapy, but have also been successfully employed in the validation of clinical rating scales.

EARLY STANDARDIZED RATINGS

One of the first widely used scales is a single-item assessment, reported by Hoehn and Yahr in a study of the natural history of Parkinson's disease (1). Although this scale was developed only as a broad classification of patients, it is very easily administered and a modified form is still widely used in practice and clinical trials. This scale, like other early scales, relies on motor signs but has elements of patient functional status in descriptions of several stages. A number of other early scales employ a general measure of independence,

for example, the Northwestern University Disability Scale (2), or a mixture of motor signs and functional status (3–5). These scales, as well as other earlier scales, are comprehensively reviewed by Martinez-Martin (6).

THE UNIFIED PARKINSONS DISEASE RATING SCALE

Description

Because of the marked variability between scales and differences in weighting signs and symptoms, a committee chaired by Fahn was created in 1984 to develop a standardized scale. This scale, the Unified Parkinson's Disease Rating Scale (UPDRS) (Fahn et al., 1987), is a composite of various previous scales and its use in the United States has largely supplanted other scales.

The UPDRS is a composite scale, consisting of six sections. Unless otherwise indicated, all items are rated from zero (normal) to four (severely affected); each item is defined by a short sentence.

Part I of the UPDRS consists of four items, assessing mentation, behavior and mood. Although helpful as a general screen, these items are inadequate to estimate the severity of dementia or depression, and other instruments should be used for their assessment.

Part II consists of 13 items, which describe the ability to perform a number activities of daily living such as bathing, dressing, using utensils, as well as ratings of any difficulty walking, tremor, and sensory symptoms. Although useful, two limitations in this section should be kept in mind. First, patient perceptions may differ considerably and it is not unusual to observe large discrepancies between subjective ratings and how the scale relates to objective measures of disease severity. A second difficulty is that functional performance may change during "on" and "off" states. As patients commonly perform certain daily activities during certain times or only during "on" periods, rating functional performance only during "on" or "off" states may be artificial and difficult for patients to accurately answer.

Part III is a 14-item rating of motor signs based largely on items in the Columbia Disability scale. In addition to ratings of tremor and an assessment of facial and generalized bradykinesia, performance on several tasks are used to rate disease severity, including any difficulty noted while repeatedly tapping the index finger against the thumb, clenching and unclenching a fist, rising from a chair, and other tasks. The definitions of difficulties with each task are straightforward, and the scale is reproducible. However, this motor scale does not take into account any interference from dyskinesias or dystonias that may downgrade motor performance in some patients.

Part IV rates complications of therapy. This includes several questions about the duration and the severity of dyskinesias and motor fluctuations, and a three-item section concerning anorexia, sleep disturbance, or orthostatic hypotension. Unlike the previous sections, some items in Part IV are rated as present or absent.

Part V is a modified version of the Hoehn and Yahr staging system; overall disease severity is divided into unilateral signs (stage I), bilateral signs without a gait or balance disorder (stage II), and bilateral disease with progressively more difficulty with mobility and balance (stage III–V); half points are allowed between stage I–II and II–III.

Part VI is a disability scale, estimating the degree of dependency in daily activities, and is a modification of an earlier scale (6).

Validation

Until recently, there was little effort to estimate the variation in either the assessments between individual raters, the reproducibility of scales over time, or the correlation between clinical scales and biologic markers of PD. Since the UPDRS has become the most commonly used scale to assess PD severity and serves as an endpoint for many studies, these issues have been extensively studied.

Validation of Clinical Ratings

Several studies have tested the UPDRS for interrater reliability. In a small study (7) 24 patients with Parkinson's disease were rated by two neurologists with experience in use of this scale. Overall, ratings closely agreed between raters (r = 0.8), suggesting good interrater reliability. Some items, such as speech (r = 0.29) and facial akinesia (r = 0.07), though, were

less reliable; this was attributed to difficulty in grading patients with equivocal hypophonia or facial masking. In another study (8), three nurse clinicians and a neurologist rated parkinsonian signs in 75 older, healthy individuals, using part III of the UPDRS; the nurses readministered the scale three weeks later. The ratings were closely correlated between different raters and over the three-week period (r = 0.7–0.9) further demonstrating that the scale has good test-retest and inter-rater reliability.

As the UPDRS is somewhat long to administer, a number of studies have addressed which items are most important and which can be omitted. In a recent study, 111 patients with Parkinson's disease were assessed using the entire UPDRS and the Hoehn and Yahr staging system, by a single rating physician (9). This study found a close correlation between these two measures, but found that some items in the UPDRS rating activities of daily living correlated poorly, and also found that some items appeared to be redundant and could be omitted without reducing the accuracy of the scale.

Another study of the UPDRS measured the variation in this scale by assessing 40 patients with multiple raters, and by assessing 127 patients, over four hospitals in different regions, by a single neurologist (10). They found good agreement between different raters (overall r = 0.98). Similar to other studies, the least reliable items were facial expression, estimating the severity of sensory symptoms, and estimating overall bradykinesia. Using the Hoehn and Yahr stage as an independent variable, this study found a significant correlation (r = 0.71) between the UPDRS and the Hoehn and Yahr stage, also noting that six items in the UPDRS accounted for most of the correlation. A shorter scale with a reduced number of items has been developed based on this and has been shown to have good interrater reliability (11).

Correlation with Biologic Markers of Disease Severity

A number of studies have compared motor ratings with in vivo markers of biochemical abnormalities observed in the basal ganglia of patients with Parkinson's disease. Several types of markers have been used. First, using 18-F-deoxyglucose, a marker of metabolism, a good correlation (r = 0.6) was found between Hoehn and Yahr stage and striatal metabolic rate (12). This study also found that measures of rigidity and bradykinesia correlated with this marker, but tremor did not.

A second approach is to use beta-CIT SPECT; this marker, an analog of cocaine, binds to dopamine presynaptic transporter sites on nerve terminals, and has been used in four studies. Significant correlations (averaging approximately 0.5) have been reported between beta–CIT uptake and Hoehn and Yahr stage, total UPDRS score, scores on part II (activities of daily living) of the UPDRS, and scores on scales of depression (13–16).

Two other markers have been used. A good correlation (r = 0.6) has been found between the motor UPDRS and striatal uptake of F-18-DOPA, another presynaptic marker (17). Similarly, another study found a very good correlation between the uptake of a radiolabelled D2 agonist and UPDDRS severity (r = 0.6 for parts I–III of the UPDRS). This study also found an even stronger correlation between measures of depression and striatal uptake (r = 0.7–0.8), illustrating the biologic basis of depression in this disorder (18).

Validation of Patient Symptom Ratings

Estimates of symptom severity have been less extensively studied. One study (9) found good correlations between part II of the UPDRS, Hoehn and Yahr stage (r = 0.7), and part III of the UPDRS (r = 0.8). This study also found that 8 of the 13 items in part II of the UPDRS accounted for most of the variability, suggesting that the scale could be shortened. Another study, which compared ratings of 30 patients with physician ratings in completing part II of the UPDRS, also found moderate to excellent agreement. This study, though, found a poor correlation with Hoehn and Yahr stage or with part VI of the UPDRS (19). Another larger study of 103 patients compared ratings of the newly designed quality of life scale with Hoehn and Yahr stage and with part VI of the UPDRS, and found a moderate correlation (r = 0.5–0.7) (20).

THE CAPIT RATING SCALE

This scale, an acronym for the Core Assessment Program for Intracerebral Transplantation (21), was devised in an attempt to standardize the ratings obtained in studies of transplantation in Parkinson's disease and is commonly used in assessing the benefits of other neurosurgical treatments.

In addition to utilizing the UPDRS, the CAPIT protocol also includes 0–5 scales for both the duration and severity of dyskinesias. Other items include diary information, timed motor tasks, and videotaped evaluation before and after an oral dose of levodopa. One useful feature is a "practically defined off" period, which is defined as the motor state in the morning after an overnight period without medications, at least one hour after arising (to avoid confounding effects of a sleep benefit).

RATINGS OF DYSKINESIAS

Several dyskinesia rating scales have been devised. The AIMS scale, which was devised for ratings of tardive dyskinesia(22), has been used in earlier studies but is not well-suited for evaluation of Parkinsons disease, in that it concentrates on cranial and oral dyskinesias, and is not recommended.

A number of very simple scales have been described. One scale, which rates the severity and the duration of dyskinesias on a 0–5 scale (but without specifying the distribution of the movements), is described in the CAPIT protocol, (21). Another simple scale rates dyskinesias in each limb, the trunk, and head and neck on a 0–4 scale (0-absent; 4-incapacitating, maximum 24) (23). These scales are very easy and quick to administer, take minimal training, and can be used for repeated examinations in pharmacologic studies.

A more detailed dyskinesia scale appropriate for Parkinson's disease was reported by Goetz et al.in 1994 (24), using a scale based on videotaped ratings of performance of motor tasks. Patients are videotaped performing four tasks (walking, drinking from a cup, putting on a coat, and buttoning), and an overall severity score is assigned (0–5). In addition, the different types and most severe dyskinesias are identified. The description of this scale also included validation measures. Videotapes of 20 patients were reviewed on two occasions by multiple raters, including physicians and study coordinators. Agreement between raters on the severity, type of dyskinesia, and severity of dyskinesia were good for both groups of raters (r = 0.8–0.9). In addition, ratings were very reproducible for individual raters.

The scale is easily performed, either by a physician or trained technician, and may be used either during an interview or from a videotape. One advantage of this scale is that the rating is clearly defined relative to physical appearance and by performance of a motor task, features which reduce subjectivity.

Although useful, there are limitations to this scale. It is relatively fast to administer, but it requires several minutes and is thus inappropriate for acute pharmacologic studies, in which dyskinetic movements may sometimes be assessed at very frequent intervals. In addition, this scale does not assess the distribution or amplitude of movements and may not be appropriate for some studies. In addition, many dyskinesias only occur at specific times of the day, and may not be readily observed during office evaluations. Finally, intensity of pain or other symptoms is not estimated on this scale.

DIARY RATINGS

Another popular instrument for assessment of motor fluctuations involves self reporting of hourly status by patients. The patient is instructed to rate motor symptoms, averaging performance over each hour or half hour. In some versions, the patient is asked to distinguish between "on" and "on with dyskinesias".

Although helpful, a number of problems are encountered with diary information. The largest problem is that in some patients, a poor correlation may be noted between their self-reports and objective assessment of parkinsonism. This may be due to several factors. First, in patients with diphasic or peak-dose dyskinesias, motor functioning may be impaired by dyskinesias and it may be difficult for patients to reliably distinguish between "on" (particularly on with dyskinesia) and "off" states. An additional problem is compliance; if patients fill out these diaries retrospectively (such as at the end of the day), their recall of performance may be inaccurate, and under controlled conditions (such as a research ward), some patient self-reports correlate poorly with nursing or physician ratings of parkinsonism. Although these problems represent a serious limitation in their usefulness, patient diaries may be a simple and effective way of reporting a number of symptoms, including prolonged "off" periods, levodopa dose failures, and severe dyskinesias that otherwise may prove difficult to quantify, and can be useful for both patient care and drug studies.

In an attempt to resolve problems related to the effect of dyskinesia on motor function, Hauser and colleagues (25,26) recently assessed the usefulness of a new diary. This diary separated dyskinesia into troublesome and nontroublesome dyskinesia. Off times and troublesome dyskinesia both were considered "bad" or disabling, whereas on without dyskinesia and on with nontroublesome dyskinesia were "good" times. This diary is currently being used in other trials. It will allow investigators to determine if a decrease in "off" time is being replaced by increased "on" time or just troublesome dyskinesias with no improvement in "on" time whatsoever.

ADMINISTRATION

The UPDRS is administered by a combination of patient interview and physical examination. It can be administered either by a physician or nurse experienced in Parkinson's disease or by a trained technician. Depending on the skill of the rater and interactions with the patient, the UPDRS requires approximately

20–30 min to administer. In practice, the motor portion of the UPDRS is the briefest to administer, particularly in mildly affected patients.

UNIFIED PARKINSON'S DISEASE RATING SCALE (UPDRS)

Mentation, Behavior, and Mood

1. Intellectual Impairment:
   0 – None.
   1 – Mild. Consistent forgetfulness with partial recollection of events and no other difficulties.
   2 – Moderate memory loss, with disorientation and moderate difficulty handling complex problems. Mild but definite impairment of function at home with need of occasional prompting.
   3 – Severe memory loss with disorientation of time and often of place. Severe impairment in handling problems.
   4 – Severe memory loss with orientation preserved to person only. Unable to make judgments or solve problems. Requires much help with personal care. Cannot be left alone at all.

2. Thought Disorder: (Due to dementia or drug intoxication)
   0 – None.
   1 – Vivid dreaming.
   2 – "Benign" hallucinations with insight retained.
   3 – Occasional to frequent hallucinations or delusions; without insight; could interfere with daily activities.
   4 – Persistent hallucinations, delusions, or florid psychosis. Not able to care for self.

3. Depression:
   0 – Not present.
   1 – Periods of sadness or guilt greater than normal, never sustained for day or weeks.
   2 – Sustained depression (1 week or more).
   3 – Sustained depression with vegetative symptoms (insomnia, anorexia, weight loss, loss of interest).
   4 – Sustained depression with vegetative symptoms and suicidal thoughts or intent.

4. Motivation/Initiative:
   0 – Normal.
   1 – Less assertive than usual; more passive.

2 – Loss of initiative or disinterest in elective (nonroutine) activities.

3 – Loss of initiative or disinterest in day to day (routine) activities.

4 – Withdrawn, complete loss of motivation.

Activities of Daily Living (Determine for "on/off")

5. Speech:
   0 – Normal.
   1 – Mildly affected. No difficulty being understood.
   2 – Moderately affected. Sometimes asked to repeat statements.
   3 – Severely affected. Frequently asked to repeat statements.
   4 – Unintelligible most of the time.

6. Salivation:
   0 – Normal.
   1 – Slight but definite excess of saliva in mouth; may have nighttime drooling.
   2 – Moderately excessive saliva; may have minimal drooling.
   3 – Marked excess of saliva with some drooling
   4 – Marked drooling, requires constant tissue or handkerchief.

7. Swallowing:
   0 – Normal.
   1 – Rare choking.
   2 – Occasional choking.
   3 – Requires soft food.
   4 – Requires NG tube or gastrostomy feeding.

8. Handwriting:
   0 – Normal.
   1 – Slightly slow or small.
   2 – Moderately slow or small; all words are legible.
   3 – Severely affected; not all words are legible.
   4 – The majority of words are not legible.

9. Cutting Food and Handling Utensils:
   0 – Normal.
   1 – Somewhat slow and clumsy, but no help needed.
   2 – Can cut most foods, although clumsy and slow; some help needed.
   3 – Food must be cut by someone, but can still feed slowly.
   4 – Needs to be fed.

10. Dressing:
    0 – Normal.
    1 – Somewhat slow, but no help needed.
    2 – Occasional assistance with buttoning, getting arms in sleeves.
    3 – Considerable help required, but can do some things alone.
    4 – Helpless.

11. Hygiene:
    0 – Normal.
    1 – Somewhat slow, but no help needed.
    2 – Needs help to shower or bathe, or very slow in hygienic care.
    3 – Requires assistance for washing, brushing teeth, combing hair, going to bathroom.
    4 – Foley catheter or other mechanical aids.

12. Turning in Bed and Adjusting Bed Clothes:
    0 – Normal.
    1 – Somewhat slow and clumsy, but no help needed.
    2 – Can turn alone or adjust sheets, but with great difficulty.
    3 – Can initiate, but not turn or adjust sheets alone.
    4 – Helpless.

13. Falling (unrelated to freezing):
    0 – None.
    1 – Rare falling.
    2 – Occasionally falls, less than once per day.
    3 – Falls an average of once daily.
    4 – Falls more than once daily.

14. Freezing When Walking:
    0 – None.
    1 – Rare freezing when walking; may have start-hesitation.
    2 – Occasional freezing when walking.
    3 – Frequent freezing. Occasionally falls from freezing.
    4 – Frequent falls from freezing.

15. Walking:
    0 – Normal.
    1 – Mild difficulty. May not swing arms or may tend to drag leg.
    2 – Moderate difficulty, but requires little or no assistance.
    3 – Severe disturbance of walking, requiring assistance.
    4 – Cannot walk at all, even with assistance.

16. Tremor:
    0 – Absent.
    1 – Slight and infrequently present.
    2 – Moderate; bothersome to patient.

3 – Severe; interferes with many activities.
4 – Marked; interferes with most activities.

17. Sensory Complaints Related to Parkinsonism:
0 – None
1 – Occasionally has numbness, tingling, or mild aching.
2 – Frequently has numbness, tingling, or aching; not distressing.
3 – Frequent painful sensations.
4 – Excruciating pain.

Motor Examination

18. Speech:
0 – Normal.
1 – Slight loss of expression, diction and volume.
2 – Monotone, slurred but understandable; moderately impaired.
3 – Marked impairment, difficult to understand.
4 – Unintelligible.

19. Facial Expression:
0 – Normal.
1 – Minimal hypomimia, could be normal "poker face."
2 – Slight but definitely abnormal diminution of facial expression.
3 – Moderate hypomimia; lips parted some of the time.
4 – Masked or fixed facies with severe or complete loss of facial expression; lips parted 1/4 inch or more.

20. Tremor at Rest:
0 – Absent.
1 – Slight and infrequently present.
2 – Mild in amplitude and persistent moderate in amplitude, but only intermittently present.
3 – Moderate in amplitude and present most of the time.
4 – Marked in amplitude and present most of the time.

21. Action or Postural Tremor of Hands:
0 – Absent.
1 – Slight; present with action.
2 – Moderate in amplitude, present with action.
3 – Moderate in amplitude, with posture holding as well as action.
4 – Marked in amplitude; interferes with feeding.

22. Rigidity: (Judged on passive movement of major joints with patient relaxed in sitting position. Cogwheeling to be ignored.)
0 – Absent.
1 – Slight or detectable only when activated by mirror or other movements.
2 – Mild to moderate.
3 – Marked, but full range of motion easily achieved.
4 – Severe, range of motion achieved with difficulty.

23. Finger Taps: (Patient taps thumb with index finger in rapid succession with widest amplitude possible, each hand separately.)
0 – Normal.
1 – Mild slowing or reduction in amplitude (11–14/5 sec).
2 – Moderately impaired. Definite and early fatiguing. May have occasional arrests in movement (7–10/5 sec).
3 – Severely impaired. Frequent hesitation in initiating movements or arrests in ongoing movement (3–6/5 sec).
4 – Can barely perform the task (0–2/5 sec).

24. Hand Movements: (Patient opens and closes hand in rapid succession with widest amplitude possible, each hand separately.)
0 – Normal.
1 – Mild slowing or reduction in amplitude.
2 – Moderately impaired. Definite and early fatiguing. May have occasional arrests in movement.
3 – Severely impaired. Frequent hesitation in initiating movements or arrests in ongoing movement.
4 – Can barely perform the task.

25. Rapid Alternating Movements of Hands: (Pronation-supination movements of hands, vertically or horizontally, with as large an amplitude as possible, both hands simultaneously.)
0 – Normal.
1 – Mild slowing or reduction in amplitude.
2 – Moderately impaired. Definite and early fatiguing. May have occasional arrests in movement.
3 – Severely impaired. Frequent hesitation in initiating movements or arrests in ongoing movement.
4 – Can barely perform the task.

26. Foot agility: (Patient taps heel on ground in rapid succession, picking up entire foot. Amplitude should be about 3 inches.)

0 – Normal.

1 – Mild slowing and/or reduction in amplitude.

2 – Moderately impaired. Definite and early fatiguing. May have occasional arrests in movement.

3 – Severely impaired. Frequent hesitation in initiating movements or arrests in ongoing movement.

4 – Can barely perform the task.

(A new version of this scale also includes the following item)

Toe tapping: subject sits in chair with or without shoes on. Knees should be flexed and legs essentially perpendicular so that heels of feet are placed comfortably about one inch forward of the perpendicular. The patient is instructed as follows: "with your heel on the ground, tap the toes of the foot and don't stop until I tell you to; keep it smooth and regular and as large and as fast as you can." The rater counts the taps to self and has the patient tap 20 times before telling him or her to stop.

0 – Normal. Height of toes off the ground should be at least 1 inch. There are no haltings or hesitations during the tapping, which is smooth and evenly spaced throughout. The normal amplitude should not decrement with continuous tapping.

1 – Mildly impaired amplitude maintained without decrementing, but there are 1-2 hesitations or irregularities in otherwise smooth tapping of toes 20 times.

2 – Moderately impaired. Able to tap the toes the full 20 times with any of the following abnormalities: (a) between 2–5 very brief hesitations; or (b) at least one longer halting period; or (c) decrementing amplitude with tapping.

3 – Severely impaired. Any of the following abnormalities; (a) cannot tap the toes 20 times but does achieve at least 10 taps; or (b) if 20 taps are achieved they are accomplished with more than five hesitations or more than one long halt; or (c) the amplitude never achieved the height of one inch or without decrementing further during the 20 taps.

4 – Markedly impaired. Cannot tap the toes 20 times.

27. Arising From Chair: (Patient attempts to arise from a straight-back wood or metal chair with arms folded across chest.)
    0 – Normal.
    1 – Slow; or may need more than one attempt.

2 – Pushes self up from arms of seat.

3 – Tends to fall back and may have to try more than one time, but can get up without help.

4 – Unable to arise without help.

28. Posture:
    0 – Normal erect.
    1 – Not quite erect, slightly stooped posture; could be normal for older person.
    2 – Moderately stooped posture, definitely abnormal; can be slightly leaning to one side.
    3 – Severely stooped posture with kyphosis; can be moderately leaning to one side.
    4 – Marked flexion with extreme abnormality of posture.

29. Gait:
    0 – Normal
    1 – Walks slowly, may shuffle with short steps, but no festination or propulsion.
    2 – Walks with difficulty, but requires little or no assistance; may have some festination, short steps, or propulsion.
    3 – Severe disturbance of gait, requiring assistance.
    4 – Cannot walk at all, even with assistance.

30. Postural Stability: (Response to sudden posterior displacement produced by pull on shoulders while patient erect with eyes open and feet slightly apart. Patient is prepared.)
    0 – Normal.
    1 – Retropulsion, but recovers unaided.
    2 – Absence of postural response; would fall if not caught by examiner.
    3 – Very unstable, tends to lose balance spontaneously.
    4 – Unable to stand without assistance.

31. Body Bradykinesia and Hypokinesia: (Combining slowness, hesitancy, decreased arm swing, small amplitude, and poverty of movement in general.)
    0 – None.
    1 – Minimal slowness, giving movement a deliberate character; could be normal for some persons. Possibly reduced amplitude.
    2 – Mild degree of slowness and poverty of movement which is definitely abnormal. Alternatively, some reduced amplitude.
    3 – Moderate slowness, poverty or small amplitude of movement.
    4 – Marked slowness, poverty or small amplitude of movement.

Complications of Therapy (in the past week)

Dyskinesias

32. Duration: What proportion of the waking day are dyskinesias present? (Historical information)
    0 – None
    1 – 1–25% of day
    2 – 26–50% of day
    3 – 51–75% of day
    4 – 76–100% of day

33. Disability: How disabling are the dyskinesia? (Historical information; may be modified by office examination.)
    0 – Not disabling
    1 – Mildly disabling
    2 – Moderately disabling
    3 – Severely disabling
    4 – Completely disabling

34. Painful Dyskinesias: How painful are the dyskinesias?
    0 – No painful dyskinesias
    1 – Slight
    2 – Moderate
    3 – Severe
    4 – Marked

35. Presence of Early Morning Dystonia: (Historical information)
    0 – No
    1 – Yes

Clinical fluctuations

36. Are any "off" periods predictable as to timing after a dose of medication?
    0 – No
    1 – Yes

37. Are any "off" periods unpredictable as to timing after a dose of medication?
    0 – No
    1 – Yes

38. Do any of the "off" periods come on suddenly, for example, over a few seconds?
    0 – No
    1 – Yes

39. What proportion of the waking day is patient "off" on average?
    0 – None
    1 – 1–25% of day
    2 – 26–50% of day
    3 – 51–75% of day
    4 – 76–100% of day

Other complications

40. Does the patient have anorexia, nausea, or vomiting?
    0 – No
    1 – Yes

41. Does the patient have any sleep disturbances, for example, insomnia or hypersomnolence?
    0 – No
    1 – Yes

42. Does the patient have symptomatic orthostasis?
    0 – No
    1 – Yes

MODIFIED HOEHN AND YAHR STAGING

Stage 0 –   No signs of disease.
Stage 1 –   Unilateral disease.
Stage 1.5 – Unilateral plus axial involvement.
Stage 2 –   Bilateral disease, without impairment of balance.
Stage 2.5 – Mild bilateral disease with recovery on pull test.
Stage 3 –   Mild to moderate bilateral disease; some postural instability; physically independent.
Stage 4 –   Severe disability; still able to walk or stand unassisted.
Stage 5 –   Wheelchair bound or bedridden unless aided.

MODIFIED SCHWAB AND ENGLAND ACTIVITIES OF DAILY LIVING SCALE

100% – Completely independent. Able to do all chores without slowness, difficulty or impairment. Essentially normal. Unaware of any difficulty.

90% –   Completely independent. Able to do all chores with some degree of slowness, difficulty and impairment. Might take twice as long. Beginning to be aware of difficulty.

80% –   Completely independent in most chores. Takes twice as long. Conscious of difficulty and slowness.

70% –   Not completely independent. More difficulty with some chores. Three to four times as long in some. Must spend a large part of the day with chores.

60% – Some dependency. Can do most chores, but exceedingly slowly and with much effort. Errors; some impossible.

50% – More dependent. Help with half, slower, et cetera. Difficulty with everything.

40% – Very dependent. Can assist with all chores, but few alone.

30% – With effort, now and then does a few chores alone or begins alone. Much help needed.

20% – Nothing alone. Can be a slight help with some chores. Severe invalid.

10% – Total dependent, helpless. Complete invalid.

0% – Vegetative functions such as swallowing, bladder and bowel functions are not functioning. Bed-ridden.

DYSKINESIA RATING SCALE (24)

Directions:
1. View the patient walk, drink from a cup, put on a coat and button clothing.
2. Rate the severity of dyskinesias. These may include chorea, dystonia, and other dyskinetic movements in combination. Rate the patient's worst function.
3. Check which dyskinesias are observed (more than one response possible).
4. Check the type of dyskinesia that is causing the most disability on the tasks seen on the tape (only one response is permitted).

Severity rating code:
0 absent;
1 minimal severity, no interference with voluntary motor acts
2 dyskinesias may impair voluntary movements but patient is normally capable of under-taking most motor acts
3 intense interference with movement control and daily life activities are greatly limited
4 violent dyskinesias, incompatible with any normal motor tasks

Dyskinesias observed (more than one choice possible): Chorea, dystonia, other most disabling dyskinesia (choose one): Chorea, dystonia, other.

REFERENCES

1. Hoehn MM, Yahr MD. Parkinsonism: Onset, progression, and mortality. *Neurology* 1967; 17:427–442.

2. Canter CJ, de la Torre R, Mier M. A method of evaluating disability in patients with Parkinson's disease. *J Nerv Ment Dis* 1961; 133:143–147.

3. Schwab RS. Progression and prognosis in Parkinson's disease. *J Nerv Ment Dis* 1960; 130:556–566.

4. Webster DD. Critical analysis of the disability in Parkinson's disease. *Mod Treat* 1968; 5:257–282.

5. Yahr MD, Duvoisin RC, Schear MJ, et al. Treatment of Parkinsonism with levodopa. *Arch Neurol* 1969; 21:343–354.

6. Martinez-Martin P. Rating scales in Parkinson's disease. In: Jankovic J, Tolosa E (eds.). *Parkinson's Disease and Movement Disorders*. Baltimore: Williams and Wilkins, 1993: pp. 281–92.

7. Richards M, Marder K, Cote L, et al. Interrater reliability of the Unified Parkinson's Disease Rating Scale Motor Examination. *Mov Disord* 1994; 9:89–91.

8. Bennett DA, Shannon KM, Beckett LA, et al. Metric properties of nurses' ratings of parkinsonian signs with a modified Unified Parkinson's Disease Rating Scale. *Neurology* 1997; 49(6):1580–1587.

9. van Hilten JJ, van der Zwan AD, Zwinderman AH, et al. Rating impairment and disability in Parkinson's disease: Evaluation of the Unified Parkinson's Disease Rating Scale. *Mov Disord* 1994; 9:84–88.

10. Martinez-Martin P, Gil-Nagel A, Gracia LM, et al. The Cooperative Multicentric Group. Unified Parkinson's Disease Rating Scale Characteristics and Structure. *Mov Disord* 1994; 9:76–83.

11. Rabey JM, Bass H, Bonuccelli U, et al. Evaluation of the Short Parkinson's Evaluation Scale: A new friendly scale for the evaluation of Parkinson's disease in clinical drug trials. *Clin Neuropharmacol* 1997; 20(4):322–337.

12. Eidelberg D, Moeller JR, Ishikawa T, et al. Assessment of disease severity in parkinsonism with fluorine-18-fluorodeoxyglucose and PET. *J Nucl Med* 1995; 36:378–383.

13. Seibyl JP, Marek KL, Quinlan D, et al. Decreased single-photon emission computed tomographic [123I]-beta-CIT striatal uptake correlates with symptom severity in Parkinson's disease. *Ann Neurol* 1995; 38(4):589–598.

14. Eising EG, Muller TT, Zander C, et al. SPECT-evaluation of the monoamine uptake site ligand [123I](1R)-2-beta- carbomethoxy-3-beta-(4-iodophenyl)-tropane ([123I]beta-CIT) in untreated patients with suspicion of Parkinson disease. *J Investig Med* 1997; 45(8):448–452.

15. Muller T, Farahati J, Kuhn W, et al. [123I]beta-CIT SPECT visualizes dopamine transporter loss in de novo parkinsonian patients. *Euro Neurol* 1998; 39(1):44–48.

16. Brucke T, Asenbaum S, Pirker W, et al. Measurement of the dopaminergic degeneration in Parkinson's disease with [123I] beta-CIT and SPECT. Correlation with clinical findings and comparison with multiple system atrophy and progressive supranuclear palsy. *J Neural Transm* 1994; Suppl:1997–24.

17. Ishikawa T, Dhawan V, Kazumata K, et al. Comparative nigrostriatal dopaminergic imaging with iodine-123-beta CIT-FP/SPECT and fluorine-18-FDOPA/PET. *J Nucl Med* 1996; 37(11):1760–1765.

18. Muller T, Eising EG, Reiners C, et al. 2-[123I]-iodolisuride SPET visualizes dopaminergic loss in de-novo parkinsonian patients: Is it a marker of striatal pre-synaptic degeneration?. *Med Comm* 1997; 18(12):1115–1121.

19. Louis ED, Lynch T, Marder K, et al. Reliability of patient completion of the historical section of the Unified Parkinson's Disease Rating Scale. *Mov Disord* 1996; 11(2):185–192.

20. Martinez-Martin P, Frades Payo B. Quality of life in Parkinson's disease: validation, study of the PDQ-39 Spanish version. The Grupo Centro for study of Movement Disorders. *J Neurol* 1998; 245(Suppl 1):S34-S38.

21. Langston JW, Widner H, Goetz CG, et al. Core Assessment Program for Intracerebral Transplantations (CAPIT). *Mov Disord* 1992; 7:2–13.

22. Guy W. AIMS. *ECDEU Assessment manual for Psychopharmacology. DHEW Publication, no. 76–338.* Washington, DC: US Government Printing Office; 1976; 534–537.

23. Nutt JG, Woodward WR, Hammerstad JP, et al. The "On-off" phenomenon in Parkinson's disease: Relation to levodopa absorption and transport. *N Engl J Med* 1984; 310:483–488.

24. Goetz CG, Stebbins GT, Shale HM, et al. Utility of an objective dyskinesia rating scale for Parkinson's disease: Inter- and intrarater reliability assessment. *Mov Disord* 1994; 9:390–394.

25. Hauser RA. Friedlander J, Zesiewicz TA, et al. Evaluation of a new home diary to assess functional status in Parkinson's disease patients with fluctuations and dyskinesia. *Mov Disord* 1997; 12:843.

26. Hauser RA, Zesiewicz TA, Friedlander J, et al. Impact of different severities of dyskinesia on patient-defined functional status in Parkinson's disease. *Mov Disord* 1997; 12:843.

15

Dementia

Karen Marder, M.D., M.P.H., and Diane M. Jacobs, Ph.D.
Columbia University College of Physicians and Surgeons, New York, New York

Although estimates of the prevalence and incidence of dementia in the setting of Parkinson's disease (PD) vary, there is little doubt that it is an important complication because of the resulting need for reduction or elimination of medications used to treat the motor manifestations and the impact on morbidity and mortality. The spectrum of cognitive impairment seen in PD may be conceptualized as a continuum. Although some patients with PD never develop cognitive impairment, the majority of patients have selective impairment in the domains of memory, executive function and visuospatial skills. A proportion of patients with isolated deficits ultimately progress to dementia. Several basic questions remain unresolved, such as (a) What is the pattern of neuropsychologic impairment in PD and how does it evolve in those who become demented? (b) What is the etiology of dementia in PD and to what extent is the dementia due to Alzheimer's disease (AD)? (c) What are the demographic characteristics, genetic, and environmental risk factors associated with dementia in PD?

DEFINING DEMENTIA IN PARKINSON'S DISEASE

The most widely used criteria for the diagnosis of dementia, from the Diagnostic and Statistical Manual of Mental Disorders, require "the development of multiple cognitive deficits ... sufficiently severe to cause impairment in occupational or social functioning (1)." The cognitive deficits must include impairment of learning or memory plus impaired language, praxis, object recognition, or executive functioning. The cognitive dysfunction must represent a decline from premorbid levels, and cannot occur exclusively during the course of delirium. Although previous editions of the Diagnostic and Statistical Manual of Mental

Disorders stated that "an underlying causative organic factor is always assumed" in cases of dementia, specification of an etiologic factor was not necessary to make the diagnosis. In the current edition of the Diagnostic and Statistical Manual of Mental Disorders (DSM-IV) (1), however, specific dementia diagnoses are assigned based on the presumed etiology; specifically, dementia of the Alzheimer's type, vascular dementia, or dementia due to other general medical conditions. Parkinson's disease is listed among the general medical conditions to which dementia can be attributed.

According to the DSM-IV, "The essential feature of Dementia Due to Parkinson's Disease is the presence of a dementia that is judged to be the direct pathophysiologic consequence of Parkinson's disease" (1). In many cases, however, it is difficult or even impossible to determine whether dementia in a patient with PD is due to a "direct pathophysiologic consequence of Parkinson's disease" or to a co-morbid dementing disorder, such as AD or dementia with Lewy bodies.

One factor to consider in determining whether dementia is due to PD is the temporal relationship between the onset of the motor and cognitive symptoms. This temporal relationship is critical in differentiating AD and dementia with Lewy bodies from PD dementia. On the basis of the consensus guidelines for the diagnosis of dementia with Lewy bodies (2), if the onset of parkinsonian motor symptoms precedes the onset of cognitive symptoms by more than 12 months, then the diagnosis of "PD with dementia" is warranted. The guidelines acknowledge, however, that the 12-month period was "arbitrarily selected to guide clinical practice but may need revision when additional information becomes available about the genetic and pathologic differences between clinical phenotypes." If, on the other hand, the cognitive and motor symptoms commence within 12 months of each other, a diagnosis of dementia with Lewy bodies should be considered.

The temporal presentation of symptoms also can be used to aid in the differential diagnosis of dementia with Lewy bodies and AD with EPS. Specifically, parkinsonism and visual hallucinations are quite common in the advanced stages of AD, however, if these symptoms are prominent early in the course of dementia, a diagnosis of dementia with Lewy bodies should be considered. Thus current diagnostic guidelines recommend that the dementia due to PD be diagnosed when the parkinsonian motor disorder is primary, and that dementia is superimposed only later in the disease course. In contrast, dementia is a central feature required for the diagnosis of dementia with Lewy bodies and the defining feature of AD. Determination of the validity of this temporal distinction, particularly between PD with dementia and dementia with Lewy bodies, awaits future clinicopathologic studies.

In an analysis of case vignettes describing 15 patients with PD, 14 with dementia with Lewy bodies, and 76 without PD, all confirmed by autopsy, PD was predicted by asymmetrical presentation (bradykinesia, tremor, and rigidity), levodopa-induced dyskinesias, and absence of cognitive impairment (3). Dementia with Lewy bodies was predicted by the presence of hallucinations, and the absence of tremor, bradykinesia, and dystonia. Clinically, dementia with Lewy bodies was under-diagnosed, and was most often misdiagnosed as AD or PD. Less likely entities that could be mistaken for dementia in PD include multi-infarct dementia, progressive supranuclear palsy, multisystem atrophy, and corticobasal degeneration.

NEUROPSYCHOLOGIC CHARACTERISTICS OF DEMENTIA IN PARKINSON'S DISEASE

Numerous studies have examined the pattern of cognitive strengths and weaknesses that characterizes dementia in patients with PD (4,5). Many investigators have compared the neuropsychologic characteristics of PD dementia with other dementias, most commonly AD. As such, in addition to the chronology of symptom presentation, the cognitive characteristics of the dementia syndrome itself may be useful in clarifying the etiology of dementia, at least in cases of mild dementia. An overview of results from these studies is presented in the Table 15-1.

Dementia associated with PD is characterized by predominant impairment of executive functions (i.e., planning, initiating, sequencing, monitoring, and shifting between responses), visuomotor and visuospatial skills, free recall memory for verbal and nonverbal material, and verbal fluency. Language functions other than verbal fluency are relatively preserved, as are orientation and cued recall and recognition memory.

Although impairment of learning or memory is a requisite criterion for the diagnosis of dementia, the characteristics of memory impairment vary somewhat depending upon the etiology of the dementia syndrome. One of the most frequently replicated observed differences between demented patients with Parkinson's and Alzheimer's disease on neuropsychologic testing is performance on tests of delayed recall and recognition memory. Both PD and AD patients are impaired

Table 15-1 *Typical Neuropsychological Test Performance of Patients with Cognitive Impairment due to Parkinson's disease, mild Parkinson's disease with dementia, and mild Alzheimer's disease.*

	PD	PD Dementia	AD
Memory			
Immediate Free Recall	Mildly Impaired	Impaired	Impaired
Delayed Free Recall	Mildly Impaired	Impaired	Severely Impaired
Delayed Recognition	Normal	Normal	Severely Impaired
Percent Retention[a]	Normal (>70 %)	Nl. – Mildly Imp. (>50 %)	Severely Impaired (<50%)
Language			
Naming	Normal	Normal – Mildly Impaired	Severely Impaired
Verbal Fluency	Impaired	Severely Impaired	Impaired
Orientation	Normal	Normal	Impaired
Visuospatial Skills	Impaired	Impaired	Impaired
Executive Functions	Impaired	Severely Impaired[b]	Severely Impaired

[a] Percent Retention = (immediate free recall/delayed free recall) X 100.
[b] Executive functions may be disproportionately impaired relative to other cognitive abilities.

in their ability to recall new information. Thus performance on tests of immediate and delayed recall memory is impaired relative to normative data for both patient groups. What distinguishes PD and AD patients is performance on delayed recall testing relative to immediate recall; that is, their retention or "savings" of new material over a delay interval differs. Patients with AD rapidly forget new information, even material that was recalled accurately on immediate memory testing (6,7) and the percentage of recently learned material that is retained after a delay interval is very low, often less than 50%. Patients with AD often are unable to recall or even recognize material that was recalled correctly several minutes earlier. In contrast, delayed recall and recognition memory in patients with PD often is commensurate with the level of recall on testing of immediate memory. Therefore, PD is associated with relatively good retention of newly acquired information over a delay interval. This difference in performance on memory testing between AD and PD patients is evident even when groups are comparable in terms of overall dementia severity, but it may be particularly pronounced in the early or mild stages of dementia. The fact that long-term retention of new material is relatively maintained in PD, but impaired in AD, supports the conclusion that the memory impairment associated with PD is primarily a retrieval deficit, whereas AD is characterized by deficient encoding or consolidation of information. The encoding deficit of AD probably reflects the prominent pathology of the hippocampus and entorhinal cortex associated with this disorder (8–10), whereas the poor retrieval of new information by PD patients may be secondary to executive dysfunction (i.e., inability to initiate a systematic search of memory) and reflects dysfunction of subcorticofrontal circuits (11).

ROLE OF DOPAMINE IN COGNITIVE DYSFUNCTION

Cognitive impairment in the absence of frank dementia occurs frequently in PD. Nevertheless the mild or relatively circumscribed cognitive dysfunction that is evident in many patients with PD does not progress to frank dementia in all affected individuals. The domains of relative impairment in nondemented PD patients, which overlap in large part with those associated with dementia in PD, include attentional and executive functions, visuospatial skills, recall memory, and verbal fluency (see Table). This pattern of impaired and preserved cognitive abilities on neuropsychologic testing is similar to that associated with damage to the frontal

lobes, particularly the prefrontal cortex (11,12), and is hypothesized to reflect dopamine deficiency and reduced neostriatal outflow to the prefrontal cortex (11). Specifically, loss of dopaminergic neurons in the substantia nigra and nigrostriatal pathway disrupts the physiologic activity of the neostriatum (13) and compromises the functioning of subcortical–cortical functional–anatomical loops.

Neuropsychologic examination of patients with MPTP-induced parkinsonism has supported the assumption that at least some of the cognitive symptoms of PD are due to loss of dopaminergic innervation of the basal ganglia. In their comparisons of patients with MPTP-induced parkinsonism to age and education matched controls, Stern and Langston (14) found that patients had impaired visuospatial and executive functions, as assessed by the Rosen Drawing (15), Stroop Color-Word (16), and verbal fluency tests (17). Similar, but less severe changes were seen in MPTP-exposed subjects who were motorically asymptomatic, suggesting that these cognitive abilities may be dopamine-specific, and deficits in these domains might be present even in the absence of parkinsonian motor impairment.

Further support for the role of dopamine in cognitive dysfunction in PD comes from examination of PD patients on and off levodopa therapy. For example, Malapani and colleagues (18) examined the ability of nondemented PD patients to process two cognitive tasks simultaneously as assessed by simple (i.e., single presentation) and complex (i.e., concurrent presentation) visual and auditory choice reaction time measures. They compared three groups of PD patients: a group receiving their usual dose of levodopa, a group of recently diagnosed untreated patients, and a group assessed at the time of maximal ("on" state) and minimal ("off" state; treatment withdrawn for 18 hours) clinical benefit of levodopa therapy. Compared to healthy, age-matched normal control subjects, PD patients receiving their standard dose of levodopa, and those tested in the "on" state performed normally on tests of simple and complex choice reactions time. In contrast, recently diagnosed untreated patients and those tested in the "off" state were impaired on complex, but not simple choice reaction time tests. These results suggest that concurrent processing of cognitive information requires adequate dopaminergic transmission (18). Similar "on-off" differences have been reported on a measure of verbal delayed recall memory (19). A report examining the cohort of patients from the original DATATOP study revealed that six months after the initiation of levodopa therapy, PD patients performed significantly higher on tests of frontal lobe function, including measures of psychomotor speed, set-shifting ability, and verbal fluency (20).

PROGRESSION OF COGNITIVE IMPAIRMENT IN PD

It is not clear what factors differentiate PD patients who develop dementia from those who remain cognitively intact or have mild or circumscribed cognitive impairments. Risk factors for dementia have been identified and discussed. Neuropsychologic predictors of later decline also have been identified. Jacobs and colleagues (21) found that the performance of nondemented patients with PD on tests of letter and category fluency was a highly sensitive neuropsychologic predictor of incident dementia. Poor verbal fluency in PD patients probably reflects poor executive function rather than an impairment of language per se. Specifically, patients are impaired in their ability to initiate a systematic retrieval of semantic stores and efficiently generate exemplars. Thus like other deficits of frontal lobe functions, the poor performance of PD patients on measures of verbal fluency may be attributable to compromised subcortical–cortical circuitry. Using a more comprehensive neuropsychologic test battery, Mahieux and colleagues (22) found that, in addition to verbal fluency, several other measures of attention and executive function (performance on the Picture Completion subtest of the Wechsler Adult Intelligence Scale – Revised (23) and the interference section of the Stroop Test (16) also were significant neuropsychologic predictors of subsequent dementia.

A growing body of evidence suggests that when cognitive impairment progresses to dementia in patients with PD, not only do the relatively circumscribed impairments seen in nondemented PD patients worsen in severity, but additional cognitive domains are affected. Specifically, there is a qualitative shift in the pattern of cognitive deficits, with substantial broadening and worsening of memory dysfunction, as dementia emerges (6). In a prospective neuropsychologic study of the evolution of cognitive changes associated with dementia in PD and AD, Stern and colleagues (24) found that performance on tests of visual confrontation naming (Boston Naming Test (25)) and delayed recall memory worsened as nondemented PD patients developed dementia. PD patients performed worse than healthy elders who subsequently developed AD on category fluency throughout the follow-up period, suggesting either that poor verbal fluency is an early manifestation of dementia in PD, but not AD, or that dementia is overlaid on this preexisting

performance deficit. In contrast, elders who subsequently developed AD consistently performed worse than PD patients on a test of delayed recognition memory, consistent with the conclusion that dementia in AD, but not PD, is characterized by an encoding deficit.

It is widely hypothesized that as dementia emerges in PD and cognitive deficits expand and worsen, so too the underlying pathology expands beyond the dopaminergic system and subcortico-frontal circuits. In some patients, a cholinergic deficit is superimposed on the dopaminergic deficit of PD. This cholinergic deficit probably reflect atrophy of cholinergic cells in the nucleus basalis of Meynart, and may occur independently of histopathologic changes indicative of AD. Other dementia patients, however, do show neuropathologic evidence of PD and AD. Finally, the contribution of cortical Lewy bodies must be considered in the differential etiology of PD dementia. The pathology of PD dementia is described more fully in the following section.

PREVALENCE OF DEMENTIA

The prevalence of dementia in the setting of PD has been reported to be as low as 8% (26) and as high as 93% (27). In an analysis of 2530 patients participating in 17 studies over a 60-year period, Brown and Marsden (28) suggested that the true prevalence of dementia was 15%. Most recent studies suggest a prevalence of approximately 20–40% (29–33). Methodological issues that have lead to this wide range of estimates include lack of uniform criteria for dementia, ascertainment from case records rather than formal neuropsychologic examination, and failure to adjust for age in many studies. For example, some of the higher estimates of dementia (34,35) may have resulted from inclusion of all forms of cognitive impairment including mild cognitive impairment, rather than including only those patients that would meet DSM-III-R criteria (36).

Ascertainment from case records may also lead to under-ascertainment compared to direct examination. A 1988 survey of case records of 339 patients from a hospital setting who did not undergo formal neuropsychologic testing yielded a prevalence estimate of 10.9% (37). In a subsequent study by the same investigators in the community of Washington Heights–Inwood in New York City, 41.3% of patients with PD, all of whom underwent neuropsychologic examination, met DSM-IIIR criteria for dementia (29). Although the sampling frames differed (service-based vs. community), this large discrepancy in prevalence suggests that dementia in the setting of PD may not be fully appreciated if targeted neuropsychologic testing is not performed. In a community-based study of 245 patients with PD in Norway, dementia was diagnosed in 27.7% (30). Although DSM-III-R criteria (36) were used to rate dementia, the mini-mental state exam (38) rather than a standardized neuropsychologic battery was used in the assessment, leading the authors to suggest that their estimate was conservative.

Lastly, many of the studies did not take into account the impact of age on the prevalence of PD. R.J. Marttila and U.K. Rinne (39) found the prevalence of dementia in those over age 70 to be almost twice that of those under 60 years of age. W.G. Reid et al. (40) found that among 107 newly diagnosed patients, 8% of those <70 and 32% of those older than 70 had dementia. In a population-based survey of 179 patients with PD in Washington Heights–Inwood, New York, the prevalence of dementia steadily rose from 0 per 100,000 for those <50 to 787.1 per 100,000 among those >80 (29). The prevalence of dementia standardized to the U.S. census estimates for 1988 among all patients was 76.0 per 100,000; 8.2 per 100,000 for ages 65 to 74 and 62.5 per 100,000 for those over age 75. In a random sample of the population over age 65 living in Gironde, France, dementia was diagnosed in 17.6% of PD patients as compared to 3.9% of individuals without PD; the age standardized ratio of dementia in PD patients compared to elders without PD was 4.6 (31). Patients over age 80 were 4.4 times as likely as those between 65 and 79 to have dementia.

INCIDENCE OF DEMENTIA

A limited number of studies have been done on the incidence of dementia in PD. Rajput et al. (41) found that over a five-year period, the cumulative probability of subsequent dementia among PD patients seen at the Mayo Clinic with incident PD was 21.1% compared to 5.7% of a sample of matched controls who attended the Mayo Clinic (p = 0.01). This increase in risk of dementia was seen only among those patients treated with levodopa, but was not believed to be attributed to the levodopa treatment itself (41). Mayeux et al. (42) in a reevaluation of the clinic-based sample five years after the prevalence date (37), determined that the incidence of dementia was 69 per 1000 person years of observation, which was almost six times that expected in an age-matched cohort, the Baltimore Longitudinal Study. The cumulative incidence of dementia by age 85 was 65%, with the highest increase in risk between ages 65 and 74. Biggins

et al. found that the incidence of dementia among 87 PD patients and 50 controls who were followed over a 54 month period was 47.6 per 1000 person-years (32). All these studies included only patients who sought medical attention and did not include extensive neuropsychologic testing.

RISK OF DEMENTIA COMPARED TO AGE-MATCHED CONTROLS

The question of whether patients with PD are at increased risk for the development of dementia compared to age-matched controls has been examined. In the community of Washington Heights–Inwood the relative risk of incident dementia over a two-year period among 140 PD patients and 572 controls, the majority of whom were over age 65, was 1.7 (95% CI 1.1–2.7) after adjustment for age, education, and gender (43). This estimate of incident dementia is lower than the registry-based estimates of Rajput et al. (risk ratio 3.7) (41) and Breteler et al. (3.0) (95%CI 2.9–3.1) (44) comparing risk of dementia among PD patients and community controls. Breteler et al. suggest that age-specific risk of dementia was highest in PD patients ages 50–54 (RR = 13.3), because of the low-baseline frequency of dementia at that age.

Echoing the findings of Rajput et al., the increased risk of dementia in the Washington Heights study (43) was confined to those PD patients who had the most severe extrapyramidal signs, suggesting that either need for treatment with levodopa or extrapyramidal findings on examination were predictors of incident dementia.

MORTALITY

The relatively high incidence rate of dementia compared to the lower prevalence rate in the hospital-based samples of Mayeux et al. (29,42) prompted the consideration that disease duration was shortened by the development of dementia. In fact, in two studies, one clinic-based (45) and the other community-based (46) the advent of dementia significantly reduced survival, after controlling for age and disease duration.

Just by virtue of having PD, there is an increased risk of death. In the Washington Heights–Inwood community study, 288 PD patients, 134 of whom were demented were compared to 1690 elderly, 436 of whom were demented. When compared to nondemented elderly, nondemented PD patients also had an elevated risk of death (rate ratio 2.7; 95%CI 1.7–4.4), but the risk for demented PD patients was even higher (risk ratio 4.9; 95%CI 3.4–7.1). When PD patients were stratified by the median motor score on the UPDRS, dementia was a predictor of mortality among those with lower scores (risk ratio 2.3;95%CI, 1.1–4.9), but it was not an independent predictor of mortality among those with higher scores (46). Numerous cross-sectional studies have shown that cognitive impairment parallels physical impairment and that demented patients have more severe motor manifestations (27,37,39,41,47–49). The more severe the extrapyramidal syndrome, the higher the likelihood of dementia and mortality.

RISK FACTORS FOR DEMENTIA IN PARKINSON'S DISEASE

Several risk factors have been associated with the development of dementia in PD. These associations have been derived from both cross-sectional studies of dementia and studies of incident dementia. Risk factors include older age at the onset of the motor manifestations of PD (30,31,37,50) severity of the extrapyramidal signs, especially bradykinesia (43,50,51), family history of dementia (52,53), depression (30,43,54) psychologic stress (e.g., holocaust) (55), and low socioeconomic or low educational attainment (50). An approach favored by epidemiologists has been to determine the risk factors for dementia in PD by following nondemented PD patients over time and determining what baseline characteristics are predictive of the development of dementia (32,43,50,54). In the Washington Heights community study (43), predictive features of incident dementia over a two-year period included motor score on the UPDRS (56) greater than 25 (relative risk 3.56 95%CI 1.4–8.9) and a Hamilton Depression Rating Scale score (57) of >10 (RR 3.55; 95%CI 1.6–7.9) at the first examination. The fact that severity of the extrapyramidal signs in nondemented patients with PD was predictive of dementia provides further evidence that dopamine deficiency may mediate, at least in part, the cognitive impairment seen in PD. Depressive symptoms may also be associated with dementia because of common dopaminergic and serotonergic deficits (58).

Recent investigations of risk factors for dementia in PD have examined whether genetic and environmental risk factors identified in AD are also associated with dementia in Parkinson's disease. A major focus has been on whether the presence of one or more Apolipoprotein (Apo) E4 alleles is associated with

dementia in PD. No association between ApoE4 and dementia in PD was seen in four studies (59–62).

A study of 43 demented PD patients and 51 nondemented PD patients found that although pesticide exposure for more than 20 days within a calendar year and the presence of a CYP2D6 29B+ allele were not independently associated with dementia, the interaction of the two was associated with a threefold increase in risk of dementia (OR 3.17 95% CI = 1.11–9.05). This is the first evidence of a gene–environment interaction for dementia in PD (63).

Family history may also be used as a marker of genetic susceptibility. Family history of dementia was six times as high among patients with PD and dementia as among nondemented PD patients (52). Demented patients were older than nondemented patients and it is likely that the relatives of demented patients were older, which may have increased the probability of dementia in the relatives of demented patients. To further evaluate the possibility of familial aggregation of AD and dementia in PD, structured family history interviews were administered to 146 nondemented PD patients, 120 patients with PD and dementia, and 903 nondemented controls from Washington Heights-Inwood. No increase in risk of AD was found among parents of patients with PD and dementia or parents of nondemented PD patients compared to parents of controls. However, siblings of demented PD patients were three times as likely (RR 3.2; 95%CI 1.1–9.4 p < 0.04)) as siblings of controls, to develop AD. When limited to siblings >65 years of age, there was a fivefold increase in risk of AD among siblings of demented PD patients compared to siblings of controls (RR 4.9; 95%CI 1.1–21.4 p < 0.03). Risk of AD was also increased for female relatives, regardless of whether the female was a relative of a demented PD patient, a nondemented PD patient, or a control. Ethnicity and ApoE genotype did not affect dementia status among relatives (53).

PATHOLOGY

No single etiology for dementia in patients with PD has been established. Neuropathologic findings in patients with PD and dementia (PDD) include the presence of concomitant AD, cortical Lewy bodies (2), degeneration of the medial substantia nigra (64), neurites in the CA2 region of the entorhinal cortex (65,66), and neuropil threads in the prelayer of entorhinal cortex (67). Currently there is no reliable way to distinguish among these etiologies either clinically or by risk factor profile.

The neuropathologic changes associated with dementia in PD have been reported in two brain bank series. In 71 clinically demented cases who met criteria for idiopathic PD based on clear depletion of brainstem pigmented neurons with Lewy bodies in the remaining cells, coexistent Alzheimer's disease was found in 29%, dementia with Lewy bodies in 10%, and vascular pathology sufficient to account for cognitive impairment in 6%. All PD cases had at least small numbers of cortical and nigral Lewy bodies. No pathologic changes to account for the dementia could be identified in half the subjects (68). In a larger series of 507 patients who met pathologic criteria for PD, 30.2% (n = 153) were demented (69). The vast majority of the 153 demented cases (85%) had concurrent Alzheimer's pathology, whereas only 5.2% had no other pathologic changes other than idiopathic PD to explain the dementia. Eight percent of the cases had associated cerebrovascular lesions. The conclusion from these studies is that pure brainstem Lewy body pathology does exist, albeit rare, and may explain a small number of cases with predominantly dopaminergic deficiency.

Dementia in the setting of PD represents the confluence of additive or synergistic effects of pathologic involvement of multiple neuronal populations. One might envision that cognitive impairment early in PD may be due to primarily dopaminergic depletion secondary to loss of dopaminergic neurons in the substantia nigra and later, a superimposition of a cholinergic deficit that might be due to degeneration of the nucleus basalis of Meynert in the setting of PD. The specific cognitive deficits seen at various stages of PD may be due to the additive effects of degeneration of the dopaminergic (ventral tegmental area and medial substantia nigra), noradrenergic (locus ceruleus), serotonergic (dorsal raphe), and cholinergic (nucleus basalis of Meynert) systems. The neuropathologic literature supports the concept of a continuum of cell loss in the ventral tegmental area and medial substantia nigra zona compacta, which is greater in nondemented PD patients than controls, and even greater in demented PD patients (70). These changes in ventral tegmental area and in prefrontal cortex may be greater in demented patients who do not have histologic changes of AD (70,71). The locus ceruleus also shows greater cell loss in demented patients compared to nondemented PD patients (72), and is more severe in demented patients without concurrent AD (70). The dorsal raphe nucleus in demented PD patients can show cell loss comparable to that seen in AD (73). Cell loss in the nucleus basalis of Meynert in demented PD patients approaches that of AD patients (50–70%) (69). In contrast, some nondemented PD patients also show significant cell loss. It has been suggested that there may be a critical threshold of 75–80% neuronal loss plus the presence of cortical Alzheimer's lesions to produce dementia (74). In summary the dementia

of PD may be due to degeneration of specific subcortical–cortical loops, and may or may not be associated with concomitant Alzheimer's pathology. The specific cognitive profiles seen may be due to individual variation in the extent and timing of the degenerative process.

Another disease entity that may account for a proportion of patients with parkinsonism and cognitive impairment, first described in 1980 by K. Kosaka et al. (75), is dementia with Lewy bodies. Controversy rages over whether dementia with Lewy bodies is a distinct entity, or whether it forms part of the spectrum of AD. A number of recent neuropathologic studies have found that 15–25% of all elderly demented patients have Lewy bodies in their brainstem or cortex compared to 2.3% of nondemented elderly. Operational criteria for defining this entity were originally published in 1992 (76) and revised in 1996 (2). Defining this condition has important treatment implications. The pathologic findings in dementia with Lewy bodies are reviewed in Chapter 20.

NEUROIMAGING

Both single photon emission computed tomography (SPECT) and positron emission tomography (PET) have been used to try to determine the neuroanatomic substrate of dementia in PD. In the mid-1980s and early 1990s, the primary distinction that investigators sought to make was between AD and PD. More recently, dementia with Lewy bodies has also been considered in the differential and the pattern on functional imaging explored. All of the studies are cross-sectional. There are no longitudinal studies of PD patients who underwent scans before and after the development of dementia.

Using SPECT, a number of investigators have demonstrated a pattern of temporoparietal hypometabolism in demented PD patients (77–79) similar to like that seen in AD compared to controls. Interestingly, nondemented PD patients did not differ significantly from controls in terms of global or regional hypoperfusion (77,79,80). There is a suggestion that in "early" PD (average of 2.5 years; stages I and II) patients with dementia, SPECT scans show significantly lower HMPAO uptake in the frontal and basal ganglia regions compared to nondemented patients (80). Sawada et al. (77) demonstrated two patterns on SPECT in 13 demented PD patients; four patients demonstrated isolated frontal perfusion, whereas nine demonstrated frontoparietal hypoperfusion. Subjects with frontoparietal hypoperfusion had lower scores on the Mini-Mental State Examination and were more prone to delirium. Frontal hypoperfusion, however, was common to all PD patients.

Using PET, investigators have shown widespread cortical global hypometabolism in PD patients compared to controls (81,82). Nondemented PD patients had cortical hypometabolism compared to controls while demented PD patients showed more severe hypometabolism in temporoparietal regions, as seen in AD (81,83). Vander Borght et al. demonstrated greater glucose reduction in the primary visual cortex in demented PD patients compared to AD (82). The authors note that these changes have also been seen in dementia with Lewy bodies and that inclusion of subjects with dementia with Lewy bodies was possible.

TREATMENT OF COGNITIVE IMPAIRMENT

Dementia is the rate-limiting step for pharmacotherapy for PD. Many medications used to treat the motor manifestations of PD must be reduced or discontinued once dementia develops to improve cognition.

No medications are available for the treatment of cognitive impairment in PD. There have been two controlled trials for treatment of dementia in PD. Sano et al. (84) showed no improvement in cognition with the nootropic piracitam. Phosphatidylserine was found to reduce anxiety, but had minimal effects on cognition (85). There have been no double-blind placebo controlled trials of any of the cholinesterase inhibitors such as tacrine or donepezil to treat the dementia associated with PD. There is a suggestion that there may be a response to cholinesterase inhibitors in patients with dementia with Lewy bodies that may be even better than in AD (86,87). The effects of estrogen replacement therapy in the setting of PD have recently been examined in 87 nondemented women with PD, 80 women with PD and dementia, and 989 community controls. Estrogen replacement therapy was protective for the development of dementia in PD (OR= 0.22, 95%CI 0.05–1) but did not affect the risk of development of PD itself (88). Therefore, a randomized clinical trial of estrogen replacement therapy in PD patients with cognitive impairment may be warranted. Selegiline, which has been shown to delay the development of functional impairment in patients with moderate AD (89), was previously examined in PD at the same dose (20). In a secondary analysis of cognitive test performance in 800 patients with early, untreated PD followed in the DATATOP study, there was no effect of either deprenyl 10 mg or tocopherol

2000 IU on test performance, although cognitive performance was relatively stable over the observation period.

The strategy most often used in patients with worsening cognitive impairment is to eliminate medications that may be exacerbating cognitive impairment. As in the treatment of psychosis (see chapter 38,43), improving mentation may occur at the expense of worsening motor function. The clinician and family must decide the optimum balance. PD patients with cognitive impairment are particularly vulnerable to the effects of medications that may exacerbate preexisting cognitive impairment. In addition to worsening domains such as memory, the medications used to treat PD may induce confusion and in particular, hallucinations. One viable management strategy is to first eliminate anticholinergic medications and medications with high anticholinergic activity. Amantadine frequently causes confusion in PD patients with cognitive impairment. If confusion does not remit, a reduction of dopaminergic agents to the lowest possible effective dose should be attempted.

DEPRESSION AND DEMENTIA

Depression is a common feature in PD (see Chapter 17). Estimates of depression range from 12 to 90% (90). In a review of 14 studies encompassing 1500 patients, Gotham et al. estimated a mean prevalence of major depression in 46% (91). Depression is probably the most common mental disorder associated with PD. In a study of 339 patients with PD, the prevalence of depression was 47% and the annual incidence of depression was 1.87 per year (92). There appears to be no relationship between depression and age, age at onset of the motor symptoms of PD, or duration of illness. The profile of depression in PD is similar but not identical to that seen in endogenous depression. Using the Beck Depression Inventory, elevated levels of dysphoria, pessimism about the future, irritability, sadness, and suicidal ideation, but little guilt, self-blame, or feelings of failure or punishment have been demonstrated.

Depression and dementia often coexist. Patients with both conditions had lower levels of 5-HIAA than either condition independently (93). In a consecutive series of 92 PD patients who underwent baseline assessment and reassessment 12 months later, those with major depression had greater cognitive decline than those with minor depression and those who were not depressed (54). In addition, PD patients with Hamilton depression rating scale score of >10 were over three times more likely to develop incident dementia, than those with lower Hamilton scores in the longitudinal study of patients in Washington Heights with PD (43). In a study comparing 44 depressed PD patients, 44 nondepressed PD patients, and 44 controls, depression was shown to exacerbate impairment on tests of memory and language associated with PD, but the effect was believed to be quantitative (depression affected the same cognitive domains affected in PD) rather than qualitative (different cognitive domains) (94).

CONCLUSION

Dementia in the setting of PD probably represents multiple pathologic substrates including PD alone, PD plus AD and dementia with Lewy bodies. Neuropsychologic, imaging, and pathologic studies suggest a common denominator referable to early dopamine deficiency. Although it has become more apparent which patients are at risk for progression to dementia, the etiologic factors leading to additional involvement of other neurotransmitter systems, with or without the pathologic changes associated with AD, deserve further investigation.

REFERENCES

1. American Psychiatric Association. *Diagnostic and Statistical Manual of Mental Disorders*, 4th ed. Washington, DC: American Psychiatric Press, 1994.
2. McKeith IG, Galasko D, Kosaka K, et al. Consensus guidelines for the clinical and pathological diagnosis of dementia with Lewy bodies (DLB): Report of the consortium on DLB international workshop. *Neurology* 1996; 47:1113–1124.
3. Litvan I, MacIntyre A, Goetz CG, et al. Accuracy of the clinical diagnoses of Lewy body disease, Parkinson's disease, and dementia with Lewy bodies; A clinicopathological study. *Arch Neurol* 1998; 55:969–978.
4. Dubois B, Boller F, Pillon B, et al. Cognitive deficits in Parkinson's disease. In: Boller F, Grafman J, eds. *Handbook of Neuropsychology*, Vol 5. Amsterdam: Elsevier, 1991: 195–240.
5. Raskin SA, Borod JC, Tweedy J. Neuropsychological aspects of Parkinson's disease. *Neuropsychol Review* 1990; 1:185–221.
6. Stern Y, Richards M, Sano M, et al. Comparison of cognitive changes in patients with Alzheimer's and Parkinson's disease. *Arch Neurol* 1993; 50:1040–1045.
7. Troster AI, Butters N, Salmon DP, et al. The diagnostic utility of savings scores: Differentiating Alzheimer's and Huntington's diseases with the Logical Memory and Visual Reproduction tests. *J Clin Exp Neuropsychol* 1993; 15:773–788.
8. Hyman BT, VanHoesen GW, Damasio AR, et al. Alzheimer's disease: cell-specific pathology isolates the hippocampal formation. *Science* 1984; 225:1168–1170.
9. VanHoesen GW, Hyman BT, Damasio AR. Entorhinal cortex pathology in Alzheimer's disease. *Hippocampus* 1991; 1:1–8.
10. Braak H, Braak E. Evolution of the neuropathology of Alzheimer's disease. *Acta Neurologica Scandinavia Supplementum* 1996; 165:3–12.
11. Taylor AE, Saint-Cyr JA, Lang AE, et al. Frontal lobe dysfunction in Parkinson's disease: The cortical focus of neostriatal outflow. *Brain* 1986; 109:845–883.
12. Bondi MW, Kaszniak AW, Bayles KA, et al. Contributions of frontal system dysfunction to memory and perceptual abilities in Parkinson's disease. *Neuropsychology* 1993; 7:89–102.
13. Penney JB, Young AB. Speculations on the functional anatomy of basal ganglia disorders. *Ann Rev Neurosci* 1983; 6:73–94.
14. Stern Y, Langston JW. Intellectual changes in patients with MPTP-induced parkinsonism. *Neurology* 1985; 35:1506–1509.
15. Rosen W. The Rosen Drawing Test. Bronx, NY:Veterans Administration Medical Center, 1981.
16. Stroop JR. Studies of interference in serial verbal reactions. *J Exp Psychol* 1935; 18:643–662.
17. Benton AL, Hamsher Kd. *Multilingual Aphasia Examination*. Iowa City: University of Iowa, 1976.
18. Malapani C, Pillon B, Dubois B, et al. Impaired simultaneous cognitive task performance in Parkinson's disease: A dopamine-related dysfunction. *Neurology* 1994; 44:319–326.
19. Mohr E, Fabbrini G, Williams J, et al. Dopamine and memory function in Parkinson's disease. *Mov Dis* 1989; 4:113–120.
20. Growdon JH, Kieburtz K, McDermott M, et al. and the Parkinson Study Group. Levodopa improves motor function without impairing cognition in mild nondemented Parkinson's disease patients. *Neurology* 1998; 50(5):1327–1331.
21. Jacobs DM, Marder K, Cote LJ, et al. Neuropsychological characteristics of preclinical dementia in Parkinson's disease. *Neurology* 1995; 45:1691–1696.
22. Mahieux F, Fenelon G, Flahault A, et al. Neuropsychological prediction of dementia in Parkinson's disease. *J Neurol Neurosurg Psychiatry* 1998; 64:178–183.
23. Wechsler D. *Wechsler Adult Intelligence Scale-Revised*. New York: The Psychological Corporation, 1981.
24. Stern Y, Tang M-X, Jacobs DM, et al. Prospective comparative study of the evolution of probable Alzheimer's disease and Parkinsons's disease dementia. *J Int Neuropsychol Soc* 1998; 4:279–284.
25. Kaplan E, Goodglass H, Weintraub S. *Boston Naming Test* Philadelphia, PA: Lea & Febiger, 1983.
26. Taylor A. Dementia prevalence in Parkinson's disease. *Lancet* 1985; 1:1037.

27. Pirozzolo FJ, Hansch EC, Mortimer JA, et al. Dementia in Parkinson disease. A neuropsychological analysis. *Brain Cog* 1982; 1:71–83.

28. Brown RG, Marsden CD. How common is dementia in Parkinson's disease? *Lancet* 1984; 1:1262–1265.

29. Mayeux R, Denaro J, Hemenegildo N, et al. A population-based investigation of Parkinson's disease with and without dementia: Relationship to age and gender. *Arch Neurol* 1992; 49:492–497.

30. Aarsland D, Tandberg E, Larsen JP, et al. Frequency of dementia in Parkinson's disease. *Arch Neurol* 1996; 53(6):538–542.

31. Tison F, Dartigues JF, Auriacombe S, et al. Dementia in Parkinson's disease: a population-based study in ambulatory and institutionalized individuals. *Neurology* 1995; 45(4):705–708.

32. Biggins CA, Boyd JL, Harrop FM, et al. A controlled, longitudinal study of dementia in Parkinson's disease. *J Neurol Neurosurg Psychiatry* 1992; 55(7):566–571.

33. Friedman A, Barcikowska M. Dementia in Parkinson's disease. *Dementia* 1994; 5:12–16.

34. Martin W, Loewenson R, Resch J, et al. Parkinson's disease. A clinical analysis of 100 patients. *Neurology* 1973; 23:783–790.

35. Mjones H. Paralysis agitans: a clinical and genetic study. *Acta Psychiatr Neurol* 1949; 54:1–195.

36. American Psychiatric Association. *Diagnostic and Statistical Manual of Mental Disorders*, Rev. 3rd ed. Washington, DC:American Psychiatric Press, 1987.

37. Mayeux R, Stern Y, Rosenstein R, et al. An estimate of the prevalence of dementia in idiopathic Parkinson's disease. *Arch Neurol* 1988; 45:260–262.

38. Folstein MF, Folstein SE, McHugh PR. 'Mini-mental State': A practical method for grading the cognitive state of patients for the clinician. *J Psychiatr Res* 1975; 12:189–198.

39. Marttila RJ, Rinne UK. Dementia in Parkinson's disease. *Acta Neurol Scand* 1976; 54:431–441.

40. Reid WG. The evolution of dementia in idiopathic Parkinson's disease: neuropsychological and clinical evidence in support of subtypes. *Int Psychogeriatr* 1992; 4 Suppl 2:147–160.

41. Rajput AH, Offord KP, Beard CM, et al. A case-control study of smoking habits, dementia, and other illnesses in idiopathic Parkinson's disease. *Neurology* 1987; 37:226–232.

42. Mayeux R, Chen J, Mirabello E, et al. An estimate of the incidence of dementia in idiopathic Parkinson's disease. *Neurology* 1990; 40:1513–1517.

43. Marder K, Tang M-X, Cote L, et al. The frequency and associated risk factors for dementia in patients with Parkinson's disease. *Arch Neurol* 1995; 52:695–701.

44. Breteler MM, deGroot RR, van Romunde LK, et al. Risk of dementia in patients with Parkinson's disease, epilepsy and severe head trauma: a register-based follow-up study. *Am J Epidemiol* 1995; 142(12):1300–1305.

45. Marder K, Leung D, Tang M, et al. Are demented patients with Parkinson's disease accurately reflected in prevalence surveys? A survival analysis. *Neurology* 1991; 41:1240–1243.

46. Louis E, Marder K, Cote L, et al. Mortality from Parkinson's disease. *Arch Neurol* 1998; 54(3):260–264.

47. Celesia GG, Wanamaker WM. Psychiatric Disturbances in Parkinson's disease. *Dis Nerv Syst* 1972; 33:577–583.

48. Mindham R. Psychiatric Syndromes in Parkinsonism. *J Neurol Neurosurg Psychiatry* 1982; 30:88–191.

49. Lieberman A, Dziatolowski M, Kupersmith M, et al. Dementia in Parkinson disease. *Ann Neurol* 1979; 6:355–359.

50. Glatt SL, Hubble JP, Lyons K, et al. Risk factors for dementia in Parkinson's disease: effect of education. *Neuroepidemiology* 1996; 15:20–25.

51. Ebmeier KP, Calder SA, Crawford JR, et al. Clinical features predicting dementia in idiopathic Parkinson's disease: A follow-up study. *Neurology* 1990; 40:1222–1224.

52. Marder K, Flood P, Cote L, et al. A pilot study of risk factors for dementia in Parkinson's disease. *Mov Disord* 1990; 5:156–161.

53. Marder K, Tang M-X, Alfaro B, et al. Risk of Alzheimer's disease in relatives of Parkinson's disease patients with and without dementia. *Neurology* 1999; (In Press)

54. Starkstein SE, Mayberg HS, Leiguarda R, et al. A prospective longitudinal study of depression, cognitive decline, and physical impairments in patients with Parkinson's disease. *J Neurol Neurosurg Psychiatry* 1992; 55:377–382.

55. Salganik I, Korczyn A. Risk factors for dementia in Parkinson's disease. In: Streifler MB, Korczyn AD, Melamed E, et al. (eds.). *Advances in Neurology*, Vol. 53: *Parkinson's Disease, Anatomy, Pathology, and Therapy*. New York: Raven Press, 1990: 343–347.

56. Stern MB, Hurting HI. The clinical characteristics of Parkinson's disease and Parkinsonian syndromes: diagnosis and assessment. In: *The Comprehensive Management of Parkinson's Disease*. New York: PMA Corp., 1978: 3–50.

57. Williams JB. A structured interview guide for the Hamilton Depression Rating Scale. *Arch Gen Psychiatry* 1988; 45:742–747.

58. Mayberg HS, Starkstein SE, Sadzot B, et al. Selective hypometabolism in the inferior frontal lobe of depressed patients with Parkinson's disease. *Ann Neurol* 1990; 26:57–64.

59. Marder K, Maestre G, Cote L, et al. The apolipoprotein epsilon 4 allele in Parkinson's disease with and without dementia. *Neurology* 1994; 44:1330–1331.

60. Koller WC, Glatt SL, Hubble JP, et al. Apolipoprotein E genotypes in Parkinson's disease with and without dementia. *Ann Neurol* 1995; 37:342–345.

61. Whitehead AS, Bertrandy S, Finnan F, et al. Frequency of the apolipoprotein E epsilon 4 allele in a case-control study of early onset Parkinson's disease. *J Neurol Neurosurg Psychiatry* 1996; 61(4):347–351.

62. Inzelberg R, Chapman J., Treves T, et al. Apolipoprotein E4 in Parkinson disease and dementia: new data and meta-analysis of published studies. *Alzheimer Dis Assoc Disord* 1998; 12(1):45–48.

63. Hubble JP, Kurth JH, Glatt SL, et al. Gene-toxin interaction as a putative risk factor of Parkinson's disease with dementia. *Neuroepidemiology* 1998; 17(2):96–104.

64. Rinne JO, Rummukainen J, Paljarvi L, et al. Dementia in Parkinson's disease is related to neuronal loss in the medial substantia nigra. *Ann Neurol* 1989; 26:47–50.

65. Churchyard A, Lees. The relationship between dementia and direct involvement of the hippocampus and amygdala in Parkinson's disease. *Neurology* 1997; 49:1570–1576.

66. Kim H, Gearing M, Mirra SS. Ubiquitin-positive CA2/3 neurites in hippocampus coexist with cortical Lewy bodies. *Neurology* 1995; 45:1768–1770.

67. Braak H, Braak E, Yilmazer D, et al. Cognitive impairment in Parkinson's disease: amyloid plaques, neurofibrillary tangles, and neuropil threads in the cerebral cortex. *J Neural Trans Basic Neurosci Neurol Sect Psychiatry Sect* 1990; 2:45–57.

68. Hughes AJ, Daniel SE, Blanston S, et al. The clinical features of Parkinson's disease: A clinicopathological study of 100 cases. *Arch Neurol* 1993; 50:140–148.

69. Jellinger K. Morphological substrates of dementia in parkinsonism. A critical update. *J Neural Trans* 1997; Suppl 51:57–82.

70. Zweig RM, Cardilio JE, Cohen M, et al. The locus ceruleus and dementia in Parkinson's disease. *Neurology* 1993; 43:986–991.

71. Agid F, Graybiel AM, Ruberg M, et al. The efficacy of levodopa treatment declines in the course of Parkinson's disease. Do non-dopaminergic lesions play a role? *Adv Neurol* 1990; 53:83–100.

72. Gaspar P, Gray F. Dementia in idiopathic Parkinson's disease. A neuropathological study of 32 cases. *Acta Neuropathol* 1984; 64:43–52.

73. Chan-Palay V, Hochli M, Jentsch B, et al. Raphe serotonin neurons in the human brain in normal controls and patients with senile dementia of the Alzheimer type and Parkinson's disease. *Dementia* 1992; 3:253–269.

74. Jellinger K. Neuropathological substrates of Alzheimer's and Parkinson's disease. *J Neural Trans* 1987; 24:109–129.

75. Kosaka K, Tsuchiya K, Yoshimura M. Lewy body disease with and without dementia: a clinicopathological study of 35 cases. *Clin Neuropath* 1988; 7:299–305.

76. McKeith IG, Perry RH, Fairbairn AF, et al. Operational criteria for senile dementia of Lewy body type (SDLT). *Psychol Med* 1992; 22:911–922.

77. Sawada H, Udaka F, Kameyama M, et al. SPECT findings in Parkinson's disease associated with dementia. *J Neurol Neurosurg Psychiatry* 1992; 55:960–963.

78. Pizzolato G, Dam G, Borsato N, et al. 99mTc-HM-PAO SPECT in Parkinson's disease. *J Cerebral Blood Flow Metab* 1988; 8 Suppl 1:101–108.

79. Spampinato U, Habert MO, Mas JL, et al. 99mTC-HM-PAO SPECT and cognitive impairment in Parkinson's disease: a comparison with dementia of the Alzheimer type. *J Neurol Neurosurg Psychiatry* 1991; 54:787–792.

80. Wang S-J, Liu R-S, Liu H-C, et al. Technetium-99m hexamethylpropylene amine oxime single photon emission tomography of the brain in early Parkinson's disease: correlation with dementia and lateralization. *Eur J Nucl Med* 1993; 20:339–344.

81. Peppard RF, Martin W, Carr GD, et al. Cerebral glucose metabolism in Parkinson's disease with and without dementia. *Arch Neurol* 1992; 49:1262–1268.

82. Vander Borght T, Minoshima S, Giordani B, et al. Cerebral metabolic differences in Parkinson's and Alzheimer's diseases matched for dementia severity. *J Nucl Med* 1997; 38:797–802.

83. Kuhl DE, Metter EJ, Riege WH. Patterns of local cerebral glucose utilization determined in Parkinson's disease by the [18F] fluorodeoxyglucose method. *Ann Neurol* 1984; 15:419–424.

84. Sano M, Stern Y, Marder K, et al. A controlled trial of piracetam in intellectually impaired patients with Parkinson's disease. *Mov Disord* 1990; 5:230–234.

85. Furigeld E, Gaggen M, Nedwidek P, et al. Double blind study with phosphatidylserine in parkinsonian patients with senile dementia of the Alzheimer's type (SDAT). *Prog Clin Biol Res* 1989; 317:1235–1246.

86. Levy R, Sahakian B. Alzheimer's disease and Lewy body dementia. *Br J Psychiatr* 1994; 164:268

87. Wilcock GK, Scott M. Tacrine for senile dementia of Alzheimer's or Lewy body type. *Lancet* 1994; 344:544

88. Marder K, Tang M-X, Alfaro B, et al. Postmenopausal estrogen use and Parkinson's disease with and without dementia. *Neurology* 1998; 50:1141–1143.

89. Sano M, Ernesto C, Thomas RG, et al. A controlled trial of Selegiline, alpha-tocopherol, or both as treatment for Alzheimer's disease. *N Engl J Med* 1997; 336:1216–1222.

90. Cummings JL. Depression and Parkinson's disease: a review. *Am J Psychiatr* 1992; 149:443–454.

91. Gotham AM, Brown RG, Marsden C. Depression in Parkinson's disease: a quantitative and qualitative analysis. *J Neurol Neurosurg Psychiatry* 1986; 49:381–389.

92. Dooneief G, Mirabello E, Bell K, et al. An estimate of the incidence of depression in idiopathic Parkinson's disease. *Arch Neurol* 1992; 49:305–307.

93. Sano M, Stern Y, Williams J, et al. Coexisting dementia and depression in Parkinson's disease. *Arch Neurol* 1989; 46:1284–1286.

94. Troster AI, Stalp L, Paolo A, et al.. Neuropsychological impairment in Parkinson's disease with and without dementia. *Arch Neurol* 1995; 52:1164–1169.

16

Dementia with Lewy Bodies, Alzheimer's Disease and Their Relationship to Parkinson's Disease

Douglas Galasko, M.D.

University of California–San Diego, San Diego, California

INTRODUCTION

The concept of Parkinson's disease (PD) as a syndrome of tremor and slowing of movement and gait is consistent with the distribution of Lewy bodies (LB), the pathologic hallmark of PD, in the substantia nigra. More recently, the clinical boundaries of PD and the regional distribution of LB have expanded. Clinically, cognitive and behavioral syndromes have gained a place in a wider spectrum of PD. Pathologically, LB may occur in cortical and limbic areas of the brain, and are not restricted only to the nigra and subcortical locations. Diffusely distributed LB are often associated with Alzheimer's disease (AD) pathology and clinically with dementia. New approaches to the clinical and pathologic classification of PD and LB are developing, incorporating these more recent findings. The relationship between PD and dementia has been discussed in detail elsewhere in this book (Chapter 15). This chapter focuses specifically on dementia syndromes associated with diffusely distributed LB.

Studies indicate that about one-third of patients with PD eventually develop dementia. Some elderly patients may develop dementia followed by parkinsonism and other features, associated with LB at widespread sites throughout the brain, and this syndrome is referred to as "dementia with Lewy bodies" (DLB) (1). DLB is a neurobehavioral syndrome and accounts for 15 to 20% of cases of dementia in several large autopsy series (2–4). Criteria for clinical and pathologic diagnoses of DLB have been published, but the syndrome and its relationship to AD remains controversial.

NEUROPATHOLOGIC FINDINGS IN DEMENTIA WITH LEWY BODIES

The existence of cortical LB and their association with dementia was described by Kosaka in 1990 (2). Classic LB, as seen in the substantia nigra, appear as hyaline intraneuronal inclusions on hematoxylin and eosin staining and usually have a clear halo surrounding the brightly eosinophilic core. Cortical LB stain as ill-defined pale eosinophilic areas and lack a halo. This makes them relatively difficult to visualize on sections with routine stains. Antibody probes against ubiquitin and α-synuclein facilitate LB identification. In the cortex, LB occur in deeper layers 5 and 6, most commonly in limbic and multi-modal association cortex. These sites of predilection of LB are consistent with many of the clinical features of DLB. For example, involvement of the hippocampus, neocortex, and cingulate may contribute to dementia. Visual hallucinations and neuropsychologic aspects, such as difficulty with visuospatial tasks, may relate to disruption of temporo-occipital circuitry.

DLB includes several other pathologic findings. Lewy neurites are abnormal processes of neurons, prominent in the hippocampus and cortex (3). Vacuolar changes in limbic cortical areas, resembling spongiform change, are prominent in 40% or more of cases (4).

Most nondemented cases of PD show at least some LB in the temporal lobe, amygdala, or other "diffuse" sites (5). In several studies the density of LB in the hippocampus and cortex in cases of PD with dementia exceeds that of PD without dementia (6,7), suggesting that LB may be a substrate of dementia in PD.

Although the coincidence of diffusely distributed LB and dementia suggests causality, two areas remain highly controversial. First, the relative scarcity of cortical LB and the lack of atrophy of areas of the brain affected by LB raise questions of whether diffuse LB are a sufficient burden of pathology to result in dementia. Second, the frequent co-occurrence of AD pathology raises questions about the relative contribution of each lesion to dementia. Regarding the first question, counts of LB in specific brain areas correlate moderately well with clinical measures of dementia severity close to the time of death in several (8,9), but not all (10), studies.

The senile plaques (SP) and neurofibrillary tangles (NFT) of AD are found in most cases of DLB or of PD with dementia (11–13). In many cases of DLB, NFT in neocortical areas are scarce. A large recent study showed that fully evolved cortical AD pathology was present in about 50% of DLB cases (13). The relative contribution of AD and DLB to dementia remains unsettled. One viewpoint is that coincident AD lesions represent pathologic aging (12,14). Another position is that AD lesions, even if less numerous than in typical AD, often contribute to dementia in DLB (11,13). Because many of the clinical features of dementia in DLB and AD overlap, the term Lewy body variant of AD has been proposed (11). Studies of well-characterized cases of "pure" DLB with negligible AD pathology indicate that LB alone can lead to dementia. Therefore it is likely that AD lesions and LB both contribute to dementia when they co-occur.

The common theme of protein aggregation into filamentous structures conceptually unites AD and DLB. LB contain aggregates of α-synuclein (15), whereas NFT comprise filaments of aggregated tau, and the amyloid cores of plaques consist of β-protein. It is possible that common mechanisms lead to the formation of LB and AD lesions. Evidence for this possibility comes from studies of brains of patients with autosomal-dominant inherited forms of AD. Even in familial AD cases, where the age of death usually ranges from 40 to 60, diffusely distributed LB are found in about 15 to 25% of cases (16). This is unlikely to be a coincidence, because the prevalence of PD is only 1 to 2% in the general population. It raises the possibility that AD pathology may predispose to widespread LB formation in some patients.

The cognitive and behavioral symptoms in DLB have several potential pathologic explanations. Cognitively important areas such as entorhinal regions, frontal-, temporal- or parietal cortex, cingulate and amygdala harbor degenerating neurons marked by LB or neurites. Neurochemical deficits in DLB include a marked reduction of acetylcholine due to LB and AD pathology in the NBM, and decreased dopamine in the basal ganglia and cortex (17,18). In addition, AD pathology may contribute to dementia.

CLINICAL FEATURES OF DEMENTIA WITH LEWY BODIES

Clinical descriptions of case series suggested that the dementia associated with diffusely distributed LB consisted of a recognizable clinical syndrome. A consensus workshop was held in 1995, at which clinical experience and earlier proposals for diagnostic criteria were discussed, and a new set of diagnostic criteria was drawn up (1), which is summarized in Table 16-1. The chief problem in diagnosing DLB is differentiating it from AD in patients who present with dementia. In patients initially diagnosed as having PD who develop dementia later in their course, the diagnosis of DLB as a likely underlying pathology does not require the DLB criteria. The criteria therefore are most useful in helping to predict pathology in patients who present with dementia. The criteria therefore are most useful in helping to predict pathology in patients who present with dementia. Whether a clinical diagnosis of DLB can be made with certainty is not clear.

Dementia is the mandatory feature of DLB. It is defined as progressive deterioration of cognition leading to impaired functional ability. Most patients have an insidious onset and show gradual progression when tracked from year to year, as is the case for AD. In some patients, fluctuation of cognition may override this gradual decline. The age at onset of DLB ranges from about 60 to 85, overlapping with AD. The duration from onset of dementia to death is variable and similar to AD. Some studies have found shorter

---

Table 16-1 Workshop Criteria for the Clinical Diagnosis of Dementia with Lewy Bodies (adapted from McKeith et al., 1995 (1))

Mandatory:
Dementia
Core features: (1 core feature = possible DLB, 2 or 3 core features = probable DLB)
Fluctuation of cognition, function or alertness
Visual hallucinations
Spontaneous Parkinsonism
Supporting features:
Repeated falls
Syncope
Transient loss of consciousness
Neuroleptic sensitivity
Systematized delusions
Nonvisual hallucinations

survival in DLB compared to AD (19,20). The explanation is not clear, but in some cases accelerated clinical progression in DLB – and even death – has followed treatment with neuroleptic medications (21). Specific psychometric aspects of the dementia syndrome may help to distinguish DLB from AD.

The DLB workshop criteria list three core features and a group of supporting features. Each of the three core features – fluctuation, spontaneous Parkinsonism, and visual hallucinations – is not unique and may be caused by a variety of other conditions. Because of the ambiguity of the core features, the presence of only one feature is designated "possible" DLB, whereas two or more features define "probable" DLB.

Fluctuation refers to marked variation in a patient's cognitive or functional abilities, or periods of confusion or decreased responsiveness that alternate with improved awareness (1). Daytime somnolence early in the course may be part of this picture. Patients with PD who later become demented show fluctuation of cognitive abilities akin to on–off motor performance. The DLB criteria acknowledge the importance of fluctuation, but also note the difficulty of characterizing how much is "significant". In patients with AD cognitive performance varies from day to day, and sundowning or nocturnal confusion and agitation is common. More dramatic variation in behavior or abilities suggests DLB. Episodes of fluctuation in DLB may last from minutes to days. When lucidity waxes and wanes over days or longer, delirium must be ruled out, and causes such as infection or medication toxicity must be considered. Fluctuation has been noted less frequently in series from centers that emphasize dementia (22–24) compared to those that emphasize geriatric psychiatry (20). One dramatic form of fluctuation, noted in several series of DLB, is the rapid onset of inattention with speech arrest usually lasting for a few minutes. When this occurs, transient cerebral ischemia or seizures may need to be ruled out.

Visual hallucinations occur in about 40 to 75% of patients with DLB (20,22,25), compared to about 5 to 20% of patients with pure AD. In DLB the hallucinations typically consist of formed images of people or animals. They are usually vivid and detailed, and often include bright colors and dramatic scenes. They occur without a provoking factor, and may recur over days, weeks or even longer periods. Some patients are indifferent to the hallucinations, whereas others find them threatening or disturbing and may incorporate them into delusional beliefs. Patients or their informants may find the hallucinations to be embarrassing, and it may require tactful history taking to elicit these symptoms. In elderly individuals, the differential diagnosis of visual hallucinations includes delirium, medication toxicity, impaired vision, and stroke. These conditions are not likely to produce hallucinations that are vivid, formed, and recurrent. As in idiopathic PD, treatment with dopaminergic medications may lead to hallucinations in DLB. However, the appearance of hallucinations in patients with dementia and Parkinsons, not yet treated with dopaminergic drugs, strongly suggests a diagnosis of DLB.

Several explanations have been proposed for the neural basis of hallucinations in DLB. Cholinergic deficiency is one candidate, because levels of cholinergic markers are markedly decreased in the temporal or parietal cortex in DLB (10), and hallucinations may improve after treatment with cholinergic drugs. Similar visual hallucinations can be provoked in normal people by anticholinergic drugs such as scopolamine. Alternatively, disruption of circuits connecting the brainstem, basal ganglia, and visual association cortex may underlie formed visual hallucinations in general (26).

Spontaneous *parkinsonism* in DLB is the clearest link to idiopathic PD. Bradykinesia, rigidity, and gait disorder are typical. Masked facies, stooped posture, and postural instability may also occur. In DLB, resting tremor is less common than in PD, found in 10 to 20% of autopsy-confirmed cases in recent autopsy series (22,23). Some series have reported higher rates of resting tremor, but included patients where PD preceded dementia (27). Postural or kinetic tremors are common in DLB, but also occur in AD and in aging.

Parkinsonian findings in DLB are often bilateral and symmetrical, although they more commonly initially show laterality or asymmetry in PD. Parkinsonism is often milder in DLB than in PD, for unclear reasons (22). The dementia and behavioral disorder predominate the picture. Possibly the later age at onset of DLB may modify the appearance of Parkinsonism. Alternatively, coexisting striatal cholinergic deficits in DLB may attenuate the acetylcholine-dopamine imbalance found in PD. Another feature relatively commonly found in DLB cases where dementia was the primary symptom is a lower rate of clinical responsiveness to levodopa (11,27).

Parkinsonian assessment measures, such as the Unified Parkinson's Disease Rating Scale (UPDRS) may be used in demented or elderly patients. In severely demented patients, scale items are often not applicable because the patients have difficulty in understanding or carrying out complex motor commands. As in idiopathic PD, bradykinesia, rigidity, and resting tremor are the most helpful signs in DLB. Findings such as masked facies, hypophonic speech, stooped posture or gait abnormalities are less specific because they may occur in many types of dementia. Also, slowed movements and stooped posture occur with aging or may result from orthopedic or other medical problems common in elderly people.

The combination of dementia and Parkinsonism is not specific to DLB or PD-dementia. The differential diagnosis most frequently includes blockade of dopaminergic receptors due to neuroleptics or other medications, and Alzheimer's disease (28). Parkinsonism and dementia also occur in degenerative disorders such as progressive supranuclear palsy, striato-nigral degeneration, cortico basal degeneration, frontotemporal dementia linked to chromosome 17, Hallervorden-Spatz disease, Parkinson–dementia complex of Guam, and Huntington's disease.

The frequency of parkinsonism in AD varies in published reports. There are two main reasons for this. First, studies have used varying definitions of parkinsonism. Second, Parkinsonism increases in association with dementia severity (28). Parkinsonism is rare early in the course of AD, but is common in institutionalized patients with severe dementia (28,29). AD with parkinsonism remains the most difficult condition to distinguish from DLB. As a rough guide, if parkinsonian findings appear late in the course of dementia, for example, when the Mini-Mental State Examination score is less than 10/30, AD is more likely. If they appear earlier, or other core features of DLB are present, DLB is more likely. There are several mechanisms for Parkinsonism in AD: pharmacologic blockade of dopamine receptors by neuroleptics, concomitant vascular lesions in the basal ganglia, or AD lesions such as neurofibrillary tangles in neurons of the substantia nigra (30).

The "supporting features" for DLB are less common or specific than the core features. They include repeated falls, syncope, transient loss of consciousness, neuroleptic sensitivity, systematized delusions, and nonvisual hallucinations. Frequent or recurrent falls early in the course of dementia without a clear explanation may be an alerting feature of DLB. However, falls can also occur in AD and other dementing disorders (early falling is especially common in PSP), or may result from orthopedic problems or frailty associated with aging, and have low specificity for DLB. Orthostasis is well recognized in PD, and syncopal episodes may occur in some patients with DLB. Transient loss of responsiveness may manifest as brief periods of apparent arrest of speech and activity, not necessarily related to syncope (10). Because these episodes may resemble transient ischemic attacks, cerebrovascular diagnostic evaluation often is needed. Delusions in DLB usually occur at a stage of moderately severe dementia. Similar delusions occur in patients with AD and also in PD–dementia. In DLB the content of the delusions may relate to visual hallucinations.

Patients with DLB are extremely sensitive to neuroleptics. Worsening of motor function, impaired level of alertness, and, in severe cases, precipitous decline requiring hospitalization, and even death have followed neuroleptic treatment. While these types of reactions were first described in association with high potency agents such as haloperidol, they also may occur after treatment with newer agents such as risperidone (31). Challenge with neuroleptics should not be considered as a diagnostically useful maneuver in DLB. The safest antipsychotic medications in patients with LB disorders are the atypical agents such as clozapine, olanzapine, and quetiapine, which have negligible D-2 receptor blocking activity.

Newer versions of DLB diagnostic criteria are likely to incorporate *REM sleep behavior disorder (RBD)*. The chief symptom is vivid dreams that patients appear to act out verbally or physically, for example, by shouting, punching or kicking, crawling, or running in bed. Polysomnography shows loss of generalized muscle atonia during REM sleep, prominent phasic muscle twitching during REM sleep, or both of these. RBD may arise spontaneously or in association with disorders such as PD, multiple system atrophy and DLB (32). Some patients who present with RBD may later develop PD (33).

PATTERNS OF COGNITIVE IMPAIRMENT IN DEMENTIA WITH LEWY BODIES

Neuropsychologic studies have shown that DLB is often associated with a recognizable profile of cognitive impairment. Several types of cognitive deficits occur to a similar degree in DLB and AD, for example impaired memory, dyscalculia, constructional and ideomotor dyspraxia and dysphasia (11,22). In fact, when dementia progresses to moderate or severe cognitive loss it may be difficult to discern patterns or profiles of impairment. Disproportionally severe deficits in tests that depend on attention, verbal fluency, and visuospatial processing are a mark of DLB. This type of profile has been described in frontal-subcortical dementias. Because many patients with DLB also have AD lesions, the clearest demonstration that LB are specifically associated with this profile of deficits comes from selected cases of dementia with "pure" DLB and negligible AD pathology (34). Even in clinical series, in which concomitant AD cannot be ruled out, DLB can be psychometrically distinguished from AD. For example, a recent study found that DLB patients matched to AD patients for overall dementia severity scored higher than AD patients on tests of recall, but worse on block design (a combined visuo-spatial and executive task) and problem solving (35). In the usual case of DLB, in which AD lesions coexist, the neuropsychologic profile shows subcortical cognitive deficits superimposed on the cortical deficits typical of AD.

NEUROIMAGING STUDIES OF DEMENTIA WITH LEWY BODIES

Attempts to develop a biologic marker for the diagnosis of DLB have recently included structural and metabolic imaging of the brain. Volumetric MRI studies have shown that temporal lobe atrophy occurs in DLB, to a lesser extent than in AD (36), but AD and DLB show much overlap. Metabolic studies show that DLB and AD share decreased metabolism in temporal and neocortical regions, but patients with DLB also have hypometabolism in the occipital lobe (37,38).

MANAGEMENT OF PATIENTS WITH DEMENTIA WITH LEWY BODIES

The management of patients and families with DLB includes social issues and medical treatment. The physician should take into account the patient's needs and wishes in conjunction with those of family members. Some key issues related to personal independence are disclosure of the diagnosis of dementia, and assessment of competence to work, drive, and manage finances. Home safety and the patient's ability to carry out basic activities of daily living should be assessed. In later stages of dementia, issues such as caregiver stress, services such as day care and institutionalization need to be considered. Acute conditions such as infections, medications, and medical comorbidity may influence the patient's symptoms and functional abilities. These should be explored when daily function or cognition suddenly declines or new behavioral symptoms such as confusion or agitation emerge.

No medication has been demonstrated to slow the progression or have neuroprotective efficacy in DLB. Medical therapy targets the motor, behavioral, and cognitive symptoms of DLB. The relative importance of each of these categories of symptoms needs to be considered before medications are prescribed. Even though reports suggest a lower likelihood of substantial motor improvement than in patients with PD, a trial of levodopa is warranted in patients with DLB. Until more

experience is gained with newer dopamine receptor agonists in DLB, Levodopa is a safer choice because it may have a lower risk of causing hallucinations.

For behavioral symptoms such as delusions, hallucinations, and agitation, medication review and a search for reversible causes such as infection or painful medical illness should precede the initiation of new medications. Nonpharmacologic strategies should be considered, for example, altering the patient's environment or routine or employing distraction when symptoms appear. Decreasing dopaminergic medications must be considered. Trazodone or valproate may be useful choices instead of neuroleptics for agitation in moderate to severe dementia. High-potency neuroleptics such as haloperidol and even newer agents such as risperidone and olanzapine may markedly worsen parkinsonism in DLB (31,38a). Atypical neuroleptics are preferable to control psychotic symptoms. Clozapine, with high affinity for D_4 receptors and weak affinity for D_1 and D_2, is relatively selective for limbic rather than striatal pathways. Although it is an effective first-line agent (39,39a), regular hematologic monitoring is needed. Quetiapine is a newer atypical antipsychotic agent that does not require hematologic monitoring. New evidence supports its efficacy and safety in AD or PD–dementia (40), and there is some published experience on efficacy in DLB.

Levels of key enzymes related to acetylcholine metabolism are profoundly decreased in the brain in DLB. This suggests that by analogy to AD, cholinergic augmentation may improve cognitive performance in DLB. To date there is scanty evidence for this. A recent short-term study of tacrine in clinically diagnosed DLB and AD patients found that about half of the patients improved to a small degree on selected cognitive tests (41). The duration of treatment was short and at best the results were weakly positive. Because tacrine has hepatotoxic side effects, its role as a cognitive enhancing agent in AD has been taken over by donepezil, an acetylcholinesterase inhibitor with an excellent side effect profile. The published experience for donepezil in DLB is limited. In a small open-label study of nine patients with DLB, donepezil led to improved cognitive scores in seven patients, and reduction in hallucinations. Parkinsonism worsened in three patients, but responded to raising the dose of levodopa (42). In another report, two DLB patients with marked cognitive fluctuation showed improvement on donepezil (43). A double-blind study of a different cholinesterase inhibitor in DLB showed positive effects on improving behavioral symptoms (44). A trial of cholinergic treatment in patients with DLB seems reasonable.

Considering that clinicopathologic studies of DLB began only in 1990, much progress has been made in mapping the clinical syndrome and treating symptoms. Further breakthroughs in understanding the biology of the Lewy body and of neuronal systems and circuits that are vulnerable in PD and DLB are needed before the ultimate goal of disease-modifying therapy can be achieved.

REFERENCES

1. McKeith IG, Galasko D, Kosaka K, et al. Consensus guidelines for the clinical and pathological diagnosis of dementia with Lewy bodies. (DLB): report of the Consortium on DLB international workshop. *Neurology* 1996; 47:1113–1124.
2. Kosaka K. Diffuse Lewy body disease in Japan. *J Neurol* 1990; 237:197–204.
3. Dickson DW, Ruan D, Crystal H, et al. Hippocampal degeneration differentiates diffuse Lewy body disease (DLBD) from Alzheimer's disease: Light and electron microscopic immunocytochemistry of CA2-3 neurites specific to DLBD. *Neurology* 1991; 41:1402–1409.
4. Hansen LA, Masliah E, Terry RD, et al. A neuropathological subset of Alzheimer's disease with concomitant Lewy body disease and spongiform change. *Acta Neuropathol* 1989; 78:194–201.
5. Hughes D, Daniel S, Blankson S, et al. A clinicopathologic study of 100 cases of Parkinson's disease. *Arch Neurol* 1993; 50:140–148.
6. Mattilla PM, Roytta, Torikka H, et al. Cortical Lewy bodies and Alzheimer-type changes in patients with Parkinson's disease. *Acta Neuropathol* 1998; 95:576–582.
7. Churchyard A, Lees AJ. The relationship between dementia and direct involvement of the hippocampus and amygdala in Parkinson's disease. *Neurology* 1997; 49:1570–1576.
8. Samuel W, Galasko D, Masliah E, et al. Neocortical Lewy body counts correlate with dementia in the Lewy body variant of Alzheimer's disease. *J Neuropathol Exp Neurol* 1996; 55:44–52.
9. Lennox G, Lowe J, Morell K, et al. Diffuse Lewy body disease: correlative neuropathology using anti-ubiquitin immunocytochemistry. *J Neurol Neurosurg Psychiatry* 1989; 52:1236–1247.
10. Perry R, McKeith I, Perry E. *Dementia with Lewy bodies*. Cambridge, UK: Cambridge University Press, 1996.
11. Hansen L, Salmon DP, Galasko D, et al. The Lewy body variant of Alzheimer's disease: a clinical and pathological entity. *Neurology* 1990; 40:1–8.
12. Perry RH, Irving D, Blessed G, et al. Senile dementia of Lewy body type: a clinically and neuropathologically distinct form of Lewy body dementia in the elderly. *J Neurol Sci* 1990; 95:119–139.

13. Gearing M, Lynn M, Mirra SS. Nurofibrillary pathology in Alzheimer Disease with Lewy bodies. Two subgroups. *Arch Neurol* 1999; 56:203–208.
14. Crystal HA, Sliwinski M, Dickson D et al. Pathological markers associated with normal aging and dementia in the elderly. *Ann Neurol* 1993; 34:566–573.
15. Trojanowski JQ, Lee VM-Y. Aggregation of neurofilaments and a-synuclein proteins in Lewy bodies: implications for the pathogenesis of Parkinson's disease and Lewy Body dementia. *Arch Neurol* 1998; 55:151–152.
16. Lippa CF, Fujiwara H, Mann DMA, et al. Lewy bodies contain altered alpha-synuclein in brains of many familial Alzheimer's disease patients with mutations in presenilin and amyloid precursor protein genes. *Am J Pathol* 1998; 153:1365–1370.
17. Langlais PJ, Thal L, Hansen L, et al. Neurotransmitters in basal ganglia and cortex of Alzheimer's disease with- and without Lewy bodies. *Neurology* 1993; 43:1927–1934.
18. Perry EK, Haroutunian V, Davis KL, et al. Neocortical cholinergic activities differentiate Lewy body dementia from classical Alzheimer's disease. *Neuro Rep* 1994; 5:747–749.
19. Olichney JM, Galasko D, Salmon DP, et al. Cognitive decline is faster in Lewy body variant than in Alzheimer's disease. *Neurology* 1998; 51:351–357.
20. McKeith IG, Fairbairn AF, Bothwell RA, et al. An evaluation of the predictive validity and inter-rater reliability of clinical diagnostic criteria for senile dementia of the Lewy body type. *Neurology* 1994; 44:872–877.
21. McKeith I, Fairbairn A, Perry R, et al. Neuroleptic sensitivity in patients with senile dementia of Lewy body type. *BMJ* 1992; 305:673–678.
22. Galasko D, Katzman R, Salmon DP. Clinical and neuropathological findings in Lewy body dementia. *Brain Cog* 1996; 31:176–185.
23. Mega MS, Masterman DL, Benson DF, et al. Dementia with Lewy bodies: reliability and validity of clinical and pathological criteria. *Neurology* 1996; 47:403–1409.
24. Weiner MF, Risser RC, Cullum CM, et al. Alzheimer's disease and its Lewy body variant: a clinical analysis of postmortem verified cases. *Am J Psychiatry* 1996; 153:1269–1273.
25. Klatka LA, Louis ED, Schiffer RB. Psychiatric features in diffuse Lewy body disease: a clinicopathologic study using Alzheimer's disease and Parkinson's disease control groups. *Neurology* 1997; 47:1148–1152.
26. Manford M, Andermann F. Complex visual hallucinations. Clinical and neurobiological insights. *Brain* 1998; 121:1819–1840.
27. Louis ED, Klatka LA, Liu Y, et al. Comparison of extrapyramidal features in 31 pathologically confirmed cases of diffuse Lewy body disease and 34 pathologically confirmed cases of Parkinson's disease. *Neurology* 1997; 48:376–380.

28. Ellis RJ, Caligiuri M, Galasko D, et al. Extrapyramidal motor signs in clinically diagnosed Alzheimer disease. *Alz Dis Assoc Disord* 1996; 10:103–114.
29. Girling DM, Berrios GE. Extrapyramidal signs, primitive reflexes and frontal lobe function in senile dementia of the Alzheimer type. *Br J Psychiatry* 1990; 157:888–893.
30. Liu Y, Stern Y, Chun MR, et al. Pathological correlates of Extrapyramidal signs in Alzheimer's disease. *Ann Neurol* 1997; 41:368–374.
31. McKeith IG, Ballard CG, Harrison RW. Neuroleptic sensitivity to risperidone in Lewy body dementia. *Lancet* 1995; 346:699.
32. Schenk CH, Bundlie SR, Mahowald MW. Delayed emergence of a parkinsonian disorder in 38% of 29 older men initially diagnosed with idiopathic rapid eye movement sleep behavior disorder. *Neurology* 1996; 46:388–393.
33. Boeve BF, Silber MH, Ferman TK, et al. REM sleep disorder and degenerative dementia: an association likely reflecting Lewy body disease. *Neurology* 1998; 52:363–370.
34. Salmon DP, Galasko D, Hansen LA, et al. Neuropsychological deficits associated with diffuse Lewy body disease. *Brain Cogn* 1996; 31:148–165.
35. Shimomura T, Mori E, Yamashita H, et al. Cognitive loss in dementia with Lewy bodies and Alzheimer disease. *Arch Neurol* 1998; 55:1547–1552.
36. Hashimoto M, Kitagaki H, Imamura T, et al. Medial temporal and whole-brain atrophy in dementia with Lewy bodies: a whole brain MRI study. *Neurology* 1998; 51:357–362.
37. Albin RL, Minoshima S, D'Amato CJ, et al. Fluoro-deoxyglucose positron emission tomography in diffuse Lewy body disease. *Neurology* 1996; 47:462–466.
38. Ishii K, Yamaji S, Kitagaki H, et al. Regional cerebral blood flow difference between dementia with Lewy bodies and AD. *Neurology* 1999; 53:413–416.
38a. Molho ES, Factor SA. Worsening of motor features of Parkinsonism with olanzapine. *Mov Disord* 1999; 14: in press.
39. Friedman JH. The management of the levodopa psychoses. *Clin Neuropharmacol* 1991; 14:283–295.
39a. The Parkinson Study Group. Low-dose clozapine for the treatment of drug-induced psychosis in Parkinson's disease. *N Engl J Med* 1999; 340:757–763.
40. Fernandez HH, Friedman JH, Jacques C, et al. Quetiapine for the treatment of drug-induced psychosis in Parkinson's disease. *Mov Disord* 1999; 14:484–487.
41. Lebert F, Pasquier F, Souliez L. Tacrine efficacy in Lewy body dementia. *Int J Geriatr Psychiatry* 1998; 13:516–519.
42. Shea C, MacKnight C, Rockwood K. Donepezil for treatment of dementia with Lewy bodies: a case series of nine patients. *Int Psychogeriatr* 1998; 10:229–238.
43. Kaufer DI, Catt KE, Lopez OL, et al. Dementia with Lewy bodies: response of delirium-like features to donepezil. *Neurology* 1998; 51:1512.
44. Grace JG, McKeith IG. The use of cholinesterase inhibitors in dementia with Lewy bodies. *Neurobiol Aging* 1998; 4S:S208.

17

Depression

Tiffany W. Chow, Donna L. Masterman, and Jeffrey L. Cummings, M.D.
Rancho Los Amigos/USC Alzheimer's Disease Center, Downey, Los Angeles, California

INTRODUCTION

Parkinson's disease (PD) is often accompanied by depression. One study reported major depression in as many as 40 to 60% of advanced and untreated PD patients, regardless of the duration of illness or degree of physical disability (1). The frequency of depression reported in PD has varied considerably depending on diagnostic methodology employed. A review of the literature in 1992 showed a mean frequency of 40% with a range of 4 to 70% in 26 reports. Lower frequencies were reported in earlier studies without standardized measures. The nine studies, which were completed later (1987–1990), demonstrated a mean frequency of 43% (range 25–70%). However, in a more recent community-based study, the numbers differed somewhat (1a). Of 235 patients, 7.7% has a major depressive episode, 5.1% were moderately to severely depressed at the time of the study, and 45% had mild depression. This report of a lower prevalence of major depression in PD was supported by another population-based study (1b), which reported a frequency of 2.7% of major depression in nondemented PD patients. Mood changes can predate the start of motor symptoms of PD as a prodromal syndrome (1,2). Although some have labeled depression in PD as a reaction to the physical disability, it most likely represents a comorbid expression of central nervous system degeneration.

Depression in PD has been classified as major depression, dysthymia, or organic mood syndrome, according to the *Diagnostic and Statistical Manual of Mental Disorders*, revised 3rd Edition, (DSM-IIIR) (3), or mood disorder due to a general medical condition, as in the *Diagnostic and Statistical Manual of Mental Disorders*, 4th edition (DSM-IV). (American Psychiatric Association, 1994 #171). Detection and treatment of depression for improvement of the quality of life and prevention of suicide are crucial issues in the management of PD patients. Studies show that PD patients with major depression have a significantly greater decline in activities of daily living than PD patients with only minor depression or no depression (4,5). In addition, in one study, patients with major depression had significantly longer duration of illness. However, when patients were matched for duration of disease and followed longitudinally, those with major depression were significantly worse (4). Although no studies to date have shown a direct effect of antidepressant therapy on delaying cognitive decline, deterioration in ADLs or motor progression, and cost-benefit analyses of antidepressant treatment in PD are definitely indicated.

Depression is difficult to recognize in the patient with PD because the signs of the two disorders overlap. Neurovegetative symptoms of depression in non-Parkinsonian and PD patients can include disturbances in sleep (6) and appetite; anhedonia; sexual dissatisfaction (7); feelings of guilt, hopelessness, and worthlessness; loss of energy; poor concentration and short term memory; the feeling that one is moving in slow motion; and suicidality. These symptoms may be accompanied by tearfulness and sadness, and the patient may or may not attribute his or her feelings to parkinsonism.

The hypomimia of PD gives the patient the appearance of having a depressed affect, whereas hypophonia and bradykinesia resemble psychomotor retardation and contribute to a saddened appearance. A patient's withdrawal from activities because of disability or social embarrassment over parkinsonism may be interpreted by others as apathy. On the basis of these features, clinicians may overdiagnose depression and undertreat parkinsonism. Screening for depression in PD patients can easily lead to false positives (1). The Beck Depression Inventory (BDI) (a self-administered scale) contains items that might appear to confound motor impairment and mood changes, however, cluster analysis supports the validity of this measure of depression in PD patients (8,8a). The Hamilton Depression Rating Scale (HDRS) (an interview-based scale) has been used more extensively in recent research.

RISK FACTORS FOR DEPRESSION IN PD

Possible risk factors for co-occurrence of depression with PD include younger age at onset (50–65 years, depending on the study design) (1), female gender (9), right-sided hemi-Parkinsonism, akinesia, increased severity of disability, anxiety, and psychosis. Younger patients experienced twice the frequency of depression than older patients (10–13) and are more likely to have experienced depression before onset of parkinsonism (2). This group of young onset PD patients is particularly vulnerable to the occurrence of a reactive depression due to the effect of illness on career, intimate relationships, financial security, and quality of life (14,15).

Studies of depression in patients with hemi-Parkinsonism have not defined a consistent right–left lateralization to correlate with mood disorder. However, Cole et al. (10) found an association of depression with right hemi-Parkinsonism. Patients with right-sided PD had significantly more depressive symptoms when depression was assessed by the HDRS, but not when assessed by Geriatric Depression Scale (10). Focal transcranial stimulation may provide additional information regarding lateralization of mood state.

The type of parkinsonism may provide another risk factor for depression. Tandberg and colleagues divided PD patients into diagnostic categories of definite, probable, or possible PD defining specificity of the clinical diagnosis. Those in the possible PD category have a higher frequency of atypical parkinsonism (16,17). Those with possible PD had depression more commonly than those with more certain diagnoses, and this might be explained by the presence of those atypical cases and higher prevalence of dementia (17). There is also a difference between rigid-dominant and tremor-dominant forms of PD. Starkstein found that akinetic PD patients had a significantly higher prevalence (38%) of major depression than tremor-dominant PD patients (15%) (18), but successful treatment of the motor manifestations of PD does not consistently relieve depression (15). Since patients with bradykinesia show hypoperfusion of medial frontal cortex (19), there may be support for a functional localization of depression in PD (18). Bradyphrenia and apathy show the strongest correlation to depression (20). Severity of disability correlates with the presence of minor depressive episodes but not sustained major depression (15,20).

Originally depression was thought to be related to the use of levodopa in the treatment of parkinsonism (1), but follow-up studies have not substantiated a causal relationship between levodopa and depression (21,22). Some patients had reactive depression when levodopa failed to show anti-parkinsonian efficacy (23). Patients with a previous history of depressive episodes rarely have been reported to make suicide attempts while on levodopa (24). These observations underscore the necessity of screening PD patients for depression and initiating appropriate treatment.

Depression in PD patients is associated with anxiety and psychosis. When compared with depressed multiple sclerosis patients, depressed PD patients differ in having a higher frequency of atypical panic and anxiety (25), which manifest as panic disorder, phobias, or generalized anxiety disorder (26). In addition, there appears to be a significant interaction between anxiety and depression in PD with up to 92% of the anxiety disorder patients also manifesting depression. In one study, patients with PD had significantly more anxiety than medical controls and 57% of the PD patients had additional depressive symptoms (26a). It has been suggested that anxiety may be secondary, in part, to the anti-parkinsonian medications and this may indicate a need for changes in pharmacologic approaches (25,27,28). Tandberg and colleagues found that PD patients with psychosis are more depressed than those without psychosis (17).

COGNITION AND DEPRESSION IN PD

Depression can exacerbate the cognitive deficits seen in nondemented PD patients (29–31). PD patients with depression have more difficulty on tasks involving shifts of cognitive set and registration memory than nondepressed PD patients (32), yet perform better on short-term memory tasks and respond well to encouragement (33). Although depression may contribute to cognitive impairment in PD, the presence of depression is equally frequent in PD with and without dementia (8). One study, however, found depression to be a risk factor for the subsequent development of dementia in PD (34). On the other hand, in another study, depression was found to be more common in patients with dementia, as measured by mini-mental status exam, 3.6% in those with a score above 20 and 25.6% in more with a score below 20 (1a). In another study (17), impaired cognitive function was considered a predictor of major depression.

RELATION OF DEPRESSION TO ON–OFF PHENOMENA

Fluctuations in mood may accompany the sudden fluctuations in motor function seen with the "on–off phenomenon" (35). Stabilization of motor symptoms may improve depression as well. Rapid cycling bipolar mood shifts have been reported during a single patient's on–off cycle (36). The pathophysiology of the on–off phenomenon may be linked to catecholaminergic systems that also determine mood states (37). Catechol-O-methyltransferase (COMT) inhibitors, developed to stabilize motor fluctuations, may have beneficial effects on mood instability.

NEUROBIOLOGIC BASIS OF DEPRESSION IN PD

Depression has been associated with deficiencies of dopamine (DA), serotonin (5-HT), and norepinephrine (NE) (1,38). Degeneration of DA neurons in ventral tegmental area (VTA), 5-HT neurons of the dorsal raphe, and NE neurons of the locus ceruleus (LC) may predispose the PD patients to depression (Table 17-1) (39).

It is the DA deficiency in the mesolimbic dopamine system which is the suspected etiology for depression in PD patients. Serotonergic neuronal of damage is not as pervasive as dopaminergic neuronal damage in PD

Table 17-1 Neurochemical Basis of Depression in Parkinson's Disease

	Dopamine (DA)	Serotonin (5-HT)	Norepinephrine (NE)
Neuropathologic Findings	Neuronal loss in the ventral tegmental area (VTA; origin of the mesolimbic dopaminergic projection); greater loss of A10 dopaminergic neurons in this area than would be expected with normal aging (14).	Neuronal loss in rostral brainstem cell groups (dorsal raphe and median raphe) (103)	Neuronal loss in rostral and caudal locus ceruleus (LC) (37); but depression in PD patients is accompanied by greater loss of LC neurons (104,105)
Biochemistry	Decreased tyrosine-hydroxylase (TH) activity in VTA -> decreased dopaminergic output to cingulate, entorhinal, and frontal cortices (106).	Abnormal binding at 5-HT uptake sites (107–109), but transcranial sonography reveals greater disruption of brainstem dorsal raphe echogenicity in depressed PD patients than nondepressed PD patients (110)	
CSF Studies	No correlation between levels of DA metabolite, homovanillic acid (HVA) and depression (81,111,112)	Lowest levels of 5-HIAA, the principal metabolite of 5-HT, in PD patients with depression (81,111,113–115), but does not correlate with the severity of depression (114,116).	Bradyphrenia correlates positively with decreased levels of norepinephrine metabolite 3-methoxy-4-hydroxyphenylene glycol (MHPG) (38).
Response to treatment	Depressed PD patients demonstrated significantly less euphoria when given intravenous methylphenidate, compared with nondepressed PD patients with equal physical disability and depressed, non-Parkinsonian patients (117); positive but nonreproducible antidepressant response to selegiline (50)	Alleviation of depression by oral 5-HTP supports the possible efficacy of 5-HT-directed antidepressant therapy. The effect was attended by a rise in level of CSF 5-HIAA (81).	Positive response to TCAs in controlled trials (118–120)

(40), and the role of 5-HT deficiency in PD-related depression has not been fully established. Similarly, deterioration of the LC in PD patients occurs with and without clinical manifestations of depression (37), leaving the contribution of norepinephrine deficiency to depression in PD unclear.

Recent studies indicate that glutamate may be involved in depression (41). N-methyl-D-aspartate (NMDA) receptor changes induced by antidepressants have been seen in animals and humans, leading some researchers to believe that the glutamate recognition site on the NMDA receptor is involved in a final common pathway of antidepressant action. There has been no evidence from studies in PD patients to indicate that there is a particular role for glutamate in depression in PD.

METABOLIC STUDIES OF DEPRESSION IN PD

Of the functional neuroimaging techniques, only positron emission tomography (PET) shows a localized abnormality in depressed PD patients. When evaluated by fluoro-deoxyglucose (FDG) PET, depressed PD patients have lower metabolism in caudate and inferior orbitofrontal cortex than both nondepressed PD patients and normal controls, and this finding correlated with the severity of patient HDRS scores (42). Orbitofrontal hypometabolism may reflect impaired dopaminergic stimulation from the ventral tegmental area (42).

Single photon emission computed tomography (SPECT) has shown no pattern of abnormality specific to depressed PD patients. Concomitant dementia in some of the PD patients tested may have confounded these studies (43). Resting state regional cerebral blood flow as measured by PET reveals bilateral reduction in the medial prefrontal cortex (Brodmann's area 9) and contiguous cingulate cortex (Brodmann's area 32). These abnormalities also were found in non-Parkinsonian, depressed patients, suggesting a common biologic substrate between endogenous depression and the depression of PD.

TREATMENT OF DEPRESSION IN PD

Anti-Parkinsonian Treatment

Mood responses to anti-Parkinsonian treatment have been limited, but monoamine oxidase inhibitors (MAO-I) and catechol-O-methyltransferase (COMT)

inhibitors show promise as antidepressants, possibly because of their combined effect on several catecholamines. Antidepressant effects of current anti-Parkinsonian agents are summarized in Table 17-2. With the exception of selegiline, their effects have not been studied in randomized, double-blind, controlled trials on PD patients with and without depression, and any evidence of positive antidepressant activity has been by case report only (14,23,28,38,44–47).

The antidepressant activity of selegiline is attributed to its MAO-I properties (48). An open-label study reported antidepressant effect (49), and a multicenter, double-blind, randomized, placebo-controlled trial showed significant improvement in HDRS scores after three months of treatment with selegiline at 10 mg/day (50), but patients entered the trial without high HDRS scores and may not have met DSM criteria for depression. Antidepressant activity of selegiline may have also been seen in a trial using the Profile of Mood States (POMS), in which the general state of psychiatric disturbance in PD patients was reduced (48).

The higher affinity for post-synaptic D3 receptors seen with the newer selective dopamine agonists, pramipexole, and ropinirole, is thought to result in antidepression effects in PD patients (51). Three different studies monitoring for adverse effects revealed that fewer PD patients taking pramipexole developed depression compared to PD patients taking placebo (52). More direct evidence for an antidepressant effect of pramipexole has been seen in an open-label study on depressed, non-Parkinsonian patients with median age 44.5 years (53), but neither drug has been studied through controlled trials in PD patients with and without depression.

Coadministration of tolcapone, a COMT inhibitor, with anti-Parkinsonian agents synergistically increases dopaminergic function and may have antidepressant effects (54). The drug is currently used for patients with fluctuating PD. One randomized, placebo-controlled study on patients with fluctuating PD showed no significant change in the UPDRS subscale for mood (55). Entacapone (a peripherally acting COMT-inhibitor) and moclobemide (MAO-$_A$ inhibitor) were tolerated well in healthy normal volunteers but did not result in elevated serum levels of NE or epinephrine and have not gone to trial in PD patients as antidepressants (56).

Response to Surgery

The response of mood state to surgery in PD have varied with the procedures. Transplantation of human fetal mesencephalic tissue for treatment of PD caused depression and nonspecific emotional and behavioral symptoms on a long-term basis, seen up to one year

Table 17-2 Antidepressant and Anti-Parkinsonian Effects of Commonly Used Medications

	Antidepressant Effect	Anti-Parkinsonian Effect
ANTI-PARKINSONIAN AGENTS		
amantadine	+	++ dopaminergic
benztropine	+	++ anticholinergic
biperiden	+	++ anticholinergic
bromocriptine	+	++ anticholinergic
L-dopa	0	+ + + dopaminergic
trihexyphenidyl	+	++ anticholinergic
tyrosine	?	+ dopaminergic
pramipexole	+	+ dopaminergic
ropinirole	?	+ dopaminergic
tolcapone	?	+ dopaminergic
MAO-Is		
selegiline*	+	+
moclobemide	?	?
nomifensine	0	+ dopaminergic
phenelzine	0	-- EPS
bifemaline	?	?
TRICYCLIC ANTIDEPRESSANTS		
amineptine (121)	?	+dopaminergic
amitriptyline	+	--- cholinergic
amoxapine (38,91)	?	---- dopamine blockade
clomipramine	-	?
desipramine (38)	++	-- tremor
imipramine (38,118,122–124)	++	+ + + dopaminergic
nortriptyline (38,80)	++	- cholinergic
protriptyline	?	--- cholinergic
SSRIs		
buspirone (38)	-	-- despite dopaminergic agonism
fluoxetine (38,63)	-	--- EPS
fluvoxamine (125)	?	?
sertraline (65,126)	+	?
trazodone	?	0
COMBINED REUPTAKE INHIBITORS		
brofaromine	?	?
mirtazapine	?	?
nefazodone	?	?
ritanserin	?	+ dopaminergic
venlafaxine	?	?
OTHER TREATMENTS		
bupropion (67)	++	++ dopaminergic
captopril	?	0
cholecystokinin	?	0
lithium	+	--- EPS
tachykinin antagonists	?	0
ECT	+	+
transcranial magnetic stimulation	+	+

*See Table 3 for outcome of selegiline in controlled trials.

+ antidepressant effect = reported to relieve depression in PD patients; ++ antidepressant effect = positive outcome after placebo-controlled trial with patients with DMS-IIR criteria for depression; -- = reported to be ineffective as an antidepressant; -- = worsens extrapyramidal signs; --- = use contraindicated in PD patients; EPS = extrapyramidal signs (rigidity, bradykinesia).

after surgery in patients without prior psychiatric histories (57). Part of this effect was accompanied by episodic, drastic worsening in patient course (57). Ventroposterior pallidotomy in 24 cognitively intact PD patients did not result in postoperative depression nor did it relieve depression (58). One of 28 PD patients had a significant decrease in Beck Depression Inventory score after words (59). Pallidal stimulation might have a similar effect (60). There is no information available about the effect of thalamotomy or subthalamic stimulation on depression. Agid reported a very interesting patient who experienced marked mood changes including depression and crying when her DBS system was activated in the region of the globus pallidus (NEJM 60a). Candidates for functional surgery should have neuropsychiatric evaluation pre- and postoperatively to facilitate identification and treatment of mood disorders.

Antidepressants

Antidepressant medications used in non-Parkinsonian patients include tricyclic antidepressants (TCAs), serotonin reuptake inhibitors (SSRIs), and combined reuptake inhibitors (CRIs) (Table 17.2). Of the antidepressants, only TCAs have been assessed in double-blind, placebo-controlled studies (summarized in Table 17-3).

Tricyclic antidepressants are primarily noradrenergic and serotonergic stimulants (38), but some tricyclic antidepressants also have dopaminergic effects. Typical adverse events pertinent to PD patients include orthostatic hypotension and anticholinergic effects (38). TCAs are useful for patients whose depressive

symptoms include insomnia and restless agitation. Agitation in PD patients may be due to multiple causes not related to depression (e.g., obsessive–compulsive behaviors or iatrogenic psychosis) and should be evaluated carefully (38).

Although SSRIs have shown efficacy in treatment of depression and CSF studies support a serotonergic hypothesis for depression in PD patients, SSRIs have not been carefully tested in depressed PD patients. Open-label studies with sertraline report efficacy in the treatment of depression in PD (60b,65). Despite a list of adverse effects including nervousness, sweating, nausea, sedation, anorexia, dry mouth, and dizziness, SSRIs offer a relatively benign side-effect profile for the elderly population (38). They do not affect cardiac conduction, do not decrease seizure threshold (61), exert minimal quinidine-like effects, and do not alter blood pressure (62). The main contraindication has to do with competition for metabolism by the cytochrome P450 system, which increases risk of toxicity in polypharmacy. Drug–drug interactions to consider when adding antidepressants to anti-Parkinsonian treatment are listed in Table 17-4.

As seen in Table 17-2, fluoxetine may worsen parkinsonism; other SSRIs may cause akathisia (63). Reversible worsening of parkinsonism due to the dopamine-antagonistic activity of fluoxetine occurs 10 to 14 days after initiation (63). Akathisia is the most common neurologic symptom caused by SSRIs in patients of any age and responds to reduction of SSRI medication or addition of propranolol at low doses (62).

The United States Food and Drug Administration recommends against giving an antidepressant (TCA or SSRI) and selegiline simultaneously to prevent the "serotonin syndrome." The syndrome consists of hyperpyrexia, tremors, agitation, restlessness, decreased mental status, and autonomic dysfunction; it has rarely proven fatal. A recent review of published case reports of adverse experiences showed that 0.24% of patients experienced nonserious symptoms possibly consistent with the serotonin syndrome (64). With the risk being low, it is not unreasonable to use antidepressants and selegiline in combination if the potential benefits outweigh the risks. The open-label study of sertraline as an antidepressant for PD patients reported that patients taking selegiline concurrently did experience more adverse effects, but none of the patients developed the serotonin syndrome (65).

Distinct from the serotonin syndrome, SSRI withdrawal has been reported. Symptoms include dizziness, lethargy, paresthesias, nausea, vivid dreams, irritability and lowered mood (66). In one study, the symptoms were more highly associated with usage of SSRIs

Table 17-3 Overview of Placebo-Controlled Antidepressant Trials for Depression in PD Patients, adapted from Klassen (80). [Reproduced with permission of the publisher.]

Study	N	Antidepressant	Outcome
Indaco & Carrieri (127)	31	amitriptyline	–
Goetz (67)	14	bupropion	+
Boer (128)	20	clomipramine	–
Laitinen (119)	39	desipramine	+
Strang (118)	38	imipramine	+
Bedard (129)	8	nomifensine	–
Andersen (120)	19	nortriptyline	+
Allain (50)	93	selegiline	+
Fischer & Baas (130)	27	selegiline	–
Lees (131)	46	selegiline	–
Przuntek & Kuhn (49)	28	selegiline	–
Hietanen (132)	18	selegiline	–

Table 17-4 Drug–Drug Interactions		
Drug 1	Drug 2	Effect
amantadine	anticholinergics	increased anticholinergic effect
fluvoxamine	TCAs	inhibited TCA metabolism, danger of toxicity (62)
L-dopa	lithium	increased extrapyramidal signs
L-dopa	MAO-Is	hypertensive reaction from increased dopamine and norepinephrine
MAO-Is	methylphenidate	hypertensive reaction from increased dopamine and norepinephrine
MAO-Is	SSRIs or TCAs	serotonin syndrome
methylphenidate	SSRIs	inhibited SSRI metabolism
nefazodone	SSRIs	inhibited metabolism of nefazodone
selegiline	SSRIs or TCAs	rare serotonin syndrome
SSRIs	TCAs	serotonin syndrome due to inhibited TCA metabolism

TCA: tricyclic antidepressant
SSRI: selective serotonin reuptake inhibitor
MAO-I: monoamine oxidase inhibitor

with shorter half-lives (i.e., fluvoxamine, paroxetine, clomipramine) (66). Although there were no significant associations with advanced age, none of the patients reported were over the age of 56 years.

Bupropion is a monocyclic antidepressant with indirect dopamine agonist properties (38). Bupropion given to PD patients on Levodopa or trihexiphenidyl improved depressive symptoms, but the response was limited (67). This medication has shown greater efficacy in treating the motor manifestations of PD than as an antidepressant (67). Side effects limit the dose administered and include elevated blood pressure (62), nausea, vomiting, restlessness, postural tremor, hallucinations, confusion, psychosis, dyskinesias (38,67), and seizures. Once epilepsy risk factors have been eliminated, the incidence of seizures approximates that of seizures caused by high doses of TCAs (exceeding 200 mg/day) (62).

A retrospective chart review found that 60% of PD patients reporting depression had marked benefit or resolution of depression during clozapine treatment (68). Concurrent use of antidepressant medications by these patients is not known, and the risk of leukopenia from clozapine make it unlikely that clozapine would be a first- or second-line antidepressant.

Electroconvulsive therapy (ECT) has some efficacy as an antidepressant and anti-Parkinsonian therapy but requires special considerations in PD patients (38,69–71). Both benefits may not be seen in the same patient after treatment. Typically, motor symptoms respond to ECT sooner than the depression, and the motor symptoms relapse more quickly (72–75). Patients with predominant rigidity respond more often with a reduction in motor and depressive symptoms than those with tremor-dominant PD after ECT (76). Unfortunately, although depression and akinesia in PD patients respond, patients are more susceptible to prolonged delirium after unilateral and bilateral ECT treatments (69,71,77). Basal ganglia injury, as indicated by T2-weighted magnetic resonance imaging (MRI) hyperintensities, specifically in the caudate, may predispose the elderly to develop a reversible, interictal delirium during a course of ECT (78). Multiple ECT treatments increase the duration of the delirium (up to 21 days), bilateral electrode placement may be less deleterious than unilateral placement (77), and preprocedural atropine may contribute to confusion (77). Despite its adverse effects (amnesia, disorientation, slurred speech, tremors, increased intraocular pressure, urinary retention, paralytic ileus (70), and worsening of tardive dyskinesia), ECT has greater efficacy and tolerability than TCAs (70,71,79).

Clinical Drug Trials

According to a meta-analysis of controlled antidepressant drug trials in PD, many trials were not successfully blinded (80). Trials testing tricyclic and monocyclic antidepressants and selegiline for treatment of depression in PD are listed in Table 17-3. Studies on SSRIs, COMT inhibitors, dopamine agonists CRIs, and often adjuvant anti-Parkinsonian medications are needed. Klaasen (80) identified clinically meaningful design criteria for future studies: randomized treatment allocation, blinded allocation procedure, enrollment of at least 75 subjects per study group, minimal bias from dropouts or dropout rates, close follow-up, no addition of cointerventions or at least comparable cointerventions in both comparison groups, adequate outcome measures, generation of a side-effect profile, and intent to treat analyses. In addition, studies that compare PD patients with controls who do not have parkinsonism or who do not have depression may not be as valid (1). Cross-sectional studies may not detect successful treatment for depression and longitudinal reporting. Of the 12 studies that were deemed at least adequate, five tested selegiline, and the rest investigated amitriptyline, clomipramine, nortriptyline, desipramine, imipramine, bupropion, and nomifensine (80). Five of 12 studies had positive outcomes, involving selegiline 10 mg, nortriptyline 100 mg, desipramine 100 mg, imipramine with age-based sliding scale dosage, and bupropion to a maximum of 450 mg (80). Longitudinal follow-up of PD patients over a mean of 2.5 years in one study revealed that depression remitted in only four of 21 patients, one spontaneously, two with standard antidepressant treatment, and one with 5-HTP (81). This indicates the necessity of developing antidepressant treatment that will be effective in PD patients over long periods of time.

Other Agents and Modalities That May Prove Useful in the Future

The SSRI citalopram is now available for use in Europe and the United States. Trials of the antidepressant effect of citalopram in elderly patients with Alzheimer's disease or after stroke have had positive results (82,83).

Newer MAO-Is (nomifensine, phenelzine) show antidepressant efficacy in animal models but have not been well-tolerated in PD (84,85). Bifemaline, an MAO-I selective for noradrenaline, shows central activity and may have potential as an antidepressant in humans (86). Moclobemide's reversible MAO_A-I activity increases central synaptic NE and 5-HT (87) in animal models of anhedonia. It has proved to be as effective as desipramine in antidepressant effect (88). Steur and Ballering found, in their six-week open-label study on PD patients with depression, that the combination of moclobemide and selegiline resulted in a larger reduction of HDRS scores than moclobemide alone (89). Brofaromine is another reversible inhibitor of MAO_A, with additional 5-HT uptake-inhibiting properties (87,90). Although it has not been tested as an antidepressant, evidence for its potential use include: (1) effects on sleep similar to those of TCA and classical MAO-Is and (2) displacement of [^{3}H]cyanoimipramine from 5-HT transporters in the rat brain (90). Neither moclobemide nor brofaromine causes hypotension in animal models and may spare

human PD patients the side effect of orthostatic hypotension (87).

Combined catecholamine reuptake inhibitor antidepressant medications venlafaxine, nefazodone, and mirtazapine, have appealing pharmacokinetic profiles and may be effective for depression in PD patients (61,91–95). Common side effects are similar to those of the SSRIs (62).

Building on the DA deficiency hypothesis of depression in PD, substance P antagonists are being investigated. Substance P–containing neurons can modulate dopaminergic cells in the substantia nigra, noradrenergic neurons in the locus coeruleus, and serotonergic neurons (96). Theoretically, substance P antagonists would allow exogenous manipulation of neurotransmitter balances, but there are doubts about the in vivo viability of peptide structures that are susceptible to enzymatic degradation (96), and there have been no investigations involving PD patients.

Transcranial magnetic stimulation (TMS) has temporarily relieved depression under experimental conditions. TMS exposes focal regions of the brain to magnetic and electrical energy, which does not cause structural change but does induce functional changes, producing transient alterations in both motor function and mood in PD (97). Setbacks to this treatment modality include very temporary therapeutic effect, muscle tension–type headache at the site of stimulation, and risk of seizures (97). Researchers have been able to induce subjective sadness while administering rapid-rate transcranial magnetic stimulation (rTMS) to left prefrontal areas, whereas happiness results from right prefrontal stimulation (97). Sandyk noted that relaxation, sleepiness, mood elevation, increased dreaming, and enhancement of alpha and beta activities in the EEG resulting from external application of picoTesla range magnetic fields, has been noted in healthy subjects taking melatonin and proposes that these effects were mediated by the pineal gland (98). While this point is speculative, there is a significant rise in prolactin after TMS, which would indicate an effect on the hypothalamic tuberoinfundibular dopaminergic system. A recent study involving older, refractory, depressed, non-Parkinsonian patients identified a significant age difference between responders and nonresponders to antidepressant rTMS; patients older than 65 years were more likely not to respond (99).

Special Considerations

Elderly Patients

Elderly patients treated with TCAs or ECT must be monitored for increased pharmacodynamic sensitivity, slower clearance of drug metabolites, and higher plasma concentrations (61). Anticholinergic effects are less well tolerated by elderly patients; they develop urinary retention, blurred vision, paralytic ileus, impaction, confusion, and dry mouth that prevents them from wearing dentures comfortably (61). In general, patients older than 75 years enjoy only modest therapeutic effect from antidepressants. This patient group also contains a subgroup of very severely depressed, refractory individuals with complicating medical illnesses, creating a further challenge for the treating physician (61).

Effects of Chronic Pain

When a patient presents with PD, depression, and chronic pain, it is advisable to consider all three entities in choosing treatment. Alleviation of the component

that troubles the patient most will impact the rest of the triad. Current literature on this issue consists of case reports. In one, buproprion was recommended for its combination of dopaminergic and antidepressant effects (100).

Algorithmic Approach to Pharmacologic Treatment of Depression in PD

1. Neuropsychiatric evaluation: rule out iatrogenic psychosis and anxiety.
2. If depressed and suicidal, treat with ECT. If depressed but not suicidal, reevaluate anti-Parkinsonian medications. Add selegiline for its antidepressant effect.
3. If inadequately treated for depression at this point, stop selegiline and begin treatment for depression (101). Apathetic depression may

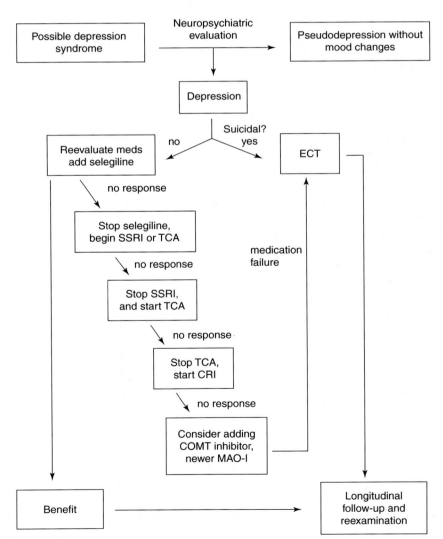

FIGURE 17-1. Treatment algorithm for depression in Parkinson's disease patients (38). See text for explanation.

be more responsive to SSRIs; patients with agitated depression have improved sleep with TCAs (101). See Table 17-5 for a listing of all antidepressants and their typical doses. More studies have focused on proving efficacy of TCAs than SSRIs, but the side-effect profile for SSRIs is more favorable for PD patients. A survey of the members of the Parkinson Study Group revealed that SSRIs were chosen as initial therapy for depression in PD more frequently than TCAs, despite the lack of evidence to support their use. The higher tolerability and presumed efficacy of SSRIs (most frequently sertraline) were motivating factors (102). Each antidepressant medication should have a six-week trial at the maximum tolerated therapeutic dose or at the appropriate plasma level (38).

4. If inadequately treated for depression with SSRIs, initiate treatment with TCAs.

5. If inadequately treated for depression, consider one of the CRIs.
6. If inadequately treated for depression, consider adding a COMT-inhibitor or newer MAO-I.
7. If inadequately treated for depression, consider ECT.
8. Once adequate antidepressant therapy has been achieved, antidepressant medications should be continued for at last six months before tapering of the drug is attempted (38). Chronic treatment may be necessary.

CONCLUSION

Depression of varying degrees commonly complicates the course of PD. The mood disorder is difficult to detect in PD patients because of overlapping symptomatology between the two disorders, but it is important to the quality of life and the course of parkinsonian illness to treat the depression. In the worst cases, patients may be suicidal. Possible risk factors for developing depression with PD include younger age at onset of parkinsonism, female gender, akinesia, increased severity of disability, anxiety, and psychosis.

Depression in PD relates neuropathologically and biochemically to DA, NE, and 5-HT deficiency. In the few placebo-controlled studies, TCAs show efficacy, and selegiline mild antidepressant properties. Nevertheless, the neurobiology of PD and depression indicates that newer medications, including serotonergic agents and COMT-inhibitors, offer potential combined anti-Parkinsonian and antidepressant treatment.

A "serotonin syndrome" has occurred frequently enough that caution should be observed with the coadministration of selegiline with SSRIs or TCAs. Multiple drug–drug interactions between anti-parkinsonian and antidepressant medications and the effects of polypharmacy on the elderly patient complicate treatment strategies. Other somatic treatments for depression in PD patients include ECT, and possibly rTMS.

An algorithmic approach to pharmacologic treatment of depression in PD calls for careful consideration of current anti-Parkinsonian medications, a trial of SSRIs, trial of TCAs, consideration of new serotonergic medications, MAO-Is, and COMT-inhibitors. There are no proven antidepressant drugs of first choice for PD patients at this time, and randomized, double-blind placebo-controlled studies are warranted.

Table 17-5 Antidepressant Medications Used in PD and Their Doses

Generic Name	Trade Name	Initial, Daily Maximum Doses (mg)
imipramine	Tofranil(®)	75, 150
amitriptyline	Elavil(®)	75, 150
doxepin	Sinequan(®)	75, 300
trimipramine	Surmontil(®)	75, 200
amoxapine	Asendin(®)	50, 300
desipramine	Norpramin(®)	25, 200
nortriptyline	Pamelor(®)	75,100
protriptyline	Vivactyl(®)	15, 60
maprotiline	Ludiomil(®)	25, 225
trazodone	Desyrel(®)	50, 600
fluoxetine	Prozac(®)	20, 60
bupropion	Wellbutrin(®)	100, 450
fluvoxamine	Luvox(®)	50, 300
paroxetine	Paxil(®)	10, 50
sertraline	Zoloft(®)	50, 200
phenelzine	Nardil(®)	45, 15
nefazodone	Serzone(®)	200, 600
venlafaxine	Effexor(®)	150, 375
mirtazapine	Remeron(®)	20, 60*
citalopram	Celexa(®)	20, 40
selegiline	Eldepryl(®), Deprenyl(®)	10, 30**

*Plasma concentrations of mirtazapine tend to be higher in the elderly (95).

**10 mg of selegiline is adequate for neuroprotective effects. 30 mg may have antidepressant activity and requires that the patient maintain a low tyramine diet.

ACKNOWLEDGMENTS

This work has been funded by an Alzheimer's Disease Center (AG15670) grant from the National Institute on Aging, the Sidell-Kagan Research Fund, and the Department of Veteran Affairs Geriatric Neurology Fellowship.

REFERENCES

1. Santamaria J, Tolosa E. Clinical subtypes of Parkinson's disease and depression. In: Huber SJ, Cummings JL (eds.). *Parkinson's Disease. Neurobehavioral Aspects.* New York: Oxford University Press, 1992: 217–228.

1a. Tandberg E, Larsen JP, Aasland D, et al. The occurrence of depression in Parkinson's disease. *Arch Neurol* 1996; 53:175–179.

1b. Hantz P, Caradoc-Davies G, Caradoc-Davies T, et al. Depression in Parkinson's disease. *Am J Psychiatry* 1994; 151:1010–1014.

2. Santamaria J, Tolosa E, Valle A. Parkinson's disease with depression: a possible subgroup of idiopathic Parkinsonism. *Neurology* 1986; 36:1130–1133.

3. American Psychiatric Association. *Diagnostic and Statistical Manual of Mental Disorders.* Washington: American Psychiatric Association, 1984.

4. Starkstein SE, Mayberg HS, Leiguarda R, et al. A prospective longitudinal study of depression, cognitive decline, and physical impairments in patients with Parkinson's disease. *J Neurol Neurosurg Psychiatry* 1992; 55:377–382.

5. Liu CY, Wang SJ, Fuh JL, et al. The correlation of depression with functional activity in Parkinson's disease. *J Neurol* 1997; 244:493–498.

6. Smith MC, Ellgring H, Oertel WH. Sleep disturbances in Parkinson's disease patients and spouses. *J Am Geriatr Soc* 1997; 45:194–199.

7. Welsh M, Hung L, Waters CH. Sexuality in women with Parkinson's disease. *Mov Disord* 1997; 12:923–927.

8. Cummings JL. Depression and Parkinson's disease: a review. *Am J Psychiatry* 1992; 149:443–454.

8a. Levin BE, Liabre MM, Weiner WJ. Parkinson's disease and depression: Psychometric properties of the beck depression inventory. *J Neural Neurosurg Psychiatry* 1988; 51:1401–1404.

9. Miyoshi K, Ueki A, Nagano O. Management of psychiatric symptoms of Parkinson's disease. *Eur Neurol* 1996; 36 Suppl 1:49–54.

10. Cole SA, Woodard JL, Juncos JL, et al. Depression and disability in Parkinson's disease. *J Neuropsychiatry Clin Neurosci* 1996; 8:20–25.

11. Kostic VS, Filipovic SR, Lecic D, et al. Effect of age at onset on frequency of depression in Parkinson's disease. *J Neurol Neurosurg Psychiatry* 1994; 57:1265–1267.

12. Starkstein SE, Berthier ML, Bolduc PL, et al. Depression in patients with early versus late onset of Parkinson's disease. *Neurology* 1989; 39:1441–1445.

13. Wagner ML, Fedak MN, Sage JI, et al. Complications of disease and therapy: a comparison of younger and older patients with Parkinson's disease. *Ann Clin Lab Sci* 1996; 26:389–395.

14. Taylor AE, Saint-Cyr JA. Depression in Parkinson's disease: reconciling physiological and psychological perspectives. *J Neuropsychiatry Clin Neurosci* 1990; 2:92–98.

15. Brown R, Jahanshahi M. Depression in Parkinson's disease: a psychosocial viewpoint. *Adv Neurol* 1995; 65:61–84.

16. Larsen JP, Dupont E, Tandberg E. Clinical diagnosis of Parkinson's disease: proposal of diagnostic subgroups classified at different levels of confidence. *Acta Neurologica Scandinavia* 1994; 89:242–251.

17. Tandberg E, Larsen JP, Aarsland D, et al. Risk factors for depression in Parkinson disease. *Arch Neurol* 1997; 54:625–630.

18. Starkstein SE, Petracca G, Chemerinski E, et al. Depression in classic versus akinetic-rigid Parkinson's disease. *Mov Disord* 1998; 13:29–33.

19. Rascol O, Sabatini U, Chollet F, et al. Supplementary and primary sensory motor area activity in Parkinson's disease. Regional cerebral blood flow changes during finger movements and effects of apomorphine. *Arch Neurol* 1992; 49:144–148.

20. Vogel H-P. Symptoms of depression in Parkinson's disease. *Pharmacopsychiatry* 1982; 15:192–196.

21. Shaw AM, Lees AJ, Stern GM. The impact of treatment with levodopa on Parkinson's disease. *Quart J Med* 1980; 49:283–293.

22. Growdon JH, Kieburtz K, McDermott MP, et al. Levodopa improves motor function without impairing cognition in mild non-demented Parkinson's disease patients. Parkinson Study Group. *Neurology* 1998; 50:1327–1331.

23. Goodwin FK. Behavioral effects of L-dopa in man. *Sem Psychiatry* 1971; 3:477–492.

24. Cherington M. Parkinsonism, L-dopa and mental depression. *J Am Geriatr Soc* 1970; 18:513–516.

25. Schiffer RB, Kurlan R, Rubin A, et al. Evidence for atypical depression in Parkinson's disease. *Am J Psychiatry* 1988; 145:1020–1022.

26. Richard IH, Schiffer RB, Kurlan R. Anxiety and Parkinson's disease. *J Neuropsychiatry Clin Neurosci* 1996; 8:383–392.

26a. Menza MA, Robertson-Hoffman DE, Bonafuee AS. Parkinson's disease and anxiety: Comorbidrty with depression. *Biol Psychiatry* 1993; 34:465–470.

27. Menza MA, Rosen RC. Sleep in Parkinson's disease. The role of depression and anxiety. *Psychosomatics* 1995; 36:262–266.

28. Factor SA, Molho ES, Podskalny GD, et al. Parkinson's disease: drug-induced psychiatric states. *Adv Neurol* 1995; 65:115–138.

29. Troester AI, Paolo AM, Lyons KE, et al. The influence of depression on cognition in Parkinson's disease: a pattern of impairment distinguishable from Alzheimer's disease. *Neurology* 1995; 45:672–675.

30. Troester AI, Stalp LD, Paolo AM, et al. Neuropsychological impairment in Parkinson's disease with and without depression. *Arch Neurol* 1995; 52:1164–1169.

31. Kuzis G, Sabe L, Tiberti C, et al. Cognitive functions in major depression and Parkinson disease. *Arch Neurol* 1997; 54:982–986.

32. Wertman E, Speedie L, Shemesh Z, et al. Cognitive disturbances in Parkinsonian patients with depression. *Neuropsychiatry Neuropsychol, Behav Neurol* 1993; 6:31–37.

33. Taylor AE, Saint-Cyr JA, Lang AE, et al. Parkinson's disease and depression. *Brain* 1986; 109:279–292.

34. Stern Y, Marder K, Tang MX, et al. Antecedent clinical features associated with dementia in Parkinson's disease. *Neurology* 1993; 43:1690–1692.

35. Friedenberg DL, Cummings JL. Parkinson's disease, depression, and the on-off phenomenon. *Psychosomatics* 1989; 30:94–99.

36. Keshavan MS, David AS, Narayanen HS, et al. "On-off" phenomena and manic-depressive mood shifts: case report. *J Clin Psychiatry* 1986; 47:93–94.

37. Sandyk R. Locus coeruleus-pineal melatonin interactions and the pathogenesis of the "on-off" phenomenon associated with mood changes and sensory symptoms in Parkinson's disease. *Internat J Neurosci* 1989; 49:95–101.

38. Silver JM, Yudofsky SC. Drug Treatment of Depression in Parkinson's Disease. In: Huber SJ, Cummings JL, (eds.). *Parkinson's Disease. Neurobehavioral Aspects*. New York: Oxford University Press, 1992:240–254.

39. Mayberg HS, Solomon DH. Depression in Parkinson's disease: a biochemical and organic viewpoint. *Adv Neurol* 1995; 65:49–60.

40. Sano M, Mayeux R. Biochemistry of Depression in Parkinson's Disease. In: Huber SJ, Cummings JL, (eds.). Parkinson's Disease. Neurobehavioral Aspects. New York: Oxford University Press, 1992:229–239.

41. Heresco-Levy U, Javitt DC. The role of N-methyl-D-aspartate (NMDA) receptor-mediated neurotransmission in the pathophysiology and therapeutics of psychiatric syndromes. *Eur Neuropsychopharmacol* 1998; 8:141–152.

42. Mayberg HS, Starkstein SE, Sadzot B, et al. Selective hypometabolism in the inferior frontal lobe in depressed patients with Parkinson's disease. *Ann Neurol* 1990; 28:57–64.

43. Bissessur S, Tissingh G, Wolters EC, et al. rCBF SPECT in Parkinson's disease patients with mental dysfunction. *J Neural Transm Suppl* 1997; 50:25–30.

44. Mindham RHS, Marsden CD, Parkes JD. Psychiatric symptoms during L-dopa therapy for Parkinson's disease and their relationship to physical disability. *Psychol Med* 1976; 6:23–33.

45. Jouvent R, Abensour P, Bonnet AM, et al. Antiparkinsonian and antidepressant effects of high doses of bromocriptine. *J Affective Disord* 1983; 5:141–145.

46. American Psychiatric Association. *Diagnostic and Statistical Manual of Mental Disorders*. Washington: American Psychiatric Association, 1994.

47. Huszonek JJ. Anticholinergic effects in a depressed parkinsonian patient. *J Geriatr Psychiatry Neurol* 1995; 8:100–102.

48. Baronti F, Davis TL, Boldry RC, et al. Deprenyl effects on levodopa pharmacodynamics, mood, and free radical scavenging. *Neurology* 1992; 42:541–544.

49. Przuntek H, Kuhn W, Draus P. The effect of P-(-)-deprenyl in de novo parkinsonian patients pretreated with levodopa and decarboxylase inhibitor correlated to depression and MHPG, HIAA, and HVA levels in the cerbrospinal fluid. *Acta Neurologica Scandinavia* 1989; 126:153–156.

50. Allain H, Pollak P, Neukirch HC. Symptomatic effect of selegiline in de novo Parkinsonian patients. The French Selegiline Multicenter Trial. *Mov Disord* 1993; 8 Suppl 1:S36–S40.

51. Piercey MF. Pharmacology of pramipexole, a dopamine D3-preferring agonist useful in treating Parkinson's disease. *Clin Neuropharmacol* 1998; 21:141–151.

52. Pogarell O, Kuenig G, Oertel WH. A non-ergot dopamine agonist, pramipexole, in the therapy of advanced Parkinson's disease: improvement of parkinsonian symptoms and treatment-associated complications. A review of three studies. *Clin Neuropharmacol* 1997; 20:S28–S35.

53. Szegedi A, Hillert A, Wetzel H, et al. Pramipexole, a dopamine agonist, in major depression: antidepressant effects and tolerability in an open-label study with multiple doses. *Clin Neuropharmacol* 1997; 20:S36–S45.

54. Mannisto PT, Lang A, Rauhala P, et al. Beneficial effects of co-administration of catechol-O-methyltransferase inhibitors and L-dihydroxyphenylalanine in rat models of depression. *Eur J Pharmacol* 1995; 274:229–233.

55. Adler CH, Singer C, O'Brien C, et al. Tolcapone Fluctuator Study Group III. Randomized, placebo-controlled study of tolcapone in patients with fluctuating Parkinson disease treated with levodopa-carbidopa. *Arch Neurol* 1998; 55:1089–1095.

56. Illi A, Sundberg S, Ojala-Karlsson P, et al. Simultaneous inhibition of catechol-O-methyltransferase and monoamine oxidase A: effects on hemodynamics and catecholamine metabolism in healthy volunteers. *Clin Pharmacol Ther* 1996; 59:450–457.

57. Price LH, Spencer DD, Marek KL, et al. Psychiatric status after human fetal mesencephalic tissue

transplantation in Parkinson's disease. *Biol Psychiatry* 1995; 38:498–505.

58. Masterman D, DeSalles A, Baloh RW, et al. Motor, cognitive, and behavioral performance following unilateral ventroposterior pallidotomy for Parkinson disease. *Arch Neurol* 1998; 55:1201–1208.

59. Perrine K, Dogali M, Fazzini E, et al. Cognitive functioning after pallidotomy for refractory Parkinson's disease [see comments]. *J Neurol Neurosurg Psychiatry* 1998; 65:150–154.

60. Troester AI, Fields JA, Wilkinson SB, et al. Unilateral pallidal stimulation for Parkinson's disease: neurobehavioral functioning before and 3 months after electrode implantation. *Neurology* 1997; 49:1078–1083.

60a. Bejjani B-P, Damier P, Arnulf I, et al. Transient acute depression induced by high frequency deep-brain stimulation. *N Engl J Med* 1999; 340:1476–1480.

60b. Shulman LM, Singer C, Lirfert R, et al. Therapeutic effects of sertraline in patients with Parkinson's disease. *Mov Disord* 1996; 11:603.

61. Drevets WC. Geriatric depression: brain imaging correlates and pharmacologic considerations. *J Clin Psychiatry* 1994; 55 Suppl A:71–81; discussion 82, 98–100.

62. Stoudemire A. New antidepressant drugs and the treatment of depression in the medically ill patient. *Psychiatr Clin North Am* 1996; 19:495–514.

63. Steur ENHJ. Increase of Parkinson disability after fluoxetine medication. *Neurology* 1993; 43:211–213.

64. Richard IH, Kurlan R, Tanner C, et al. Parkinson Study Group. Serotonin syndrome and the combined used of deprenyl and an antidepressant in Parkinson's disease. *Neurology* 1997; 48:1070–1077.

65. Hauser RA, Zesiewicz TA. Sertraline for the treatment of depression in Parkinson's disease. *Mov Disord* 1997; 12:756–759.

66. Coupland NJ, Bell CJ, Potokar JP. Serotonin reuptake inhibitor withdrawal. *J Clin Psychopharmacol* 1996; 16:356–362.

67. Goetz CG, Tanner CM, Klawans HL. Bupropion in Parkinson's disease. *Neurology* 1984; 34:1092–1094.

68. Trosch RM, Friedman JH, Lannon MC, et al. Clozapine use in Parkinson's disease: a retrospective analysis of a large multicentered clinical experience. *Mov Disord* 1998; 13:377–382.

69. Moellentine C, Rummans T, Ahlskog JE, et al. Effectiveness of ECT in patients with parkinsonism. *J Neuropsychiatry Clin Neurosci* 1998; 10:187–193.

70. Rasmussen KG, Abrams R. The role of electroconvulsive therapy in Parkinson's disease. In: Huber SJ, Cummings JL, (eds.). *Parkinson's Disease. Neurobehavioral Aspects*. New York: Oxford University Press, 1992:255–270.

71. Douyon R, Serby M, Klutchko B, et al. ECT and Parkinson's disease revisited: a "naturalistic" study. *Am J Psychiatry* 1989; 146:1451–1455.

72. Lebensohn ZM, Jenkins RB. Improvement of Parkinsonism in depressed patients treated with ECT. *Am J Psychiatry* 1975; 132:283–285.

73. Asnis G. Parkinson's disease, depression, and ECT: a review and case study. *Am J Psychiatry* 1977; 134:191–195.

74. Holcomb HH, Sternberg DE, Heninger GR. Effects of electroconvulsive therapy on mood, Parkinsonism, and tardive dyskinesia in a depressed patient: ECT and dopamine systems. *Biol psychiatry* 1983; 18:865–873.

75. Burke WJ, Peterson J, Rubin EH. Electroconvulsive therapy in the treatment of combined depression and Parkinson's disease. *Psychosomatics* 1988; 29:341–346.

76. Fromm GH. *Observations on the effect of electroshock treatment on patients with Parkinsonism.* Bulletin of Tulane University 1959; 18:71–73.

77. Figiel GS, Hassen MA, Zorumski C, et al. ECT-induced delirium in depressed patients with Parkinson's disease. *J Neuropsychiatry Clin Neurosci* 1991; 3:405–411.

78. Figiel GS, Coffey CE, Djang WT, et al. Brain magnetic resonance imaging findings in ECT-induced delirium. *J Neuropsychiatry Clin Neurosci* 1990; 2:53–58.

79. Balldin J, Granerus A, Linstedt G, et al. Predictors for improvement after electroconvulsive therapy in parkinsonian patients with on-off symptoms. *J Neural Trans* 1981; 52:199–211.

80. Klaassen T, Verhey FRJ, Sneijders GHJM, et al. Treatment of depression in Parkinson's disease: a meta-analysis. *J Neuropsychiatry Clin Neurosci* 1995; 7:281–286.

81. Mayeux R, Stern Y, Sano M, et al. The relationship of serotonin to depression in Parkinson's disease. *Mov Disord* 1988; 3:237–244.

82. Nyth AL, Gottfries CG, Lyby K, et al. A controlled multicenter clinical study of citalopram and placebo in elderly depressed patients with and without concomitant dementia. *Acta Psychiatrica Scandinavica* 1992; 86:138–145.

83. Nyth AL, Gottfries CG. The clinical efficacy of citalopram in treatment of emotional disturbances in dementia disorders. A Nordic multicentre study. *Br J Psychiatry* 1990; 157:894–901.

84. Brown AS, Gershon S. Dopamine and depression. *J Neural Trans* 1993; 91:75–109.

85. Harvey NS. Psychiatric disorders in parkinsonism: 1. Functional illnesses and personality. *Psychosomatics* 1986; 27:91–103.

86. Moryl E, Danysz W, Quack G. Potential antidepressive properties of amantadine, memantine and bifemelane. *Pharmacol Toxicol* 1993; 72:394–397.

87. Lavian G, Finberg JPM, Youdim MBH. The advent of a new generation of monoamine oxidase inhibitor antidepressants: pharmacologic studies with

moclobemide and brofaromine. *Clin Neuropharmacol* 1993; 16:S1–S7.

88. Haefely W, Burkard WP, Cesura A, et al. Pharmacology of moclobemide. *Clin Neuropharmacol* 1993; 16:S8–S18.

89. Steur EN, Ballering LA. Moclobemide and selegeline in the treatment of depression in Parkinson's disease [letter]. *J Neurol Neurosurg Psychiatry* 1997; 63:547.

90. Waldmeier PC, Glatt A, Jaekel J, et al. Brofaromine: a monoamine oxidase-A and serotonin uptake inhibitor. *Clin Neuropharmacol* 1993; 16:S19–S24.

91. Cunningham LA. Depression in the medically ill: choosing an antidepressant. *J Clin Psychiatry* 1994; 55 Suppl A:90–97; discussion 98–100.

92. Fontaine R, Ontiveros A, Elie R, et al. A double-blind comparison of nefazodone, imipramine, and placebo in major depression. *J Clin Psychiatry* 1994; 55:234–241.

93. Kasper S. Clinical efficacy of mirtazapine: a review of meta-analyses of pooled data. *Int Clin Psychopharmacol* 1995; 10 Suppl 4:25–35.

94. Marttila M, Jaaskelainen J, Jarvi R, et al. A double-blind study comparing the efficacy and tolerability of mirtazapine and doxepin in patients with major depression. *Eur Neuropsychopharmacol* 1995; 5:441–446.

95. Montgomery SA. Efficacy in long-term treatment of depression. *J Clin Psychiatry* 1996; 57 Suppl 2:24–30.

96. Khawaja AM, Rogers DF. Tachykinins: receptor to effector. *Int J Biochem Cell Biol* 1996; 28:721–738.

97. George MS, Wassermann EM, Post RM. Transcranial magnetic stimulation: a neuropsychiatric tool for the 21st century. *J Neuropsychiatry Clin Neurosci* 1996; 8:373–382.

98. Sandyk R, Derpapas K. The effects of external picoTesla range magnetic fields on the EEG in Parkinson's disease. *Int J Neurosci* 1993; 70:85–96.

99. Figiel GS, Epstein C, McDonald WM, et al. The use of rapid-rate transcranial magnetic stimulation (rTMS) in refractory depressed patients. *J Neuropsychiatry Clin Neurosci* 1998; 10:20–25.

100. Stein WM, Read S. Chronic pain in the setting of Parkinson's disease and depression. *J Pain Symptom Manage* 1997; 14:255–258.

101. Lieberman A. Managing the neuropsychiatric symptoms of Parkinson's disease. *Neurology* 1998; 50:S33–S38; discussion S44–S48.

102. Richard IH, Kurlan R. A survey of antidepressant drug use in Parkinson's disease. Parkinson Study Group. *Neurology* 1997; 49:1168–1170.

103. Sano M, Stern Y, Cote L, et al. Depression in Parkinson's disease: a biochemical model. *J Neuropsychiatry Clin Neurosci* 1990; 2:88–92.

104. Chan-Palay V, Asan E. Alterations in catecholamine neurons of the locus coeruleus in senile dementia of the Alzheimer type and in Parkinson's disease with and without dementia and depression. *J Compar Neurol* 1989; 287:373–392.

105. Chan-Palay V. Depression and dementia in Parkinson's disease. Catecholamine changes in the locus ceruleus, a basis for therapy. *Adv Neurol* 1993; 60:438–446.

106. Javoy-Agid F, Agid Y. Is the mesocortical dopaminergic system involved in Parkinson disease? *Neurology* 1980; 30:1326–1330.

107. Schneider LS, Chui HC, Severson JA, et al. Decreased platelet 3H-imipramine binding in Parkinson's disease. *Biol Psychiatry* 1988; 24:348–351.

108. Cash R, Raisman R, Ploska A, et al. High and low affinity [3H]imipramine binding sites in control and Parkinsonian brains. *Eur J Pharmacol* 1985; 117:71–80.

109. D'Amato RJ, Zweig RM, Whitehouse PJ, et al. Aminergic systems in Alzheimer's disease and Parkinson's disease. *Ann Neurol* 1986; 22:229–236.

110. Becker T, Becker G, Seufert J, et al. Parkinson's disease and depression: evidence for an alteration of the basal limbic system detected by transcranial sonography. *J Neurol Neurosurg Psychiatry* 1997; 63:590–596.

111. Mayeux R, Stern Y, Cote L, et al. Altered serotonin metabolism in depressed patients with Parkinson's disease. *Neurology* 1984; 34:642–646.

112. Wolfe N, Katz DI, Albert ML, et al. Neuropsychological profile linked to low dopamine in Alzheimer's disease, major depression, and Parkinson's disease. *J Neurol Neurosurg Psychiatry* 1990; 53:915–917.

113. Mena MA, Aguado EG, de Yebenes JG. Monoamine metabolites in human cerebrospinal fluid. HPLC/ED method. *Acta Neurologica Scandinavia* 1984; 69:218–225.

114. Mayeux R, Stern Y, Williams JBW, et al. Clinical and biochemical features of depression in Parkinson's disease. *Am J Psychiatry* 1986; 143:756–759.

115. Kostic VS, Djuricic BM, Covickovic-Sternic N, et al. Depression and Parkinson's disease: possible role of serotonergic mechanisms. *J Neurol* 1987; 234:94–96.

116. Chia LG, Cheng FC, Kuo JS. Monoamines and their metabolites in plasma and lumbar cerebrospinal fluid of Chinese patients with Parkinson's disease. *J Neurol Sci* 1993; 116:125–134.

117. Cantello R, Aguggia M, Gilli M, et al. Major depression in Parkinson's disease and the mood response to intravenous methylphenidate: possible role of the "hedonic" dopamine synapse. *J Neurol Neurosurg Psychiatry* 1989; 52:724–731.

118. Strang RR. Imipramine in treatment of parkinsonism: a double-blind placebo study. *Br Med J* 1965; 2:33–34.

119. Laitinen L. Desipramine in treatment of Parkinson's disease. *Acta Neurologica Scandinavica* 1969; 45:109–113.

120. Andersen J, Aabro E, Gulmann N, et al. Antidepressive treatment in Parkinson's disease: a controlled trial of the effect of nortriptyline in patients with Parkinson's disease treated with L-dopa. *Acta Neurologica Scandinavia* 1980; 62:210–219.

121. Garattini S. Pharmacology of amineptine, an antidepressant agent acting on the dopaminergic system: a review. *Internat Clin Psychopharmacol* 1997; 12:S15–S19.

122. Mandell AJ, Markham C, Fowler W. Parkinson's syndrome, depression and imipramine: a preliminary report. *Calif Med* 1961; 95:12–14.

123. Denmark JC, David JDP, McComb SG. Imipramine hydrochloride (Tofranil) in Parkinsonism: a preliminary report. *Br J Clin Prac* 1961; 15:523–524.

124. Gillhespy RO, Mustard DM. The evaluation of imipramine in the treatment of Parkinson's disease. *Br J Clin Prac* 1963; 17:205–208.

125. McCance-Katz EF, Marek KL, Price LH. Setonergic dysfunction in depression associated with Parkinson's disease. *Neurology* 1992; 42:1813–1814.

126. Meara RJ, Bhowmick BK, Hobson JP. An open uncontrolled study of the use of sertraline in the treatment of depression in Parkinson's disease. *J Serotonin Res* 1996; 4:243–249.

127. Indaco A, Carrieri PD. Amitriptyline in the treatment of headache in patients with Parkinson's disease. *Neurology* 1988; 38:1720–1722.

128. Boer BH, Erdman RAM, Onstenk HJVC, et al. Clomipramine, depresie en de ziekte van Parkinson. *Tijdchrift voor Psychiatrie* 1976; 28:499–509.

129. Bedard P, Parkes JD, Marsden CD. Nomifensine in Parkinson's disease. *Br J Clin Pharmacol* 1977; 4:187S–190S.

130. Fischer PA, Baas H. Therapeutic efficacy of R-(-) deprenyl as adjuvant therapy in advanced parkinsonism. *J Neural Tran* 1987; Suppl 25:137–147.

131. Lees A, Shaw KM, Kohout LJ, et al. Deprenyl in Parkinson's disease. *Lancet* 1977; 2:791–795.

132. Hietanen MH. Selegiline and cognitive function in Parkinson's disease. *Acta Neurol Scand* 1991; 84:407–410.

18

Anxiety and Panic

Irene Hegeman Richard, M.D., and Roger Kurlan, M.D.

University of Rochester Medical School, Rochester, New York

INTRODUCTION

Dementia and depression have been recognized as the two major behavioral disorders typically associated with Parkinson's disease (PD). However, recent evidence suggests that there is a third behavioral condition that also represents an important characteristic of the illness, anxiety. This chapter focuses on available information that supports a relationship between PD and anxiety. This relationship may be important in elucidating pathogenetic mechanisms and improving therapy. Treatment of anxiety is addressed but the lack of available clinical research data will be readily apparent. It is hoped that the new millennium will bring advances in our knowledge regarding effective treatments for anxiety and other psychiatric symptoms occurring in PD.

Anxiety is a state characterized by a vague and unpleasant sense of apprehension, often accompanied by autonomic symptoms such as palpitations and dry mouth. Anxiety may serve as a beneficial alerting signal that can warn off impending danger and stimulate the taking of appropriate measures, but it may also be pathologic if the symptoms are prolonged or excessive or if they occur at inappropriate times. An anxiety disorder connotes the presence of significant dysfunction due to anxiety. There are many different anxiety disorders, which are distinguished from one another by their constellation of symptoms, response to medications, and, in some cases, presumed etiologic mechanisms. DSM-IV (1) includes the categories of anxiety disorders listed in Table 18-1. The specific criteria for a panic attack as outlined in DSM-IV is listed in Table 18-2.

ANXIETY IN PD

Prevalence of Anxiety

One of the first formal studies of anxiety in PD was conducted by Rubin et al. (2). The authors used a standardized questionnaire and DSM-III-R (3) criteria for anxiety and affective disorders to evaluate 16 PD patients who reported marked episodic anxiety (out of a total PD population of 210 patients). Eight patients (4% of the total population) met criteria for panic-anxiety disorder and 6 simultaneously met criteria for major depression or dysthymia. The rate for panic-anxiety disorder was noted to be greater than that estimated for the general population. Other subsequent studies have also observed that anxiety in patients with PD occurs more frequently than expected. Stein and coworkers (4) systematically evaluated 24 PD patients for the presence of DSM-III-R Axis I syndromes. Nine subjects (38%) had a clinically significant anxiety disorder, a rate that is much greater than the incidence in the general population (5%–15%), in primary care clinics (10%), and in patients with chronic medical conditions (11%). Vazquez et al. (5) found that 31 of 131 PD patients (24%) had experienced recurrent panic attacks that fulfilled most DSM-111-R criteria (3) for panic disorder.

In addition to exceeding prevalence rates in the general population, anxiety disorders in PD have been found to be more common than in other neurologic or medical illnesses. Schiffer et al. (6) carried out structured clinical psychiatric interviews for 16 depressed PD patients and 20 depressed multiple sclerosis patients and found that anxiety disorders were more common in the patients with PD. Seventy-five percent of the patients with PD met criteria for past or present generalized anxiety disorder (GAD) or panic disorder, whereas only 10% of patients with multiple sclerosis met these criteria.

Menza et al. (7) compared 42 patients with PD and 21 matched medical control subjects (patients with chronic debilitating osteoarthritis matched for age and length of illness) by using DSM-111-R criteria and a variety of psychiatric rating scales. Twelve PD patients (29%), but only one medical control subject (5%), had

Table 18-1 Categories of Anxiety Disorders in DSM-IV

Panic disorder with and without agoraphobia
Agoraphobia without a history of panic disorder
Specific and social phobias
Obsessive–compulsive disorder
Posttraumatic stress disorder and acute stress disorder
Generalized anxiety disorder
Anxiety disorder due to a general medical condition
Substance-induced anxiety disorder
Anxiety disorder not otherwise specified (including mixed anxiety-depressive disorder)

Table 18-2 Possible Symptoms of Panic Attack in DSM-IV

1.	Palpitations, pounding heart, or accelerated heart rate
2.	Sweating
3.	Trembling or shaking
4.	Sensations of shortness of breath or smothering
5.	Feeling of choking
6.	Chest pain or discomfort
7.	Nausea or abdominal distress
8.	Feeling dizzy, unsteady, lightheaded, or faint
9.	Derealization (feelings of unreality) or depersonalization (being detached from oneself)
10.	Fear of losing control or going crazy
11.	Fear of dying
12.	Paresthesias (numbness or tingling sensations)
13.	Chills or hot flushes

the subjective concomitants of autonomic failure and that this might lead to an overdiagnosis of these psychiatric disorders in the PD population. Given the fact that "significance persisted after the autonomic items were removed from the Hamilton scales," it would appear more likely that patients with PD have a common neurobiological abnormality that can result in both emotional and autonomic dysfunction.

Thus most studies have shown that anxiety occurs commonly in patients with PD at a higher rate than in normal or other disease comparison populations.

Clinical Features of Anxiety Disorders

In many studies the type of anxiety disorder was not specified by the authors. However, other studies have reported a wide range of anxiety disorders in patients with PD. In the study by Stein and coworkers (4), of the nine PD subjects with a clinically significant anxiety disorder, one had GAD, two had panic disorder, one had long-standing panic disorder with recent onset of a superimposed major depressive episode, one had panic disorder and social phobia, three had social phobia alone, and one had anxiety disorder not otherwise specified. The authors judged that three additional patients had symptoms of social phobia that appeared to be secondary to self-consciousness about PD symptoms. These patients were not considered to have a clinically significant anxiety disorder because they did not meet DSM-111-R (3) diagnostic criteria for social phobia (where it was specified that a diagnosis of social phobia could not be made if the fear is related to symptoms of a medical disorder); these patients would now meet DSM-IV (1) criteria for anxiety disorder not otherwise specified. Vazquez et al. (5) described only panic disorder, whereas Schiffer et al. (6) reported the presence of panic disorder and GAD. Menza et al. (7) noted that anxiety diagnoses in PD patients are clustered among panic disorder, phobic disorder, and GAD.

Lauterbach and Duvoisin (11) described anxiety disorders in patients with familial parkinsonism and noted the following rates: simple phobia, 34.27%; agoraphobia, 15.8%; obsessive–compulsive disorder (OCD), 13.2 %; panic disorder, 7.9%; GAD and social phobia, each 5.3%. The authors noted that their observed rate of GAD was similar to that reported by Stein et al. (4) in their study of patients with PD, whereas a lower rate of panic disorder and higher rates of social phobia and OCD were identified in their familial parkinsonism subjects.

Thus a wide range of anxiety disorders may occur in patients with PD. Further studies involving larger patient populations and standard psychiatric

a formal anxiety disorder. In a subsequent study of 104 PD patients and 61 medical control subjects with equal disability, Menza and Mark (8) noted that PD patients scored higher than control subjects on measures of depression and anxiety. In another study, Gotham et al. (9) found that the frequency of anxiety in PD exceeded that of healthy control subjects but was not greater than that in patients with chronic arthritis. One study revealed that PD patients experienced more complaints related to autonomic function (e.g., postural dizziness, urinary frequency, dry mouth) than controls (10). The authors concluded that some PD patients diagnosed with anxiety or depression may, in fact, be experiencing interviews are needed to further clarify the relative frequencies of the various anxiety disorder types.

Time of Onset of Anxiety

Although one study that involved patients with familial parkinsonism reported that the onset of anxiety typically preceded the appearance of Parkinsonian motor symptoms (11), most investigators who have assessed patients with idiopathic PD have observed that anxiety symptoms tend to appear after the diagnosis of PD has been established (4,5,12). DSM-IV, under the category "Anxiety Disorder, Not Otherwise Specified," indicates that symptoms of social phobia can occur in PD because patients are embarrassed about their PD symptoms (such as tremor) (1) Lauterbach and Duvoisin (11) noted 5 of 28 patients who experienced embarrassment about PD symptoms but found that 12 of their familial parkinsonism patients diagnosed with social phobia experienced anxiety symptoms before the diagnosis of the motor features. Stein et al. (4) found that of the nine PD patients with anxiety disorders, two had the onset of anxiety before and seven after the diagnosis of PD. The authors did not specifically comment about the time of onset of social phobia but they did note that the four patients in whom they diagnosed social phobia had self-consciousness that was not related to their PD symptoms. Thus although there appear to be some patients who have social phobia directly related to their PD symptoms, others have more diffuse social phobia unrelated to, and at times even predating, the diagnosis of PD. These observations suggest that anxiety symptoms in PD may not simply be related to psychological and social difficulties in adapting to the illness, but rather may be due to specific neurobiological processes occurring in PD.

Relationship of Anxiety to Anti-Parkinsonian Medications

The issue of whether anti-Parkinsonian medications might be responsible for some of the anxiety symptoms seen in PD patients remains unsettled. R. Henderson et al. (12) noted that for PD subjects taking levodopa and reporting anxiety, 44% had the onset of anxiety before beginning levodopa and 56% had it after treatment was initiated. Stein et al. (4) found no significant difference between anxious and nonanxious patients with PD with regard to the cumulative dose of levodopa. The authors did note, however, that many subjects were taking other anti-parkinsonian medications, such as anticholinergics, amantadine, and bromocriptine and that a potential influence of these drugs could not be excluded.

Siemers and coworkers (13) studied the anxiety state and motor performance in 19 patients with idiopathic PD. All 19 patients were taking levodopa or carbidopa, and most were also receiving adjunctive anti-parkinsonian medications, including dopamine receptor agonists, selegiline (deprenyl), and anticholinergics. Two patients were taking benzodiazepines. The authors found no statistical differences in motor, depression, or anxiety scores based on the presence or absence of the additional medications. In the study by Menza and coworkers (7), levodopa dose did not significantly correlate with anxiety measures. The authors also found that there was no difference in measures of anxiety for patients receiving or not receiving selegiline or pergolide. In distinction to the above reports, Vazquez et al. (5) concluded that panic attacks were related to levodopa therapy but not to other agonist drugs. The authors found that 24% of PD patients under chronic levodopa therapy had experienced recurrent panic attacks. It was noted that the PD patients with panic were put on levodopa earlier than the PD patients without panic and needed higher dosages. Rondot and coworkers (14) found that anxious PD patients received similar doses of levodopa when compared to the general PD population and therefore concluded that anxiety was not caused by chronic treatment with levodopa. However, they noted that anxiety is seen in certain individuals as an acute mental disorder associated with the taking of levodopa. Thus whether treatment with anti-parkinsonian medications might influence anxiety symptoms in PD patients remains an unsettled issue.

Relationship of Anxiety to Motor Symptoms

The majority of past studies have shown that depression in PD is not closely correlated with the severity of motor symptoms or the degree of disability (15), thus supporting the notion that this behavioral disorder is not a reaction to the illness but is more likely related to central biochemical disturbances that accompany PD. Recent studies have examined the relationship between anxiety and PD motor symptoms. Most studies have identified no significant difference in disability ratings between PD patients with and those without anxiety (4,7).

Some authors have reported higher degrees of anxiety in patients who experience "on-off" motor fluctuations (7,12,16), whereas others have failed to confirm this relationship (4,11,17). One could conjecture that the unpredictable nature of the on-off states might result in anxiety behavior similar to that which occurs in laboratory animals after they are exposed to unpredictable aversive stimuli (18). Riley and Lang (19) include anxiety as one of the psychiatric disturbances that vary with Parkinsonian motor fluctuations. Most authors have noted that in patients who do experience the on-off phenomenon, anxiety tends to occur most often during the "off" phase (4,5,12,13). It is interesting that as early as 1976, Marsden and Parkes (20) commented that "the off period may be accompanied by panic, flushing and sweating, and leg pain," although they did not specifically discuss the relationship between anxiety and Parkinsonian mobility states. One study revealed that in most patients, mood or anxiety improved significantly from "off" to "on," but then worsened again in the "on" state when dyskinesias appeared (21). In their levodopa infusion studies, Maricle et al. (22) found that mood, anxiety, and motor fluctuations tended to correlate in that patients experienced greater anxiety and depression during periods of poor mobility and vice versa. They did not find that patients had a recurrence of anxiety and depression with the onset of dyskinesias. Other studies have found a relationship between mood, arousal or psychic activation, and mobility changes during on-off fluctuations but did not specifically address anxiety (23,24). Lauterbach and Duvoisin (11) noted that for patients with familial parkinsonism who had panic attacks before the diagnosis of the movement disorder, the symptoms lessened as the disease advanced and particularly when "freezing" episodes (sudden immobility that can render a patient motionless) appeared.

A variety of questions have been raised regarding the exact relationship between anxiety and motor function. Does decreased mobility cause anxiety? Can anxiety cause decreased mobility? Are both anxiety and decreased mobility the result of common central neurochemical disturbances? Routh et al. (25) described a patient with PD and anxiety characterized by both social phobia and agoraphobia or panic disorder. The patient's motor symptoms could not be controlled by levodopa during periods of increased anxiety, leading the authors to conclude that anxiety may indeed worsen Parkinsonian motor features. Arguing against such causality would be the finding that even during experimental yohimbine-induced panic attacks and anxiety (26) (described later under "Neurobiology"), patients had no measured worsening of their Parkinsonian motor symptoms. To determine how CNS dopaminergic activity may relate to mood and anxiety, Menza et al. (21) assessed 10 patients with PD and motor fluctuations for mood and anxiety changes during discrete "off", "on," and "on with dyskinesias" periods. Only one patient rated his moods as consistently improving from "off" to "on" to "on with dyskinesias," paralleling presumed increasing

striatal and limbic dopaminergic activity. Most of the patients, however, felt depressed and anxious when they were "off" and when they were "on with dyskinesias," leading the authors to conclude that the behavioral responses of most patients probably reflect an emotional reaction to their motor symptoms. An alternative explanation might be that there is an optimal level of dopamine that is necessary to prevent depressed mood and anxiety. In the levodopa infusion study conducted by Maricle and colleagues (22), the emotional changes generally preceded the motor changes by several minutes, thereby making it unlikely that the anxiety and depression represented an emotional reaction to motor impairment. It seems more likely that CNS levodopa depletion resulted in both mood and motor changes but that the time course of effects might be slightly different.

Some authors have suggested that changes in other neurotransmitters that may occur during Parkinsonian motor fluctuations may play a role in the occurrence of anxiety. Siemers et al. (13) postulated that an alteration in serotonin may be responsible for the increase in anxiety symptoms related to motor performance (as measured by the Spielberger State-Trait Anxiety Inventory). Vazquez et al. (5) suggested that norepinephrine may play a primary role in panic attacks in PD. Further studies are needed to clarify the relationship between motor state and anxiety in PD and to uncover pathogenetic mechanisms.

Epidemiology of Anxiety

Because anxiety occurring in PD involves a population of older-age individuals, it is of interest that anxiety disorders in psychiatric patients characteristically begin by young adulthood. Thus the onset of anxiety in late age, in association with PD, is contrary to the expected natural course of this condition and favors an etiologic link between the two disorders. This notion is further supported by current data, indicating that anxiety disorders are less common in the elderly when compared with younger adults (27). Anxiety in a substantial portion of patients with PD exceeds the expected prevalence rates in this age group and also favors a pathogenetic relationship. It should be noted, however, that some authors believe that an underdiagnosis of anxiety in late life may contribute to low prevalence estimates in the elderly population (28,29). In reviewing the epidemiology and comorbidity of anxiety disorders in the elderly, A.J. Flint (27) concluded that GAD and phobias account for most anxiety in late life and that panic disorder is rare, which is in contrast to the rather frequent occurrence of panic disorder in patients with PD. It was noted that when panic disorder did occur in elderly patients, females accounted for all the cases. In contrast to these observations in elderly subjects, it is interesting to note that panic disorder occurring in the setting of PD involves both males and females.

B.A. Raj et al. (30) suggested that late-onset panic disorder may be more common than previously thought, and they also noted that this group of patients was more likely to have coexistent medical disorders such as chronic obstructive pulmonary disease (COPD), vertigo, and PD. The authors speculated that medical disorders such as COPD and PD might have a role in the onset of late-life panic disorder.

Relationship Between Anxiety and Depression

It is well known that in psychiatric populations, anxiety and depressive disorders commonly coexist. In a review of coexisting depression and anxiety, Lydiard (31) notes that up to 60% of patients with depressive symptoms also have anxiety and that 20%–30% of patients with major depression meet criteria for panic disorder. Between 21% and 91% of patients meeting criteria for panic disorder experience an episode of major depression one or more times during their lives. He also notes that patients with combined panic disorder and major depression are more significantly impaired than patients with either disorder alone.

There appears to be a relationship between anxiety and depression in PD as well. In a review of depression in PD, Cummings (15) notes that the depression in PD is distinguished from other depressive disorders by greater anxiety and less self-punitive ideation. After discovering that the diagnoses of anxiety and panic disorder were significantly more frequent among depressed patients with PD than depressed patients with multiple sclerosis, Schiffer et al. (6) suggested that PD patients may experience an atypical depression. One study showed that 92% of PD patients who had an anxiety disorder also had a depressive disorder and that 67% of those with a depressive disorder also had an anxiety disorder (7). Another study compared PD patients with age-matched healthy spouse controls and noted that the report of depression plus panic or anxiety (as compared with either condition alone) best distinguished the two populations (12). Although other studies have also shown a close correlation between depression and anxiety in PD (5,32), anxiety can clearly occur in the absence of depression. A study by Lin et al. (33) revealed that, although the degrees of anxiety and depression assessed via standardized rating scales were generally correlated, 14 of 58 PD patients determined to be free of depressive symptoms fulfilled DSM-III-R criteria for GAD.

Because most patients with PD are elderly, it is important to look at comorbidity in this age group. It was pointed out by Flint (27), in his review of anxiety in the elderly, that studies show considerable comorbidity of anxiety disorders and depression in late life. The rate of comorbidity for GAD and phobias with depression in old age is similar to that quoted for younger patients. However, the depressed elderly appear to have a lower risk for developing panic attacks (27). The frequent occurrence of depression coexisting with panic in PD is of particular interest and suggests that these behavioral responses may be etiologically related to the neurobiological changes that accompany PD.

Relationship Between Anxiety and Dementia

Although there is some evidence for an increased rate of anxiety in primary dementia disorders (34), the relationship between anxiety and dementia in PD is not clear. Depression appears to be equally frequent in PD with and without dementia (15). Iruela et al. (35) hypothesized that anxiety may actually lessen in PD patients if they become demented; there is a significant decrease in brain levels of norepinephrine in demented PD patients (36), and (as noted below under "Neurobiology") an abnormal activity of noradrenergic cells in the locus ceruleus has been hypothesized to cause anxiety. Addressing this issue, however, Lauterbach (37) studied 38 patients with familial Parkinsonism and found no relationship between dementia and anxiety symptoms. Most of the studies that examined anxiety in patients with PD either failed to comment on the cognitive status of the patients (6,12) or deliberately excluded patients with dementia (4,7,13), so definite conclusions cannot be reached regarding a relationship between anxiety and cognitive decline in this illness. S. Fleminger (32) noted that two groups of patients with PD who differed with regard to the presence of anxiety did not differ on their performance on two tests of cognitive function (National Adult Reading Test and Information, Memory, and Concentration Test). Vazquez et al. (5) found that anxious and nonanxious PD patients did not differ with respect to their severity of dementia as assessed by the Unified Parkinson's Disease Rating Scale (UPDRS) but noted that more formal measures of cognitive function were not performed and also that the degree of mental impairment was low in both groups.

Neurobiology of Anxiety as It Relates to Parkinson's Disease

Significant advances have been made in uncovering some of the possible biologic mechanisms of anxiety.

Examining these findings along with the known neurobiological alterations in PD may shed light on common mechanisms that might be responsible for the apparent clinical relationship between the two conditions.

The main neurotransmitters implicated in the pathogenesis of anxiety include nor-epinephrine, serotonin, and gamma-aminobutyric acid (GABA) (38,39). There is strong evidence implicating noradrenergic dysfunction, particularly of the alpha-2 adrenergic receptors, and perhaps of the locus coeruleus itself, in the development of primary anxiety disorders, especially panic disorder (38–44). Interestingly, many abnormalities of the noradrenergic system have also been discovered in PD patients (45). The dorsal ascending noradrenergic pathway is particularly affected. This pathway originates in the locus coeruleus and projects to the cerebral cortex, amygdala, hippocampus, and septum (46). Studies have demonstrated catecholaminergic cell loss in the locus coeruleus in PD (47,48). The loss appears to correlate with the presence of dementia (36,49,50). There appear to be changes in both central and peripheral adrenergic receptors in PD. Studies have shown that alpha-2 receptors are decreased in number in the cerebral cortex (51). Other studies have noted a decrease in alpha-2 adrenoceptors (52) and decreased yohimbine-binding sites (53), in platelets of untreated PD patients. Bernal and coworkers (54) suggested that untreated PD is associated with a significant reduction in alpha-2 adrenergic sensitivity. It is possible that patients with PD are more vulnerable to panic attacks because they have an alteration of alpha-2 adrenergic receptors. It is also possible that the locus ceruleus is disinhibited in PD secondary to changes in other neurotransmitter systems. Lauterbach (37), Lauterbach and Duvoisin (11), and Vazquez and coworkers (5) independently provided data in PD suggesting that locus ceruleus disinhibition may lead to secondary panic attacks, whereas locus ceruleus degeneration and subsequent incompetence might explain attenuation of primary panic attacks.

Further support for a noradrenergic role in anxiety associated with PD comes from our pilot study of experimental yohimbine-induced panic. Oral yohimbine (an alpha-2 antagonist) was administered to six patients with PD who had a history of anxiety or depression, two parkinsonian patients without psychiatric illness, and two normal controls. Parkinsonian patients with a history of anxiety developed panic attacks at frequencies comparable to primary psychiatric patients with panic disorder. Regardless of their history of anxiety and/or depression, parkinsonian patients demonstrated a vulnerability to yohimbine-induced somatic symptoms (26,55).

Alterations in the serotonin neurotransmitter system have also been postulated to play a role in anxiety disorders, particularly OCD but also social phobia (56,57), posttraumatic stress disorder, GAD, and perhaps panic disorder (58). Some abnormalities of the serotonergic system have been noted in PD. Studies have demonstrated a loss of large neurons in the median (59) and dorsal (60) raphe nucleus. There is decreased serotonin concentration in the putamen, caudate, globus pallidus, substantia nigra, hypothalamus, and frontal cortex. Less severe declines occur in other areas as well (61). A decrease in the density of binding sites in the putamen for the serotonin-specific reuptake inhibitors has been shown (62,63). It is therefore possible that alterations in serotonergic function may be playing a role in anxiety disorders associated with PD, although the role of serotonin in specific disorders has not been established. It is possible that interactions between noradrenergic and serotonergic systems may be relevant to the expression of certain anxiety disorders, since serotonin can decrease locus coeruleus firing by 5-HT2 serotonin receptors (58).

The potential role of GABA in the genesis of anxiety is suggested by the efficacy of benzodiazepines for the treatment of panic disorder and GAD; these drugs produce their effects by activating GABA receptors in the brain (58). In most of the PD brains examined, an increased concentration of GABA in putamen and pallidum and a decreased concentration in cortical areas have been observed (45).

There is some evidence suggesting that dopamine may be involved in the development of anxiety. Some authors have postulated a dopaminergic dysregulation in social phobia (64) and panic disorder (65,66). It has been suggested that both dopamine and serotonin systems may be involved in OCD (67,68). If an abnormality of dopaminergic function does result in anxiety, it is not surprising that patients with PD have a greater than expected frequency of anxiety disorders. The levodopa infusion studies in patients with PD that were performed by Maricle et al. (22) clearly implicate a dopaminergic deficiency state in anxiety, at least that which is associated with motor fluctuations. Tomer et al. (69) hypothesized that reduced dopaminergic activity in the striatum may be responsible for obsessive-compulsive symptoms in PD. It has been noted that dopamine decreases the firing rate of the locus coeruleus (70). Several investigators have hypothesized that the dopamine deficiency of PD might result in an alteration of noradrenergic systems and could be responsible for certain anxiety disorders in patients with this illness (5,35,37).

Aside from classic neurotransmitter systems, neuropeptides may also play a role in anxiety. It is of interest that abnormalities of corticotropin-releasing factor (CRF) have been related to anxiety and depression, possibly via influences on the locus coeruleus (71). Thus a disturbance of CRF in PD, which has not yet been investigated, might explain the combination of anxious and depressive symptoms.

There is some evidence suggesting that lateralized cerebral factors may be important in the genesis of anxiety. Imaging studies have revealed right hemispheric abnormalities in panic disorders (72). No imaging studies such as these have been reported that specifically examined anxiety in PD. There is evidence, however, for greater involvement of the right side of the brain in PD patients with anxiety. Fleminger (32) examined 17 patients with PD that was worse on the right side of the body (RHP) and 13 patients whose symptoms were worse on the left side of the body (LHP). Present State Examination symptoms that were more common in the LHP group were panic with autonomic features, depressed mood, and social withdrawal. Similarly, Rubin et al. (2) noted that panic-anxiety disorder in PD patients was associated with early left-right asymmetry of PD motor features. Tomer et al. (69) noted highly significant correlations between severity of left-sided motor symptoms and obsessive-compulsive symptomatology in patients with PD.

Brain imaging studies in psychiatric patients with anxiety have shown abnormalities in the basal ganglia (73–75). Potts and coworkers (75) found no statistically significant differences between social phobia patients and normal control subjects with regard to cerebral, caudate, putamen, and thalamic volumes but noted an age-related reduction in putamen volumes in patients with social phobia. The authors conjectured that social phobia might be a manifestation of a dopamine-deficiency state and that some social phobic patients as they age may be at greater risk of developing the manifestations of parkinsonism. Neuropsychological testing has also demonstrated that patients with OCD and PD have deficits attributable to basal ganglia dysfunction (76,77). These findings suggest that basal ganglia disturbances in PD might explain the development of anxiety in patients suffering from this illness.

There appear to be many demonstrated biologic abnormalities in PD that not only may explain the frequent occurrence of anxiety in this disorder, but may also contribute to our understanding of the mechanisms of anxiety in psychiatric patients.

Treatment of Anxiety in Parkinson's Disease

If anxiety occurs exclusively during the "off" period, it would be reasonable to first try to minimize "off" time with adjustment of the antiparkinsonian medication regimen. There have also been some preliminary studies suggesting that the dopamine agonist pramipexole might be effective in alleviating depressive symptoms (78–80). Effects of this medication on anxiety have not yet been studied. However, one will need to consider treating the anxiety with psychotherapy and/or psychotropic medications.

Commonly used drugs to treat anxiety disorders include tricyclic antidepressants (TCAs), selective serotonin reuptake inhibitors (SSRIs), atypical cyclic antidepressants (e.g., trazadone), nonselective monoamine oxidase inhibitors (MAOIs), benzodiazepines, and buspirone. There are very few clinical trials of medication treatment for anxiety in the elderly (81), and there are no studies that specifically address the optimal treatment of anxiety in patients with PD.

Stein et al. (4) comments that anxiety disorders in PD may respond to pharmacotherapy with antidepressants and benzodiazepines. Lauterbach and Duvoisin (11) cautioned, however, that benzodiazepines can at times worsen Parkinsonian symptoms. Benzodiazepines can also be problematic with regard to impairment in arousal, cognition, and balance. Benzodiazepines can provide relief of symptoms associated with panic, GAD, and social phobia but are not indicated for OCD. Alprazolam was shown to be effective for anxiety symptoms in mixed anxiety-depressive disorder in patients who are more than 60 years old and who had just undergone bypass surgery (29).

Buspirone can be effective for GAD but is unlikely to help panic, OCD, or social phobia (29). A study of buspirone in PD patients designed to investigate possible antiparkinsonian effects of the drug noted that the agent was well tolerated in doses up to 60 mg but actually caused increased anxiety and worsening of motor function at doses of 100 mg/day. Antianxiety effects at the well-tolerated doses were not observed, but patients were not selected for the presence of anxiety (82). Another study investigating the efficacy of buspirone for dyskinesias in PD revealed no change in depression or anxiety scores at a dosage of 20 mg/day. However, patients were not selected on the basis of psychological symptoms (83).

One should keep in mind that specific aspects of PD, especially the use of antiparkinsonian medications, may importantly influence the choice of medications used to treat anxiety in patients with this illness. For instance, nonselective MAOIs are contraindicated in patients receiving levodopa because of the risk of hypertensive crisis. Selegiline (deprenyl, eldepryl) is a selective MAO type B inhibitor when used at low doses, and it does not induce hypertensive crisis in PD patients treated with dopaminergic agents. The drug is commonly used in PD to prolong the duration of levodopa action in patients with motor fluctuations and also because of controversial reports that this drug may slow the progression of disease. The drug has been found to be an effective antidepressant agent in psychiatric populations, but only at higher doses where its MAO-B selectivity is lost. Although selegiline has not been specifically tested for its antianxiety effects, it was noted that depressed patients with anxiety or panic actually responded less well to selegiline than those without anxiety symptoms (84). The manufacturer of selegiline cautions against the combined use of a TCA or an SSRI with this medication because of potentially serious central nervous system (CNS) toxicity that may represent the serotonin syndrome.

Manifestations of the serotonin syndrome vary but may include changes in mental status, motor, and autonomic function. Based on our survey of members of the Parkinson Study Group (PSG), and our review of published case reports and adverse experiences reported to the U.S. Food and Drug Administration and the manufacturer of Eldepryl, it appears as though serious adverse experiences resulting from the combined use of deprenyl and antidepressants in patients with PD are quite rare and the frequency of the true "serotonin syndrome" is even rarer (85). One patient treated with selegiline developed hypertensive crisis when given buspirone (83). A conservative approach would be to avoid selegiline in any PD patient who requires a TCA, an SSRI, or, perhaps, buspirone for treatment of anxiety or depression. We believe that careful monitoring of patients on this combination is important and that patients should be informed of potential risks. We would not, however, consider the risks unacceptable if the patient could benefit from the combination of deprenyl and an antidepressant medication (85). We did not formally explore the issue of combined therapy with deprenyl and buspirone and could only recommend that physicians monitor blood pressure carefully if they decide to coprescribe these agents.

SSRIs are generally well tolerated and can be effective for almost all types of anxiety, including panic, OCD, and social phobia. Their role in the treatment of GAD is less clear (29). There are, however, case reports of SSRIs increasing the level of motor disability in patients with PD (86–88), although other authors have reported that the drug does not appear to be associated with exacerbations of parkinsonian signs and symptoms (89–91). It is advisable to use an SSRI

if deemed appropriate but to monitor motor function and discontinue the SSRI (via gradual taper to avoid a possible withdrawal syndrome) if it appears to have been associated with a worsening motor status. The issue of whether SSRIs result in motor dysfunction awaits a formal clinical trial, which would also address the issue of antidepressant and perhaps anxiolytic efficacy of these generally well-tolerated agents in patients with PD.

Elderly patients may be more sensitive to anxiolytic medications by virtue of their altered metabolism, tendency toward falls and oversedation, and concomitant medical conditions (29,92,93).

The full effect that surgical therapies for PD may have on psychiatric symptoms is not clear. In one study of unilateral pallidotomy's effect on cognition, it was noted that patients reported significantly fewer symptoms of anxiety after surgery (94).

CONCLUSION

Although few studies have specifically investigated anxiety in patients with PD, some preliminary conclusions can be drawn.

Anxiety disorders frequently occur in association with PD and may be important causes of morbidity. Actual prevalence rates are uncertain, but estimates suggest that up to 40% of patients with PD experience significant anxiety. This frequency is greater than expected, particularly for an elderly population. In addition, the age at onset of anxiety in PD patients is later than what would be expected from current information regarding the natural course of anxiety disorders. It should be noted that most psychiatric rating instruments used to assess anxiety may present some difficulties in interpretation when applied to PD patients, and this could confound prevalence studies. Some of the somatic symptoms of anxiety, such as tremor, may be difficult to distinguish from symptoms of the underlying disease.

Virtually all of the types of anxiety disorders have been described in PD, but panic disorder, GAD, and social phobia appear to be the ones most commonly encountered. The frequency of panic disorder, in particular is high.

Anxiety usually appears after the diagnosis of PD is established, but it can also develop before the motor features. The latter observation suggests that anxiety may not represent psychologic and social difficulties in adapting to the illness but rather may be linked to specific neurobiological processes occurring in PD. It is possible that anxiety might represent the first sign of illness for some patients with PD (36). Whether anti-parkinsonian medications themselves contribute to anxiety needs clarification.

Although anxiety in PD does not appear to be simply a reaction to degree of disability, there does appear to be a strong relationship between motor state and anxiety. In particular, most patients experience greater anxiety during the "off" phase of their motor fluctuations. It is still not clear whether anxiety is an emotional reaction to motor impairment, whether anxiety might worsen motor function, or whether anxiety and motor dysfunction occur together as the result of common central neurochemical mechanisms. The fact that levodopa infusions resulted in increased anxiety several minutes before motor impairment makes the first less tenable (22).

Anxiety and depression frequently coexist in PD. It remains to be determined whether anxiety in patients with PD reflects one of the following: (a) an underlying depressive mood disorder, (b) represents a particular subtype of depression (atypical depression, anxious or agitated depression), or (c) occurs as an independent psychiatric disturbance. The association between depression and panic disorder, which is commonly observed in PD patients, is less common in the general elderly population and does suggest a unique relationship in PD.

The relationship between anxiety and dementia in PD is not clear, but current evidence suggests that cognitive dysfunction is not related to the presence of anxiety symptoms in this disorder.

Current information supports the view that specific neurobiological processes associated with PD may be responsible for the development of anxiety in patients with this illness. Most evidence points to disturbances in central noradrenergic systems, but other neurotransmitters or neuropeptides maybe involved as well. Studies suggest that right hemispheric disturbances may be particularly important for the genesis of anxiety, especially panic and OCD.

The optimal pharmacologic treatment for anxiety in patients with PD has not been established. Clinicians should be aware that some anxiolytic agents may be contraindicated in PD and others may worsen symptoms of the illness.

REFERENCES

1. American Psychiatric Association. *Diagnostic and Statistical Manual of Mental Disorders*. 4th ed. Washington, DC: American Psychiatric Association, 1994.
2. Rubin AJ, Kurlan R, Schiffer R, et al. Atypical depression and Parkinson's disease (abstract). *Ann Neurol* 1986; 20:150.
3. American Psychiatric Association. *Diagnostic and Statistical Manual of Mental Disorders*. 3rd ed. Washington, DC: American Psychiatric Association, 1987.
4. Stein M, Henser IJ, Juncos JL, et al. Anxiety disorders in patients with Parkinson's disease. *Am J Psychiatry* 1990; 147:217–220.
5. Vázquez A, Jiménez-Jiménez FJ, Garcia-Ruiz P, et al. "Panic attacks" in Parkinson's disease: A long-term complication of levodopa therapy. *Acta Neurol Scand* 1993; 87:14–18.
6. Schiffer RB, Kurlan R, Rubin A, et al. Evidence for atypical depression in Parkinson's disease. *Am J Psychiatry* 1988; 145:1020–1022.
7. Menza MA, Robertson-Hoffman DE, Bonapace AS. Parkinson's disease and anxiety: Comorbidity with depression. *Biol Psychiatry* 1993; 34:465–470.
8. Menza MA, Mark MH. Parkinson's disease and depression: The relationship to disability and personality. *J Neuropsychiatry Clin Neurosci* 1994; 6:165–169.
9. Gotham A-M, Brown RG, Marsden CD. Depression in Parkinson's disease: A quantitative and qualitative analysis. *J Neurol Neurosurg Psychiatry* 1986; 49:381–389.
10. Berrios GE, Campbell C, Politynska. Autonomic failure, depression and anxiety in Parkinson's disease. *Brit J Psychiatry* 1995; 166:789–792.
11. Lauterbach EC, Duvoisin RC. Anxiety disorders and familial Parkinsonism (letter). *Am J Psychiatry* 1992; 148:274.
12. Henderson R, Kurlan R, Kersun JM, et al. Preliminary examination of the comorbidity of anxiety and depression in Parkinson's disease. *J Neuropsychiatry Clin Neurosci* 1992; 148:274.
13. Siemers ER, Shekhar A, Quaid K, et al. Anxiety and motor performance in Parkinson's disease. *Mov Disord* 1993; 8:501–506.
14. Rondot P, deRecondo J, Colgnet A, et al. Mental disorders in Parkinson's disease after treatment with L-dopa. *Adv Neurol* 1984:40.
15. Cummings JL. Depression and Parkinson's disease: A review. *Am J Psychiatry* 1992; 149:443–454.
16. Factor SA, Molho ES, Podskalny GD, et al. Parkinson's disease: Drug-induced psychiatric states. In: Weiner WJ and Lang AE (eds.). Behavioral Neurology of Movement Disorders, *Advances in Neurology* Vol 65. New York: Raven Press, 1995:115–138.
17. Nissenbaum H, Quinn NP, Brown RG, et al. Mood swings associated with the "on-off" phenomenon in Parkinson's disease. *Psychol Med* 1987; 17:899–904.
18. Seligman MEP. Chronic fear produced by unpredictable shock. *J Comp Physiol psychol* 1968; 66:402–411.
19. Riley DE, Lang AE. The spectrum of levodopa-related fluctuations in Parkinson's disease. *Neurology* 1993; 43:1459–1464.
20. Marsden CD, Parkes JD. "On-off" effects in patients with Parkinson's disease on chronic levodopa therapy. *Lancet* 1976; 1:292–296.

21. Menza MA, Sage J, Marshall E, et al. Mood changes and "on-off" phenomena in Parkinson's disease. *Mov Disord* 1990; 5:148–151.

22. Maricle RA, Nutt JG, valentine RJ, et al. Dose-response relationship of levodopa with mood and anxiety in fluctuating Parkinson's disease: A double-blind, placebo controlled study. *Neurology* 1995; 45:1757–1760.

23. Brown RG, Marsden CD, Quinn N, et al. Alterations in cognitive performance and affect-arousal state during fluctuations in motor function in Parkinson's disease. *J Neurol Neurosurg Psychiatry* 1984; 47:454–465.

24. Cantello R, Gilli M, Riccio A, et al. Mood changes associated with "end-of-dose deterioration" in Parkinson's disease: A controlled study. *J Neurol Neurosurg Psychiatry* 1986; 49:1182–1190.

25. Routh LC, Black JL, Ahlskog JE. Parkinson's disease complicated by anxiety. *Mayo Clin Proc* 1987; 62:733–735.

26. Kurlan R, Lichter D, Schiffer RB. Panic/anxiety in Parkinson's disease: Yohimbine challenge (abstract). *Neurology* 1989; 39(Suppl 1):421.

27. Flint AJ. Epidemiology and comorbidity of anxiety disorders in the elderly. *Am J Psychiatry* 1994; 151:640–649.

28. Palmer BW, Jeste DV, Sheikh JI. Anxiety disorders in the elderly: DSM-IV and other barriers to diagnosis and treatment. *J Affect Disord* 1997; 46(3):183–190.

29. Small GW. Recognizing and treating anxiety in the elderly. *J Clin Psychiatry* 1997; 58:41–17.

30. Raj BA, Corvea MH, Dagon EM. The clinical characteristics of panic disorder in the elderly: A retrospective study. *J Clin Psychiatry* 1993; 54:150–155.

31. Lydiard RB. Coexisting depression and anxiety: Special diagnostic and treatment issues. *J Clin Psychiatry* 1991; 52(suppl 6):48–54.

32. Fleminger S. Left-sided Parkinson's disease is associated with greater anxiety and depression. *Psychol Med* 1991; 21:629–638.

33. Liu CY, Yang SJ, Fuh JL, et al. The correlation of depression with functional activity in Parkinson's disease. *J Neurol* 1997; 244:493–498.

34. Wands K, Merskey H, Hachinski VC, et al. A questionnaire investigation of anxiety and depression in early dementia. *J Am Geriatr Soc* 1990; 38:535–538.

35. Iruela LM, Ibañez-Rojo V, Inmaculada P, et al. Anxiety disorders and Parkinson's disease (letter). *Am J Psychiatry* 1992; 149:719–720.

36. Cash R, Dennis T, L'Heureux R, et al. Parkinson's disease and dementia: Norepinephrine and dopamine in locus ceruleus. *Neurology* 1987; 37:42–46.

37. Lauterbach EC. The locus ceruleus and anxiety disorders in demented and nondemented familial parkinsonism (letter). *Am J Psychiatry* 1993; 150:994.

38. Nutt D, Lawson C. Panic attacks: a neurochemical overview of models and mechanisms. *Br J Psychiatry* 1992; 160:165–178.

39. Heninger GR, Charney DS. Monoamine receptor systems and anxiety disorders. *Psychiatr Clin North Am* 1988; 11:309–326.

40. Charney DS, Heninger GR, Brief A. Noradrenergic function in panic anxiety: Effects of yohimbine in healthy subjects and patients with agoraphobia and panic disorder. *Arch Gen Psychiatry* 1984; 41:751–763.

41. Charney DS, Woods SW, Goodman WK, et al. Neurobiological mechanisms of panic anxiety: Biochemical and behavioral correlates of yohimbine-induced panic attacks. *Am J Psychiatry* 1987; 144:1030–1036.

42. Nutt DJ. Altered alpha-2-adrenoceptor sensitivity in panic disorder. *Arch Gen Psychiatry* 1989; 46:165–169.

43. Uhde T, Stein MB, Vittone BJ, et al. Behavioral and physiologic effects of short-term and long-term administration of clonidine in panic disorder. *Arch Gen Psychiatry* 1989; 46:170–177.

44. Charney DS, Heninger GR. Abnormal regulation of noradrenergic function in panic disorders: Effects of clonidine in healthy subjects and patients with agoraphobia and panic disorder. *Arch Gen Psychiatry* 1986; 43:1042–1054.

45. Agid Y, Cervera P, Hirsch E, et al. Biochemistry of Parkinson's disease 28 years later: A critical review. *Mov Disord* 1989; (suppl 1):5126–5144.

46. Weiner WJ, Lang AE. *Movement Disorders: A Comprehensive Survey.* Mount Kisco, NY: Futura, 1989.

47. Patt S, Gerhard L. A study of human locus ceruleus in normal brains and in Parkinson's disease. *Neuropathol Appl Neurobiol* 1993; 19:519–523.

48. German DC, Manaye KF, White CL III, et al. Disease-specific patterns of locus ceruleus cell loss. *Ann Neurol* 1992; 32:667–676.

49. Chan-Palay V. Depression and dementia in Parkinson's disease: Catecholamine changes in the locus ceruleus, a basis for therapy. *Adv Neurol* 1993; 60:438–446.

50. Zweig RM, Cardillo JE, Cohen M, et al. The locus ceruleus and dementia in Parkinson's disease. *Neurology* 1993; 43:986–991.

51. Cash R, Ruberg M, Raisman R, et al. Adrenergic receptors in Parkinson's disease. *Brain Res* 1984; 322:269–275.

52. Villeneuve A, Berlan M, Lafontan M, et al. Platelet alpha-2-adrenoceptors in Parkinson's disease: Decreased number in untreated patients and recovery after treatment. *Eur J Clin Invest* 1985; 15:403–407.

53. Montastruc J-L, Villeneuve A, Berlan M, et al. Study of platelet alpha-2-adrenoceptors in Parkinson's disease. *Adv Neurol* 1986; 45:253–258.

54. Bernal M, Rascol O, Belin J, et al. Alpha-2 adrenergic sensitivity in Parkinson's disease. *Clin Neuropharmacol* 1989; 12:138–144.

55. Richard IH, Kurlan R, Lichter D, et al. Parkinson's disease: A preliminary study of yohimbine challenge in patients with anxiety. *Clin Neuropharmacol*, 1999, 22:172–175.

56. Insel TR, Zohar J, Benkelfat C, et al. Serotonin in obsessions, compulsions, and the control of aggressive impulses. *Ann NY Acad Sci* 1990; 600:574–585.

57. Miner CM, Davidson JR. Biological characterization of social phobia (review). *Eur Arch Psychiatry Clin Neurosci* 1995; 244:304–308.

58. Charney DS, Woods SW, Krystal JH, et al. Serotonin function and human anxiety disorders. *Ann NY Acad Sci* 1990; 600:558–572.

59. Halliday GM, Blumbergs PC, Cotton RG, et al. Loss of brainstem serotonin and substance P-containing neurons in Parkinson's disease. *Brain Res* 1990; 5120:104–107.

60. Jellinger K. The pathology of parkinsonism. In: Marsden CD, Fahn S (eds.). *Movement Disorders.* Vol 2. (International Medical Reviews, Neurology; Vol 7). London: Butterworth, 1987:124–165.

61. Agid Y, Javoy-Agid F, Ruberg M. Biochemistry of neurotransmitters in Parkinson's disease. In: Marsden CD, Fahn S (eds.). *Movement Disorders.* Vol 2. (International Medical Reviews, Neurology; Vol 7). London: Butterworth, 1987:166–230.

62. Raisman R, Cash R, Agid Y. Parkinson's disease: Decreased density 3H-imipramine and 3H-paroxetine binding sites in putamen. *Neurology* 1986; 36:556–560.

63. D'Amato RJ, Zweig RM, Whitehouse PJ, et al. Aminergic systems in Alzheimer's disease and Parkinson's disease. *Ann Neurol* 1987; 22:229–236.

64. Potts NLS, Davidson JRT. Social phobia: Biological aspects and pharmacotherapy. *Prog Neuropsychopharmacol Biol Psychiatry* 1992; 16:635–646.

65. Pitchot W, Ansseau M, Gonzalez Moreno A, et al. Dopaminergic function in panic disorder: Comparison with major and minor depression. *Biol Psychiatry* 1992; 32:1004–1011.

66. Argyl N. Panic attacks in chronic schizophrenia. *Br J Psychiatry* 1990; 157:430–433.

67. McDougle CJ, Goodman WK, Price LH. Dopamine antagonists in tic-related and psychotic spectrum obsessive compulsive disorder (literature review). *J Clin Psychiatry* 1994; 55(suppl):24–31.

68. Marazziti D, Hollander E, Lensi P, et al. Peripheral markers of serotonin and dopamine function in obsessive-compulsive disorder. *Psychiatry Res* 1992; 42:41–51.

69. Tomer R, Levin BE, Weiner WJ. Obsessive-compulsive symptoms and motor asymmetries in Parkinson's disease. *Neuropsychiatry Neuropsychol Behav Neurol* 1993; 6:26–30.

70. Cedarbaum JM, Aghajanian GK. Catecholamine receptors on locus ceruleus neurons: Pharmacological characterization. *Eur J Pharmacol* 1977; 44:375–385.

71. Owens MJ, Nemeroff CB. The role of corticotropin-releasing factor in the pathophysiology of affective and anxiety disorders: Laboratory and clinical studies. *Ciba Found Symp* 1993; 172:296–308.

72. Fontaine R, Breton G, Dery R, et al. Temporal lobe abnormalities in panic disorder: An MRI study. *Biol Psychiatry* 1990; 27:304–310.

73. Faulstich ME, Sullivan DC. Positron emission tomography in neuropsychiatry. *Invest Radiol* 1991; 26:184–194.

74. Davidson JRT, Krishnan KRR, Charles HC, et al. Magnetic resonance spectroscopy in social phobia: Preliminary findings. *J Clin psychiatry* 1993; 54(suppl 12):19–24.

75. Potts NLS, Davidson JRT, Krishnan KRR, et al. Magnetic resonance imaging in social phobia. *Psychiatry Res* 1994; 52:35–42.

76. Hollander E, Cohen L, Richards M, et al. A pilot study of the neuropsychology of obsessive-compulsive disorder and Parkinson's disease: Basal ganglia disorders. *J Neuropsychiatry Clin Neurosci* 1993; 5:104–107.

77. Saint-Cyr JA, Taylor AE, Nicholson K. Behavior and the basal ganglia (literature review). *Adv Neurol* 1995; 65:1–28.

78. Pogarell O, Kunig G, Oertel WH. A non-ergot dopamine agonist, pramipexole, in the therapy of advanced Parkinson's disease: Improvement of parkinsonian symptoms and treatment-associated complications. A review of three studies. *Clin Neuropharmacol* 1997; 20:S28–S35.

79. Corrigan M, Evans. *Pramipexole, a Dopamine Agonist, in the Treatment of Major Depression.* Abstract presented at Annual American Society of Neuropsychology Meeting, 1997, Honolulu, HI.

80. Szegedi A, Hillert A, Wetzel H, et al. Pramipexole, a dopamine agonist, in major depression: Antidepressant effects and tolerability in an open-label study with multiple doses. *Clin Neuropharmacol* 1997; 20:S36–S45.

81. Pearson JL. Research in late-life anxiety. Summary of a National institute of Mental Health Workshop on Late-Life Anxiety. *Psychopharmacol Bull* 1998; 34:127–138.

82. Ludwig CL, Weinberger DR, Bruno G, et al. Buspirone, Parkinson's disease, and the locus ceruleus. *Clin Neuropharmacol* 1986; 9:373–378.

83. Bonifati V, Fabrizio E, Cipriani R, et al. Buspirone in levodopa-induced dyskinesias. *Clin Neuropharmacol* 1994; 17:73–82.

84. Mann JJ, Aarons SF, Wilner PJ, et al. A controlled study of the antidepressant efficacy and side effects of (-)-deprenyl. *Arch Gen Psychiatry* 1989; 46:45–50.

85. Richard IH, Kurlan R, Tanner C, et al. and the Parkinson Study Group. Serotonin syndrome and the combined use of deprenyl and an antidepressant in Parkinson's disease. *Neurology* 1997; 48:1070–1077.

86. Steur ENHJ. Increase in Parkinson disability after fluoxetine medication. *Neurology* 1993; 43:211–213.

87. Chouinard G, Sultan S. A case of Parkinson's disease exacerbated by fluoxetine. *Human Psychopharmacol* 1992; 7:63–66.

88. Jiménez-Jiménez FJ, Tejeiro J, Martínez-Junquera G, et al. Parkinsonism exacerbated by paroxetine. *Neurology* 1994; 44:2406.

89. Caley CF, Friedman JH. Does fluoxetine exacerbate Parkinson's disease? *J Clin Psychiatry* 1992; 53:278–282.

90. Shulman LM, Singer C, Liefert R, et al. Therapeutic effects of Seratraline in patients with Parkinson's disease. *Mov Disord* 1996; 11:603.

91. Montastruc J-L, Fabre N, Blin O, et al. Does fluoxetine aggravate Parkinson's disease? A pilot prospective study. *Mov Disord* 1995; 10:355–357.

92. Stoudemire A, Moran MG. Psychopharamacologic treatment of anxiety in the medically ill elderly patient: Special considerations. *J Clin Psychiatry* 1993; 54(suppl 5):27–33.

93. Salzman C. Anxiety in the elderly: Treatment strategies. *J Clin Psychiatry* 1990; 51(suppl 10):18–21.

94. Troster AI, Fields JA, Wilkinson SB, et al. Unilateral pallidal stimulation for Parkinson's disease: Neurobehavioral functioning before and 3 months after electrode implantation. *Neurology* 1997; 49:1078–1083.

95. Richard IH, Schiffer RB, Kurlan R. Anxiety and Parkinson's disease. *J Neuropsychiatr Clin Neurosci* 1996; 8:383–392.

19

Apathy and Amotivation

Lisa M. Shulman, M.D.

University of Maryland School of Medicine, Baltimore, Maryland

Take a few moments to think about the role that qualities such as creativity, ambition, imagination, and perseverance play in your life. What kind of an impact would a reduction of energy, drive, and initiative have on your career, on your personal life, and on your general sense of fulfillment? It is easy to overlook the capacity that apathy and amotivation have to reduce our productivity and self-satisfaction. Cognitive dysfunction and depression are increasingly regarded as significant sources of functional impairment in Parkinson's disease (PD), but the contribution of loss of motivation to disability is generally not acknowledged. The study of apathy in PD and other medical conditions is in its infancy; in total there have been about 500 papers about apathy in the medical literature over the last ten years, while 50,000 papers about depression appeared during the same time interval. We are only beginning to explore the pathophysiology and management of amotivation, and there is still much to be learned about the associations between apathy and the range of motor and nonmotor symptoms of PD. This chapter reviews our current understanding of apathy in the setting of PD, focusing on issues of definition, recognition, clinical correlates, pathophysiology, and treatment.

The word *apathy* is derived from the Greek *pathos* or passions and is defined most simply as loss of motivation. Apathy may contribute to disability in a broad range of medical and psychiatric conditions, yet it may also pose a problem in healthy adults, especially the elderly. Since amotivation is commonly an intrinsic personality trait, it is important for the clinician to evaluate a patient's level of motivation relative to the individual's previous level of functioning and the standards of his/her age and culture (1). Silva and Marin (1,2) described three spheres of evidence of the syndrome of apathy including diminished goal-directed behavior, diminished goal-directed cognition, and diminished emotional concomitants of goal-directed behavior. Reduced goal-directed behavior is manifest by a lack of effort, initiative, and perseverance. A change in goal-directed cognition is evidenced by a lack of interest in experiencing or learning new things and a lack of concern about one's health or functional disability. Lastly, emotional evidence of apathy includes flat affect or indifference. Loss of motivation may dominate a clinical presentation or may be subordinated by the presence of more overt symptomotology such as dementia or depression.

There is a complex relationship between emotional intensity and apathy. An absence of emotional intensity is an important element of apathy, yet apathy frequently coexists with depression, which by definition is accompanied by despair and emotional pain. Neurologic disorders such as PD result in disruption of motor function, facial expressivity, body language and communication that can all interfere with our perception of the patient's emotional state. The patient with PD may appear disinterested, while remaining profoundly concerned with his/her goals and responsibilities (3). Neurology is replete with symptoms and signs that may confound the accurate assessment of apathy including abulia, anhedonia, aprosodia, psychomotor retardation, and bradyphrenia.

CLINICAL CORRELATES OF APATHY IN PARKINSON'S DISEASE

Marsden and Parkes (4) observed in 1977 that some PD patients manifest a "blunting of interest and drive, amounting to apathy." The study of apathy in PD, however, awaited the development of a reliable and valid scale by Marin in the 1990s (5,6) (Table 19-1). There are two version of the scale – one that is

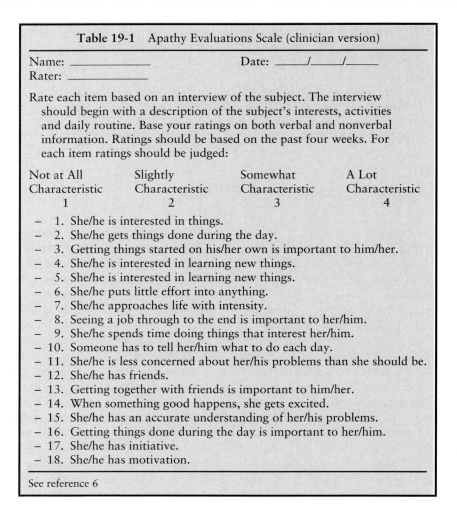

Table 19-1   Apathy Evaluations Scale (clinician version)

Name: _____   Date: _____/_____/_____
Rater: _____

Rate each item based on an interview of the subject. The interview should begin with a description of the subject's interests, activities and daily routine. Base your ratings on both verbal and nonverbal information. Ratings should be based on the past four weeks. For each item ratings should be judged:

Not at All Characteristic 1	Slightly Characteristic 2	Somewhat Characteristic 3	A Lot Characteristic 4

– 1. She/he is interested in things.
– 2. She/he gets things done during the day.
– 3. Getting things started on his/her own is important to him/her.
– 4. She/he is interested in learning new things.
– 5. She/he is interested in learning new things.
– 6. She/he puts little effort into anything.
– 7. She/he approaches life with intensity.
– 8. Seeing a job through to the end is important to her/him.
– 9. She/he spends time doing things that interest her/him.
– 10. Someone has to tell her/him what to do each day.
– 11. She/he is less concerned about her/his problems than she should be.
– 12. She/he has friends.
– 13. Getting together with friends is important to him/her.
– 14. When something good happens, she gets excited.
– 15. She/he has an accurate understanding of her/his problems.
– 16. Getting things done during the day is important to her/him.
– 17. She/he has initiative.
– 18. She/he has motivation.

See reference 6

self-administered and one scored by the clinician. In 1992, Starkstein et al. (7) administered an abridged version of Marin's Apathy Evaluation Scale along with scales measuring depression, anxiety, cognitive function, and PD severity to 50 patients with PD. Forty-two percent of patients had significant apathy. 12 percent of those with apathy were not depressed, and 30% had both apathy and depression. An additional 26% had depression but no apathy and 32% had neither apathy nor depression. There was no difference in the level of apathy between depressed and nondepressed patients.

Anxiety scores were significantly higher in depressed patients as compared with those with apathy. Apathetic patients (with and without depression) showed a poorer performance on tests of verbal memory and time-dependent tasks. There was no difference between PD patients with and without apathy in terms of age, gender, level of education, PD duration, or severity. The presence of apathy was also not associated with the severity of akinesia or rigidity. The poor performance of PD patients with apathy on time-dependent cognitive

tasks suggests a relationship between the concepts of bradyphrenia and apathy.

CAUSES OF APATHY

Like many common behavioral symptoms such as depression or anxiety, apathy may be a significant determinant of behavior either as an inherent feature of the adult personality or as an acquired symptom associated with neurologic, psychiatric, or medical conditions. Apathetic behavior can be analyzed from a strictly organic biochemical perspective or from a psychologic perspective.

Where does motivation reside in the brain? The limbic system has been traditionally viewed as being central to emotion and motivation. In particular, the amygdala is thought to play the role of a "motivational rheostat" (8) filtering environmental stimuli and influencing goal-directed behavior. Duffy (8) proposed four different neuronal circuits, all with limbic input, that are involved in generating motivational valence and translating motivation into behavior. This motivational circuitry makes important connections with the basal ganglia. Key structures of the motivation circuits are believed to be the nucleus accumbens, the ventral pallidum, and the ventral tegmental area. Levy et al. (9) suggested that apathy occurs when the cortex is functionally disconnected from key limbic input and Mayeux et al. (10) proposed that bradyphrenia arises from neuronal depletion of the locus ceruleus.

Apathy syndromes have been described in a range of neurologic disorders that provide a glimpse of the localization of motivation in the brain. In addition to PD, apathy is a common feature of basal ganglia disorders including progressive supranuclear palsy, Huntington's disease, Wilson's disease, carbon monoxide poisoning, dementia pugilistica, and lacunar stroke (11). Diminished motivation ranging from apathy to akinetic mutism arises from prefrontal syndromes following lesions of the mesiofrontal cortex and its connections to the anterior cingulate cortex. These syndromes result from trauma, meningioma, hydrocephalus, and aneurysm or stroke affecting the anterior cerebral circulation. Lesions of the dorsolateral frontal region related to frontotemporal dementia, Alzheimer's disease, alcoholic dementia, tumor, or subdural hematoma give rise to diminished cognitive flexibility, concrete thinking, perseveration, and impersistence that result in amotivational behavior. In a single photon emission computed tomography (SPECT) imaging study of Alzheimer's patients, the presence of apathy was correlated with decreased right temperoparietal perfusion, whereas loss of insight was correlated with decreased right temperooccipital perfusion (12).

Cerebral infarction of the posterior limb of the internal capsule has been associated with apathy, psychic akinesia, motor neglect, and akinetic mutism (13,14). Starkstein et al. (13) described neural pathways between the internal pallidum and the pedunculopontine nucleus with relays in the posterior limb of the internal capsule and the substantia nigra that may result in bradyphrenia and apathy. Thalamic infarction has also been associated with motivational disorders (11).

Neuropathology of the deep white matter including subcortical encephalomalacia, human immunodeficiency virus, multiple sclerosis, diffuse axonal injury, radiation injury, and postanoxic encephalopathy may result in behavioral changes that include amotivation (11). In particular, subcortical encephalomalacia is increasingly recognized as a significant factor in late-onset depression (15) and is likely to also be an important cause of apathy in the elderly. Injury to the limbic system related to herpes simplex encephalitis, anoxic encephalopathy, and carbon monoxide are also associated with amotivational states.

The prefrontal cortex is instrumental to real-life decision making. Individuals with damage to the prefrontal cortex fail to act according to their understanding of the consequences of their actions and thus appear oblivious to the future (16). Apathy and amotivation may be reflections of an underactivated approach system. The left prefrontal cortex may play a role in setting positive goals and when this region is underactivated or dysfunctional, apathy is likely to occur (17). Data from position emission tomography (PET) and functional magnetic resonance imaging (MRI) indicates lateralization of cerebral hemispheric functions of goal-directed behavior. Functional imaging demonstrates an association between positive goal attainment and activity in the left prefrontal cortex. In general, the left prefrontal cortex is associated with positive, expansive, and optimistic emotions, whereas the right prefrontal cortex is associated with more negative and withdrawn behaviors (18,19).

Dopamine is the principle neurotransmitter of goal-directed behavior, modulating motivation, arousal, motor response, and sensorimotor integration (8). There is abundant evidence of the impact of dopaminergic input on goal-directed behavior including the effects of amphetamines that initially give rise to enhanced focus and motivation but with chronic usage later result in stereotypic behaviors. Chronic neuroleptic administration is often associated with apathetic behavior. PD patients frequently describe improved arousal and motivation with the use of dopaminergic medications that is not solely explained by the antiparkinsonian motor response. A number of other neurotransmitters modify dopamine's effects on motivation including N-methyl-D-aspartate, AMPA, neurotensin, and substance P as well as agonists of the nicotinic and opioid receptors. Cholinergic and serotonergic pathways also play a neuromodulatory role in the motivational circuitry. A rare dominantly inherited syndrome of apathy, central hypoventilation, and parkinsonism is characterized by deficiences of multiple neurotransmitters including dopamine, serotonin, glutamate, and GABA with severe neuronal loss and gliosis of the substantia nigra (20).

Another approach to understanding apathy and its association with PD is derived from theories of personality. Cloninger's theory of personality describes three heritable major dimensions of personality: novelty seeking, harm avoidance, and reward dependence (21). Novelty seeking is believed to be modulated by dopamine and is associated with behavioral activation, exploratory behavior, and avoidance of monotony.

Harm avoidance is believed to be determined by serotonergic activity and reward dependence by norepinephrine. Scientific evidence of dopamine's role in novelty-seeking behavior includes the reduction of spontaneous investigatory behavior of animals following dopamine-depleting lesions (22), increased novelty-induced motor activity following dopamine microinjection in the ventral pallidum and nucleus accumbens (23), and the appearance of self-stimulation behavior secondary to electrode placement in the dopaminergic pathways (24,25).

When Cloninger's Tridimensional Personality Questionnaire (TPQ) was administered to patients with PD, they showed significantly reduced novelty-seeking behavior as compared with a group of age and disability-matched rheumatologic and orthopedic patients (26,27). There was no significant difference between patient groups on the harm-avoidance or reward-dependence ratings. These results confirm the notion of a discrete set of personality traits associated with PD patients that has been commonly described as rigid, serious, cautious, and introverted (28–30). Speculation that these personality traits precede the diagnosis of PD led Menza et al. (26) to repeat a questionnaire asking the PD patient and spouse to complete the questions as they would have 20 years ago. The PD patients persisted in scoring lower on novelty seeking based on the premorbid ratings. Novelty-seeking behaviors were negatively correlated with advanced age in agreement with the TPQ normative data that indicated that the total novelty-seeking score declined one point per decade (31). This finding is consistent with the common observation of increased passivity and amotivation among the elderly and may be related to the reduction of dopaminergic tone with advancing age. Two studies demonstrated an intriguing association between novelty-seeking behavior and the dopamine D4 receptor alleles (32,33), whereas two follow-up studies failed to replicate these results (34,35).

APATHY VS. DEPRESSION

Apathy has been traditionally viewed as a feature of depression. Criteria for depression including poor concentration, difficulty making decisions, low self-esteem, markedly diminished interest, and feelings of hopelessness and fatigue are commonly manifest as loss of motivation (36). It is fair to question whether apathy can be clearly differentiated from depression and whether this distinction holds clinical relevance.

Marin et al. (37) explored the discriminability of apathy and depression by rating five patient subgroups (healthy elderly adults, left hemispheric stroke, right hemispheric stroke, Alzheimer's disease, and major depression) with both the Apathy Evaluation Scale and the Hamilton Rating Scale for Depression. The results suggest that the relationship between apathy and depression varies according to diagnosis. Mean apathy scores were significantly higher than healthy elderly scores in right hemispheric stroke, Alzheimer's disease, and major depression. Elevated apathy scores were associated with low depression in Alzheimer's disease, high depression in major depression, and intermediate scores for depression in right hemispheric stroke. The prevalence of elevated apathy scores ranged from 73% in Alzheimer's disease, 53% in major depression, 32% in right hemispheric stroke, 22% in left hemispheric stroke, and 7% in normal subjects. The prevalence of an apathy syndrome, characterized by high apathy and low depression was 55% in Alzheimer's disease and 23% in right hemispheric stroke. Between-group differences in education and income were not correlated with apathy scores. The authors suggest that the discriminability of apathy and depression between diagnoses suggests possible differences in mechanisms and management of apathy.

Syndromes of high apathy with relatively low depression were also described in frontotemporal dementia and progressive supranuclear palsy using the Neuropsychiatric Inventory (38,39). Levy et al. (9) again used this scale to study the discriminability of apathy and depression in 154 patients with five different neurodegenerative disorders: PD, Alzheimer's disease, frontotemporal dementia, Huntington's disease, and progressive supranuclear palsy. The prevalence of apathy (with and without depression) was extremely high in nearly all the patient subgroups, 91% in progressive supranuclear palsy, 90% in frontotemporal dementia, 80% in Alzheimer's disease, 59% in Huntington's disease, and 33% in PD. It should be noted that this sample of PD patients had relatively higher functional status and relatively less cognitive impairment than the other patient subgroups. The severity of apathy was disproportionately high as compared with the severity of depression in progressive supranuclear palsy, Alzheimer's disease, and frontotemporal dementia, whereas the severity of apathy and depression were quite similar in the PD and Huntington's disease patients. Apathy, but not depression, correlated with increased cognitive impairment in the patients with PD and Alzheimer's disease, but not with those with progressive supranuclear palsy or Huntington's disease. There was no correlation between the presence of apathy and depression in the total sample, and the authors concluded that apathy is a distinct behavioral syndrome from depression.

Comorbidity between apathy and depression poses a conundrum: how to reconcile the presence of one disorder characterized by loss of interest, emotion, and flattening of affect (apathy) with a disorder characterized by considerable emotional distress (depression). Level of insight may be one factor that determines the association of apathy with depression. Ott et al. (12) studied apathy and loss of insight in Alzheimer's patients, a disorder characterized by high apathy and low depression. Apathy was measured with the Apathy Evaluation Scale and awareness of dementia with the Clinical Insight Rating Scale. The presence of problem behaviors that cause distress to the caregiver was measured with the Dementia Behavior Disturbance Scale. Increased apathy was highly correlated with loss of insight (p < 0.005) but not with general cognitive impairment. Problem behaviors were highly correlated with apathy (p < 0.005) but not with level of insight or level of cognitive impairment. These results suggest that the presence of apathy may increase the likelihood of caregiver distress. This may "ring a bell" for clinicians caring for patients with PD, who frequently hear the concerns of caregivers who are less prone to complain about motor symptoms than to report that the patient "no longer wants to do anything."

APATHY IN MEDICAL, NEUROLOGIC, AND PSYCHIATRIC DISORDERS

Apathy poses a problem in many diverse medical conditions (11,40). Endocrinopathies including hypothyroidism (41), Cushing's syndrome (42), and Addison's disease (43) may be associated with amotivational states that could be difficult to distinguish from primary behavioral disorders. Human immunodeficiency virus (HIV) is an important cause of cognitive dysfunction and impaired motivation when associated with the AIDS-dementia complex (44). The overlap between behavioral symptoms and chronic fatigue syndrome is substantial, with frequent common symptoms of fatigue, depression, and amotivation (45).

In addition to depression, apathy is commonly observed as a component of the "negative symptoms" of schizophrenia (46). Impaired motivation often accompanies substance abuse in addition to appearing as an adverse effect of many prescription drugs. Routine administration of sedatives, catecholamine-depleting drugs (reserpine, tetrabenazine), and dopamine receptor antagonists (neuroleptics) may result in apathy. Chronic alcoholism and long-term marijuana usage may also be associated with amotivational states (47,48).

In addition to PD, neurologic disorders associated with apathy include cerebrovascular disease, dementia, traumatic brain injury, and sleep disorder. Starkstein et al. (13) evaluated 80 patients within ten days of a cerebral infarction with a battery of tests measuring apathy, depression, anxiety, cognitive function, and physical impairment. Apathy was demonstrated in 22.5% of the patients, half of whom had both apathy and depression. Patients with apathy were older, had more significant cognitive impairment, and more significant functional impairment. The subgroup with mixed apathy and depression had the most severe impairment of their functional status. Neither lesion size nor lesion side correlated with the presence of apathy or depression; however, patients with apathy had a higher frequency of lesions involving the posterior limb of the internal capsule.

Traumatic brain injury frequently results in damage to the prefrontal region and the deep white matter tracts. Consequently, it is not surprising that amotivation is a significant component of the behavioral syndrome that follows closed head injury. Kant et al. (49) found that 71% of patients exhibited apathy following traumatic brain injury. Sleep disorders such as obstructive sleep apnea are also accompanied by amotivation along with excessive daytime sleepiness and irritability (50).

RECOGNITION OF APATHY AND AMOTIVATION

Nonpsychiatrists require a high index of suspicion to recognize behavioral disorders during routine office visits. Depression has a much higher profile than the symptoms of apathy and amotivation, yet when the physician's recognition of depression is compared to standardized testing, the physician has a mean diagnostic accuracy of only 30–40% (51–54). Shulman et al. (55) studied the diagnostic accuracy of the treating neurologist for the detection of depression, anxiety, fatigue, or sleep disturbance in patients with PD. The neurologist's impression following a routine office visit was compared to the patient's performance on the Beck Depression Inventory, Beck Anxiety Inventory, Fatigue Severity Scale, and the Pittsburgh Sleep Quality Inventory. The neurologist's diagnostic accuracy was 35% for depression, 42% for anxiety, 25% for fatigue, and 60% for sleep disturbance.

In the absence of clinical studies of physician recognition of apathy, one can speculate that physician awareness and diagnostic accuracy is likely to be considerably lower than that seen in depression. The patient suffering from extreme apathy is particularly unlikely to spontaneously report this problem to a physician. Indeed, the patient's insight into the changes in his/her own behavior may be impaired as well. The training of physicians has tended to emphasize disorders of emotion over disorders of motivation (2). Recognition of behavioral symptoms is also affected by the time constraints of the office visit, preoccupation of the physician with the medical pathology, and the physician's general level of comfort with discussion and treatment of behavioral symptoms.

Amotivation is more likely to be observed in patients with other behavioral symptoms. Covington (56) conceptualized a feedback loop in which behavioral and organic symptoms along with inactivity, deconditioning, and loss act synergistically to increase suffering and disability (Figure 19-1). In a study of the comorbidity of nonmotor symptoms in PD that included depression, anxiety, fatigue, sleep disturbance, and sensory symptoms, 60% of patients had two or more nonmotor disorders and 25% had four or more (57). The index of suspicion for comorbid behavioral disorders such as apathy should be increased when other nonmotor symptoms are identified.

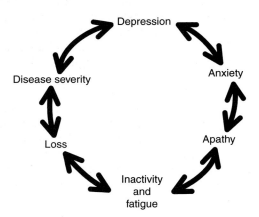

FIGURE 19-1. The interrelationships between disease severity and behavioral symptoms generate a vicious cycle of increasing symptom severity and loss of function.

The failure to recognize the emergence of an amotivational state commonly leads to the misattribution of the patient's behavior as lazy, uncaring, self-centered, or as evidence of cognitive impairment (58). Family members may become resentful and angry as the patient becomes increasingly withdrawn. Health professionals may find the care of the apathetic patient unrewarding since the patient is likely to be more passive, less interested in their condition, and less compliant. It is common for both the health care staff and family to lose sight of the fact that behavioral symptoms including apathy, depression, and anxiety are frequently endogenous to the organic pathology of the disorder, rather than evidence of maladjustment or "being difficult."

In particular, the phenomenology of parkinsonism contributes to the nonrecognition of behavioral symptoms. How can the clinician differentiate PD signs and symptoms of masking of facial expression, akinesia, bradyphrenia, stooping of posture, hypophonia, and cognitive dysfunction from the common clinical signs of apathy and depression? (Table 19-2) Focused interviewing skills are critical in improving the detection of behavioral symptoms in all patients, especially patients with extrapyramidal disorders. Simple and straightforward questions such as "What do you do for fun?" or "What do you enjoy doing these days?" in order to assess anhedonia or apathy are deceptively simple, yet often neglected (59).

In some situations family members will be reassured to simply learn that facial masking is a common symptom in parkinsonians, or that apathy is itself a common symptom of PD. In a symposium attended by patients with PD where the topic of coping with PD symptoms was under discussion, a gentleman with PD volunteered that he frequently tells new friends and acquaintances that the blankness of his face does not mean that he is not interested in what they are saying. Perhaps as clinicians we have neglected the simple approach of explaining to the patient and family the variety of motor and behavioral symptoms in PD and the manner in which they may interfere with communication and social interaction.

Table 19-2	Apathy and Amotivation in Parkinson's Disease	
Apathy/Amotivation	*Signs/Symptoms*	*Parkinson's Disease*
Indifference	Absence of facial animation	Masked facial expression
Lack of effort	Paucity of body language	Bradykinesia
Flat effect	Monotone speech	Hypophonia
Passivity	Reduced spontaneous speech	Cognitive dysfunction
Withdrawn behavior	Reduced socialization	Bradyphrenia
	Reduced interest in hobbies	

THE MANAGEMENT OF APATHY AND AMOTIVATION

The understanding of the clinical management of apathy and amotivation is still in its infancy, resting primarily on case reports rather than well-designed clinical research studies. It is important to note the potential for "ethical pitfalls" in the care of patients with apathy (60). Patients with apathy may be less likely to question recommendations from the physician; however, passive compliance is not equivalent to informed consent. Thorough discussion of the rationale and goals of therapy with the patient and family as well as careful documentation is important to alleviate concerns that the patient was not informed.

Early attempts to treat apathy involved the use of methylphenidate in demented or depressed elderly patients. Amphetamines are still occasionally prescribed by physicians for symptoms of amotivation and/or fatigue with inconsistent results (61–64). Dopaminergic agents including levodopa, dopamine receptor agonists, selegiline, and amantadine have all been reported to have benefit in selected cases (58,65).

Rational pharmacotherapy for apathy rests on the traditional foundations of accurate recognition and diagnosis as well as exclusion of reversible medical, pharmacologic, or psychosocial factors. A review of case reports involving the pharmacologic treatment of apathy yields a number of general observations. Dopamine receptor agonists are believed to be the most effective treatment for apathy. The therapeutic dose range used in nonparkinsonians is variable but has often been fairly high (bromocriptine: mean 10 mg/d, range 2.5–60 mg/d, pergolide mean 3 mg/d, range 1–5 mg/d) (58). A newer dopamine receptor agonist, pramipexole, has been suggested to have particular efficacy for depression and apathy (66), and a prospective, double-blind, placebo-controlled study is in progress to evaluate the behavioral effects of this agonist in patients with PD. It has been observed that apathy uncomplicated by cognitive dysfunction tends to respond better to pharmacotherapy. This may in part be related to the increased incidence of adverse effects in cognitively impaired patients under treatment with dopaminergic medications.

In PD patients apathy should be considered along with the other parkinsonian symptoms that may respond to dopaminergic therapy. If apathy persists when the motor symptoms are adequately treated, introduction of a dopamine agonist or elevation of the dosages of the dopaminergic medications should be considered. In patients with Alzheimer's disease (AD), apathy may contribute to poor cognitive performance and the cholinesterase inhibitor tacrine has been reported to improve motivation in these patients (67).

Patients with mixed apathy and depression may benefit from combined therapy with dopaminergic and antidepressant medication. Theoretically, antidepressants with stimulant properties (bupropion, protryptilline, venlafaxine, sertraline) are indicated, although little data is available to guide the clinician.

THE EFFECT OF MOTIVATION ON LIVING WITH CHRONIC ILLNESS

Both aging and chronic illness may have profound effects on an individual's perception of control, competency, and autonomy. While self-determination depends upon the belief that outcomes are controllable, amotivation is associated with a perceived disconnection of behavior from outcomes (68). Vallerand et al. studied the relationship between level of motivation and quality of life in elderly nursing home residents. Intact intrinsic motivation was correlated with increased self-esteem, satisfaction with life, fulfillment, feelings of control, and less depression. Conversely, the presence of amotivation was correlated with reduced self-esteem, decreased satisfaction with life, the perception of loss of control, and reduced general health status. This vicious cycle of organic illness, depression, apathy, and helplessness (Figure 19-1) is often intractable to medical intervention, even when other disabling symptoms are relieved.

Motivational status is an important determinant of successful adjustment to stressful life events and illness. Patients with self-determination and motivation are more likely to deal with health problems in a more constructive manner. It is instructive to observe the common behaviors of PD patients with and without apathy syndromes. Patients with intact motivation are more likely to be proactive, searching out current information about medical and surgical interventions as well as new clinical research opportunities. These patients are more likely to expect to be consulted regarding clinical decision making and will often provide more detailed historical information. They may follow instructions more reliably and will often provide better feedback regarding their response to therapy. The motivated patient is more likely to seek out specialty consultation, to practice preventative medicine, and to make lifestyle choices regarding exercise, nutrition, and stress management that are designed to enhance their feelings of well-being. Conversely, the consequences of amotivation on self-management, lifestyle, socialization, family interaction, and community involvement are likely to result in a greater loss of functional status (69). Increased scrutiny of the relationships between apathy, disease severity, and quality of life may indeed identify apathy as a "red flag" associated with a poorer prognosis.

CONCLUSION

The determinants of an individual's motivational tendencies are likely to be a combination of factors: intrinsic personality traits (heredity), experiential learning (environment), and acquired conditions such as PD. Motivational behavior is an ongoing construct, continuously being remodeled by all of these influences. Clinical research studies are needed to identify effective therapies for apathy and amotivation associated with PD. Both pharmacologic and nonpharmacologic interventions are likely to be effective.

Management styles that foster autonomy and choice may accentuate the individual's sense of personal responsibility and control while authoritative styles may promote passivity and a sense of incompetence. The expectation of a person's active role in their daily management and long-range decision making preserves the individual's dignity and sense of self. As we become increasingly aware of the factors that determine quality of life, we are likely to discover that restoration of motor function is only one facet of restoring quality of life for patients with PD.

REFERENCES

1. Silva SJ, Marin RS. Apathy in neuropsychiatric disorders. *CNS Spectrums* 1999; 4:31–50.
2. Marin RS. Differential diagnosis of apathy and related disorders of diminished motivation. *Psychiatr Ann* 1997; 27:30–33.
3. Marin RS. Apathy: A neuropsychiatric syndrome. *J Neuropsychiatry Clin Neurosci* 1991; 3:243–254.
4. Marsden CD, Parkes JD. Success and problems of long-term levodopa therapy in Parkinson's disease. *Lancet* 1977; 1:345–349.
5. Marin RS. Differential diagnosis and classification of apathy. *Am J Psychiatry* 1990; 147:22–30.
6. Marin RS, Biedrzycki RC, Firinciogullari S. Reliability and validity of the apathy evaluation scale. *Psychiatry Res* 1991; 38:143–162.
7. Starkstein SE, Mayberg HS, Preziosi TJ, et al. Reliability, validity and clinical correlates of apathy in Parkinson's disease. *J Neuropsychiatry Clin Neurosci* 1992; 4:134–139.
8. Duffy JD. The neural substrates of motivation. *Psychiatr Ann* 1997; 27:24–29.
9. Levy ML, Cummings JL, Fairbanks LA, et al. Apathy is not depression. *J Neuropsychiatry Clin Neurosci* 1998; 10:314–319.
10. Mayeux R, Stern Y, Sano M, et al. Clinical and biochemical correlates of bradyphrenia in Parkinson's disease. *Neurology* 1987; 37:1130–1134.
11. Duffy JD, Kant R. Apathy secondary to neurologic disease. *Psychiatr Ann* 1997; 27:39–43.
12. Ott BR, Noto RB, Fogel BS. Apathy and loss of insight in Alzheimer's disease: A SPECT imaging study. *J Neuropsychiatry Clin Neurosci* 1996; 8:41–46.
13. Starkstein SE, Federoff JP, Price TR, et al. Apathy following cerebrovascular lesions. *Stroke* 1993; 24:1625–1630.
14. Helgason C, Wilbur A, Weiss A, et al. Acute pseudobulbar mutism due to discrete bilateral capsular infarction in the territory of the anterior choroidal artery. *Brain* 1988; 111:507–519.
15. Salloway SP, Malloy PF, Rogg J, et al. MRI and neuropsychological differences in early- and late-life-onset geriatric depression. *Neurology* 1996; 46:1567–1574.
16. Bechara A, Tranel D, Damasio H, et al. Failure to respond autonomically to anticipated future outcomes following damage to prefrontal cortex. *Cereb Cortex* 1996; 6:215–25.
17. Davidson RJ. Internet communication: *Washingtonpost. com.* Live online, 11/2/99.
18. Davidson RJ, Coe CC, Dolski I, et al. Individual differences in prefrontal activation asymmetry predict natural killer cell activity at rest and in response to challenge. *Brain Behav Immun* 1999; 13:93–108.
19. Davidson RJ, Abercrombie H, Nitschke JB, et al. Regional brain function, emotion and disorders of emotion. *Curr Opin Neurobiol* 1999; 9:228–234.
20. Perry TL, Wright JM, Berry K, et al. Dominantly inherited apathy, central hypoventilation, and Parkinson's syndrome: Clinical, biochemical, and neuropathologic studies of 2 new cases. *Neurology* 1990; 40:1882–1887.
21. Cloninger CR. A systematic method for clinical description and classification of personality variants: A proposal. *Arch Gen Psychiatry* 1987; 44:573–588.
22. Stellar JR, Stellar E. *The Neurobiology of Motivation and Reward.* New York: Springer-Verlag New York, 1985.
23. Hooks MS, Kalivas PW. Involvement of dopamine and excitatory amino acid transmission in novelty-induced motor activity. *J Pharmacol Exp Ther* 1994; 269:976–988.
24. Crow TJ. A map of rap mesencephalon for electrical self-stimulation. *Brain Res* 1972; 36:265–273.
25. Fray P, Dunnett S, Iverson S, et al. Nigral transplants reinnervating the dopamine-depleted neostriatum can sustain intracranial self-stimulation. *Science* 1983; 219:416–419.

26. Menza MA, Forman NE, Goldstein HS, et al. Parkinson's disease, personality and dopamine. *J Neuropsychiatry Clin Neurosci* 1990; 2:282–287.

27. Menza MA, Golbe LI, Cody RA, et al. Dopamine-related personality traits in Parkinson's disease. *Neurology* 1993; 43:505–508.

28. Todes CJ, Lees AJ. The pre-morbid personality of patients with Parkinson's disease. *J Neurol Neurosurg Psychiatry* 1985; 48:97–100.

29. Estough VM, Kempster PA, Stern GM, et al. Premorbid personality and idiopathic Parkinson's disease. In: Streifler MB, Korzyn AD, Melamed E, et al. (eds.). Parkinson's disease: anatomy, pathology, and therapy. *Advances in neurology* Vol 53. New York: Raven Press, 1990:335–337.

30. Poewe W, Karamat E, Kemmler GW, et al. The premorbid personality of patients with Parkinson's disease: A comparative study with healthy controls and patients with essential tremor. In: Streifler MB, Korczyn AD, Melamed E, et al. (eds.). Parkinson's disease: Anatomy, pathology and therapy. *Advances in neurology* Vol 53. New York: Raven Press, 1990:339–342.

31. Cloninger CR, Przybeck TR, Svrajuc DM. The tridimensional personality questionnaire: U.S. normative data. *Psychol Rep* 1991; 69:1047–1057.

32. Ebstein RP, Novick O, Umansky R, et al. Dopamine D4 receptor (D4DR) exon III polymorphism associated with the human personality trait of novelty seeking. *Nat Genet* 1996; 12:78–80.

33. Benjamin J, Li L, Patterson C, et al. Population and familial association between the D4 dopamine receptor gene and measures of novelty seeking. *Nat Genet* 1996; 12:81–84.

34. Jonsson EG, Nothen MM, Gustavsson P, et al. Lack of evidence for allelic association between personality traits and the dopamine D4 receptor gene polymorphisms. *Am J Psychiatry* 1997; 154:697–699.

35. Sullivan PF, Fifield WJ, Kennedy MA, et al. No association between novelty seeking and the type 4 dopamine receptor gene (DRD4) in two New Zealand samples. *Am J Psychiatry* 1998; 155:98–101.

36. American Psychiatric Association. *Diagnostic and Statistical Manual of Mental Disorders*, 4th ed., Washington, DC: American Psychiatric Association, 1994.

37. Marin RS, Firinciogullari S, Biedrzycki RC. Differences in the relationship between apathy and depression. *J Nerv Ment Dis* 1994; 182:235–239.

38. Levy ML, Miller BL, Cummings JL, et al. Alzheimer's disease and frontotemporal dementias: Behavioral distinctions. *Arch Neurol* 1996; 53:687–690.

39. Litvan I, Mega MS, Cummings JL, et al. Neuropsychiatric aspects of progressive supranuclear palsy. *Neurology* 1996; 47:1184–1189.

40. Krupp BH, Fogel BS. Motivational impairment in primary psychiatric and medical illness. *Psychiatr Ann* 1997; 27:34–38.

41. Gold MS, Pearsall HR. Hypothyroidism – or, is it depression? *Psychosomatics* 1983; 24:646–656.

42. Starkman MN, Schteingart DE. Neuropsychiatric manifestations of patients with Cushing's syndrome. *Arch Intern Med* 1981; 141:215–219.

43. Varadaraj R, Cooper AJ. Addison's disease presenting with psychiatric symptoms. *Am J Psychiatry* 1986; 143:553–554.

44. Navia BA, Jordan BD, Price RN. The AIDS-dementia complex I: Clinical features. *Ann Neurol* 1986; 19:517–524.

45. Holmes FP, Kaplan JE, Ganz NM, et al. Chronic fatigue syndrome: A working case definition. *Ann Intern Med* 1988; 108:387–389.

46. Andraeson NC. Negative symptoms in schizophrenia. *Arch Gen Psychiatry* 1982; 39:784–788.

47. Duffy JD. The neurology of alcoholic denial: Implications for assessment and treatment. *Can J Psychiatry* 1995; 40:257–263.

48. Gersten SP. Long term adverse effects of brief marijuana use. *J Clin Psychiatry* 1980; 41:60–61.

49. Kant R, Duffy JD, Pivovarnik A. Apathy following closed head injury. *J Neuropsychiatry Clin Neurosci* 1995; 7:425.

50. Berlin RM, Litovitz GL, Diaz M, et al. Sleep disorders on a psychiatric consultation service. *Am J Psychiatry* 1984; 141:582–584.

51. Katon W, Berg A, Robins AJ, et al. Depression: Medical utilization and somatization. *Western J Med* 1986; 144:564–568.

52. Perez-Estable EJ, Miranda J, Munoz RF, et al. Depression in medical patients. *Arch Intern Med* 1990; 150:1083–1088.

53. Schulberg HC, Saul M, McClelland M. Assessing depression in primary medical and psychiatric practices. *Arch Gen Psychiatry* 1985; 12:1164–1170.

54. Simon GE, Von Korff M. Recognition, management, and outcomes of depression in primary care. *Arch Fam Med* 1995; 4:99–105.

55. Shulman LM. Singer C, Leifert R, et al. The diagnostic accuracy of neurologists for anxiety, depression, fatigue and sleep disorders in Parkinson's disease. *Mov Disord* 1997; 12(suppl 1):127.

56. Covington EC. Depression and chronic fatigue in the patient with chronic pain. *Primary Care* 1991; 18:341–358.

57. Shulman LM, Singer C, Leifert R, et al. The comorbidity of the nonmotor symptoms of Parkinson's disease. *Ann Neurol* 1996; 40:536.

58. Campbell JJ, Duffy JD. Treatment strategies in amotivated patients. *Psychiatr Ann* 1997; 27:44–49.

59. Cole S, Raju M. Making the diagnosis of depression in the primary care setting. *Am J Med* 1996; 101(suppl 6A):10S–17S.

60. Krupp BH. Ethical considerations in apathy syndromes. *Psychiatr Ann* 1997; 27:50–54.

61. Jaffe GV. Depression in general practice: A clinical trial of a new psychomotor stimulant. *Practitioner* 1961; 186:492–495.

62. Darvill FT, Wooley S. Double-blind evaluation of methylphenidate (Ritalin) hydrochloride: Its use in

the management of institutionalized geriatric patients. *JAMA* 1959; 169:1739–1741.

63. Chiarello RJ, Cole JO. The use of psychostimulants in general psychiatry: A reconsideration. *Arch Gen Psychiatry* 1987; 44:286–295.

64. Masand PS, Tesar GE. Use of stimulants in medically ill. *Psychiatr Clin North Am* 1996; 19:515–547.

65. Marin RS, Fogel BS, Hawkins J, et al. Apathy: A treatable syndrome. *J Neuropsychiatry Clin Neurosci* 1995; 7:23–30.

66. Szegedi A, Hilbert A, Wetzel H, et al. Pramipexole, a dopaminergic agonist in major depression: Antidepressant effects and tolerability in an open label study with multiple doses. *Clin Neuropharmacol* 1997; 20:S36–S45.

67. Kaufer DI, Cummings JL, Christine D. Effect of tacrine on behavioral symptoms in Alzheimer's disease: An open-label study. *J Geriatr Psychiatry Neurol* 1996; 9:1–6.

68. Vallerand RJ, O'Connor BP, Hamel M. Motivation in later life: Theory and assessment. *Int J Aging Human Dev* 1995; 41:221–238.

69. Webster J, Grossberg G. Disinhibition, apathy, indifference, fatigability, complaining and negativism. *Int Psychogeriatr* 1996; 8(suppl 3):403–408.

20

Pathology

Kevin D. Barron, M.D.

Albany Medical College, Albany, New York

The histopathology of Parkinson's disease (paralysis agitans) (PD) is characterized by (1) a loss of neurons in the pigmented nuclei of the brainstem, particularly affecting the subnucleus (pars) compactus of the substantia nigra (SN), and (2) the occurrence, in nerve cells of the degenerating nuclei, of laminated cytoplasmic inclusions named after F.H. Lewy, who described them in 1912 (1). Nigral neuronal loss and the occurrence of Lewy bodies define the disease. The account that follows does not use the term *arteriosclerotic* parkinsonism since, in the opinion of the author and others too numerous to enumerate (2,3), there is no such entity. Postencephalitic parkinsonism, which is no longer seen, and certain conditions that do occur and may resemble Parkinson's disease clinically will be treated briefly. The term *Parkinson's disease* (PD) will be applied to both the idiopathic and the genetically determined examples of the disorder. The present state of our knowledge and experience indicate that familial cases of PD account for only a small minority (10–15%) of the total (4).

HISTORICAL DEVELOPMENT

Greenfield (5) relates that Meynert suggested in 1871 that parkinsonian tremor might be due to a lesion of the basal ganglia. In 1895 Brissaud postulated that the SN was the site of the lesion responsible for parkinsonism (5). Lewy (1), who discovered the characteristic intracytoplasmic inclusions and related them to PD, did not mention their occurrence in the SN (he actually found them initially in the substantia innominata and dorsal motor nucleus of vagus) but rather emphasized a finding of degeneration of the caudate and lenticular nuclei in parkinsonian brains. Tretiakoff reported his histopathologic investigations on idiopathic and postencephalitic parkinsonism in 1919 (6). He asserted the constancy of nigral lesions in both paralysis agitans (PD) and the postencephalitic form of parkinsonism. The latter disorder had appeared on the world scene with the outbreak of von Economo's encephalitis (encephalitis lethargica) during 1916–1917. There has been no verified recurrence of this form of encephalitis since 1930. It rarely produced an exact clinical replica of PD since tics and dystonic movements, long tract signs, oculogyric crises, and intellectual deficits were regular sequelae of the infection. Neurofibrillary degeneration of surviving nigral neurons was prominent in postencephalitic cases and Lewy bodies were absent. Also in postencephalitic Parkinsonism, although the substantia nigra (both pars reticulata and pars compacta) was particularly devastated, overt brain lesions were widespread and included the globus pallidus. These histopathologic differences between paralysis agitans and postencephalitic Parkinsonism notwithstanding, the possibility that PD had a basis in a subclinical encephalitis became popular and the importance of the Lewy body in defining paralysis agitans was contested for several decades (2). Lewy noted the usefulness of Mann and hematoxylin-eosin stains for microscopic visualization of his cytoplasmic bodies, and one wonders whether reliance by neuropathologists on the basic dyes of the Nissl technique hindered the early recognition of Lewy inclusions and subsequent appreciation of their importance.

In earlier literature, much was made of alteration in the caudate and lenticular nuclei in PD, such as diminution in number and size of the large neurons (5) of these structures. However, there is agreement today that basal ganglion histology in PD does not differ from that of age-matched controls (2,5), despite the fact that dopamine depletion in the caudoputamen is both the paramount neurochemical abnormality of PD and a signature of the progressive deterioration of the dopaminergic nigrostriatal pathway that constantly accompanies the disease. The papers of Beheim-Schwarzbach in 1952 (7) and Greenfield and

Bosanquet in 1953 (2) established the essentiality of the lesion of the SN and the occurrence of Lewy bodies in the neuropathologic definition of paralysis agitans.

HISTOPATHOLOGY

Nerve Cell Death and Neuroglial Reaction

The constant lesion (2,7,8), manifest to qualitative microscopic scanning, lies in the subnucleus pars compactus of the substantia nigra where there is an evident loss of the melanin-bearing, pigmented nerve cells and an apparent increase in the neuroglial population (Figures 20-1, 20-2). The loss of pigmented neurons causes, in cases of moderate or greater duration and severity, a readily recognized diminution of the ordinarily dark, highly visible coloration of the substantia nigra (SN) and locus ceruleus (LC). Pallor of the SN and LC characterizes the macroscopic appearance of the parkinsonian brain (Figures 20-1, 20-4). Microscopically, astrocytes in affected areas are enlarged and fibril-rich while microglial nuclei (Figure 20-5) are markedly increased in number (9). Other histologic features include melanin granules, which lie extracellularly in the neuropil or within macrophages, and the occurrence of neuropilar axonal spheroids (Figure 20-5), sometimes associated with hemosiderin granules. The microglia are of the activated-reactive type (9,10) and express MHC Class II antigens. The potential of this cell for cytotoxic activity is notable (10) and may contribute to the neuronal loss that, in the compact

subnucleus, has been estimated to range from 50 to 85% (4,11,12). If the microglial response is indicative of a harmful, immunologically determined inflammatory response, therapeutic intervention for its suppression might have beneficial impact on the course of PD. Astrocytic changes in the SN of PD also are noteworthy because of the importance of astrocyte–neuron interactions for the survival of the latter (13).

The neuronal loss referred to above is pertinent to consideration of aging as a contributory factor in the causation of PD. McGeer and colleagues (14) reported that aging was associated with a significant loss of nigral neurons. However, the refined counting methods applied by B. Pakkenberg et al. (12) did not confirm the findings of McGeer's laboratory.

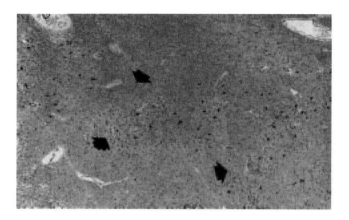

FIGURE 20-2.

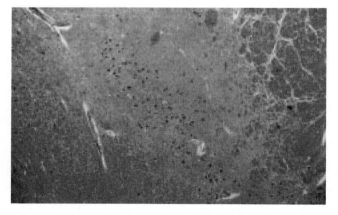

FIGURE 20-3. Figures 20-2 and 20-3 were made from paraffin section of, respectively, normal and parkinsonian brain stained with hematoxylin-eosin. The pigmented neurons of SN, subnucleus compactus, are readily visible at this low magnification. In parkinsonian tissue, note areas of neuronal loss and gliosis (arrows); and close examination will show minute dark clusters of free pigment in the neuropil, e.g., proximate to the large right hand arrow. 50x approx.

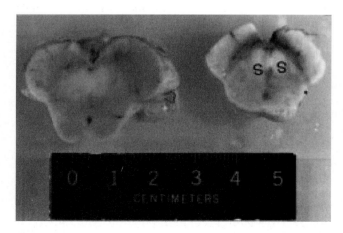

FIGURE 20-1. The normal brain slice lies on the right and the dark line of the substantia nigra (S), subnucleus compactus, is readily visible, but on the left side the midbrain slice of a parkinsonian brain has virtually no dark nigral pigmentation to display.

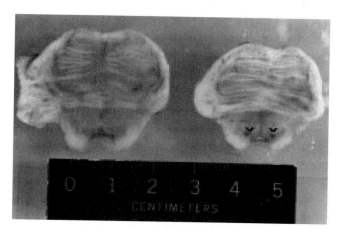

FIGURE 20-4. The locus ceruleus of the right hand brain slice (arrows) through the rostral pons is readily apparent, but there is virtually no grossly visible pigmentation on the left side where a brain slice at the some pontine level derives from a PD brain.

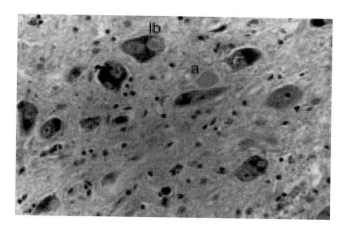

FIGURE 20-5. Compact subnucleus, paraffin section, PD tissue. Note Lewy body (lb) and axonal spheroid (a). One Marinesco body is marked (arrow) and many dark elongated microglial nuclei are present. Hematoxylin-eosin. Approx 450x.

Neuronal loss in PD is not limited to brainstem aggregates of pigmented neurons. The nonpigmented zona reticulata of the SN is also depleted severely of nerve cells as is the dorsal raphe nucleus, the basal nucleus of Meynert (substantia innominata), and the dorsal motor nucleus of the vagus (4,11,12,15,16). In the vagal nucleus, indeed, pigmented and sensory neurons are spared – only motor nerve cells are involved (15). Zweig and colleagues (17) reported loss of cholinergic neurons from the pedunculopontine nucleus. There the degree of nerve cell diminution paralleled that observed in the pigmented neuronal population of the nigral zona compacta. From the list given it should be apparent that, although the

biochemical hallmark of the neurochemical pathology of PD is depletion of dopamine in the corpus striatum, neuronal populations affected in the disease are all of dopaminergic, noradrenergic, serotoninergic, and cholinergic types. Hypothalamic dopaminergic neurons are however, spared (18).

The Lewy Body

These cytoskeletal, cytoplasmic inclusions, although present in normal aging (7,19), occur invariably in the brainstem of cases of PD where their presence in neurons of LC and SN is a sine qua non for the diagnosis. Even when they are present in brains of people presumed to have been neurologically asymptomatic during life, their occurrence raises the possibility that they represent a preclinical pathologic change. Indeed, search of the clinical records of Forno's 50 "incidental cases" found reference to extrapyramidal phenomena in more than 1/5 of her autopsied subjects (19).

The archetype of the Lewy body occurs in brainstem sites. It is round or spherical in shape, generally 5 to 30 μm in diameter and characterized by a central hyaline core, which is acidophilic in hematoxylin−eosin stains, and is surrounded by a pale halo (Figure 20-5). Lewy bodies may be multilamellated (Figure 20-6). In sites other than the brainstem and diencephalon, where the typical lamellated appearance predominates, a peripheral halo may be absent, the shape of the body may be cylindrical, and the location may be intraaxonal or intradendritic. Rarely, the bodies are extracellular. denHartog Jager and Bethlem (20) list 21 nuclei in which they found Lewy bodies. Rarely two or more Lewy bodies occurred within a single

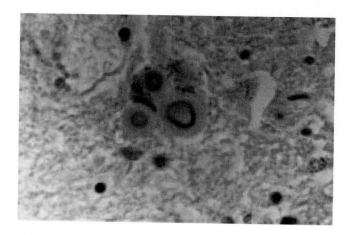

FIGURE 20-6. A nigral neuron of a PD brain contains three Lewy bodies that are trilaminated. Hematoxylin-eosin, paraffin section. Approx 900x.

neuron (Figure 20-6). In the brainstem, Lewy bodies are by no means limited to pigmented neurons. In the dorsal motor nucleus of the vagus, Lewy bodies occur predominantly in nonpigmented neurons (15,19). Lewy bodies occur also in the cerebral cortex (Figure 20-7) and the lateral horn of the thoracic spinal cord (20,21). In the cerebral cortex, the cingulate gyrus, the superior temporal gyrus and the subiculum and adjacent temporal gray matter are favored sites. In cortical locations Lewy bodies may lack a halo and appear as rounded homogeneously acidophilic structures. Additionally, Lewy bodies are numerous in the peripheral autonomic ganglia and alimentary nerve plexuses where they take a more serpiginous form (20,22,23). They have been described also in peripheral autonomic nerve fibers (24). In PD, cytoplasmic inclusions also occur in cells of the adrenal medulla referred to as "adrenal bodies." These inclusions are said to be "virtually specific" for the disease, although they are different histochemically from Lewy bodies (25). They contain sphingomyelin, free fatty acids, and polysaccharides.

Lewy bodies are usually unstained with basic dyes, such as toluidine blue and thionin although they may display metachromatic reactions with basic dyes when wet-mounted (2). They differ from Pick bodies in that the latter have no central core and, in contrast to Lewy bodies, are strongly argyrophilic; Lewy bodies stain faintly with silver methods or not at all. In trichrome stains Lewy bodies have a brilliantly red central core. Histochemical studies indicate the presence of sphingomyelin (26). Staining reactions for carbohydrates, including the PAS method, and for nucleic acids are negative (8). Histochemical reactions do indicate the presence of proteins containing aromatic alpha amino acids.

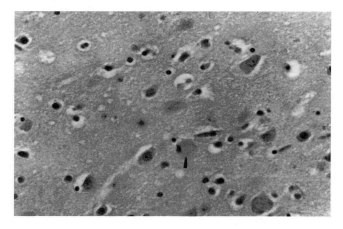

FIGURE 20-7. A neuron of the cingulate cortex of a PD brain contains a Lewy body. Hematoxylin-eosin, paraffin section. Approx 300x.

Electron microscopically, Lewy bodies in the brainstem have an electron-dense amorphous core surrounded by randomly arranged or outward-radiating filaments and, most external in location, melanin granules. Ultrastructural features of the bodies were first described by Duffy and Tennyson (27). The filaments vary in diameter between 7–12 nm and may appear fragmented. Circular profiles, electron-lucent vesicles, and dark granules may be included in the core. The Lewy bodies of peripheral autonomic structures vary considerably in structural composition and are often located within neurites (22,23,24). Inclusion of "twisted tubules" (paired helical filaments) in the periphery of Lewy bodies is described in locus ceruleus of aged human brain (28) and in nerve cell processes of hypothalamus in a case of presenile dementia (29).

The immunohistochemistry of Lewy bodies is of major interest and importance. Galloway et al. examined immunostaining properties of Lewy bodies for cytoskeletal proteins (30). In contrast to senile plaques and neurofibrillary tangles, Lewy bodies are tau negative, effectively. They react readily with most antibodies to neurofilament and microtubular proteins (including microtubule-associated proteins, or MAPs, and tubulin) and also react with monoclonal antibodies that recognize neurofibrillary tangles (30). Positivity of Lewy bodies in stains for neuronal cytoskeletal proteins is marked by a dense ring of staining. Both phosphorylated and nonphosphorylated neurofilament antigens of the three major subtypes of neurofilament protein are recognized. Ubiquitin antibodies stain Lewy inclusions intensely and diffusely and provide an excellent histologic method for their routine display (Figure 20-8).

The discovery that families with PD have a mutation in the alpha-synuclein gene (31) may prove to have crucial significance. In sporadic and familial PD, Lewy bodies contain immunohistochemically demonstrable alpha synuclein but not the beta form of this cytoskeletal protein (32,33). The exact mechanism by which alpha synuclein accumulation relates to neuronal degeneration in PD (and Lewy body dementia) is obscure presently but research on the matter is aggressively being pursued. The function of alpha synuclein is not known. In normal brain it is localized at axonal terminals (33).

Commentary on the cytology of Lewy bodies will conclude with brief reference to other cytoplasmic neuronal inclusions. The protein-rich cytoplasmic bodies described in perikarya and dendrites of SN and LC neurons by Issidorides and coworkers (35) are stained metachromatically and intensely by a

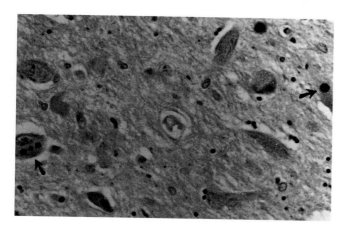

FIGURE 20-8. Neurons of nucleus basalis, PD brain, paraffin section stained for ubiquitin. Note densely stained Lewy bodies in neurons (arrows) at margins of field. Three are present in one cell. Approx 400x.

phosphotungstic acid technique that detects proteins rich in free basic amino acid groups. The cores of Lewy bodies may stain similarly. The PTAH-positive structures occur in abundance in normal SN but their numbers are notably reduced in Parkinsonian tissue. Marinesco bodies (36) are brightly eosinophilic, nonlamellated, intranuclear inclusions (Figure 20-5) of no known pathologic significance. They are differentiated easily from Lewy bodies. The colloid bodies of normal neuronal cytoplasm are homogeneously eosinophilic proteinaceous structures that may distend the cell body (37). They are commonly encountered in motor nerve cells, especially those of the hypoglossal nucleus.

Platelet Pathology

Blood platelets have characteristics that are similar to catecholaminergic neurons because of their ability to manufacture, store, and release monoamines. Morphologic abnormalities have been described in platelets in PD using electron microscopy that may have some specificity (62). In both treated and untreated patients large intracytoplasmic vacuoles formed from the open canulicular system were the main changes. Morphometric measures of the area and volume percent of the platelets that these vacuoles encompassed supported the conclusion that these abnormalities were significant when compared to non Parkinsonian controls. There were no abnormalities in the mitochondria, storage granules, or glycogen. In addition to these morphologic changes, alterations in platelet mitochondrial complex I and MAO B activities as well as alterations in dopamine reuptake have been described (62). Although structural changes in platelets

have been described in Alzheimer's disease (62a), they were clearly different from those described in PD.

Neurochemical Pathology

The discovery in 1960 that dopamine levels are reduced in the corpus striatum in PD (38) led to the first rational therapy for the disease. Tyrosine hydroxylase and levodopa-decarboxylase activities and the markers for the dopamine transporter are also reduced (39). Greater reduction of dopamine levels in putamen than in the caudate nucleus reflects the fact that there is greater loss of neurons in the laterally placed nuclei of the SN. These normally project to the putamen, whereas more medially placed neurons of the zona compacta project to the caudate nucleus. It is estimated that dopamine levels must be reduced by more than 60 to 80% from the normal before clinical expression of PD results. With severe dopamine depletion of more than 90%, the number of D2 dopamine receptor sites in the PD striatum increases (39) – a fact that may relate to the usefulness of D2 receptor agonist treatment even in late stages of the disease. In addition to dopamine, other neurotransmitter levels are reduced in PD brain. Choline acetylase and acetylcholine levels are significantly lower in cerebral cortex and nucleus basalis while neuropeptide concentrations are lowered in the striatum and there are variable losses of norepinephrine and serotonin (4,39). GABA levels are increased (39). The loss of acetylcholine in the cerebral cortex is a result of degeneration of the widely projecting cholinergic neurons of the nucleus basalis.

An intriguing abnormality of the Parkinsonian brain is an overall increase in iron content that occurs despite a generalized reduction in brain ferritin. Specifically, the ferritin content of SN is reduced although iron content is increased (41). Ferritin-bound iron is chemically inactive. Non-ferritin-bound iron is potentially toxic and capable of catalyzing free radical formation thereby promoting oxidative stress. The finding in parkinsonian brain of a decrease in nigral reduced glutathione levels coupled with an increase in iron and products of lipid peroxidation supports the oxidant stress hypothesis of the causation of PD (42). Systemic iron metabolism may also be abnormal (43). (See Chapter 28 for details of this process).

Modern cytochemical methods for in situ examination of tissue deoxyribonucleic acid (DNA) have been applied to the question of whether apoptosis is a mechanism of cell death in PD (see Chapter 29 for details). In situ end-labeling of DNA fragments such as is demonstrable during apoptotic cell death was found by Tompkins and Hill (44) in neurons of the SN of PD brains. An antiubiquitin antibody for colocalization of Lewy bodies was applied in conjunction with the in situ DNA method. Apoptotic-like changes occurred in neurons independently of the presence of Lewy bodies and were found in SN in both normal and diseased brain (45). Using fluorescent double-labeling methods, Tatton et al. (46) also found indication that dopaminergic neurons of the SN die via apoptosis in PD. However, Banati et al. (47) found no evidence of nigral neuronal apoptosis. They used in situ end-labeling of DNA fragments and employed biotinylated dUTP and terminal deoxynucleotidyl transferase (TdT) and studied 10 brains with pathologically proven PD. They stressed the prominence of microglial activation in the SN in PD. Microglial reactivity was independent of the disease duration and was florid even in the presence of severe nerve cell loss.

DEMENTIA AND PD

The emphasis that James Parkinson placed on "the senses and intellects being uninjured" (48) in PD cannot be supported by modern experience (49). For a detailed discussion of dementia and parkinsonism, see chapters 15 and 16. The pathoanatomic basis for the frequency of dementia, especially in the later stages of the disorder, is varied. A major cause is the apparent increased incidence of Alzheimer's disease (AD) in parkinsonians (3,50). About 25% of brains with histopathologic features sufficient by accepted criteria for the neuropathologic diagnosis of Alzheimer's disease have Lewy bodies in cortical and subcortical distribution (50,51). Conversely, a majority of brains with a diffuse distribution of Lewy bodies has a burden of neuritic and diffuse neocortical plaques sufficient by CERAD (Consortium to Establish a Registry for Alzheimer's Disease) criteria to allow a diagnosis of Alzheimer's disease (52). Even allowing for the facts that (1) Parkinson's disease and Alzheimer's disease are common afflictions of the senium and thus may occur together by chance and (2) Lewy bodies occur in the "normal" senile cerebrum, there is still a significant association between Alzheimer's and Parkinson's diseases. The overlap between both clinical and histopathologic features of these conditions (50) appears to account for most cases of dementia in PD. However, a proportion of cases of progressive degenerative dementia with Parkinsonian features have cortical and brain stem Lewy bodies but show senile plaque counts no greater than age-matched controls (52). These account for a postulated separate entity, diffuse Lewy body disease (52,53). Neurofibrillary tangles, an important histopathologic correlate of dementia in AD, are less frequent in the diffuse Lewy body group (52,54). The issue of whether diffuse Lewy body disease and Alzheimer's dementia with Lewy bodies are separate entities is discussed in Chapter 16.

Another cause of dementia in PD is neuronal loss in the medial SN and adjacent ventral tegmental area (49,55,56). For these cases, Torack and Morris suggested the term *mesolimbocortical dementia* because of the particular affection of medial mesencephalic dopaminergic neurons, especially those of the ventral tegmental area, that project to the hippocampus, amygdala, and entorhinal and cingulate cortex, and orbitofrontal area (55). Four of the six cases described in the 1988 report (56), all autopsied, lacked Lewy bodies.

CAUSATION

Environmental Toxins

A major event in the search for an etiology of PD was the discovery that the pyridine compound 1-methyl-4-phenyl-1,2,3,6-tetrahydropyridine (MPTP), a byproduct of illicit synthesis of meperidine, is a neurotoxin that selectively destroys the substantia nigra in humans and primates and produces a parkinsonian syndrome quite similar to PD (57,58). The metabolite, MPP+, a product of the enzymatic action of monoamine oxidase B on MPTP, is the direct agent of the neurotoxic effect of MPTP (59) and acts as a mitochondrial poison. Systemic administration of MPTP to monkeys induces a parkinsonian state that, with appropriate dosage schedules, involves both SN and locus ceruleus and produces eosinophilic bodies within neurons (58, 60) that resemble Lewy bodies both in their distribution within the brain and in their ultrastructure. However, the constituent filaments of the MPTP-induced bodies are arranged in bundles rather than randomly oriented as in PD (60).

The MPTP story has raised the possibility that an environmental toxin may be responsible for sporadic PD. Even in genetically determined cases an environmental factor may be at work (61). Alterations in blood platelet morphology and function that accompany PD (62) might also indicate the presence of an environmental agent that acts to produce the disease. Chronic occupational exposure to metals, including combinations of lead-copper, lead-iron, and iron-copper seem to be significantly associated with paralysis agitans (63). The oxidant stress hypothesis of PD causation (42) is compatible with the theory that an environmental toxin is primary. Biochemical phenomena that accompany oxidant stress include decreased activity of the mitochrondrial enzyme NADH-CoQ reductase that occurs also in MPTP poisoning where it is associated with increased superoxide anion radical formation that is damaging to tissue (42,59). Chapter 30 provides details on MPTP intoxication and the syndrome that results.

Heredity

Another recent finding important to the understanding of the etiology of PD is the identification of large kindreds that exhibit inheritance of the disease in autosomal dominant fashion (61). The familial PD patients at autopsy have brain pathology typical of cases of sporadic occurrence of the disease including the presence of Lewy bodies in the usual locations. The families referred to derive from Contursi, Italy, and Greece. The mutation that accounts for the disease resides in the gene encoding for alpha synuclein, located on chromosome 4q (31). Also described recently is an autosomal-recessive chromosome 6q-linked juvenile form of parkinsonism with neuronal loss and gliosis limited to the SN and LC. Lewy bodies are absent (64). This gene has been referred to as "Parkin" (62a). Gibb et al. (65) have described a familial case of juvenile-onset parkinsonism with nigral degeneration and intraneuronal Lewy bodies. Inheritance was probably autosomal dominant. Hereditary PD accounts for 10 to 15% of cases of the disease (4). For further details on the familial forms of PD, see Chapter 52.

Trauma and Other Causes

Whether head trauma can cause or provoke the onset of PD (as distinct from parkinsonism) or permanently aggravate the symptoms and signs of PD is a medicolegally and societally significant problem in our litigious country. Parkinson (48) considered a traumatic etiology but believed the site and source of the trauma to locate at the upper cervical spine and to affect the spinal cord and medulla oblongata. The subject of posttraumatic Parkinsonism has been reviewed by Factor (66). One can reasonably conclude that Parkinsonism must rarely indeed be induced by head trauma (66,67), although the neurologic sequelae of head trauma may include parkinsonian features, particularly bradykinesia, rigidity, dysarthria, and gait impairment. Often, however, tremor is absent and clinical phenomena such as Babinski signs, dystonia, and limb ataxia, are unlike those encountered in PD. Similarly, there is no evidence that trauma can produce permanent worsening of preexistent PD. The author however has seen one case of head trauma with unconsciousness occurring at about the age of 30, where complete recovery of consciousness ensued in 20 minutes to be followed three months later by hemi-parkinsonian rigidity and tremor. There was gradual progression thereafter to a clinical state indistinguishable from sporadic PD including

motor fluctuations and dyskinesia. The man's bilateral parkinsonian condition has been levodopa responsive and unassociated with long tract signs, dementia, and atacia and he remains ambulatory more than 25 years after the traumatic event. Pugilistic parkinsonism has typically a resting tremor in addition to bradykinesis, rigidity, and postural changes dysarthria but Babinski signs, cerebellar ataxia, dementia, and seizures are often present and together with the history of pugilism allow ready diagnosis. In the brains of affected pugilists, neurofibrillary tangle formation, absence of Lewy bodies, and cell loss in the SN are significant findings (66,67).

Rarely, mass lesions and infarcts of vascular origin that involve the SN (5,68) may cause a neurologic deficit very similar to but not identical with PD. Neurologic deficits may be on the same side as the nigral lesion.

OTHER DISEASES ASSOCIATED WITH PARKINSONIAN SYMPTOMATOLOGY

Parkinsonism-Dementia Complex of the Mariana Islands

Histopathologically, the Parkinsonism-dementia complex of Guam differs from PD in the absence of Lewy bodies, the presence of cell loss throughout the medial and lateral portions of the SN, the widespread occurrence of neurofibrillary tangles, which invariably affect nigral neurons, and an obvious loss of nerve cells from the globus pallidus evident to qualitative light microscopic study (69). Senile plaques were originally reported to be few or absent but this aspect may need reappraisal (70). The disorder is commonly associated with a syndrome indistinguishable clinically from amyotrophic lateral sclerosis and may be related to an environmental toxin (71).

Progressive Supranuclear Palsy (PSP)

PSP (Steele-Richardson-Olszewski syndrome) is readily distinguished from PD histopathologically. Although the SN is severely affected by neuronal loss and astrogliosis in this disease, the conspicuous nerve cell loss and glial reaction in the pallidum, tectum, and periaqueductal gray and the characteristic argyrophilic, intracytoplasmic, globose neurofibrillary tangles in surviving neurons readily identify the disorder (72). Lewy bodies are absent. Clinically, at onset, PSP may mimic PD without tremor. However, supranuclear ophthalmoplegia is a defining accompaniment of the disease (72) and, together with early balance problems allows clinical diagnosis early in the course.

Multiple System Atrophy (MSA)

MSA is a disorder that is associated separately or concurrently with (1) olivopontocerebellar atrophy (OPCA), (2) degeneration of craniospinal and peripheral autonomic nuclei (with OPCA constituting Shy-Drager syndrome) and (3) striatonigral degeneration. MSA may, at onset, mimic PD without tremor but typically is unresponsive to levodopa therapy. All three components of MSA are not necessarily present in a given brain. When striatonigral degeneration is present, magnetic resonance imaging studies may show signal abnormality in the lenticular nuclei indicative of iron deposition, thus aiding clinical diagnosis. MSA is largely, but not exclusively, sporadic. In the striatonigral form of MSA, the formalin-fixed brain shows pallor of the SN accompanied by shrinkage and green discoloration of the lenticular nuclei. The SN, putamen, and caudate are sites of severe neuronal loss and fibrillary astrogliosis. Especially when OPCA is present, highly (but not exclusively) characteristic cytoplasmic inclusions abound in oligodendroglia and some neurons (73). Primarily cytoplasmic, although sometimes observed in cell nuclei and processes, these so called inclusions are ubiquitinated, argyrophilic, and tau- and alpha and beta tubulin-positive immunohistochemically (73). They also contain alpha-synuclein (74,75). These characteristic bodies do occur in hereditary cases (74). Ultrastructurally, the inclusions consist of tubular profiles that have a "fuzzy cover" and side extensions similar to the cytoplasmic structures encountered in motor neuron disease (73). In the putamen in striatonigral degeneration, hypertrophied astroglia contain iron-positive lipofuscin granules that probably account for the green color of the striatum after formalin fixation (76).

Miscellany

Huntington's disease is a genetically determined, progressive, and degenerative condition inherited in autosomal dominant pattern. The defective gene lies on the short arm of chromosome 4 (3). This disease may cause a rigid akinetic syndrome but factors such as familial occurrence, early age of onset, concurrent dementia, and neuroimaging evidence of neostriatal atrophy should permit its identification clinically. The neurohistology is remarkably different from PD. There is striking neuronal loss and reactive fibrillary astrogliosis in the caudoputamen. Cerebral cortex, subthalamic body, and other sites are also affected (37). Microglial hypertrophy and hyperplasia are remarkably absent. Huntington's disease is another example of the strikingly different responses of microglial and astroglial cells in different degenerative diseases of the brain.

Carbon monoxide intoxication can produce a clinical syndrome indistinguishable from PD (77) as this author's own experience has several times attested, but this is a very rare occurrence and the pathology consists of nigropallidal cavitary necrosis in the absence of Lewy bodies.

At onset, Wilson's disease may present parkinsonian features, such as rigidity, tremor, and disorder of gait, but the addition of other features, such as dystonia, Kayser-Fleischer ring, and the youth of the patient together with hepatic abnormalities and a low serum ceruloplasmin level should promptly lead to diagnosis. The distinctive pathology of Wilson's disease (37) includes cavitary necrosis of the lenticular nuclei and proliferation of Alzheimer type II astroglia in gray matter throughout the brain.

Lubag, an X-linked recessive disorder of dystonia and parkinsonism with onset between the second and sixth decade is another example of Parkinsonism plus. It has been characterized as a progressive neurodegenerative disease and Parkinsonian features include tremor, rigidity, bradykinesia, and postural instability. The dystonia is usually craniocervical in distribution but can involve any muscle group. Pathology is characteristic and consists of a mosaic pattern of gliosis with neuronal loss in the gliotic strands and normal islands of tissue between them in the neostriatum. The large striatal neurons are spared in the affected regions (14). The substantia nigra is unaffected by this disease. Lubag can be easily distinguished clinically and pathologically from PD.

REFERENCES

1. Lewy FH. Paralysis agitans. I. Pathologische Anatomie. In: Lewandowsky M (ed.). *Handbuch der neurologie.* Berlin: Springer J, 1912:920–933.
2. Greenfield JG, Bosanquet FD. The brain-stem lesions in Parkinsonism. *J Neurol Neurosurg Psychiatry* 1953; 16:213–226.
3. Adams RD, Victor M. Parkinson disease (Paralysis agitans) In: Ropper AH (eds.). *Principles of Neurology.* 6th ed. New York: McGraw-Hill, 1997:1067–1075.
4. DeArmond SJ, Dickson DW, DeArmond B. Degenerative diseases of the nervous system. In: Davis RL, Robertson DM (eds.). *Textbook of Neuropathology.* 3rd ed. Baltimore: Williams and Wilkins, Baltimore, 1997:1063–1178.
5. Greenfield JG. The pathology of Parkinson's disease. In: Critchley M (ed.). *James Parkinson (1755–1824).* London: MacMillan & Co., 1955:219–243.
6. Tretiakoff C. Contribution a l'etude de l'anatomie pathologic du locus niger de soemmering avec quelques deductions relative a la pathogenie des

troubles du tonus musculaire et de la maladie de Parkinson. *These pour le doctorat en Medicine.* Paris: These de Paris, 1919:1–24.

7. Beheim-Schwarzbach D. Uber zelleib-veranderungen in nucleus coeruleus bei Parkinson-symptomen. *J Nerv Ment Dis* 1952; 116:619–632.

8. Bethlem J, denHartog-Jager WA. The incidence and characteristics of Lewy bodies in idiopathic paralysis agitans (Parkinson's disease). *J Neurol Neurosurg Psychiatry* 1960; 23:74–80.

9. McGeer PL, Kawamata T, Walker DG, et al. Microglia in degenerative neurological disease. *Glia* 1993; 7:84–92.

10. Barron KD. The microglial cell. A historical review. *J Neurol Sci* 1995; 134 (Suppl):57–68.

11. Jellinger K. Overview of morphological changes in Parkinson's disease. *Adv Neurol* 1986; 45:1–18.

12. Pakkenberg B, Moller A, Gundersen HJG, et al. The absolute number of nerve cells in substantia nigra in normal subjects and in patients with Parkinson's disease estimated with an unbiased stereological method. *J Neurol Neurosurg Psychiatry* 1991; 54:30–34.

13. Factor SA, Barron KD. Mosaic pattern of gliosis in the neostriatum of a North American man with a craniocervical dystonia and Parkinsonism. *Mov Disord* 1997; 12:783–789.

14. McGeer PL, McGeer EG, Suzuki JS. Aging and extrapyramidal function. *Arch Neurol* 1977; 34:33–35.

15. Eadie MJ. The pathology of certain medullary nuclei in Parkinsonism. *Brain* 1963; 86:781–792.

16. Nakano I, Hirano A. Parkinson's disease: Neuron loss in the nucleus basalis without concomitant Alzheimer's disease. *Ann Neurol* 1984; 15:415–418.

17. Zweig RM, Jankel WR, Hedreen JC, et al. The pedunculopontine nucleus in Parkinson's disease. *Ann Neurol* 1989; 26:41–46.

18. Matzuk MM, Saper CB. Preservation of hypothalamic dopaminergic neurons in Parkinson's disease. *Ann Neurol* 1985; 18:552–555.

19. Forno LS. Concentric hyalin intraneuronal inclusion of Lewy type in the brains of elderly persons (50 incidental cases); Relationship to Parkinsonism. *J Am Geriatr Soc* 1969; 17:557–575.

20. denHartog-Jager WA, Bethlem J. The distribution of Lewy bodies in the central and peripheral autonomic nervous systems in idiopathic paralysis agitans. *J Neurol Neurosurg Psychiatry* 1960; 23:283–290.

21. Pollanen MS, Dickson DW, Bergeron C. Pathology and biology of the Lewy body. *J Neuropathol Exp Neurol* 1993; 52:183–191.

22. Forno LS, Norville RL. Ultrastructure of Lewy bodies in the stellate ganglion. *Acta Neuropathol* 1976; 34:183–197.

23. Wakabayashi K, Takahashi H, Takeda S, et al. Parkinson's disease: The presence of Lewy bodies in Auerbach's and Meissner's plexuses. *Acta Neuropathol* 1988; 76:217–221.

24. Iwanaga K, et al. Lewy-body type degeneration in cardiac plexus in Parkinson's and incidental Lewy body disease. *Neurology* 1999; 52:1269–1271.

25. denHartog-Jager WA. Histochemistry of adrenal bodies in Parkinson's disease. *Arch Neurol* 1970; 23:528–533.

26. denHartog-Jager, WA. Sphingomyelin in Lewy inclusion bodies in Parkinson's disease. *Arch Neurol* 1969; 21:615–619.

27. Duffy PE, Tennyson VM. Phase and electron microscopic observations of Lewy bodies and melanin granules in the substantia nigra and locus coeruleus in Parkinson's disease. *J Neuropathol Exp Neurol* 1965; 24:398–414.

28. Tomonaga M. Neurofibrillary tangles and Lewy bodies in the locus ceruleus neurons of the aged brains. *Acta Neuropathol* 1981; 53:165–168.

29. Forno LS, Barbour PJ, Norville RL. Presenile dementia with Lewy bodies and neurofibrillary tangles. *Arch Neurol* 1978; 35:818–822.

30. Galloway PG, Grundke-Iqbal I, Iqbal K, et al. Lewy bodies contain epitopes both shared and distinct from Alzheimer neurofibrillary tangles. *J Neuropathol Exp Neurol* 1988; 47:654–663.

31. Polymeropoulos MH, Lavedan C, Leroy E, et al. Alpha-synuclein gene identified in families with Parkinson's disease. *Science* 1997; 724:1197–1199.

32. Spillantini MG, Schmidt LL, Lee VM-Y, et al. Mutation in the alpha-synuclein in Lewy bodies. *Nature* 1997; 338:839–840.

33. Trojanowski JQ, Lee VM-Y. Aggregation of neurofilament and alpha-synuclein proteins in Lewy bodies. *Arch Neurol* 1998; 55:151–152.

34. Goedert M. The awakening of alpha-synuclein. *Nature* 1997; 338:232–233.

35. Issidorides MR, Mytilineou C, Whetsell WO Jr, et al. Protein-rich cytoplasmic bodies of substantia nigra and locus ceruleus. A comparative study in Parkinsonian and normal brain. *Arch Neurol* 1978; 35:633–637.

36. Leestma JE, Andrews JM. The fine structure of the Marinesco body. *Arch Pathol* 1969; 88:431–436.

37. Nelson JS, Parisi JE, Schochet SS, Jr. *Principles and Practice of Neuropathology.* St. Louis: Mosby, 1993.

38. Ehringer H, Hornykiewicz O. Verteilung von noradrenalin und dopamin (3-hydroxytyramin) ingehirn des menschen und ihr verhalten bei erkrankungen des extrapyramidalen systems. *Klin Wochenschr* 1960; 38:1236–1239.

39. Hornykiewicz O. Biochemical aspects of Parkinson's disease. *Neurology* 1998; 51 (Suppl 2):S2–S9.

40. Scherman D, Desnos C, Darchen F, et al. Striatal dopamine deficiency in Parkinson's disease: Role of aging. *Ann Neurol* 1989; 26:551–557.

41. Dexter DT, Carayan A, Javoy-Agid F, et al. Alterations in the level of iron, ferritin and other trace metals in Parkinson's disease and other neurodegenerative diseases affecting the basal ganglia. *Brain* 1991; 114:1953–1975.

42. Fahn S, Cohen G. The oxidant stress hypothesis in Parkinson's disease: Evidence supporting it. *Ann Neurol* 1992; 32:804–812.

43. Logroscino G, Marder K, Graziano J, et al. Altered systemic iron metabolism in Parkinson's disease. *Neurology* 1997; 49:714–717.

44. Tompkins MM, Hill WD. Contribution of somal Lewy bodies to neuronal death. *Brain Res* 1997; 775:24–29.

45. Tompkins MM, Basgall EJ, Zamrini E, et al. Apoptotic-like changes in Lewy-body-associated disorders and normal aging in substantia nigral neurons. *Am J Pathol* 1997; 150:119–131.

46. Tatton NA, Maclean-Fraser A, Tatton WG, et al. A fluorescent double-labeling method to detect and confirm apoptotic nuclei in Parkinson's disease. *Ann Neurol* 1998; 44(Suppl 1):S142–S148.

47. Banati RB, Daniel SE, Blunt SB. Glial pathology but absence of apoptotic nigral neurons in long-standing Parkinson's disease. *Mov Disord* 1998; 13:865–870.

48. Parkinson J. *An Essay on the Shaking Palsy.* London: Sherwood, Neely, and Jones, 1817:66.

49. Rinne JO, Rummukainen J, Pajarvi L, et al. Dementia in Parkinson's disease is related to neuronal loss in the medial substantia nigra. *Ann Neurol* 1989; 26:47–50.

50. Brown DF, Dababo MA, Bigio E, et al. Neuropathologic evidence that the Lewy body variant of Alzheimer's disease represents coexistence of Alzheimer's disease and idiopathic Parkinson's disease. *J Neuropathol Exp Neurol* 1998; 57:39–46.

51. Brown DF, Risser RC, Bigio EH, et al. Neocortical synapse density and Braak stage in the Lewy body variant of Alzheimer's disease: A comparison with classic Alzheimer's disease and normal aging. *J Neuropathol Exp Neurol* 1998; 57:955–960.

52. Samuel W, Alford M, Hofstetter R, et al. Dementia with Lewy bodies versus pure Alzheimer's disease: Differences in cognition, neuropathology, cholinergic dysfunction and synapse density. *J Neuropathol Exp Neurol* 1997; 56:499–508.

53. Sima AAF, Clark AW, Sternberger NA, et al. Lewy body dementia without Alzheimer's changes. *Can J Neurol Sci* 1986; 13:490–497.

54. Gearing M, Lynn M, Mirra SS. Neurofibrillary pathology in Alzheimer's disease with Lewy bodies. Two subgroups. *Arch Neurol* 1999; 56:203–208.

55. Torack RM, Morris JC, Mesolimbocortical dementia: A clinicopathologic case study of a putative disorder. *Arch Neurol* 1986; 43:1074–1078.

56. Torack RM, Morris JC. The association of central tegmental area histopathology with adult dementia. *Arch Neurol* 1988; 45:497–501.

57. Langston JW, Irwin I, Langston EB, et al. 1-methyl-4-phenylpyridinium ion (MPP+): Identification of a metabolite of MPTP, a toxin selective to the substantia nigra. *Neurosci Lett* 1984; 48:87–92.

58. Forno LS, Langston JW, DeLanney LE, et al. Locus ceruleus lesions and eosinophilic inclusions in MPTP-treated monkeys. *Ann Neurol* 1986; 20:449–455.

59. Kinemuchi H, Fowler CJ, Tipton KF. The neurotoxicity of 1-methyl-4-phenyl-1,2,3,6 tetrahydropyridine (MPTP) and its relevance to Parkinson's disease. *Neurochem Int* 1987; 11:359–373.

60. Forno LS, DeLanney LE, Irwin I, et al. Electron microscopy of Lewy bodies in the amygdala-parahippocampal region. Comparison with inclusion bodies in the MPTP-treated squirrel monkey. *Adv Neurol* 1996; 69:217–228.

61. Golbe LI, DiIorio G, Bonavita V, et al. A large kindred with autosomal dominant Parkinson's disease. *Ann Neurol* 1990; 27:276–282.

62. Factor SA, Ortof E, Dentinger MP, et al. Structural alterations of platelets in Parkinson's disease. An electron microscopic study. *J Neurol Sci* 1994; 122:84–89.

62a. Zubenko GS, Malinacova I, Chojnacki B. Proliferation of internal membranes in platelets from patients with Alzheimer's disease. *J Neuropathol Exp Neurol* 1987; 46:407–418.

63. Gorell JM, Johnson CC, Rybicki BA, et al. Occupational exposure to metals as risk factors for Parkinson's disease. *Neurology* 1997; 48:650–658.

64. Mori H, Kondo T, Yokochi M, et al. Pathologic and biochemical studies of juvenile Parkinsonism linked to chromosome 6q. *Neurology* 1998; 51:890–892.

65. Gibb WRG, Narabayashi H, Yokochi M, et al. New pathologic observations in juvenile onset Parkinsonism with dystonia. *Neurology* 1991; 41:820–822.

66. Factor SA. Posttraumatic Parkinsonism. In: Stern MB, Koller WC (eds.). *Parkinsonian Syndromes.* New York: Marcel Dekker, 1993:95–110.

67. Jankovic J. Post-traumatic movement disorders: Central and peripheral mechanisms. *Neurology* 1994; 44:2006–2014.

68. Hunter R, Smith J, Thomson T, et al. Hemiparkinsonism with infarction of the ipsilateral substantia nigra. *Neuropathol Appl Neurobiol* 1978; 4:297–301.

69. Hirano A, Malamud N, Kurland LT. Parkinsonism-Dementia complex, an endemic disease on the island of Guam-II. Pathological features. *Brain* 1961; 84:662–679.

70. Hirano A. Amyotrophic lateral sclerosis and Parkinsonism-dementia complex on Guam: Immunohistochemical studies. *Keio J Med* 1992; 41:1–5.

71. Spencer PS, et al. Guam amyotrophic lateral sclerosis-parkinsonism-dementia linked to a plant excitant neurotoxin. *Science* 1987; 237:517–522.

72. Steele JC, Richardson JC, Olszewski J. Progressive supranuclear palsy: A heterogeneous degeneration involving the brain stem, basal ganglia and cerebellum with vertical gaze and pseudobulbar palsy, nuchal dystonia, and dementia. *Arch Neurol* 1964; 10:333–359.

73. Papp MI, Lantos PL. Accumulation of tubular structures in oligodendroglial and neuronal cells as the basic alteration in multiple system atrophy. *J Neurol Sci* 1992; 107:172–182.

74. Gilman S, Sima AAF, Junek L, et al. Spinocerebellar ataxia type I with multiple system degeneration and glial cytoplasmic inclusions. *Ann Neurol* 1996; 39:241–255.

75. Wakabayashi K, Hayashi S, Kakita A, et al. Accumulation of alpha-synuclein/NACP is a cytopathological feature common to Lewy body disease and multiple system atrophy. *Acta Neuropathol* 1998; 96:445–452.

76. Koeppen AH, Barron KD, Cox JF. Striatonigral degeneration. *Acta Neuropathol* 1971; 19:10–19.

77. Ringel SP, Klawans HL, Jr. Carbon monoxide-induced Parkinsonism. *J Neurol Sci* 1972; 16:245–251.

21

Neurochemistry

Jose Martin Rabey, M.D.

Chairman, Department of Neurology, Assaf Harofe Medical Center, Sackler School of medicine, Tel Aviv University, Israel

and

Richard Stanley Burns, M.D.

Director, Movement Disorders Clinic, Department of Neurology, SIU School of Medicine Springfield, Illinois

ANATOMY OF THE BASAL GANGLIA AND RELATED CIRCUITS

It is known that the motor features of Parkinson's disease (PD) result from altered basal ganglia function. The basal ganglia include the caudate nucleus and putamen (collectively referred to as the striatum), the globus pallidus (pars interna and pars externa [Gpi and Gpe]), the subthalamic nucleus (STN), and the substantia nigra (pars reticulata and pars compacta [SNr and SNc]) (1). Other structures considered part of the basal ganglia circuitry and which play an important role in extrapyramidal motor function include premotor cortex, primary motor cortex, and thalamus. A somatotopic organization of motor function exists within the basal ganglia and its circuits (2) (Figure 21-1).

The principal afferents to the basal ganglia arising from extrinsic neuronal groups include projections from the neocortex to the caudate and putamen, from the nonspecific nuclei of the thalamus to the striatum, from the locus ceruleus to the substantia nigra, and from the raphe nuclei to the striatum and substantia nigra (SN). The principal efferent pathways from the basal ganglia to external neuronal groups project from the Gpi and SNr to the thalamus and from the SNr to the superior colliculus, brainstem reticular formation, and spinal cord. Intrinsic connections between basal ganglia structures include projections from the striatum to both segments of the globus pallidus and reciprocal connections between the SN and the striatum. In addition, the STN receives afferents from the Gpe and projects to both the Gpi and the SNr (3). The principal intrinsic and extrinsic connections of the

nerve cell groups that comprise the basal ganglia and their neurotransmitters are depicted in Figure 21-2.

The input to the putamen from the neocortex is excitatory and involves glutamate as a neurotransmitter. The putamen in turn projects to the Gpi via two pathways, the so-called "direct" and "indirect" pathways. The one neuron "direct" pathway from the putamen to the Gpi involves gamma-aminobutyric acid (GABA)-substance P (Sub P) neurons, and is considered to be primarily inhibitory in nature. The three neuron "indirect" pathway is more complex and involves two other nuclei, the Gpe and STN. The primary projection from the putamen to the Gpe via GABA-enkephalin neurons and the secondary projection from the Gpe to the STN via GABA neurons are both inhibitory in nature. The tertiary projection from the STN to the Gpi is excitatory and involves glutamatergic neurons. The output from Gpi to the thalamus occurs via inhibitory GABAergic neurons. The thalamus in turn projects to the cortex via excitatory glutamatergic neurons (4). Dopaminergic neurons from the SNc project to the putamen leading to excitation of the striatal output neurons that are the origin of the "direct" pathway and inhibition of the striatal output neurons of the "indirect" pathway and, thus, modulate activity in both pathways Figure 21-2.

DOPAMINERGIC SYSTEMS

Several dopaminergic pathways have been identified in the central nervous system. One of the most important heterogeneous populations of dopaminergic cells

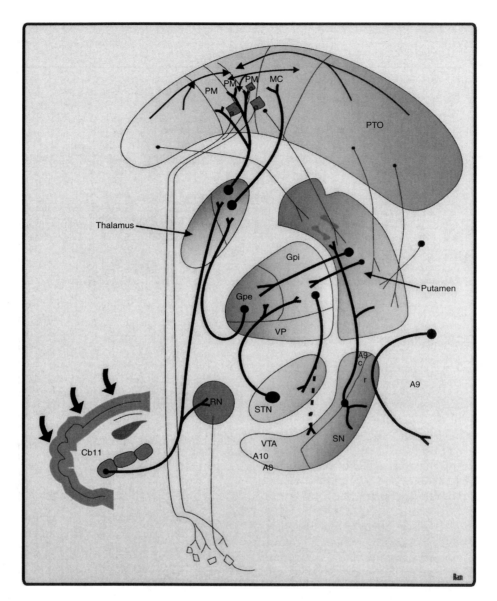

FIGURE 21-1. Schematic representation of extrapyramidal motor system. Pallido-thalamo-cortical and cerebello-thalamo-cortical pathways in heavy lines. Also shown in heavy lines are inputs to globus pallidus from the striatum and the putamen and the pallido subthalamo-pallidal loop. MC, motor cortex; PM, premotor cortex; PF, prefrontal cortex; PTO, parieto-temporo-occipital association cortex; GP, globus pallidus; SN, substantia nigra AQ, dopaminergic cells comprising substantia nigra compacta; STN, subthalamic nucleus. RN red nucleus, VP ventral pallidus, VTH ventral tegmental area, Cb11, cerebellum.

are located in the midbrain (it is estimated that there are about 15,000 to 20,000 cells on each side of the brain stem, whereas the number of noradrenergic neurons in the entire brainstem is about 5000 on each side) (5). On the basis of retrograde tracing techniques (6), the dopaminergic systems that have been identified include: (1) ultrashort systems: such as the interplexiform amacrine-like neurons located in the outer plexiform layers of the retina and the periglomerular dopamine (DA) cells of the olfactory

bulb; (2) intermediate length systems: these systems include the (i) tuberoinfundibular DA cells that project from the arcuate and periventricular nuclei to the intermediate lobe of the hypophysis and the median eminence (the tuberoinfundibular dopaminergic system), (ii) incertohypothalamic neurons that link the dorsal and posterior hypothalamus with the dorsal anterior hypothalamus and lateral septal nuclei, and (iii) medullary periventricular group that includes those DA cells in the dorsal motor nucleus of the vagus, the

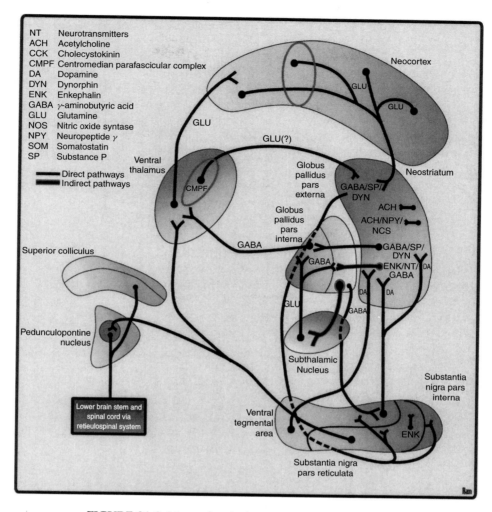

FIGURE 21-2. Neurochemical anatomy of the neostriatum.

nucleus tractus solitarius, and the cells dispersed in the tegmental radiation of the periaqueductal grey matter; and, (c) long-length systems: these systems include the long projections linking the ventral tegmental and SN dopaminergic cells with three principal set of target nuclei: the neostriatum (caudate nucleus and putamen); the limbic cortex (medial prefrontal, cingulate and entorhinal areas); and, other limbic structures (septum, olfactory tubercle, nucleus accumbens septi, amygdala complex, and piriform cortex). The first of these long-length systems is referred to as the nigrostriatal dopaminergic system and the latter two as the mesocortical and mesolimbic dopaminergic systems, respectively.

DOPAMINE METABOLISM

Levodopa, the precursor of dopamine, must be transported across the blood-brain barrier. The conversion of L-tyrosine to L-dihydroxyphenylalanine (L-DOPA) by the enzyme tyrosine hydroxylase (TH) is the rate-limiting step in DA synthesis. DOPA is subsequently converted to DA by the enzyme L-aromatic amino acid decarboxylase (LAAD) (Figure 21-3).

Several endogenous mechanisms have been identified for the regulation of DA synthesis that involve modulation of TH activity. DA and other catecholamines act as end-product inhibitors of TH by competing with the cofactor tetrahydrobiopterin (BH-4) for its binding site on the enzyme. The availability of BH-4 also plays a role in the regulation of TH activity. TH exists in two kinetic forms that exhibit different affinities for BH-4. The conversion of TH from the low to high-affinity form involves phosphorylation of the enzyme. Presynaptic DA receptors also modulate TH activity. These receptors (autoreceptors) are activated by DA released from the nerve terminals, resulting in feedback inhibition of DA synthesis. DA synthesis also depends on the rate of impulse flow in the nigrostriatal

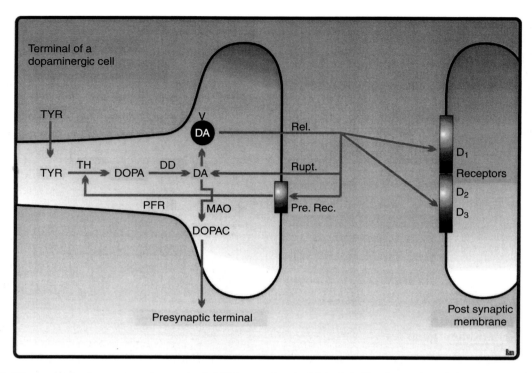

FIGURE 21-3. Diagram of a dopaminergic terminal. TYR, tyrosine; DOPA, 3,4-dihydroxyphenylalanine; DA, dopamine; TH, tyrosine hydroxylase; DD, dopa-decarboxylase; V, vesicles; REL. release; RUPT. re-ptake; PRE. REC. presynaptic receptor; PFR, presynaptic feedback regulation; DOPAC, 3,4-dihydroxphenylacetic acid; MAO, monoamine oxidase.

pathway. During increased impulse flow, TH activity is increased primarily through kinetic activation of TH, which increases its affinity for BH-4 and decreases its affinity for the normal end-product inhibitor DA.

DOPAMINE, NEUROMELANIN, AND TYROSINE HYDROXYLASE

Once synthesized, DA is sequestered in storage vesicles. The membrane of the vesicles contains a high affinity, energy dependent (Na$^+$-pump), carrier-mediated transport system that concentrates DA within the vesicles. The release of DA from the vesicles at synaptic terminals occurs by a Ca^{++}-dependent mechanism. DA released into the synaptic cleft can interact with specific, membrane-bound, cell surface receptors (DA receptors) on a second neuron (postsynaptic heteroreceptors) or on the same neuron from which it is released (autoreceptors). DA released into the synaptic cleft is inactivated primarily by a high-affinity, stereospecific, carrier-mediated reuptake process. The membrane carrier is capable of transporting DA in either direction, depending on the existing concentration gradient. The DA transporter plays an important physiologic role in the inactivation and recycling of DA released into the synaptic cleft.

Considering that platelets can be considered relatively good peripheral models for the study of catecholaminergic cells Rabey et al. (7) studied DA incorporation by platelet granules in PD patients. DA incorporation into the platelet granules was found to be altered in naive PD patients and partially improved after treatment with levodopa.

After its reuptake into nerve terminals, DA is inactivated by enzymatic conversion to dihydroxyphenlylacetic acid (DOPAC) by the action of monoamine oxidase, type B (MAO-B), located within the mitochondria. Released DA that diffuses out of the synapse is converted to homovanillic acid (HVA) outside the neuron by the sequential action of catechol-O-methyltransferase (COMT) and MAO; both enzymes are located primarily in glial cells. The principal metabolite of DA in humans is HVA in its free form, which results from the deamination and 3-O-methylation of DA and the 3-O-methylation of DOPAC at an extraneuronal site (5).

Since the levels of L-tyrosine in the brain are relatively high (above the Km for tyrosine hydroxylase), it is not feasible to increase DA synthesis in the brain by increasing the availability of L-tyrosine. The activity of LAAD in dopaminergic neurons is very high under normal conditions and, as a result Levodopa levels in the brain are negligible. LAAD is also present in nondopaminergic neurons such as serotonergic neurons (5). Exogenous Levodopa is converted to DA within dopaminergic neurons by LAAD; the activity of LAAD in DA terminals within the striatum remains relatively high in Parkinson's disease (PD).

Exogenous levodopa is transported across the endothelial cells of cerebral vessels into the brain by the L-transport system for neutral amino acids. The L-system is stereospecific, bidirectional, saturable, and competitively inhibited. The L-system is also involved in the transport of other L-neutral amino acids including phenylalanine, tyrosine, tryptophane, leucine, isoleucine, methionine, valine, and histadine. The reversal of the motor effects of Levodopa by the ingestion of proteins containing these other amino acids is thought to occur at the blood-brain barrier by competitive inhibition (8,9).

The existence of morphologic changes in the SN, consisting primarily of a loss of neurons combined with decreased neuromelanin, had already been described in PD at the beginning of the twentieth century (10,11). In 1957, DA was discovered to be a neurotransmitter in the brain by Carlsson et al. (12,13), who applied the newly developed histofluorescence method. This finding was important for the future

isolation of DA in human postmortem brain (14) and for the identification of the loss of DA in the striatum in PD (15) (Table 21-1). Shortly after that discovery, W. Birkmayer and O. Hornykiewicz (16,17) discovered that DOPA (the racemic mixture of L- and D-DOPA), the amino acid precursor of DA, was able to reduce the symptoms of PD. Monoamine oxidase (MAO) inhibitors intensified the effects and D-DOPA (the dextrorotatory isomer) and 5-hydroxytryptophane (5-HTP) were found to be the ineffective. Together, these findings demonstrated that DA was the primary neurotransmitter in the nigrostriatal tract, and they gave a clearer picture about the biochemical characteristics of PD. The finding of a dramatic decrease in striatal and nigral DA concentrations in PD indicated that these cells corresponded to the nigrostriatal dopaminergic system.

A link between the vulnerability of nigral neurons and their prominent pigmentation, although long suspected, was not proven until Hirsch et al. (18) performed a quantitative analysis of neuromelanin-containing, pigmented neurons in the midbrain in control and PD brains. He and his colleagues demonstrated that DA-containing cell groups in the normal human midbrain differ markedly from

Table 21-1   DA and HVA Concentration in Selected Brain Regions in Parkinsonian Patients and Controls

	DA	HVA	DA/HVA
Putamen (a)			
controls	5.06 ± 0.39 (17)	4.92 ± 0.32 (16)	1.03
PD patients	0.14 ± 0.13 (3)	0.54 ± 0.13 (3)	0.26
Caudate nucleus (a)			
controls	4.06 ± 0.47 (18)	2.92 ± 0.37 (19)	1.39
PD patients	0.2 ± 0.19 (3)	1.19 ± 0.10 (3)	0.17
Nucleus accumbens (b)			
controls	3.79 ± 0.82 (8)	4.38 ± 0.64 (8)	0.86
PD patients	1.61 ± 0.28 (4)	3.13 ± 0.13 (3)	0.51
Parolfactory gyrus (b)			
controls	0.35 ± 0.09 (4)	0.98 (2)	0.35
PD patients	<0.03 (2)		
Lateral hypothalamus (b)			
controls	0.51 ± 0.08 (4)	1.96 ± 0.28 (3)	0.26
PD patients	<0.03 (2)		
		1.03 ± 0.23 (3)	
Substantia nigra (c,d)			
controls	0.46 ± (13)	2.32 (7)	0.20
PD patients	0.07 (10)	0.41 (9)	0.17

Results are expressed as mean ± S.E.M; numbers of cases are in parentheses.
a) Ref 20;
b) Ref 93;
c) Ref 92;
d) Ref 94.

each other in the percentage of neuromelanin-containing neurons. In addition, they showed a significant positive correlation between the cell loss in different brainstem nuclei and the percentage of neuromelanin-containing neurons normally present in those nuclei. They also showed that in PD there was a relative sparing of nonpigmented neurons compared to pigmented neurons within each cell group. This evidence suggested a "selective vulnerability of the neuromelanin-pigmented subpopulation of DA-containing mesencephalic neurons in PD."

The loss of dopaminergic neurons in the nigrostriatal pathway follows an identifiable topographic pattern: the decrease of DA is greater in the rostral than caudal striatum (19), and the putamen is more severely affected than the caudate nucleus (15). The later finding is thought to be related to the fact that cell loss is more severe in the caudal and internal portions of the SN that preferentially project to the putamen.

The degree of neuronal loss in the SN correlates with the loss of activity of TH in the striatum (see Table 21-2) (20,21). These changes are associated with a marked decrease in the DA content and the concentrations of its metabolites, DOPAC and HVA, in the striatum. The loss of DA is more pronounced

than that of HVA (22). It is generally considered that DA loss in the striatum must be reduced by about 70–80% before the triad of PD symptoms (akinesia, rigidity, rest tremor) becomes apparent.

The loss of TH activity is one of the most prominent findings in PD. Because TH is highly localized in catecholamine neurons, it is often utilized as a specific marker for DA neurons. Biochemical analysis and immunocytochemistry have shown a substantial loss of TH in the ventral tegmental area (VTA) and in the nucleus paranigralis, in addition to the loss of TH in the SN (23–25).

PROTEIN SYNTHESIS

A dearrangement in protein synthesis in the SN and locus ceruleus have been demonstrated (26) and histologic studies indicate that this may be an important component in the pathogenesis of PD (27). The loss of TH activity, which constitutes one of the hallmarks in PD seems to be due to reduced TH protein synthesis. The hypothesis of a role for TH in the pathophysiology of PD is supported by findings

Table 21-2 Enzyme Activities in Selected Brain Areas from Parkinsonian Patients and Controls				
Brain Region	Tyrosine hydroxylase (TH)	Dopa-Decarboxylase (DDC)	Catechol-0-methyl transferase (COMT)	Monoamine-Oxidase (MAO)
Putamen				
control	$17.4 \pm 2.4(3)$	$432 \pm 109(18)$	$24.1 \pm 2.5(11)$	$1520 \pm 127(11)$
PD patients	$3.1 \pm 1.2\ (3)(a)$	$32 \pm 7\ (13)(b)$	$19.8 \pm 3.7\ (9)$	$1648 \pm 128\ (10)$
Caudate nucleus				
control	$18.7 \pm 2.0\ (3)$	$364 \pm 95\ (19)$	$25.4 \pm 2.8\ (10)$	$1726 \pm 149\ (10)$
PD patients	$3.2 \pm 0.5\ (2)(a)$	$54 \pm 14\ (13)(b)$	$17.8 \pm 3.8\ (9)$	$1742 \pm 197\ (10)$
Substantia nigra				
control	$17.4\ (1)$	$549 \pm 294\ (15)$	$26.4 \pm 4.7\ (5)$	$1828 \pm 200\ (5)$
PD patients	$6.1 \pm 1.5\ (3)$	$21 \pm 6\ (10)$	$21.7 \pm 10.2\ (9)$	$1477 \pm 284\ (4)$
Frontal cortex				
control	$3.7\ (2)$	$32 \pm 4\ (6)$	$24.1 \pm 4.4\ (9)$	
PD patients	$2.5 \pm 0.2\ (3)$	$10 \pm 2\ (3)(a)$	$28.7 \pm 4.1\ (7)$	
Hypothalamus				
control	$4.4\ (2)$	$149 \pm 53\ (9)$	$29.4 \pm 4.5\ (3)$	
PD patients	$2.7\ (2)$	$63 \pm 17(5)$		

Results are expressed as mean $\pm$ S.E.M; numbers of cases shown in parentheses.
Differs from control $p < 0.02$.
Differs from control $p < 0.01$
Data derived from ref 18
TH: (nmol / CO_2 / 30 min / 100 mg protein)
DDC: (nmol / CO_2 / 2hr / 100 mg protein)
COMT: (nmol / NMN / hr 100 mg protein)
MAO: (nmol / PPA / 30 min / 100 mg protein)
Source: ref 18.

indicating that TH antisera stain the characteristic Lewy bodies in catecholaminergic neurons (28).

Cyclic adenosine monophosphate (cAMP)–dependent protein kinase activity is reduced in the brains of patients with PD (29). Moreover, TH synthesis measured in the putamen from PD patients shows supersensitivity to stimulation by CAMP-dependent protein kinase in vitro (30). These findings and the increase in histones H1, H2B, and H4 in the SN, but not in the striatum and frontal cortex, indicate disturbances in protein phosphorylation and protein synthesis. It appears, that degeneration of dopaminergic neurons is connected with a reduction in the transcription rate, as indicated by the increase in histones (31). It also seems likely that protein synthesis in the central nervous system is influenced by the synaptic activity, that is, the stimulatory capacity of adenylate cyclase–dependent processes. Functional disturbances at the synaptic level are thought to cause changes in the conformation of chromatin and a reduction in the transcription rate and RNA content, with changes in the ratio of RNA to DNA (32). These processes show an age-dependent decline, with increased vulnerability within time.

DOPAMINE METABOLITES

The metabolites of DA, DOPAC, and HVA, are decreased in the SN and the striatum in PD (20,22,33). However, the metabolites of DA are reduced to a lesser degree than DA itself (34). This may in part be explained by: (a) postmortem diffusion of DA from its storage sites and subsequent catabolism by endogenous enzymes that are still active. Monoamine oxidase, type A (MAO-A), and type B (MAO-B) activity (the latter more specific for DA), and COMT activity are not affected by the disease (Table 21-2). These enzymes are located primarily outside dopaminergic neurons. (b) Another hypothesis to explain the difference between the degree of DA deficiency and the levels of its metabolites, is that it results from an increase in the turnover of DA in surviving neurons (35).

Compensatory changes in dopaminergic neurotransmission in remaining Nissl cells with functional overactivity have been described. The HVA (concentration) to DA (content) ratio (HVA/DA ratio) can be used as an index of the presynaptic activity of the surviving dopaminergic neurons. The level of HVA has been considered to be a good measure of the amount of DA released and the density of the DA terminals is indicated by the DA content. Thus the HVA/DA ratio provides an index of the rate of DA turnover in the remaining dopaminergic nerve terminals. This has been

confirmed by experimental lesions in animals. Partial nigral lesions in animals do not produce a significant change in the HVA/DA ratio; with lesions of 70–85%, changes in the release of DA from surviving dopaminergic nerve terminals are able to compensate functionally for the derangement. When lesions exceed 90%, DA receptors become hypersensitive and a change in behavioral response is observed (36,37).

In PD, the HVA/DA ratio is significantly increased in the putamen, caudate nucleus, and nucleus accumbens, but not in the hippocampus and frontal cortex (Table 21-1). These findings suggest that the lesion of the mesocortical pathway are not severe enough to induce compensatory changes in DA turnover. Another possibility is that the DA neurons that project to the cortex and hippocampus, compared to the nigral DA neurons, lack the capability to increase their synthesis and turnover of DA (38).

DOPAMINE RECEPTORS

Five distinct types of DA receptors (see Chapter 23) have been identified (39). They are classified into a D1-family (D1 and D2 receptors) and a D2-family (D2, D3 and D4 receptors) based on similarities in their structural and pharmacologic properties. The dopamine receptors consist of a polypeptide chain of 387–477 amino acids with variable carbohydrate chains and an overall size range of 90–120 kD. They belong to the G-protein-coupled receptor family with 7 transmembrane domains and G-protein coupling sites in the 3rd cytoplasmic loop. The subtypes of dopamine receptors differ in their extracellular and intracellular loops but are highly homologous in their transmembrane domains. The 3rd cytoplasmic loop is short in the dopamine receptors, which belong to the D1-family and long in those that belong to the D2-family. The D1-family of dopamine receptors with a short 3rd loop are coupled to stimulatory G-proteins (Gs), which activate adenylate cyclase. The D2-family of dopamine receptors with a long 3rd loop are coupled to Gi or Go proteins, which inhibit adenylate cyclase or are inactive, respectively, and to Gq proteins that couple with phospholipase C. As a general biochemical property, the D1-family of receptors (D1 and D5 receptors) stimulate adenylate cyclase leading to an increase in the formation of cAMP, whereas the D2-family of dopamine receptors either inhibit adenylate cyclase (D2 receptor) or do not modify its activity (D3 and D4 receptors). The effects of the D2 receptor on second messenger systems are complex and include an increase in phosphatidyl inositol metabolism, the release of arachnidonic acid and the activation of K^+ channels, in addition to the inhibition of adenylate cyclase.

The genes that code for the five subtypes of DA receptors are located on different chromosomes: D1 receptor at 5q34–35; D2 receptor at 11q22–23; D3 receptor at 3q13.3; and D4 and D5 receptors at 4p16. The genes that code for the D1-family of dopamine receptors have no introns in contrast to the genes for the D2-family of receptors, which possess introns in their coding regions: the D2 receptor gene has 6 introns; the D3 receptor gene has 5 introns; and, the D4 receptor gene has 4 introns.

D1 receptors are present on striatal GABA-Sub P output neurons (which project to the Gpi and SNr-so called "direct pathway") and at terminal regions of neurons in the SN. In contrast, D2 receptors are present on striatal GABA-enkephalin output neurons (which project to the Gpe so called "indirect pathway") and on DA neurons of the SNc (auto receptors). The D1 and D2 receptors are the most abundant subtypes in the striatum; D3 receptors are expressed at low levels and D4 receptors at very low levels in the striatum. Most of the DA receptors in the SNc are of the D2 subtype with a small number of the D3 subtype. All five subtypes of dopamine receptors are expressed in the cortex with a greater number of D4 and D5 receptors than of D3 receptors. The D3 receptor has the highest affinity (nM range) for the natural ligand DA.

D1 and D2 receptors are thought to play a central role in the motor disturbances in PD. The number of D2 receptors in the striatum have been found to be increased in the early stages of PD; the number of D1 receptors remain unchanged in this disease. DA generated from exogenous Levodopa acts at all of the DA receptor subtypes (40,41).

DOPAMINE TRANSPORTER

Dopamine transporters terminate dopaminergic neurotransmission by actively pumping extracellular DA back into the presynaptic nerve terminal (Na^+ and Cl^--dependent) (42,43). DA uptake is accomplished by a membrane carrier that is capable of transporting DA in either direction, depending on the concentration gradient.

A complementary DNA encoding a rat DA transporter (DAT) has been isolated with high sequence homology with the previously cloned norepinephrine and gamma-aminobutyric acid transporters. DAT is a 619 amino acid protein with 12 hydrophobic putative membrane spanning domains and is a member of the family of Na/Cl-dependent plasma membrane transporters. Using the energy provided by the Na gradient generated by the Na/K-transporting ATPase, DAT recaptures DA soon after its release, modulating its concentration in the synapse and its time-dependent interaction with both pre- and postsynaptic DA receptors (44).

Studies of the binding of tritiated alpha-dihydrotetrabenazine ([3H] TBZOH) (a specific ligand for the vesicular monoamine transporter) in the striatum in postmortem brains from 49 controls and 57 patients with PD suggested that parkinsonian symptoms appear when the degeneration of the striatal dopamine terminals is greater than 50% of normal innervation (45). The expression of the DA transporter messenger RNA (mRNA) assessed by in situ hybridization in individual pigmented neurons of the SNc in sections of the midbrain from 7 PD and 7 control brains showed that DA transporter mRNA expression in surviving SNc neurons was only 57% of normal control levels in PD (46). The authors speculated that the decrease in the level of DA transporter mRNA expression in the remaining neurons in the SNc of PD patients reflected neuronal dysfunction. They added, "conceivably it might also reflect differential vulnerability of those neurons that initially expressed higher levels of DA transporter to the insult of parkinsonism" (46).

NIGROSTRIATAL DOPAMINE SYSTEM AND PARKINSONIAN SYMPTOMS

Deficiency of DA in the striatum plays a major role in the motor symptoms of PD. However, it is less clear whether all of these symptoms result from DA deficiency alone or if other neurotransmitters are involved. A strong correlation has been found between the severity of akinesia and the decrease in striatal DA and degree of neuronal loss in the SN (22). Moreover, akinesia has been found to be more severe on the side of the body contralateral to the greatest degree of cell loss in the SN (22). DA depletion may also influence tremor. Monkeys with combined lesions of the nigrostriatal DA system and the rubro-olivocerebellar rubral loop exhibit rest tremor (47). Rigidity is thought to result from hyperactive alpha-motoneurones of supraspinal origin. The role of the derangement of DA systems in the occurrence of rigidity is less clear (48). The freezing gait is another feature that appears to be unrelated to DA loss. It occurs randomly and unrelated to dopaminergic therapy. Later onset postural instability also appears to be at least partially related to other transmitters.

OTHER NEUROTRANSMITTERS AND RECEPTORS

Other brainstem nuclei (locus ceruleus, raphe nuclei, nucleus basalis of Meynert) have been found to be affected in PD (49–52); these nuclei are the origin of the noradrenergic, serotonergic, and cholinergic systems, respectively.

Noradrenergic Systems

Two ascending noradrenergic pathways have been identified in the rat: a dorsal system originating in the locus ceruleus and projecting to the whole neocortex and the limbic forebrain (amygdala, septum, hippocampus); and a ventral system extending from the lower brainstem to the hypothalamus and the nucleus interstitialis terminalis. An additional descending noradrenergic pathway inervates the spinal cord. (53). In human brain, the highest levels of norepinephrine (NE) are found in the nucleus accumbens and hypothalamus, with low levels in the cortex and undetectable amounts in the striatum, suggesting a similar organization in the rat and human brain (54).

In PD, the level of NE is reduced in the locus ceruleus and this is associated with a loss of pigmented neurons and the formation of Lewy body inclusions. Moreover, NE concentrations in the neocortex, nucleus accumbens, amygdala, and hippocampus are 40–70% lower than normal (55,56). In limbic regions, the level of the major metabolite of NE, 3-methoxy-4-hydroxyphenylglicol (MHPG), is also reduced (56). These changes suggest that the dorsal NE system degenerates in PD.

Nagatsu et al. (57) reported a reduction in MHPG and dopamine beta-hydroxylase (DBH) activity (the enzyme that converts DA to NE in noradrenergic neurons) in the CSF of PD patients suggesting a more general noradrenergic deficiency.

Depressive features commonly observed in patients with PD might be related to a central NE deficiency (58), as administration of NE reuptake blockers (59,60) improves depression in these patients.

It has been postulated that NE might affect the motor system by a dual effect, indirectly through the modulation of the activity of dopaminergic cells (61) as well as directly. For example, freezing episodes have been attributed to a deficiency of NE. This symptom has been reportedly alleviated by the administration of dihydroxyphenylserine (DOPS), a specific precursor of NE (62). However, this observation has not been replicated.

Although some studies suggest that NE deficiency might play a role in the motor symptoms and mood changes in PD, the exact mechanism has not yet been clarified.

Serotonergic Systems

Two major serotonergic systems have been demonstrated in the central nervous system: an ascending pathway from the mesencephalic raphe nuclei to the forebrain and a descending pathway from the pontine raphe nuclei to the spinal cord (63). The highest concentrations of serotonin (5HT) and its metabolite, 5-hydroxyindole acetic acid (5-HIAA), are found in the SN, striatum, amygdala, and spinal cord. The levels are lower in the neocortex and hippocampus (64).

In PD, 5HT concentrations are reduced in several areas of the forebrain including the basal ganglia, hipppocampus, and cerebral cortex (43). They are also reduced in the lumbar spinal cord and the hypothalamus. These biochemical changes are not uniformly distributed, reflecting selective damage to some cell groups in the raphe nuclei (43). In the caudate nucleus and frontal cortex, 5HT itself (a marker of serotonergic nerve terminals) is reduced more than 5-HIAA (a marker of 5HT metabolism). The increase in the 5-HIAA /5HT ratio probably reflects a compensatory increase in the turnover of 5HT in surviving serotonergic neurons.

Although DA transmission in both the SN and the striatum are known to be under the inhibitory control of ascending serotonergic systems, at the present time there is no evidence of a relationship between the motor symptoms of parkinsonism and the changes in the serotonergic systems. However, some reports suggest that low 5HT levels might play a role in the occurrence of depressive features in PD. Lower levels of 5-HIAA were found in the CSF of PD patients with depression compared to that seen in PD subjects without depression (65).

Cholinergic Systems

The cholinergic system can be divided into groups of short neurons intrinsic to particular brain regions (located in the basal ganglia and cortex) and long fiber systems extending from the brainstem and basal forebrain to subcortical and cortical regions. In the striatum, acetylcholine (ACh) is released predominantly from the large aspiny interneurons. The principal cholinergic fibers projecting to forebrain areas (olfactory bulb, hippocampus, amygdala, thalamus, cortex) originate from large neurons with long axons. The fibers innervating the neocortex are located mainly in the substantia innominata, in particular the nucleus basalis of Meynert, but there is also in input from the mesencephalic nuclei (pedunculopontine nucleus). The fibers innervating the hippocampus are located in the septum (66).

Studies in animals indicate that the nigrostriatal dopaminergic neurons make synapses with cholinergic neurons in the striatum, inhibiting their activity (67–69). Choline acetyltransferase (CAT), a marker of cholinergic neurons, does not seem to be affected in PD (70). Therefore, it is generally accepted that the striatal cholinergic neurons are released from the inhibitory influence of dopaminergic neurons in PD and, as a consequence, are hyperactive. The effects of degeneration of the nigrostriatal dopaminergic projection neurons in PD might be counter-balanced by the use of anticholinergic drugs. This hypothesis, which suggests a beneficial effect of anticholinergic drugs in PD, has proven to be correct in clinical practice. The therapeutic effects of muscarinic receptor antagonists in PD are thought to be due to inhibition of M1 receptor-mediated excitation of striatal GABA-enkephalin neurons (that project via the "indirect" pathway to the Gpe) and of M4 receptor-mediated inhibition of GABA-Sub P neurons (that project via the "direct" pathway to the Gpi and SNr) (71).

Several studies have shown severe neuronal loss and subnormal CAT activity in the substantia innominata (especially the nucleus of Meynert) in PD supporting the contention that the innominatocortical cholinergic system is deranged in patients with PD and associated cognitive impairment (72–74). More intriguing is the fact that a diffuse cortical cholinergic deficiency has also been found in PD patients without mental deterioration (mainly in frontal and occipital lobes) (73,74). This fact suggests that degeneration of subcortical cholinergic systems might precede the appearance of intellectual deterioration in PD. Subnormal levels of CAT activity have also been described in the septohippocampal cholinergic system and in the pedunculpontine nucleus (75). The significance of this diffuse degeneration of cholinergic neurons in the basal forebrain in PD is not clearly understood.

Gabaergic Systems

Long GABAergic striatopallidal, striatonigral, pallidothalamic pathways, and intrinsic striatal GABAergic neurons have been identified using an assay that measures the activity of the GABA-synthesizing enzyme glutamate decarboxylase (GAD) (76) Figures 21-1 and 21-2.

Although some studies have been nonconclusive regarding the integrity of GABAergic systems in PD (77–79), others using brain samples that were carefully matched for age and pre- and postmortem conditions have found no significant changes in the content of GABA in brain in PD (80).

The critical issue concerning the GABAergic system is whether GABA turnover is altered and, if so, in which neuronal groups. It would be unlikely, however, that up or down regulation of GABA activity might occur as a consequence of DA depletion in the striatum.

Adenosine A$_{2A}$ Receptor

The adenosine A$_{2A}$ receptor, one of four cloned adenosine receptors, is a member of the G-protein-coupled receptor family, and when activated, stimulates adenylate cyclase. It is highly concentrated in the striatum; it is copresent with D2 receptors on striatal GABA-enkephalin output neurons and present on striatal cholinergic interneurons. The adensoine A$_{2A}$ receptor is thought to modulate the neuronal activity of striatal GABA-enkephalin output neurons, which project to the Gpe via the "indirect" pathway. Striatal GABA-enkephalin neurons are excited by inputs from cortical glutamatergic neurons and cholinergic interneurons and inhibited by inputs from nigral dopaminergic neurons via D2 receptors and recurrent neurons and collaterals via GABA receptors. Antagonism at the adenosine A$_{2A}$ receptor is thought to result in a decrease in the stimulation of GABA-enkephalin output neurons by striatal cholinergic interneurons and an increase in the GABA-mediated recurrent inhibition of these neurons. Antagonist activity at adenosine A$_{2A}$ receptors in the striatum might effectively compensate for the lack of dopamine-mediated inhibition of these neurons in PD (81).

Neuropeptides

The distribution of neuropeptides in the brain is heterogeneous. Cholecystokinin-8 (CCK-8) and vasointestinal peptide (VIP) are most abundant in cortical areas, whereas methionine (Met) and leucine (Leu)-enkephalins, Sub P and thyrotropin-releasing factor (TRH) are most abundant in the basal ganglia (82). Subnormal concentrations of various neuropeptides have been reported in various brain regions in PD using radioimmunoassay (RIA) methods. These changes have not always been confirmed by immunocytochemical techniques (83). The role of these peptides in the symptomatology of PD is not clear.

Hokfelt et al. (84) reported that CCK-8 is colocalized with DA in dopaminergic neurons in the SNc and the VTA. The level of CCK-8 in the SNc has been found to be decreased by 30% in PD subjects. However, normal levels of CCK-8 have been found (85) in the caudate nucleus, putamen, amygdala, cerebral cortex, and hippocampus using RIA methods. The decrease in CCK-8 in the SN might result from selective degeneration of CCK-8-containing neurons or of CCK-8 afferent fibers of unknown origin. The functional consequences of the nigral CCK-8 deficiency are not known. This peptide apparently has an excitatory effect on nigral dopaminergic neurons (86). However, CCK-8 also has been shown to decrease DA release in the striatum (87).

Mauborgne et al. (88) reported reduced Sub P levels in the basal ganglia in PD based on the RIA method (3). Grafe et al. (89), using an immunocytochemical technique, did not confirm these findings. If confirmed, the observed decrease in Sub P concentrations might indicate a change in the turnover rate due to the loss of regulatory input from depaminergic cell loss rather than the primary loss of Sub P–containing neurons.

The highest concentration of dynorphin in the brain is found in the SN (90). Its levels are unchanged in PD (90).

Met-enkephalin levels are reduced by 70% in the SN and VTA and by 30 to 40% in the putamen and globus pallidus in PD. They are similar to controls in the nucleus accumbens, caudate nucleus, amygdala, cerebral cortex, and hippocampus (91,92). If Met-enkephalin modulates the activity of DA neurons in the SN, changes in its levels might influence the turnover of DA at the cell body level. In PD, Leu-enkephalin levels are reduced by 30 to 40% in the putamen and the globus pallidus. In the SN and VTA, the concentrations of this peptide are similar to control values (92).

Somatostatin levels in the basal ganglia of PD patients are similar to those of control subjects (93). However, in demented PD subjects, somatostatin levels are reduced in the frontal cortex, entorhinal cortex and hippocampus when compared to nondemented PD patients.

At the present time, there is not enough data to support the hypothesis that an alteration in the concentration of neuropeptides plays a primary role in the pathogenesis of PD.

LEWY BODIES

The chemical composition of the Lewy body is complex. The classical cytoplasmic, eosinophilic inclusions found in brainstem nuclei are composed mainly of neurofilament proteins and ubiquitin (see Chapter 20). In addition to all three molecular forms of neurofilament proteins (NF-H; NF-M; NF-L) in both the phosphorylated and nonphosphorylated state, Lewy bodies have been found to contain protein kinases (Ca^{++}-calmodulin-dependent protein kinase II), high molecular weight microtubule-associated proteins and tubulin, ubiquitin carboxyl terminal hydrolase (PGP-9), gelsolin and amyloid precursor protein. Cortical Lewy bodies are distinct in containing alpha-B-crystalline and tropomysin (94). More recently, it was discovered that Lewy bodies also contain the alpha-synuclein protein (36).

CONCLUSION

Although a tremendous amount of information has accumulated over the past several years as the result of advances in biochemical techniques, the pathophysiology of PD is still not fully understood. The selective loss of dopaminergic cells in the nigrostriatal system explains part of the motor symptomatology but there are a number of features of the disease that apparently are not related to the deficiency of DA in the striatum. For example, the midline symptoms of the disease (speech, postural stability and freezing gait) are not responsive to treatment with exogenous levodopa. Moreover, other ascending neurotransmitter systems are also damaged in PD: the noradrenergic ceruleocortical, the serotonergic projections from the raphe nuclei, the dopaminergic mesocorticolimbic, and the innominatocortical and septohippocampal cholinergic systems. Alterations in the integrity of these systems would be expected to contribute to the disruption of circuits responsible for the motor and cognitive features of PD. The application of the new methods of molecular biology together with new biochemical (PET, SPECT, MRS) and functional (fMRI) neuroimaging techniques will undoubtedly lead to a better understanding of the pathophysiology of PD in the next decade.

REFERENCES

1. Anthoney TR. Neuroanatomy and the neurologic exam. *Ann Arbor CRC*, 1994:106–109.
2. Cote L, Crutcher MD. The basal ganglia (Chap. 42). In: Kandel E, James H Schwartz, Thomas M.G (eds.). *Principles of Neural Science*. 3rd edition. Elsevier, New York: 1991:647–659.

3. Alexander GE, Crutcher MD. Functional architecture of basal ganglia circuits: neural substrates of parallel processing. *Trends Neurosci* 1990; 13:266–271.

4. De Long MR. Primates models of movement disorders of basal ganglia origin. *Trends Neurosci* 1990; 13:231–285.

5. Cooper JR, Bloom FE, Roth RH. Dopamine. In: Cooper JR, Bloom FE, Roth RH (eds.). *Biochemical Basis Neuropharmacology* (7th edition) Oxford: University Press, 1996:292–351. (Chapter 9)

6. Björklund A, Lindvall O. Dopamine-containing systems in the CNS. In: Björklund A, Hökfelt T (ed.). *Handbook of Chemical Neuroanatomy, Vol 2: Clinical Transmitters in the CNS.* Elsevier, Amsterdam: 1984:55–122.

7. Rabey JM, Shabtai H, Graff E, et al. (^{3}H) Dopamine uptake by platelet storage granules in Parkinson's disease. *Life Sci* 1993; 53(23):1753–1761.

8. Cancilla PA, Bready J, Berliner J. Brain endothelial–astrocyte interactions. In: Pardridge WM, (eds.). *The Blood-Brain Barrier; Cellular and Molecular Biology.* New York: Raven Press, 1993:25–46.

9. Eriksson R, Graneros A, Linde A, et al. "On-off" phenomenon in Parkinson's disease: Relationship between dopa and other large neutral amino acids in plasma. *Neurology* 1988; 38:1245–1248.

10. Tretiakoff C. *Contribution a l' etude de l' anatomia pathologique du locus niger.* These. University of Paris 1919.

11. Hassler R. Zur Pathologie der Paralysis agitans und des postenzephalitischen Parkinsonism. *J. Psychol Neurol (Lpz)* 1938; 48:387–476.

12. Carlsson A, Lindquist M, Magnusson T. 3-4 dihydroxyphenylalanine and 5-hydroxy-tryptophan as reserpine antagonists. *Nature* (Lond) 1957; 180:1200.

13. Carlsson A, Lindquist M, Magnusson T, et al. On the presence of 3-hydroxy-tyramine in brain. *Science* 1958; 127:471.

14. Sano I, Gamo T, Kakimoto Y, et al. Distribution of catechol compounds in human brain. *Biochem Biophys Acta* 1959; 32:586–587.

15. Ehringer H, Hornykiewicz O. Verteilung von Noradrenalin und Dopamin im Gehirn des Menschen und ihr Verhalten bei Erkrankungen des extrapyramidalen Systems. *Wien Klin Wschr* 1960; 38:1236–1239.

16. Birkmayer W, Hornykiewicz O. Der L-3-4-Dioxyphenylalanin (=DOPA). Effeckt bei Parkinson Akinese. *Wien Klin Wschr* 1961; 73:787–788.

17. Birkmayer W, Hornykiewicz O. Der L-Dioxyphenylalanin (=DOPA). *Effekt beim Parkinson-Syndrom des Menschen Arch Psych Nervenkr* 1962; 203:560–574.

18. Hirsch E, Graybiel AM, Javoy-Agid A. Melanized dopaminergic neurons are differentially suceptible to degeneration in Parkinson's disease. *Nature* 1988; 334:345–348.

19. Fahn S, Libsch IR, Cuttler RW. Monoamines in the human neostriatum. Topographic distribution in normals and in Parkinson's disease and their role in akinesia, rigidity, chorea and tremor. *J Neurol Sci* 1971; 14:427–455.

20. Lloyd KG, Davidson L, Hornykiewicz O. The neurochemistry of Parkinson's disease: effect of L-Dopa therapy. *J Pharmacol Exp Ther* 1975; 195:453–464.

21. Riederer P, Rausch WD, Birkmayer W, et al. CNS modulation of adrenal tyrosine hydroxylase in Parkinson's disease and metabolic encephalophathies. *J Neural Transm* (Suppl) 1978; 14:121.

22. Bernheimer H, Birkmayer W, Hornykiewicz O, et al. Brain dopamine and the syndromes of Parkinson's and Huntington's: clinical morphological and neurochemical correlation. *J Neurol Sci* 1973; 20:415–455.

23. Riederer P, Wuketich S. Time course of nigrostriatal degeneration in Parkinson's disease. *J Neural Transm* 1976; 38:277–301.

24. Nakashima S, Kumanishi T, Ikuta F. Immunohistochemistry on tyrosine hydroxylase in the substantia nigra of human autopsied cases. *Brain Nerve* 1983; 35:1023–1029.

25. Pearson J, Goldstein M, Markey K, et al. Human brain catecholamine neuronal anatomy as indicated by immunocytochemistry with antibodies to tyrosine hydroxylase. *Neuroscience* 1983; 8:3–32.

26. Issidorides MR, Mytilineou C, Whetsell WO, et al. Protein-rich cytoplasmic bodies of substantia nigra and locus coeruleus. *Arch Neurol* 1978; 35:633–637.

27. Jacob H. Klinische Neuropathologie des Parkinsonismus. In Ganshirt H (eds.). Pathophysiologie, Klinik und Therapie des Parkinsonismus. *Roche Basel* 1983:5–18.

28. Nakashima S, Ikuta F. Tyrosine hydroxylase proteins in Lewy bodies of Parkinsonism and senile brain. *J Neurol Sci* 1984; 66:91–96.

29. Kato T, Nagatsu T, Iizuka R, et al. Cyclic AMP-dependent protein kinase activity in human brain: Values in parkinsonism. *Biochem Med* 1979; 21:141.

30. Rausch WD, Hirata Y, Nagatsu T, et al. Human brain tyrosine hydroxylase; in vitro effects of iron and phosphorylating agents in the CNS of controls, Parkinson's disease and schizophrenia. *J Neurochem* 1988; 50(1); 202–208.

31. Crapper-Mc Lachlan DR, Bebon U. Models for the study of pathological neural aging. In Terry RD, Bolis CL, Toffano G (eds.). *Neural Aging and Its Implications in Human Neurological Pathology.* (Aging, Vol. 18). New York: Raven Press, 1982:61–71.

32. Ringborg U. Composition of RNA in neurons of rat hippocampus at different ages. *Brain Res* 1966; 2:296–298.

33. Bokobza B, Ruberg M, Scatton B, et al. (^{3}H) spiperone binding, dopamine and HVA concentrations in

Parkinson's disease and supranuclear palsy. *Europ J Pharmacol* 1984; 99:167–175.

34. Scatton B, Monfort JC, Javoy-Agid F, et al. Neurochemistry of monoaminergic neurons in Parkinson's disease. In: Alan R (ed.). *Catecholamines: Neuropharmacology and Central Nervous System. Therapeutic Aspects.* New York: Liss Inc., 1984:43–52.

35. Hornykiewicz O. Compensatory biochemical changes at the striatal dopamine synapse in Parkinson's disease. Limitations of L-dopa therapy. *Adv Neurol* 1979; 24:275–281.

36. Melamed E, Hefti F, Wurtman RJ. Compensatory mechanism in the nigrostriatal dopaminergic system in Parkinson's disease studies in an animal model. *Israel J Med Sci* 1982; 18(1):159–163.

37. Creese I, Snyder SH. Nigrostriatal lesions enhance striatal (^{3}H) apomorphine and (^{3}H) spiroperidol binding. *Europ J Pharmacol* 1979; 56:277–281.

38. Javoy-Agid F, Ruberg M, Taquet H, et al. Biochemical neuropathology of Parkinson's disease. *Adv Neurol* 1984; 40:189–198.

39. Ogawa N. Molecular and chemical neuropharmacology of dopamine receptor subtypes. *Acta Med Okayama* 1995; 49(1):1–11.

40. Sokoloff P, Schwartz J-C. Novel dopamine receptors half a decade later. *Trends Pharmacol Sci* 1995; 16(8):270–275.

41. Meador-Woodruff JH. Neuroanatomy of dopamine receptor gene expression: Potential substrates for neuropsychiatric illness. *Clin Neuropharmacol* 1995; 18, Suppl.1:S14–24.

42. Horn AS. Dopamine uptake: A review of progress in the last decade. *Prog Neurobiol* 1990; 34:397–400.

43. Iversen LL. Role of transmitter uptake mechanisms in synaptic neurotransmission. *Br J Pharmacol* 1971; 41:571–591.

44. Giros B, Caron MG. Molecular characterization of the dopamine transporter. *TIPS* 1993; 14(2):43–49.

45. Scherman D, Desnos C, Darchen F, et al. Striatal dopamine deficiency in Parkinson's disease: Role of aging. *Ann Neurol* 1989; 26:551–557.

46. Uhl G, Walther D, Mash D, et al. Dopamine transporter messenger RNA in Parkinson's disease and control substantia nigra neurons. *Ann Neurol* 1994; 35:494–498.

47. Jenner P, Marsden CD. Neurochemical basis of parkinsonian tremor. In: Findley LJ, Capildeo R (eds.). *Movement Disorders: Tremor.* London: Macmillan, 1984:305–319.

48. Ellenbroeck B, Schwarcz M, Sontag KH, et al. Muscular rigidity and delineation of a dopamine-specific neostriatal subregion: Tonic EMG activity in rats. *Brain Res* 1985; 345:132–140.

49. Jellinger K. Pathology of parkinsonism In: Fahn S, Marsden CD, Jenner P, et al. (eds.). *Recent Development in Parkinson's Disease.* New York: Raven Press, 1986:33–66.

50. Hornykiewicz O. Die topische lokalization und das verhalten von noradrenalin und dopamin (3-Hydroxytyramin) in der substantia nigra des normalen und parkinsonkranken menschen. *Wien Klin Wochenschr* 1963; 75:309–312.

51. Price KS, Farley U, Hornykiewicz O. Neurochemistry of Parkinson's disease. Relation between striatal and limbic dopamine. *Adv Biochem Psychopharmacol* 1978; 19:293–300.

52. Bernheimer H, Hornykiewicz O. Herabgesetzte konzentration der homovaillinsaure im gehirn von parkinsonkranken menschen als ausdruck der storung des zentralen dopaminestroffwechsels. *Klin Wochenschr* 1965; 43:711–715.

53. Lindvall O, Björklund A. Organization of catecholamine neurons in the rat central nervous system. In: Iversen LI, Iversen SD, Snyder SH (eds.). *Handbook of Psychopharmacology* Vol. 9, New York: Plenum Press, 1978:139–231.

54. Farley IJ and Hornykiewicz O. Noradrenaline in subcortical brain regions of patients with Parkinson's disease and control subjects. In: Birkmayer W, Hornykiewicz O, (eds.). *Advances in Parkinsonism* Basel: Roche 1976:178-185

55. Scatton B, Javoy-Agid F, Rouquier L, et al. Reduction of cortical dopamine, noradrenaline, serotonin and their metabolites in Parkinson's disease. *Brain Res* 1983; 275:321–328.

56. Riederer P, Birkmayer W, Seeman D, et al. Brain-noradrenaline and 3-methoxy-hydroxyphenylglycol in Parkinson's syndrome. *J Neural Transm* 1977; 41:241–251.

57. Nagatsu T, Wakui Y, Kato TJ, et al. Dopamine beta-hydroxylase activity in cerebrospinal fluid of parkinsonian patients. *Biomed Res* 1982; 3:395–398.

58. Mayeaux R, Williams JBW, Stern Y, et al. Depression and Parkinson's disease. *Adv Neurol* 1984; 40:241–250.

59. Strang RR. Imipramine in the treatment of parkinsonism: A double-blind placebo study. *Br J Med* 1965; 2:33–34.

60. Anderson J, Aabro E, Gulman N, et al. Antidepressant treatment of Parkinson's disease. *Acta Neurol Scand* 1980; 62:210–219.

61. Hornykiewicz O. Parkinson's disease. In: Crow TJ (eds.). *Disorders of Neurohumoral Transmission* London: Academic Press, 1982:121–143.

62. Narabayashi H, Kondo T, Hayashi A, et al. L-threo-3, 4-Dyhydroxyphenylserine treatment for akinesia and freezing of parkinsonism. *Proc J Acad* 1981; 3:395–398.

63. Steinbusch HWM. Serotonin-immunoreactive neurons and their projection in the CNS. In: Björklund A, Hökfelt T, Kuhar ML (eds.). *Classical Transmitters and Receptors in the CNS. Part II. Handbook of*

Chemical Neuroanatomy. Vol. 3. Amsterdam: Elsevier, 1984:68–126.

64. Forno LS. Pathology of Parkinson's disease. In: Marsden CD, Fahn S (eds.). Movement Disorders Neurology 2, London: Butterworths, 1982:40–85.

65. Mayeaux R, Stern Y, Cote L, et al. Altered serotonin metabolism in depressed patients with Parkinson's disease. Neurology 1984; 34:642-646.

66. Woolf NJ, Butcher LL. Central cholinergic systems: Synopsis of anatomy and overview of pharmacology and pathology. In: Scheibel AB, Wechsler AF (eds.). The Biological Substrates of Alzheimer's Disease, New York: Academic Press, 1989:73–78.

67. Agid Y, Javoy F, Guyenet P, et al. Effects of surgical and pharmacological manipulation of the dopaminergic nigrostriatal neurons on the activity of the neostriatal cholinergic system in the rat. In: Boissier JR, Hippius H, Pichot P (eds.). Neuropsychopharmacology. Amsterdam: Excerpta Medica, 1975:480–486.

68. Javoy-Agid F, Ploska A, Agid Y. Microtopography of TH, CAT and GAD activity in the substantia nigra and ventral tegmental area of control and parkinsonian human brain. Neurochemistry, 1982; 37:1221–1227.

69. Hattori T, Singh VK, Mc Geer EG, et al. Immunohistochemical localization of choline acetyltransferase containing neostriatal neurons and their relationship with dopaminergic synapses. Brain Res 1976; 102:164–173.

70. Mc Geer PL, Mc Geer EG. Enzyme associated with the metabolism of catecholamines, acetylcholine and GABA in human controls and patients with Parkinson's disease and Huntington's chorea. J Neurochem 1976; 26:65–76.

71. Mayorga AJ, Cousins MS, Trevitt JT, et al. Characterization of the muscarinic receptor subtype mediating pilocarpine – induced tremulous jaw movements in rats. Eur J Pharmacol 1999; 364:7–11.

72. Candy JM, Perry RH, Perry EK, et al. Pathological changes in the nucleus of Meynert in Alzheimer's and Parkinson's disease. J Neurol Sci 1983; 54:277–289.

73. Dubois B, Ruberg M, Javoy-Agid F, et al. A sub-cortico-cortical cholinergic system is affected in Parkinson's disease. Brain Res 1983; 288:213–218.

74. Perry EK, Curtis M, Dick DJ, et al. Cholinergic correlates of cognitive impairment in Parkinson's disease: Comparison with Alzheimer's disease. J Neurol Neurosurg Psychiatry 1985; 48:413–421.

75. Ruberg M, Ploska A, Javoy-Agic F, et al. Muscarinic binding and choline acetyltransferase activity in parkinsonian subject with reference to dementia. Brain Res 1982; 232:129–139.

76. Javoy Agid F, Ruberg M, Hirsch E, et al. Recent progress in the neurochemistry of PD. In: Fahn S (eds.). Recent Developments in PD. New York: Raven Press, 1986:67–83.

77. Lloyd KG, Hornykiewicz O. L-glutamic acid decarboxylase in Parkinson's disease. Effects of L-dopa therapy. Nature 1973; 243:521–523.

78. Laaksonen H, Rinne UK, Sonninen V, et al. Brain GABA neurons in Parkinson's disease. Acta Neurol Scand 1978; 57(Suppl 67):282–283.

79. Perry TL, Javoy-Agid F, Agid Y, et al. Striatal GABA-ergic neuronal activity is not reduced in Parkinson's disease. J Neurochem 1983; 40:1120–1123.

80. Monfort JE, Javoy-Agid F, Hauw JJ, et al. Brain glutamate decarboxylase and "premortem severity index" with a special reference to Parkinson's disease. Brain 1985; 108(2):301–303.

81. Richardson PJ, Kase H, Jenner PG. Adenosine A2A receptor antagonists as new agents for the treatment of Parkinson's disease. Trends Pharmacol Sci 1997; 18:338–344.

82. Bartfai T. Presynaptic aspects of the coexistence of classical neurotransmitters and peptides. Trends Pharmacol Sci 1985; 6(7):331–334.

83. Agid Y and Javoy-Agid F. Peptides and Parkinson's disease. Trends Neurosci 1985; 8:30–35.

84. Hökfelt T, Skirboll l, Rehfeld JF, et al. A subpopulation of mesencephalic dopamine neurones projecting to limbic areas contains a cholesystokinin-like peptide: Evidence from immunohistochemistry combines with retrograde tracing. Neuroscience 1980; 5:2093–2124.

85. Studler JM, Javoy-Agid F, Cesselin F, et al. CCK-8 immunoreactivity distribution in human brain: Selective decrease in the substantia nigra from parkinsonian patients. Brain Res 1982; 243:176–179.

86. Skirboll LR, Grace AA, Hommer DW, et al. Peptide-monoamine coexistence: Studies of the actions of cholecystokinin-like peptide on the electrical activity of mid-brain dopamine neurons. Neuroscience 1981; 6:2111–2124.

87. Markstein R and Hökfelt T. Effects of cholecystokinin-octopeptide on dopamine release from slices of cat caudate nucleus. J Neurosci 1984; 4:570–575.

88. Mauborgne A, Javoy-Agid F, Legrand JC, et al. Decrease of substance P-like immunoreactivity in the substantia nigra and pallidum of parkinsonian brains. Brain Res 1983; 268:167–170.

89. Grafe MR, Forno LS, Eng LF. Immunocytochemical studies of substance P and Met-enkephalin in the basal ganglia and substantia nigra in Huntington's, Parkinson's and Alzheimer's diseases. J Neuropathol Exp Neurol 1985; 44:47–59.

90. Taquet H, Javoy-Agid F, Giraud P, et al. Dynorphin levels in parkinsonian patients; Leu-enkephalin production from either proenkephalin A or prodynorphin in human brain. Brain Res 1985; 341:390–392.

91. Taquet H, Javoy-Agid F, Cesselin F, et al. Microtopography of methionine-enkephalin dopamine and noradrenaline in the ventral mesencephalon of human

control and parkinsonian brains. *Brain Research* 1982; 235:303–314.

92. Taquet H, Javoy-Agid F, Hamon M, et al. Parkinson's disease affects differently Met[5] and Leu[5]-enkephalin production in the human brain. *Brain Res* 1983; 280:379–382.

93. Epelbaum J, Ruberg M, Moyse E, et al. Somatostatin and dementia in Parkinson's disease. *Brain Res* 1983; 278:376–378.

94. Lowe J. Lewy bodies. In: Calne DB (eds.). *Neurodegenerative Diseases*. Philadelphia: W.B. Saunders Company, 1994:51–69.

22

Basal Ganglia Anatomy and Physiology

Thomas Wichmann, M.D., Ph.D., Yoland Smith, Ph.D., and Jerrold L. Vitek, M.D., Ph.D.
Emory University, Atlanta, Georgia

INTRODUCTION

Research in the past decade has led to major insights into the structure and function of the basal ganglia and into the pathophysiologic basis of basal ganglia disorders, such as Parkinson's disease (PD) (1–8). This discussion will summarize current concepts of the anatomy and physiology of the basal ganglia as well as the pathophysiology of PD.

STRUCTURE AND FUNCTION OF BASAL GANGLIA CIRCUITS

The basal ganglia (see Figure 22-1) are a group of functionally related subcortical nuclei that include the striatum (comprised of the caudate nucleus and the putamen), the external globus pallidus (GPe), the internal globus pallidus (GPi), the substantia nigra, which includes the dopaminergic neurons in the pars compacta (SNc) and the GABAergic (gamma-amino butyric acid) neurons in the pars reticulata (SNr), and the subthalamic nucleus (STN). Anatomically and physiologically, these structures are integrally related to large portions of the cerebral cortex. The striatum, and, to a lesser extent, the STN, are the main entries for cortical information to the basal ganglia circuitry. From the striatum and the STN, cortical information is conveyed to the basal ganglia output nuclei, GPi and SNr. Basal ganglia outflow is directed at a variety of targets, among which are frontal areas of the cerebral cortex (via the ventrolateral thalamus), various brainstem structures (superior colliculus, lateral habenular nucleus, pedunculopontine nucleus, parvicellular reticular formation), and the striatum (via connections with thalamostriatal neurons in the caudal intralaminar nuclei).

Sources of Input to the Basal Ganglia

The Corticostriatal Projection

The corticostriatal projection terminates in a strict topographical organization that imposes on the striatum a segregation of functional territories (9–11). In primates the somatosensory, motor, and premotor cortices project somatotopically to the postcommissural region of the putamen (12–15) and the associative cortical areas project to the caudate nucleus and the precommissural putamen (16–20), whereas the limbic cortices, the amygdala, and the hippocampus terminate preferentially in the ventral striatum, which includes the nucleus accumbens and the olfactory tubercle (21–24).

Processing and integration of functionally related information in these striatal territories is probably governed by both convergence and segregation of cortical inputs. For instance evidence that associative areas of the cerebral cortex, which have reciprocal cortico-cortical projections, innervate common regions of the caudate nucleus in Rhesus monkeys (17,25) is opposed by studies demonstrating that projections from linked associative cortical areas were either completely segregated or minimally overlapping in the monkey striatum (18). Even more complex patterns of intrastriatal organization have been described for projections from sensorimotor cortical areas (14,15,26).

The striatum is composed of two main populations of neurons: the medium-sized spiny projection neurons that account for more than 90% of the total neuronal population, and aspiny neurons that are much less abundant and generally considered as interneurons (27–29). Dendritic spines of output neurons are, by far, the main targets of corticostriatal afferents (30), although GABAergic interneurons also receive significant cortical inputs (31).

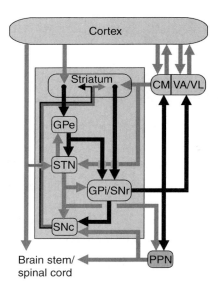

FIGURE 22-1. Schematic diagram of the basal ganglia-thalamocortical circuitry under normal conditions. Inhibitory connections are shown as filled arrows, excitatory connections as open arrows. Gpe = External segments of the globus pallidus; Gpi = internal segment of the globus pallidus; SNr = substantia nigra, pars reticulata; SNc = substantia nigra, pars compacta; STN = subthalamic nucleus; VL = ventrolateral thalamus.

The Thalamostriatal Projection

The intralaminar thalamic nuclei are a major source of excitatory afferents to the striatum (30,32–34). In primates, the caudal intralaminar nuclear group, the centromedian (CM) and the parafascicular (PF) nuclei, provide inputs that largely terminate in different functional territories in the striatum (34–36). The CM projects to the postcommissural sensorimotor part of the putamen, whereas the PF innervates predominantly the associative part of the caudate nucleus and the ventral striatum (34–36). CM and PF inputs innervate preferentially the dendritic shafts of specific striatal output neurons (33,34,37,38). Striatal interneurons immunoreactive for choline acetyltransferase, parvalbumin, and somatostatin also receive inputs from CM in monkeys (38).

The Cortico- and Thalamo-Subthalamic Projections

Anatomic evidence indicates that the corticosubthalamic projection is exclusively ipsilateral (39,40). In contrast to the corticostriatal projection that arises from the entire cortical mantle, the corticosubthalamic projection is largely derived from the primary motor cortex, with a minor contribution from prefrontal and premotor cortices (12,39–41). Afferents from the primary motor cortex are confined to the dorsolateral part of the STN (39,41), while afferents from premotor and supplementary motor areas innervate mainly the medial third of the nucleus (13,39,41,42). The prefrontal-limbic cortices project to the medialmost tip of the STN (39,40,43,44). Anatomic and physiologic evidence indicates that, like the cortical input to the striatum, the corticosubthalamic projection from M1 is somatotopically organized with the face area projecting laterally, the arm area centrally, and the leg area medially (12,39,41,45). Input from the supplementary motor area (SMA) to the STN appears to show a somatotopy that is reversed to the one from M1 (41). It is worth noting, however, that STN neurons in rats have long dendrites that may cross the boundaries of functional territories imposed by cortical projections (46).

A second major source of excitatory inputs to the STN arises from the caudal intralaminar thalamic nuclei (34,47,48). The thalamosubthalamic and thalamostriatal projections arise largely from segregated sets of neurons in the parafascicular nucleus of the thalamus in rats (48), although neurons that project to both structures were also found (49). Cortical and thalamic inputs are thought to be excitatory on STN neurons, resulting in faster transmission of cortical information to the basal ganglia output structures than via striato fugal pathways (44,50,51).

Intrinsic Basal Ganglia Connections

Direct and Indirect Striatofugal Projections

Over the last few years a model of the functional connectivity of the basal ganglia has emerged that describes how cortical information is conveyed from the striatum to the output nuclei of the basal ganglia (GPi and SNr) (see Figure 22-1). Most authors agree that the intrinsic organization of striatofugal projections impose the striatal organization into motor, limbic, associative, and oculomotor territories on the other basal ganglia structures (9). This organizational principle results in the formation of distinct motor, associative, limbic, and oculomotor cortico-basal ganglia-thalamo-cortical circuits that remain segregated through their subcortical course (9). Within the boundaries of each of these circuits, striatofugal pathways are divided into the so-called *direct* and *indirect* striatofugal pathways (3,52,53). The direct pathway arises from a subpopulation of neurons that project directly to neurons of the output nuclei, whereas the indirect pathway arises from a separate population of spiny neurons that project to GPe (57). In turn, GPe conveys the information either directly, or via the intercalated STN, to GPi and SNr. The direct GABAergic GPe → GPi projection terminates predominately on the proximal part of GPi and SNr neurons. In monkey, GPe terminals account for almost 50% of the total number of terminals in contact with the perikarya of GPi neurons (53,54).

Although the degree of segregation of striatofugal neurons is still a matter of debate (55–57), it appears that the subpopulation of striatal neurons that gives rise to the direct pathway can be further characterized by the presence of the neuropeptides substance P and dynorphin and by the preferential expression of the dopamine D1-receptors, while the subpopulation that gives rise to the indirect pathway expresses preferentially enkephalin and dopamine D2 receptors (58–60). The axons of striatal output neurons tend to form distinct bands of termination (55,57,61–63) that are highly specific (62,63). It appears that thalamic inputs from the centromedian nucleus of the thalamus target prefrentially neurons of the direct pathway, whereas sensorimotor cortical inputs influence preferentially indirect pathway neurons (38,64).

STN Projections

The main projection sites of the STN are GPi (EP in the rat) and SNr. The STN also provides a dense feedback projection to the GPe (46,65–70). Additional projections to the striatum (35,71,72), the SNc (68,73,74), the pedunculopontine nucleus (72,73,75) and the spinal cord (76) have also been described. STN output is highly collateralized in the rat (77,78) but is thought to be far more specific in primates (43,70,72,78,79,56,63).

Several recent studies have demonstrated highly ordered and specific relationships between neurons of the GPe, STN, and GPi (54,70,80). Thus populations of neurons within sensorimotor, cognitive and limbic territories in the GPe are reciprocally connected with populations of neurons in the same functional territories of the STN and the neurons in each of these regions, in turn, innervate the same functional territory of the GPi (54,70). It is possible, however, that additional, more divergent, circuits may exist (54,70,80,81).

Output Projections of the Basal Ganglia

Information flowing through the basal ganglia-thalamocortical circuitry probably remains segregated throughout their subcortical course (9), and structural convergence and functional integration are more likely to occur within than between the separate basal ganglia-thalamocortical circuits (9).

Nigrofugal Pathways

SNr neurons project to the thalamus, superior colliculus, pedunculopontine nucleus (PPN), and medullary reticular formation. Studies in rats suggest that SNr neurons may also project to the striatum (82). Nigrocollicular fibers terminate mainly on tectospinal neurons in the intermediate layer of the superior colliculus and play a critical role in the control of visual saccades (83). Nigrotegmental neurons terminate predominantly on noncholinergic neurons in the medial two-thirds of the PPN (84, 85). Many PPN neurons send projections back to the basal ganglia nuclei, including the SNr. The nigroreticular projection terminates in the parvicellular reticular formation, a region whose neurons are directly connected with orofacial motor nuclei (86–88).

At the thalamic level, inputs from the medial part of the SNr terminate mostly in the medial magnocellular division of the ventral anterior nucleus (VAmc) and the mediodorsal nucleus (MDmc) that, in turn, innervate anterior regions of the frontal lobe including the principal sulcus (Walker's area 46) and the orbital cortex (Walker's area 11) in monkeys (89). On the other hand, neurons in the lateral part of the SNr project preferentially to the lateral posterior region of the VAmc and to different parts of the MD. These areas of the thalamus are predominately related to posterior regions of the frontal lobe including the frontal eye field and areas of the premotor cortex, respectively (89). The striatonigral projections and output neurons in the rat SNr appear to be organized in a laminar pattern allowing for functionally segregated corticostriatal information to be channeled to separate thalamic, tectal, and brainstem targets (90,91). Based on the arrangement of striatal inputs and nigral outputs, the SNr in rats can be subdivided into a dorsolateral sensorimotor and a ventromedial associative territory (91), further supporting the hypothesis of a broad organization of the basal ganglia into segregated channels (9).

Pallidofugal Pathways

Current anatomic models view the GPi as a largely segregated structure, in which the ventrolateral two-thirds, the dorsal third, and the rostromedial pole of the GPi receive afferents arising from striatal territories innervated predominantly by sensorimotor, associative, and limbic cortical areas, respectively (11). The segregation is maintained in the pallidothalamic projection (92); sensorimotor information appears to be conveyed almost exclusively to the posterior part of the ventrolateral nucleus (VLo in macaques) and the associative GPi projects preferentially to the parvocellular part of the ventral anterior (VA) and the dorsal VL (VLc in macaques) (92–94). Projections from associative and limbic portions of GPi were found to innervate the same thalamic nuclei, suggesting that emotional and cognitive information from the basal ganglia may be integrated at the level of individual thalamocortical neurons.

Sensorimotor output from GPi is projected toward the supplementary motor area (SMA) (95–97), the primary motor cortex (M1) (97–103), and premotor (PM) cortical area (99). Virus transport studies have suggested that the outflow from basal ganglia motor areas, directed at cortical areas M1, PM, and SMA, arise from segregated populations of pallidothalamic neurons in macaques (99). Basal ganglia output related to associative and limbic functions, on the other hand, may be transmitted in a less specific manner to prefrontal cortical areas (104,105) as well as motor and supplementary motor regions (97,106).

Most GPi neurons that project to VA or VLo also send axon collaterals to the caudal intralaminar nuclear group (CM/PF), which in turn projects predominantly to the striatum, as mentioned earlier; (92). Neurons in the sensorimotor territory of the GPi project exclusively to CM, whereas associative and limbic areas predominantly reach PF. Therefore the functional segregation imposed upon the GPi by striatal afferents appears to be maintained at the level of the CM or PF in monkeys.

In monkeys a large proportion of neurons that project to the VA or VLo will also send axon collaterals to the noncholinergic portion of the PPN (107–111). The PPN gives rise to descending projections to the pons, medulla, and spinal cord as well as prominent ascending projections to the basal ganglia, the thalamus, and the basal forebrain (112). Besides the obvious potential for the basal ganglia to influence brainstem and spinal cord territories via the PPN, this nucleus may also integrate neuronal input from different functional territories of the GPi (107), which returns projections to the basal ganglia circuitry via its massive projection to the dopaminergic neurons of the SNc (113–118).

Functional Considerations

Feedback Circuits

The basal ganglia circuitry outlined above incorporates several potentially closed subcortical circuits. These closed subcortical circuits introduce a high degree of complexity into the models of basal ganglia function. These circuits include local loops consisting of axon collaterals within the basal ganglia nuclei,

as well as connections between them, such as reciprocal connections between STN and GPe (negative feedback), and GPe and GPi (positive feedback). Other feedback loops involve structures outside of the basal ganglia. For example, feedback loops may exist that involve the PPN; PPN output may directly affect basal ganglia output (Gpi $\xrightarrow{-}$ PPN $\xrightarrow{+}$ STN $\xrightarrow{+}$ GPi, negative feedback), or may indirectly affect basal ganglia activity via the intercalated SNc (GPi $\xrightarrow{+}$ PPN $\rightarrow$ SNc $\rightarrow$ striatum $\rightarrow$ direct, indirect pathway $\rightarrow$ GPi, positive feedback) (85,119–121). The thalamic nucleus CM may be involved in at least two separate feed back loops (Gpi $\xrightarrow{-}$ CM $\xrightarrow{+}$ STN $\xrightarrow{+}$ GPi (negative feedback), and Gpi $\xrightarrow{-}$ CM $\xrightarrow{+}$ putamen $\xrightarrow{+}$ GPi (positive feedback)). Another feedback loop may involve the habenula (Gpi $\xrightarrow{-}$ lateral habenula-raphé nuclei SNc $\rightarrow$ striatum $\rightarrow$direct, indirect pathway GPi).

The functional importance of these feedback systems is not clear, but it is obvious that basal ganglia output is very tightly controlled. Abnormal discharge in the basal ganglia output nuclei in movement disorders will affect the activity not only in the feedback loops but also in the primary targets. Positive feedback loops, such as the one involving PPN and the STN, or the pathway through CM and the putamen will tend to aggravate the abnormalities of discharge in the basal ganglia output nuclei associated with movement disorders, whereas negative feedback circuits, such as the one involving CM and STN, could serve to normalize neuronal discharge in the basal ganglia output nuclei. The possible role of these feedback loops in the pathogenesis of movement disorders will be considered.

Convergence vs Segregation in Basal Ganglia Circuits

The anatomic organization of the basal ganglia suggests that the basal ganglia-thalamocortical circuits are a highly specific system in which territories related to motor and to nonmotor functions remain segregated throughout the subcortical course. This anatomic concept is strongly supported by evidence from electrophysiologic recording studies that have demonstrated that each basal ganglia structure can be physiologically divided into distinct regions. Each region contains neurons that respond selectively to a narrow range of specific inputs or behaviors (at least within the experimental framework studied). For instance the sensorimotor portions of the basal ganglia contain specific areas with neurons that are concerned with active or passive limb movements (45,122–139). This region is anatomically separated from other areas, in which neuronal function is, for instance, related to eye movements (oculomotor circuit-140–144). Although the striatal interneuronal arrangement and the pallidal organization of neurons with large disklike dendritic trees that are traversed by multiple striatal efferent fibers suggest that at least some convergence takes place in the basal ganglia circuitry, physiologic studies to date have generally failed to demonstrate correlated discharge of neighboring striatal or pallidal cells (45,145,146). Furthermore, functional neurosurgical studies have demonstrated that lesions in the sensorimotor portion of the GPi alleviate the motor signs associated with Parkinsonism without affecting cognitive functions, whereas lesions outside of this region do not improve motor function but may affect cognition (147,148). Conceivably, one of the actions of dopamine (and other neuromodulators) may be to maintain functional segregation and to modulate the synaptic strength of collaterals and interneurons. This may occur particularly at the level of the striatum, as demonstrated through studies investigating the degree of (nonsynaptic) dye-coupling in the striatum (149–151) and studies in dopamine-depleted animals in which specificity of neuronal responses to stimuli appears to break down (146,152–158).

The Role of the Basal Ganglia in Motor Control

In functional terms, voluntary movements appear to be initiated at the cortical level of the motor circuit with simultaneous output to the brainstem and spinal cord, as well as to multiple subcortical targets, including the thalamus, putamen, and the STN. According to the model, an intended movement should depend on activation of specific portions of the direct pathway (resulting in appropriate reduction of inhibitory basal ganglia output), disinhibition of targeted thalamocortical neurons, and *facilitation* of the intended movement. By contrast, activation of the indirect pathway would lead to increased basal ganglia output and to *suppression* of unintended movement. Because the most common change in discharge in GPi output neurons during movement is an increase in activity, suppression of unintended or competing movement may be a particularly important role of the basal ganglia. Since the functions of the direct and indirect pathways appear to be distinctly different, it is possible that selective dysfunction of one or the other pathway may result in distinct clinical disturbances.

Based on clinical and experimental studies it has been widely accepted that the basal ganglia play a role in specifying the amplitude or velocity of movement (159). The combination of information traveling via the direct and the indirect pathways of the motor circuit has been proposed to > scale = or > focus = movements (10,160). To achieve scaling and termination of movements, striatal output would first inhibit specific neuronal populations in GPi/SNr via the direct pathway, facilitating movement, followed after a delay by disinhibition of the same GPi/SNr neuron via inputs over the indirect pathway, leading to an inhibition of the ongoing movement. In the focusing model, by contrast, inhibition of relevant pallidal or nigral neurons via the direct pathway would allow intended movements to proceed, whereas unintended movements would be suppressed by concomitant increased excitatory input via the indirect pathway in other GPi or SNr neurons. Similar models have been proposed for the generation of saccades in the oculomotor circuit (142). Direct anatomic support for either of these functions is lacking, because it is uncertain whether the direct and indirect pathways (emanating from neurons that are concerned with the same movement) converge on the same or separate neurons in GPi or SNr (56,161–163), and thus, whether > focusing = or > scaling = would be anatomically possible.

Although changes in discharge in most movement-related neurons in the basal ganglia occurs too late to influence the initiation of movement, changes in discharge could influence the amplitude or focus of ongoing movements (45,164). Conceivably, neurons with shorter onset latencies or with > preparatory = activity may indeed play such a role (101,165–173). Recent PET studies have reported that basal ganglia activity is modulated in relation to low-level parameters of movement, such as force or movement speed (174,175), thus supporting a scaling function of the basal ganglia.

Other proposed motor functions of the basal ganglia include roles in self-initiated (internally generated) movements in motor learning and in movement sequencing (176–178). For instance, both dopaminergic nigrostriatal neurons and tonically active neurons in the striatum have been shown to develop transient responses to sensory conditioning stimuli during behavioral training in classical conditioning tasks (178–181). This supports a role of these cells, and of basal ganglia areas whose activity they influence, in motor learning. Shifts in the response properties of striatal output neurons during performance of a maze task that involved learning were indeed recently demonstrated in the rat (182).

Lesion studies have yielded conflicting evidence regarding the motor functions of the basal ganglia. Most studies have found either no or only short-lived effects on skilled fine movements or mild bradykinesia after such lesions (183–193). A notable exception to this is a study by Mink and Thach (160,194,195) in which co-contractions were observed after lesioning or inactivation of GPi, although this may have been due to inadvertent involvement of GPe in these experiments. Given the relative paucity of motor side-effects of pallidal lesions in animals and humans, it could be concluded that, under normal conditions, basal ganglia output may not play a significant role in movement initiation or execution (176). When output from these structures is deranged (as is the case in movement disorders) the disruption of otherwise normal motor systems produces major abnormalities of movement.

It is also possible that the motor system may be sufficiently redundant so that loss of basal ganglia function after lesioning is compensated for by other neuronal mechanisms. The striking lack of motor side-effects *immediately* after pallidotomy argues against this possibility, because it could be expected that reorganization and changes in synaptic strength in other areas would require time to develop.

PATHOPHYSIOLOGY OF PARKINSON'S DISEASE

Parkinson's disease is characterized by the cardinal motor signs of akinesia, bradykinesia, muscular rigidity, and tremor at rest. The salient pathologic feature of idiopathic PD is relatively selective degeneration of neurons in the pars compacta of the substantia nigra (SNc) that give rise to dopamine-producing nigrostriatal fibers (196–198). In the earlier stages of PD, dopamine depletion appears to be greatest in the sensorimotor territory of the striatum, that is, the postcommissural portion of the putamen, suggesting that the motor circuit is preferentially involved in Parkinsonian pathophysiology (199).

The study of pathophysiologic changes in the basal ganglia that result from striatal dopamine loss has been facilitated by the discovery that primates treated with the neurotoxin 1-methyl-4-phenyl-1,2,3,6-tetrahydropyridine (MPTP) develop behavioral and anatomic changes that closely mimic the features of PD in humans (200–206). Physiologic changes in the striatopallidal pathways were first documented in biochemical studies, which indicated that in MPTP-induced Parkinsonism in primates the metabolic activity (as measured with the 2-deoxyglucose technique) is increased in both pallidal segments (207–213). This data was interpreted as evidence for increased activity of the striatum-GPe connection and the STN-GPi pathway, or, alternatively, as evidence for increased activity via the

projections from the STN to both pallidal segments. Later it was shown directly with microelectrode recordings of neuronal activity that MPTP-induced Parkinsonism in primates is associated with reduced tonic neuronal discharge in GPe, and increased mean discharge rates in the STN and GPi, as compared to normal controls (152–154,214,215) (see Figure 22-3). In Parkinsonian patients undergoing pallidotomy it has also been shown that, similar to findings in Parkinsonian animals, the discharge rates in GPe are significantly lower than those in GPi (216–219), although, of course, there has been no recording in normal controls for comparison. These findings have been interpreted as indicating that striatal dopamine depletion leads to increased activity of those striatal neurons that give rise to the projection to GPe, supressing neuronal discharge in GPe and resulting in disinhibition of STN and GPi via the indirect pathway. Loss of dopamine in the striatum is also postulated to lead to reduced activity via the inhibitory direct pathway (see Figure 22-2). However, this has not been directly demonstrated.

Reciprocal changes in the indirect and in the direct pathways following dopamine depletion should have the same net effect, that is, increased activity in GPi or SNr, leading to increased basal ganglia output to the thalamus and excessive inhibition of thalamocortical neurons. Two-deoxy-glucose studies demonstrated increased (synaptic) activity in the VA and VL nucleus of the thalamus (207–211), presumably reflecting increased inhibitory basal ganglia output to these subnuclei. Consistent with this are PET studies in parkinsonian patients, which have consistently shown reduced activation of motor and premotor areas in such patients (220–222) that are at least partially reversed after neurosurgical interventions designed to reduce GPi output, such as pallidotomies (223–225) or stimulation of the STN or GPi (226,227). Alterations of cortical activity in motor cortex and supplementary motor areas have also been demonstrated with single-cell recording in hemi-Parkinsonian primates (228).

The fact that the thalamic nucleus CM is tightly linked to the basal ganglia structures makes it highly likely that abnormal GPi output to CM may also play a role in parkinsonism. Increased inhibition of CM would not only lead to reduced activation of the CM-cortical pathway but could also lead to a further reduction of activity in the direct pathway, (i.e., CM → striatum → GPi/SNr), resulting in increased (inhibitory) output from GPi and SNr.

The PPN may also be involved in the development of parkinsonian signs. It has been shown that lesions of this nucleus in normal monkeys can lead to a hemi-Parkinsonian syndrome, possibly by reducing

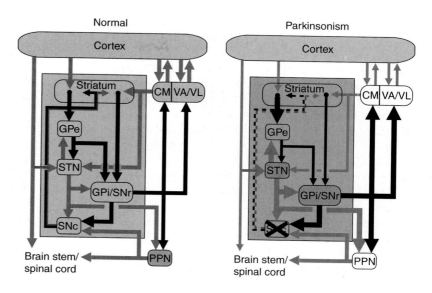

FIGURE 22-2. Schematic diagram of the basal ganglia-thalamocortical circuitry under normal and parkinsonian conditions. Parkinsonism leads to differential changes in the two striatopallidal projections, which are indicated by the thickness of the connecting arrows. Basal ganglia output to the thalamus is increased. Same abbreviations as in Figure 22-1.

excitation of SNc neurons by input from the PPN (229). Conceivably, in PD, activity in the PPN is inhibited by increased basal ganglia output, with the detrimental consequence that SNc activity would be further reduced, leading to worsening of parkinsonian signs.

Strong evidence for the importance of increased basal ganglia output in the development of parkinsonian motor signs comes from lesion studies. Specifically, lesions of the STN in MPTP-treated primates have been shown to reverse all of the cardinal motor signs of parkinsonism, probably by reducing GPi activity, but possibly also by normalizing the pattern of pallidal output (230–233). Recently, STN lesions have been shown to reverse Parkinsonian signs in PD patients (234,235). Stereotactic lesions of the motor portion of GPi have been reintroduced in human patients as treatment for medically intractable parkinsonism and have shown to be effective against all major parkinsonian motor signs and against drug-induced dyskinesias (191–193,236,237) (see Chapter 49). PET studies in such patients have shown that frontal motor areas whose metabolic activity was reduced in the parkinsonian state were again active following pallidotomy (223–225,236).

From the inception of the early model of the pathophysiology of parkinsonism, it was clear that it represented a gross oversimplification, as it was well recognized that lesions of the motor thalamus that abolish thalamocortical output from the motor circuit do not result in akinesia or bradykinesia and that GPi lesions do not result in excessive movement. The model also did not incorporate the prominent changes in discharge patterns of basal ganglia output neurons that are seen in Parkinsonian animals and humans and did not provide a satisfactory link between increased

basal ganglia output and the development of specific Parkinsonian motor signs.

Neuronal responses to passive limb manipulations in STN, GPi, and thalamus (152–155) have been shown to occur more often, to be more pronounced, and to have widened receptive fields after treatment with MPTP and the development of Parkinsonian motor signs. Cross-correlation studies have also revealed that a substantial proportion of neighboring neurons in globus pallidus and STN discharge in unison in MPTP-treated primates (146,154). This is in contrast to the virtual absence of synchronized discharge of such neurons in normal monkeys (45). Finally, the proportion of cells in STN, GPi, and SNr that discharge in oscillatory or nonoscillatory bursts is greatly increased in the parkinsonian state (152–154,214,219,238–241). Oscillatory burst discharge patterns are often seen in conjunction with tremor. The question of whether this is simply a reflection of tremor-related proprioceptive input or of active participation of the basal ganglia in the generation of tremor is still unsettled.

The importance of altered phasic discharge patterns is underlined by a consideration of the effects of selective ablations of key structures in parkinsonism. According to the simple rate-based model, a further reduction of thalamic activity should lead to increased Parkinsonian signs. It is therefore striking that lesions of the thalamus do not lead to parkinsonism but are, in fact, beneficial in the treatment of both tremor (cerebellar-receiving areas of thalamus) and rigidity (basal ganglia-receiving areas of thalamus). Lesions of GPi in the setting of parkinsonism lead to improvement in all aspects of PD without any obvious detrimental effects as long as lesions are

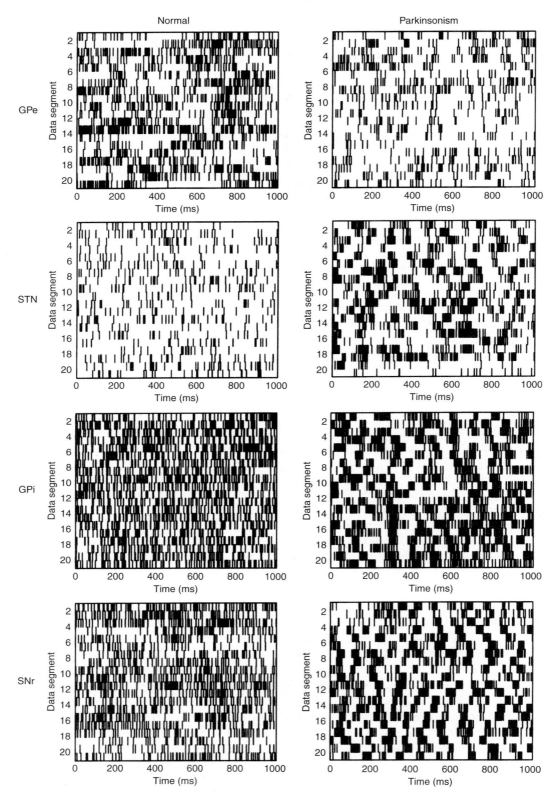

FIGURE 22-3. Raster display of spontaneous neuronal activity from different structures within the basal ganglia circuitry in the normal and parkinsonian state. SNr = substantia nigra pars reticulata. All other abbreviations are the same as Figure 22-1.

restricted to the sensorimotor portion of GPi. These results suggest that parkinsonism may not be simply due to an overall increase in basal ganglia output but instead may result from altered gain, abnormal timing, patterning, and synchronization of discharge in the basal ganglia that introduces specific errors into the thalamocortical signal. For instance, increased phasic activity in the basal ganglia may erroneously signal excessive movement or velocity to precentral motor areas, leading to a slowing or premature arrest of ongoing movements and to greater reliance upon external cues during movement. Alternatively, phasic alteration of discharge in the basal ganglia may simply introduce nonspecific noise into thalamic output to the cortex that is detrimental to cortical operations. The fact that both hypo- and hyperkinetic disorders (in which pallidal output is decreased) are relieved by pallidotomy strongly argues for the role of deranged rather than just increased or decreased basal ganglia output in the pathogenesis of these disorders.

A significant challenge to the proposed pathophysiologic model of parkinsonism has arisen from histochemical studies on the amount of mRNA for GAD_{67}, one of the enzymes synthesizing GABA in basal ganglia neurons. In contrast to GAD itself, which is found in neuronal cell bodies or terminals, the messenger RNA (mRNA) for the enzyme is thought to be contained exclusively in cell bodies. In these studies the GAD mRNA activity in a given nucleus is therefore taken as a parameter for the level of activity of GABAergic neurons in the structure under study. Experiments in parkinsonian primates have shown that, as expected from the above-mentioned model, GAD_{67} mRNA activity is increased in GPi neurons (242–244) and was reversible with levodopa administration. Although GAD_{67} mRNA activity in the GPi of humans with Parkinsonism was similar to that in controls, probably because these patients were chronically treated with levodopa (243,244).

Some of the findings regarding GAD mRNA in GPe, however, are at odds with the above-mentioned model in which the activity of GABAergic neurons in GPe is decreased. In rats, primates, and humans, GAD_{67} mRNA in GPe was either unchanged in the Parkinsonian state or even increased (5,243–246). These results have been interpreted as evidence that GPe and GPi function may not be as tightly linked via the indirect pathway, as proposed by the model outlined above and that observed activity changes in the basal ganglia may in fact primarily be due to altered activity via the cortico-subthalamic projection or dopaminergic inputs to the STN itself. These inputs, by changing STN activity, may cause the neuronal activity in both nuclei to increase, possibly due to a greater

tendency of neurons to discharge in bursts (247). However, the clear and consistent finding of decreased GPe discharge in MPTP-treated animals (153) and Parkinsonian patients are difficult to reconcile with the lack of change in GAD_{67} mRNA in GPe. Conceivably, GAD_{67} mRNA levels may reflect something other than neuronal discharge rates (248,249) or may be greatly influenced by the emergence of burst discharges.

Pathophysiology of Individual Parkinsonian Motor Signs

Parkinsonian signs, that is, tremor, rigidity, akinesia, and bradykinesia can occur independent of each other in patients. For instance, patients with severe akinesia or bradykinesia do not necessarily exhibit tremor, and akinetic patients may not experience significant bradykinesia or rigidity. This suggests that these different signs may depend on different pathophysiologic mechanisms or involve different portions of the cortico-subcortical circuitry. The physiologic basis of the cardinal Parkinsonian motor signs (2,99,250,251) will be briefly considered in the following:

Akinesia Akinesia, the hallmark of hypokinetic disorders such as PD is characterized by a global impairment of movement initiation. Patients typically report a normal or even increased desire to move but are unable to do so effectively. Although there is some evidence that certain aspects of akinesia may be related to abnormal activity along the brainstem projections of the basal ganglia output nuclei (229), most workers attribute akinesia to changes in cortical processing due to altered basal ganglia output. Discharge rates in the basal ganglia output nuclei probably have a significant impact on the amount of movement. Discharge rates in GPi or SNr are determined, at least in part, by the amount and distribution of striatal dopamine, which in turn determines the balance between overall discharge in the direct and indirect pathways. There are many possible ways in which increased basal ganglia output could lead to akinesia. For instance, increased tonic inhibition of thalamocortical neurons by excessive output from GPi or SNr may reduce the responsiveness of cortical mechanisms involved in motor control and prevent transmission of phasic reductions in activity that occur during movement execution. This may, in turn, interfere with the normal scaling of movement. Increased tonic inhibition of thalamocortical neurons may also render precentral motor areas less responsive to other inputs normally involved in initiating movements or could interfere with "set" functions that have been shown to be highly dependent on the integrity of basal ganglia pathways (52).

Although there has been at least one study in which large bilateral lesions of the VA territory in primates induced transient problems with akinesia and more long-term problems with motor learning (252), by and large, lesions of the basal ganglia-receiving and cerebellar-receiving areas of thalamus (VLo, and VPLo, respectively) do not induce akinesia. This is a strong argument against the view that increased tonic pallidal output and resulting inhibition of the thalamocortical neurons is the sole reason for the development of akinesia. Altered discharge patterns in the basal ganglia output to the thalamus may therefore be more important than rate changes alone. Alternatively, akinesia may develop as a consequence of abnormally reduced activity in the PPN nucleus and descending brainstem projections.

Akinesia is the best example of a parkinsonian sign whose development appears to depend on discharge abnormalities in specific subcircuits of the motor loop. PET studies of cortical activation in akinesia-predominant Parkinsonism suggest that the supplementary (SMA) and dorsal prefrontal motor areas are hypoactive in such patients (253,254). Further evidence for abnormal activity in these areas comes from studies of the Bereitschaftspotential (readiness potential), a slow negative cortical potential that precedes self-paced movements and is thought to reflect the neural activity in SMA (255). The early portion of the Bereitschaftspotential is smaller in Parkinsonian patients than in age-matched controls (256,257), suggesting a deficit in the normal function of the SMA in the early stages of preparation for self-initiated movements. Thus, akinesia may be related to abnormal discharge in a subcircuit with mostly "preparatory" activity (101,166–173), interfering with the planning and early execution stages of movement. A disorganization of preparatory activity in SMA neurons were indeed identified with electrophysiologic methods in hemi-parkinsonian primates (228) and is consistent with this proposal.

Bradykinesia Although bradykinesia is usually associated with akinesia, these two signs can be strikingly dissociated in some patients. The pathophysiology of bradykinesia may be closely associated with the postulated scaling function of basal ganglia output (as mentioned earlier) (258–265) and is probably also dependent on abnormal processing in prefrontal cortical areas that are strongly influenced by increased basal ganglia output. In normal monkeys, neurophysiologic studies, and, more recently, PET studies investigating cerebral blood flow, have described an influence of velocity and amplitude on the discharge of neurons in these premotor cortical areas (132–139,174,175,266).

Conceivably, abnormally increased phasic GPi or SNr output during movement may signal excessive speed and/or amplitude of ongoing movement, leading to a corrective reduction in cortical motor output. PET studies measuring cerebral blood flow in human Parkinsonian patients investigated before and during deep brain stimulation of GPi have revealed that stimulation that improved bradykinesia lead to an increase in blood flow in the ipsilateral premotor cortical areas (227). A recent PET study has shown a significant correlation between movement speed and basal ganglia activation (175), which is lost in PD (Turner et al. personal communication). Furthermore, recent studies in Parkinsonian monkeys have demonstrated a direct correlation between the severity of bradykinesia and mean discharge rates of neurons in GPi (267). Neuronal data from Parkinsonian patients has also demonstrated that patients whose predominant symptoms were bradykinesia and akinesia had higher mean discharge rates in GPi than those patients who were tremor predominant and had mild bradykinesia (268). Thus there are several independent lines of evidence supporting the role of the basal ganglia motor circuitry in the scaling of movement and the disruption of this in diseases such as PD.

Rigidity Parkinsonian rigidity is characterized by a uniform increase in resistance to passive movements about individual joints. The pathophysiology of rigidity is elusive, but it must ultimately result from changes at the spinal cord level. It has been suggested that altered basal ganglia output mediated via the PPN and its output to the pontine nucleus gigantocellularis and the dorsal longitudinal fasciculus of the reticulospinal projection may lead to increased inhibition of Ib interneurons that in turn may disinhibit $\forall$-motoneurons (269–271). Abnormalities of long-latency reflexes (LLRs) may also play a role in abnormal $\forall$-motoneuron excitability (272–274), although the velocity-independence of rigidity suggests that it is not a reflex phenomenon *per se*. The finding that rigidity is abolished by both pallidal and thalamic ablation strongly suggests that pallidal output leads to rigidity via the thalamocortical route rather than directly via brainstem projections.

Tremor Parkinsonian tremor is typically a 4–5 Hz tremor at rest that is suppressed by movement. Parkinsonian tremor has been shown to be critically dependent on the integrity of the thalamic nucleus ventralis intermedius (Vim) and that lesions of Vim abolish tremor. It has been demonstrated that Vim contains neurons that exhibit oscillatory discharges at the tremor frequency (275–281). It has also been proposed that oscillatory discharge in these thalamic cells may be induced by hyperpolarization of these neurons induced by increased inhibitory basal ganglia output (282), which increases the likelihood that these cells will discharge in bursts (283–288).

It is also possible that tremor arises primarily from oscillatory discharge originating within the basal ganglia. This notion is based on the finding of oscillatory discharge patterns in the STN and GPi in Parkinsonian patients and animals (154,218,239,268,289–291). It has been speculated that intrinsic membrane properties of basal ganglia neurons are conducive to the development of oscillatory discharge (292) in basal ganglia neurons themselves or may contribute to the generation of oscillatory discharge in the thalamus (2,293–295) that may then be transmitted to the cortex.

Support for the concept that altered basal ganglia discharge is important in tremor development comes from lesion studies showing that Parkinsonian tremor in MPTP-treated African green monkeys and in patients with Parkinsonism is ameliorated by lesions of the STN and GPi (53,192,218,237,294). It has been suggested that loss of *extrastriatal* dopamine may contribute to the development of tremor, because primates in which MPTP treatment affects the dopamine supply to GPi (African green monkeys) tend to develop tremor, whereas species in which the dopamine supply to GPi is not as severely affected (Rhesus monkeys) rarely develop Parkinsonian tremor (296). Furthermore, in a postmortem study it was found that the degree of dopamine loss in the striatum did not correlate with the extent of tremor in Parkinsonian patients, whereas the degree of dopamine loss in the pallidum did (197).

CONCLUSIONS

The basal ganglia are part of cortico-subcortical circuits that may be involved in a large variety of motor as well as nonmotor functions. Parkinsonism emerges as a complex disorder in which striatal dopamine depletion results in increased and disordered discharge in motor areas of basal ganglia thalamocortical loops. It is likely that individual Parkinsonian motor signs are caused by distinct abnormalities in basal ganglia discharge and by involvement of specific subcircuits related to distinct cortical targets.

The current models of basal ganglia anatomy, physiology, and pathophysiology clearly need further refinement. Most pertinently, changes in the firing pattern, degree of synchronization, and receptive field properties of neurons in the basal ganglia and thalamus need to be better incorporated along with new anatomic connections into future models of basal

ganglia pathophysiology. A greater emphasis needs to be placed on the manner in which thalamic, brainstem, and cortical neurons utilize basal ganglia output as we continue to define and develop concepts of basal ganglia function.

REFERENCES

1. DeLong MR. Primate models of movement disorders of basal ganglia origin. *Trends Neurosci* 1990; 13:281–285.
2. Wichmann T, DeLong MR. Functional and pathophysiological models of the basal ganglia. *Curr Opin in Neurobiol* 1996; 6:751–758.
3. Albin RL, Young AB, Penney JB. The functional anatomy of basal ganglia disorders. *Trends Neurosci* 1989; 12:366–375.
4. Albin RL. The pathophysiology of chorea/ballism and parkinsonism. *Parkinsonism Rel Disord* 1995; 1:3–11.
5. Chesselet MF, Delfs JM. Basal ganglia and movement disorders: An update. *Trends Neurosci* 1996; 19:417–422.
6. Brooks DJ. The role of the basal ganglia in motor control: Contributions from PET. *J Neurol Sci* 1995; 128:1–13.
7. Graybiel AM. Basal ganglia: New therapeutic approaches to Parkinson's disease. *Curr Biol* 1996; 6(4):368–371.
8. Graybiel AM, et al. The basal ganglia and adaptive motor control. *Science* 1994; 265(5180):1826–1831.
9. Alexander GE, DeLong MR, Strick PL. Parallel organization of functionally segregated circuits linking basal ganglia and cortex. *Ann Rev Neurosci* 1986; 9:357–381.
10. Alexander GE, Crutcher MD, DeLong MR. Basal ganglia-thalamocortical circuits: Parallel substrates for motor, oculomotor, 'prefrontal' and 'limbic' functions. *Prog Brain Res* 1990; 85:119–146.
11. Parent A. Extrinsic connections of the basal ganglia. *Trends Neurosci* 1990; 13:254–258.
12. Kunzle H. Bilateral projections from precentral motor cortex to the putamen and other parts of the basal ganglia. An autoradiographic study in macaca fascicularis. *Brain Res* 1975; 88:195–209.
13. Kunzle H. An autoradiographic analysis of the efferent connections from premotor and adjacent prefrontal regions (areas 6 and 9) in macaca fascicularis. *Brain Behav Evol* 1978; 15:185–234.
14. Flaherty AW, Graybiel AM. Corticostriatal transformations in the primate somatosensory system. Projections from physiologically mapped body-part representations. *J Neurophysiol* 1991; 66:1249–1263.
15. Flaherty AW, Graybiel AM. Two input systems for body representations in the primate striatal matrix: Experimental evidence in the squirrel monkey. *J Neurosci* 1993; 13:1120–1137.

16. Goldman PS, Nauta WJH. An intricately patterned prefronto-caudate projection in the rhesus monkey. *J Comp Neurol* 1977; 171:369–386.

17. Yeterian EH, VanHoesen GW. Cortico-striate projections in the rhesus monkey: The organization of certain cortico-caudate connections. *Brain Res* 1978; 139:43–63.

18. Selemon LD, Goldman-Rakic PS. Longitudinal topography and interdigitation of cortico-striatal projections in the rhesus monkey. *J Neurosci* 1985; 5:776–794.

19. Yeterian EH, Pandya DN. Prefrontostriatal connections in relation to cortical architectonic organization in rhesus monkeys. *J Comp Neurol* 1991; 312(1):43–67.

20. Yeterian EH, Pandya DN. Corticostriatal connections of the superior temporal region in rhesus monkeys. *J Comp Neurol* 1998; 399(3):384–402.

21. Russchen FT, et al. The amygdalostriatal projections in the monkey. An anterograde tracing study. *Brain Res* 1985; 329:241–257.

22. Alheid GF, Heimer L. New perspectives in basal forebrain organization of special relevance for neuropsychiatric disorders: The striatopallidal, amygdaloid, and corticopetal components of substantia innominata. *Neuroscience* 1988; 27(1):1–39.

23. Kunishio K, Haber SN. Primate cingulostriatal projection: Limbic striatal versus sensorimotor striatal input. *J Comp Neurol* 1994; 350:337–356.

24. Haber SN, et al. The orbital and medial prefrontal circuit through the primate basal ganglia. *J Neurosci* 1995; 15:4851–4867.

25. Parthasarathy HB, Schall JD, Graybiel AM. Distributed but convergent ordering of corticostriatal projections: Analysis of the frontal eye field and the supplementary eye field in the macaque monkey. *J Neurosci* 1992; 12(11):4468–4488.

26. Malach R, Graybiel AM. Mosaic architecture of the somatic sensory-recipient sector of the cat's striatum. *J Neurosci* 1986; 6(12):3436–3458.

27. Smith Y, Bolam JP. The output neurones and the dopaminergic neurones of the substantia nigra receive a GABA-containing input from the globus pallidus in the rat. *J Comp Neuro* 1990; 296(1):47–64.

28. Kawaguchi Y, et al. Striatal interneurones: Chemical, physiological and morphological characterization [published erratum appears in Trends Neurosci 1996 Apr;19(4):143]. *Trends Neurosci* 1995; 18(12):527–535.

29. Wilson CJ. Basal ganglia. In: Shepherd GM (ed.). *The Synaptic Organization of the Brain*, Oxford: Oxford University Press, 1990.

30. Kemp JM, Powell TPS. The connections of the striatum and globus pallidus: Synthesis and speculation. *Phil Trans R Soc Lond* 1971; 262:441–457.

31. Lapper SR, et al. Cortical input to parvalbumin-immunoreactive neurones in the putamen of the squirrel monkey. *Brain Res* 1992; 580(1–2):215–224.

32. Wilson CJ, Chang HT, Kitai ST. Origins of post synaptic potentials evoked in spiny neostriatal projection neurons by thalamic stimulation in the rat. *Exp Brain Res* 1983; 51:217–226.

33. Dube L, Smith AD, Bolam JP. Identification of synaptic terminals of thalamic or cortical origin in contact with distinct medium-size spiny neurons in the rat neostriatum. *J Comp Neurol* 1988; 267:455–471.

34. Sadikot AF, et al. Efferent connceions of the centromedian and parafascicular thalamic nuclei in the squirrell monkey: A light and electron microscopic study of the thalamostriatal projection in relation to striatal heterogeneity. *J Comp Neurol* 1992; 320:228–242.

35. Smith Y, Parent A. Differential connections of caudate nucleus and putamen in the squirrel monkey (Saimiri Sciureus). *Neuroscience* 1986; 18:347–371.

36. Nakano K, et al. Topographical projections from the thalamus, subthalamic nucleus and pedunculopontine tegmental nucleus to the striatum in the Japanese monkey, Macaca fuscata. *Brain Res* 1990; 537(1–2):54–68.

37. Smith Y, et al. Synaptic relationships between dopaminergic afferents and cortical or thalamic input in the sensorimotor territory of the striatum in monkey. *J Comp Neurol* 1994; 344:1–19.

38. Sidibe M, Smith Y. Differential synaptic innervation of striatofugal neurones projecting to the internal or external segments of the globus pallidus by thalamic afferents in the squirrel monkey. *J Comp Neurol* 1996; 365(3):445–465.

39. Hartmann-von Monakow K, Akert K, Kunzle H. Projections of the precentral motor cortex and other cortical areas of the frontal lobe to the subthalamic nucleus in the monkey. *Exp Brain Res* 1978; 33:395–403.

40. Afsharpour S. Topographical projections of the cerebral cortex to the subthalamic nucleus. *J Comp Neurol* 1985; 236(1):14–28.

41. Nambu A, et al. Dual somatotopical representations in the primate subthalamic nucleus: Evidence for ordered but reversed body-map transformations from the primary motor cortex and the supplementary motor area. *J Neurosci* 1996; 16(8):2671–2683.

42. Nambu A, et al. Corticosubthalamic input zones from forelimb representations of the dorsal and ventral divisions of the premotor cortex in the macaque monkey: Comparison with the input zones from the primary motor cortex and the supplementary motor area. *Neurosci Lett* 1997; 239(1):13–16.

43. Berendse HW, Groenewegen HJ. The connections of the medial part of the subthalamic nucleus in the rat. Evidence for a parallel organization. In: Bernardi G, et al. (eds.). *The Basal Ganglia II*. New York: Plenum Press, 1989:89–98.

44. Maurice N, et al. Relationships between the prefrontal cortex and the basal ganglia in the rat: Physiology of the corticosubthalamic circuits. *J Neurosci* 1998; 18(22):9539–9546.

45. Wichmann T, Bergman H, DeLong MR. The primate subthalamic nucleus. I. Functional properties in intact animals. *J Neurophysiol* 1994; 72:494–506.

46. Bevan MD, Clarke NP, Bolam JP. Synaptic integration of functionally diverse pallidal information in the entopeduncular nucleus and subthalamic nucleus in the rat. *J Neurosci* 1997; 17(1):308–324.

47. Sugimoto T, et al. Direct projections from the centre median-parafascicular complex to the subthalamic nucleus in the cat and rat. *J Comp Neurol* 1983; 214:209–216.

48. Feger J, Bevan M, Crossman AR. The projections from the parafascicular thalamic nucleus to the subthalamic nucleus and the striatum arise from separate neuronal populations: A comparison with the corticostriatal and corticosubthalamic efferents in a retrograde double-labelling study. *Neuroscience* 1994; 60(1):125–132.

49. Deschenes M, et al. A single-cell study of the axonal projections arising from the posterior intralaminar thalamic nuclei in the rat. *Eur J Neurosci* 1996; 8(2):329–343.

50. Ryan LJ, Clark KB. The role of the subthalamic nucleus in the response of globus pallidus neurons to stimulation of the prelimbic and agranular frontal cortices in rats. *Exp Brain Res* 1991; 86(3):641–651.

51. Kita H. Physiology of two disynaptic pathways from the sensorimotor cortex to the basal ganglia output nuclei, New ideas and data on structure and function, Percheron G, McKenzie JS, Feger J (eds.). *The Basal Ganglia IV*. New York and London: Plenum Press, 1994:263–276.

52. Alexander GE, Crutcher MD. Functional architecture of basal ganglia circuits: neural substrates of parallel processing. *Trends Neurosci* 1990; 13:266–271.

53. Bergman H, Wichmann T, DeLong MR. Amelioration of Parkinsonian Symptoms by Inactivation of the Subthalamic Nucleus (STN) in MPTP Treated Green Monkeys. First International Congress of Movement Disorders Abstracts, 1990.

54. Smith Y, et al. Microcircuitry of the direct and indirect pathways of the basal ganglia. *Neuroscience* 1998; 86(2):353–387.

55. Kawaguchi Y, Wilson CJ, Emson PC. Projection subtypes of rat neostriatal matrix cells revealed by intracellular injection of biocytin. *J Neurosci* 1990; 10(10):3421–3438.

56. Parent A, Hazrati L-N. Functional anatomy of the basal ganglia. I. The cortico-basal ganglia-thalamo-cortical loop. *Brain Res Rev* 1995; 20:91–127.

57. Gerfen CR, Wilson CJ. The Basal Ganglia. In: Björkland A, Hökfeld T, Swanson L (eds.). Amsterdam: Elsevier, 1996:396.

58. Gerfen CR, et al. D1 and D2 dopamine receptor-regulated gene expression of striatonigral and striatopallidal neurons. *Science* 1990; 250:1429–1432.

59. LeMoine C, et al. Dopamine receptor gene expression by enkephalin neurons in rat forebrain. *Proc Natl Acad Sci USA* 1990; 182:611–612.

60. Surmeier DJ, Song WJ, Yan Z. Coordinated expression of dopamine receptors in neostriatal medium spiny neurons. *J Neurosci* 1996; 16(20):6579–6591.

61. Chang HT, Wilson CJ, Kitai ST. Single neostriatal efferent axons in the globus pallidus: A light and electron microscopic study. *Science* 1981; 213:915–918.

62. Gerfen CR. The neostriatal mosaic. I. Compartmental organization of projections from the striatum to the substantia nigra in the rat. *J Comp Neurol* 1985; 236:454–476.

63. Parent A, Hazrati L. Anatomical aspects of information processing in primate basal ganglia. *Trends Neurosci* 1993; 16(3):111–116.

64. Parthasarathy HB, Graybiel AM. Cortically driven immediate-early gene expression reflects influence of sensorimotor cortex on identified striatal neurons in the squirrel. *J Neurosci* 1997; 17:2477–2491.

65. Nauta HJ, Cole M. Efferent projections of the subthalamic nucleus: An autoradiographic study in monkey and cat. *J Comp Neurol* 1978; 180(1):1–16.

66. Carpenter MB, et al. Interconnections and organization of pallidal and subthalamic nucleus neurons in the monkey. *J Comp Neurol* 1981; 197:579–603.

67. Moriizumi T, et al. Ultrastructural analyses of afferent terminals in the subthalamic nucleus of the cat with a combined degeneration and horseradish peroxidase tracing method. *J Comp Neurol* 1987; 265(2):159–174.

68. Smith Y, Hazrati LN, Parent A. Efferent projections of the subthalamic nucleus in the squirrel monkey as studied by PHA-L anterograde tracing method. *J Comp Neurol* 1990; 294:306–323.

69. Shink E, Smith Y. Differential synaptic innervation of neurons in the internal and external segments of the globus pallidus by the GABA- and glutamate-containing terminals in the squirrel monkey. *J Comp Neurol* 1995; 358(1):119–141.

70. Shink E, et al. The subthalamic nucleus and the external pallidum: Two tightly interconnected structures that control the output of the basal ganglia in the monkey. *Neuroscience* 1996. in press.

71. Beckstead RM. A reciprocal axonal connection between the subthalamic nucleus and the neostriatum in the cat. *Brain Res* 1983; 275(1):137–142.

72. Parent A, Smith Y. Organization of efferent projections of the subthalamic nucleus in the squirrel monkey as revealed by retrograde labeling methods. *Brain Res* 1987; 436:296–310.

73. Kita H, Kitai ST. Efferent projections of the subthalamic nucleus in the rat: Light and electron microscope analysis with the PHA-L method. *J Comp Neurol* 1987; 260:435–452.

74. Smith ID, Grace AA. Role of the subthalamic nucleus in the regulation of nigral dopamine neuron activity. *Synapse* 1992; 12(4):287–303.

75. Hammond C, et al. Anatomical and electrophysiological studies on the reciprocal projections between the

subthalamic nucleus and nucleus tegmenti pedunculopontinus in the rat. *Neuroscience* 1983; 9:41–52.

76. Takada M, Li ZK, Hattori T. Long descending direct projection from the basal ganglia to the spinal cord: A revival of the extrapyramidal concept. *Brain Res* 1987; 436(1):129–135.

77. Deniau JM, et al. Electrophysiological properties of identified output neurons of the rat substantia nigra (pars compacta and pars reticulata): Evidences for the existence of branched neurons. *Exp Brain Res* 1978; 32(3):409–422.

78. Van Der Kooy D, Hattori T. Single subthalamic nucleus neurons project to both the globus pallidus and substantia nigra in rat. *J Comp Neurol* 1980; 192(4):751–768.

79. Haber SN, Lynd-Balta E, Mitchell SJ. The organization of the descending ventral pallidal projections in the monkey. *J Comp Neurol* 1993; 329:111–128.

80. Smith Y, Shink E, Sidibe M. Neuronal circuitry and synaptic connectivity of the basal ganglia. *Neurosurg Clin North Am* 1998; 9(2):203–222.

81. Joel D, Weiner I. The connections of the primate subthalamic nucleus: Indirect pathways and the open-interconnected scheme of basal ganglia-thalamocortical circuitry. *Brain Res-Brain Res Reviews* 1997; 23(1–2):62–78.

82. Rodriguez M, Gonzalez-Hernandez T. Electrophysiological and morphological evidence for a GABAergic nigrostriatal pathway. *J Neurosci* 1999; 19(11):4682–4694.

83. Wurtz RH, Hikosaka O. Role of the basal ganglia in the initiation of saccadic eye movements. *Prog Brain Res* 1986; 64:175–190.

84. Spann BM, Grofova I. Origin of ascending and spinal pathways from the nucleus tegmenti pedunculopontinus in the rat. *J Comp Neurol* 1989; 283:13–27.

85. Grofova I, Zhou M. Nigral innervation of cholinergic and glutamatergic cells in the rat mesopontine tegmentum: Light and electron microscopic anterograde tracing and immunohistochemical studies. *J Comp Neurol* 1998; 395(3):359–379.

86. Chandler SH, et al. The effects of nanoliter ejections of lidocaine into the pontomedullary reticular formation on cortically induced rhythmical jaw movements in the guinea pig. *Brain Res* 1990; 526(1):54–64.

87. von Krosigk M, et al. Synaptic organization of gabaergic inputs from the striatum and the globus pallidus onto neurons in the substantia nigra and retrorubral field which project to the medullary reticular formation. *Neuroscience* 1993; 50:531–549.

88. Mogoseanu D, Smith AD, Bolam JP. Monosynaptic innervation of facial motoneurones by neurones of the parvicellular reticular formation. *Exp Brain Res* 1994; 101(3):427–438.

89. Ilinsky IA, Jouandet ML. Goldman-Rakic PS. Organization of the nigrothalamocortical system in the rhesus monkey. *J Comp Neurol* 1985; 236:315–330.

90. Deniau JM, Chevalier G. The lamellar organization of the rat substantia nigra pars reticulata: Distribution of projection neurons. *Neuroscience* 1992; 46(2):361–377.

91. Deniau JM, Thierry AM. Anatomical segregation of information processing in the rat substantia nigra pars reticulata. *Adv Neurol* 1997; 74:83–96.

92. Sidibe M, et al. Efferent connections of the internal globus pallidus in the squirrel monkey: I. Topography and synaptic organization of the pallidothalamic projection. *J Comp Neurol* 1997; 382(3):323–347.

93. Kim R, et al. Projections of the globus pallidus and adjacent structures: An autoradiographic study in the monkey. *J Comp Neurol* 1976; 169(3):263–290.

94. DeVito JL, Anderson ME. An autoradiographic study of efferent connections of the globus pallidus in Macaca mulatta. *Exp Brain Res* 1982; 46(1):107–117.

95. Schell GR, Strick PL. The origin of thalamic inputs to the arcuate premotor and supplementary motor areas. *J Neurosci* 1984; 4:539–560.

96. Strick PL. How do the basal ganglia and cerebellum gain access to the cortical motor areas? *Behav Brain Res* 1985; 18(2):107–123.

97. Inase M, Tanji J. Thalamic distribution of projection neurons to the primary motor cortex relative to afferent terminal fields from the globus pallidus in the macaque monkey. *J Comp Neurol* 1995; 353(3):415–426.

98. Nambu A, Yoshida S, Jinnai K. Projection on the motor cortex of thalamic neurons with pallidal input in the monkey. *Exp Brain Res* 1988; 71:658–662.

99. Hoover JE, Strick PL. Multiple output channels in the basal ganglia. *Science* 1993; 259:819–821.

100. Hoover JE, Strick PL. The organization of cerebellar and basal ganglia outputs to primary motor cortex as revealed by retrograde transneuronal transport of herpes simplex virus type 1. *J Neurosci* 1999; 19(4):1446–1463.

101. Jinnai K, et al. The two separate neuron circuits through the basal ganglia concerning the preparatory or execution proceses of motor control. In: Mamo M, Hamada I, DeLong MR (eds.). *Role of the cerebellem and Basal Ganglia in Volumatry Movement*. Elsevier Science, 1993:153–161.

102. Rouiller EM, et al. Cerebellothalamocortical and pallidothalamocortical projections to the primary and supplementary motor cortical areas: A multiple tracing study in macaque monkeys. *J Comp Neurol* 1994; 345(2):185–213.

103. Kayahara T, Nakano K. Pallido-thalamo-motor cortical connections: An electron microscopic study in the macaque monkey. *Brain Res* 1996; 706(2):337–342.

104. Goldman-Rakic PS, Porrino LJ. The primate mediodorsal (MD) nucleus and its projection to the frontal lobe. *J Comp Neurol* 1985; 242:535–560.

105. Middleton FA, Strick PL. Anatomical evidence for cerebellar and basal ganglia involvement

in higher cognitive function. *Science* 1994; 266(5184):458–461.

106. Darian-Smith C, Darian-Smith I, Cheema SS. Thalamic projections to sensorimotor cortex in the macaque monkey: Use of multiple retrograde fluorescent tracers. *J Comp Neurol* 1990; 299:17–46.

107. Shink E, Sidibe M, Smith Y. Efferent connections of the internal globus pallidus in the squirrel monkey: II. Topography and synaptic organization of pallidal efferents to the pedunculopontine nucleus. *J Comp Neurol* 1997; 382(3):348–363.

108. Harnois C, Filion M. Pallidofugal projections to thalamus and midbrain: A quantitative antidromic activation study in monkeys and cats. *Exp Brain Res* 1982; 47:277–285.

109. Parent A, De Bellefeuille L. Organization of efferent projections from the internal segment of globus pallidus in primate as revealed by flourescence retrograde labeling method. *Brain Res* 1982; 245:201–213.

110. Rye DB, et al. Medullary and spinal efferents of the pedunculopontine tegmental nucleus and adjacent mesopontine tegmentum in the rat. *J Comp Neurol* 1988; 269(3):315–341.

111. Steininger TL, Rye DB, Wainer BH. Afferent projections to the cholinergic pedunculopontine tegmental nucleus and adjacent midbrain extrapyramidal area in the albino rat. I. Retrograde tracing studies. *J Comp Neurol* 1992; 321(4):515–543.

112. Inglis WL, Winn P. The pedunculopontine tegmental nucleus: Where the striatum meets the reticular formation. *Prog Neurobiol* 1995; 47:1–29.

113. Jackson A, Crossman AR. Nucleus tegmenti pedunculopontinus: Efferent connections with special reference to the basal ganglia, studied in the rat by anterograde and retrograde transport of horseradish peroxidase. *Neuroscience* 1983; 10:725–765.

114. Moon-Edley S, Graybiel AM. The afferent and efferent connections of the feline nucleus tegmenti pedunculopontinus, pars compacta. *J Comp Neurol* 1983; 217:187–215.

115. Lee HJ, et al. Cholinergic vs. noncholinergic efferents from the mesopontine tegmentum to the extrapyramidal motor system nuclei. *J Comp Neurol* 1988; 275(4):469–492.

116. Lavoie B, Parent A. Pedunculopontine nucleus in the squirrel monkey: Projections to the basal ganglia as revealed by anterograde tract-tracing methods. *J Comp Neurol* 1994; 344(2):210–231.

117. Oakman SA, et al. Distribution of pontomesencephalic cholinergic neurons projecting to substantia nigra differs significantly from those projecting to ventral tegmental area. *J Neurosci* 1995; 15(9):5859–5869.

118. Charara A, Smith Y, Parent A. Glutamatergic inputs from the pedunculopontine nucleus to midbrain dopaminergic neurons in primates: Phaseolus vulgaris-leucoagglutinin anterograde labeling combined with postembedding glutamate and GABA immunohistochemistry. *J Comp Neurol* 1996; 364(2):254–266.

119. Futami T, Takakusaki K, Kitai ST. Glutamatergic and cholinergic inputs from the pedunculopontine tegmental nucleus to dopamine neurons in the substantia nigra pars compacta. *Neurosci Res* 1995; 21(4):331–342.

120. Smith Y, Charara A, Parent A. Synaptic innervation of midbrain dopaminergic neurons by glutamate-enriched terminals in the squirrel monkey. *J Comp Neurol* 1996; 364(2):231–253.

121. Kitai ST. Afferent control of substantia nigra compacta dopamine neurons: Anatomical perspective and role of glutamatergic and cholinergic inputs. *Adv Pharmacol* 1998; 42:700–702.

122. DeLong MR, Activity of pallidal neurons during movement. *J Neurophysiol* 1971; 34:414–427.

123. DeLong MR, Strick PL. Relation of basal ganglia, cerebellum, and motor cortex units to ramp and ballistic limb movements. *Brain Res* 1974; 71:327–335.

124. DeLong MR, Crutcher MD, Georgopoulos AP. Relations between movement and single cell discharge in the substantia nigra of the behaving monkey. *J Neurosci* 1983; 3:1599–1606.

125. Crutcher MD, DeLong MR. Single cell studies of the primate putamen. I. Functional organization. *Exp Brain Res* 1984; 53:233–243.

126. Crutcher MD, DeLong MR. Single cell studies of the primate putamen. II. Relations to direction of movement and pattern of muscular activity. *Exp Brain Res* 1984; 53:244–258.

127. DeLong MR, Crutcher MD, Georgopoulos AP. Primate globus pallidus and subthalamic nucleus: Functional organization. *J Neurophysiol* 1985; 53:530–543.

128. Magarinos-Ascone C, Buno W, Garcia-Austt E. Activity in monkey substantial nigra neurons related to a simple learned movement. *Exp Brain Res* 1992; 88:283–291.

129. Allum JHJ, Anner-Baratti REC, Hepp-Raymond MC. Activity of neurons in the motor thalamus and globus pallidus during the control of isometric finger force in the monkey, In: Paillard MJ, Schultz W, Wiesendanger M (eds.). *Neural coding of motor performance. Exp Brain Res Suppl.* 7 New York: Springer, 1983:194–203.

130. Apicella P, et al. Neuronal activity in monkey striatum related to the expectation of predictable environmental events. *J Neurophysiol* 1992; 68:945–960.

131. Schultz W. Activity of pars reticulata neurons of monkey substantia nigra in relation to motor, sensory, and complex events. *J Neurophysiol* 1986; 4:660–677.

132. Ashe J, Georgopoulos AP. Movement parameters and neural activity in motor cortex and area 5. *Cereb Cortex* 1994; 4(6):590–600.

133. Bauswein E, et al. Phasic and tonic responses of premotor and primary motor cortex neurons to torque changes. *Exp Brain Res* 1991; 86:303–310.

134. Crutcher MD, Alexander GE. Movement-related neuronal activity selectively coding either direction or

muscle pattern in three motor areas of the monkey. *J Neurophysiol* 1990; 64:151–163.

135. Fu QG, Suarez JI, Ebner TJ. Neuronal specification of direction and distance during reaching movements in the superior precentral premotor area and primary motor cortex of monkeys. *J Neurophysiol* 1993; 70(5):2097–2116.

136. Hepp-Reymond MC, et al. Force-related neuronal activity in two regions of the primate ventral premotor cortex. *Can J Physiol Pharmacol*, 1994; 72(5):571–579.

137. Kurata K. Premotor cortex of monkeys: Set- and movement-related activity reflecting amplitude and direction of wrist movements. *J Neurophysiol* 1993; 69(1):187–200.

138. Smith AM. The activity of supplementary motor area neurons during a maintained precision grip. *Brain Res* 1979; 172:315–327.

139. Werner W, Bauswein E, Fromm C. Static firing rates of premotor and primary motor cortical neurons associated with torque and joint position. *Exp Brain Res* 1991; 86(2):293–302.

140. Hikosaka O, Wurtz RH. Visual and oculomotor functions of monkey substantia nigra pars reticulata. I. Relation of visual and auditory responses to saccades. *J Neurophysiol* 1983; 49:1230–1253.

141. Hikosaka O, Sakamoto M, Usui S. Functional properties of monkey caudate neurons. I. Activities related to saccadic eye movements. *J Neurophysiol* 1989; 61:780–798.

142. Hikosaka O, et al. Role of basal ganglia in initiation and suppression of saccadic eye movements, in *Role of the cerebellum and basal ganglia in voluntary movement*, Mano N, Hamada I, DeLong MR (eds.). 1993, Elsevier: Amsterdam. 213–220.

143. Kato M, et al. Eye movements in monkeys with local dopamine depletion in the caudate nucleus. I. Deficits in spontaneous saccades. *J Neurosci* 1995; 15:912–927.

144. Kori A, et al. Eye movements in monkeys with local dopamine depletion in the caudate nucleus. II. Deficits in voluntary saccades. *J Neurosci* 1995; 15:928–941.

145. Jaeger D, Kita H, Wilson CJ. Surround inhibition among projection neurons is weak or nonexistent in the rat neostriatum. *J Neurophysiol* 1994; 72(5):2555–2558.

146. Nini A, et al. Neurons in the globus pallidus do not show correlated activity in the normal monkey, but phase-locked oscillations appear in the MPTP model of parkinsonism. *J Neurophysiol* 1995; 74(4):1800–1805.

147. Vitek JL, et al. Lesion location related to outcome in microelectrode-guided pallidotomy. American Neurological Association, 1994.

148. Gross RE, et al. Lesion location and outcome following pallidotomy: Support for multiple output channels in the human pallidum. *Mov Disord* 1998; 13(Suppl. 2):262.

149. Onn SP, Grace AA. Repeated treatment with haloperidol and clozapine exerts differential effects on dye coupling between neurons in subregions of striatum and nucleus accumbens. *J Neurosci* 1995; 15(11):7024–70236.

150. Onn SP, Grace AA. Dye coupling between rat striatal neurons recorded in vivo: Compartmental organization and modulation by dopamine. *J Neurophysiol* 1994; 71(5):1917–1934.

151. O'Donnell P, Grace AA. Different effects of subchronic clozapine and haloperidol on dye-coupling between neurons in the rat striatal complex. *Neuroscience* 1995; 66(4):763–767.

152. Filion M, Tremblay L, Bedard PJ. Abnormal influences of passive limb movement on the activity of globus pallidus neurons in parkinsonian monkeys. *Brain Res* 1988; 444:165–176.

153. Miller WC, DeLong MR. Altered tonic activity of neurons in the globus pallidus and subthalamic nucleus in the primate MPTP model of parkinsonism, In: Carpenter MB, Jayaraman A (eds.). *The Basal Ganglia II*. New York: Plenum Press, 1987:415–427.

154. Bergman H, et al. The primate subthalamic nucleus. II. Neuronal activity in the MPTP model of parkinsonism. *J Neurophysiol* 1994; 72:507–520.

155. Vitek JL, et al. Altered somatosensory response properties of neurons in the 'motor' thalamus of MPTP treated parkinsonian monkeys. *Soc Neurosci Abstr* 1990;16:425.

156. Raz A, et al. Neuronal synchronization of tonically active neurons in the striatum of normal and parkinsonian primates. *J Neurophysiol* 1996. in press.

157. Filion M, Tremblay L, Bedard P. Effects of dopamine agonists on the spontaneous activity of globus pallidus neurons in monkeys with MPTP-induced parkinsonism. *Brain Res* 1991; 547:152–161.

158. Tremblay L, Filion M, Bedard PJ. Responses of pallidal neurons to striatal stimulation in monkeys with MPTP-induced parkinsonism. *Brain Res* 1989; 498:17–33.

159. Georgopoulos AP, DeLong MR, Crutcher MD. Relations between parameters of step-tracking movements and single cell discharge in the globus pallidus and subthalamic nucleus of the behaving monkey. *J Neurosci* 1983; 3:1586–1598.

160. Mink JW, Thach WT. Basal ganglia motor control. III. Pallidal ablation: Normal reaction time, muscle cocontraction, and slow movement. *J Neurophysiol* 1991; 65:330–351.

161. Bevan MD, Bolam JP, Crossman AR. Convergent synaptic input from the neostriatum and the subthalamus onto identified nigrothalamic neurons in the rat. *Eur J Neurosci* 1994; 6(3):320–334.

162. Bolam JP, Smith Y. The striatum and the globus pallidus send convergent synaptic inputs onto single cells in the entopeduncular nucleus of the rat: A double anterograde labelling study combined with postembedding immunocytochemistry for GABA. *J Comp Neurol* 1992; 321(3):456–476.

163. Hazrati L, Parent A. Convergence of subthalamic and striatal efferents at pallidal level in primates: An anterograde double-labeling study with biocytin and PHA-L. *Brain Res* 1992; 569:336–340.

164. Jaeger D, Gilman S, Aldridge JW. Neuronal activity in the striatum and pallidum of primates related to the execution of externally cued reaching movements. *Brain Res* 1995; 694(1–2):111–127.

165. Jaeger D, Gilman S, Aldridge JW. Primate basal ganglia activity in a precued reaching task: Preparation for movement. *Exp Brain Res* 1993; 95:51–64.

166. Alexander GE, Crutcher MD. Preparatory activity in primate motor cortex and putamen coded in spatial rather than limb coordinates. *Soc Neurosci Abstr* 1987; 13:245.

167. Alexander GE, Crutcher MD. Coding in spatial rather than joint coordinates of putamen and motor cortex preparatory activity preceding planned limb movements, In: Sambrook MA, Crossman AR (eds.). *Neural mechanisms in disorders of movement*, London: Blackwell, 1989:55–62.

168. Anderson M, et al. Movement and preparatory activity of neurons in pallidal-receiving areas of the monkey thalamus. Role of Cerebellum and Basal Ganglia in Voluntary Movement, 1992:39.

169. Apicella P, Scarnati E, Schultz W. Tonically discharging neurons of monkey striatum respond to preparatory and rewarding stimuli. *Exp Brain Res* 1991; 84:672–675.

170. Boussaoud D, Kermadi I. The primate striatum: Neuronal activity in relation to spatial attention versus motor preparation. *Eur J Neurosci* 1997; 9(10):2152–2168.

171. Crutcher MD, Alexander GE. Supplementary motor area (SMA): Coding of both preparatory and movement-related neural activity in spatial rather than joint coordinates. *Soc Neurosci Abstr* 1988; 14:342.

172. Kubota K, Hamada I. Preparatory activity of monkey pyramidal tract neurons related to quick movement onset during visual tracking performance. *Brain Res* 1979; 168:435–439.

173. Schultz W, Romo R. Role of primate basal ganglia and frontal cortex in the internal generation of movement. I. Preparatory activity in the anterior striatum. *Exp Brain Res* 1992; 91:363–384.

174. Dettmers C, et al. Relation between cerebral activity and force in the motor areas of the human brain. *J Neurophysiol* 1995; 74(2):802–815.

175. Turner RS, et al. Motor subcircuits mediating the control of movement velocity: A PET study. *J Neurophysiol* 1998; 80(4):2162–2176.

176. Marsden CD, Obeso JA. The functions of the basal ganglia and the paradox of stereotaxic surgery in Parkinson's disease. *Brain* 1994; 117:877–897.

177. Joel D, Weiner I. The organization of the basal ganglia-thalamocortical circuits: Open interconnected rather than closed segregated. *Neuroscience* 1994; 63(2):363–379.

178. Graybiel AM. Building action repertoires: Memory and learning functions of the basal ganglia. *Curr Opin Neurobiol* 1995; 5:733–741.

179. Schultz W. The phasic reward signal of primate dopamine neurons. *Adv Pharmacol* 1998; 42:686–690.

180. Aosaki T, Kimura M, Graybiel AM. Temporal and spatial characteristics of tonically active neurons of the primate striatum. *J Neurophysiol* 1995; 73:1234–1252.

181. Aosaki T, et al. Responses of tonically active neurons in the primate's striatum undergo systematic changes during behavioral sensory-motor conditioning. *J Neurosci* 1994; 14:3969–3984.

182. Jog MS, et al. Building neural representations of habits. *Science* 1999; 286(5445):1745–1749.

183. Hore J, Villis T. Arm movement performance during reversible basal ganglia lesions in the monkey. *Exp Brain Res* 1980; 39:217–228.

184. Inase M, Buford JA, Anderson ME. Changes in the control of arm position, movement, and thalamic discharge during local inactivation in the globus pallidus of the monkey. *J Neurophysiol* 1996; 75(3):1087–1104.

185. Kato M, Kimura M. Effects of reversible blockade of basal ganglia on a voluntary arm movement. *J Neurophysiol* 1992; 68(5):1516–1534.

186. Horak FB, Anderson ME. Influence of globus pallidus on arm movements in monkeys. II. Effects of stimulation. *J Neurophysiol* 1984; 52:305–322.

187. Horak FB, Anderson ME. Influence of globus pallidus on arm movements in monkeys. I. Effects of kainic-induced lesions. *J Neurophysiol* 1984; 52:290–304.

188. Alamy M, et al. A defective control of small-amplitude movements in monkeys with globus pallidus lesions: An experimental study on one component of pallidal bradykinesia. *Behav Brain Res* 1995; 72(1–2):57–62.

189. Alamy M, et al. Globus pallidus and motor initiation: The bilateral effects of unilateral quisqualic acid-induced lesion on reaction times in monkeys. *Exp Brain Res* 1994; 99(2):247–258.

190. DeLong MR, Georgopoulos AP. Motor functions of the basal ganglia, In: Brookhart JM, et al. (eds.). *Handbook of Physiology. The Nervous System. Motor Control. Sect II Vol. II. Pt. 2.* Bethesda: American Physiological Society, 1981:1017–1061.

191. Laitinen LV. Pallidotomy for Parkinson's diesease. *Neurosurg Clin North America* 1995; 6:105–112.

192. Baron MS, et al. Treatment of advanced Parkinson's disease by GPi pallidotomy: 1 year pilot-study results. *Ann Neurol* 1996; 40:355–366.

193. Lozano AM, et al. Effect of GPi pallidotomy on motor function in Parkinson's disease. *Lancet* 1995; 346(8987):1383–1387.

194. Mink JW, Thach WT. Basal ganglia intrinsic circuits and their role in behavior. *Curr Opin Neurobiol* 1993; 3(6):950–957.

195. Mink JW. The basal ganglia: Focused selection and inhibition of competing motor programs. *Prog Neurobiol* 1996; 50(4):381–425.

196. Ehringer H, Hornykiewicz O. Verteilung von Noradrenalin und Dopamin (3-Hydroxytyramin) im Gehirn des Menschen und ihr Verhalten bei Erkrankungen des extrapyramidalen Systems. *Klin Wschr* 1960; 38:1236–1239.

197. Bernheimer H, et al. Brain dopamine and the syndromes of Parkinson and Huntington. *J Neurol Sci* 1973; 20:415–455.

198. Hornykiewicz O, Kish SJ. Biochemical pathophysiology of Parkinson's disease. *Adv Neurol* 1987; 45:19–34.

199. Kish SJ, Shannak K, Hornykiewicz O. Uneven pattern of dopamine loss in the striatum of patients with idiopathic Parkinson's disease. *New Engl J Med* 1988; 318:876–880.

200. Burns RS, et al. A primate model of parkinsonism: Selective destruction of dopaminergic neurons in the pars compacta of the substantia nigra by N-methyl-4-phenyl-1,2,3,6-tetrahydropyridine. *Proc Natl Acad Sci USA* 1983; 80:4546–4550.

201. Burns RS, et al. The clinical syndrome of striatal dopamine deficiency. *New Engl J Med* 1985; 312(22):1418–1421.

202. Bankiewicz KS, et al. Hemiparkinsonism in monkeys after unilateral internal carotid artery infusion of 1-methyl-4-phenyl-1,2,3,6-tetrahydropyridine (MPTP). *Life Sci* 1986; 39:7–16.

203. Forno LS, et al. Locus ceruleus lesions and eosinophilic inclusions in MPTP-treated monkeys. *Ann Neurol* 1986; 20:449–455.

204. Forno LS, et al. Similarities and differences between MPTP-induced parkinsonism and Parkinson's disease. *Adv Neurol* 1993; 60:600–608.

205. Irwin I, et al. The evolution of nigrostiratal neurochemical changes in the MPTP-treated squirrel monkey. *Brain Res* 1990; 531(1–2):242–252.

206. Langston JW. In: Marsclen CD, Fahn S (eds.). *Movement Disorders* 2. London: Butterworths & Co., 1987:73–90.

207. Crossman AR, Mitchell IJ, Sambrook MA. Regional brain uptake of 2-deoxyglucose in N-methyl-4-phenyl-1,2,3,6-tetrahydropyridine (MPTP)-induced parkinsonism in the macaque monkey. *Neuropharmacology* 1985; 24(6):587–591.

208. Mitchell IJ, et al. Neural mechanisms mediating 1-methyl-4-phenyl-1,2,3, 6-tetrahydropyridine-induced parkinsonism in the monkey: Relative contributions of the striatopallidal and striatonigral pathways as suggested by 2-deoxyglucose uptake. *Neurosci Lett* 1986; 63(1):61–65.

209. Mitchell IJ, et al. Neural mechanisms underlying parkinsonian symptoms based upon regional uptake of 2-deoxyglucose in monkeys exposed to 1-methyl-4-phenyl-1,2,3,6-tetrahydropyridine. *Neuroscience* 1989; 32(1):213–226.

210. Schwartzman RJ, Alexander GM. Changes in the local cerebral metabolic rate for glucose in the 1-methyl-4-phenyl-1,2,3,6-tetrahydropyridine (MPTP) primate model of Parkinsons disease. *Brain Res* 1985; 358(1–2):137–143.

211. Schwartzman RJ, et al. Cerebral metabolism of parkinsonian primates 21 days after MPTP. *Exp Neurol* 1988; 102:307–313.

212. Palombo E, et al. Local cerebral glucose utilization in monkeys with hemiparkinsonism induced by intracarotid infusion of the neurotoxin MPTP. *J Neurosci* 1990; 10(3):860–869.

213. Porrino LJ, et al. Changes in local cerebral glucose utilization associated with Parkinson's syndrome induced by 1-methyl-4-phenyl-1,2,3,6-tetrahydropyridine (MPTP) in the primate. *Life Sci* 1987; 40:1657–1664.

214. Filion M, Tremblay L. Abnormal spontaneous activity of globus pallidus neurons in monkeys with MPTP-induced parkinsonism. *Brain Res* 1991; 547(1):142–151.

215. Boraud T, et al. Effects of L-DOPA on neuronal activity of the globus pallidus externalis (GPe) and globus pallidus internalis (GPi) in the MPTP-treated monkey. *Brain Res* 1998; 787(1):157–160.

216. Dogali M, et al. Anatomic and physiological considerations in pallidotomy for Parkinson's disease. *Stereotact Funct Neurosurg* 1994; 62(1–4):53–60.

217. Lozano A, et al. Methods for microelectrode-guided posteroventral pallidotomy. *J Neurosurg* 1996; 84(2):194–202.

218. Taha JM, et al. Tremor control after pallidotomy in patients with Parkinson's disease: Correlation with microrecording findings. *J Neurosurg* 1997; 86(4):642–647.

219. Vitek JL, et al. Neuronal activity in the internal (GPi) and external (GPe) segments of the globus pallidus (GP) of parkinsonian patients is similar to that in the MPTP-treated primate model of parkinsonism. *Soc Neurosci Abstr* 1993; 19:1584.

220. Brooks DJ. Detection of preclinical Parkinson's disease with PET. *Neurology* 1991; 41(suppl. 2):24–27.

221. Calne D, Snow BJ. PET imaging in Parkinsonism. *Adv Neurol* 1993; 60:484.

222. Eidelberg D, et al. The metabolic topography of Parkinsonis. *J Cereb Blood Flow Metab* 1994; 14:783–801.

223. Ceballos-Bauman AO, et al. Restoration of thalamocortical activity after posteroventrolateral pallidotomy in Parkinson's disease. *Lancet* 1994; 344:814.

224. Grafton AT, et al. Pallidotomy increases activity of motor association cortex in Parkinson's disease: A positron emission tomographic study. *Ann Neurol* 1995; 37:776–783.

225. Samuel M, et al. Pallidotomy in Parkinson's disease increases supplementary motor area and prefrontal activation during performance of volitional movements an H2(15)O PET study. *Brain*, 1997; 120(Pt 8):1301–1313.

226. Limousin P, et al. Changes in cerebral activity pattern due to subthalamic nucleus or internal pallidum stimulation in Parkinson's disease. *Ann Neurol* 1997; 42(3):283–291.

227. Davis KD, et al. Globus pallidus stimulation activates the cortical motor system during alleviation of parkinsonian symptoms. *Nat Med* 1997; 3(6):671–674.

228. Watts RL, Mandir AS. The role of motor cortex in the pathophysiology of voluntary movement deficits associated with parkinsonism. *Neurol Clin* 1992; 10(2):451–469.

229. Kojima J, et al. Excitotoxic lesions of the pedunculopontine tegmental nucleus produce contralateral hemiparkinsonism in the monkey. *Neurosci Lett* 1997; 226(2):111–114.

230. Bergman H, Wichmann T, DeLong MR. Reversal of experimental parkinsonism by lesions of the subthalamic nucleus. *Science* 1990; 249:1436–1438.

231. Aziz TZ, et al. Lesion of the subthalamic nucleus for the alleviation of 1-methyl-4-phenyl-1,2,3,6-tetrahydropyridine (MPTP)-induced parkinsonism in the primate. *Mov Disord* 1991; 6:288–292.

232. Guridi J, et al. Subthalamotomy improves MPTP-induced parkinsonism in monkeys. *Stereotact Funct Neurosurg* 1994; 62(1–4):98–102.

233. Kaneoke Y, Vitek JL. Normalization of altered spontaneous neuronal activity in the motor thalamus in parkinsonian monkeys following lesioning of the subthalamic nucleus. *J Neurophysiol* 2000; submitted.

234. Gill SS, Heywood P. Bilateral dorsolateral subthalamotomy for advanced Parkinson's disease [letter]. *Lancet* 1997; 350(9086):1224.

235. Gill SS, Heywood P. Bilateral subthalamic nucleotomy can be accomplished safely. *Mov Disord* 1998; 13(Suppl 2):201.

236. Dogali M, et al. Stereotactic ventral pallidotomy for Parkinson's disease. *Neurology* 1995; 45:753–761.

237. Vitek JL, et al. Randomized clinical trial of GPi pallidotomy versus best medical therapy for Parkinson's disease. *Ann Neurol* 2000; submitted.

238. Vitek JL, et al. Physiologic properties and somatotopic organization of the primate motor thalamus. *J Neurophysiol* 1994; 71:1498–1513.

239. Wichmann T, Bergman H, DeLong MR. Comparison of the effects of experimental parkinsonism on neuronal discharge in motor and non-motor portions of the basal ganglia output nuclei in primates. *Soc Neurosci Abstr* 1996; 22:415.

240. Filion M, Tremblay L, Bedard PJ. Excessive and unselective responses of medial pallidal neurons to both passive movements and striatal stitmulation in monkeys with MPTP-induced Parkinsonism. London: John Libbey, 1989:157–164.

241. Filion M, Boucher R, Bedard P. Globus pallidus unit activity in the monkey during the induction of parkinsonism by 1-methyl-4-phenyl-1,2,3,6,-tetrahydropyridine (MPTP). *Soc Neurosci Abstr* 1985; 11:1160.

242. Soghomonian JJ, et al. Increased glutamate decarboxylase mRNA levels in the striatum and pallidum of MPTP-treated primates. *J Neurosci* 1994; 14(10):6256–6265.

243. Herrero MT, et al. Glutamic acid decarboxylase mRNA expression in medial and lateral pallidal neurons in the MPTP-treated monkeys and patients with Parkinson's disease. *Adv.Neurol* 1996; 69:209–216.

244. Herrero MT, et al. Consequence of nigrostriatal denervation and L-dopa therapy on the expression of glutamic acid decarboxylase messenger RNA in the pallidum. *Neurology* 1996; 47:219–224.

245. Soghomonian JJ, Chesselet MF. Effects of nigrostriatal lesions on the levels of messenger RNAs encoding two isoforms of glutamate decarboxylase in the globus pallidus and entopeduncular nucleus of the rat. *Synapse*, 1992; 11(2):124–133.

246. Delfs JM, Anegawa NJ, Chesselet MF. Glutamate decarboxylase messenger RNA in rat pallidum: Comparison of the effects of haloperidol, clozapine and combined haloperidol-scopolamine treatments. *Neuroscience* 1995; 66(1):67–80.

247. Levy R, et al. Re-evaluation of the functional anatomy of the basal ganglia in normal and Parkinsonian states. *Neuroscience* 1997; 76(2):335–343.

248. Martin DL, Rimvall K. Regulation of gamma-aminobutyric acid synthesis in the rat brain. *J Neurochem* 1993; 60:395–407.

249. Rimvall K, Martin DL. The level of GAD67 protein is highly sensitive to small increases in intraneuronal gamma-aminobutyric acid levels. *J Neurochem* 1994; 62:1375–1381.

250. Miller WC, DeLong MR. Parkinsonian symptomatology: An anatomical and physiological analysis. *Ann N Y Acad Sci*, 1988; 515:287–302.

251. Wichmann T, DeLong MR. Pathophysiology of parkinsonian motor abnormalities, In: Narabayashi H et al. (eds.). *Advances in Neurology*. Vol. 60. New York: Raven Press, 1993:53–61.

252. Canavan AG, Nixon PD, Passingham RE. Motor learning in monkeys (Macaca fascicularis) with lesions in motor thalamus. *Exp Brain Res*, 1989; 77(1):113–126.

253. Brooks DJ. PET and SPECT studies in Parkinson's disease. *Baillieres Clin Neurol* 1997; 6(1):69–87.

254. Jenkins IH, et al. Impaired activation of the supplementary motor area in Parkinson's disease is reversed when akinesia is treated with apomorphine. *Ann Neurol* 1992; 32(6):749–757.

255. Deecke L. Cerebral potentials related to voluntary actions: Parkinsonism and normal subjects, In: Delwaide PJ, Agnoli A (eds.). *Clinical Neurophysiology in Parkinsonism*. Amsterdam and Oxford: Elsevier, 1985:91–105.

256. Dick JPR, et al. The Bereitschaftspotential is abnormal in Parkinson's disease. *Brain* 1989; 112:233–244.

257. Obeso JA, et al. The mechanism of action of pallidotomy in Parkinson's disease (PD): Physiological

and imaging studies. *Soc Neurosci Abstr* 1995; 21:1982.

258. Berardelli A, et al. Single-joint rapid arm movements in normal subjects and in patients with motor disorders. *Brain* 1996; 119(Pt 2):661–674.

259. Hallett M, Khoshbin S. A physiological mechanism of bradykinesia. *Brain* 1980; 103:301–314.

260. Jordan N, Sagar HJ, Cooper JA. A component analysis of the generation and release of isometric force in Parkinson's disease. *J Neurol* Neurosurgery & Psychiatry, 1992; 55(7):572–576.

261. Kunesch E, et al. Altered force release control in Parkinson's disease. *Behav Brain Res* 1995; 67(1):43–49.

262. Praamstra P, et al. Movement preparation in Parkinson's disease. Time course and distribution of movement-related potentials in a movement precueing task. *Brain* 1996. 119(Pt 5):1689–1704.

263. Stelmach GE, et al. Force production characteristics in Parkinson's disease. *Exp Brain Res* 1989; 76(1):165–172.

264. Thompson PD, et al. The coexistence of bradykinesia and chorea in Huntington's disease and its implications for theories of basal ganglia control of movement. *Brain* 1988; 111(Pt 2):223–244.

265. Wascher E, et al. Responses to cued signals in Parkinson's disease. Distinguishing between disorders of cognition and of activation. *Brain* 1997; 120(Pt 8):1355–1375.

266. Winstein CJ, Grafton ST, Pohl PS. Motor task difficulty and brain activity: Investigation of goal-directed reciprocal aiming using positron emission tomography. *J Neurophysiol* 1997; 77(3):1581–1594.

267. Zhang J, et al. The effect of GPe lesions on GPi cell activity and motor behavior in the MPTP-treated monkey. *Soc Neurosc* 1997; 23:542.

268. Chockkan V, et al. A comparison of discharge pattern of internal segment neurons of the globus pallidus (GPi) in akinetic and tremor parkinsonian patients (PD). *Soc Neurosci* (abstract), 1997; 23:470.

269. Delwaide PJ, Pepin JL. Maertens de Noordhout A. Short-latency autogenic inhibition in patients with parkinsonian ridigity. *Ann Neurol* 1991; 30:83–89.

270. Hyland B, et al. What is the role of the supplementary motor area in movement initiation? *Prog Brain Res* 1989; 80:431–436; discussion 427–430.

271. Delwaide PJ, Pepin JL. Maertens de Noordhout A. Contribution of reticular nuclei to the pathophysiology of parkinsonian rigidity. *Adv Neurol* 1993; 60:381–385.

272. Lee RG, Murphy JT, Tatton WG. Long-latency myotatic reflexes in man: Mechanisms, functional significance, and changes in patients with Parkinson's disease or hemiplegia, In: Desmedt JE (ed.). *Motor Control Mechanisms in Health and Disease.* New York: Raven Press, 1983:489–507.

273. Berardelli A, Sabra A, Hallett M. Physiological mechanisms of rigidity in Parkinson's disease. *J Neurol Neurosurg Psychiatry* 1983; 46:45–53.

274. Tsai CH, Chen RS, Lu CS. Reciprocal inhibition in Parkinson's disease. *Acta Neurologica Scandinaviae* 1997; 95(1):13–18.

275. Lenz FA, et al. Cross-correlation analysis of thalamic neurons and EMG activity in parkinsonian tremor. *Appl Neurophysiol* 1985; 48:305–308.

276. Lenz FA, et al. Single unit analysis of the human thalamic ventral nuclear group: Correlation of thalamic "tremor cells" with the 3–6 Hz component of parkinsonian tremor. *J.Neurosci* 1988; 8:754–764.

277. Lenz FA, et al. Functional classes of "tremor cells" in the ventral tier of lateral thalamic nuclei of patients with parkinsonian tremor, In: Brock M (ed.). *Modern Neurosurgery.* Berlin: Springer Verlag, 1989: 205–217.

278. Lenz FA, et al. Single unit analysis of the human ventral thalamic nuclear group: The 3–6 Hz component of tremor synchronous activity in functionally identified cells. *J Neurosci* 1989; in preparation.

279. Ohye C, et al. Recording and stimulation of the ventralis intermedius nucleus of the human thalamus. *Conf Neurol* 1975; 37:258.

280. Narabayashi H, Ohye C. Parkinsonian tremor in nucleus ventralis intermedius of the human thalamus, In: Desmedt JE (ed.). *Progress in clinical Neurophysiology: Physiological tremor, pathological tremors and clonus* New york: S. Karger, 1978:165–172.

281. Ohye C, Narabayashi H. Physiological study of presumed ventralis intermedius neurons in the human thalamus. *J Neurosurg* 1979; 50:290–297.

282. Pare D, Curro'Dossi R, Steriade M. Neuronal basis of the parkinsonian resting tremor: A hypothesis and its implications for treatment. *Neuroscience* 1990; 35:217–226.

283. Steriade M, Jones EG, Llinas RR. Thalamic Oscillations and Signaling. 1990, New York: Wiley-Interscience, 1990.

284. Steriade M, McCormick DA, Sejnowski TJ. Thalamo-cortical oscillations in the sleeping and aroused brain. *Science* 1993; 262(5134):679–685.

285. Llinas R, Jahnsen H. Electrophysiology of mammalian thalamic neurones in vitro. *Nature* 1982; 29:406–408.

286. Jahnsen H, Llinas R. Ionic basis for the electro-responsiveness and oscillatory properties of guinea-pig thalamic neurones in vitro. *J Physiol* 1984; 349:227–247.

287. Jahnsen H, Llinas R. Electrophysiological properties of guinea-pig thalamic neurones: An in vitro study. *J Physiol* 1984; 349:205–226.

288. Kim U, Sanchez-Vives MV, McCormick DA. Functional dynamics of GABAergic inhibition in the thalamus. *Science* 1997; 278(5335):130–134.

289. Lenz FA, Vitek JL, DeLong MR. Role of the thalamus in parkinsonian tremor: Evidence from studies in patients and primate models. *Stereotact Funct Neurosurg* 1993; 60:94–103.

290. Dogali M, et al. Anatomic and physiological considerations in pallidotomy for Parkinson's disease. *Acta Neurochirurgica - Supplementum* 1995; 64:9–12.

291. Karmon B, Bergman H. Detection of neuronal periodic oscillations in the basal ganglia of normal and parkinsonian monkeys. *Israeli J Med Sci* 1993; 29:570–579.

292. Nambu A, Llinas R. Electrophysiology of the globus pallidus neurons: An in vitro study in guinea pig brain slices. *Soc Neurosci Abstr* 1990; 16:428.

293. Vitek JL, Wichmann T, DeLong MR. Current concepts of basal ganglia neurophysiology with respect to tremorgenesis, In: Findley LJ, Koller W (eds.).

New York, Basal, Hong Kong: Marcel Decker, 1994:37–50.

294. Wichmann T, Bergman H, DeLong MR. The primate subthalamic nucleus. III. Changes in motor behavior and neuronal activity in the internal pallidum induced by subthalamic inactivation in the MPTP model of parkinsonism. *J Neurophysiol* 1994; 72:521–530.

295. Vitek J, Giroux M. The physiology of hypokinetic and hyperkinetic movement disorders: A model for the dyskinesias. *Ann Neurol* 1999; In press (Supplement).

296. Bergman H, et al. Physiology of MPTP tremor. *Mov Disord* 1998; 13(Suppl. 3):29–34.

23

Dopamine Receptor Diversity

Deborah C. Mash

University of Miami School of Medicine, Miami, Florida

INTRODUCTION

Dopamine plays a role not only in the execution of movement but also in higher order cognitive processes, including motor planning and sequencing, motor learning, and motivational drives and affect. Of the many slow-acting neurotransmitters in the central nervous system, dopamine has been the best studied. The actions of dopamine are segregated into specific neuronal circuits within a diffuse axonal projection system. For example, dopamine in the nigrostriatal pathway is involved in the generation and execution of voluntary movement. In this function, dopamine is a prime modulator of various other basal ganglia neurotransmitters implicated in motor control, including GABA, acetylcholine, glutamate, enkephalin, and substance P. Dopamine in the mesolimbic pathway plays a role in the control of various cognitive functions, including reinforcement, attention, instrumental avoidance, and in the addiction to psychostimulant drugs.

The central effects of dopamine are mediated by five different molecular receptor subtypes that are members of the large G-protein coupled receptor superfamily. Dopamine receptors are divided into two major subclasses; D_1-like and D_2-like receptors, which differ in their pharmacology, and messenger transduction systems and anatomic locations. The cloning of these receptors and their genes in the last decade has led to the identification of multiple molecular receptor subtypes termed D_1, D_2, D_3, D_4, and D_5. The molecular D_1 and D_5 subtypes of dopamine receptors exhibit overlapping functional and pharmacologic properties that are related to the D_1 receptor (D_1-like), whereas the remaining members of this receptor family share pharmacologic characteristics that are in keeping with the D_2 receptor subtype (D_2-like). The two receptor subclasses have overlapping but distinct neuroanatomical distributions as determined by radioligand binding autoradiography. Thus the various functions of dopaminergic neurotransmission appear to be mediated by the expression of different receptor proteins.

Studies on dopamine neurotransmission have been an important research focus for decades because it is known that alterations in dopamine function are involved in many different neurodegenerative and psychiatric brain disorders. Degeneration of the nigral dopamine-containing neurons contributes to the pathogenesis of Parkinson's disease (PD) (1). Dopamine receptor agonists acting at multiple receptors, but primarily D_2, are used to treat the dopamine deficiency of this disease (2). The chorea of Huntington's disease is related to a deterioration of the dopaminoceptive cells localized in the striatum. Schizophrenia and other psychotic disorders are thought to be due to an imbalance in corticolimbic dopamine signaling (3). Dopamine receptor antagonists are used for the clinical management of these disorders (3–5). Chronic dopamine receptor blockade leads to a dysregulation of dopaminergic tone and the development of extrapyramidal syndromes including parkinsonism and chorea, whereas involuntary movements and psychosis are observed with chronic administration of the indirect-acting agonist levodopa in PD (2). Although none of the dopamine receptor subtypes have been linked to the etiology of schizophrenia, the distinct regional locations of D_3 and D_4 receptors in cerebral cortical and associated subcortical limbic brain areas have led to the suggestion that subtype-selective neuroleptics that lack extrapyramidal side effects can be developed. Clozapine, an antipsychotic that antagonizes the D_4 receptor, is a perfect example of this possibility.

MOLECULAR CHARACTERIZATION OF DOPAMINE RECEPTORS

The molecular characterization of dopamine receptor heterogeneity was advanced by the recognition that all G-protein coupled receptors are evolutionarily related (6). The existence of a G protein coupled receptor supergene was proposed based on the reported sequences for rhodopsin and β_2 adrenergic receptors (7). Both of these receptors have a membrane typology of highly conserved amino acid residues that form seven transmembrane spanning domains. Several structural features are common to the catecholamine receptors, including the specific aspartate and serine residues that interact with the neurotransmitter (agonist recognition sites), sites for N-linked glycosylation located on putative extracellular regions, and consensus sites for phosphorylation by protein kinase A or C found on putative intracellular domains (Figure 23-1). The recognition of these similarities led to the assumption that all G-protein coupled receptors had similar structural characteristics, a suggestion that was further strengthened by the cloning and sequencing of the m2 muscarinic receptor (8). The identification of shared amino acid sequence similarities among all G-protein coupled receptors promoted the development of technical approaches for first the cloning of the D_2 receptor (9) and then the D_1 receptor (10,11) subtypes.

The D_2 receptor cDNA was first isolated in 1988 (9), and subsequently alternative splice variants were identified (12,13). The cDNA for the D_2 receptor encodes a protein of 415 amino acids, with three glycosylation sites in the N-terminus, a large third intracellular loop between transmembrane regions 5 and 6, and a short C-terminus. The D_3 receptor was isolated by screening rat libraries with the known D_2 sequence followed by polymerase chain reaction extension (14). The topography of the D_3 receptor includes a glycoprotein of 400 amino acids with a glycosylation site in the N-terminus and a short C-terminus. The D_4 receptor was cloned by screening a library from the human neuroblastoma cell line SK-N-MC (15). The D_4 glycoprotein is 387 amino acid residues in length with the characteristic seven transmembrane spanning domains, a large third intracellular loop, and a short C-terminus. The dopamine D_1 (or D_{1a}) receptor was independently cloned by four separate groups of investigators (10,11,16,17). The isolation of cDNAs or genes from rat or human DNA libraries was done by either homology screening with a D_2 receptor probe or by PCR with degenerate primers. Both the rat and human D_1 receptor genes encode a protein that is 91 percent homologous for amino acid sequence. The second member of the D_1-like receptor family, D_5 was isolated using the sequence of the D_1 receptor (18). The coding region for the carboxy terminal of the protein is about seven times longer for D_1-like than for D_2-like receptors (19). The cloned D_1 and D_5 receptors are 446 residues in length and exhibit 91 percent amino acid sequence homology within the highly conserved seven transmembrane spanning region.

The analysis of the gene structure of D_2 receptors demonstrated that the coding region contains six introns, the D_3 receptor contains five, and the D_4 has three introns (19,20). The presence of introns within the coding region of the D_2 receptor family allows generation of receptor variants. For example, alternative splicing of the D_2 receptor at the exon between introns 4 and 5 results in functional D_{2S} and D_{2L} isoforms (12,13). Nonfunctional proteins encoded by alternative splice variants of the D_3 receptor have been demonstrated (21–23). The human D_4 receptor gene, located on the short arm of chromosome 11, has eight different polymorphic variants. The existence of polymorphic variations within the coding sequence of the D_4 receptor demonstrated a 48 base pair sequence in the third cytoplasmic loop that exists with multiple-repeated sequences (24). The number of repeated

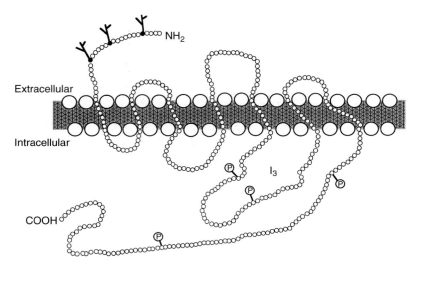

FIGURE 23-1. Dopamine receptor structure. Proposed structure of D_1-like dopamine receptor. The seven transmembrane domains have highly conserved amino acid sequences. Potential glycosylation sites are shown on the NH_2 terminal. The intracellular loop 3 and the carboxy terminus have multiple phosphorylation sites. The coupling of the receptor to G proteins occurs through the interactions of the proteins at sites on the carboxy-terminus and the third cytoplasmic loop (l_3) to activate second messenger signaling pathways.

sequences is related to ethnicity, with most humans (70%) having four repeats. Nonfunctional, truncated isoforms of the D_5 receptor have been reported on human chromosomes 1 and 2 (20,25).

NEUROANATOMIC LOCALIZATION OF DOPAMINE RECEPTOR PROTEIN AND mRNA

The dopaminergic systems in brain comprise three distinct pathways, including the nigrostriatal, mesocortical, and mesolimbic projections (26). The nigrostriatal pathway originates in the substantia nigra pars compacta and terminates in the striatum. The mesolimbic pathway originates in the ventral tegmental area (VTA) and projects to the limbic sectors of the striatum, amygdala, and olfactory tubercle. The mesocortical pathway originates in the VTA and terminates within particular sectors of the cerebral cortical mantle, including the prefrontal, cingulate, and entorhinal cortices.

D_1-like and D_2-like receptors and their mRNAs are abundant in the CNS, having a widespread distribution within the different dopaminergic systems (20). The neuroanatomic localization of D_1 receptors correlates with DA-stimulated adenylyl cyclase activities and radioligand binding. High densities of radioligand binding sites are found within the caudate and putamen, and nucleus accumbens with lower levels in the

thalamus and cerebral cortical sectors (Figure 23-2a). D_1 receptor mRNA has been localized to medium-sized neurons of the striatonigral projection that also express substance P (27). D_5 mRNA is distributed in a more restricted pattern than D_1 mRNA with the highest expression seen in limbic and cortical brain areas Very low levels of D_5 mRNA are found within the striatum (20).

Radioligand binding and mRNA studies have confirmed a good correlation for the D_2-like receptors. D_2 receptors and message are found in the striatum and substantia nigra of the rat and human brain (Figure 23-2b). The globus pallidus, a major efferent projection system of the striatum, has high densities of D_2 receptors (28). However, neurons expressing D_2 receptor mRNA are lower in the globus pallidus than in the caudate and putamen. D_2 receptor mRNA is colocalized with enkephalin in many brain areas, including the periaquaductal gray, suggesting a role for these sites in the modulation of analgesia (27).

Radioligand binding to D_3 receptors in human brain demonstrates a distinct localization pattern and a less widespread distribution than D_2-binding sites (Figure 23-2). The highest densities are seen over limbic brain regions, with very low levels over the ventromedial sectors of the striatum (28). The highest levels of message expression are found within the telencephalic areas receiving mesocortical dopaminergic inputs, including the islands of Calleja, bed nucleus of the stria terminalis, hippocampus,

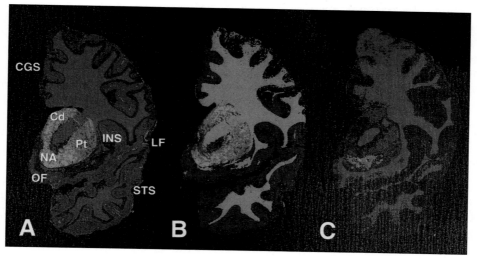

FIGURE 23-2. Autoradiographic localization of the distribution of D_1 and D_2 receptors in representative coronal half-hemisphere sections of the human brain. Panels show pseudocolor autoradiograms (red = high densities; green = intermediate densities; purple = low densities) for a control subject (Male, age 28 yr.). Panel A illustrates the distribution of D_1 receptors with 1 nM [^{3}H]SCH 23390 in the presence of 10nM mianserin to occlude labeling of the 5-HT$_2$ receptor. Panel B shows the distribution of D_2 receptors labeled with 2 nM [^{3}H] raclopride. Panel C illustrates the distribution of D_3 receptors labeled with [^{3}H]7OH DPAT. Abbreviations: Cd, caudate; CGS, cingulate sulcus; INS, insular cortex; LF, lateral fissure; NA, nucleus accumbens; Pt, putamen; STS, superior temporal sulcus.

and hypothalamus. In the cerebellum, Purkinje cells in lobules IX and X express abundant D_3 mRNA, whereas binding sites are found only in the molecular layer (28,30). Since no dopaminergic projections are known to exist in these areas, it has been suggested that the D_3 receptor may mediate the nonsynaptic (paracrine) actions of dopamine (30). D_4 receptor message is localized to dopamine cell body fields of the substantia nigra and VTA. This pattern suggests that the D_4 receptor protein may function as presynaptic autoreceptors in dendrites and/or presynaptic terminals (15). The highest areas of D_4 expression are found in the frontal cortex, amygdala, and brain stem areas. The very low levels of D_4 receptor message in the striatum are in keeping with the lack of extrapyramidal side effects observed following treatment with putative D_4 selective atypical neuroleptics (31).

Previous studies suggested that D_1-like and D_2-like receptors may be colocalized in a subpopulation of the same neostriatal cells (32). This hypothesis has been questioned by recent data from Gerfen and Keefe (33), which suggested that the interactions may occur at an intercellular level as opposed to an intracellular level with second messenger integration. This latter hypothesis suggests that the D_1-like and D_2-like receptor proteins are on distinct populations of neurons with extensive axon collateral systems subserving the integration across neural subfields. However, the evidence indicating that direct cointegration may occur at the single cell level from anatomic and electrophysiologic studies, is considerable (32). This anatomic arrangement would afford D_1-mediated cooperative–synergistic control of D_2-mediated motor activity and other psychomotor behaviors. Most studies have demonstrated opposing roles of D_1 and D_2 receptor-mediated actions in the striatum resulting from the stimulation and inhibition of adenylyl cyclase, respectively (34). Although more studies are needed to clarify the precise nature and extent of these functional interactions on cAMP second messenger systems, species-specific differences may limit the extrapolation of rodent studies to monkeys and humans (35).

Second Messenger Pathways

Dopamine receptors transduce their effects by coupling to specific heterotrimeric GTP binding proteins (i.e., G proteins) consisting of α, β, and γ subunits (36). Within the dopamine receptor family, the adenylyl cyclase stimulatory receptors include the D_1 and D_5 subtypes. Although the D_1 and D_5 share sequence homology that is greater than 80 percent, the receptors display 50 percent overall homology at the amino acid level (19). D_5 receptors have been suggested to have higher

affinity toward dopamine and lower affinity for the antagonists (+) butaclamol (20,37). However, when the D_1 and D_5 subtypes are expressed in transfected cell lines derived from the rat pituitary, both D_1 and D_5 receptors stimulate adenylyl cyclase and have identical affinities for agonists and antagonists (38). Studies done in transfected cell lines are complicated by the fact that transfection systems may not express the relevant compliment of G proteins as in the native tissue environment. In the primate brain, there is a overlap in the regional brain expression of D_1 and D_5 receptors. Thus, because of the identical affinities of D_1 and D_5 receptors for agonists and antagonists and the lack of subtype selective drugs that fully discriminate between these receptor subtypes, it is not yet possible to assign with certainty specific functions to D_1 versus D_5 receptor activation.

Although G protein–coupled receptors were initially believed to selectively activate a single effector, they are now known to have an intrinsic ability to generate multiple signals through an interaction with different α subunits (39). D_1 and D_5 receptors have been shown by a variety of methodologies to couple to the Gsα subunit of G proteins. The Gsα subunit has been linked to the regulation of Na^+, Ca^+, and K^+ channels, suggesting that D_1 receptor activation affects the functional activity of these ion channels. To complicate this picture, D_1 receptors inactivate a slow K^+ current in the resting state of medium spiny neurons in the striatum (40) through an activation of Goα in the absence of D_1 receptor Gsα coupling (38,41). These studies provide evidence for the involvement of this G protein subunit in the D_1-mediated regulation of diverse ion channels.

The ability of the D_5 receptor to stimulate adenyl-cyclase predicts that this subtype couples to Gsα. D_5 receptors inhibit catecholamine secretion in bovine chromaffin cells (42). The negligible dopamine-stimulation of adenyl-cyclase demonstrated in these cells suggests the possibility that this activity of D_5 receptor is mediated by a different G protein. Recent studies have demonstrated that the D_5 receptor can couple to a novel G protein termed $G_{z\alpha}$ (43), which is abundantly expressed in neurons. Thus, despite similar pharmacologic properties, differential coupling of D_1 and D_5 receptors to distinct G proteins can transduce varied signaling responses by dopamine stimulation. However, since the precise function of Gzα has not been established, the molecular implications of D_5/Gz α coupling is not yet known. Activation of Gzα has been shown to inhibit adenyl cyclase activity in certain cell types (44). Although it is not clear which signaling pathways are linked to D_5/Gz α coupling, the colocalization of D_5, Gzα, and specific cyclase subtypes may provide a clue to the physiologic relevance. For example, $G_{z}\alpha$ inhibits adenyl cyclase types I and V (44). Both type V cyclase and D_1 receptors are expressed in very high amounts in striatum, which has dense dopaminergic input (45). D_1 receptor activation in the striatum is known to stimulate the activity of adenyl cyclase type V (46). In contrast, the hippocampus is rich in D_5 but not in D_1 receptors, and type I cyclase is abundantly expressed in this brain region (47). Taken together, these studies suggest the functional relevance of colocalization of specific cyclases with a particular member of the D_1-like receptor family.

D_2, D_3, and D_4 receptors have introns in their coding region and exist in various forms by alternate splicing in the region of the third cytoplasmic loop. These receptors produce rapid physiologic actions by two major mechanisms, *involving either* the activation of inward K^+ channels or the inhibition of a voltage-dependent Ca^+ channels, *or involving* activation of Gi/Go proteins to inhibit adenylcyclase activity (20). D_2 and D_4 receptors inhibit adenylcyclase by coupling to inhibitory G proteins of the Gi/Go family (19,20), whereas D_3 receptors demonstrate weak inhibition of adenyl cyclase activity (48). This weak effect on inhibiting cAMP production led to the conclusion that the D_3 receptor does not couple to G proteins (20,48). Both isoforms of the D_2 receptor inhibit adenyl cyclase activity, although the short isoform requires lower concentrations of agonist to cause half maximal inhibition than the long isoform expressed in transfected cell lines (49,50). The short D_2 receptor isoform couples to K+ currents via a pertussis-toxin insensitive mechanism (51), whereas the long isoform couples to the same current via a pertussis-toxin-sensitive mechanism (52). Thus D_2 receptors, if expressed by the same cells, can influence transmembrane currents in similar ways but through independent transduction pathways. D_2-like receptors that couple to G proteins modulate a variety of other second messenger pathways, including ion channels, Ca^+ levels, K^+ currents, arachidonic acid release, phosphoinositide hydrolysis, and cell growth and differentiation (53).

PHARMACOLOGIC SELECTIVITY

Central dopamine systems have properties that make them unique in comparison to other neurotransmitter systems. For example, dopaminergic projections are mainly associated with diffuse neural pathways. This anatomic arrangement argues for dopamine to act as a neuromodulatory molecule in addition to its role as a neurotransmitter in brain. Dopamine neurons are highly branched with elongated axons capable of releasing neurotransmitter from many points along their terminal networks en route to the striatum (54). This mode of volumetric transmission of action potentials suggests that dopamine release mediates paracrine (i.e., neurohumoral) signals across the network. This view is supported by the observation that dopamine is released by axon terminals and dendrites, providing a double polarity for regulating basal ganglia function, simultaneously gating signaling at nigral, striatal, and pallidal levels. These properties have important implications in the clinical expression of human disorders involving dopamine neuron dysfunction.

The members of the D_1 receptor subfamily have several characteristics that distinguish them from the D_2 subfamily. All members of the D_1 subfamily bind-benzazapines with high affinity and butyrophenones and benzamides with low affinity (18). Subtypes in the D_1 family have approximately 50 percent homology overall and 80 percent homology in the highly conserved transmembrane region. All of the receptors in this family have short third intracellular loops and a long carboxy terminus. These regions are important for the generation of second messenger signals as explained earlier. D_5 and the rat D_1b are species homologs because they map to the same chromosomal locus (55). D_5 and D_1b have a 10-fold higher affinity for dopamine, suggesting that D_5 receptors are activated at neurotransmitter concentrations that are subthreshold for the D_1 receptor (20,56). The D_2-like receptors bind butyrophenones and benzamides with high affinity and bind *benzazepines* with low affinity [57].

The pharmacologic distinction of dopamine receptor subtypes holds tremendous potential for treatment of nervous system dysfunction. Dopamine receptors are the primary targets for the pharmacologic treatment of PD, schizophrenia, and several other nervous system disorders. Presently used drugs have significant limitations that are in part due to their nonselective binding to many receptor subtypes. For example, drug-related side effects, including dyskinesias and psychosis, are frequent and important problems in parkinsonian patients receiving levodopa or dopamine agonist therapy. These adverse effects result from stimulation of dopamine receptors in motor and cognitive circuits, respectively (59). Conversely, treatment of schizophrenia with dopaminergic antagonists, although intended to selectively block receptors in cortical and limbic circuits, may induce parkinsonian symptoms or even permanent dyskinesias by interaction with dopamine receptor subtypes in motor pathways. Clearly, drugs aimed at molecular subtypes of dopamine receptors offer the potential for specific therapeutic interventions for motor and psychiatric disorders of the nervous system.

Although there are agonists and antagonists that are selective and can discriminate between D_1-like and D_2-like receptor subfamilies, there are few agents that are highly selective for any of the individual receptor subtypes (Table 23-1). Some progress has been made in the development of antagonists for the D_2 receptor family. For the D_1/D_5 receptor subtypes, there are currently no compounds that exhibit high selectivity. Thus, the high overall sequence homology between dopamine receptors of the same subfamily have made it difficult to develop specific ligands that do not interact with related receptors. The high affinity of the "atypical" neuroleptic clozapine for D_4 receptors and the low level of D_4 receptor expression in the striatum and high levels in the cerebral cortex and certain limbic brain areas led to the suggestion that the antipsychotic properties of the neuroleptics may be mediated through blockade of D_4 receptors, whereas the side effects may be mediated through blockade of D_2 receptors (14,60). This hypothesis was strengthened by the low incidence of extrapyramidal side effects for clozapine. However, clozapine at therapeutic doses also blocks many other types of receptors in addition to D_4 receptors, making it difficult to draw definitive conclusions. For example, clozapine binds to muscarinic acetylcholine receptors and is 20- to 50-fold more potent at these sites than at D_2 receptors (61).

Recently it has been suggested that clozapine and other related antipsychotic drugs that elicit little or no parkinsonism, bind more loosely than dopamine to brain D_2 receptors yet have high occupancy of these receptors (61). By determining fractional occupancies of receptors bound at therapeutic drug levels, these authors demonstrate that the dominant factor for deciding if a particular antipsychotic drug will elicit parkinsonism is whether it binds more tightly or more loosely than dopamine at the D_2 receptor subtype. Thus, for those antipsychotic drugs that elicit little or no parkinsonism, it appears that the high endogenous dopamine in the human striatum must outcompete the more loosely bound neuroleptic at the striatal D_2 receptor subtype. Dopamine less readily displaces the more hydrophobic radioligands of the haloperidol type, providing an additional correlate between the magnitude of in vivo competition with endogenous agonist and parkinsonism. The separation of antipsychotic drugs into "loose" and "tight" binding to D_2 receptors is consistent with the observation that catalepsy induced by olanzepine and loxapine (more loosely bound than dopamine), but not haloperidol (more tightly bound than dopamine to D_2 receptors), was fully reversible (61). Taken together, these observations suggest that D_2 blockade may be necessary for achieving antipsychotic action. This suggestion is in keeping with the observation that many patients will suddenly relapse when stopping clozapine, perhaps due to a sudden pulse of endogenous dopamine arising from emotional or physical activity that displaces the loosely bound neuroleptic from the receptor. Clinical dosing schedules can be adjusted to obtain sufficient but low occupancies of D_2 receptors in order to minimize the development of parkinsonism. The psychosis caused by levodopa or bromocriptine can be readily treated by low doses of either clozapine

Receptor Subtype	D₁-like D_1	D_5	D₂-like D_2	D_3	D_4
Amino acids	446	477	443	400	387
Chromosome	5q35.1	4p15.1-16.1	11q22-23	3p13.3	11p15.5
Second messenger	$\uparrow$cAMP	$\uparrow$cAMP	$\downarrow$cAMP K^+ channel Ca^+ channel	K^+ channel Ca^+ channel	$\downarrow$cAMP K^+ channel
mRNA	Striatum	Hippocampus Kidney	Striatum	Nucleus Accumbens	Cerebral Cortex
Selective agonists	SKF38393	SKF38393	Bromocriptine Butaclamol Pergolide Ropinirole	7-OH-DPAT Pramipexole Ropinirole	–
Selective antagonists	SCH23390	SCH23390	Spiperone Raclopride Sulpiride	Spiperone Raclopride Sulpiride	Spiperone Clozapine

Table 23-1   Properties of Dopamine Receptor Subtypes

(62) or remoxipride (63), as there is very little endogenous dopamine to compete with the antagonist. Further studies are needed to determine whether newer antipsychotic drugs with low affinity for D_2 receptors and with low risk for parkinsonism will also cause less tardive dyskinesia.

The success of treating parkinsonian symptoms with the dopamine precursor amino acid levodopa is due to its ability to reverse the dopamine deficiency. Unfortunately, treatment complications emerge shortly after beginning levodopa therapy. In the DATATOP study (64), almost half of the patients developed wearing-off (loss of efficacy toward the end of a dosing interval), about one-third showed dyskinesias, and about one-fourth were showing early signs of freezing (sudden loss of capacity to move) with a mean duration of treatment of only 18 months. Modern pharmacologic treatment of PD has been advanced by the increased understanding of the complexity of dopamine receptor pharmacology and the ability to screen drug candidates in vitro against cloned and expressed human dopamine receptor subtypes. New treatment approaches are aimed at developing subtype-selective, direct-acting agonists to restore dopaminergic function (2).

Symptoms of parkinsonism in primate models are treated with agonists that activate the D_2-like receptor subfamily. D_2 agonists with long half-lives can relieve parkinsonism in these animals with little risk of motor side effects, whereas repetitive levodopa doses will induce motor fluctuations and dyskinesias [65]. In dyskinetic animals that had received levodopa doses, D_2 agonists that had few side effects on their own now elicit dyskinesias. These observations suggest that repetitive coactivation of denervated striatal dopamine receptor subtypes initiates the development of these movements by nonselective activation of postsynaptic D_1 and D_2/D_3 receptors.

Pramipexole is a novel dopamine agonist with preferential affinity for D_3 receptors (Table 23-1). It has little affinity for the D_1-like receptors, and within the D_2 receptor subfamily, it exhibits its highest affinity at the D_3 receptor subtype distinguishing it from all other dopamine agonists currently used for the treatment of PD [66]. Dopamine normally inhibits striatal GABAergic cells of the indirect pathway by acting on D_2 receptors and stimulates GABAergic cells of the direct pathway by stimulating D_1 and D_3 receptors (67). These effects result in the inhibition of the globus pallidus (GPi, internal segment). In PD, when dopamine innervation has been lost, the GPi fires at very high rates to inhibit thalamic relay neurons resulting in bradykinesia (66). Pramipexole stimulates D_3 receptors, which directly inhibit GPi neurons, removing its inhibitory gate on thalamocortical motor pathways, and stimulates D_2 receptors to indirectly inhibit GPi neurons (68). Thus pramipexole has two synergistic mechanisms to mimic dopamine and restore function in PD. Although D_3 receptors have a lower density in the striatum as compared with D_2 receptors (Figure 23-2), chronic administration of indirect-acting agonists may cause an upregulation in the number of D_3 binding sites in this region. In keeping with this suggestion, chronic cocaine abusers have elevated densities of D_3 receptor sites in limbic sectors of the striatum and nucleus accumbens (69). It is not known if this regulatory change occurs in the denervated striatum, early in the course of agonist replacement for PD. Pramipexole also has shown efficacy for the treatment of depression in PD, in keeping with its postsynaptic effects on limbic targets (70). Thus the antidepressant activity of pramipexole for treating moderate depression, may be a property that is possibly tied to its preferential binding to the D_3 receptor subtype (66).

Whether other subtypes of dopamine receptors exist is not known. However, rapid advances in molecular cloning may reveal additional heterogeneity in the expression of synaptic proteins involved in dopaminergic neurotransmission. At this time, five cloned and expressed dopaminergic receptor proteins provide a complex molecular basis for a variety of neural signals mediated by a single neurotransmitter.

REFERENCES

1. Hornykiewicz O. Dopamine and brain function *Pharmacol Res* 1966; 18:925–964.

2. Factor SA. Dopamine agonists. *Med Clin North Am* 1999; 83(2):415–443.

3. Carlsson A. The current status of the dopamine hypothesis of schizophrenia. *Neuropsychopharm* 1988; 1:179–186.

4. Creese I, Burt DR, Snyder SH. Dopamine receptor binding predicts clinical and pharmacologic potencies of antischizophrenic drugs. *Science* 1976; 192:481–483.

5. Seeman P, Lee T, Chan-Wong M, et al. Antipsychotic drug doses and neuroleptic/dopamine receptors. *Nature* 1976; 261:717–719.

6. Dohlman HG, Caron MG, Lefkowitz RJ. A family of receptors coupled to guanine nucleotide regulatory proteins. *Biochemistry* 1987; 26:2657–2664.

7. Dixon RA, Koblika BK, Strader DJ, et al. Cloning of the gene and cDNA for mammalian b-adrenergic receptor and homology with rhodopsin. *Nature* 1986; 321:75–79.

8. Kubo T, Maeda A, Sugimoto, et al. Primary structure of porcine cardiac muscarinic acetylcholine receptor

deduced from the cDNA sequence. *FEBS Lett* 1986; 209:367–372.

9. Bunzow JR, Van Tol HHM, Grandy DK, et al. Cloning and expression of a rat D_2 dopamine receptor cDNA. *Nature* 1988; 336:783–787.

10. Dearry A, Gingrich JA, Falardeau P, et al. Molecular cloning and expression of the gene for a human D_1 dopamine receptor. *Nature* 1990; 347:72–76.

11. Monsma FJ Jr, Mahan LC, McVittie LD, et al. Molecular cloning and expression of a D_1 dopamine receptor linked to adenylyl cyclase activation. *Proc Natl Acad Sci USA* 1990; 87(17):6723–6727.

12. Dal Tosos R, Sommer B, Ewart M, et al. The dopamine receptor: Two molecular forms generated by alternative splicing. *EMBO J* 1989; 8:4025–4034.

13. Monsuma FJ, McVittie LD, Gerfen CR, et al. Multiple D_2 dopamine receptors produced by alternative RNA splicing. *Nature* 1989; 324:926–929.

14. Sokoloff P, Giros B, Martres MP, et al. Molecular cloning and characterization of a novel dopamine receptor (D-3) as a target for neuroleptics. *Nature* 1990; 347:146–151.

15. Van Tol HHM, Bunzow JR, Guan H-C, et al. Cloning of the gene for a human dopamine D_4 receptor with high affinity for the antipsychotic clozapine. *Nature* 1991; 350:610–614.

16. Sunahara RK, Niznik HB, Weiner DM, et al. Human dopamine D_1 receptor encoded by an intronless gene on chromosome 5. *Nature* 1990; 347:80–83.

17. Zhou QY, Grandy DK, Thambi L, et al. Cloning and expression of human and rat D_1 dopamine receptors. *Nature* 1990; 347:76–80.

18. Sunhara RK, Guan H-C, O'Dowd BF, et al. Cloning of the gene for a human dopamine D_5 receptor with higher affinity for dopamine than D_1. *Nature* 1991; 350:614–619.

19. O'Dowd BF. Structures of dopamine receptors. *J Neurochem* 1993; 60:804–816.

20. Lachowicz J, Sibley DR. Molecular characteristics of mammalian dopamine receptors. *Pharmacol Toxicol* (Mini Review) 1997, 81:105–113.

21. Snyder LA, Roberts JL, Sealfon SC. Alternative transcripts of the rat and human dopamine D_3 receptor. *Biochem Biophys Res Commun* 1991; 180(2):1031–1035.

22. Fishburn CS, Belleli D, David C, et al. A novel short isoform of the D_3 dopamine receptor generated by alternative splicing in the third cytoplasmic loop. *J Biol Chem* 1993; 268(8):5872–5878.

23. Giros B, Martres MP, Pilon C, et al. Shorter variants of the D_3 dopamine receptor produced through various patterns of alternative splicing. *Biochem Biophys Res Commun* 1991; 176(3):1584–1592.

24. Van Tol HH, Wu CM, Guan HC, et al. Multiple dopamine D_4 receptor variants in the human population. *Nature* 1992; 358(6382):149–152.

25. Weinshank RL, Adham N, Macchi M, et al. Molecular cloning and characterization of a high affinity dopamine receptor (D_1 b) and its pseudogene. *J Biol Chem* 1991; 266(33):22427–22435.

26. Bjorklund A, Lindvall O. Dopamine-containing systems in the CNS. In: Bjorklund A, Hokfelt T. (eds.). *Handbook of Chemical Neuroanatomy*, Vol 2, *Classical Transmitters in the CNS Part I* 1994:55–122.

27. Le Moine C, Normand E, Guitteny AF, et al. Dopamine receptor gene expression by enkephalin neurons in rat forebrain. *Proc Natl Acad Sci USA* 87(1):230–234.

28. Diaz J, Levesque D, Griffon N, et al. Opposing roles for dopamine D_2 and D_3 receptors on neurotensin mRNA expression in nucleus accumbens. *Eur J Neurosci* 1994; 6(8):1384–1387.

29. Diaz J, Levesque D, Lammers CH, et al. Phenotypical characterization of neurons expressing the dopamine D_3 receptor in the rat brain. *Neuroscience* 1995; 65(3):731–745.

30. Bouthenet ML, Souil MP, Martes P, et al. Localization of dopamine D_3 mRNA in the rat brain using in situ hybridization histochemistry: Comparision with D_2 dopamine receptor. *Brain Res* 1991: 564:203–219.

31. Le Moine C, Bloch B. Anatomical and cellular analysis of dopamine receptor gene expression. In: Ariano MA, Surmeir DJ (eds.). *Molecular and Cellular Mechanisms of Neostriatal Function*. New York: Springer-Verlag, 1995:45–58.

32. Surmier DJ, Eberwine J, Wilson CJ, et al. Dopamine receptor subtypes colocalize in rat striatonigral neurons. *Proc Natl Acad Sci USA* 1992; 89:10178–10182.

33. Gerfen CR, Keefe KA, Steiner H. Dopamine-mediated gene regulation in the striatum. *Adv Pharmacol* 1998; 42:670–673.

34. Waddington JL, O'Boyle KM, Drugs acting on brain dopamine receptors: A conceptual reevaluation five years afer the first selective D_1 antagonist. *Pharmacol Ther* 1989; 43:1–52.

35. Loschmann PA, Smith LA, Lange KW, et al. Motor activity following the administration of selective D-1 and D-2 dopaminergic drugs to normal common marmosets. *Psychopharmacology* 1991; 105(3):303–309.

36. Hepler JR, Gilman AG. G proteins. *Trends Biochem Sci* 1992;17(10):383–387.

37. Grandy DK, Zhang Y, Bouvier C, et al. Multiple human D_5 dopamine receptor genes, a functional receptor and two pseudogenes. *Proc Natl Acad Sci USA* 1991; 88:9175–9179.

38. Sidhu A. Coupling of D_1 and D_5 dopamine receptors to multiple G proteins: Implications for understanding the diversity in receptor-G protein coupling. *Mol Neurobiol* 1998; 16(2):125–134.

39. Birnbaumer L, Abramowitz J, Brown AM. Receptor-effector coupling by G proteins. *Biochim Biophys Acta* 1990; 1031(2):163–224.

40. Kitai ST, Surmeier DJ. Cholinergic and dopaminergic modulation of potassium conductances in neostriatal neurons. *Adv Neurol* 1993; 60:40–52.

41. Kimura K, White BH, Sidhu A. Coupling of human D_1 dopamine receptors to different guanine nucleotide binding proteins. Evidence that D_1 dopamine receptors

can couple to both Gs and G(o). *J Biol Chem* 1995; 270:14672–14678.

42. Dahmer MK, Senolges SE. Dopaminergic inhibition of catecholamine secretion from chromaffin cells: Evidence that inhibition is mediated by D4 and D5 dopamine receptors. *J Neurochem* 1996; 66:222–232.

43. Sidhu A. Regulation and expression of D-1, but not D-5, dopamine receptors in human SK-N-MC neuroblastoma cells. *J Recep Res/Sig Trans* 1997; 17:777–784.

44. Kozasa T Gilman AG. Purification of recombinant G proteins from Sf9 cells by hexahistidine tagging of associated subunits: Characterization of α12 and inhibition of adenylyl cyclase by Gzα. *J Biol Chem* 1995; 270:1734–1741.

45. Glatt CE, Snyder SH. Cloning and expression of an adenylyl cyclase localized to the corpus striatum. *Nature* 1993; 361:536–538.

46. Yoshimurea M, Ikeda H, Tabakoff B. Opioid receptors inhibit dopamine-stimulated activity of type V adenylyl cyclase and enhance dopamine-stimulated activity of type VII adenylyl cyclase. *Mol Pharmacol* 1996; 50:43–51.

47. Cooper DMF, Mons N, Karpen JW. Adenylyl cyclases and the interaction between calcium and cAMP signalling. *Nature* 1995; 374:421–424.

48. McAllister G, Knowles MR, Ward-Booth SM, et al. Functional coupling of human D2, D3, and D4 dopamine receptors in HEK293 cells. *J Recept Signal Trans Res* 1995; 15:267–281.

49. Hayes G, Biden TJ, Selbie LA, et al. Structural subtypes of the dopamine D2 receptor are functionally distinct: Expression of the cloned D2A and D2B subtypes in a heterologous cell line. *Mol Endocrinol* 1992; 6:920–926.

50. Montmaueur J-P, Borelli E. Transcription mediated by a cAMP-responsive promoter element is reduced upon activation of dopamine D2 receptors. *Proc Natl Acad Sci USA* 1991; 7:161–170.

51. Castellano MA, Liu LX, Monsma FJ Jr, et al. Transfected D2 short dopamine receptors inhibit voltage-dependent potassium current in neuroblastoma x glioma hybrid (NG108-15) cells. *Mol Pharmacol* 1993; 44(3):649–656.

52. Liu L-X, Monsma FJ Jr, Sibley DR, et al. Coupling of D2-long receptor isoform to K+ currents in neuroblastoma x glioma (NG108-15) cells. *Soc Neurosci* 1993; 19:79.

53. Jaber M, Robinson SW, Missale C, et al. Dopamine receptors and brain function. *Neuropharm* 1996; 35(11):1503–1519.

54. Levey AI, Hersch SM, Rye DM, et al. Localization of D1 and D2 receptors in brain with subtype-specific antibodies. *Proc Nat Acad Sci USA* 1993; 90:8861–8865.

55. Tiberi M, Jarvie KR, Silvia C, et al. Cloning, molecular characterization and chromosomal assignment of a gene endocing a second D1 dopamine receptor subtype: Differential expression pattern in rat brain compared with the D1 receptor. *Proc Natl Acad Sci USA* 1991, 88:7491–7495.

56. Jarvie KR, Tiberi M, Silvia C, Gingrich JA, Caron MG. Molecular cloning, stable expression and desensitization of the human dopamine D1b/D5 receptor. *J Recept Res* 1993; 13:573–590.

57. Bunzow JR, Van Tol HH, Grandy DK, et al. Cloning and expression of a rat D2 dopamine receptor cDNA. *Nature* 1989; 336(6201):783–787.

58. Van Tol HH, Bunzow JR, Guan HC, et al. Cloning of the gene for a human dopamine D4 receptor with high affinity for the antipsychotic clozapine. *Nature* 1991; 350(6319):610–614.

59. Sokoloff P, Giros B, Martress M-P, et al. Molecular cloning and characterization of a novel dopamine receptor (D3) as a target for neuroleptics. *Nature* 1990; 347:146–151.

60. Gerlach J, Behnkek K, Heltberg J, et al. Sulpiride and haloperidol in schizophrenia: A double-blind cross-over study of therapeutic effect, side effects and plasma concentrations. *Br J Psychiatry* 1985; 147:283–288.

61. Seeman P, Tallerico T. Antipsychotic drugs which elicit little or no parkinsonism bind more loosely to brain D2 receptors, yet occupy high levels of these receptors. *Mol Psychiatry* 1998; 3:123–134.

62. Rabey JM, Reves TA, Nuefeld MY, et al. Low dose clozapine in the treatment of levodopa-induced mental disorders in Parkinson's disease. *Neurology* 1995; 48:432–434.

63. Sandor P, Lang AE, Singal S, et al. Remoxipride in the treatment of levodopa-induced psychosis. *J Clin Psychopharmacol* 1996; 18:395–399.

64. Parkinson Study Group. Impact of deprenyl and tocopherol treatment in progression of disability in early Parkinson's disease. *N Engl J Med* 1993; 328:176–183.

65. Blanchet PJ, Calon F, Martel JC, et al. Continuous administration decreases and pulsatile administration increases behavioral sensitivity to a novel dopamine D2 agonist (U-91356A) in MPTP-exposed monkeys. *J Pharmacol Exp Ther* 1995; 272:854–859.

66. Bennett JP Jr, Piercey MF. Pramipexole – a new dopamine agonist for the treatment of Parkinson's disease. *J Neurol Sci* 1999; 163:25–31.

67. Piercey MF, Hyslop DK, Hoffman WE. Excitation of type II anterior caudate neurons by stimulation of D3 receptors. *Brain Res* 1997; 762:19–28.

68. Staley JK, Mash DC. Adaptive increase in D3 dopamine receptors in the brain reward circuits of human cocaine fatalities. *J Neurosci* 1996; 16(19):6100–6106.

69. Szegedi A, Wetzel J, Hillert A, et al. Pramipexole, a novel selective dopamine agonist in major depression. *Mov Disord* 1996; 11(Suppl 1):266.

24

Problems in Diagnosis

Andrew J. Lees, M.D.

The National Hospital for Neurology and Neurosurgery, London, United Kingdom

Most physicians acknowledge Parkinson's disease as a discrete clinically recognizable malady. However, like the chimera, its clinical picture has altered as our concepts of the underlying cause and pathology have evolved. The most disabling component is an insidious slowness, with an associated reduction in amplitude of individual movements during repetitive motor tasks. Patients usually describe this difficulty as clumsiness, weakness, or awkwardness during dexterous activities; a complaint of being unable to do two tasks at once is less common but characteristic. A dilapidation of motor planning and programming underlies many of these early deficits and is due to dysfunction within the circuitry of the basal ganglia. A slightly worried poker face, absent arm swing, quiet monotonous speech, hang-dog appearance, and leaden shuffle are other clinical hallmarks that may instantly suggest the diagnosis. However, it is usually a quiver or shake of the fingers or less commonly the leg or jaw that cannot be explained away as "getting old" or "being tired" that brings the patient to the doctor. This may only be present when yawning, laughing, or straining at stool. Muscle rigidity, a sign first appreciated by Charcot, which leads to complaints of painful stiffness, is another feature that is readily detected on physical examination and may be commented on by family or physical therapists.

This triad of cardinal signs makes up what we now perceive to constitute Parkinson's disease, and when all three are present the diagnosis should be seriously entertained. If, in addition, there is a sustained improvement to levodopa treatment with the eventual emergence of interdose dyskinesias and motor fluctuations, then the diagnosis is probable.

In the absence of a biologic marker or laboratory test for Parkinson's disease the diagnosis can only be made with certainty at autopsy. The histopathologic criteria for the diagnosis of Parkinson's disease have developed somewhat independently and there are very few studies where detailed clinical description is combined with scrupulous pathologic examination.

Most neurologists, however, consider a severe loss of neuromelanin-containing neurons in the pars compacta of the substantia nigra and locus coeruleus with Lewy bodies in surviving neurons in the absence of any alternative pathology as minimum confirmatory postmortem criteria (see Chapter 20).

If one accepts these pathologic diagnostic criteria as the gold standard for the diagnosis, then it is now evident that even seasoned physicians will make clinical errors, especially in the early phases of the disease. Careful attention to nuances in the history of the presenting complaint and recognition of distinctive constellations of physical signs can, however, narrow the margin of error. The differential diagnosis of Parkinson's disease is a growing list of considerations that are provided in Table 24-1.

RECENT CLINICOPATHOLOGIC STUDIES

The United Kingdom Parkinson's Disease Society Brain Research Center at the National Hospital for Neurology and Neurosurgery in London started to receive bequests of brain tissue about 10 years ago. Clinical data has been prospectively collected from 1500 donors with Parkinson's and postmortem tissue obtained from 710. Although most cases of idiopathic Parkinson's disease are correctly diagnosed during life, neuropathologic series have shown that even in specialist centers, a substantial proportion of patients prove to have alternative pathologies. The first 100 brains of patients diagnosed as Parkinson's disease in life on the basis of the presence of at least two of the three cardinal signs – an improvement of some sort with levodopa and the absence of an alternative neurologic diagnosis – were examined at the United Kingdom brain bank. The mean age of disease onset in this group was 64.5 years (range 31–85 years) with a mean disease duration at the time of death of 11.9 years

Table 24-1

Parkinson Syndromes

Common
    Neuroleptic – provoked
    Diffuse cerebrovascular disease
    Progressive supranuclear palsy (atypical presentations)
    Multiple system atrophy (strionigral variant)
    Benign tremulous Parkinson's disease

Rare
    Neurodegenerations:
        Corticobasalganglionic degeneration, Alzheimer's disease,
        Pick's disease, Hallervorden-Spatz disease
    Neurogenetic:
        Huntington's disease, SCA mutations, Dentate-rubro-pallido-luysian atrophy,
        Wilson's disease, hereditary acoeruloplasminaemia, neuro-acanthocytosis
    Trauma:
        Striatal variant of dementia pugilistica
        Chronic subdural haematoma, mid-brain trauma
    Metabolic:
        Hypoxia, acquired hepato-cerebral syndrome, familial basal ganglia calcification,
        extrapontine myelinolysis
    Toxic:
        Carbon monoxide, cyanide, alcohol, carbon disulphide, hydrocarbons,
        MPTP, manganese, solvents
    Tumours:
        Supratentorial and brain-stem neoplasms, arteriovenous malformation
    Infections:
        Postencephalitic (Von Economo, Japanese B, Western equine, Echo,
        coxsackie, measles, AIDS, prion disease, TB, neurosyphilis)
    Other Parkinson syndromes:
        Communicating hydrocephalus
        Hemi-atrophy-hemiparkinson syndrome

(range 2–35 years). Only 76 had Parkinson's disease, but interestingly, all of these had some Lewy bodies in the cerebral cortex. The clinical records of the 24 false positive diagnoses were then scrutinized and even with the eye of hindsight, based on the clinical picture, Parkinson's disease seemed highly likely in 16.

Neurofibrillary degeneration was the commonest pathologic finding in the misdiagnosed cases (1). Similar levels of error (10 of 41) occurred in a smaller series in one hospital in Canada where all cases had been examined in life by a opinion leader in Parkinson's disease (2). Based on these studies, more stringent clinical diagnostic criteria have been developed and used widely in research (3). If selected criteria (asymmetrical onset, no atypical features, and no other possible aetiology for another Parkinson syndrome) were applied to the United Kingdom Parkinson's Disease Society Brain Research Center data, then the proportion of true Parkinson's disease cases was increased to 93%, but 32% of pathologically confirmed cases would be rejected on this basis.

These observations indicate that studies based even on Parkinson's specialists' diagnosis using standard criteria will include cases other than Parkinson's disease leading to some distortion in epidemiologic studies and clinical trials. The use of additional criteria can reduce misdiagnosis, but at the cost of excluding genuine Parkinson's disease cases (4). A further problem is that perhaps as many as 10% of patients who have a predominant parkinsonian syndrome in life and fulfil pathologic criteria for Parkinson's disease at autopsy have atypical clinical features such as early severe dementia, supranuclear vertical gaze palsies, or a negative response to large doses of levodopa (5,6). Encouragingly, only 16% of the last 100 clinically diagnosed cases of Parkinson's disease had incompatible pathology (7), suggesting that greater awareness of diagnostic alternatives to Parkinson's disease had occurred among British neurologists over the five years since the original publication. In this second series, the commonest diagnostic errors were neurofibrillary degeneration (PSP) in seven cases, cerebrovascular disease in the absence of alternative pathology in four cases, and multiple system atrophy in three cases, with no demonstrable pathology in the other two. Alternative criteria for the diagnosis have also been proposed, but these have not developed out of prospective clinicopathologic studies (8,9).

HELPFUL CLINICAL POINTERS FOR THE DIAGNOSIS OF PARKINSON'S DISEASE

A coarse 6 Hertz rest tremor of the fingers, legs, or jaw in a patient with an asymmetrical bradykinetic-rigid syndrome is a good pointer to the diagnosis of Parkinson's disease, provided iatrogenic disease has been eliminated. There are, however, a significant number of patients who present with a severe rest tremor, often with an additional postural tremor, who have some rigidity and no or minimal bradykinesia, and who seem to respond relatively poorly or not at all to levodopa and progress extremely slowly (10). These cases are often hard to characterize with certainty. A number of patients with essential tremor may also have mild limb rigidity and a reduced arm swing, and the tremor when severe may resemble a rest tremor. Other patients with Parkinson's disease have essential tremor that may precede the onset of the malady by many years (11).

Parkinson's disease is of extremely gradual onset and the emergence of motor symptoms is invariably asymmetrical and often initially unilateral. Clumsiness of one hand leading to difficulties with writing, dressing, bathing, and household chores is a common early sign; common early complaints include difficulties with top buttons, cleaning teeth, shampooing hair, beating eggs, getting small objects out of back pockets, and turning a key in a lock. Later on, problems rising from a low chair, getting in and out of bed or the bath, and turning in a confined space intrude. Other patients start to drag one leg when tired, but a presentation with falls due to postural instability or unsteadiness or blocking while walking would be exceptional. Prodromal complaints of pain in the spine or shoulder, fatigue, disturbances of temperature regulation, depression, pins and needles, and impaired smell appreciation are quite common but by no means invariable. Nevertheless, their presence, once the diagnosis of Parkinson's syndrome is suspected, favours Lewy body pathology.

Parkinson's disease spreads slowly from limb to limb, and there is usually a delay of two to three years before patients start noticing disturbances of movement on the second side (12). Significant impairment of balance with falls is only exceptionally present in the first five years after diagnosis. Eye movements are normal on bedside testing even late in the course of the illness, and the presence of corticospinal signs or cerebellar ataxia is incompatible with a diagnosis of Parkinson's disease. A striatal dystonic toe, on the other hand, may be seen early in young onset Parkinson's disease (13). Characteristic clinical features that point

Table 24-2	
Parkinson Plus Syndromes	
Disorder	Distinguishing Features
Progressive supranuclear palsy (Steele-Richardson-Olszewski)	Slowness or reduction of downgaze Early falls backwards Frontal lobe signs Growling dysarthria Symmetrical axial onset
Diffuse cerebrovascular disease (Binswanger, leuko-araiosis, pseudo-parkinsonism)	Broad-based shuffling gait Cognitive dysfunction Gait ignition failure Facial expression Often preserved
Multiple system atrophy (strio-nigral degeneration)	Impotence, urinary incontinence Syncope Nasal dysphonia Early gait unsteadiness
Corticobasalganglionic degeneration	Unilateral presentation Cortical sensory deficits Jerky myoclonic jerks Eye movement disorder

to the diagnosis of other Parkinson plus syndromes are listed in Table 24-2.

More than 95% of patients respond gratifyingly to levodopa therapy. Some symptoms improve more than others and speech and balance problems become more prominent as the years pass. Levodopa remains effective for decades. Although undesirable, the emergence of generalized interdose dyskinesias and motor fluctuations are a useful marker for the diagnosis of Parkinson's disease. An acute diagnostic challenge with levodopa solution or subcutaneously administered apomorphine is useful if there is doubt about dopaminergic responsiveness and whether dyskinesias is present (14).

THE NEUROLOGIC EXAMINATION

In the early stages of the disease there are relatively few physical signs. As the patient enters the consulting room, a slightly staring impassive face with infrequent blinking may suggest the diagnosis; a severe reduction of arm swing on one side with a mild scuffing of the sole on walking may be present. Tremor at rest may be restricted to a single finger and may be present only occasionally. The motor disturbance in the limbs is best brought out by asking the patient to touch the fingers of both hands as quickly as possible with the thumbs. In Parkinson's disease a slight delay in starting the movements and a progressive reduction in amplitude of each finger movement is characteristic. The patient may maintain the hand in the posture adopted for the test for a short time afterwards. Repetitive tapping of the thumb and index finger is another useful test, and three or four lines of script should always be obtained to look for micrographia. Tapping of the foot on the floor as fast as possible may bring out early difficulties in one leg. Cogwheel rigidity at the wrist can be brought out by Froment's maneuver in which the wrist is put through a full range of passive movement while the patient voluntarily moves the other arm. Lead pipe rigidity is better appreciated at the shoulder and in the leg. Although marked asymmetry of physical signs is usual, careful examination will usually detect mild motor deficits even on the apparently unaffected side. A slight flexion at the wrist, elbow, and knee with a scoliosis is sometimes appreciated early on. Variations in normal speech are so wide that subtle alterations of prosody and intonation may only be apparent to those who know the patient well, and the initial consultation should whenever possible be conducted in the presence of a family member or close friend. Subtle slowness may be detected by watching the patient undress, dress, and walk down the street.

An unnatural stillness when seated in company and a reduction in nonverbal communication are other useful early telltale signs.

Later in the course of the illness, walking difficulties become more striking with a narrow-based festinant shuffle interrupted by freezing in doorways or on turning in confined spaces. By this stage the posture is simian, the body is rigid and moves en bloc, and a tendency to break into a trot following mild forward displacement becomes irresistible. Balance becomes increasingly precarious with start hesitation, blocking, and retropulsion, triggering falls. At this stage disability will be bilateral but still asymmetrical, and facial expression is frozen. Dribbling of saliva and a greasy skin may be detected. Speech is quiet, slurred, slow, and at times difficult to decipher.

LEWY BODY DEMENTIA

Although first described in Japan by Okazaki in 1961 (15), it is only in the last 15 years that it has been generally recognized that a neuropsychiatric syndrome may be the presenting feature of Lewy body pathology. Fluctuating memory loss combined with visual hallucinations, confusional states and depression, anxiety, and paranoid psychosis may antecede the emergence of signs of Parkinson's syndrome by several years, effectively reversing the picture seen in Parkinson's disease where clinical signs of dementia and psychosis usually emerge after more than 10 years of motor disease (16). Some patients with numerous neocortical Lewy bodies also present with a dementing illness similar to Alzheimer's disease. In these patients, Lewy bodies, which can be demonstrated with ubiquitin or synuclein stains, are most numerous in the limbic system, particularly the entorhinal, inferior temporal, parahippocampus, insular, and anterior cingulate cortex. In the neocortex they are mostly found in the deeper cortical layers in small and medium pyramidal neuron. In addition to Lewy bodies in the cerebral cortex and brain-stem, most of these patients also have many beta-amyloid plaques with dystrophic neurites in the CA2-3 hippocampal sectors. Neurofibrillary tangles are usually sparse unless there is coexistent Alzheimer's disease. It is believed to be the second commonest cause of dementia, and many authorities now consider it a discrete clinicopathologic entity (17). However, it is important to recognize that all patients with Parkinson's disease have some neocortical Lewy bodies irrespective of whether they had dementia in life. Furthermore, all patients with Lewy body dementia have nigral cell loss and Lewy bodies, even when signs of Parkinson's disease were not reported in life; molecular biology is likely to resolve this controversy in the future. If an Alzheimer-type dementia is present in a patient with otherwise typical Parkinson's disease, a number of diagnostic possibilities exist in addition to Lewy body pathology. Coexistent Alzheimer's disease or diffuse cerebrovascular disease are the first alternatives to consider, but there are a number of other rare neurodegenerations where the two may be seen together.

ANCILLARY INVESTIGATIONS

Progress in functional neuroimaging continues to occur and it is now possible to quantify dopamine in the central nervous system (18) See Chapters 25 and 26. Single photon-emission computed tomography (SPECT) using dopamine transporter radioligands (e.g., B-CIT) is already proving useful in clinical practice as an aid in distinguishing essential tremor and neuroleptic-induced parkinson's in (19); it can also be helpful in confirming a suspected diagnosis of psychogenic parkinson's in (19a). Nonetheless, at the present time it is not possible to differentiate, with certainty, Parkinson plus syndromes from Parkinson's disease by magnetic resonance imaging, spectroscopy, or positron emission tomography. Other tests claimed to be of value include clonidine challenge tests with growth hormone estimations (20), urethral and anal sphincter electromyography (21), autonomic function laboratory testing for multiple system atrophy (22), electro-oculography (23), neuropsychology (24), startle reflex examination (25) for progressive supranuclear palsy, and a metabolic regional blood flow SPECT brain scan for cortico-basal degeneration (26).

Abnormalities of odor discrimination of a particular type have also been reported as occurring in Parkinson's disease (27). At present none of these tests are sensitive and specific enough to be recommended as reliable diagnostic aids, and findings have not been correlated with pathologic confirmation of the diagnosis.

CONCLUDING REMARKS

For the practising physician, the critical division of Parkinson syndromes is into those who will respond with functional benefit to levodopa and those who will not (Table 24-3). The large majority of patients with Lewy body Parkinson's disease respond in a sustained fashion to dopaminergic treatment with the eventual emergence of oscillations in motor performance and dyskinesias. There may, however, be more patients who are hyporesponsive to levodopa than is acknowledged at present, and it has recently been suggested that Afro-Caribbeans and Indians with Parkinson's disease may have a suboptimal response (28,29). There is a small group of patients in the author's own practice who fulfill all diagnostic criteria for Parkinson's disease but do not benefit from levodopa. About 50% of patients with strio-nigral degeneration (MSA) have a beneficial response initially to therapy, but the accelerated course of the illness compared with Parkinson's disease, the emergence of levodopa-induced dystonia with a predilection for the head and face, and the relatively rare occurrence of the on-off syndrome are helpful distinguishing features (30). Patients with postencephalitic and MPTP-induced parkinsonism are now very rare, and the diagnosis is usually straightforward. Both conditions respond rapidly and strikingly to levodopa with the early appearance of dyskinesias and motor fluctuations. Young onset Huntington's and Wilson's disease with parkinsonian presentations may also improve to some extent but diagnostic testing for both disorder's is available. The assessment of dopaminergic responsiveness in parkinsonian syndromes is often difficult, particularly in the first few years of the disease when disability may be relatively mild and a long-duration levodopa response occurs. Most patients receiving 300 mg or more of levodopa will improve within seven days of starting therapy, but delayed responses can occur, and a few patients need at least 600 mg a day to see benefit. After six weeks of levodopa therapy, if there is doubt on the part of the physician and/or the patient, either a

Table 24-3		
L-DOPA Responsiveness in Parkinson Syndromes		
Good and sustained	Moderate and less sustained	No response
Parkinson's disease	Multisystem atrophy	Progressive supranuclear palsy
Postencephalitic Parkinson	Posttraumatic Parkinsonism	Corticobasalganglionic
	Huntington's disease (rigid form)	degeneration
MPTP-induced parkinsonism	Cerebrovascular disease	Neuroleptic-induced
		Parkinson's disease

drug holiday with reassessment after a week or an acute levodopa or apomorphine challenge can be helpful (14). It has been claimed that even one dose of levodopa is sufficient to kindle dyskinesias and that all patients should start on dopamine agonist therapy. As it is even more difficult to determine responsiveness to an agonist and as almost all patients will be receiving levodopa within three years of the diagnosis, a single levodopa challenge may be helpful in encouraging patients to persist with incremental build-up of the agonist.

Accurate diagnosis of Parkinson's disease is, in the majority of cases, possible after one or two years of continued observation. Difficulties arise in a substantial number either in levodopa responsive patients with one or two atypical features or in levodopa unresponsive patients who have none of the additional findings associated with Parkinson plus syndromes. The identification of two mutations in the gene for the cytoskeletal protein alpha synuclein in autosomal dominant Lewy body Parkinson's disease and the presence of alpha synuclein in brain-stem and cortical Lewy bodies in sporadic Parkinson's disease brings Parkinson's disease closer to multiple system atrophy where synuclein has been identified in glial cytoplasmic inclusions. A second gene abnormality called "parkin" in autosomal-recessive young onset parkinsonism has also been identified. These newly identified genetic disorders together with overlap pathologic and clinical syndromes will be increasingly diagnosed, suggesting that our concepts of what constitutes Parkinson's disease may again be in a state of flux.

REFERENCES

1. Hughes AJ, Daniel SE, Kilford L, et al. The accuracy of clinical diagnosis of idiopathic Parkinson's disease: A clinicopathological study of 100 cases. *J Neurol Neurosurg Psychiatry*, 1991; 55:181–184.

2. Rajput AH, Rozdilsky B, Rajput A, et al. Levodopa efficacy and pathological basis of Parkinson syndrome. *Clin Neuropharmacol* 1990; 13:553–558.

3. Gibb WRG, Lees AJ. The relevance of the Lewy body to the pathogenesis of idiopathic Parkinson's disease. *J Neurol Neurosurg Psychiatry* 1988, 51:745–752.

4. Hughes AJ, Ben-Shlomo Y, Daniel S, et al. What features improve the accuracy of clinical diagnosis in Parkinson's disease: A clinico-pathologic study. *Neurology* 1992, 42:1142–1146.

5. Hughes AJ, Daniel SE, Blankson SJ, et al. A clinico-pathologic study of 100 cases of Parkinson's disease. *Arch Neurol* 1993, 50:140–148.

6. Sage JL, Miller DC, Golbe LI, et al. Clinically atypical expression of pathologically typical Lewy body parkinsonism. *Clin Neuropharmacol* 1990; 13:36–47.

7. Ansorge O, Lees AJ, Daniel SE. The neuropathological spectrum of clinically diagnosed idiopathic Parkinson's disease. *Neuropath Appl Neurobiol* 1997; 23:181 (Abstr).

8. Larsen JP, Dupont E, Tandberg E. Clinical diagnosis of Parkinson's disease. Proposal of diagnostic subgroups classified at different levels of confidence. *Acta Neurol Scand* 1984; 89:242–251.

9. Gibb DJ, Oliver E, Gilman S. Diagnostic criteria for Parkinson's disease. *Arch Neurol* 1999; 56:33–59.

10. Hoehn MM, Yahr MD. Parkinsonism, onset, progression and mortality. *Neurology* 1967, 17:427–442, 1436.

11. Brooks DJ, Playford ED, Ibanez V, et al. Isolated tremor and description of the nigrostriatal dopaminergic system. An F^{18}dopa PET study. *Neurology* 1992; 42:1554–1560.

12. Poewe WH, Wenning GK. The natural history of Parkinson's disease. *Ann Neurol* 1998; Sep 44(3 suppl.1):51–59.

13. Lees AJ, Hardie RJ, Stern GM. Kinesigenic foot dystonia as a presenting feature of Parkinson's disease. *J Neurol Neurosurg Psychiatry* 1984; 47:Vol 885.

14. Hughes AJ, Lees AJ, Stern GM. The apomorphine test to predict dopaminergic responsiveness in parkinsonian syndrome. *Lancet* 1990, 336:32–34.

15. Okazaki H, Lipkin LE, Aronson SM. Diffuse intracytoplasmic ganglionic inclusions (Lewy type) associated with progressive dementia and quadriparesis in flexion. *J Neuropath Exp Neurol* 1961; 20:237–244.

16. Byrne EJ, Lennox G, Lowe J, et al. Diffuse Lewy body disease: clinical features in 15 cases. *J Neurol Neurosurg Psychiatry* 1989; 52:709–717.

17. McKeith I, Galasko D, Kasaka K, et al. Consensus guidelines for the clinical and pathological diagnosis of dementia with Lewy bodies (SLB). Report of the consortium on DLB International Workshop. *Neurology* 1996; 47:1113–1124.

18. Brooks DJ. The early diangosis of Parkinson's disease. *Ann Neurol* 1998; 44(3 suppl.1): S10–S18.

19. Seibyl JP, Marek KL, Quinlan D, et al. Decreased single-photon emission computed tomographic [123I] beta-CIT striatal uptake correlates with symptom severity in Parkinson's disease. *Ann Neurol* 1995; 38:589–598.

19a. Factor SA, Seibyl J, Innis R, et al. Pshychoqeric parkinsonism: confirmation of diagnosis with β-CIT SPECT Scans. *Mov Disord* 1998; 13:860.

20. Kimber JR, Watson L, Mathias CJ. Distinction of idiopathic Parkinson's disease from multiple system atrophy by stimulation of growth hormone release with clonidine. *Lancet* 1997; 349:1877–1881.

21. Eardley I, Quinn NP, Fowler CJ, et al. The value of urethral sphincter electromyography in the differential diagnosis of Parkinsonism. *Brit J Urol* 1989; 64:360–362.

22. Mathias CJ. Autonomic disorders and their recognition. *New Eng J Med* 1997; 336:721–724.

23. Rascol O, Sabatini U, Simonetta-Morcau M, et al. Square wave jerks in Parkinsonian syndromes. *J Neurol Neurosurg Psychiatry* 1991; 54:599–602.

24. Pillon B, Dubois B, Agid Y. Testing cognition may contribute to the diagnosis of movement disorders. *Neurology* 1996; 46:329–334.

25. Vidailhet M, Rothwell JC, Thompson PD, et al. The auditory startle response in the Steele-Richardson-Olszewski syndrome and Parkinson's disease. *Brain* 1992; 115:1181–1192.

26. Markus HS, Lees AJ, Lennox G, et al. Patterns of regional cerebral blood flow in corticobasal degeneration studied using HMPAO SPECT comparison with Parkinson's disease and normal controls. *Mov Disord* 1995; 10:179–187.

27. Hawkes CH, Shephard BC, Daniel SE. Olfactory dysfunction in Parkinson's disease. *J Neurol Neurosurg Psychiatry* 1997; 62:435–446.

28. Caparros-Lefebvre D, Lees AJ, Tolosa E. Phenomenological study of Parkinsonism in the French West Indies. *Neurology* 1999; 52:A224.

29. Hu MTM, Richards M, Agapito C, et al. Parkinsonism in immigrant Afro-Caribbean and Indian subjects living in the United Kingdom. *J Neurol Neurosurg Psychiatry* 1999; 66:258–259.

30. Hughes AJ, Colosimo C, Kleedorfer B, et al. The dopaminergic response in mulple system atrophy. *J Neurol Neurosurg Psychiatry* 1992; 55:1009–1013.

25

Single Photon Emission Tomography and Dopamine Transporter Imaging

Kenneth Marek, M.D.

Institute for Neurodegenerative Disorders, New Haven, Connecticut

In his description of the "shaking palsy" in 1817, James Parkinson noted that understanding this newly described disorder was limited by a lack of objective pathologic data and specifically that "unaided by previous inquiries immediately directed to the disease, and not having the advantage in a single case of that light, which anatomical examination yields, opinion and not facts can only be offered (1)." He could not have predicted that now almost two hundred years later, the developing technology of in vivo imaging has opened an increasingly clear window on the neurochemical pathophysiology of Parkinson's disease (PD) and more specifically on the onset, progression, and physiology of the degenerative process. As we are poised on the brink of new protective and restorative therapies for PD, the potential of imaging to teach us about in vivo brain neurochemistry offers both promise and challenge.

In vivo functional imaging uses specific chemical ligands as tags or markers to neurochemically dissect the dopaminergic deficit in PD and related disorders. The strengths and limitations of in vivo functional imaging studies depend on the imaging technology used to measure brain neurochemistry and the ligand or biochemical marker used to tag a specific brain neurochemical system. Positron emission tomography (PET) and Single Photon Emission Computerized Tomography (SPECT) have been the primary techniques used to study the dopaminergic system in PD and related disorders (2,3). PET cameras usually have better resolution than SPECT cameras, but SPECT studies may be technologically and clinically more feasible. PET radionuclides have short half lives (e.g., ^{11}C, T1/2 20 min) and must be produced with an on-site cyclotron. In contrast, SPECT radionuclides have longer half lives (e.g., ^{123}I, T1/2 13 hr) and can be commercially supplied. The resolution of a state-of-the-art PET camera is 3–5 mm and that of a SPECT camera is 6–7 mm full width at half maximum (FWHM) in all three axes measured with a point source in air. Both PET and SPECT methods correct for tissue attenuation and for photon scatter. Recent use of three dimensional imaging coupled with statistical parametric mapping (SPM) analysis rather than a region of interest analysis has further enhanced PET resolution and promises to enhance SPECT technology as well. A major advantage of SPECT imaging over PET imaging in human studies is that SPECT cameras are much more widely available and studies are simpler and less expensive to accomplish. Both SPECT and PET are sensitive methods of measuring in vivo neurochemistry. The choice of imaging modality is ultimately determined by the specific study questions and study design.

Specific markers for the dopaminergic system have been widely used to evaluate patients with PD. Dopaminergic ligands may be divided into those that target the presynaptic dopaminergic neuron and those that bind to the postsynaptic dopamine receptor. [^{18}F]FDOPA imaged via PET was the first widely used presynaptic dopaminergic ligand. [^{18}F]FDOPA imaging is dependent on conversion of [^{18}F]FDOPA to [^{18}F]FDopamine and therefore is a measure of dopaminergic nerve function. Several studies have shown that [^{18}F]FDOPA activity is correlated with nigral dopaminergic neuron number and clinical severity of disease (4–7). More recently several ligands have been developed that bind to the dopamine transporter (8–12). The dopamine transporter is a protein that is located on the dopamine presynaptic nerve terminal. Therefore these SPECT and PET ligands directly measure dopamine terminal integrity and degeneration.

This chapter will focus on the recent studies using [^{123}I]ß-CIT (2ß-carboxymethoxy-3ß(4-iodophenyl) tropane), also known as DOPASCAN™, and SPECT to image the dopamine transporter. [^{123}I]ß-CIT has

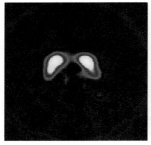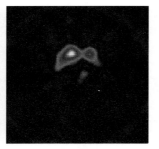

Healthy Subject   Parkinson's Disease

FIGURE 25-1. SPECT [^{123}I]ß-CIT images from a patient with mild PD and from an age-matched healthy subject. Note the asymmetric reduction in [^{123}I]ß-CIT uptake more marked in the putamen than caudate in the patient. Regions of interest were drawn based on coregistered MRI. Levels of SPECT activity are color-encoded from low (black) to high (yellow/white). Courtesy of J. Seibyl, Yale Neurospect Center.

been the most widely used and well-validated dopamine transporter marker (Figure 25-1) (13,14). Several other transporter ligands including FP-CIT, Altropane, and Trodat are in earlier stages of development (12, 15–17). The high specific striatal uptake and the unusual binding kinetics of [^{123}I]ß-CIT are unique and have enabled it to be used to quantify changes in dopamine transporter density. After a bolus injection of [^{123}I]ß-CIT, striatal activity reaches a plateau in about 18 hours, changing less than 1%/h thereafter through the thirtieth hour. Occipital and cerebellar activity peak at about 30–45 min, then is stabilized 100 to 200 minutes after injection. The midbrain activity reaches a plateau after four hours. The slow striatal uptake of [^{123}I]ß-CIT is caused, in part, by the exceptionally slow clearance of the tracer from the plasma. The terminal half-life of plasma clearance is greater than 48 h, which causes a state of near equilibrium binding conditions on the day after injection. Kinetic modeling of arterial input function and brain activity for the first eight hours after injection of [^{123}I]ß-CIT in eight healthy subjects demonstrated that equilibrium distribution volumes from these day one data closely matched the results obtained from day two imaging in these same individuals (18,19). These results provide strong support for the simple calculation of striatal uptake as the ratio of specific to nondisplaceable uptake (termed V3") and calculated as (striatal–occipital)/occipital activity. The value of V3" = (Bmax/KD)/V2; where Bmax is transporter density, I/KD is affinity, and V2 is the nonspecific volume of distribution (e.g., occipital) (18). Thus this relatively simple outcome measure is linearly related to the density of dopamine transporters and can be used

as the primary outcome measure for imaging studies using [^{123}I]ß-CIT. The reliable and easy quantitation of [^{123}I]ß-CIT uptake has been critical to its development as a quantitative biomarker for PD. These kinetics are unique among known dopamine transporters and make [^{123}I]ß-CIT the ligand of choice for quantitative studies of the dopamine transporter deficit in PD and related disorders.

DIAGNOSIS AND DISEASE SEVERITY

The first question regarding an imaging marker is whether it reliably distinguishes between subjects with and without known pathology. Studies with [^{123}I]ß-CIT discriminated between individuals with PD and healthy subjects with a sensitivity of >95% (13). These studies take advantage of the relatively greater dopaminergic loss in the putamen to enhance the discriminant function. Furthermore, the reduction in dopamine transporter density correlated with well-defined clinical rating scales of PD severity (Figure 25-2) (12,13,20). Interestingly, when specific PD symptoms are compared, the loss of dopaminergic activity measured by imaging correlated with bradykinesia, but not with tremor. Cross-sectional studies show that severity of bradykinesia measured by clinical rating scales reflects the severity of the nigrostriatal dopamine neuron loss. Therefore, in vivo dopaminergic imaging provides a biomarker, both for the presence of

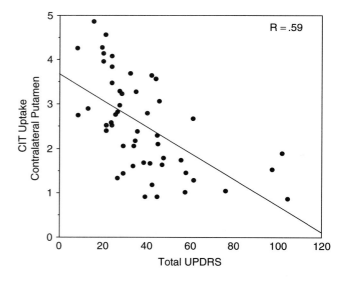

FIGURE 25-2. Correlation of [^{123}I]ß-CIT uptake in the putamen contralateral to initial symptoms with Total UPDRS measured after 12 hours off medicine in the defined off state. The reduction in [^{123}I]ß-CIT uptake correlates with the increasing severity of clinical scores in this cohort.

disease and for the severity of the pathologic process (12,13,20).

In clinical practice, diagnosis is most difficult at the onset of symptoms. In studies focussed on early PD, at the threshold of their illness, in vivo imaging demonstrated a 50% reduction in [^{123}I]ß-CIT uptake in the putamen contralateral to the symptomatic side (20,21). Similar data have been obtained using PET FDOPA or PET dopamine transporter ligands (22,23). Parkinson's disease generally presents as a unilateral motor disorder and progresses during a variable period of 3 to 6 years to effect both sides although frequently remaining asymmetric . The unilateral motor presentation reflects the asymmetric dopaminergic pathology which is, in turn, demonstrated (Figure 25-1) by in vivo dopaminergic imaging (21–23).

Another difficult diagnostic problem is the distinction between the more specific diagnosis of PD and other neurodegenerative disorders categorized as Parkinsonism or Parkinson's syndrome. While PD is the most common cause of Parkinsonism, other neurodegenerative disorders including progressive supranuclear palsy, multisystem atrophy, corticobasal ganglionic degeneration, and diffuse Lewy body disease may account for about 15 to 20% of patients with Parkinson's syndrome. Parkinsonism is characterized by significant nigrostriatal neuronal loss, which is demonstrated by reduction in in vivo presynaptic dopaminergic imaging. While the severity of the reduction in [^{123}I]ß-CIT uptake does not discriminate between PD and other causes of Parkinson's syndrome, the pattern of loss in Parkinson's syndrome is less region-specific (putamen and caudate equally effected) and more symmetric than PD. This strategy discriminates between PD and other causes of Parkinson's syndrome with a sensitivity of about 75 to 80% (24). In addition, the more widespread pathology associated with Parkinson's syndrome may be reflected in abnormalities of postsynaptic dopamine receptor imaging and metabolic imaging, which are not seen in PD (8,24–26). Therefore the pattern of dopamine transporter loss may be coupled with postsynaptic dopamine receptor imaging or metabolic imaging to distinguish PD from other Parkinsonian syndromes.

PARKINSON'S DISEASE PROGRESSION

The rate of clinical progression of PD is highly variable and unpredictable (27). Several clinical studies have followed large cohorts for several years, but these studies lack an objective measure of disease progression. Clinical rating scales are extremely useful, but ratings may be investigator-dependent and are frequently confounded by changes in treatment. Pathologic studies investigating rate of progression have been limited and rely entirely on cross-sectional data (28,29). These studies have in general mainly considered patients with severe illness of long duration. In vivo imaging studies provide the opportunity to evaluate patients longitudinally from early to late disease using an objective biomarker for dopaminergic degeneration.

Before using imaging to assess disease progression the outcome measure must be thoroughly validated in sequential studies. The reliability of [^{123}I]ß-CIT uptake was examined in a test/retest study in seven healthy human subjects (age range 19–74 years) and five PD patients (30). SPECT images were obtained at 18, 21, and 24 h after the bolus injection of [^{123}I]ß-CIT. Repeat [^{123}I]ß-CIT SPECT scans were performed 7–10 days after the initial study. Specific:nondisplaceable uptake ratios were compared within subjects across the two test sessions using the average difference calculation; (abs[test-retest])/[test+retest]/2) expressed as a percent. All healthy controls and PD subjects demonstrated unchanging striatal activity over the six h imaging interval with a mean change in striatal activity of 0.4% /h ± 0.05%). All healthy subjects showed excellent test-retest reproducibility for specific:nondisplaceable uptake (mean = 6.8%). Similarly, PD patients demonstrated low-difference scores between test and retest scans on both outcome measures (mean reproducibility specific:nondisplaceable uptake = 12.3%) (30). These data establish the high degree of reproducibility of the outcome measure obtained at 18–24 hours post [^{123}I]ß-CIT injection and support the feasibility of performing serial SPECT measurements in humans for detecting alterations in [^{123}I]ß-CIT binding in striatum.

A second issue that must be addressed before studying PD progression is the age-related degeneration of the dopamine system in healthy subjects. In vitro studies of human tissue demonstrate a decline in dopamine transporters with age of approximately 6 to 8% per decade (31,32). In a study of 28 healthy subjects (14 males, 14 females, age range 19–75 years) [^{123}I]ß-CIT imaging demonstrated similar reductions of 8% per decade in striatal CIT uptake (33). This study has been extended to a total of approximately 100 healthy subjects showing a comparable decline of about 8% per decade. These data must be considered in assessing the change in dopamine transporter density in PD patients in long-term studies.

Finally, a third practical issue that must be resolved before monitoring PD progression is the effect of PD medication on the imaging outcome measure used to assess neuronal degeneration. Even if patients with PD are initially evaluated on no medications, as their disease progresses, medication will be required to treat their progressive disability. In several studies the effect of levodopa, selegiline, and pergolide on [^{123}I]ß-CIT has been examined. Six patients were evaluated with [^{123}I]ß-CIT at baseline, after treatment with levodopa for six weeks up to a dose of 750 mg, and again off levodopa for 48 hours. There was no change in [^{123}I]ß-CIT uptake in these patients. All patients responded clinically to levodopa therapy (34). In a similar study design, eight patients were evaluated before, while on, and after discontinuing selegiline 10 mg, again without any effect on [^{123}I]ß-CIT striatal uptake (34). A study of 12 patients treated with pergolide and imaged before, on treatment, and subsequent to discontinuation of treatment also showed no significant change in [^{123}I]ß-CIT striatal uptake (35).

With these important validation studies completed, [^{123}I]ß-CIT uptake has been evaluated as a biomarker for dopamine neuron degeneration in studies of PD progression. Sequential dopamine transporter imaging in 32 PD patients and 21 healthy subjects imaged with a mean interval of 24.5 months and 19.9 months, respectively demonstrated a mean annual reduction in [^{123}I]ß-CIT striatal uptake of $11.09 \pm 8.6\%$ in the PD patients and $0.8 + 7.8\%$ in the healthy subjects (36) (Figure 25-3). These data are very similar to data obtained in sequential [^{18}F]FDOPA/PET studies (37). Evidence from studies of hemi-PD subjects provide further insight into the rate of progression of disease. In early hemi-PD There is a reduction in [^{123}I]ß-CIT uptake of about 50% in the effected putamen and of 25 to 30% in the unaffected putamen. As most patients will progress clinically from unilateral to bilateral in 3 to 6 years, it is therefore likely that the loss of these in vivo imaging markers of dopaminergic degeneration

in the previously unaffected putamen will progress at about 5 to 10% per annum (21,23).

Progression studies have begun to provide important new insights into the onset and natural history of PD. For example, given the assumption that progression is linear, it is possible to back extrapolate from sequential imaging data and reported symptom duration to estimate the level of reduction in dopaminergic activity at symptom onset and the duration of the preclinical phase of PD (Figure 25-4). Data from longitudinal imaging studies using both [^{18}F]FDOPA and dopamine transporter imaging have been remarkably consistent with estimated disease onset at 70 to 75% of normal dopaminergic activity and a preclinical phase of 3 to 10 years (36,38). These data are consistent with estimates of duration of the preclinical phase from pathology studies of 4.7 years derived from cross-sectional data (29). While the data available to calculate estimates of preclinical phase must be viewed as preliminary, data acquired using two different imaging methods measuring different components of the dopaminergic system and data from a pathology study suggest a relatively brief preclinical phase of less than a decade for PD. If correct, this has tremendous implications for understanding disease etiology and for developing strategies for disease screening and treatment. For example, if preclinical disease is relatively short, repetitive screening might be required to identify effected individuals in an at risk

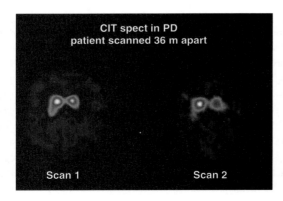

FIGURE 25-3. Sequential SPECT [^{123}I]ß-CIT images in PD subjects demonstrating the progression of dopaminergic degeneration during the scanning interval. Levels of SPECT activity are color-encoded from low (black) to high (yellow/white). Courtesy of J. Seibyl, Yale Neurospect Center.

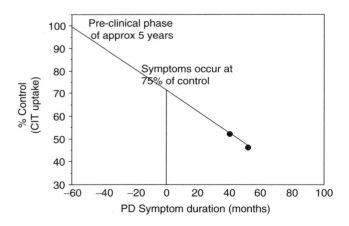

FIGURE 25-4. Estimate of preclinical phase of Parkinson's disease. Schematic representation based on data from two separate cohorts demonstrating relative loss of ß-CIT uptake in sequential SPECT scans. The data points (●) indicated are the means of the relative reduction from controls of ß-CIT uptake with mean scan interval of approximately 24 months. If linear progression of disease is assumed, the progression of disease based on extrapolation of these data suggest that the percent loss of ß-CIT uptake at the start of symptoms is approximately 25% and the estimated duration of the preclinical phase approximately five years.

population. Furthermore, as potential preventive or restorative therapies are developed, these treatments might be directed to the time period from onset of degeneration to onset of symptoms.

Longitudinal imaging studies provide a tool to objectively assess potential neuroprotective and restorative therapies for PD. Prior studies examining putative neuroprotective agents have been flawed because of lack of a biomarker of progression and reliance solely on clinical measures of disease (38a,38b). Future studies of possible neuroprotective agents will require the addition of an objective biomarker to establish disease protection especially in the context of possible symptomatic benefit of the study medication. Estimates from completed imaging progression studies suggest that sample sizes required for appropriately powered studies evaluating a neuroprotective agent are feasible, but depend on the effect size of the intervention (Table 25-1) (36,37). At present $[^{123}I]\beta$-CIT SPECT imaging is being used to assess the rate of progression of PD in two large multicenter studies coordinated by the Parkinson Study Group, the CALM-PD study (comparing pramipexole to levodopa in early patients) and the ELLDOPA study (comparing various doses of levodopa to placebo) (39,40). Similarly, therapeutic interventions such as cell-replacement therapies, growth factor treatments, or gene therapy will require an objective biomarker to assess efficacy.

Although progression studies are provocative and exciting, a number of questions regarding the data are unresolved. For example, some dopaminergic imaging studies suggest that the rate of progression in PD may be greater in the early as compared to late stages, consistent with a nonlinear rate of dopaminergic degeneration . The effect of aging on the dopaminergic nigrostriatal system is also an important component to understanding PD progression. Pathologic studies have demonstrated that neuron number and dopamine transporter density decrease with aging by about

1%/year. Dopamine transporter imaging and SPECT demonstrate a similar reduction of 6–8%/ decade (33). Furthermore, data also indicates that younger patients may develop symptoms of PD at dopamine transporter densities that may be normal for older subjects (13). These data suggest that Parkinsonian symptoms do not arise out of a threshold loss of dopaminergic neurons but that a variety of as yet poorly-understood compensatory mechanisms may exist, which influence the onset and progression of disease. Understanding these compensatory mechanisms will provide additional insight to the factors that determine the rate of progression of disease, an essential issue for patients with PD.

PRECLINICAL PARKINSON'S DISEASE

One goal that must be realized for every neurodegenerative disorder is the development of biomarkers to identify individuals at risk for disease prior to onset of symptoms. Preclinical identification of at risk subjects is particularly important if intervention exists, which may delay or prevent progression of disease. Although clearly effective treatment to prevent PD currently exists, many putative neuroprotective therapies are under investigation and are likely to be tested in clinical trials in the next three to five years. Both clinical and imaging data from longitudinal studies of PD patients suggests that a preclinical phase of several years duration exists, when neurodegeneration is occurring but symptoms have not developed. It is during this time when a neuroprotective agent might be effective.

Several lines of evidence demonstrate that in vivo dopaminergic imaging provides a possible method to identify subjects during that preclinical phase of their disease. The most extensive preclinical data is from studies imaging patients with hemi-PD. In several imaging studies there is a significant reduction in putamen dopamine transporter uptake of about 25–30% in the "presymptomatic" striatum. These patients are known to progress to bilateral disease (21–23). Other attempts at identifying preclinical disease using imaging methods have focused at risk populations such as family members or unaffected twins of PD patients. Studies in these groups using FDOPA have demonstrated that, in several well-characterized kindreds, 11 of 32 asymptomatic relatives had reduced FDOPA uptake and three of these subjects subsequently developed symptomatic PD (41). Several asymptomatic cotwins who also showed a reduction in FDOPA activity later developed Parkinsonian symptoms, although the concordance

Table 25-1 *Sample Size to Assess Neuroprotection.* Estimates of total sample size required to show neuroprotection using sequential neuroimaging with ß-CIT SPECT with 80% power and *p* < .05 (36).

	Scan Interval		
	1 year	2 years	5 years
Protection (Effect size)			
100%	56–68	16–20	6–10
50%	208–260	57–68	14–22
25%	798–1034	208–260	44–48

rate for monozygotic and dyzygotic twins remains uncertain. Similar studies are underway with [^{123}I]ß-CIT SPECT imaging. As we face the millennium the identification of new genes associated with PD will provide additional opportunity to evaluate the progression of preclinical nigrostriatal loss.

FUTURE DIRECTIONS

In vivo dopaminergic imaging of the nigrostriatal system with [^{123}I]ß-CIT/SPECT has provided unique and useful data as a biomarker for PD diagnosis, disease severity, and disease progression. Future studies using these techniques will have practical clinical applications such as assessing drugs that may be neuroprotective, and theoretical neuroscientific implications such as assessing when neuronal degeneration occurs in a genetically at risk cohort. As new ligands develop, future studies will also explore nondopaminergic, extrastriatal abnormalities in PD including, freezing gait, depression, and psychosis. As the underlying molecular neurobiology of this disease is elucidated, in vivo imaging will continue to expand its role as a window to the neurochemical pathophysiology of PD and related disorders.

REFERENCES

1. Parkinson J. *An Essay on the Shaking Palsy*. London: Sherwood, Neely, and Jones, 1817.
2. Phelps M. Positron emission tomography (PET). In: Mazziota J, Gilman S, (eds.). *Clinical brain imaging: Principles and Applications*. Philadelphia: F.A. Davis, 1992: 71–107.
3. Lassen N, Holm S. Single photon emission computerized tomography (SPECT). In: Mazziota J, Gilman S, (eds.). Clinical brain imaging: Principles and Applications. Philadelphia: F.A. Davis, 1992: 108–134.
4. Brooks DJ. Functional imaging in relation to parkinsonian syndromes. *J Neurol Sci* 1993; 115:1–17.
5. Calne DB, Langston JW, Martin WRW, et al. Positron emission tomography after MPTP: Observations relating to the cause of Parkinson's disease. *Nature* 1985; 317:246–248.
6. Leenders K, Salmon EP, Tyrrell P, et al. The nigrostriatal dopaminergic system assessed in vivo by positron emission tomography in healthy volunteer subjects and patients with Parkinson's disease. *Arch Neurol* 1990; 47:1290–1298.
7. Nahmias C, Garnett ES, Firnau G, et al. Striatal dopamine distribution in parkinsonian patients during life. *J Neurol Sci* 1985; 69:223–230.
8. Tatsch K, Schwarz J, Mosley P, et al. Relationship between clinical features of Parkinson's disease and presynaptic dopamine transporter binding assessed with [^{123}I]IPT and single-photon emission tomography. *Eur J Nucl Med* 1997; 24:415–421.
9. Innis RB, Seibyl JP, Scanley BE, et al. Single photon emission computed tomographic imaging demonstrates loss of striatal dopamine transporters in Parkinson disease. *Proc Natl Acad Sci USA* 1993; 90:11965–11969.
10. Fischman A, Bonab A, Babich J, et al. Rapid detection of Parkinson's disease by SPECT with altropane: a selective ligand for dopamine transporters. *Synapse* 1998; 29:128–141.
11. Frost JJ, Rosier AJ, Reich SG, et al. Positron emission tomography imaging of the dopamine transporter with ^{11}C-WIN 35,428 reveals marked decline in mild Parkinson's disease. *Ann Neurol* 1993; 34:423–431.
12. Booij T, Tissingh G, Boer G. [^{123}I]FP-SPECT shows a pronounced decline of striatal dopamine transporter labelling in early and advanced Parkinson's disease. *J Neurol Neurosurg Psychiatry* 1997; 62:133–140.
13. Seibyl J, Marek K, Quinlan D, et al. Decreased SPECT [^{123}I]ß-CIT striatal uptake correlates with symptom severity in idiopathic Parkinson's disease. *Ann Neurol* 1995; 38:589–598.
14. Brücke T, Asenbaum S, Pirker W, et al. Measurement of the dopaminergic degeneration in Parkinson's disease with [^{123}I]ß-CIT and SPECT. *J Neural Trans* 1997; Suppl 50:9–24.
15. Seibyl J, Marek K, Sheff K, et al. Within-subject comparison of [^{123}IFP-CIT and [^{123}I]B-CIT for SPECT imaging of dopamine transporters in Parkinson's disease. *Neurology* 1996; 46:A456.
16. Kushner S, McElgin W, Kung M, et al. Kinetic modeling of [99mTc]TRODAT-1: a dopamine transporter imaging agent. *J Nucl Med* 1999; 40:150–158.
17. Fischman A, Bonab A, Babich J, et al. Rapid detection of Parkinson's disease by SPECT with altropane: A selective ligand for dopamine transporters. *Synapse* 1998; 29:128–141.
18. Laruelle M, Wallace E, Seibyl JP, et al. Graphical, kinetic, and equilibrium analyses of in vivo [^{123}I]ß-CIT binding to dopamine transporters in healthy human subjects. *J Cereb Blood Flow Metab* 1994; 14:982–994.
19. Laruelle M, Giddings S, Zea-Ponce Y, et al. Methyl 3ß-(4-[125+I]Iodophenyl)Tropane-2ß-Carboxylate In Vitro Binding to Dopamine and Serotonin Transporters Under "Physiological" Conditions. *J Neurochem* 1994; 62:978–986.
20. Asenbaum S, Brucke T, Pirker W, et al. Imaging of dopamine transporters with iodine-123-B-CIT and SPECT in Parkinoson's disease. *J Nucl Med* 1997; 38:1–6.
21. Marek K, Seibyl J, Scanley B, et al. [I-123]CIT Spect Imaging demonstrates bilateral loss of dopamine transporters in hemi-Parkinson's disease. *Neurology* 1996; 46:231–237.

22. Morrish P, Sawlw G, Brooks D. Clinincal and [18F]dopa PET findings in early Parkinson's disease. *J Neurol Neurosurg Psychiatry* 1995; 59:597–600.

23. Guttman M, Burkholder J, Kish S, et al. [11C]RTI-32 PET studies of the dopamine transporter in early dopa-naive Parkinson's disease. *Neurology* 1997; 48:1578–1583.

24. Ichise M, Kim Y, Ballinger J, et al. SPECT imaging of the pre and postsynaptic alterations in L-dopa-untreated PD. *Neurology* 1999; 52:

25. Brooks D, Ibanez V, Sawle G, et al. Differing patterns of striatal 18F-DOPA uptake in Parkinson's disease, multiple system atrophy and progressive supranuclear palsy. *Ann Neurol* 1990; 28:547–555.

26. Pirker W, Asenbaum S, Wenger S, et al. Iodine-123-epidepride-SPECT: studies in Parkinson's disease, multiple system atrophy and Huntington's disease. *J Nucl Med* 1997; 38:1711–1717.

27. Hoehn MM, Yahr MD. Parkinsonism: Onset, progression and mortality. *Neurology* 1967; 17:427–442.

28. McGeer PL, Itagaki S, Akiyama S, et al. Rate of cell death in Parkinsonism is an active neuropathological process. *Ann Neurol* 1988; 24:574.

29. Fearnley J, Lees A. Ageing and Parkinson's disease: substantia nigra regional selectivity. *Brain* 1991; 114:2283–2301.

30. Seibyl J, Marek K, Sheff K, et al. Test/retest reproducibility of [123I]B-CIT SPECT brain measurement of dopamine transporters in Parkinson's disease patients. *J Nucl Med* 1997; 38:1453–1461.

31. Zelnik N, Angel I, Paul SM, et al. Decreased density of human striatal dopamine uptake sites with age. *Eur J Pharmacol* 1986; 126:175–176.

32. De Keyser JD, Ebinger G, Vauquelin G. Age-related changes in the human nigrostriatal dopaminergic system. *Ann Neurol* 1990; 27:157–161.

33. van Dyck C, Seibyl J, Malison R, et al. Age-related Decline in Dopamine Transporter Binding in Human Striatum with [123I]ß-CIT SPECT. *J Nucl Med* 1995; 36:1175–1181.

34. Innis R, Marek K, Sheff K, et al. Treatment with carbidopa/levodopa and selegiline on striatal transporter imaging with [123I]B-CIT. *Mov Disord* 1999; 14:436–443.

35. Ahlskog J, Ryan J, O'Connor M, et al. The effect of dopmine agonist therapy on dopamine transporter imaging in Parkinson's disease. *Mov Disord* 1999; 14:940–950.

36. Marek K, Seibyl J, Innis R. [123I] ß-CIT/SPECT: Assessment of determinants of variability in progression of Parkinson's disease. *Neurology* 1999; 52:A91–A92.

37. Morrish P, Sawle G, Brooks D. An [18F]dopa-PET and clinical study of the rate of progression in Parkinson's disease. *Brain* 1996; 119:585–591.

38. Morrish P. Parkinson's disease is not a long-latency illness. *Mov Disord* 1997; 849–854.

38a. Parkinson Study Group. Effect of deprenyl on the progression of disability in early Parkinson's disease. *N Engl J Med* 1989; 321: 1364–1371.

38b. Parkinson Study Group. Effects of tocopherol and deprenyl on the progression of disability in early Parkinson's disease. *N Engl J Med* 1993; 328: 176–183.

39. Parkinson Study Group. Design of a clinical trial comparing pramipexole to levodopa in early PD (CALM-PD). *Clin Neuropharmacol* in press;

40. Fahn S. Parkinson Disease, the effect of levodopa, and the ELLDOPA trial. *Arch Neurol* 1999; 56:529–535.

41. Piccini P, Morrish P, Turjanski N, et al. Dopaminergic function in familial Parkinson's disease: A clinical and 18F-Dopa positron emission tomography study. *Ann Neurol* 1997; 41:222–229.

26

Positron Emission Tomography

Mark Guttman, M.D., F.R.C.P.C.

Department of Medicine (Division of Neurology) and
Department of Psychiatry, University of Toronto, Ontario, Canada

INTRODUCTION

A number of new imaging technologies are being developed to assess patients with Parkinson's disease (PD) and related disorders. Positron emission tomography (PET) is one of the emerging techniques that shows promise as a tool that can confirm the diagnosis of parkinsonism. As a research tool, PET has provided useful insights into the pathophysiology of PD over the last decade or more. In the future, will the role of PET change and will it be used to confirm the diagnosis of PD? Will the previous high standards of a neurologist's bedside clinical acumen for an accurate diagnosis of PD be displaced by PET studies ordered by a primary care physician? This chapter reviews this rapidly changing field and offers a view to the future as to how PET may affect the neurologist's role once the technology becomes widely available.

Neuroscience research has identified important biochemical alterations that are responsible for the signs and symptoms of PD. Most of this work has been performed on postmortem samples from patients with PD. These patients are typically are in the end stages of the condition. These postmortem biochemical observations are not relevant to the earlier stages of PD. There are many problems in correlating postmortem observations and clinical findings. Investigators are unable to perform studies that prospectively evaluate the biochemical changes related to the different stages of the disease, the response to medication, and alterations due to medication side effects. Now, with PET, there is the potential to evaluate these biochemical changes during life.

PET METHODOLOGY

The aim of PET scanning is to provide a quantitative in vivo analysis of regional brain chemistry, blood flow, and metabolism. A number of steps are required to perform and interpret these studies. They include production of unstable positron-containing atoms, on-site radiochemistry to synthesize ligands that will label specific neurochemical systems, intravenous injection of the ligand to the subject, sophisticated cameras to detect the radioactivity, and complex data analysis to provide the quantitative measurement.

A positron is part of the atom's nucleus that usually couples with an electron to form a neutron. When an uncoupled positron is part of the nucleus, the atom becomes unstable. The positron leaves the nucleus and collides with an electron in orbit of other atoms in the surrounding area. The collision of the positron and electron results in two coincident photons of energy that originate from the place of collision. These photons emerge at 180 degrees in opposite directions and have specific energy characteristics.

PET cameras have been developed to detect the coincident photons and create a tomographic image that identifies where in space they emerged. PET cameras have crystal detectors arranged in rings and connected to computer systems to analyze the radioactive events. The cameras have become more sophisticated over time, evolving from a single ring of detectors that could create a single tomographic image to detectors that acquire three-dimensional data that can create more than 30 slices of data simultaneously. PET cameras have specific characteristics that influence their performance. The resolution of the latest generation cameras is now close to 3 mm. The images must be filtered, and different corrections are made that usually reduce the final image resolution. Ultimately, the resolution is less than that of magnetic resonance imaging (MRI) or CT but much better than SPECT images. PET images show the chemistry of the brain but not the anatomy. It therefore is necessary to have a method of referencing the regions of interest in the PET studies with anatomic images. There is no standard way of dealing with this. Many PET groups will attempt to coregister PET images with resliced MRI images lined up with the PET scans to choose regions of interest.

A number of positron-emitting isotopes are being used in PET studies for PD. The most common isotopes are ^{18}F, which has a half-life of 110 minutes; ^{11}C with a 20 minute half-life; and ^{15}O, which has only a two-minute half-life. These isotopes are made in medical cyclotrons, which must be located either on site or in close proximity to the camera. This is an important difference compared with SPECT, which uses radioisotopes with much longer half-lives. The cyclotron operation is labor-intensive and requires expert operators who work closely with the radiochemistry staff. Different targets are used in the cyclotron for different isotopes, and for practical reasons it may be difficult to make multiple ligands on a single day.

After radiosynthesis of the desired ligand for a PET study, the compound is intravenously injected, as either a bolus or infusion, into the patient. There are many ways of performing a PET study, but the most common is to have the patient placed in the camera at the time of the injection and to take sequential scans of increasing time lengths. A typical example at our PET Centre is a [11C]RTI-32 scan to assess dopamine-transporter concentration in the brain. The patient has a bolus injection of ligand with a series of 39 emission scans over a 90-minute period. For image reconstruction, an attenuation correction scan is performed before the ligand administration to correct for skull thickness. To reduce head movement the patient's head is held in place by various methods including thermoplastic masks or stereotactic head-holding devices.

After the scan is performed, regions of interest are placed on the images and time activity curves are generated. These decay-corrected plots show the amount of radioactivity in the area over the time course of the study. The final step is to perform data analysis, which may involve compartmental modeling with plasma-input function and estimates of rate constants to obtain biologically meaningful data.

The steps necessary for a successful PET study are therefore complex and varied. It is very time consuming, and in busy centres it may be possible to study two or three subjects a day. The actual cost of a scan depends on a number of issues but can be as high as $4,000 if one takes into consideration equipment costs, personnel, and expendables. This is one of the reasons PET has not become as popular as predicted years ago.

PET LIGANDS TO STUDY PARKINSON'S DISEASE

There are an infinite number of possible compounds that can be used in the study of PD with PET. Ligand development is an enormous undertaking, which involves preclinical testing of compounds to assess their pharmacology, as well as potential toxicity in patients. All compounds require pyrogenicity and toxicity studies, as well as radiation dosimetry testing before human PET studies are possible. Many groups perform preliminary studies on primates before embarking on these costly studies, which are required by research and ethics committees.

Ligands may be divided into compounds that assess cerebral blood flow and metabolism, presynaptic dopaminergic function, postsynaptic dopaminergic function, and other striatal neurochemical systems (see Table 26-1, p. 264).

Oxygen Studies

Oxygen studies with $[^{15}O_2]$ have been performed both with steady-state inhalation and water bolus techniques. Hemiparkinsonian patients have increased cerebral blood flow and oxygen utilization in the contralateral basal ganglia (1). Some investigators found increased blood flow to the globus pallidus in these patients. L-dopa administered to parkinsonian patients has produced a reversal of the pallidal changes (2). Bilateral parkinsonian patients have reduced global blood flow but no changes in oxygen metabolism (1).

Cerebral Glucose Metabolism

Cerebral metabolic changes may be assessed with FDG and PET. Glucose metabolism is increased in the contralateral basal ganglia in hemiparkinsonian patients (3). Other investigators found increased glucose utilization in the basal ganglia and normal cortical metabolism in bilaterally affected individuals (4). PD patients with dementia in addition to their parkinsonian features have reduced cortical metabolism in a similar pattern to Alzheimer patients (5). This suggested that the dementia seen in PD may be due to concomitant Alzheimer's disease rather than a feature of the primary disorder.

Presynaptic Dopaminergic Studies in PD

6-FD is an analogue of L-dopa. The cerebral radioactivity measured after the administration of 6-FD is a function of uptake of the isotope into the brain and its subsequent decarboxylation to dopamine and storage in vesicles (6). Patients with hemiparkinsonism have reduced accumulation of radioactivity in the contralateral striatum (7). The putamen is more severely affected compared to the caudate, in agreement with postmortem biochemical observations in PD (8). Similar findings have been observed in bilaterally affected individuals. The reduced 6-FD influx correlates with the severity of disease. A number of analysis procedures have been applied to this technique. One involves a graphical analysis of striatal 6-FD uptake called Ki.

Other tracers have been synthesized to study the presynaptic nigrostriatal system. Cocaine-like agents have been used to label the dopamine transporter. These include WIN, CIT, FPCIT, and RTI-32. We have used [^{11}C]RTI-32 to assess early PD patients. In these drug-naive, unilaterally affected subjects, the posterior putamen had a 50 percent reduction compared with controls. This suggests that individuals must exceed a threshold of 50 percent depletion in nigrostriatal presynaptic terminals before symptoms result (9). These subjects are clearly separated from age-matched controls.

The Ann Arbor, Michigan, group has employed the vesicular monoamine transporter agent [^{11}C]dihydrotetrabenazine to study patients with PD (10). They found reduced striatal binding in PD patients. This ligand does not appear to be regulated by drugs used to treat PD and may be useful in the longitudinal assessment of PD as a marker of disease progression.

It is possible to study individuals who have preclinical nigrostriatal dopamine dysfunction with PET. In Vancouver, British Columbia, asymptomatic subjects who self-administered MPTP were shown to have a reduced striatal 6-FD uptake (11). Studies of identical twins in which one had parkinsonism and the other was asymptomatic have shown that many preclinical subjects have a progressive reduction in 6-FD Ki over time (12). In asymptomatic subjects with pallido-ponto-nigral degeneration there is reduced 6-FD striatal uptake, thus providing another example of presymptomatic detection of nigrostriatal damage (13). The use of PET in screening individuals to detect preclinical dopamine depletion may become more important after neuroprotective drugs become available.

POSTSYNAPTIC DOPAMINERGIC STUDIES IN PARKINSON'S DISEASE

Dopamine D2 PET Studies

[^{11}C]raclopride is a substituted benzamide that is very selective and specific for D2 sites. The Finnish group found the striatum: cerebellum ratio is increased in the contralateral hemisphere in nontreated patients with early hemiparkinsonism (14). Antonini and colleagues followed patients longitudinally with [^{11}C]raclopride binding. They observed the initial increase in binding but found that the raclopride binding reduced over time (15). Results of PET studies of D2 receptors have confirmed that untreated patients have increased D2 binding, which is similar to that seen in postmortem studies (16). The increased binding seems to be reversed over the course of the disease.

Dopamine D1 PET Studies

A PET study of five untreated patients with early PD with [^{11}C]SCH23390 did not show changes in mean striatum/cerebellum ratio compared with controls (17). The same patients underwent [^{11}C]raclopride studies. There was a significant increase in striatum: cerebellum ratio in the hemisphere contralateral to the symptoms for this D2 ligand.

The Vancouver, British Columbia, group assessed individuals with either a stable response to levodopa, a fluctuating response, or dyskinesias. There was no systematic change in the D1 or D2 PET binding (Stoessl, personal communication).

DIFFERENTIAL DIAGNOSIS OF PD WITH PET

Patients with other forms of parkinsonism have been studied with FDG and PET. Studies in patients with progressive supranuclear palsy (PSP) have shown reduced striatal metabolism (18). Subjects with multiple system atrophy (MSA) with the striatal nigral degeneration (SND) variant have frontal lobe reduction and reduced striatal metabolism. Patients with the Olivopontocerebellar atrophy (OPCA) variant have reduced glucose utilization in the brain stem and cerebellum. Corticobasal ganglionic degeneration (CBGD) has a pattern of cortical reduction in glucose utilization in the parietal lobes that is usually asymmetric. This combined with reduced 6-FD uptake in the striatum is thought to be specific to CBGD.

6-FD PET studies have been employed to assess patients with other types of parkinsonism (19). These patients were shown to have a more diffuse reduction in 6-FD uptake compared with patients with PD. The caudate was equally as affected as the putamen in patients with the amyotrophic lateral sclerosis–parkinsonism dementia complex of Guam, PSP, MSA, symptomatic MPTP subjects, SND, and CBGD. Brooks and colleagues reported that in patients with MSA the striatal D2 binding with [^{11}C]raclopride is also reduced (20).

Shinotoh and colleagues employed a novel cholinergic marker that labels acetylcholinesterase activity (21). They found that there was a significant reduction in cortical uptake in PD subjects. In PSP there was a significant reduction in thalamic k3. The authors suggest that this pattern may be useful in differentiating the two conditions by PET. Frost and coworkers also studied PSP patients with PET but used WIN to assess dopamine-transporter binding (22). They found PD subjects had an uneven distribution of transporter reduction with the maximal loss in the posterior putamen. In PSP, however, the reduction was similar in all striatal areas. It is, however, not feasible to confirm the diagnosis of typical or atypical parkinsonism based solely on the PET pattern since it has not been subject to a proper prospective clinicopathologic evaluation.

PET MEASUREMENTS TO ASSESS THERAPEUTICS IN PARKINSON'S DISEASE

Eidelberg and colleagues recently reported pre- and postsurgical FDG PET studies in subjects undergoing stereotactic pallidotomies. They found significant increases in frontal metabolism and reduction in the ipsilateral lentiform nucleus metabolism after the surgery. They suggest that FDG PET studies are useful in identifying the metabolic correlates of the surgical outcome after the stereotactic procedures (23).

6-FD PET studies were performed in parkinsonian subjects who have undergone various transplantation procedures to control their symptoms. Patients treated with autologous adrenal implants did not have clinical and PET indices of improvement (24). Human fetal tissue graft recipients were studied at a number of centres. The clinical improvement in some patients is associated with an increase in the 6-FD uptake in the striatum. This has provided an objective measure to assess the viability of fetal tissue transplants (25).

6-FD studies have also been employed to examine the effectiveness of new PD drugs. Entacapone is a catechol-O-methyltransferase inhibitor, which reduces the peripheral metabolism of levodopa (26) (see Chapter 36). A number of studies showed that the coadministration of this drug with 6-FD increases the delivery of 6-FD to the brain and its bioavailability.

Tedroff and colleagues reported an interesting finding with [^{11}C]dopa that may help clarify some of the questions about the mechanisms of late complications of PD (27). They studied early and

late PD subjects before and after the infusion of levodopa. They found early subjects had reduced decarboxylation of [^{11}C]dopa after levodopa, which suggests that the enzyme is downregulated with increased synaptic dopamine. In more advanced subjects, there was an increase in decarboxylation of [^{11}C]dopa after levodopa. A later study confirmed the reduced decarboxylation of [^{11}C]dopa after apomorphine injection in early PD but lack of change in advanced PD (28). These findings suggest a change in autoreceptor function in advancing PD, which may be important in the pathogenesis of motor fluctuations.

Many investigators are very interested in using PET to investigate the progression of PD. Eidelberg and Feigin cover this in Chapter 13. PET might be used as a surrogate marker to assess neuroprotective strategies. Many trials are being designed to examine this possibility.

CONCLUSIONS

At present, physicians treating PD have the challenge of appropriately using both new and longstanding therapies to improve the quality of life of their patients. Exciting new research is being developed that hopefully will lead to further advances in treatment that may slow the progression of PD or reverse nigrostriatal dopaminergic dysfunction. Where does PET fit into this rapidly evolving field?

Despite earlier predictions, I do not think PET will play a meaningful role in the routine diagnosis of PD in the near future. I believe a detailed neurologic examination, the response to treatment, and the evolution of the clinical features over time will still be the enabling factors for a clinician to determine the correct diagnosis. It will be possible to use PET as a supplemental examination to add information for the diagnosis of patients with other Parkinsonian syndromes. The pattern of PET abnormalities in these conditions is certainly not specific. Furthermore, there is no evidence that PET scans with various ligands are a sensitive tool in determining the differential diagnosis. Until the positive predictive value of these tests is well documented, the potential advantages of using sophisticated imaging tests for the initial diagnosis of PD and other Parkinsonian syndromes is rather low relative to their cost.

The future of PET lies clearly in research applications. With the potential to use different drugs as neuroprotective agents, we will need an objective marker of the progression of PD. PET certainly has the potential to do this. Many pharmaceutical companies are planning to perform clinical trials with PET as an outcome measure. Important questions relating to the choice of the optimal ligand, scanning protocol and study designs are being formulated. It is hoped that there will be consensus in the near future that will permit easy comparisons of future studies. New pharmaceutical products can also be evaluated with PET to identify details of their mechanism of action, occupancy at receptor sites, and distribution in the brain. In my view, PET will continue to be an important research tool for the study of PD and hopefully will play a major role in the search for a cause and cure for this disorder.

BIBLIOGRAPHY

1. Wolfson LI, Leenders KL, Brown LL, Jones T. Alterations of regional cerebral blood flow and oxygen metabolism in Parkinson's disease. *Neurology* 1985; 35:1399–1405.
2. Perlmutter JS, Raichle ME. Regional blood flow in hemiparkinsonism. *Neurology* 1985; 35:1127–1134.
3. Martin WRW, Beckman JH, Calne DB. et al. Cerebral glucose metabolism in Parkinson's disease. *Can J Neurol Sci* 1984; 11:169.
4. Eidelberg D, Moeller JR, Ishikawa T, et al. Assessment of disease severity in parkinsonism with fluorine-18-fluorodeoxyglucose and PET. *J Nucl Med* 1995; 36:378–383.
5. Peppard RF, Martin WRW, Carr GD, et al. Cerbral glucoce metabolism in Parkinson's disease with and without dementia. *Arch Neurol* 1992; 49:1262–1268.
6. Garnett ES, Firnau G, Nahmias C. Dopamine visualized in the basal ganglia of living man. *Nature* 1983; 305:137–138.
7. Morrish PK, Sawle GV, Brooks DJ. Clinical and [18F]dopa PET findings in early Parkinson's disease. *J Neurol Neurosurg Psychiatry* 1995; 59:597–600.
8. Kish SJ, Shannak K, Hornykiewicz O. Uneven pattern of dopamine loss in the striatum of patients with idiopathic Parkinson's disease. *N Engl J Med* 1988; 318:876–880.
9. Guttman M, Burkholder J, Kish SJ, et al. PET studies of the dopamine transporter in early dopanaive Parkinson's disease: Implications for the symptomatic threshold. *Neurology* 1997; 48:1578–1582.
10. Frey KA, Koeppe RA, Kilbourn MR, et al. Presynaptic monoaminergic vesicles in Parkinson's disease and normal aging. *Ann Neurol* 1996; 40:873–884.
11. Calne DB, Langston JW, Martin WRW, et al. Positron emission tomography after MPTP: Observations relating to the cause of Parkinson's disease. *Nature* 1985; 317:246–248.
12. Piccini P, Burn DJ, Ceravolo R, Maraganore D, Brooks DJ. The role of inheritance in sporadic Parkinson's disease: Evidence from a longitudinal study of dopaminergic function in twins. *Ann Neurol* 1999; 45:577–582.
13. Kishore A, Wszolek ZK, Snow BJ, et al. Presynaptic nigrostriatal function in genetically tested asymptomatic relatives from the pallido-ponto-nigral degeneration family. *Neurology* 1996; 47:1588–1590.
14. Rinne JO, Laihinen A, Ruottinen H, et al. Increased density of dopamine D2 receptors in the putamen, but not in the caudate nucleus in early Parkinson's disease: A PET study with [11C]raclopride. *J Neurol Sci* 1995; 132:156–161.
15. Antonini A, Schwarz J, Oertel WH, Pogarell O, Leenders KL. Long-term changes of striatal dopamine D2 receptors in patients with Parkinson's disease: A study with positron emission tomography and [11C]raclopride. *Mov Disord* 1997; 12:33–38.
16. Guttman M, Seeman P. L-dopa reverses the elevated density of D2 dopamine receptors in Parkinson's disease striatum. *J Neural Transm* 1985; 64:93–103.
17. Rinne JO, Laihinen A, Nagren K, et al. PET demonstrates different behaviour of striatal D1 and D2 receptors in early Parkinson's disease. *J Neurosci Res* 1990; 27:494–499.
18. Antonini A, Kazumata K, Feigin A, et al. Differential diagnosis of parkinsonism with[18F]fluorodeoxyglucose and PET. *Mov Disord* 1998; 13:268–274.
19. Brooks DJ, Ibanez GV, Sawle GV, et al. Differing patterns of striatal 18F-dopa uptake in Parkinson's disease, multiple system atrophy and progressive supranuclear palsy. *Ann Neurol* 1990; 28:547–555.
20. Brooks DJ, Ibanez GV, Sawle GV, et al. Striatal D2 receptor status in Parkinson's disease, striatonigral degeneration, and progressive supranuclear palsy, measured with 11C-raclopride and PET. *Ann Neurol* 1992; 31:184–192.
21. Shinotoh H, Namba H, Yamaguchi M, et al. Positron emission tomograhic measurement of acetylcholinesterase activity reveals differential loss of ascending cholingergic systems in Parkinson's disease and progressive supranuclear palsy. *Ann Neurol* 1999; 46:62–69.
22. Ilgin N, Zubieta J, Reich SG, et al. PET imaging of the dopamine transporter in progressive supranuclear palsy and Parkinson's disease. *Neurology* 1999; 52:1221–1226.
23. Eidelberg D, Moeller JR, Ishikawa T, et al. Regional metabolic correlates of surgical outcome following unilateral pallidotomy for Parkinson's disease. *Ann Neurol* 1996; 39:450–459.
24. Guttman M, Martin WRW, Peppard RF, et al. PET studies of Parkinsonian patients treated with autologous adrenal implants. *Can J Neurol Sci* 1989; 16:305–309.
25. Freeman TB, Olanow CW, Hauser RA, et al. Bilateral fetal nigral transplantation into the postcomissural putamen in Parkinson's disease. *Ann Neurol* 1995; 38:379–388.
26. Guttman M, Leger G, Reches A, et al. Administration of the new COMT inhibitor OR-611 increases striatal uptake of fluorodopa. *Mov Disord* 1993; 8:298–304.

27. Torstenson R, Hartvig P, Langstrom B, Westerberg G, Tedroff J. Differential effects of levodopa on dopaminergic function in early and advanced Parkinson's disease. *Ann Neurol* 1997; 41:334–340.

28. Ekesbo A, Rydin E, Torstenson R, et al. Dopamine autoreceptor function is lost in advanced Parkinson's disease. *Neurology* 1999; 52:120–125.

Table 26-1   PET Ligands Used to Study PD

Type	Class	Ligand
Nonspecific	Blood Flow	$H_2{}^{15}O$
	Metabolism	[^{18}F]uorodeoxyglucose (FDG)
Pre-synaptic dopaminergic	Dopa decarboxylase	[^{18}F]uorodopa (FD)
		[^{11}C]dopa
	Dopamine transporter	[^{11}C]RTI-32
		[^{11}C]CFT/[^{11}C]WIN35,428 (WIN)
		[^{11}C]CIT
		[^{11}C]methylphenidate
		[^{18}F]FPCIT
		[^{11}C]nomifensine
		[^{11}C]GBR-13119
	Vesicular monoamine transporter (2)	[^{11}C]Dihydrotetrabenazine
Post-synaptic dopaminergic	Dopamine D_2 receptor	[^{11}C]raclopride
		[^{11}C]N-methylspiperone
	Dopamine D_1 receptor	[^{11}C]SCH-23390
Cholinergic	Acetylcholinesterase activity	[^{11}C]N-methyl-piperidyl acetate (MP4A)

27

Etiology: The Role of Environment and Genetics

Caroline M. Tanner, M.D., Ph.D.

The Parkinson's Institute, Sunnyvale, California

INTRODUCTION

During the last century, theories regarding the causes of Parkinson's disease (PD) regularly cycled between heredity and environment. More recently, multifactorial theories of gene–environment interaction have emerged (1,2). Whatever the prevailing theory, epidemiologic observations – that is, the distribution of PD in human populations and associated risk factors identified in these groups – were cited as providing, supporting, or detracting evidence. Yet only a few distinct forms of parkinsonism have been described. The causes of the majority of cases remain unexplained.

This chapter provides an intellectual framework for the clinical investigation of the determinants of PD. First, the challenges particular to the investigation of the cause(s) of PD are reviewed. Second, parkinsonisms of known cause are discussed briefly, and particular attention is given to the degree to which investigation of these unique and, so far, rare disorders can guide the study of typical PD. Third, etiologic clues provided by epidemiologic studies are presented. Finally, some speculation regarding the most fruitful next steps is considered.

CHALLENGES IN INVESTIGATING PARKINSON'S DISEASE

The interpretation of the epidemiologic studies discussed in the section must be tempered by the limitations imposed by the current state of knowledge regarding the clinical entity known as Parkinson's disease. The first step in understanding the cause of PD is to define the disorder. Although on the surface this appears to be a straightforward task, there are many potential difficulties.

First, the clinical definition of PD has evolved over the past 50 years. Thus knowledge of the diagnostic criteria used in a given study is critical to interpretation of its results. In the middle of the twentieth century, the term *Parkinson's disease* was often applied to the syndrome of parkinsonism without distinguishing etiology. Thus postencephalitic parkinsonism, parkinsonism secondary to dopamine-receptor blocking drugs, or neurodegenerative parkinsonism of any type would not be distinguished in epidemiologic or clinical reports. Over the last three to four decades, distinct causes of parkinsonism have increasingly been identified. As the causes of different parkinsonian syndromes have been understood, studies have incorporated more precise diagnostic criteria, excluding parkinsonism of known etiology, such as drug-induced disease, and clinical syndromes thought to reflect a different pathologic substrate than "idiopathic" parkinsonism (such as progressive supranuclear palsy or multiple system atrophy). Most recently, two rare genetic forms of parkinsonism have been identified. To date, no epidemiologic study published has distinguished these genetic parkinsonisms from "idiopathic" disease. Over time more causes of the syndrome will surely be identified. To be most useful, descriptive epidemiologic studies should enumerate these different forms of parkinsonism separately. In analytic studies, failure to study parkinsonism of known cause separately from the "idiopathic" disorder lessens the ability to identify potential causative factors unless all cases have the same cause. In this chapter, the term *Parkinson's disease* is reserved for that component of parkinsonism that as yet has no known cause. This includes those cases with the syndrome of bradykinesia, muscle rigidity, resting tremor, and postural tremor, reflecting underlying degeneration of pigmented brainstem neurons, and characteristic neuronal intracytoplasmic inclusions (Lewy bodies) staining for alpha-synuclein are observed. Parkinsonism with known causes is identified separately whenever possible.

Variations in diagnostic criteria make it difficult to compare studies performed at different times or in different areas. In reports from earlier in this century, cases were classified as "arteriosclerotic parkinsonism" that today might be considered typical PD (3,4). Other reports grouped secondary parkinsonism, such as drug-induced parkinsonism and postencephalitic parkinsonism, along with PD in determining incidence or prevalence rates, although these disorders are etiologically and pathologically distinct (3,5). Many of the "atypical" parkinsonian syndromes were widely recognized only in the last several decades. These disorders probably would have been classified as PD in earlier reports. Most recently, two genetic forms of parkinsonism have been described (see subsequent section). These genetic forms of disease probably represent just a fraction of all parkinsonism, but the clinical characteristics of these forms, particularly younger onset make them likely to be disproportionately included in clinical studies.

A further challenge when investigating PD is the lack of a diagnostic test. Diagnosis is entirely dependent on the neurologic history and examination. This forced reliance on clinical diagnostic methods provides a potential source of error. Variations in the experience of diagnosticians can affect diagnostic accuracy. For example, a different neurologic disorder, essential tremor, may be confused with PD. Up to 40% of the diagnoses of PD gleaned from public health registries were false-positives, largely comprised of essential tremor cases (6). Because in many cases essential tremor is found in a familial pattern consistent with autosomal dominant inheritance, inclusion of such cases could lead to the conclusion that much of PD is dominantly inherited. Conversely, bona fide PD may be misdiagnosed, particularly in the very elderly, thus underestimating the pattern of disease in these age groups. In the older age groups, slowness and tremor may be considered "normal" by some. Other common disorders, including Alzheimer's disease, hypothyroidism, depression, arthritis, and stroke may not always be easily distinguished from PD. A further difficulty is presented by people with both parkinsonism and dementia, who may be classified as either primary disorder in different epidemiologic surveys. The common use of neuroleptics in institutionalized elderly, especially those with cognitive impairment, can further confound diagnosis in this age group.

There is no clinical criterion that predicts with absolute certainty the pathologic changes typical of PD.

Surveys of postmortem findings in cases clinically diagnosed as PD found typical postmortem neuropathology in only 80% of cases (7,8). These results probably overestimate the actual misdiagnosis rate, however, because autopsy most likely is performed when there is a question of clinical diagnosis (9). The identification of individuals with early disease presents additional uncertainties because at least 50% of substantia nigra pars compacta (SNPC) cells are believed to be lost before the symptoms prompt medical attention (10). In autopsy series, the pathologic changes of PD are identified in the brains of people who were not diagnosed during life; these "asymptomatic Lewy body" cases increase with increasing age of the population surveyed and may represent clinically presymptomatic PD (11). Postmortem validation of clinical diagnosis, although ideal, has not been systematically available in any epidemiologic investigation of PD.

The uncertainty of clinical diagnosis is an important factor in the design and critical analysis of studies of the etiology of PD. Inclusion of patients who do not have typical disease serves to increase estimates of disease frequency, whereas excluding early disease has the opposite effect. Either type of misclassification could alter demographic patterns. In case-control studies, including people who do not actually have PD usually lowers the precision of the study, decreasing the ability to find a risk factor for disease. If many such patients were included in a study, however, it is possible that a risk factor identified with the non-PD cases might erroneously be associated with PD. In genetic studies, inclusion of such cases would usually lower the likelihood of finding an association of a gene or chromosome marker with PD. Moreover, the mode of inheritance of a genetic defect could be misinterpreted, particularly if a disorder frequently misclassified as PD were inherited.

Finally, PD is a relatively rare disorder. As a result, even studies of large populations will find relatively few cases, and the potential error in any single study may be significant. In analytic studies, this can be particularly problematic if the cause(s) of disease differ across populations.

PARKINSONISM OF KNOWN CAUSE

Current theories of the pathogenic mechanisms underlying PD is derived largely from investigations of the forms of parkinsonism with identifiable causes (both genetic and environmental) and the pursuit of the mechanisms of these disorders in the laboratory. Although it is popular to pose debates supporting a purely genetic or environmental cause

was derived only from medical databases, potentially causing an underestimate of concordance. To address these concerns, the authors compared concordance for PD in MZ and DZ twins, in a long-established cohort of elderly male twins, unselected for diseases of late life, using direct assessment by a movement disorders specialist (91). Overall, concordance for PD in MZ and DZ pairs was similar. This finding is not consistent with a significant genetic cause of PD. The exception was those few pairs with at onset early age (under age 50), in whom concordance was much higher in MZ twins, suggesting strong genetic determinants in younger onset disease.

Although these results appear clear-cut, twins were evaluated at a single point in time, and new cases occurring after this examination may have been missed. Recently two small follow-up studies highlighted this concern. In the first, a study of 34 twin pairs, concordance for decreased putamenal ^{18}F-DOPA uptake was higher in MZ twins than in DZ twin pairs. Higher MZ concordance was most evident in the 19 pairs in whom longitudinal follow-up was possible, particularly when concordance was further defined to include an increased rate of loss of putamenal ^{18}F-DOPA (103). These findings were interpreted to strongly support a genetic cause of PD. In contrast, follow-up of 23 twin pairs for eight years did not find differences in clinical concordance when comparing MZ twins and DZ twins (104). In this study, twins with prior decreased ^{18}F-DOPA uptake on PET had not developed clinical PD. Because both studies are small in number and subject to selection and other possible biases, a final interpretation of these different findings awaits confirmation in a larger, unselected population. Moreover, the radiographic finding itself is of uncertain clinical and prognostic significance and will require further investigation. To address these concerns, a second evaluation of the National Academy of Sciences/National Research Council (NAS/NRC) World War II veteran twins cohort is under way, using both clinical examination and β-CIT SPECT (single photon-emission computed tomography) imaging. Other researchers are using a different research strategy to investigate a genetic determinant of PD, the investigation of affected sibling pairs (105). These studies should do much to clarify the contribution of genetic factors to PD.

Case-Control Studies of Genetic Risk Factors

Case-control studies compare the rates of a proposed risk (or protective) factor between people with the disease and people in the general population without the disease. Genetic risk factors for PD that have been studied using this method include family history of PD, specific genetic polymorphisms, and interaction of genes and other exposures. Case-control studies can demonstrate an association between a specific factor and disease. However, association does not prove causation. The significance of any association observed must be determined using other methods.

Case-control studies that compared the rate of PD in family members of cases and controls have also implicated a genetic contribution to the cause of the disease. On an average, reported rates reflect those first described by Gowers (88) – approximately 10 to 15% of cases selected from clinics report a first-degree relative with PD. In some studies based in specialty clinics, much higher rates of PD and isolated tremor in relatives are reported (106–108). Because attendance at such clinics may be more likely if there are unusual characteristics to the illness, such as a familial pattern, these findings may not be generalizable to the population at large.

A recent community-based study (109) also found a significantly increased risk of PD in first-degree relatives of PD patients, but the magnitude of risk was considerably less. After controlling for sex, ethnicity, and relationship to proband, first-degree relatives of cases were 2.3 times more likely to develop PD than relatives of controls, and male relatives were at twice the risk as female relatives. The lifetime incidence (to age 75) in first-degree relatives of patients was only two percent versus one percent in control families, suggesting that, although there is a significant familial component, PD is probably not due to simple Mendelian inheritance. A similar 2.5-fold increased risk was also found in a recent prospective community-based study among people reporting a family history of PD (110).

Others have used a case-control method to investigate whether specific genetic polymorphisms alter the risk of PD. So far, polymorphisms of several genes have been associated with PD in some studies, but no finding is consistent across populations. These associations have been proposed to be directly or indirectly related to disease etiology. Many of the specific genes associated with PD encode enzymes involved in xenobiotic metabolism. If PD is multifactorial, resulting from both genetic factors and environmental factors, risk from various environmental factors could be influenced by metabolizing enzymes. An interaction of genetic factors with these exposures could result in a high level of disease risk. Differences in the activity of enzymes metabolizing xenobiotics might result in toxicity in one person but not affect another. Polymorphisms of several genes involved in xenobiotic metabolism have been associated with increased PD risk, including cytochrome P 450 2D6, cytochrome P 450 1A1, glutathione transferase, N-acetyl transferase, the dopamine transporter MAO-B, paraoxonase, alpha 1 antichymotrypsin, and ubiquitin carboxy-terminal hydrolase L1, but results are not consistent (111–127).

The inconsistent nature of these associations with PD risk could represent spurious findings. Factors such as differences in ethnicity, presence of other diseases, or survival could cause control populations to differ from case populations in genetic makeup independent of disease-specific factors. However, inconsistent results may also be observed if gene–environment interactions are the determinant of PD (128); that is, these variants might only result in an increased risk if an individual were exposed to certain environmental factors, resulting in toxic effects from levels of compounds that might not otherwise be toxic. Enzymatic variability could result in decreased detoxification of toxic compounds or increased bioactivation of otherwise nontoxic compounds. One such gene–environment interaction is the observation by one group that the inverse association of smoking and PD is present only in those with a specific MAO-B allele (129). The combined effects of multiple genes, alone or in combination with exposures, may also be important (130). Whether the inconsistent results of studies to date are because of design differences or reflect a true absence of an important gene environment or gene–gene interaction in PD cannot be determined. Most investigators agree that further investigation in this area is clearly warranted (131).

Environmental Risk Factors

More than 20 case-control studies have evaluated the role of environmental factors in the etiology of PD (2,132) Many of these have implicated agricultural or industrial chemical exposures but have focused on broad groupings of agents or classes of chemicals rather than on specific exposures. Although these categories provide important leads, they have been too broad to pinpoint causal agents. The major findings are summarized in the following sections.

Agriculture and Related Factors

Rural living, farming, gardening, pesticide use, or well water drinking have been associated with PD in almost every study (2,132–135). The consistency of these findings in many populations contributed to interest in the relationship between farming and PD. Pesticide exposure (defined as including herbicides and fungicides) was associated with an increased PD risk in 14 studies. The risk was increased from 1.6 to 7 times in those exposed. The structural and mechanistic

resemblance of some common agricultural chemicals to MPTP and the potential of others to cause oxidative stress make this association particularly intriguing.

On the other hand, specific pesticides or chemical classes have been identified in only a few of these studies. In Taiwan, PD risk was more than six times greater in people using paraquat for 20 years or more (136). Paraquat use was also associated with an increased risk in univariate, but not multivariate, analyses in two Canadian studies (137,138). In Germany, organochlorines were associated with a 5.8-fold increased risk of PD, and using alkylated phosphates or carbamates had a 2.5-fold increase if cases were compared with regional controls but not if neighborhood controls were used (139). In other studies, chlorphenoxy and thiocarbamate herbicides and organophosphates are associated with increased PD risk in univariate but not multivariate analyses (136,137). In a postmortem comparison of organochlorine pesticide concentrations in the brains of PD patients, people with Alzheimer's disease, and controls, the organochlorine insecticide dieldrin was associated with an elevated risk of PD (42). So far, no study in humans has investigated the combined effects of several agents, although combined exposure is the norm in an agricultural setting. In support of the importance of pursuing such questions, in an animal model, combined exposure to the herbicide paraquat and the fumigant maneb caused greater damage to dopamine systems than exposure to either agent alone (140). Although none of this evidence is conclusive regarding possible causative agents in PD, these investigations certainly point to specific compounds that should be included in future studies.

Other Occupational Risk Factors

Several other occupational exposures have been associated with an increased risk of PD. Gorell and coworkers (141) reported significant associations with prolonged occupational exposure to copper and manganese and from combined exposures to lead–copper, lead–iron, and iron–copper. Odds ratios rose with duration of exposure to 2.5 for copper and to over 10 for manganese among workers with 20 or more years of employment (133). Interestingly, at least one group has reported that manganese can result in progressive parkinsonism (142). Ecological studies have reported increased parkinsonism in proximity to areas in which iron ore mining and wood pulp and paper manufacture have occurred (13). In addition to these specific agents, some very broad categories of chemicals or specific occupations have been associated with PD in case-control studies, including organic solvent exposure, chemical manufacturing, metal working, carpentry (men only), and cleaning (women only) (2,132–134). Although these are less helpful in formulating a more focused effort on finding specific compounds that may contribute to PD, they add support to the proposition that environmental factors are at play in the disease.

Lifestyle-Associated Risk Factors

Lifestyle-associated factors such as habits and diet have also been investigated as risk factors for PD. The most consistent association in this category is the inverse association between cigarette smoking and PD (see Chapter 46). Cigarette smoking has been associated with a lower risk of PD in numerous prevalent case-control studies in a wide variety of populations, but whether this association is due to a biologic effect of tobacco or is the result of some other factor remains controversial (2,132). Although alternative explanations for the association have been put forth, including a higher mortality in smokers with PD (143) and a conservative preparkinsonian personality (144), there is compelling support for a biologic effect of tobacco based on a number of studies that used rigorous methodology. For example, an inverse dose-response relationship between cigarette smoking and PD has been found in both prevalent and incident case-control investigations, as well as in a prospective cohort study (141,145,146). Furthermore, laboratory studies support a direct effect of nicotine, the major bioactive component of cigarette smoke. For example, nicotine has been found to protect against transection-induced and MPTP-induced dopaminergic neuronal cell loss in rodent substantia nigra (147–150).

Although the laboratory evidence supporting a neuroprotective effect of nicotine is compelling, the possibility still remains that drinking coffee or alcohol, behaviors that are commonly associated with cigarette smoking, might actually be the risk factor(s) responsible for the observed inverse association between cigarette smoking and PD risk. For example, a recent longitudinal study and two case-control studies of incident PD cases provide provocative new evidence that coffee drinking may also be inversely associated with PD risk. In a longitudinal study of Japanese-American men, greater consumption of coffee was inversely associated with PD risk in a dose-dependent fashion (151). A very provocative finding in the same cohort was that greater intake of coffee was inversely associated with incidental Lewy bodies at postmortem (152). A similar dose-dependent inverse association between coffee drinking and PD was observed in two prospective studies (153,154) and retrospectively in

an incident case-control study in northern California (146). In each case, the inverse association between PD and coffee drinking continued to be observed in multivariate analyses adjusting for cigarette smoking, alcohol use, and other potential confounders. Similar associations had previously been reported in a few case-control studies of prevalent cases, but these results were inconsistent and a dose-response gradient was not described (2,132). Caffeine is an antagonist at the adenosine A2A receptor, a pharmacologic action proposed to be of benefit in treating PD (155). This action may underlie the observed inverse association of caffeine and PD. Alternatively, both cigarette use and coffee drinking may instead reflect an underlying premorbid personality (156). Several studies have also found that consumption of alcohol is inversely associated with PD risk (133,146,157,158), but others have failed to observe this effect (154,159–161). Furthermore, in most studies to date, the possible confounding effects of cigarette smoking or coffee drinking cannot be assessed definitively.

A diet that is high in antioxidants has been proposed to lower the risk of PD, but to date such a diet has not been consistently associated with this lower risk (133, 162–166). On the other hand, positive associations of PD with animal fat consumption and with a diet that is high in iron have been reported (141,163,164,167). High dietary intake of these foods may increase oxidative stress. Thus these observations again raise the possibility that oxidative damage may contribute to nigral cell degeneration in PD.

Infectious Risk Factors

The observation that encephalitis lethargica often resulted in parkinsonism during the influenza pandemic of the early 1900s suggested a possible infectious etiology for PD. Since that time, however, clinical and neuropathologic criteria have clearly differentiated postencephalitic parkinsonism from typical idiopathic PD. Although many subsequent studies have been unable to identify an infectious agent in PD (168–171), a number of studies have continued to suggest that infection may play a role in the cause of PD. Also, rather than reflecting exposure to a chemical, the increased risk of developing PD associated with rural residence may reflect exposure to an infectious agent.

Mattock and coworkers (172) suggested that exposure to influenza virus in utero may result in damage to fetal substantia nigra, predisposing to the occurrence of PD in adulthood, but this observation was not confirmed (173). Fazzini and coworkers (174) found increased cerebrospinal fluid antibody titers to coronaviruses in PD patients, whereas Hubble and colleagues (175) and Kohbata and Shimokawa (176) found increased *Nocardia* antibody titers. Although elevated *Nocardia* titers were not found in a subsequent case-control study (171), *Nocardia* has a specific affinity for substantia nigral neurons and has been shown to cause a levodopa-responsive movement disorder in mice (177,178). Martyn and Osmond (179) found that PD patients were more likely to report childhood infection with diphtheria and croup than controls, but there were no reported differences in the frequency of other lifetime infections. Conversely, Sasco and Paffenbarger (180) found an inverse association between most childhood viral infections and PD, and a significant inverse association with childhood measles was reported. Rather than a protective effect, this may reflect a relatively greater risk associated with subclinical or adult measles infection.

Trauma

Several case-control studies have reported that head trauma is associated with an increased risk for PD (1,161,181,182,182a), including a recent report showing a dose-dependent increase associated with more frequent or more severe injuries (183). Because parkinsonism and dementia can follow repeated head injury, as is experienced by boxers, this result is interesting. However, an equally plausible explanation for this association is that of recall bias; that is, those with the disease are more likely to remember past injuries than nondiseased controls, and those with brain disease are more likely to remember head injuries in particular. In a prospective study, recall is not a factor. In the only study reported to date using prospectively collected information on head trauma, no association between head trauma and PD was observed (184). There are several explanations for the association between head trauma and PD. It could be a recall bias because subjects with PD are more likely to remember some significant events, especially when it occurs to the head. On the other hand, laboratory studies have suggested that chronic head injuries could affect the delivery of oxygen and cause defective energy metabolism and subsequently excitotoxicity in certain susceptible areas of the brain, including the nigrostriatal system. Additional well-designed studies (particularly perspective studies) are needed to clarify this association.

Emotional Stress

There are two reports indicating that people experiencing the extreme emotional and physical hardships of concentration camp imprisonment during the holocaust or a war have been shown to have an increased risk for developing PD (185–187). Whether these observations reflect an accelerated nigral injury as the result of stress-related increase in dopamine turnover with resultant increased oxidative injury (188), nutritional deficiencies of dietary protective agents (see previous section) or other factors cannot be determined. Evaluation of the relationship of less-severe emotional or physical stress to the development of PD poses significant methodologic challenges.

Personality

It has been reported that certain premorbid personality traits may predispose individuals to PD. Several studies suggest that people who are characterized as introverted, shy, timid, subordinate, less outgoing, nervous, responsible, morally rigid, and law-abiding have a higher risk of developing PD (156,189–191). This finding was explained by a potential illness-related distortion of recall bias. However, it could also reflect genetically determined endogenous individual differences in dopamine metabolism and in biochemical capacity to detoxify certain xenobiotics.

CONCLUSION

Although both genetic and environmental causes of parkinsonism have been identified, these causes, taken together, account for only a small fraction of patients with the disease. Many risk factors have been associated with PD in some studies, but few are consistently observed. Of these, increasing age, male gender, and not cigarette smoking are found in nearly every population studied. More controversial, but also frequently associated with PD, are not drinking coffee, farming-associated exposures, and head trauma. Parkinson's disease probably has many determinants, both within an individual and among members of a population. Many of these exposures associated with disease may be capable of triggering similar mechanisms, independently, in combination, or only in the presence of specific genetic susceptibility factors. These pathogenetic mechanisms then could result in the final process of nerve cell degeneration in the substantia nigra that produces PD. More sophisticated methods of investigation are needed to arrive at an answer. These will include prospective investigations of large populations, use of incident cases in case-control studies, and the study of populations with known exposures, in addition to the studies described in this chapter. In each case, close collaboration with basic scientists involved in laboratory investigations of disease mechanisms will be critical in guiding the questions addressed in these populations.

REFERENCES

1. Semchuk K, Love E, Lee R. Parkinson's disease: A test of the multifactorial etiologic hypothesis. *Neurology* 1993; 43:1173–1180.
2. Tanner C, Goldman S. Epidemiology of Parkinson's disease. *Neurol Clin* 1996; 14:317–335.
3. Kurland LT. Descriptive epidemiology of selected neurologic and myopathic disorders with particular reference to a survey in Rochester, Minnesota. *J Chron Dis* 1958; 8(4):378–418.
4. Gudmundsson KR. A clinical survey of parkinsonism in Iceland. *Acta Neurol Scand* 1967; 33:9–61.
5. Schoenberg BS, Anderson D, WHaerer **Name OK?** AF. Prevalence of parkinson's disease in the biracial population of Copiah County, Mississippi. *Neurology* 1985; 35:841–845.
6. Mutch W, et al. Parkinson's disease in a Scottish city. *Br Med J* 1986:534–536.
7. Rajput AH, Calne D, BLang **Name OK?** AE. National conference on Parkinson's disease. *Can J Neurol Sci* 1991; 18:87–92.
8. Hughes AJ, et al. A clinicopathologic study of 100 cases of Parkinson's disease. *Arch Neurol* 1993; 50:140–148.
9. Maraganore D, et al. Autopsy patterns for Parkinson's disease and related disorders in Olmsted County, Minnesota. *Neurology* 1999; 53(6):1342–1344.
10. Bernheimer H, et al. Brain dopamine and the syndromes of Parkinson and Huntington: Clinical, morphological, and neurochemical correlations. *J Neurol Sci* 1973; 20:415-455.
11. Gibb WR, Lees AJ. Anatomy, pigmentation, ventral, and dorsal subpopulations of the substantia nigra, and differential cell death in Parkinson's disease. *J Neurol Neurosurg Psychiatry* 1991; 54(5):388–396.
12. Goetz C. *Neurotoxins in Clinical Practice*. New York. 1985.
13. Tanner CM. *Occupational and Environmental Causes of Parkinsonism*. Philadelphia. 1992; 503–513.
14. Langston JW, et al. Chronic Parkinsonism in humans due to a product of meperidine analog synthesis. *Science* 1983; 219:979–980.
15. Irwin I, DeLanney LE, Langston JW. MPTP and aging: *Studies in the C57BL/6 Mouse*. New York. 1993; (197–206). **(INCOMPLETE)**.
16. Tipton K, Singer T. Advances in our understanding of the mechanisms of the neurotoxicity of MPTP and related compounds. *J Neurochem* 1993; 61:1191–1206.
17. McCrodden JM, Tipton KF, Sullivan JP. The neurotoxicity of MPTP and the relevance to Parkinson's disease. *Pharmacol Toxicol* 1990; 67(1):8–13.
18. Salach JI, et al. Oxidation of the neurotoxic amine 1-methyl-4-phenyl-1, 2, 3, 6-tetrahydropyridine (MPTP) by monoamine oxidases A and B and suicide inactivation of the enzymes by MPTP. *Biochem Biophys Res Comm* 1984; 125:831–835.
19. Javitch JA, Snyder SH. Uptake of MPP(+) by dopamine neurons explains selectivity of Parkinsonism-inducing neurotoxin, MPTP. *Eur J Pharmacol* 1985; 106:455–456.
20. Ramsay R, et al. Energy driven uptake of MPP+ by brain mitochondria mediates the neurotoxicity of MPTP. *Life Sci* 1986; 39:581–588.
21. Nicklas WJ, Vyas I, Heikkila RE. Inhibition of NADH-linked oxidation in brain mitochondria by 1-methyl-4- phenyl-pyridine, a metabolite of the neurotoxin, 1-methyl-4-phenyl- 1, 2, 5, 6-tetrahydropyridine. *Life Sci* 1985; 36(26):2503–2508.
22. Di Monte DA, Smith MT. Free radicals, lipid peroxidation and 1-methyl-4-phenyl-1, 2, 3, 6-tetrahydropyridine (MPTP)-induced Parkinsonism. *Rev Neurosci* 1988; 2(1):67–81.
23. Singer T, et al. Biochemical events in the development of Parkinsonism induced by MPTP. *J Neurochem* 1987; 49(1):1–8.
24. Cassaret and Doull. Cassaret and Doull's Toxicology: *The Basic Science of Poisons*. New York. 1996.
25. McNaught KS, et al. Isoquinoline derivatives as endogenous neurotoxins in the aetiology of Parkinson's disease. *Biochem Pharmacol* 1998; 56(8):921–933.
26. Di Monte DA, Chan P, Sandy MS. Glutathione in Parkinson's disease: A link between oxidative stress and mitochondrial damage. *Ann Neurol* 1992; 32 (Suppl):S111–S115.
27. Ames BN, Shigenaga MK, Hagen TM. Mitochondrial decay in aging. *Biochim Biophys Acta* 1995; 1271(1):165–170.
28. Ames BN, Shigenaga MK, Hagen TM. Oxidants, antioxidants, and the degenerative diseases of aging. *Proc Natl Acad Sci USA* 1993; 90:7915–7922.
29. Olanow CW, Arendash GW. Metals and free radicals in neurodegeneration. *Curr Opin Neurol* 1994; 7(6):548–558.
30. Simonian NA, Coyle JT. Oxidative stress in neurodegenerative diseases. *Annu Rev Pharmacol Toxicol* 1996; 36:83–106.
31. Facchinetti F, Dawson VL, Dawson TM. Free radicals as mediators of neuronal injury. *Cell Mol Neurobiol* 1998; 18(6):667–682.
32. Amdur M, Doull J, Klaasen C. *The Basic Science of Poisons*. New York. 1991;
33. Sanchez-Ramos JR, Hefti F, Weiner WJ. Paraquat and Parkinson's disease. *Neurology* 1987; 37:728.
34. Sechi GP, et al. Acute and persistent Parkinsonism after use of diquat. *Neurology* 1992; 42:261–263.

35. Makino Y, et al. Presence of tetrahydroisoquinoline and 1-methyl-tetrahydro-isoquinoline in foods: Compounds related to Parkinson's disease. *Life Sci* 1988; 43:373–378.

36. Niwa T, et al. Presence of tetrahydroisoquinoline, a Parkinsonism-related compound, in foods. *J Chromatogr* 1989; 493:347–352.

37. Williams AC, et al. *N-methylation of Pyridines and Parkinson's disease.* New York, 1993; (194–196).

38. Tipton KF, McCrodden JM, Sullivan JP. Metabolic aspects of the behavior of MPTP and some analogues. *Adv Neurol* 1993; 60:186–193.

39. Naoi M, et al. *N-methylated tetrahydroisoquinolines as dopaminergic neurotoxins.* New York. 1993; (212–217).

40. Ansher SS, et al. Role of N-methyltransferases in the neurotoxicity associated with the metabolites of 1-methyl-4-phenyl-1, 2, 3, 6-tetrahydropyridine (MPTP) and other 4-substituted pyridines present in the environment. *Biochem Pharmacol* 1986; 35:3359–3363.

41. Niwa T, et al. Presence of tetrahydroisoquinoline-related compounds, possible MPTP-like neurotoxins, in Parkinsonian brain. New York. 1993; (234–23).

42. Fleming L, et al. Parkinson's disease and brain levels of organochlorine pesticides. *Ann Neurol* 1994; 36:100–103.

43. Friedrich M. Pesticide study aids Parkinson research. *JAMA* 1999; 282:2200.

44. Polymeropoulos MH, Higgins JJ, Golbe LI, et al. Mapping of a gene for Parkinson's disease to chromosome 4q–21.q23. *Science* 1996; 274:1197–1199.

45. Papadimitriou A, Veletza V, Hadjigeorgiou GM, et al. Mutated alpha-synuclein gene in two Greek kindreds with familial PD: Incomplete penetrance? *Neurology* 1999; 52(3):651–654.

46. Golbe LI, et al. Clinical genetic analysis of Parkinson's disease in the Contursi kindred. *Ann Neurol* 1996; 40:767–775.

47. Kruger R, et al. Ala30Pro mutation in the gene encoding alpha-synuclein in Parkinson's disease [letter]. *Nat Genet* 1998; 18(2):106–108.

48. Chan D, et al. Genetic and environmental risk factors for Parkinson's disease in a Chinese population. *J Neurol Neurosurg Psychiatry* 1998; 65(5):781–784.

49. Vaughan J, et al. The alpha-synuclein Ala53Thr mutation is not a common cause of familial Parkinson's disease: A study of 230 European cases. European Consortium on Genetic Susceptibility in Parkinson's Disease. *Ann Neurol* 1998; 44(2):270–273.

50. Conway K, Harper J, Lansbury P. Accelerated in vitro fibril formation by a mutant alpha-synuclein linked to early-onset Parkinson disease. *Nat Med* 1998; 4:1318–1320.

51. Irizarry M, et al. Characterization of the precursor protein of the non-A beta component of senile plaques (NACP) in the human central nervous system. *J Neuropathol Exp Neurol* 1996; 55:889–895.

52. Feany M, Bender W. A drosophila model of Parkinson's disease. *Nature* 2000; 404:394–400.

53. Spillantini M, et al. Alpha-synuclein in filamentous inclusions of Lewy bodies from Parkinson's disease and dementia with Lewy bodies. *Proc Natl Acad Sci USA* 1998; 95:6469–6473.

54. Matsumine H, et al. Localisation of a gene for autosomal recessive form of juvenile Parkinsonism to chromosome 6q–25.2-27. *Am J Hum Genet* 1997; 60:588–596.

55. Kitada T, et al. Mutations in the parkin gene cause autosomal recessive juvenile Parkinsonism (see comments). *Nature* 1998; 392(6676):605–608.

56. Hattori N, et al. Point mutations (Thr240Arg and Ala311Stop) in the Parkin gene. *Biochem Biophys Res Comm* 1998; 249:754–758.

57. Abbas N, et al. A wide variety of mutations in the Parkin gene are responsible for autosomal recessive Parkinsonism in Europe. *Hum Mol Genet* 1999; 8(4):567–574.

58. Yamamura Y, et al. Paralysis agitans of early onset with marked diurnal fluctuations of symptoms. *Neurology* 1973; 23:239–244.

59. Takahashi H, et al. Familial juvenile Parkinsonism: Clinical and pathologic study in a family. *Neurology* 1994; 44:437–441.

60. Lucking C, et al. Association between early-onset Parkinson's disease and mutations in the Parkin gene. *New Engl J Med* 2000; 342(21):1560–1567.

61. Nelson L, et al. Incidence of idiopathic Parkinson's disease (PD) in a health maintenance organization (HMO): Variations by age, gender, and race/ethnicity. *Neurology* 1997:A334.

62. Harada H, Nishikawa S, Takahashi K. Epidemiology of Parkinson's disease in a Japanese city. *Arch Neurol* 1983; 40:151–154.

63. Mayeux R, et al. A population-based investigation of Parkinson's disease with and without dementia: Relationship to age and gender. *Arch Neurol* 1992; 49:492–497.

64. Morgante L, et al. Prevalence of Parkinson's disease and other types of Parkinsonism: A door-to-door survey in three Sicilian municipalities. *Neurology* 1992; 42:1901–1907.

65. Rosati G, et al. The risk of Parkinson disease in Mediterranean people. *Neurology* 1980; 30:250–255.

66. Sutcliffe RLG, et al. Parkinson's disease in the district of Northampton Health Authority, United Kingdom. A study of prevalence and disability. *Acta Neurol Scand* 1985; 72:363–379.

67. Mayeux R, et al. The frequency of idiopathic Parkinson's disease by age, ethnic group, and sex in northern Manhattan, 1988–1993. *Am J Epidemiol* 1995; 142:820–827.

68. Granieri E, et al. Parkinson's disease in Ferrara, Italy, 1967 through 1987. *Arch Neurol* 1991; 48:854–857.

69. Morens DM, White LR, Davis JW. Re: "The frequency of idiopathic Parkinson's disease by age, ethnic group, and sex in northern Manhattan, 1988–1993." *Am J Epidemiol* 1996; 144(2):198–199.

70. Ashok PP, et al. Epidemiology of Parkinson's disease in Benghazi, Northeast Libya. *Clin Neurol* 1986; 88(2):109–113.

71. D'Allessandro R, et al. Prevalence of Parkinson's disease in the republic of San Marino. *Neurology* 1987; 37:1679–1682.

72. Jenkins AC. Epidemiology of Parkinsonism in Victoria. *Med J Australia* 1966; 2:496–502.

73. Kessler II. Epidemiology study of Parkinson's disease. *Am J Epidemiol* 1972; 96:242–254.

74. Rajput AH, et al. Epidemiology of Parkinsonism: Incidence, classification, and mortality. *Ann Neurol* 1984; 16:278–282.

75. Svenson LW, Platt GH, Woodhead SE. Geographic variations in the prevalence rates of Parkinson's disease in Alberta. *Can J Neurol Sci* 1993; 20:307–311.

76. Imaizumi Y. Geographical variations in mortality from Parkinson's disease in Japan, 1977–1985. *Acta Neurol Scand* 1995; 91:311–316.

77. Kurtzke JF, Murphy FM. The changing patterns of death rates in Parkinsonism. *Neurology* 1990; 40:42–49.

78. Chia L-GLiu L-H. Parkinson's disease in Taiwan: An analysis of 215 patients. *Neuroepidemiology* 1992; 11:113–120.

79. Li SC, et al. A prevalence survey of Parkinson's disease and other movement disorders in the People's Republic of China. *Arch Neurol* 1985; 42:655–657.

80. Tanner CM, et al. Environmental factors and Parkinson's disease: A case-control study in China. *Neurology* 1989; 39:660–664.

81. Wang SJ, et al. Parkinson's disease in Kin-Hu, Kinmen: A community survey by neurologists. *Neuroepidemiology* 1994; 13:69–74.

82. Morens DM, et al. Epidemiologic observations on Parkinson's disease: Incidence and mortality in a prospective study of middle-aged men. *Neurology* 1996; 46:1044–1050.

83. Kuopio A, et al. Changing epidemiology of Parkinson's disease in southwestern Finland. *Neurology* 1999; 52(2):302–308.

84. Chan P, et al. Prevalence of Parkinson's disease in Beijing, China. *Neurology* 2000; 54(7)(Suppl 3):A348.

85. Riggs J. The environmental basis for rising mortality from Parkinson's disease. *Arch Neurol* 1993; 50:653–656.

86. Parkinson J. *An Essay on the Shaking Palsy*. London. 1817.

87. Charcot J. Lectures on the diseases of the nervous system. London. 1878; (1)

88. Gowers W. Diseases of the nervous system. Philadelphia. 1888.

88a. Calne S, et al. Familial Parkinson's disease: Possible role of environmental factors. *Can J Neurol Sci* 1987; 14:303–305.

89. Swerdlow R, et al. Matrilineal inheritance of complex I dysfunction in a multigenerational Parkinson's disease family. *Ann Neurol* 1998; 44(6):873–881.

90. Zweig RM, et al. The locus ceruleus and dementia in Parkinson's disease. *Neurology* 1993; 43:986–991.

91. Tanner C, et al. Parkinson disease in twins: An etiologic study. *JAMA* 1999; 281:341–346.

92. Farrer M, et al. A chromosome 4q haplotype segregating with Parkinson's disease and postural tremor. *Hum Mol Genet* 1999; 8:81–85.

93. Gasser T, et al. A susceptibility locus for Parkinson's disease maps to chromosome 2p–13. *Nat Genet* 1998; 18:262–265.

94. Wszolek Z, et al. Danish–American family (family E) with "Parkinson's disease": Pitfalls of genetic studies. *Parkinsonism Related Disord* 1996; 2(1):47–49.

95. Dwork A, et al. Dominantly inherited, early-onset Parkinsonism: Neuropathology of a new form. *Neurology* 1993; 43:69–74.

96. Mizutani Y, Yokochi M, Oyanagi S. Juvenile Parkinsonism: A case with first clinical manifestation at the age of six years and with neuropathological findings suggesting a new pathogenesis. *Clin Neuropathol* 1991; 10(2):91–97.

97. Roy EP III, et al. Familial Parkinsonism, apathy, weight loss, and central hypoventilation: Successful long-term management. *Neurology* 1988; 38:637–639.

98. Denson MA, Wszolek ZK. Familial Parkinsonism: Our experience and review. *Parkinsonism Related Disord.* 1995; 1(1):35–46.

99. Pembrey ME. Discordant identical twins. II. Parkinsonism. *Practitioner* 1972; 209:240–243.

100. Duvoisin R, et al. Twin study of Parkinson disease. *Neurology* 1981; 31:77–80.

101. Johnson WG, Hodge SE, Duvoisin RC. Twin studies and the genetics of Parkinson's disease. *Mov Disord* 1990; 5(3):187–194.

102. Burn DJ, et al. Parkinson's disease in twins studied with 18F-dopa and positron emission tomography. *Neurology* 1992; 42:1894–1900.

103. Piccini P, Brooks D. Etiology of Parkinson's disease: Contributions from 18F-DOPA positron emission tomography. 45. 1999; 5:577–582.

104. Vieregge P, et al. Parkinson's disease in twins – A follow-up study. *Neurology* 1999; 53(3):566–572.

105. Hubble JP, Weeks CC, Nance M, et al. Parkinson's disease: Clinical features in sibships. *Neurology* 1999; 52(Suppl 2):A13.

106. Payami H, et al. Increased risk of Parkinson's disease in parents and siblings of patients. *Ann Neurol* 1994; 36:659–661.

107. Vieregge P, Heberlein I. Increased risk of Parkinson's disease in relatives of patients. *Ann Neurol* 1995; 37:685.

108. De Michele G, et al. Environmental and genetic risk factors in Parkinson's disease: A case-control study in Southern Italy. *Mov Disord* 1996; 11(1):17–23.

109. Marder K, et al. Risk of Parkinson's disease among first-degree relatives: A community-based study. *Neurology* 1996; 47:155–160.

110. de Rijk MC, et al. Prevalence of Parkinsonism and Parkinson's disease in Europe: The EUROPARKINSON collaborative study. *J Neurol Neurosurg Psychiatry* 1997; 62:10–15.

111. Smith CAD, et al. Debrisoquine hydroxylase gene polymorphism and susceptibility to Parkinson's disease. *Lancet* 1992; 339:1375–1377.

112. Armstrong M, et al. Mutant debrisoquine hydroxylase genes in Parkinson's disease. *Lancet* 1992; 339:1017–1018.

113. Tsuneoka Y, et al. A novel cytochrome P450IID6 mutant gene associated with Parkinson's disease. *J Biochem* 1993; 114:263–266.

114. Akhmedova A, et al. Frequency of a specific cytochrome P4502-6. (CYP2-6.) mutant allele in clinically differentiated groups of patients with Parkinson's disease. *Biochem Mol Med* 1995; 54:88–90.

115. Lucotte G, et al. Mutation frequencies of the cytochrome CYP2-6.gene in Parkinson's disease patients and in families. *Am J Med Gen* 1996; 67:361–365.

116. Sandy MS, et al. CYP2-6.allelic frequencies in young onset Parkinson's disease. *Neurology* 1996; 47:225–230.

117. Bordet R, et al. Debrisoquine hydroxylation genotype in familial forms of idiopathic Parkinson's disease. *Adv Neurol* 1996; 69:97–100.

118. Kurth J, et al. Lack of association of CYP3-6.and MAO-B alleles with Parkinson's disease in a Kansas cohort. *Neurology* 1995; 45(Suppl 4):A429.

119. Diederich N, et al. Genetic variability of the *CYP 2D6* gene is not a risk factor for sporadic Parkinson's disease. *Ann Neurol* 1996; 40:463–465.

120. Bandmann O, et al. Sequence of the superoxide dismutase 1(SOD1) gene in familial Parkinson's disease. *J Neurol Neurosurg Psychiatry* 1995; 59:90–91.

121. Stroombergen MCMJ, et al. Determination of the *GSTM1* gene deletion frequency in Parkinson's disease by allele specific PCR. *Parkinsonism and Related Disord* 1996; 2(3):151–154.

122. Kurth JH, et al. Association of a monoamine oxidase B allele with Parkinson's disease. *Ann Neurol* 1993; 33:368–372.

123. Hotamisligil GS, et al. Hereditary variations in monoamine oxidase as a risk factor for Parkinson's disease. *Mov Disord* 1994; 9(3):305–310.

124. Nicholl DJ, et al. A study of five candidate genes in Parkinson's disease and related neurodegenerative disorders. *Neurology* 1999:1415–1421.

125. Munoz E, et al. Alphal-antichymotryspin gene polymorphism and susceptibility to Parkinson's disease. *Neurology* 1999; 52(2):297–301.

126. Maraganore D, Farrer M, Hardy J, et al. Case-control study of the ubiquitin carboxy-terminal hydrolase *L1* gene in Parkinson's disease. *Neurology* 1999; 53(8):1858–1860.

127. Lincoln S, et al. Low frequency of pathogenic mutations in the ubiquitin carboxyterminal hydrolase gene in familial Parkinson's disease. *NeuroReport* 1999; 10(2):427–429.

128. Landi MT, et al. Gene–environment interaction in Parkinson's disease – the case of *CYP2D6* gene polymorphisms. *Adv Neurol* 1996; 69:61–72.

129. Checkoway H, et al. A genetic polymorphism of MAO-B modifies the association of cigarette smoking and Parkinson's disease. *Neurology* 1998; 50:1458–1461.

130. Bon M, et al. Neurogenetic correlates of Parkinson's disease: Apolipoprotein-E and cytochrome P450 2-6.genetic polymorphism. *Neurosci Lett* 1999; 266(2):149–51.

131. Markopoulou K, Langston J. Candidate genes and Parkinson's disease – Where to next? *Neurology* 1999; 53(7):1382–1383.

132. Checkoway H, Nelson L. Epidemiologic approaches to the study of Parkinson's disease etiology. *Epidemiology* 1999; 10(3):327–336.

133. Fall PA, et al. Nutritional and occupational factors influencing the risk of Parkinson's disease: A case-control study in southeastern Sweden. *Mov Disord* 1999; 14(1):28–37.

134. Smargiassi A, et al. A case-control study of occupational and environmental risk factors for Parkinson's disease in the Emilia-Romagna region of Italy. *Neurotoxicology* 1998; 19(4–5.:709–712.

135. Tuchsen F, Jensen A. Agricultural work and the risk of Parkinson's disease in Denmark, 1981–1993. *Scand J Work Environ Health* 2000 (in press).

136. Liou HH, et al. Environmental risk factors and Parkinson's disease: A case-control study in Taiwan. *Neurology* 1997; 48(6):1583–1588.

137. Semchuk KM, Love EJ, Lee RG. Etiology of Parkinson's disease: A test of the multifactorial hypothesis. *Can J Neurol Sci* 1992; 19(2):251.

138. Hertzman C, et al. A case-control study of Parkinson's disease in a horticultural region of British Columbia. *Mov Disord* 1994; 9(1):69–75.

139. Seidler A, et al. Possible environmental, occupational, and other etiologic factors for Parkinson's disease: A case-control study in Germany. *Neurology* 1996; 46:1275–1284.

140. Thiruchelram M, et al. Potentiated and preferential effects of combined paraquat and maneb on nigrostriatal dopamine systems: Environmental risk factors for Parkinson's disease. 2000.

141. Gorell J, et al. A population-based case-control study of nutrient intake in Parkinson's disease. *Neurology* 1997; 48:A298.

142. Huang C, et al. Long-term progression in chronic manganism: Ten years of follow-up. *Neurology* 1998; 50(3):698–700.

143. Ellenberg JH. Differential postmorbidity mortality in observational studies of risk factors for neurologic disorders. *Neuroepidemiology* 1994; 13:187–194.

144. Poewe WH, et al. Premorbid personality of Parkinson patients. *J Neural Transm* 1983; (Suppl 19) 215–224.

145. Grandinetti A, et al. Prospective study of cigarette smoking and the risk of developing idiopathic Parkinson's disease. *Am J Epidemiol* 1994; 139:1129–1138.

146. Nelson L, et al. Association of alcohol and tobacco consumption with Parkinson's disease: A population-based study. *Neurology* 1999:A538–539.

147. Janson AM, Fuxe K, Goldstein M. Differential effects of acute and chronic nicotine treatment on MPTP-(1-methyl-4-phenyl-1, 2, 3, 6-tetrahydropyridine) induced degeneration of nigrostriatal dopamine neurons in the black mouse. *Klin Wochenschr* 1992; 70:232–238.

148. Janson AM, Moller A. Chronic nicotine treatment counteracts nigral cell loss induced by a partial mesodiencephalic hemitransection: An analysis of the total number and mean volume of neurons and glia in substantia nigra of the male rat. *Neuroscience* 1993; 57:931-941.

149. Janson A, et al. Chronic nicotine treatment counteracts dopamine D2 receptor upregulation induced by a partial meso-diencephalic hemitransection in the rat. *Brain Res* 1994; 655(1–2.:25–32.

150. Prasad C, et al. Chronic nicotine intake decelerates aging of nigrostriatal dopaminergic neurons. *Life Sci* 1994; 54:1169–1184.

151. Ross G, et al. Association of coffee and caffeine intake with the risk of Parkinson disease. *JAMA* 2000; 283(20):2674–2679.

152. Ross G, et al. Lack of association to midlife smoking or coffee consumption with presence of Lewy bodies in the locus ceruleus or substantia nigra at autopsy. *Neurology* 1999; 52(Suppl 2):A539.

153. Willems-Giesbergen P, et al. Smoking, alcohol, and coffee consumption and the risk of PD: Results from the Rotterdam Study. *Neurology* 2000; 54(7 Suppl 3):A347.

154. Benedetti M, et al. Smoking, alcohol, and coffee consumption preceding Parkinson's disease. *Neurology* 2000 (in press).

155. Richardson P, Kase H, Jenner P. Adenosine A2A receptor antagonists as new agents for the treatment of Parkinson's disease. *Trends Pharmacol Sci* 1997; 18:338–344.

156. Todes CJ, Lees AJ. The pre-morbid personality of patients with Parkinson's disease. *J Neurol Neurosurg Psychiatry* 1985; 48:97–100.

157. Jimenez-Jimenez F, Mateo D, Gimenez-Roldan S. Premorbid smoking, alcohol, consumption, and coffee drinking habits in Parkinson's disease: A case-control study. *Mov Disord* 1992; 7:339–344.

158. Hellenbrand W, et al. Diet and Parkinson's disease. II: A possible role for the past intake of specific nutrients. Results from a self-administered food-frequency questionnaire in a case-control study [see comments]. *Neurology* 1996; 47(3):644–650.

159. Baumann RJ, et al. Cigarette smoking and Parkinson's disease: I. A comparison of cases with matched neighbors. *Neurology* 1980; 30:839–843.

160. Lang AE, et al. Early onset of the "on-off" phenomenon in children with symptomatic Parkinsonism. *J Neurol Neurosurg Psychiatry* 1982; 45:823–825.

161. Bharucha NE, et al. A case-control study of twin pairs discordant for Parkinson's disease: A search for environmental risk factors. *Neurology* 1986; 36:284–288.

162. Hellenbrand W, et al. Diet and Parkinson's disease. I: A possible role for the past intake of specific foods and food groups. Results from a self-administered food- frequency questionnaire in a case-control study. *Neurology* 1996; 47(3):636–643.

163. Logroscino G, et al. Dietary lipids and antioxidants in Parkinson's disease: A population-based, case-control study. *Ann Neurol* 1996; 39:89–94.

164. Anderson KC, et al. Dietary factors in Parkinson's disease: The role of food groups and specific foods. *Mov Disord* 1999; 14(1):21–27.

165. Morens DM, et al. Case-control study of idiopathic Parkinson's disease and dietary vitamin E intake. *Neurology* 1996; 46:1270–1274.

166. Tanner CM. The role of environmental toxins in the etiology of Parkinson's disease. *TINS* 1989; 12:49–54.

167. Logroscino G, Mayeux R. Diet and Parkinson's disease [letter; comment]. *Neurology* 1997; 49(1):310–311.

168. Elizan TS, Casals J. The viral hypothesis in Parkinson's disease and Alzheimer's disease: A critique. New York. 1987; (47–59).

169. Marttila RJ, et al. Viral antibodies in the sera from patients with Parkinson's disease. *Eur Neurol* 1977; 15:25–33.

170. Wang W, et al. A case-control study on the environmental risk factors of Parkinson's disease in Tianjin, China. *Neuroepidemiology* 1993; 12:209–218.

171. Hubble JP, et al. *Nocardia* species as an etiologic agent in Parkinson's disease: Serological testing in a case-control study. *J Clin Microbiol* 1995; 33(10):2768–2769.

172. Mattock C, Marmot MG, Stern GM. Could Parkinson's disease follow intra-uterine influenza – a speculative hypothesis? *J Neurol Neurosurg Psychiatry* 1988; 51:753–756.

173. Ebmeier K, et al. Does idiopathic Parkinsonism in Aberdeen follow intrauterine influenza? *J Neurol Neurosurg Psychiatry* 1989; 52:911–913.

174. Fazzini E, Fleming J, Fahn S. Cerebrospinal fluid antibodies to coronaviruses in patients with Parkinson's disease. *Neurology* 1990; 40 (Suppl 1):169.

175. Hubble J, et al. *Nocardia* serology in Parkinson's disease. *Mov Disord* 1992; 7:292.

176. Kohbata S, Shimokawa K. Circulating antibody to *Nocardia* in the serum of patients with Parkinson's disease. *Adv Neurol* 1993; 60:355–357.

177. Kohbata S, Beaman BL. L-dopa-responsive movement disorder caused by *Nocardia* asteroids localized in the brains of mice. *Infect Immun* 1991; 59:181–191.

178. Beaman BL. *Nocardia* as a pathogen of the brain: Mechanisms of interactions in the murine brain – A review. *Gene* 1992; 115:213–217.

179. Martyn C, Osmond C. Parkinson's disease and the environment in early life. *J Neurol Sci* 1995; 132:201–206.

180. Sasco AJ, Paffenbarger JRS. Measles infection and Parkinson's disease. *Am J Epidemiol* 1985; 122:1017–1031.

181. Tanner CM, et al. Environmental factors in the etiology of Parkinson's disease. *Can J Neurol Sci* 1987; 14:419–423.

182. Stern MB. Head trauma as a risk factor for Parkinson's disease. *Mov Disord* 1991; 6(2):95–97.

182a. Factor SA, Weiner WJ. Prior history of head trauma in Parkinson's disease. *Mov Disord* 1991; 6:225–229.

183. Van Den Eeden S, et al. The risk of Parkinson's disease associated with head injury and depression: A population-based case-control study. *Neurology* 2000; 54(7)(Suppl 3):A347.

184. Rajput A, et al. Epidemiology of Parkinsonism. Incidence, classification and mortality. *Ann Neurol* 1984; 16:278–282.

185. Gibberd FB, Simmonds JP. Neurological disease in exDFar-East prisoners of war. *Lancet* 1980; 2:135–137.

186. Treves TA. Parkinson's disease mortality: Preliminary report. *Adv Neurol* 1990; 53:411–415.

187. Page W, Tanner C. Parkinson's disease and motorneuron disease in former prisoners-of-war. *Lancet* 2000; 355(9206):843.

188. Spina MB, Cohen G. Dopamine turnover and glutathione oxidation: Implications for Parkinson disease. *Proc Nat Acad Sci USA* 1989; 86:1398–1400.

189. Paulson G, Dadmehr N. Is there a premorbid personality typical for Parkinson's disease? *Neurology* 1991; 41(Suppl 2):73–76.

190. Menza MA, Robertson-Hoffman DE, Bonapace AS. Parkinson's disease and anxiety: Comorbidity with depression. *Biological Psychiatry* 1993; 34:465–470.

191. Hubble J, Venkatesh R, Hassanein R, et al. Personality and depression in Parkinson's disease. *J Nerv Ment Dis* 1993; 181:657–662.

28

Pathogenesis: Oxidative Stress, Mitochondrial Dysfunction, and Excitotoxicity

David K. Simon, M.D., Ph.D.

Beth Israel Deaconess Medical Center, Boston, Massachusetts

and

M. Flint Beal, M.D.

Massachusetts General Hospital, Boston, Massachusetts

Parkinson's disease (PD) is associated with progressive loss of neurons in the substantia nigra (SN). Numerous agents effective in treating the symptoms of PD are available, but no agent has yet been definitively shown to slow the progression of the underlying disease. However, an expanding knowledge of the basic mechanisms of neuronal death in PD is guiding the emergence of potential neuroprotective strategies. A great deal of recent research has focused on the interrelated mechanisms of oxidative stress, mitochondrial dysfunction, and excitotoxicity.

THE OXIDATIVE STRESS HYPOTHESIS

Oxidative stress due to increased exposure to, or increased susceptibility to, free radicals is hypothesized to play a significant role in the pathogenesis of PD (1,2). Oxidative stress refers to the production of free radicals capable of damaging DNA, proteins, or lipids. Free radicals are molecules containing one or more unpaired electrons, such as superoxide ($\cdot O_2^-$), hydroxyl ($\cdot OH$), and nitric oxide ($NO\cdot$). Free radicals are highly reactive and induce oxidative damage to neighboring molecules by extracting electrons. The major intracellular site of free radical generation is the mitochondria, where oxidative phosphorylation occurs in association with ATP production (3). Oxidative phosphorylation is the transfer of electrons to oxygen via the electron transport chain of the inner mitochondrial

membrane. The electron transport chain consists of five multisubunit complexes (I–V). Impaired function of the electron transport chain results in increased free radical generation and thus causes oxidative stress (4–9). This chapter outlines the evidence for a role for oxidative stress, mitochondrial dysfunction, and excitotoxicity in the pathogenesis of PD.

MARKERS OF OXIDATIVE DAMAGE IN PARKINSON'S DISEASE

Direct evidence of oxidative stress in PD patients comes from analyses of levels of biochemical markers for oxidative damage in postmortem brains. Postmortem analyses of PD SN reveal increased levels of malondialdehyde and other markers of oxidative damage to lipids (10–12). The increase in oxidative damage to lipids in the substantia nigra occurs within pigmented neurons, based on increased immunostaining for 4-hydroxynonenal (10), a marker of membrane lipid peroxidation (13). PD brains also have elevated levels of oxidative damage to proteins, based on a diffusely distributed increase in protein carbonyls (14) and an increase in nitrotyrosine within melanized neurons in the SN (15). Oxidative damage to DNA also has been identified in the SN of PD patients in studies of postmortem tissue (16). In vivo studies of PD patients have yielded variable results. Ahlskog et al. (17) found no increase in malondialdehyde in plasma of PD patients.

In contrast, C. Mariani et al. (18) found increased lipid peroxidation in platelets of PD patients, which indicated the presence of systemic oxidative damage. T. Ilic et al. (19) recently reported that, compared with controls, the cerebrospinal fluid concentrations of malondialdehyde in PD patients is elevated more than fivefold, although this finding remains to be confirmed.

Several factors contribute to an increase in oxidative damage in PD. These include dysfunction of the mitochondrial electron transport chain, impaired antioxidant mechanisms, increased exposure to environmental or endogenous sources of oxidative stress, and excitotoxicity. These mechanisms are outlined in this chapter.

IMPAIRED ENERGY METABOLISM IN PARKINSON'S DISEASE

Functional Imaging Reveals Defects in Energy Metabolism in Parkinson's Disease

Imaging studies reveal impaired energy metabolism in the brains of PD patients. [18F]fluorodeoxyglucose positron emission tomography (^{18}F-FDG/PET) reveals decreased glucose utilization in the cortex (20) and basal ganglia (21,22). In addition, increased lactate has been demonstrated in the occipital cortex (23) and striatum (24) of PD patients using proton magnetic resonance spectroscopy.

Complex I Defects

The activity of complex I of the mitochondrial electron transport chain decreases with age (24,25). However, in PD patients, complex I activity is decreased in the brain to a greater extent than that accounted for by normal aging (26–30). Most studies also find a decrease in complex I activity in platelets (31–35) suggesting a systemic defect, although this finding has not been consistent in all studies (29,36). In the brain, the decrease in complex I activity is specific for the substantia nigra (28,29). Reports of complex I activities in muscle (37) and lymphocytes (32,38,39) of PD patients have been variable. Multiple system atrophy patients, who also develop degeneration of the substantia nigra, have normal complex I activity, suggesting that the decrease in PD patients is not a nonspecific secondary consequence of neurodegeneration (28,34). The complex I defect is not secondary to levodopa therapy, as it does not correlate with levodopa dosage and is absent in multiple system atrophy patients taking levodopa (28,34). This is confirmed by the presence of decreased complex I

activity in platelets of early PD patients who had never been treated with levodopa (35).

The finding of a complex I defect raises the question of whether dysfunction of the mitochondrial electron transport chain plays a causal role in PD. In support of this hypothesis, the mitochondrial toxin 1-methyl-4-phenyl-1,2,3,6-tetrahydropyridine (MPTP) inhibits complex I and induces clinical and pathologic features similar to those of PD when it is systemically administered to man or nonhuman primates (40). This suggests that complex I deficiency can be a primary cause of neuronal degeneration. However, doubts as to the mechanism of MPTP toxicity have been raised by the finding of MPP+ (the toxic metabolite of MPTP) toxicity in "Rho-0" cells, which are mutant cells lacking mitochondrial electron transport activity (41). Furthermore, in addition to its inhibition of complex I, MPTP also inhibits alpha-ketoglutarate dehydrogenase (KGDH) (42). KGDH catalyzes the rate-limiting step in the Krebs cycle (43). Immunohistochemical staining of KGDH is decreased in postmortem PD substantia nigra (44), and a polymorphism in a the E2 subunit of KGDH occurs at increased frequency in PD patients (45). Thus, the relative roles of complex I and KGDH inhibition in MPTP toxicity and in PD remain uncertain. A recent report indicates that chronic infusion of low-dose rotenone, a specific inhibitor of complex I, like MPTP, can reproduce a PD-like syndrome in rats (46). The demonstration of two distinct complex I inhibitors both of which induce a Parkinsonian syndrome emphasizes the importance of further investigation of complex I dysfunction as a potential pathogenic mechanism in PD.

Consequences of Complex I Dysfunction

Complex I inhibition probably results in oxidative stress because of impaired energy metabolism (Figure 28-1) (8,9). Systemic administration of MPTP or intrastriatal injection of MPP+ results in depletion of striatal ATP (47,48). In vitro studies demonstrate that MPTP induces the production of free radicals including superoxide (4–7). Complex I deficiency also is associated with increased production of free radicals in patients with various clinical syndromes (49). MPTP stimulates increased levels of nitrotyrosine with a time course that parallels MPTP-induced neuronal death, supporting a role for oxidative damage in MPTP toxicity (41). The damage induced by MPTP in the brains of mice that are genetically deficient in mitochondrial superoxide dismutase (MnSOD), an antioxidant enzyme, is greater than that in normal mice (8), whereas mice overexpressing MnSOD show less dam-

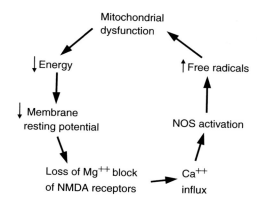

FIGURE 28-1. Cycle of mitochondrial dysfunction and excitotoxicity. Mg^{++} = magnesium. NMDA = N-methyl-D-aspartate. NOS = nitric oxide synthase. Ca^{++} = calcium.

age (50,51). These data suggest that superoxide radical formation plays a key role in MPTP toxicity. The relevance of these data to PD is suggested by studies of "cybrid" cell lines expressing mitochondrial DNA from PD patients. These cell lines exhibit complex I deficiency and show increased susceptibility to MPP+ and increased production of free radicals (52). Thus oxidative stress due to complex I deficiency may play a key role in PD.

Oxidative stress due to mitochondrial dysfunction may lead to cell death by the induction of apoptosis. Apoptotic neurons are reported in some studies to be present at increased frequencies in the substantia nigra of PD patients, although others have not reproduced this finding (53). Opening of the mitochondrial permeability transition pore resulting in loss of the mitochondrial membrane potential is one of the earliest events in apoptosis (54), and this is associated with the release of activators of apoptosis, including apoptosis-inducing factor (AIF) and cytochrome c (55). Thus mitochondrial dysfunction and oxidative stress may be important triggers and mediators of apoptosis in PD (53).

Origin of the Complex I Defect

Both environmental and genetic factors may contribute to the complex I defect in PD patients. The identification of MPTP led to the hypothesis that other MPTP-like toxins may be present in the environment. Several epidemiologic studies have suggested an association between certain environmental factors (for example, rural living) and the risk of PD (see Chapter 28) (56,57). Endogenous MPP+ analogs have been identified in the cerebrospinal fluid of PD patients (56–60), and they can induce Parkinsonism in nonprimate animals (61). Thus environmental and endogenous mitochondrial toxins may partially account for the complex I defect in PD patients.

Genetic factors, both nuclear and mitochondrial, also appear to play a role in the complex I deficiency in PD. A polymorphism in a nuclear-encoded gene for a subunit of complex I (the NDUFV2 gene) was reported to occur at increased frequency in PD patients in a Japanese population, suggesting that it may be a risk factor for PD (62). Recent data suggests that the complex I defect in PD patients is at least partially accounted for by mutations in mitochondrial DNA (mtDNA). In these studies, platelet mtDNA was transferred from PD patients (or controls) to cell lines devoid of endogenous mtDNA to create "cybrids" (cytoplasmic hybrids), and this resulted in the transfer of complex I deficiency to the cybrids, indicating that the complex I deficiency in PD patients results from mtDNA mutations (52,63).

Attempts to identify the specific mutations have been inconclusive (64,65). A study of the mitochondrial genome sequence in five PD patients revealed several missense mutations, but each either involved a nonconserved amino acid or was also identified in a control patient, making the association of these variants with PD uncertain (66). Reports of a link between PD and a mitochondrial transfer RNA polymorphism (at nucleotide position 4336) (67) or a mtDNA deletion (68) could not be replicated by others (69,70). A recent study of complex 1 and tRNA genes in PD patients failed to reveal significant mtDNA mutations in the majority of patients (70a).

It remains unclear if the putative mutations are acquired or inherited. A tendency towards maternal inheritance would be predicted if inherited mtDNA mutations play a major role in PD. Evidence for maternal inheritance has been reported in PD (71), although this remains a controversial issue (72). A family with atypical Parkinsonism and neuronal loss in the substantia nigra was recently found to harbor a missense mtDNA mutation at position 11778 of the ND4 subunit of complex I (72a). The same mutation was earlier identified as the most common cause of Lebers hereditary optic neuropathy (LHON) (73), although this family lacked clinical features of LHON. Although the disorder in this family is distinct from idiopathic PD, this finding demonstrates that a specific inherited mtDNA mutation can cause parkinsonism and substantia nigra neuronal death.

OTHER POTENTIAL SOURCES OF OXIDATIVE STRESS

MAO-b

Complex I deficiency probably results in increased free radical production. Other mechanisms may also contribute to oxidative stress in PD. Dopamine metabolism by monoamine oxidase B (MAO-b) is associated with the generation of hydrogen peroxide (H_2O_2), which normally is inactivated in a reaction with glutathione. However, if excess H_2O_2 reacts in a "Fenton reaction" with ferrous iron, a highly reactive hydroxyl radical (·OH) is produced, which is capable of initiating damaging lipid peroxidation (Figure 28-2) (1). Therefore, inhibition of MAO-b, might prevent oxidative stress associated with dopamine metabolism. MAO-b activity is also required to convert MPTP to MPP^+, its active metabolite (74). Thus, inhibition of MAO-b may also prevent the activation of endogenous or environmental MPTP-like compounds (58–60). A number of studies in vitro and in animal models of PD provide evidence of neuroprotection against MPTP or other toxins by the MAO-b inhibitor deprenyl (selegiline) (75). The possibility that MAO-b might be important in PD is supported by findings of an association of MAO-b gene polymorphisms and PD (76–78), although not all studies find this association (79,80). Furthermore, inhibition of MAO-b is hypothesized to account for the apparent "protective" effect of tobacco smoking on PD risk (81), although other explanations for the inverse association of smoking and PD have been suggested (82) (see Chapter 46).

A large, multicenter, placebo-controlled clinical trial(Deprenyl and Tocopherol Antioxidant Therapy of Parkinsonism, or "DATATOP") was conducted to determine if deprenyl could slow disease progression in early PD patients (83–85). Although deprenyl clearly exerted a symptomatic effect, a clear effect on disease progression could not be demonstrated. A second smaller study by Olanow et al. (86) reported sustained benefits from deprenyl even after a two-month wash-out period. The question of whether deprenyl has any truly "protective" effects remains controversial, but it

- DA $\xrightarrow{\text{MAO-b}}$ DOPAC + NH_3 + H_2O_2

- H_2O_2 $\xrightarrow{\text{Fe}^{2+}}$ OH^- + ·OH

- H_2O_2 $\xrightarrow{\text{GSH-Px}}$ H_2O + O_2

- NO· + ·$O2^-$ $\longrightarrow$ $ONOO^-$ + H+ $\longrightarrow$ NO_2· + ·OH

FIGURE 28-2. Multiple factors contribute to oxidative stress and excitotoxicity in PD. Abbreviations: DA = dopamine. MAO-b = monoamine oxidase type b. DOPAC = 3, 4-dihydroxyphenylacetic acid. NH_3 = ammonia. H_2O_2 = hydrogen peroxide. Fe^{2+} = iron. OH− = hydroxyl anion. ·OH = hydroxyl radical. GSH-Px = glutathione peroxidase. NO· = nitric oxide. ·O2− = superoxide radical. ONOO− = peroxynitrite. NO_2· = nitrogen dioxide.

is clear that if there is an effect, the magnitude is modest at best.

Iron

Iron can act as a catalyst in the formation of hydroxyl radicals from hydrogen peroxide (87). Several studies have demonstrated increased amounts of iron (88–91) and decreased ferritin (92) in the brain of PD patients. Ferritin binding of iron renders it incapable of catalyzing oxidative reactions. Therefore the finding of decreased ferritin in PD suggests that the iron may be present in its reactive form. However, the finding of increased iron accumulation in the substantia nigra of 6-hydroxydopamine-treated rats (93) and in MPTP-treated monkeys (94) indicates that iron can accumulate secondarily rather than as a primary cause of PD. This does not rule out the possibility that increased iron content in the substantia nigra of PD patients can contribute to disease progression secondarily by increasing oxidative stress.

Antioxidant Mechanisms

In addition to increased *exposure* to free radicals due to mitochondrial dysfunction, dopamine metabolism, and increased iron content, neurons in the substantia nigra may have increased *susceptibility* to oxidative stress. Glutathione is an important antioxidant that can detoxify hydrogen peroxide, preventing the formation of hydroxyl radicals. Levels of reduced glutathione are decreased in the substantia nigra of PD patients (90,95,96). A depletion of glutathione may be secondary to excessive production of hydrogen peroxide in the mitochondria and result in a predisposition to further oxidative damage (97). Glutathione depletion in newborn rats results in abnormal mitochondrial ultrastructure and decreased activity of mitochondrial enzymes (98). Glutathione depletion in PCIZ cells specifically impairs complex I activity (98a). Therefore glutathione depletion may predispose to free radical-induced mitochondrial damage in the substantia nigra of PD patients. There is evidence to suggest that glutathione depletion may occur early, possibly first in the cascade of events (98b).

Impaired antioxidant mechanisms may be important in the pathogenesis of PD in patients carrying the alpha-synuclein mutation that has been recently identified in a family with PD (99). Expression of mutant alpha-synuclein is associated with a threefold increase in susceptibility to free radicals compared with cells expressing wild-type alpha-synuclein (100). Susceptibility was not increased to several other toxic stimuli, suggesting that the alpha-synuclein mutation is associated with a specific vulnerability to oxidative stress.

EXCITOTOXICITY

Mitochondrial Dysfunction and Excitotoxicity

Glutamate is a prominent excitatory neurotransmitter in the brain. However, excessive glutamate exposure can be toxic to neurons (101). A form of "weak excitotoxicity" has been proposed as a potential mechanism in late-onset neurodegenerative diseases (2,102). At normal resting potential, calcium influx through NMDA receptor channels is blocked by magnesium. Maintenance of this resting potential is energy-dependent. Defects in energy metabolism may therefore lead to reduction in the membrane potential resulting in calcium influx due to loss of the voltage-dependent magnesium blockade of NMDA receptor channels (Figure 28-1). Calcium influx through these channels may then reach a sufficient concentration to induce mitochondrial generation of free radicals (103). Increased intracellular calcium also activates nitric oxide synthase (NOS) (104). This results in increased production of nitric oxide (NO·) and superoxide radicals ($O_2 \cdot ^-$), which can then react to form peroxynitrate ($ONOO^-$) (Figure 28-2) (105,106). Peroxynitrite can mediate oxidative damage to proteins, lipids, or DNA and can break down to form highly reactive hydroxyl radicals (OH·). Thus excitotoxicity can lead to an increase in oxidative stress and mitochondrial damage.

Mitochondrial dysfunction, in turn, can result in an increased susceptibility to excitotoxicity. Intracellular energy depletion in cultured rat cerebellar neurons by omission of glucose or oxygen, or inhibition of oxidative phosphorylation or sodium-potassium ATPase activity results in an increased sensitivity to excitotoxic damage from glutamate exposure (107). Cyanide (a complex IV inhibitor) also increases susceptibility of cultured retinal (108), hippocampal, or cortical (109) cells to excitotoxicity. A cycle of mitochondrial damage resulting in impaired energy metabolism c, which causes increased susceptibility to excitotoxicity, which then induces further mitochondrial damage can be envisioned (Figure 28-1).

Another consequence of calcium sequestration by the mitochondria is the opening of the permeability transition pore complex, resulting in the release of cytochrome c and other apoptosis inducing factors (53). Inhibition of mitochondrial calcium uptake reduces glutamate-induced cell death despite enhancement of glutamate-stimulated increases in intracellular calcium concentrations (110). Thus the toxicity of glutamate-induced increases in intracellular calcium depends on calcium sequestration in the mitochondria. The potential importance of this mechanism in PD is highlighted by the finding of impaired calcium buffering by mitochondria in PD cybrids (111).

Excitotoxicity in Parkinson's Disease

Mitochondrial dysfunction is a well-established feature in the substantia nigra of PD patients, and this may lead to enhanced sensitivity to excitotoxicity in PD, which could contribute to disease progression. Substantia nigra neurons contain NMDA receptors (112) and receive excitatory (glutamate) input from the subthalamic nucleus. As substantia nigra neurons are lost, disinhibition of the subthalamic nucleus may induce further excitotoxic damage in the substantia nigra, contributing to the ongoing loss of nigral neurons (113).

There is little direct evidence of excitotoxicity in PD. MPTP toxicity may in part reflect excitotoxic mechanisms. MPTP induces increased glutamate release (114) and decreased glutamate uptake by glial cells (115). Some studies have found protection in vitro and in vivo against MPTP toxicity using NMDA receptor antagonists, but this remains a controversial issue (116). Riluzole, which blocks glutamate release, protects against MPTP toxicity in rodents (117,118) and primates (119,120), although the precise mechanism of action of riluzole remains uncertain (121). NOS inhibitors protect against MPTP toxicity in mice (122) and baboons(123). Substantia nigra neurons of mice lacking the neuronal NOS gene are resistant to MPP^+-induced toxicity (124). Thus excitotoxicity and NO-mediated toxicity may be important in the mechanism of MPTP-induced neuronal death. Direct evidence that these mechanisms play a role in PD remains to be demonstrated.

CONCLUSIONS

A growing body of evidence indicates a central role for mitochondrial dysfunction and the related mechanisms of oxidative stress and excitotoxicity in the pathogenesis of PD. Patients with PD have decreased complex I activity in the substantia nigra. Toxins that inhibit mitochondrial complex I induce a parkinsonian syndrome in humans and experimental animals. Markers of oxidative stress are elevated in the PD brain. Several strategies to block oxidative stress and excitotoxicity are effective in animal models of PD. However, effective neuroprotective strategies in PD patients remain elusive (see Chapter 43). PD clearly is a complex multifactorial disorder. An individual's susceptibility to developing PD probably involves a combination of nuclear genetic, mitochondrial genetic, and environmental factors (Figure 28-3). A better understanding of these mechanisms will help to guide future attempts to alter the course of this disease.

57. Rajput AH. Environmental causation of Parkinson's disease. *Arch Neurol* 1993; 50:651–652.

58. Moser A, Kompf D. Presence of methyl-6,7-dihydroxy-1,2,3,4-tetrahydroisoquinolines, derivatives of the neurotoxin isoquinoline, in Parkinsonian lumbar CSF. *Life Sci* 1992; 50:1885–1891.

59. Matsubara K, Kobayashi S, Kobayashi Y, et al. beta-Carbolinium cations, endogenous MPP+ analogs, in the lumbar cerebrospinal fluid of patients with Parkinson's disease. *Neurology* 1995; 45:2240–2245.

60. Hao R, Norgren RB, Jr., Lau YS, et al. Cerebrospinal fluid of Parkinson's disease patients inhibits the growth and function of dopaminergic neurons in culture. *Neurology* 1995; 45:138–142.

61. Matsubara K, Gonda T, Sawada H, et al. Endogenously occurring beta-carboline induces Parkinsonism in nonprimate animals: A possible causative protoxin in idiopathic Parkinson's disease. *J Neurochem* 1998; 70:727–735.

62. Hattori N, Yoshino H, Yanaka M, et al. Genotype in the 24-kDa subunit gene (NDUFV2) of mitochondrial complex I and susceptibility to Parkinson disease. *Genomics* 1998; 49:52–58.

63. Gu M, Cooper JM, Taanman JW, et al. Mitochondrial DNA transmission of the mitochondrial defect in Parkinson's disease. *Ann Neurol* 1998; 44:177–186.

64. Parker WD, Jr. Mitochondrial genetics '98: Mitochondrial dysfunction in idiopathic Parkinson disease. *Am J Hum Genet* 1998; 62:758–762.

65. Bandemann O, Marsden CD, Wood NW. Genetic aspects of Parkinson's disease. *Mov Disord* 1998; 13:203–211.

66. Ikebe S-i, Tanaka M, Ozawa T. Point mutations of mitochondrial genome in Parkinson's disease. *Mol Brain Res* 1995; 28:281–295.

67. Shoffner JM, Brown MD, Torroni A, et al. Mitochondrial DNA variants observed in Alzheimer disease and Parkinson disease patients. *Genomics* 1993; 17:171–184.

68. Ikebe S, Tanaka M, Ohno K, et al. Increase of deleted mitochondrial DNA in the striatum in Parkinson's disease and senescence. *Biochem Biophys Res Commun* 1990; 170:1044–1048.

69. Mayr-Wohlfart U, Rodel G, Henneberg A. Mitochondrial tRNA(Gln) and tRNA(Thr) gene variants in Parkinson's disease. *Eur J Med Res* 1997; 2:111–113.

70. Bandmann O, Sweeney MG, Daniel SE, et al. Mitochondrial DNA polymorphisms in pathologically proven Parkinson's disease. *J Neurol* 1997; 244:262–265.

70a. Simon DK, Mayeux R, Marder K, et al. Mitochondrial DNA mutations in complex I and tRNA genes in parkinson's disease, *Neurology* 2000; 54:703–709.

71. Wooten GF, Currie LJ, Bennett JP, et al. Maternal inheritance in Parkinson's disease. *Ann Neurol* 1997; 41:265–268.

72. Duvoisin RC. Role of genetics in the cause of Parkinson's disease. *Mov Disord* 1998; 13:7–12.

72a. Simon DK, Pulst SM, Sutton JP et al. Familial multisystem degeneration with parkinsonism associated with the 11778 mitochondrial DNA mutation. *Neurology* 1999; 53:1787–1793.

73. Wallace DC, Singh G, Lott MT, et al. Mitochondrial DNA mutation associated with Leber's hereditary optic neuropathy. *Science* 1988; 242:1427–1430.

74. Singer TP, Castagnoli N, Jr., Ramsay RR, et al. Biochemical events in the development of Parkinsonism induced by 1-methyl-4-phenyl-1,2,3,6-tetrahydropyridine. *J Neurochem* 1987; 49:1–8.

75. Gerlach M, Youdim MB, Riederer P. Pharmacology of selegiline. *Neurology* 1996; 47:S137–S145.

76. Kurth JH, Kurth MC, Poluslo SE, et al. Association of a monoamine oxidase B allele with Parkinson's disease. *Ann Neurol* 1993; 33:368–372.

77. Hotamisligil GS, Girmen AS, Fink JS, et al. Hereditary variations in monoamine oxidase as a risk factor for Parkinson's disease. *Mov Disord* 1994; 9:305–310.

78. Costa P, Checkoway H, Levy D, et al. Association of a polymorphism in intron 13 of the monoamine oxidase B gene with Parkinson disease. *Am J Med Genet* 1997; 74:154–156.

79. Ho SL, Kapadi AL, Ransden DB, et al. An allelic association study of monoamine oxidase B in Parkinson's disease. *Ann Neurol* 1995; 37:403–405.

80. Plante-Bordeneuve V, Taussig D, Thomas F, et al. Evaluation of four candidate genes encoding proteins of the dopamine pathway in familial and sporadic Parkinson's disease: Evidence for association of a DRD2 allele. *Neurology* 1997; 48:1589–1593.

81. Fowler JS, Volkow ND, Wang G-J, et al. Inhibition of monoamine oxidase B in the brains of smokers. *Nature* 1996; 379:733–736.

82. Mayeux R, Tang MX, Marder K, et al. Smoking and Parkinson's disease. *Mov Disord* 1994; 9:207–212.

83. Effects of tocopherol and deprenyl on the progression of disability in early Parkinson's disease. The Parkinson Study Group [see comments]. *N Engl J Med* 1993; 328:176–183.

84. Impact of deprenyl and tocopherol treatment on Parkinson's disease in DATATOP subjects not requiring levodopa. Parkinson Study Group [see comments]. *Ann Neurol* 1996; 39:29–36.

85. DATATOP: A multicenter controlled clinical trial in early Parkinson's disease. Parkinson Study Group. *Arch Neurol* 1989; 46:1052–1060.

86. Olanow CW, Hauser RA, Gauger L, et al. The effect of deprenyl and levodopa on the progression of Parkinson's disease [see comments]. *Ann Neurol* 1995; 38:771–777.

87. Olanow CW. An introduction to the free radical hypothesis in Parkinson's disease. *Ann Neurol* 1992; 32:S2–S9.

88. Earl KM. Trace metals in Parkinsonian brains. *J Neuropathol Exp Neruol* 1968; 27:1–14.

attainment of support and result in induced death. This does occur; intrastriatal injection of 6-OHDA in developing animals results in the induction of apoptotic death in dopamine neurons of the SNpc (30). This ability of intrastriatal 6-OHDA to induce apoptotic death, like early target injury, is developmentally dependent, with a major induction of death during the first two postnatal weeks and smaller effects at later postnatal times. Interestingly, at later postnatal times intrastriatal 6-OHDA induces two different morphologies of cell death in the SNpc, apoptotic and nonapoptotic, as demonstrated by suppressed silver staining (30). Although we have emphasized the interpretation that 6-OHDA induces apoptosis in developing animals by interfering with target support, it is also theoretically possible that the toxin itself acts directly to induce apoptosis; 6-OHDA has been shown in vitro to induce apoptosis in (PC12) cells (31).

Another important model of human Parkinsonism is dopamine neuron death induced by the neurotoxin MPTP (1-methyl-4phenyl-1,2,3,6-tetrahydropyridine), which is capable of inducing in humans a clinical syndrome that is virtually indistinguishable from idiopathic Parkinson's disease (32) and a profound loss of dopamine neurons of the SNpc (33) (see Chapter 30). Administration of MPTP to primates (34) or mice (35) similarly results in a loss of dopamine neurons and a reduction in biochemical markers for these neurons in both SNpc and striatum. A number of investigators have shown that MPP+ (the active metabolite of MPTP) can induce apoptosis in vitro. B. Dipasquale and colleagues first showed that MPP+ can induce apoptotic morphology and DNA fragmentation in postnatal cerebellar granule cells in culture (36). Subsequently, others have shown that MPP+ induces apoptosis in embryonic mesencephalon culture (37); in PC12 cells, both differentiated (38) and undifferentiated (39); and in a human neuroblastoma cell line (40). In the first study of MPTP in a living mouse model, apoptotic cell death was not observed in SN by either silver staining or end-labeling techniques at any point of time following injection of any of three doses – 80, 60, or 40 mg/kg (41). This study was performed in an acute MPTP model in which the drug was given in four separate doses and administered every two hours. Subsequently, Tatton and Kish demonstrated apoptosis in phenotypically defined dopamine neurons in a chronic model in which MPTP was administered as 30 mg/kg each day for five days (42). The possibility that cell death in the MPTP model may be mediated by the mechanisms of PCD is also suggested by the demonstration that MPTP treatment of mice induces an increase in Bax mRNA and Bax protein immunoreactivity in SN neurons (43).

Bax, a protein homologue of Bcl-2, is capable of heterodimerizing with Bcl-2 and mediating apoptotic cell death (44). Additional evidence for a possible role for PCD in the MPTP model is that mice containing a null mutation for the tumor suppressor gene *p53* appear to be relatively resistant to dopamine neuron loss (45). In a number of models, *p53* has been shown to participate in PCD. (46–47)

MOLECULAR CORRELATES OF APOPTOSIS IN SNPC NEURONS

Much remains to be known of the molecular basis of PCD in defined dopamine neurons of the SNpc in living brain. To study this process, we can be guided by the rapid advances being made in our understanding of PCD in simpler in vitro systems, both neural and nonneural. The molecular events underlying PCD are conceptualized as occurring in three phases: an initial signaling phase, an effector or execution phase, and a late phase in which the cell and its constituents undergo the structural alterations characteristic of apoptosis (48). In relation to the initial signaling phase, the transcription factor c-jun has been proposed to play a role. In an in vitro model of apoptotic death in sympathetic neurons induced by NGF withdrawal, c-jun mRNA expression was increased and neurons were protected from death by intracellular microinjection of neutralizing antibodies to c-jun (49). In the same model, other investigators have shown that NGF withdrawal induced increased levels of c-jun protein and c-jun phosphorylation (50). These investigators showed that transfection with a dominant negative mutant of c-jun protected neurons from apoptotic death. Expression of c-jun has also been observed during PCD in living animals, in cerebellar neurons undergoing apoptotic death following exposure to ionizing radiation (51), and during natural cell death in brain (52).

Phosphorylation of c-jun at Ser63 and Ser73 results in increased transcriptional activation (53). This phosphorylation is mediated by c-jun N-terminal kinase (JNK) (also known as stress-activated protein kinase, or SAPK) (53). JNK is a member of the mitogen-activated protein kinase (MAPKs) family of kinases, which includes p38 MAP and the ERKs (53). JNK and p38 have both been implicated in mediating PCD in PC12 cells following NGF withdrawal, and their action opposes the ERKs (54). The role of JNK in PCD in PC12 cells was confirmed by Park et al., who also demonstrated that JNK activation occurs either upstream to or in an independent path relative to activation of the caspases (55). JNK activation is likely to be a common mediator of PCD in neural cells because it is also upregulated in sympathetic ganglia following NGF withdrawal (56–58). In the study by Deckwerth et al., it was proposed to be upstream to activation of the caspases (58). These investigators also showed that induction of death is accompanied by phosphorylation of c-jun on Ser63.

Relatively little is known about expression of JNK and c-jun phosphorylation in living animal models of PCD. In an adult ischemia model, Herdegen and colleagues have shown that Ser73-phosphorylated c-jun is induced following injury and that this labeling in some instances colocalizes at a cellular level with TUNEL (59). In the target-injury model of induced death in SNpc, we have shown that the occurrence of PCD in the model correlates regionally and temporally with protein expression of c-jun, Ser63-phosphorylated c-jun, and JNK. Cellular colocalization of JNK protein expression with apoptotic morphology (60) has been demonstrated. Thus data suggests an important role for JNK and c-jun as initiators of PCD in SN neurons. However, studies thus far in the target-injury model have only been correlational, and a functional analysis will be required.

Many important new insights into the molecular mechanisms of PCD have been derived from studies of developmental cell death in the nematode *C. elegans* (1). One of the genes necessary for cell death in this organism is *ced-3* (1), which is homologous to mammalian (ICE), a cysteine protease (61). Other aspartate-specific cysteine proteases (caspases) have been subsequently identified (14,62). Evidence implicating these proteases in PCD includes observations that their ectopic expression in cell lines induces apoptotic death (63) and that their inhibition either by viral proteins, such as CrmA (64,65) or by specific peptide inhibitors based on the cleavage site, such as YVAD (65,66) inhibits apoptotic death. All of the caspases are synthesized in a proenzyme form, which is cleaved at an aspartate to yield a larger (p17–p20) and a smaller subunit (p10–p12), which heterodimerize to form an active enzyme form. Among the caspases, caspase-3(CPP32/Yama/Apopain) (64,67,68) is of particular interest in relation to neuronal death. It is activated in vitro upon induction of PCD in postnatal cerebellar granule neurons (69,70) and embryonic mouse neurons (71). Strong evidence for a role for caspase-3 in mediating developmental neuronal death in vivo is derived from observations made in knockout mice, which demonstrate hyperplastic brains due to supernumerary cells (16). There is also evidence of caspase-3 activation in vivo in models of induced retinal ganglion cell death following axotomy (72) and acute brain injury either due to trauma (73) or

due to stroke (74,75). It has been shown that the activated form of caspase-3 is expressed in apoptotic neurons in the SN during natural cell death and in death induced either by early target or by terminal injury (17). However, this was strictly a correlational study, and a functional analysis will be required.

APOPTOSIS IN PARKINSON'S DISEASE: DOES IT PLAY A ROLE IN NEURON DEATH?

There have been a number of reports of evidence for apoptotic cell death in the SN in postmortem PD brain. One report identified possible apoptotic profiles by electron microscopy in the SN of three patients (76). In this report, electron-dense intranuclear aggregates were identified, but there has been concern that the characteristic features of apoptotic chromatin clumps, that is, a uniform increase in electron density with sharply delineated edges (9), were not clearly identified. In addition, observations were not made in controls, so the pathologic significance of the findings was not clear. Nevertheless, although apoptotic morphology was not definitively demonstrated, some of the morphologic findings, such as relative preservation of mitochondria and cellular membranes, may be compatible with other morphologies of PCD. Another report identified positive TUNEL labeling in the SN of four of seven patients with typical late-onset PD (77). Although this report clearly demonstrated free 3'-end labeling in neurons of the SN, it was not clear that the morphology was apoptotic. The potential problem of false-positive TUNEL labeling can be excluded only by a clear definition of apoptotic morphology. A study by Tompkins et al. examined postmortem brain tissue from patients with Alzheimer's disease, PD, and diffuse Lewy body disease (DLBD) in comparison to neurologically normal controls, using in situ end-labeling, propidium iodide nuclear staining, and ultrastructural analysis (78). Some of the micrographs, particularly some representing a case of DLBD, clearly show in situ end-labeling with apoptotic morphology in neuromelanin-containing neurons of the SNpc. Thus this study presents clear evidence of apoptotic morphology in neurons in a degenerative disorder related to PD. In addition, these authors present evidence for the presence of apoptotic bodies, identified by ultrastructural analysis, in the SNpc of patients with PD and DLBD (78). Similar evidence has been presented by Tatton et al. by using a fluorescent double-labeling technique and confocal microscopy to demonstrate both DNA fragmentation and apoptotic morphology in neuromelanin-bearing neurons of the SN in PD patients, thus fulfilling the most rigorous criteria for demonstration of apoptosis (79).

However, not all studies have been positive. Kosel et al. (80) examined the brains of 22 pathologically confirmed cases of PD using in situ end-labeling and did not identify definitive apoptotic morphology in a single neuron. Approximately 80 neurons per brain were examined. Some end-labeling was observed in glia in about 50% of PD patients, and a reticular labeling pattern was observed in some neurons, but none showed definitive apoptotic morphology (80). Banati and colleagues examined 10 patients with proven PD, using TUNEL labeling (81). No evidence of apoptotic neuronal death was observed in the SN of any of these patients.

Thus, there is mixed evidence on whether apoptotic morphology can be identified in the brains of patients with PD or related disorders. In evaluating this evidence, it is important to keep several points in mind. First, PD and the related disorders are caused because of neuronal degeneration that takes place over years. In all of the experimental models studied to date, apoptotic cell death takes place within a brief period of time. Thus, it may be exceedingly difficult to identify this morphology in a chronic, degenerative disease. Second, it is very difficult to perform high-quality ultrastructural studies on human postmortem material because it is impossible to control many variables related to the quality of tissue preservation. Thus it becomes difficult to use the "gold standard" morphologic technique in evaluating human tissue. Third, it is important to recognize that apoptotic morphology is only one of the morphologies of PCD; inability to identify its features does not definitively exclude a possible role for PCD, defined in the broadest sense as a genetically regulated form of cell death. What is clearly needed are better biochemical markers for the PCD process and reagents to identify those markers. For example it may be very informative to investigate the expression of the caspases in PD and related disorders.

RELEVANCE OF APOPTOSIS TO OTHER ASPECTS OF PARKINSON'S DISEASE

Whether or not PCD is determined to play a direct role, or even a secondary role, in the neuron death of PD, it may be relevant to other aspects of the pathogenesis and treatment. For example, a new approach to the treatment of PD is that of transplantation of fetal mesencephalic dopaminergic neurons (82). Although preliminary clinical results support transplantation

as a promising approach, very few transplanted dopaminergic neurons survive (83). Although it has been assumed in the past that the death of implanted cells is mediated by exogenous factors such as tissue handling, local trauma, or the lack of a vascular supply, it has been shown that implanted mesencephalic tissue undergoes apoptotic cell death (84,85). Such findings would suggest that if the factors that regulate natural cell death in the SN can be identified, they could then be used to augment cell survival in transplants.

PCD may also be relevant to the effects of chronic levodopa treatment on the Parkinson brain. The subject is quite controversial, but there is some clinical evidence suggesting that levodopa may aggravate some aspects of PD. On theoretical grounds, if the metabolism of dopamine leads to oxidative stress, augmentation of dopamine availability by ingestion of levodopa might be expected to worsen the underlying disease process. It has been shown in vitro that either dopamine or levodopa is capable of inducing apoptosis. Ziv and colleagues have shown that dopamine induces apoptosis in cultured embryonic chick sympathetic neurons (86). Walkinshaw and Waters have demonstrated that levodopa, in micromolar concentrations, induces apoptosis in PC12 cells (87). The relationship between these findings and the human disease remains unclear.

CONCLUSIONS

PCD can occur within dopamine neurons of the SN; it does so during the normal natural cell death of these neurons. There is also no question that PCD can occur in these neurons in pathologic states induced by toxin models of parkinsonism. The likelihood of toxins to induce apoptotic, rather than necrotic, death depends on the age of the animal, the dose, timing, and route of administration. Whether PCD actually occurs within the human Parkinson brain remains controversial, and this possibility has been neither confirmed nor definitively excluded. It is fair to say that we have probably learned as much as we can on the basis of classic morphologic techniques, and what is now required is an investigation of the expression of molecular markers of PCD in parkinson brains. Whether or not PCD is ultimately shown to mediate neuron death in PD it will remain an important process to define for dopamine neurons, because an understanding of this process will aid the development of novel therapeutic methods, including stem cell and neurotrophic factor approaches. Clearly, the more we understand about the factors that control the life and death of dopamine neurons, the better we will be able to protect and sustain them in human disease.

Acknowledgments

The author is supported by grants from the NIH (NS 26836), The Smart Family, and the Lowenstein Foundations. The author would especially wish to acknowledge The Parkinson's Disease Foundation for its loyal support.

REFERENCES

1. Ellis RE, Yuan J, Horvitz HR. Mechanisms and functions of cell death. *Annu Rev of Cell Biol* 1991; 7:663–698.
2. Martin SJ, Green DR. Protease activation during apoptosis: Death by a thousand cuts? *Cell* 1995; 82:349–352.
3. Korsmeyer SJ. Regulators of cell death. *Trends Genet* 1995; 11:101–105.
4. Martin DP, Schmidt RE, DiStefano P, et al. Inhibitors of protein synthesis and RNA synthesis prevent neuronal death caused by nerve growth factor deprivation. *J Cell Biol* 1988; 106:829–844.
5. Oppenheim RW, Prevette D, Tytell M, et al. Naturally occurring and induced neuronal death in the chick embryo in vivo requires protein and RNA synthesis: Evidence for the role of cell death genes. *Dev Biol* 1990; 138:104–113.
6. Kerr JFR, Wyllie AH, Currie AR. Apoptosis: A basic biological phenomenon with wide-ranging implications in tissue kinetics. *Br J Cancer* 1972; 26:239–257.
7. Clarke PGH. Developmental cell death: Morphological diversity and multiple mechanisms. *Anat Embryol* 1990; 181:195–213.
8. Schwartz LM, Smith SW, Jones MEE, et al. Do all programmed cell deaths occur via apoptosis? *Proc Natl Acad Sci USA* 1993; 90:980–984.
9. Kerr JFR, Gobe GC, Winterford CM, et al. Anatomical methods in cell death. In: Schwartz LM, Osborne BA (eds). *Methods in Cell Biology: Cell Death*. New York: Academic Press, 1995:1–27.
10. Clarke PGH, Oppenheim RW. Neuron death in vertebrate development: In vivo methods. In: Schwartz LM, Osborne BA (eds). *Methods in Cell Biology: Cell Death*. New York: Academic Press, 1995:277–321.
11. Janec E, Burke RE. Naturally occurring cell death during postnatal development of the substantia nigra of the rat. *Mol Cell Neurosci* 1993; 4:30–35.
12. Gavrieli Y, Sherman Y, Ben-Sasson SA. Identification of programmed cell death in situ via specific labeling of nuclear DNA fragmentation. *J Cell Biol* 1992; 119:493–501.
13. Grasl-Kraupp B, Ruttkay-Nedecky B, Koudelka H, et al. In situ detection of fragmented DNA (TUNEL assay) fails to discriminate among apoptosis, necrosis, and autolytic cell death: A cautionary note. *Hepatology* 1995; 21:1465–1468.
14. Alnemri ES. Mammalian cell death proteases: A family of highly conserved aspartate-specfic cysteine proteases. *J Cell Biochem* 1997; 64:33–42.
15. Kidd VJ. Proteolytic activities that mediate apoptosis. *Annu Rev Physiol* 1998; 60:533–573.
16. Kuida K, Zheng TS, Na S, et al. Decreased apoptosis in the brain and premature lethality in CPP32-deficient mice. *Nature (London)* 1996; 384:368–372.
17. Jeon BS, Kholodilov NG, Oo TF, et al. Activation of caspase-3 in developmental models of programmed cell death in neurons of the substantia nigra. *J Neurochem* 1999;
18. Srinivasan A, Roth KA, Sayers RO, et al. In situ immunodetection of activated caspase-3 in apoptotic neurons in the developing nervous system. *Cell Death Differ* 1998; 5:1004–1016.
19. Burke RE, Macaya A, DeVivo D, et al. Neonatal hypoxicischemic or excitotoxic striatal injury results in a decreased adult number of substantia nigra neurons. *Neuroscience* 1992; 50:559–569.
20. Macaya A, Burke RE. Effect of striatal lesion with quinolinate on the development of substantia nigra dopaminergic neurons: A quantitative morphological analysis. *Dev Neurosci* 1992; 14:362–368.
21. Prochiantz A, Di Porzio U, Kato A, et al. In vitro maturation of mesencephalic dopaminergic neurons from mouse embryos is enhanced in presence of their striatal target cells. *Proc Natl Acad Sci USA* 1979; 76:5387–5391.
22. Hemmendinger LM, Garber BB, Hoffmann PC, et al. Target neuron-specific process formation by embryonic mesencephalic dopamine neurons in vitro. *Proc Natl Acad Sci USA* 1981; 78:1264–1268.
23. Hoffmann PC, Hemmendinger LM, Kotake C, et al. Enhanced dopamine cell survival in reaggregates containing target cells. *Brain Res* 1983; 274:275–281.
24. Tomozawa Y, Appel SH. Soluble striatal extracts enhance development of mesencephalic dopaminergic neurons in vitro. *Brain Res* 1986; 399:111–124.
25. Barde YA. Trophic factors and neuronal survival. *Neuron* 1989; 2:1525–1534.
26. Clarke PGH. Neuronal death in the development of the vertebrate nervous system. *Trends Neurosci* 1985; 8:345–349.
27. Oo TF, Burke RE. The time course of developmental cell death in phenotypically defined dopaminergic neurons of the substantia nigra. *Dev Brain Res* 1997; 98:191–196.
28. Tepper JM, Damlama M, Trent F. Postnatal changes in the distribution and morphology of rat substantia nigra dopaminergic neurons. *Neuroscience* 1994; 60:469–477.
29. Macaya A, Munell F, Gubits RM, et al. Apoptosis in substantia nigra following developmental striatal excitotoxic injury. *Proc Natl Acad Sci USA* 1994; 91:8117–8121.

30. Marti MJ, James CJ, Oo TF, et al. Early developmental destruction of terminals in the striatal target induces apoptosis in dopamine neurons of the substantia nigra. *J Neurosci* 1997; 17:2030–2039.
31. Walkinshaw G, Waters CM. Neurotoxin induced cell death in neuronal PC12 cells is mediated by induction of apoptosis. *Neuroscience* 1994; 63:975–987.
32. Langston JW, Ballard PA, Tetrud JW, et al. Chronic Parkinsonism in humans due to a product of meperidine- analog synthesis. *Science* 1983; 219:979–980.
33. Davis GC, Williams AC, Markey SP, et al. Chronic Parkinsonism secondary to intravenous injection of meperidine analogs. *Psychiatry Res* 1979; 1:249–254.
34. Burns RS, Chiueh CC, Markey SP, et al. A primate model of Parkinsonism: Selective destruction of dopaminergic neurons in the pars compacta of the substantia nigra by N-methyl-4- phenyl-1,2,3,6-tetrahydropyridine. *Proc Natl Acad Sci USA* 1983; 80:4546–4550.
35. Heikkila RE, Hess A, Duvoisin RC. Dopaminergic neurotoxicity of 1-methyl-4-phenyl-1,2,5,6- tetrahydropyridine in mice. *Science* 1984; 224:1451–1453.
36. Dipasquale B, Marini AM, Youle RJ. Apoptosis and DNA degradation induced by 1-methyl-4-phenylpyridinium in neurons. *Biochem Biophys Res Commun* 1991; 181:1442–1448.
37. Mochizuki H, Nakamura N, Nishi K, et al. Apoptosis is induced by 1-methyl-4-phenylpyridinium ion (MPP+) in ventral mesencephalic striatal co-culture in rat. *Neurosci Lett* 1994; 170:191–194.
38. Mutoh T, Tokuda A, Marini AM, et al. 1-methyl-4-phenylpyridinum kills differentiated PC12 cells with a concomitant change in protein phosphorylation. *Brain Res* 1994; 661:51–55.
39. Hartley A, Stone JM, Heron C, et al. Complex I inhibitors induce dose dependent apoptosis in PC12 cells relevance to Parkinsons Disease. *J Neurochem* 1994; 63:1987–1990.
40. Itano Y, Nomura Y. 1-Methyl-4-phenyl-pyridinium ion (MPP(+)) causes DNA fragmentation and increases the Bcl-2 expression in human neuroblastoma, SH-SY5Y cells, through different mechanisms. *Brain Res* 1995; 704:240–245.
41. Jackson-Lewis V, Jakowec M, Burke RE, et al. Time course and morphology of dopaminergic neuronal death caused by the neurotoxin 1-methyl-4-phenyl-1,2,3,6-tetrahydropyridine. *Neurodegen* 1995; 4:257–269.
42. Tatton NA, Kish SJ. In situ detection of apoptotic nuclei in the substantia nigra compacta of 1-methyl-4-phenyl-1,2,3,6-tetrahydropyridine-treated mice using terminal deoxynucleotidyl transferase labelling and acridine orange. *Neuroscience* 1997; 77:1037–1048.
43. Hassouna I, Wickert H, Zimmermann M, et al. Increase in Bax expression in substantia-nigra following 1-methyl-4-phenyl-1,2,3,6-tetrahydropyridine (MPTP) treatment of mice. *Neurosci Lett* 1996; 204:85–88.
44. Oltvai ZN, Milliman CL, Korsmeyer SJ. Bcl-2 heterodimerizes in vivo with a conserved homolog, Bax, that accelerates programed cell death. *Cell* 1993; 74:609–619.
45. Trimmer PA, Smith TS, Jung AB, et al. Dopamine neurons from transgenic mice with a knockout of the p53 gene resist MPTP neurotoxicity. *Neurodegen* 1996; 5:233–239.
46. Lane DP, Lu X, Hupp T, et al. The role of p53 protein in the apoptotic response. *Philos Trans R Soc Lond Ser A* 1994; 345:277–280.
47. Yonish-Rouach E, Grunwald D, Wilder S, et al. p53-Mediated cell death: Relationship to cell cycle control. *Mol Cell Biol* 1993; 13:1415–1423.
48. Goldstein P. Controlling cell death. *Science* 1997; 275:1081–1082.
49. Estus S, Zaks WJ, Freeman RS, et al. Altered gene expression in neurons during programmed cell death identification of c-jun as necessary for neuronal apoptosis. *J Cell Biol* 1994; 127:1717–1727.
50. Ham J, Babij C, Whitfield J, et al. A c-jun dominant negative mutant protects sympathetic neurons against programmed cell death. *Neuron* 1995; 14:927–939.
51. Ferrer I, Olive M, Blanco R, et al. Selective c-Jun overexpression is associated with ionizing radiation-induced apoptosis in the developing cerebellum of the rat. *Mol Brain Res* 1996; 38:91–100.
52. Ferrer I, Olive M, Ribera J, et al. Naturally occurring (programmed) and radiation-induced apoptosis are associated with selective c-jun expression in the developing rat brain. *Eur J Neurosci* 1996; 8:1286–1298.
53. Davis RJ. MAPKs: New JNK expands the group. *TIBS* 1994; 19:470–473.
54. Xia Z, Dickens M, Raingeaud J, et al. Opposing effects of ERK and JNK-p38 MAP kinases on apoptosis. *Science* 1995; 270:1326–1331.
55. Park DS, Stefanis L, Yan CYI, et al. Ordering the cell-death pathway – differential-effects of Bcl-2, an interleukin-1β-converting enzyme family protease inhibitor, and other survival agents on JNK activation in serum nerve growth factor-deprived PC12 cells. *J Biol Chem* 1996; 271:21898–21905.
56. Virdee K, Bannister AJ, Hunt SP, et al. Comparison between the timing of JNK activation, c-jun phosphorylation, and onset of death commitment in sympathetic neurons. *J Neurochem* 1997; 69:550–561.
57. Eilers A, Whitfield J, Babij C, et al. Role of the jun kinase pathway in the regulation of c-jun expression and apoptosis in sympathetic neurons. *J Neurosci* 1998; 18:1713–1724.
58. Deckwerth TL, Easton RM, Knudson CM, et al. Placement of the Bcl-2 family member Bax in the death pathway of sympathetic neurons activated by trophic factor deprivation. *Exp Neurol* 1998; 152:150–162.
59. Herdegen T, Claret FX, Kallunki T, et al. Lasting N-terminal phosphorylation of c-jun and activation of c-jun N-terminal kinases after neuronal injury. *J Neurosci* 1998; 18:5124–5135.

60. Oo TF, Henchcliffe C, James D, et al. Expression of c-fos, c-jun, and c-jun N-terminal kinase (JNK) in a developmental model of induced apoptotic death in neurons of the substantia nigra. *J Neurochem* 1999; 72:557–564.

61. Yuan J, Shaham S, Ledoux S, et al. The *C. elegans* cell death gene *ced-3* encodes a protein similar to mammalian interleukin-1β-converting enzyme. *Cell* 1993; 75:641–652.

62. Alnemri ES, Livingston DJ, Nicholson DW, et al. Human ICE/CED-3 protease nomenclature. *Cell* 1996; 87:171.

63. Miura M, Zhu H, Rotello R, et al. Induction of apoptosis in fibroblasts by IL-1 beta-converting enzyme, a mammalian homolog of the *C. elegans* cell death gene *ced-3*. *Cell* 1993; 75:653–660.

64. Tewari M, Quan LT, O'Rourke K, et al. Yama/ CPP32β, a mammalian homolog of CED-3, is a CrmA-inhibitable protease that cleaves the death substrate poly(ADP-ribose) polymerase. *Cell* 1995; 81:801–809.

65. Enari M, Hug H, Nagata S. Involvement of an ICE-like protease in Fas-mediated apoptosis. *Nature* 1995; 375:78–81.

66. Milligan CE, Prevette D, Yaginuma H, et al. Peptide inhibitors of the ICE protease family arrest programmed cell death of motoneurons in vivo and in vitro. *Neuron* 1995; 15:385–393.

67. Fernandes-Alnemri T, Litwack G, Alnemri ES. CPP32, a novel human apoptotic protein with homology to *C. elegans* cell death protein *ced-3* and mammalian interleukin-1β-converting enzyme. *J Biol Chem* 1994; 269:30761–30764.

68. Nicholson DW, Ali A, Thornberry NA, et al. Identification and inhibition of the ICE/CED-3 protease necessary for mammalian apoptosis. *Nature* 1995; 376:37–43.

69. Armstrong RC, Aja TJ, Hoang KD, et al. Activation of the CED-3/ICE-related protease CPP32 in cerebellar granule neurons undergoing apoptosis but not necrosis. *J Neurosci* 1997; 17:553–562.

70. Du Y, Bales KR, Dodel RC, et al. Activation of a caspase 3-related cysteine protease is required for glutamate-mediated apoptosis of cultured cerebellar granule neurons. *Proc Natl Acad Sci USA* 1997; 94:11657–11662.

71. Keane RW, Srinivasan A, Foster LM, et al. Activation of CPP32 during apoptosis of neurons and astrocytes. *J Neurosci Res* 1997; 48:168–180.

72. Kermer P, Klocker N, Labes M, et al. Inhibition of CPP32-like proteases rescues axotomized retinal ganglion cells from secondary cell death in vivo. *J Neurosci* 1998; 18:4656–4662.

73. Yakovlev AG, Knoblach SM, Fan L, et al. Activation of CPP32-like caspases contributes to neuronal apoptosis and neurological dysfunction after traumatic brain injury. *J Neurosci* 1997; 17:7415–7424.

74. Namura S, Zhu J, Fink K, et al. Activation and cleavage of caspase-3 in apoptosis induced by experimental cerebral ischemia. *J Neurosci* 1998; 18:3659–3668.

75. Chen J, Nagayama T, Jin K, et al. Induction of caspase-3-like protease may mediate delayed neuronal death in the hippocampus after transient cerebral ischemia. *J Neurosci* 1998; 18:4914–4928.

76. Anglade P, Vyas S, Javoy-Agid F, et al. Apoptosis and autophagy in nigral neurons of patients with Parkinson's disease. *Histo Histopathol* 1997; 12:25–31.

77. Mochizuki H, Goto K, Mori H, et al. Histochemical detection of apoptosis in Parkinson's disease. *J Neurol Sci* 1996; 137:120–123.

78. Tompkins MM, Basgall EJ, Zamrini E, et al. Apoptotic-like changes in Lewy-body-associated disorders and normal aging in substantia nigral neurons. *Am J Pathol* 1997; 150:119–131.

79. Tatton NA, Maclean-Fraser A, Tatton WG, et al. A fluorescent double-labeling method to detect and confirm apoptotic nuclei in Parkinson's disease. *Ann Neurol* 1998; 44:S142–S148.

80. Kosel S, Egensperger R, von Eitzen U, et al. On the question of apoptosis in the Parkinsonian substantia nigra. *Acta Neuropathol* 1997; 93:105–108.

81. Banati RB, Daniel SE, Blunt SB. Glial pathology but absence of apoptotic nigral neurons in long-standing Parkinson's disease [In Process Citation]. *Mov Disord* 1998; 13:221–227.

82. Lindvall O, Brundin P, Widner H, et al. Grafts of fetal dopamine neurons survive and improve motor function in Parkinson's disease. *Science* 1990; 247:574–577.

83. Yurek DM, Sladek JR. Dopamine cell replacement: Parkinson's disease. *Annu Rev Neurosci* 1990; 13:415–440.

84. Mahalik TJ, Hahn WE, Clayton GH, et al. Programmed cell death in developing grafts of fetal substantia nigra. *Exp Neurol* 1994; 129:27–36.

85. Zastrow DJ, Zawada WM, Clarkson ED, et al. Preincubation with growth factors improves survival of early mesencephalic grafts in hemi-Parkinsonian rats. *Soc Neurosci Abstr* 1996; 22:1493(Abstract).

86. Ziv I, Melamed E, Nardi N, et al. Dopamine induces apoptosis-like cell death in cultured chick sympathetic neurons: A possible novel pathogenetic mechanism in Parkinsons disease. *Neurosci Lett* 1994; 170:136–140.

87. Walkinshaw G, Waters CM. Induction of apoptosis in catecholaminergic PC12 cells by L-dopa. *J Clin Invest* 1995; 95:2458–2464.

30

The Impact of MPTP on Parkinson's Disease Research: Past, Present, and Future

J. William Langston, M.D.

The Parkinson's Institute, Sunnyvale, California

INTRODUCTION

Recognition of the biologic effects of MPTP (1-methyl-4-phenyl-1,2,3,6-tetrahydropyridine), an event that occurred in 1983, has proved to be a fertile step in the history of Parkinson's disease (PD) research. This observation applies to many levels of work and thought, ranging from its influence on etiologic concepts to the creation of a new animal model of the disease. This chapter reviews the discovery of this fascinating compound, and current knowledge regarding its mechanism of action is summarized. The major focus will be on areas where MPTP has had a significant impact on PD research, with an emphasis on its use as a tool to investigate the cause and treatment of the disease. Wherever possible, future directions of research are highlighted with a goal of furthering the already prolific scientific career of this novel and interesting compound.

THE DISCOVERY OF THE BIOLOGIC EFFECTS OF MPTP

MPTP was not discovered in the environment, but emerged from a pharmaceutical laboratory in 1947 (1), in which it was first synthesized as part of a search for novel narcotic analgesics. Although it was used primarily as a building block for the synthesis of other chemicals, in a remarkable harbinger of things to come, the compound was actually tested in rodents and primates as a possible therapeutic agent for PD (2). The studies on MPTP were abandoned, at least in part, because of the compound's toxic profile, but it remains a mystery to this day why its potential as a tool to study PD was not recognized at the time.

Over the next 35 years, MPTP continued to have some use in the chemical industry, primarily as a chemical building block for other compounds. In fact, in 1983, when its parkinsonogenic effects were finally recognized, MPTP was commercially available through a specialty supplier of chemical products (3). Unfortunately, however, it probably first caused parkinsonism in humans well before this time in a number of chemists who were using MPTP for legitimate purposes. Exposure in these cases probably occurred either through cutaneous absorption or vapor inhalation (4–6). At least one case of MPTP-neurotoxicity through self-administration (by an individual who made a tainted batch of a "synthetic narcotic") was published in 1979, but the identity of the offending agent was not clearly determined at the time (7).

Final recognition that MPTP induces parkinsonism would have to await a dramatic outbreak of parkinsonism among relatively young drug-abusers in northern California in 1982 (3). This occurred after a clandestine chemist in Morgan Hill, California, began making and selling a meperidine analog known as 1-methyl-4-phenyl-4-proprionoxy-piperidine (MPPP). This synthetic narcotic was sold under the name of "China White," and was selling quite well until the chemist used either too much heat or acid and made a bad batch of the drug. When this "tainted heroin" reached the streets, its users began experiencing a myriad of untoward effects (8), the worst of which was enduring and profoundly disabling parkinsonism. On the basis of the analysis of heroin bindles used by these patients, their clinical picture, and an autopsy study of the earlier reported case, it seemed clear that MPTP was the culprit, and that it was selectively toxic to the substantia nigra (3), something which has since been confirmed in both human (9) and nonhuman primates (10–16), as well as in other species, including mice (17).

WHAT HAVE WE LEARNED FROM MPTP INDUCED-PARKINSONISM IN HUMANS?

Since the first observations that MPTP caused parkinsonism in these young addicts, a great deal has been learned that provides a better understanding of the idiopathic form of the disease. First, observations in these patients have made it quite clear that all of the motor symptoms of PD, including tremor, can result from a lesion of the substantia nigra (18). This conclusion is based on two findings: (1) our patients with MPTP-induced parkinsonism exhibit all of the motor features of PD, including rest tremor and (2) we now have clear-cut pathologic evidence that MPTP induces a selective lesion of the zona compacta of the substantia nigra in humans (9). The observation regarding tremor is particularly important, because there has been substantial controversy over the years regarding the neuroanatomic origins of rest tremor and whether a purely nigral lesion can induce it (19). Observations in these patients also allows us to draw the conclusion that some of the nonmotor aspects of PD result from a nigral dopaminergic deficit, which includes the more subtle cognitive deficits seen in nondemented patients with the disease (20,21) and facial seborrhea (18). The fact that a primary nigrostriatal dopaminergic deficit can cause most if not all of the signs and symptoms of PD has enormous therapeutic consequences for those attempting to restore dopaminergic function using cellular replacement techniques.

A second observation in patients with MPTP-induced parkinsonism relates to the side effects of therapy. Our original patients were not only dramatically responsive to dopaminergic therapy as might be expected (18), but they also experienced all of the side effects typically encountered with chronic levodopa treatment (13). Furthermore, complications of levodopa therapy were seen surprisingly early in the course of treatment. For example, in several cases, a short duration response was seen almost immediately after starting treatment and dyskinesias were encountered within days of initiating treatment, which suggests that severity of disease may be more important than duration of treatment, at least for these particular complications of levodopa. As a qualifier to this statement, however, it must be pointed out that a second variable cannot be controlled in this group,

and that is age of onset. Dyskinesias are well known to begin earlier in younger patients (22), and the MPTP patients were much younger than is typical for the idiopathic form of the disease. However, the short duration response is not known to be age-dependent, therefore it can be concluded that it is related to disease severity, an observation that is consistent with the hypothesis that diminishing storage at the level of the synaptic vesicles may be a key feature underlying this phenomenon.

Although the forgoing observations have been available to the scientific community for some time, a fascinating new observation has emerged from neuropathologic studies in two of the original MPTP cases and a third more recent case from New Hampshire (9). The time from exposure to MPTP until death in these three cases ranged from three to 14 years. Surprisingly, in each of these individuals there was neuropathologic evidence of active, ongoing nerve cell death. Specific findings included microglia proliferation and clustering with clear-cut neuronophagias, and in two of the cases, abundant extraneuronal melanin. The mechanism of this active neuropathologic process is presently not clear, but could include enhanced oxidative stress from increased dopamine turnover in remaining dopaminergic neurons or an active inflammatory process. The latter is supported by the surprising degree of microglia proliferation. One interesting possibility is that neuromelanin is playing a role in triggering an ongoing autoimmune phenomenon, perhaps being toxic itself, or possibly by accumulating neurotoxic agents such as MPP+ after MPTP exposure (23). In any case, these observations may be precedent setting, as they provide compelling evidence that a time-limited exposure to an exogenous toxin can induce an active neurodegenerative process that can persist for many years. The working hypothesis is that this process may be due to chronic inflammation, perhaps through an autoendocrine inflammatory loop. A number of groups, which include our own, are exploring this hypothesis experimentally. For example, in MPTP mouse model, it is shown that there is a nigrostriatal inflammatory response after MPTP, which can be suppressed with dexamethasone (24). The further development of such models to explore the inflammatory hypothesis of PD could have important therapeutic implications by raising the possibility that anti-inflammatory agents slow or halt the process of disease progression.

An Animal Model for Parkinson's Disease

When viewed from a broad perspective, the discovery of MPTP opened at least three new research avenues:

(1) it gave immediate promise for the development of a new animal model for PD, (2) it provided an entirely new tool to investigate mechanisms of nigral cell degeneration and to test new protective strategies to block that degeneration, and (3) it focused attention on the hypothesis that environmental toxins play a causative role in the disease. This section reviews, the first of these new avenues.

MPTP remains unusual among experimental compounds in that its toxic effects were serendipitously discovered in humans who self-administered the compound, but this has had some powerful scientific consequences. For example, there is a remarkably clear picture of just how faithfully MPTP replicates the idiopathic disorder in humans, an observation that gave birth to an immediate search for new animal models for PD. And indeed, the drug has been given to animals ranging from monkeys (14,25) to the goldfish (26). However, the models that have found the most favor over the years are the mouse and the nonhuman primate. But these two species have proved to be quite different. In spite of inducing substantial nigrostriatal damage in mice, this species fails to develop behaviorally evident parkinsonism (27,28). Surprisingly, rats were found to be almost impervious to the toxic effects of the compound after systemic administration (29). Indeed, only human and nonhuman primates develop full-blown, characteristic parkinsonism after MPTP exposure. Therefore, when it comes to investigating the therapeutic benefit of antiparkinsonian agents, or exploring the aspects of nigrostriatal circuitry that are deranged in the parkinsonian state, this model has proved not only invaluable, but also a necessity, because only in this model can one directly observe the effects of any manipulations on clinically overt parkinsonism. And indeed this model has been used intensively to investigate new pharmacologic and surgical approaches to the treatment of PD. As is evident in this chapter, if there is one consistent theme that has emerged from MPTP-related research, it is that this model has been highly predictive and reflective of the human condition, its physiology, and responses to therapy.

The Role of the Subthalamic Nucleus (STN)

It should not be surprising, then, that critical advances have been made using the animal model. One of the most important of these came from the work of DeLong and his colleagues (30–35), who carefully investigated the neurophysiologic changes in basal ganglia circuitry in primates with MPTP-induced parkinsonism. In 1990, they made the seminal observation that lesioning of the subthalamic nucleus resulted in a reversal of motor deficits on the contralateral side in primates rendered parkinsonian by MPTP, including akinesia, rigidity, and tremor (31). This experiment came after painstaking neurophysiologic work indicating that the lesioning of the substantia nigra with MPTP resulted in a decrease in striatal inhibitory output, with subsequent disinhibition of the STN. Because the output of the STN to internal segment of the pallidum is excitatory, this appears to cause over-stimulation of the globus pallidus, thus altering outflow to the thalamus and cortex. Blocking this pallidal over stimulation appears to correct many of the features of PD.

The impact of these experimental observations is enormous. They first led to renewed interest in pallidotomy, a procedure that was first attempted half a century ago (see Chapter 47). However, with the advent of deep brain stimulation, which can be done bilaterally, and implanted directly into the STN, interest has increasingly turned to this procedure (see Chapter 49). And indeed, high frequency stimulation of the STN in MPTP-lesioned parkinsonian monkeys has been shown to reverse parkinsonism (36,37). These new surgical procedures offer perhaps the most immediate hope for patients no longer enjoying satisfactory control from current forms of medical therapy. As is true with most good science, this story began with a series of careful and thoughtful experiments to understand the underlying pathophysiology, which in turn rested on the shoulders of an accurate and stable animal model of the disease, a model that was not available before the advent of MPTP.

Neurotransplantation

The other surgical approach to the treatment of PD for which the MPTP model has been very helpful is neural transplantation. Although a huge amount of the original work laying the foundation for this approach has been carried out in rodents (38), the lack of clinically identifiable parkinsonism in this species kept it a step short of being an ideal model to transition this basic research to humans with PD. The MPTP-lesioned primate, however, with its full array of parkinsonian features, has proved an excellent testing ground for the effectiveness of this approach. Indeed, many groups have been able to demonstrate clear-cut therapeutic benefits of neural grafting in this model (39–42). It has also been used for a wide variety of related investigations, which include autologous superior cervical ganglion grafting (43), intracerebral adrenomedullary grafting (44), polymer-encapsulated PC12 cells (45), and the use of genetically ex vivo and in vivo gene therapy (46). Furthermore, using this model, it has been possible to show the effects of grafts at the neuropharmacologic level. For example, Elsworth and colleagues (47) have shown that D2 receptors (which are upregulated after MPTP-induced nigrostriatal denervation) are downregulated after neural grafting, suggesting a return to normal synaptic function, and others have shown that there is extensive graft reinervation and interaction with surrounding tissue in primates with MPTP-induced parkinsonism (48). Such studies have been invaluable in transitioning this potentially curative therapeutic approach to humans in terms of showing feasibility, potential efficacy, and safety.

In the late 1980s this fetal grafting procedure was extended to three human cases of MPTP-induced parkinsonism. All three subjects traveled to Lund, Sweden, where they underwent neural grafting, and all three subjects experienced substantial improvement. Two of the three have been reported in detail (49). Interestingly, these patients seem to have done slightly better than patients with the idiopathic disease, possibly because of their age, the amount of tissue transplanted, or because they have more selective lesions of the substantia nigra. Although this area of research has not proceeded as rapidly as originally hoped, it still remains an important part of the long-term search for a cure for this disease, which may ultimately depend on finding alternative tissue sources for transplantation. A review of the current status of neural transplantation can be found in Chapter 50.

Dopamine Receptors

The MPTP-lesioned monkey provided an excellent opportunity to understand the dopamine receptor system better in the presence of nigrostriatal denervation and behaviorally overt parkinsonism. After lesioning with MPTP, dopamine receptor studies (using D1 and D2 specific radioligands) have typically shown that D2 receptors are upregulated (denervation supersensitivity). On the other hand, D1 receptors have been reported to be either unchanged, increased, or decreased after denervation (50–54). The parkinsonian primate has been used for a wide variety of approaches to pharmacologic therapy, which includes the study of D1 and D2 agonists, and their value in the treatment of PD. The antiparkinsonian effects of D2 agonists have been consistently demonstrated as predicted from both clinical experience and the dopamine receptor studies in MPTP-lesioned monkeys (55,56). However, results of studies using D1 agonists have not always been consistent (possibly reflecting the variable results of studies on D1 receptors after MPTP lesioning), with some groups demonstrating antiparkinsonian effects

(57–59), but others failing to see any benefit (60–62). At least one group has reported that D1 agonists may exhibit fairly rapid desensitization with a shorten duration of response (63). Interestingly, one selective D1 agonist has also been shown to improve cognition in a chronic model of MPTP intoxication (64).

Dopa-Dyskinesias

Another important area relates to the study of side-effects of dopaminergic therapy, particularly levodopa. As expected from the experience with humans, monkeys with MPTP-induced parkinsonism were quickly found to develop classic dopa-dyskinesias (65–67), something that to date seems to be unique to primates. Thus, this model has found increasing use, and indeed, has become the "gold standard" for investigating this troubling and dose-limiting side effect of levodopa therapy. Several studies have suggested that the more severe the lesion, the more likely animals are to develop dyskinesias (68,69). Somewhat surprisingly, it is often difficult to obtain a therapeutic response without also encountering dyskinesias (68). The reason for this is not clear, but it may be related to the high-dose acute regimens of levodopa that most investigators use. Another potentially important observation is that these animals never develop dyskinesias on their first dose of levodopa, thus confirming the need for so-called "priming," something that may hold a clue as to their cause, but for which there has not previously been an adequate model (Di Monte, in press).

There is no doubt that DA receptors play a role in dyskinesias as D1, D2, and D3 dopamine receptor subtype-selective agonists have all been shown to induce dyskinetic movements in MPTP-lesioned monkeys (58,62,70–76). When given in combination, D1 and D2 agonists cause dyskinesias more prominently than either alone, perhaps because they simulate the effect of levodopa more completely (77). However, dopamine agonists when given individually seem less likely to induce dyskinesias than levodopa, even when given at an apparently equivalent therapeutic dose (78). In a head to head match, D1 agonists were less likely to cause dyskinesias than either levodopa or a D2 agonist in levodopa-primed animals (79). Not surprisingly, apomorphine has been found to induce dyskinesias in this model (80). It has also been reported that pulsatile administration of D1 and D2 agonists is more likely to cause dyskinesias than constant administration (81,82). Despite these compelling observations on the importance of dopamine receptors in the generation of dyskinesias, neither D1 nor D2 receptor changes in the striatopallidal complex have been found to correlate with their occurrence (81,83–85). Our own work with D3 receptors and dopa-dyskinesias has demonstrated that D3 receptors decline after MPTP lesioning only in the caudate, and that in levodopa-treated dyskinetic animals D3 receptors return to normal (Quik et al., in press). Thus, we have not been able to establish that an abnormality of this receptor population is related to dyskinesias.

Recently there has been increasing interest in the possibility that NMDA receptors mediate dopa-dyskinesias, and indeed, similar to observations in humans with PD, the administration of NMDA receptor antagonists attenuates dopa-dyskinesias in the MPTP-lesioned monkey (86–90), which suggests excessive activity at NMDA glutamatergic receptors may be playing a role. However, the molecular mechanisms by which glutamate receptors are activated and in turn contribute to dopa-dyskinesias remains unknown, although rodent studies have suggested that alterations in certain levodopa-induced motor responses may be linked to modifications in the phosphorylation state of the NR2A and NR2B subunits of the NMDA receptor (91,92).

Preproenkephalin (PPE) has been investigated as a link in the sequence of events that lead to dyskinesias. Nigral dopaminergic neurons are thought to tonically inhibit striatopallidal output through activation of D2 receptors located on enkephalin containing GABAergic striatal neurons in the striatum. Lesioning of the nigrostriatal system in rodents is shown to increase in PPE mRNA in these neurons (93–97). Striatal PPE mRNA levels are also shown to increase in MPTP-lesioned monkeys (98–101). However, these elevations do not appear to be appreciably changed in MPTP-lesioned monkeys with dopa-dyskinesias (99,100). On the other hand, Morissette et al. (101) found that these elevations were corrected in animals treated with a D2 agonist at a dose that corrected the parkinsonism, but did not cause dyskinesias, whereas D1 agonist treatment at a level that induced dyskinesias further elevated PPE mRNA. Further studies are indicated to see if this peptide is marking one or more important cellular changes in the sequence of events that lead to dopa-dyskinesias.

This model has also been employed in the search for pharmacologic agents that might block or lessen dopa-dyskinesias. Among those that have been reported to ameliorate dyskinesias in parkinsonian primates are CCK (102), (-)-OSU 6160 (a D2 receptor selective compound) (103), 17 beta-estradiol (104), and the alpha2-adrenergic receptor antagonist idazoxan (97,105). Exploring new pharmacologic approaches to minimize or even prevent dyskinesias may be one of the more fruitful ways to learn more about their underlying

pathophysiology and, at a more practical level, is the quickest way to find approaches for their prevention. Given the number of compounds tested to date, we are already off to a good start, and indeed, there are few advances that could have more of an immediate impact on the successful long-term treatment of PD.

Before leaving the subject of dyskinesias, two interesting observations warrant note. The first relates to the neurophysiology of the internal segment of the globus pallidus (GPi). Quite early after the MPTP-model was developed, Crossman and colleagues (106) observed that 2-deoxyglucose use was markedly increased in the GPi in MPTP-lesioned parkinsonian animals but markedly decreased when the animals were experiencing dopa-dyskinesias. Their observations now appear to be confirmed physiologically by Papa and colleagues (107), who found that cellular firing in the internal segment of the globus pallidus is almost completely suppressed in animals with dopa-dyskinesias. This may be a key change in the cascade of events that lead to dyskinesias, and certainly warrants further study. However, one of the first tasks ahead is to explain the paradox as to why pallidotomy, which might be expected to do nearly the same thing, clearly has an antidyskinetic effect.

The other, and perhaps one of the most provocative observations to emerge from work using primates to study dopa-dyskinesias, relates to the conventional wisdom that a loss of nigrostriatal terminals is required for their development. This generally accepted convention is based not only on clinical observation, but also a substantial body of experimental literature. For example, using a dose of 40 mg/kg of levodopa, Boyce et al. (69) reported that animals with an intact nigrostriatal system became hyperactive, but did not show typical dopa-dyskinesias, whereas animals with lesioned nigrostriatal system developed peak-dose dyskinesias that were choreoathetoid in nature. Alexander et al. (52,108) were also unable to induce dyskinesias in animals with an intact nigrostriatal system. However, R.K. Pearce et al. (109) have recently challenged this view by reporting that normal monkeys that received extremely high doses of levodopa (80 mg/kg) over many months do exhibit dyskinesias. Recent observations revealed dyskinesias in normal monkeys receiving short-term levodopa. Because of the importance of this issue, a prospective, blinded study using the Global Primate Dyskinesia Scale, which has been tested for both reliability and validity, was initiated (110,111). The results of this experiment were dramatic, as all of the nonlesioned levodopa-treated animals developed dyskinesias that were indistinguishable from dyskinesias in animals with MPTP-induced parkinsonism (Togasaki et al., submitted for publication). A careful review of the literature revealed that, in one of the original experimental studies of levodopa in monkeys in 1973, Mones (112) reported that normal animals develop involuntary choreiform movements of the limbs along with hyperactivity and orofacial movements when very high doses of levodopa were given (200–400 mg/kg). What is different about the recent prospective study is that far lower doses of levodopa were given (15 mg/kg), which are much closer to the range used in humans with PD.

This new model offers an entirely new strategy in which to explore the pathophysiology of dyskinesias because it is now possible to investigate changes in basal ganglia that lead to dopa-dyskinesias in a setting that is not confounded by the severe derangement in basal ganglia circuitry that occurs after MPTP lesioning. Perhaps by using both the parkinsonian and nonparkinsonian models of dopa-dyskinesias in a complimentary fashion, it may finally be possible to unlock the mysteries as to why levodopa induces this rather bothersome complication.

Variations on the MPTP Model in Primates

It should be noted that there are a number of variations of the MPTP model that have been developed. These include the hemi-lesioned model, which uses unilateral MPTP intracarotid injection (113), the bilateral intra-carotid model (114), the so-called over-lesioned model (unilateral intracarotid lesioning followed by low-dose systemic injection), and a low-dose chronic model (115). The advantages and disadvantages of each of these models has been reviewed in detail elsewhere (116).

Summary

The MPTP model continues to be used for the testing of new therapeutic strategies in PD and to understand better the complications of therapy, because monkeys lesioned with MPTP exhibit not only the clinical consequences of a nigrostriatal dopaminergic deficit, that is clinically overt parkinsonism, but almost all of the underlying neurophysiologic changes that seem to occur in the idiopathic disease. For these reasons, it is clear that one can expect this model to be highly predictive of the therapeutic responses that will be observed in humans with the disease, and will continue to provide invaluable opportunities for transitioning new therapies from the laboratory to patients.

Mechanism of Action of MPTP: The Beginning of the Age of Neuroprotection

After it became clear that MPTP was capable of inducing parkinsonism in humans, by virtue of selectively killing nigral neurons (3), there was a tremendous surge in research activity, both to document beyond doubt that this was the case and to unravel its mechanism of action (117). There was tremendous interest in understanding exactly how a compound could be so selectively toxic to the neurons of the substantia nigra. This research has also led to a myriad of new strategies to protect against MPTP toxicity, which have been tested at almost every level of biologic complexity, ranging from tissue culture to patients with PD. These studies have helped usher in a new age of research on neuroprotective strategies aimed at slowing the progress of PD.

The Biotransformation of MPTP: The Monoamine Oxidase Story

The first major step in unraveling the mechanism of action of MPTP was the discovery that MPTP itself is not toxic. Rather, it required biotransformation to a toxic metabolite, 1-methyl-4-phenylpyridinium ion or MPP+ (15,28). A clue that monoamine oxidase might be responsible for this biotransformation came from B. Parsons and T.C. Rainbow (118), who astutely observed that the distribution of MPTP binding in the rodent brain corresponded closely to the known distribution of MAO. However, definitive evidence that MAO (and specifically MAO B) was the enzyme mediating the bioactivation of MPTP came from Chiba and colleagues (119), who demonstrated that the MAO B inhibitors, deprenyl and pargyline, blocked the conversion of MPTP to its toxic metabolite. It was quickly shown that blocking MAO B prevented dopamine depletion in mice (27,28), and nigral cell degeneration in primates (11). This transition almost certainly is taking place in glia, not intraneuronally (120–123).

These observations have several interesting implications, both practical and theoretical. First, they triggered a mini-renaissance of interest in MAO, and its role in the human nervous system (124). Generally thought to be a housekeeping enzyme, these new data raised the possibility that MAO might have other less well-known biologic functions. Second, the potential therapeutic implications were immediately obvious. If deprenyl could be used to block the neurodegenerative effects of MPTP, might this drug be used to slow or halt the progression of PD? For this reason we initiated a prospective controlled trial in patients with PD to assess the effect of deprenyl on disease progression (125).

Shortly thereafter, planning for a much larger trial was initiated, which was also designed to assess alpha-tocopherol in addition to deprenyl. In 1988 the results of both of these studies were published (125,126), and both showed that levodopa therapy could be substantially delayed with the initiation of early deprenyl therapy in de novo patients. Furthermore, based on clinical evaluation, the drug appeared to slow disease progression by about 50 percent. However, these findings became controversial when the larger study showed that a very small but definite and statistically significant symptomatic benefit was derived from deprenyl, which could have confounded the results. Although this debate can never be unequivocally resolved until there is a way to monitor nigral cell degeneration in living humans, deprenyl has continued to enjoy substantial use in clinical practice. Furthermore, this compound seems to have had a second life as a neuroprotective agent after the discovery that it may also have a "rescue effect" independent of MAO B inhibition (see Section entitled: The Deprenyl Story: Part II).

The MAO-mediated biotransformation of MPTP to MPP+, which is presently well documented, could have broader implications for neurodegenerative disease. This is because it provides an example of a nontoxic compound being converted to a neurotoxin by the brain's own enzymatic machinery – to at least some degree, this is precedent setting, and could represent a metabolic "Achilles' heel" of the brain. Xenobiotics are frequently metabolized into reactive compounds that can then be conjugated and excreted. However, in this instance, something has gone wrong because MPP+ cannot be further metabolized and is toxic. This failure of the xenobiotic metabolic pathway could have implications for PD and other neurodegenerative processes, and has generated an entire field of research on genetically determined abnormalities of xenobiotic metabolism as potential risk factors for neurodegenerative disease.

Uptake of MPP+

The mystery of the remarkable selectivity of MPTP was at least partially solved when it was found that MPP+ (but not MPTP) is selectively taken up via the dopamine transporter, thus accounting for its selective accumulation in dopaminergic neurons (127). Uptake inhibitors were quickly shown to protect against MPTP toxicity in rodents (128–130), but protection in primates was more difficult to achieve (131), probably because of the long half-life of MPP+, and difficulties in maintaining constant uptake inhibition with currently available agents. Perhaps for this reason there has yet to be serious consideration of a neuroprotective trial in

PD using dopamine-uptake inhibitors. More recently, in an elegant study using transgenic mice, Bezard and colleagues (132) showed that animals that lack the dopamine transporter were completely protected from MPTP-induced cell loss.

If one considers this aspect of MPTP toxicity, it could be argued that it exemplifies a remarkable sequence of events. First, the brain (more specifically glia) converts a nontoxic substance into a toxin that cannot be further metabolized or conjugated. Next the dopaminergic uptake system recognizes this potentially toxic compound as a friendly substance (i.e., dopamine or a dopamine-like compound) and transports it intracellularly, where it can cause cell death. The vast abundance of uptake systems in the brain accounts for the need for a tight barrier between the blood and the brain, but in this instance the blood-brain barrier is circumvented in the form of MPTP, a nontoxic and lipophilic compound. The system is then undone from within by the creation of MPP+. Certainly one of the more interesting questions to address is whether this remarkable sequence of events is a rare aberration, or is it a much more common scenario that plays a role in one or more human neurodegenerative diseases.

MPP+: A Mitochondrial Toxin

Once in nigral neurons, MPP+ accumulates as much as 40-fold in mitochondria (133,134). This is apparently due to the energy-dependent electrical gradient that is maintained across the mitochondria membrane. Once accumulated in mitochondria, MPP+ inhibits Complex I of the electron transport chain (135,136), at or near the rotenone sensitive site. Di Monte and colleagues (137) demonstrated the functional consequences of this effect when they showed that MPTP induced a dramatic depletion of ATP in isolated hepatocytes. These observations led to the search for similar deficits in PD, where a Complex I deficiency was found (138–140).

The mitochondrial hypothesis of PD, which was largely precipitated by MPTP-related discoveries, continues. However, there is still much that is not known. Although there is near universal agreement that a Complex I deficit is present in the substantia nigra of patients with PD (141), whether a similar deficit is present in other tissues, such as muscle and platelets, remains controversial (142–147). Nor do we know if the mitochondrial deficit is primary or secondary. If primary, what causes the deficit in the first place? Perhaps the strongest argument against mitochondria DNA playing a major role in PD is the paucity of evidence for maternal inheritance (148), as would be expected if mitochondrial DNA were involved. On the other hand, Shapira and colleagues (141) have shown that, at least in a subset of patients, this deficit in Complex I activity does appear to be determined by mitochondrial DNA, a conclusion that was based on an elegant series of experiments using rho cybrid cells that carried mitochondrial DNA from patients with PD (149).

Regardless of the answers to these questions, interest in the energy-depleting effects of MPTP, which have now been confirmed in vivo experimentally (150), has led to intensive investigations that focus on blocking these effects using a variety of approaches. Fructose was shown to be neuroprotective in isolated hepatocytes (151). In models of mild MPTP-toxicity (i.e., modest MPTP-induced striatal dopamine depletions in the mouse) a combination of coenzyme Q10 and nicotinamide (both thought to improve mitochondrial function) protected against toxicity (152). Oral administration of creatine or cyclocreatine, which may increase phosphocreatine or cyclophosphocreatine buffering against ATP depletion, also protect against MPTP-induced striatal dopamine depletion in mice. Here again is an example of basic science having direct implications for PD, as a controlled clinical trial is currently under way to determine if Co-enzyme Q, a promoter of mitochondrial function, can be used to slow or halt the progression of the disease (153). This important clinical trial was largely based on the observations that originated from the MPTP model.

Oxidative Stress

Although evidence that MPP+ is a mitochondrial toxin is incontrovertible, it is certainly not the only mechanism that has been proposed to explain how MPTP/MPP+ kills cells. The foremost of the other theories relates to oxidative stress. Although it was originally proposed that MPP+ undergoes redox cycling in a manner similar to paraquat, this concept has long since been abandoned (154,155). However, there are a myriad of other ways that this compound could induce oxidative stress, including disruption of the electron transport chain (156), and there is now abundant literature on the effects of MPTP administration and the generation of potentially damaging oxyradicals.

One of the most common approaches used to investigate the "free radical hypothesis" is to use antioxidants to protect against MPTP toxicity, but these studies have been frustratingly contradictory. Alpha-tocopherol (157), beta-carotene (157), and ascorbic acid (157,158) have been reported to protect against MPTP-induced striatal dopamine depletions in the mouse, but not all investigators have seen this

effect (159,160). Furthermore, investigations in the nonhuman primate using alpha-tocopherol and beta-carotene (161), as well as ascorbic acid (162) have failed to show a neuroprotective effect. Blanchet and colleagues (163) used OPC-14117, a potent antioxidant, to block MPTP-induced parkinsonism in a chronic model of MPTP intoxication (a model which attempts to closely mimic the slow progression of PD), but it failed.

More recently, spin trapping agents such as alpha-phenyl-ter-butyl-nitrone (PBN) (164), azulenyl nitrone (165), MDL 101,002 (166) have been reported to be at least partially neuroprotective in the mouse model of MPTP toxicity, but Ferger and colleagues (167) were unable to make an association between the hydroxyl radical savaging effect of PBN and MPTP neurotoxicity. In yet another study, bromocriptine was found to block MPTP toxicity in the mouse (168). Because this drug was also effective in blocking striatal glutathione depletion, the possibility was raised that this dopamine agonist was acting by stimulating antioxidant activity in the brain. Melatonin, an endogenous antioxidant, has been shown to inhibit a loss of tyrosine hydroxylase (TH) immunoreactivity in the mouse striatum presumably through a similar mechanism (169). Another interesting agent that has been found to ameliorate the effects of MPTP is apomorphine, which could be working as a radical scavenger (170).

Metallothioneins have also been studied as a way to investigate the free radical hypothesis of MPTP neurotoxicity since they scavenge free radicals. In 1997, Rojas and Rios (171) reported that inducers of metallothionein provided significant protection against MPTP-induced striatal dopamine depletions in the mouse. MPTP alone produced a 50% reduction in striatal metallothionein. However, in a later study, metallothionein-I and metallothionein-II knockout mice were not found to be more sensitive to MPTP, which suggests that these proteins are not directly involved in blocking the effects of MPTP (172). Because iron may be involved in the process of free radical generation, chelators of iron have been tested for neuroprotective effects. Ferger and colleagues (173) showed that cytosine is an effective chelator of iron, and that it significantly protected against MPTP-induced striatal dopamine depletions in the mouse.

In a study by Aubin and colleagues (174), salicylate, aspirin, and aspergic were all found to prevent MPTP neurotoxicity. These investigators also demonstrated that cyclo oxygenase inhibitors or agents that inhibited NF-kappB did not have this effect, and also demonstrated that this effect of salicylates was not due to either inhibition of MAO B or dopamine uptake. In a separate study, this same group reported that hydroxylated salicylate metabolites were present in the brains of MPTP and salicylate treated mice, suggesting that hydroxyl radical savaging may be the mechanism underlying this neuroprotective effect (174). Subsequently, Ferger and colleagues (175) have shown that salicylate blocks the MPTP-induced decline in TH-positive cells in the mouse substantia nigra, further suggesting that salicylate is neuroprotective.

Another way to investigate the role of oxidative stress is to search for evidence of reactive oxygen species in the brain of animals exposed to MPTP. For example, Sriram and colleagues (176), used both sagittal slices of mouse brain exposed directly to MPTP and mice exposed via systemic administration of MPTP and found that there were significant increases in both reactive oxygen species and lipid peroxidation products and declines in glutathione. Because these changes preceded Complex I inhibition, they suggested that free radical generation was the primary event leading to toxicity. Ali and colleagues (177) identified the generation of reactive oxygen species in older, but not young mice given MPTP, and a number of investigators have reported evidence that MPTP alone induces hydroxyl radical formation (178–180). In cell culture systems, it has been shown that cell lines deficient in catalase activity are more sensitive to the effects of MPP+ than those with higher levels (181). On the other hand, in a series of experiments using a murine dopaminergic cell line comparing 6-hydroxydopamine and MPTP, Choi and colleagues (182) found that reactive oxygen radicals seemed to play an essential role in 6-OHDA-mediated apoptosis, but there was no evidence of this in the setting of MPP+-induced necrosis.

Transgenic mice have also been used to investigate the possible role of oxidative stress in MPTP toxicity. For example, mice over-expressing the mitochondrial form of dysmutase superoxide seem to be at least partially protected from MPTP (183,184) and mice over-expressing Bcl-2, which may protect against free radicals, were found to be partially protected against MPTP toxicity (185,186).

In summary, there is a diverse literature on the possible role of free radicals in MPTP neurotoxicity, but some of this literature is conflicting. At least part of the problem relates to the use of different models, animal strains, and experimental paradigms. Also contributing to the confusion may be the fact that other actions of putative antioxidants, such as inhibition of MAO B or blocking the dopamine transporter, were not ruled out as contributing to their possible "neuroprotective" effects. Finally, many of these studies relied on striatal dopamine concentrations as the primary measure of nigrostriatal integrity, and therefore may not have actually been assessing the process of neuronal degeneration. Adding to the complexity of this problem is that any process that affects the mitochondrial respiratory chain and energy production will probably cause leakage or generation of oxyradicals and subsequent oxidative stress, so that the two processes are probably inexorably linked (187). A role for oxidative stress in the cascade of events that lead to toxicity seems to be established, and will probably continue to be an important and challenging area of investigation, and one that continues to have implications for the cause and treatment of PD.

Although interest in the so-called "free-radical" hypothesis of PD long antedated the discovery of MPTP (188), it took the MAO B inhibitor trial to precipitate an antioxidant trial in PD, as alpha-tocopheral was added as an additional component to the DATATOP trial that tested deprenyl (126). This arm of the trial showed no evidence of neuroprotection, somewhat dampening hopes that antioxidants might be able to slow disease progression. However, it is not known if adequate levels of alpha-tocopherol were ever achieved in the CNS, so it is difficult to known how much weight to place on a negative result. Successful neuroprotection against MPTP neurotoxicity in experimental models, particularly in the primate, could well lead to a second attempt for forestall progression of PD in humans using effective antioxidant therapy.

Nitric Oxide

During the last decade, nitric oxide (NO) has come to the forefront as a possible endogenous toxin that could play a role in the process of neurodegeneration in a variety of diseases (189). PD has proved to be no exception. To some degree this interest is a result of studies using the MPTP model. This began when several investigators reported that inhibiting NO synthetase (NOS) was partially protective against MPTP neurotoxicity in mice (190,191) and the baboon (192). It was also shown in the baboon that MPTP-induced increase in nigral perxoynitrite was prevented by inhibiting NOS (193). Furthermore, MPTP administration causes upregulation of iNOS in the substantia nigra and iNOS knockouts have been reported to be less sensitive to the effects of MPTP by one group (194), but not another (195).

The importance of NO in MPTP toxicity was questioned when several groups, including our own, found that the most commonly used NOS inhibitor, 7-nitroindazole (7-NI), also inhibited MAO B (196–198), which suggests, rather than by blocking the synthesis of NO, inhibition of MAO might explain at least some of the effects of 7-NI in protecting against MPTP toxicity. The next step was to examine other NOS inhibitors to see if they blocked MPTP toxicity as well. Although Matthews et al. (199) reported that S-methylthiocitruline, a relatively selective inhibitor of NOS, protected mice against MPTP-induced striatal dopamine depletion, MacKenzie and colleagues (200) were unable to inhibit MPTP toxicity in the monkey using another NOS inhibitor (L-NGnitro-arginine methyl ester or L-NAME).

The reasons for these disparate results regarding a role for NO in MPTP toxicity are not clear. However, it seems likely that the effects of 7-NI on MAO B have confounded at least some of the studies. In a study by Tsai and Lee (201) NO donors actually appeared to protect astrocytes from MPP+-induced damage. More recently, S. Rose and colleagues (202), using intracerebral microdialysis in rats, found that NO appeared to be involved in the MPP+-induced production of hydroxyl radical, but not MPP+-induced dopamine release.

At the moment, one can only say that transition of experimental studies with NO and NOS inhibitors to PD is a work in progress. The only primate study done to date, which used a NOS inhibitor other than 7-NI, failed to show a neuroprotective effect. Although there have been some hints of a role for NO in PD (203,204), the exact role of NO in the disorder is far from established (189). Another problem is that the clinical effects of NOS inhibitors remain unknown (205). Should new evidence of the importance of NO in MPTP toxicity be forthcoming in primates, there might well be a revitalization of research interest in NOS inhibitors as neuroprotective agents for PD.

Excitotoxicity

Unraveling the importance of excitotoxicity as a mechanism that underlies neurotoxicity has proved to be a more complex endeavor in the investigation of MPTP. Whereas NMDA antagonists were first used in an attempt to induce symptomatic improvement in the MPTP-lesioned monkey with variable results (206–208), they were also used to protect against MPTP toxicity. In the study by Turski and colleagues (209), and several others that followed (210,211), NMDA antagonists were shown to protect against MPTP/MPP+ toxicity, including actual nigral cell degeneration. However, the waters were

clouded by a rapid succession of reports that NMDA antagonists provided only partial (212,213) or no protection (214–216) in mice. Similar results were reported using rat mesencephalic cell cultures (217). On the other hand, Srivastava and colleagues (218) found that decortication (a procedure that removes glutamateric input to the striatum) or MK-801, a prototype NMDA antagonist, blocked MPP+ induced cell loss in the rat using direct intra-striatal injections of MPP+. Clonidine, an alpha 2-agonist that is thought to block glutamate overflow, has been shown to partially protect mice against MPTP-induced dopamine depletions (219).

Our own group found that MK-801 did protect against MPTP-induced striatal dopamine depletions in the mouse, but this protection was only transient, lasting less than 12 hours. The drug did not block degeneration of dopaminergic neurons (216). However, MK-801 was found to delay elimination of MPP+ from the brain. Since sequestration of MPP+ in synaptic vesicles has been shown to protect neurons from its toxic effects (220), one possibility is MK-801 is at least temporarily promoting vesicular storage. In support of this possibility is the observation that MK-801 inhibits MPP+-induced striatal dopamine release (221), although whether this is related to an effect on vesicular release is not known.

Although the mixed results described may have tempered enthusiasm, there continues to be abundant interest in exploring the possibility that NMDA receptor antagonists might be neuroprotective in PD. One agent that has come under close scrutiny is the NMDA-inhibitor riluzole. Although there has been great interest in this drug as a potential neuroprotective agent in ALS, it has also been found to block MPTP-induced striatal dopamine depletions in mice (222) and monkeys (223,224). In 1998 a clinical trial specifically designed to test its potential neuroprotective effects in PD began. A clinical trial has also been completed with remacemide, another glutamate antagonist (225).

Growth Factors

The use of trophic factors to treat PD is a very attractive possibility, because they could theoretically achieve the same goals as surgery. This is because current evidence suggests that, although dopamine depletions in the disease exceed the 80 percent threshold required to cause parkinsonian signs and symptoms, cell loss is more in the range of 60 percent. This suggests that there may be a substantial number of "dormant" or nonfunctional neurons still present. If these could be coaxed back into service, it is theoretically possible that trophic factors could be used not only slow or halt disease progression, but actually reverse signs and symptoms if enough cells could be rejuvenated. This represents one of the most exciting options for the future, but it may well prove to be one of the most challenging.

MPTP models have provided a vigorous testing ground for trophic factors in PD. Indeed, fibroblast growth factor (FGF) (226–229), glial-derived neurotrophic factor (GDNF) (230,231), epidermal growth factor (EGF) (232), brain-derived neurotrophic factor (BDNF) (233–235), and even nerve growth factor (NGF) (234) have all been tested in the MPTP model. However, the results of these studies have not always been consistent. For example, although FGF was effective in the mouse model, it was not found to be neuroprotective in tissue culture (236). When studies with this trophic factor were extended to primates, no effect was seen on the nigrostriatal system (237). With higher intraventricular doses, ependymal and choroids plexus overgrowth was observed. In some instances this led to hydrocephalus, reminding us that this approach is not without hazard.

It is important to note that at least two strategies have been employed in the testing of growth factors. The first can be described as a neuroprotective strategy, in which the trophic factor is given before or around the time of MPTP administration to block or ameliorate toxicity. The other strategy, which is typically carried out in vivo, is to give the trophic factor after an animal has been lesioned in an attempt to induce recovery. Studies on GDNF illustrate these two approaches. This neurotrophic factor burst on the dopaminergic scene in 1995, when it was shown to both protect against MPTP-induced striatal dopamine depletion and nigral cell loss in the mouse, as well as at least partially restoring nerve fiber densities and dopamine levels when given after MPTP administration (230). Investigations were quickly extended to primates, where GDNF was found to improve bradykinesia, rigidity, and postural instability, as well as increase nigral dopamine levels (231). This restorative effect of GDNF has been shown to be effective in old as well as young mice (238), an important observation if this approach is to be used in PD. One puzzling but fascinating feature about GDNF is its apparent ability to improve dopaminergic function at the level of the substantia nigra, but not at the level of nigrostriatal terminals (239). This is a unique effect, and suggests that, because these animals improve, the events occurring at the level of the substantia nigra deserve more attention in regard to their neurophysiologic role in movement.

In 1996 the first human trial using GDNF for the treatment of PD began. One problem was the fact that, because trophic factors are large molecules, delivery to the CNS represents a major challenge. Because animal studies have shown that GDNF reaches the substantia nigra after intraventricular administration (240), this offered one route by which to administer the drug, but this approach requires the use of an intraventicular cannulae. Results of this study have yet to be reported, but one potential future solution to the delivery problem is to use ex vivo or in vivo gene therapy. This has been attempted by Kojima and colleagues (241), who used a recombinate adenovirus vector to deliver GDNF directly to the brain and found that these animals were partially protected against MPTP-induced striatal dopamine depletions.

More recently, a novel class of trophic factors has appeared. These are potentially neurotrophic molecules that are small enough to cross the blood-brain barrier known as neuroimmunophilins. In 1997, one of these compounds, GPI-1046, was shown to induce regenerative sprouting of surviving dopaminergic neurons after MPTP lesioning in mice (242). Subsequently, another immunophilin (V-10,367) was reported to completely protect against MPTP-induced loss of TH staining in the mouse striatum (243), again suggesting that this class of compounds may be effective in protecting and possibly even restoring dopaminergic neurons. Although primate studies have yet to be reported, given the potential of this class of drugs to treat PD, ease of administration, and the impressive data in the MPTP-treated mouse, clinical trials seemed a logical next step. In 1999, trials with the oral neuroimmunophilin NIL-A to treat PD began.

Does MPTP Cause Apoptosis and/or Necrosis?

Not only are many of the theories on the mechanism of action of MPTP highly reflective of current theories on PD, but also, so are many of the controversies. Nowhere has this been more evident than when it comes to determining the role of apoptosis in cell death. This possibility was raised by Mochizuki and colleagues (244) when they reported morphologic and histochemical evidence of apoptotic cell death in mesencephalic-striatal co-cultures exposed to MPTP. However, a year later, using an acute dose in vivo paradigm in mice, Jackson-Lewis and colleagues (245) failed to find any evidence of apoptosis (although, interestingly, they did note that MPTP can induce a loss of TH immunoreactivity without causing neuronal degeneration, an important caveat for anyone working in the field). Subsequent studies, however, have found evidence of apoptosis, including experiments involving the exposure of PC12 cells in tissue culture to the 2'-ethylphenyl analog of MPTP (246), SH-SY5Y human neuroblastoma cells to MPP+ (247), and also in mice given systemically administered MPTP (248,249). On the other hand, another investigation using PC 12 cells failed to find evidence apoptosis (250), and Choi et al. (182), a murine dopaminergic cell line, and found that MPP+ (in contrast to 6-OHDA) caused noncaspase-dependent necrosis rather than apoptosis. Thus, there continues to be a lack of consensus on the role apoptosis in MPTP-induced neurotoxicity. Much the same controversy continues to brew in regard to apoptosis in PD (251,252).

Deprenyl – Part Two

The original deprenyl story seemed straightforward enough, in that the drug appeared to prevent MPTP toxicity simply by blocking the conversion of MPTP to its toxic metabolite MPP+ by inhibiting MAO B. However, there was one loose end that appeared quite early. In 1985, Mytilineou and colleagues (253) reported the curious observation that deprenyl prevented neurotoxicity of MPP+ in rat mesencephalic cultures, an observation that was later repeated in another cell system (and linked to apoptosis) (254). This early finding hinted that deprenyl might have other neuroprotective actions besides simply inhibiting MAO B. In 1991, Tatton et al. (255) reported that deprenyl could at least partially protect against the neurodegenerative effects of MPTP in mice, even when given for up to five days after MPTP administration, apparently "rescuing" neurons that were destined for destruction. Further evidence that deprenyl had other actions besides its effect on MAO came from a study by Wu and colleagues (256). These investigators found that dopamine release and hydroxyl radical formation produced by the infusion of MPP+ into the striatum of rats declined significantly when deprenyl was added to the perfusate. Later, this same group also provided evidence of a rescue effect using a very different paradigm, one that involved lesioning the nigrostriatal system by infusing MPP+ directly into the substantia nigra (257). When deprenyl was given for four days following the infusion, it partially protected against even high doses of MPP+. These investigators suggested that deprenyl was acting as an antioxidant, because similar results were obtained when 2-methylaminochromans (an inhibitor of iron-catalyzed lipid peroxidation) and DSMO (a hydroxyl radical scavenger) (258) were given instead of deprenyl.

In 1996, Magyar and colleagues (259) reported that deprenyl was a potent inhibitor of MPTP-induced apoptosis in PC12 cells, and Hassouna et al. (260) demonstrated that bax expression was increased in the substantia nigra of MPTP lesioned mice. Tatton and colleagues (248,261) have shown that one of the metabolites of deprenyl, desmethyldeprenyl appears to mediate an anti-apoptotic action, and that it alters expression of SOD 1 and 2, BCL-, BCL-XL, NOS, c-JUN and nicotinamides in a variety of cell systems; this anti-apoptotic effect appears to be associated with reduction of the mitochondrial membrane potential, an early stage in the evolution of apoptosis, possibly by binding to glyceraldehyde-3-phosphate dehydrogenase (GAPDH). Although apoptosis is still controversial in regard to MPTP toxicity, these findings certainly suggest there are properties of the drug that still have yet to be fully elucidated in spite of the fact that it has been almost 20 years since it was first introduced as a treatment for PD (262).

Poly(ADF-ribose) Polymerase (PARP)

A recent and perplexing observation relates to the role of poly(ADF-ribose) polymerase (PARP) in the cascade of events that lead to MPTP neurotoxicity. PARP is an enzyme repair system for DNA that catalyzes the attachment of ADP ribose units (from NAD) to nuclear proteins after DNA damage, a process that consumes considerable energy. In 1996 Cosi et al. (263) reported that a variety of PARP inhibitors partially protected against MPTP-induced striatal dopamine depletions (and cortical noradrenalin depletions as well) in the mouse. PARP inhibitors were subsequently found to block MPTP-induced ATP depletions (264). In accordance with this observation, these investigators reported that MPTP reduced AND levels, which could also be blocked with PARP inhibition (265). More recently it has been reported that PARP knockout mice are almost completely resistant to MPTP (266). This striking result, which is not fully understood, certainly deserves further exploration. However, neuronally derived NO seems to be essential for this process, an observation that may tie in with earlier studies on NO. In view of the evidence that an energy deficit may be important in PD, these findings may have implications for the idiopathic disease itself. In the MPTP model, it could be that the energy deficit induced by this mitochondrial toxin is simply not enough to kill the cell, but rather that an additional oxygen-depleting event is necessary to administer the "coup de gras" to the cell, that event being PARP activation in response to free radical–induced DNA damage. Studies in primates represent a logic next step in the evaluation of the importance of PARP activation in MPTP toxicity, and perhaps PD.

GM1 as a Neuroprotective Agent

Interest in GM1 was first sparked by Hadji-constantinou and colleagues (267) in 1986 when they reported that its administration largely restored striatal dopamine levels in mice with MPTP-induced dopamine depletion. They later showed that GM1 also restored normal morphology to remaining dopaminergic neurons (268) and corrected MPTP-induced D2 receptor supersensitivity (269). Although concerns were originally expressed that systemically administered GM1 is unlikely to reach the target areas in the CNS, it has since been shown to at least reach the CSF (270). Date et al. (271) reported similar reversal of dopamine depletion in young but not older mice, but others have observed at least some recovery in older mice as well (272). On the other hand, Fazzini et al. (273) found the effects of GM1 were only transient in the MPTP model.

Schneider and colleagues (274) have shown that there is a return of TH immunoreactivity in MPTP-lesioned GM1-treated mice, and suggested that the compound could cause regenerative sprouting in the damaged nigrostriatal system, an observation that was supported by later studies, which indicate that both mazindole-binding and KCL-induced striatal dopamine release are improved in lesioned mice after GM1 administration (275). GM1 treatment may also improve the ability of remaining dopaminergic neurons to convert levodopa to dopamine (276), which of course could have implications for treating PD. Recently, it has been shown that a synthetic form of GM1 is more effective in aged mice, and actually works in mice with very extensive MPTP-induced lesions not responsive to GM1 itself (277).

Finally, GM1 has been reported to facilitate behavioral and neurochemical recovery after MPTP exposure in both cats (278) and monkeys (Macaca fascicularis) (279). On the other hand, Herrrero and colleagues (280) reported that GM1 did not protect against either striatal neurochemical changes or nigral cell loss in cynomolgus monkeys, although it did seem to enhance TH cellular content in the substantia nigra. They suggested this compound might be a "palliative" approach to PD.

The GM1 story represents another example of basic research with MPTP-stimulating clinical trials in PD. On the basis of the promising work in mice, and their own studies in primates, Schneider and colleagues initiated an open-label trial in parkinsonian patients, and reported promising if not dramatic results in 1995 (281). The results of a double-blind, controlled study were subsequently reported in 1998, and a significant difference in UPDRS motor scores was found at 16 weeks. The ADL scores in off periods were also improved, as were timed motor tests of arm, hand, foot movements, and walking. These encouraging results have now lead to a five-year double-blind, placebo-controlled trial using 100 patients to examine symptomatic improvement with GM1-treatment over a 6-month period, as well as long-term effects on disease and symptom progression (Jay Schneider, personal communication).

Other Neuroprotective Agents to Emerge from the Study of MPTP

A variety of other agents have been identified as possible inhibitors of MPTP toxicity. Pai et al. (282), using lactic acid release in striatal tissue slices as a marker of toxicity, reported that inhibitors of cytochrome P450 at least partially protect against MPTP toxicity. Bodis-Wollner and colleagues (283) observed that neither parkinsonism nor electroretinograph features of MPTP toxicity were seen in primates pretreated with acetyl-levo-carnitine. The very robust epidemiologic findings that cigarette smoking protects against PD have also been pursued in the MPTP model. In fact one group actually tested cigarette smoke directly, and found that it partially protected against MPTP-induced striatal dopamine depletion (284), an effect that was associated with inhibition of MAO. Nicotine, when given in an acute intermittent, but not a chronic continuous, fashion partially protects against MPTP-induced striatal dopamine depletions in the mouse (285). Thalidomide has also been shown to protect again MPTP-induced striatal dopamine depletion in the mouse, presumably by blocking the inflammatory component of the response (286). Agents that stimulate dopamine receptor activity may be neuroprotective in the mouse model (287), and adenosine A1 agonists prevent MPTP-induced striatal dopamine depletion in mice both when given before and up to five hours after MPTP administration (288). Finally, coadministration of the vigilance promoting drug modafinil has been reported to block MPTP-induced loss of both TH-positive and TH-negative neurons using stereologic counting techniques in the mouse (289), but the mechanism by which this occurs has yet to be determined. These bits and pieces may all be providing interesting new leads for the future as we continue our quest to find neuroprotective agents to test for PD.

Exacerbation of MPTP Toxicity

Although the preceding section focused almost exclusively on ways to prevent toxicity, there has been a parallel, though perhaps less vigorous, effort focusing on ways to enhance toxicity. In 1985 Corsini

and that subpopulations of neurons higher in DAT were actually more sensitive to MPTP (329). Their observations raise the possibility that the lack of a dopamine transporter might explain why these neurons are less vulnerable to MPTP/MPP+. Similarly, there is now evidence that low levels of DAT in the ventral tegmental area may explain the long-standing mystery as to why this dopaminergic area is less sensitive to the effects of MPTP than the zona compacta of the substantia nigra (330). These observations are supported by the work of Airaksinen and colleagues (331), who found that calbindin null-mutant mice exposed to MPTP were not more sensitive to the effects of MPTP, as would have been predicted if calbindin itself was neuroprotective in some manner. This re-focusing on the dopamine transporter as a key to selective vulnerability within the nigra could also be quite relevant to the etiopathogenesis of PD. This is because a similar pattern of intranigral vulnerability has been seen in humans with the disorder, possibly representing a clue that selective uptake of an exogenous or endogenous toxin may be important.

EPIDEMIOLOGIC INVESTIGATIONS

The discovery of the biologic effects of MPTP had at least three major scientific implications, the third of which was its impact on thinking regarding the environmental hypothesis of PD. The fact that such a simple compound could induce virtually all of the motor (and even non-motor) features of PD raised the dramatic possibility that one or more environmental agents might play a role in the causing or triggering the idiopathic disease. This possibility was further stimulated by the similarities between MPP+ and the herbicide paraquat, although their basic mechanisms action were quickly shown to be different (154,155). Although earlier studies failed to show that paraquat was not toxic to the dopaminergic system in mice (332,333), recently Brooks et al. (334) have reported that this herbicide causes dopamine depletion and actual degeneration of nigrostriatal neurons after systemic injection.

Armed with knowledge of the biologic effects MPTP, and the results of a twin study that was also published in 1983 (335) that failed to show a genetic influence on PD, investigators initiated a wide variety of epidemiologic studies aimed at finding environmental risk factors in PD, and indeed many such factors, including rural living, pesticide exposure, well water consumption, and excessive exposure to metals have all been reported to apparently increase the risk.

Another line of research enhanced by MPTP relates to the metabolism of xenobiotics and the risk for PD. Simply put, the hypothesis is that inherited defects in xenobiotic metabolism could enhance the susceptibility to toxicity from exogenous agents, and thereby increase the risk for PD. This concept was fostered by earlier observations suggesting that inherited abnormalities in the cytochrome P450 system could enhance the risk for PD. This has since become a fascinating and complex literature (336). Finally, it is worth mentioning that a recently published twin study (337), which is the largest twin study ever done in PD, once again points to the importance of the environment.

CONCLUSIONS

The discovery of the biologic effects of MPTP has had a remarkably diverse impact on research in PD. Indeed, knowledge of the very existence of such a compound ushered in a research renaissance on the disease, with new initiatives ranging from those focused on basic mechanisms of cell death to large epidemiologic studies. In regard to mechanisms of neurodegeneration, it is striking to see how each step in the cascade of events that lead to MPTP toxicity have in some way or another been implicated in PD. Perhaps the most impressive outcome of this research is the number of clinical trials that have been generated from basic science on MPTP and its mechanisms. However, this impact has undoubtedly been equaled by its usefulness in the primate model in unraveling basal ganglia circuitry. It is now possible to say that this model has stood the test of time in terms of relevance to the idiopathic disease, at least when it comes to neuropharmacologic and neurophysiologic changes in the basal ganglia that occur in parkinsonism. The model has therefore proved to be a widely used testing ground, even a "gold standard," for investigating new pharmacologi and surgical forms of therapy. Finally, almost all aspects of research on MPTP have fostered new investigations directed at finding the cause or causes of PD.

What can we expect in the new millennium from MPTP-related research? Undoubtedly, new compounds will continue to be tested for their symptomatic and/or neuroprotective effects in MPTP-induced models of the disease. Although neuroprotective studies will be performed in a variety of settings and models, symptomatic forms of therapy will ultimately rely on primate studies, as they are the only species to manifest full-blown and behaviorally typical parkinsonism. This model is proving equally valuable in the investigation of side effects of therapy, particularly dopa-dyskinesias.

From a basic research standpoint, there remain an abundance of controversies to be resolved regarding various aspects of the mechanism of action of MPTP. Furthermore, there are many unsolved mysteries – such as the question of why the primate brain has such difficulty eliminating MPP+, while the rodent brain can do it in a matter of hours. Also, it seems almost certain that, as new theories regarding cell death in PD emerge, they will probably explored using MPTP. The recent identification of alpha-synuclein represents an excellent example. The relevance of this protein to PD came about as the result of identification of the A53T mutation in the region encoding for the protein α-synuclein in a large Italian kindred with an autosomal dominant form of parkinsonism (338). While it is still a mystery as to how this mutation orchestrates both nigral cell degeneration and Lewy body formation (although theories abound), interest in α-synuclein was further enhanced with the discovery that this protein is a major component of the Lewy body, not only in typical PD (339), but also in all Lewy body diseases (340). As might have been predicted, MPTP is already being used to study alpha-synuclein. For example, MPTP administration has now been shown to upregulate α-synuclein in the substantia nigra of mice (341). In the baboon, MPTP causes a relocation for alpha-synuclein from its normal presynaptic location to the cell bodies were it aggregates (342). These investigators suggest that this models Lewy body formation, which in turn could represent a fundamental step in PD. There will undoubtedly be many more studies investigating the interaction between MPTP (and other putative environmental agents) and alpha-synuclein. The fundamental importance of these is that, because few if any patients with sporadic PD have a mutation in the region encoding for alpha-synuclein, other factors must be involved in precipitating pathologic aggregation of this protein, and MPTP (and other toxicants) represent a logical place to start from an experimental standpoint.

In closing, it seems reasonable to ask the rhetorical question: Will MPTP-related research eventually solve the complex riddle that we call PD? Certainly, it has had an enormous impact on research and will likely do so in the future. There is little doubt that it will continue to be used as a readily accessible tool to explore new hypotheses on the cause and treatments of the disease. Certainly, research on this disease has never been at a higher level, and there is reason for optimism. But science must continue at its own pace. If and when the disease is solved, it seems MPTP will likely be allowed to take a bow as a member of the cast, even if it is not as the player with the leading role.

REFERENCES

1. Ziering ABL, Heineman SD, Lee J. Piperidine derivatives. III. 4-Arylpiperidines. *J Org Chem* 1947; 12:894–903.
2. Langston J, Palfremann J. *The Case of the Frozen Addicts.* New York: Random House; 1995.
3. Langston JW, Ballard P, Tetrud JW, et al. Chronic parkinsonism in humans due to a product of meperidine-analog synthesis. *Science* 1983; 219(4587):979–980.
4. Langston JW, Ballard PA, Jr. Parkinson's disease in a chemist working with 1-methyl-4-phenyl-1,2,5,6-tetrahydropyridine [letter]. *N Engl J Med* 1983; 309(5):310.
5. Barbeau A, Roy M, Langston JW. Neurological consequence of industrial exposure to 1-methyl-4-phenyl-1,2,3,6-tetrahydropyridine. *Lancet* 1985; 1(8431):747.
6. Burns RS, LeWitt PA, Ebert MH, et al. The clinical syndrome of striatal dopamine deficiency. parkinsonism induced by 1-methyl-4-phenyl-1,2,3,6-tetrahydropyridine (MPTP). *N Engl J Med* 1985; 312(22):1418–1421.
7. Davis GC, Williams AC, Markey SP, et al. Chronic parkinsonism secondary to intravenous injection of meperidine analogues. *Psychiatry Res* 1979; 1(3):249–254.
8. Langston JW. MPTP neurotoxicity: an overview and characterization of phases of toxicity. *Life Sci* 1985; 36(3):201–206.
9. Langston JW, Forno LS, Tetrud J, et al. Evidence of active nerve cell degeneration in the substantia nigra of humans years after 1-methyl-4-phenyl-1,2,3,6-tetrahydropyridine exposure. *Ann Neurol* 1999; 46(4):598–605.
10. Burns RS, Chiueh CC, Markey SP, et al. A primate model of parkinsonism: Selective destruction of dopaminergic neurons in the pars compacta of the substantia nigra by N-methyl-4-phenyl-1,2,3,6-tetrahydropyridine. *Proc Natl Acad Sci USA* 1983; 80(14):4546–4550.
11. Langston JW, Irwin I, Langston EB, et al. Pargyline prevents MPTP-induced parkinsonism in primates. *Science* 1984; 225(4669):1480–1482.
12. Langston JW, Langston EB, Irwin I. MPTP-induced parkinsonism in human and non-human primates – clinical and experimental aspects. *Acta Neurol Scand Suppl* 1984; 100:49–54.
13. Langston JW, Ballard P. Parkinsonism induced by 1-methyl-4-phenyl-1,2,3,6-tetrahydropyridine (MPTP): implications for treatment and the pathogenesis of Parkinson's disease. *Can J Neurol Sci* 1984; 11(Suppl 1):160–165.
14. Langston JW, Forno LS, Rebert CS, et al. Selective nigral toxicity after systemic administration of 1-methyl-4-phenyl-1,2,3,6-tetrahydropyridine (MPTP) in the squirrel monkey. *Brain Res* 1984; 292(2):390–394.

15. Langston JW, Irwin I, Langston EB, et al. 1-Methyl-4-phenylpyridinium ion (MPP+): identification of a metabolite of MPTP, a toxin selective to the substantia nigra. *Neurosci Lett* 1984; 48(1):87–92.

16. Jenner P, Rupniak NM, Rose S, et al. 1-Methyl-4-phenyl-1,2,3,6-tetrahydropyridine-induced parkinsonism in the common marmoset. *Neurosci Lett* 1984; 50(1–3):85–90.

17. Gerlach M, Riederer P, Przuntek H, et al. MPTP mechanisms of neurotoxicity and their implications for Parkinson's disease. *Eur J Pharmacol* 1991; 208(4):273–286.

18. Ballard PA, Tetrud JW, Langston JW. Permanent human parkinsonism due to 1-methyl-4-phenyl-1,2,3,6-tetrahydropyridine (MPTP): Seven cases. *Neurology* 1985; 35(7):949–956.

19. Tetrud JW, Langston JW. Tremor in MPTP-induced parkinsonism. *Neurology* 1992; 42(2):407–410.

20. Stern Y, Langston JW. Intellectual changes in patients with MPTP-induced parkinsonism. *Neurology* 1985; 35(10):1506–1509.

21. Stern Y, Tetrud JW, Martin WR, et al. Cognitive change following MPTP exposure. *Neurology* 1990; 40(2):261–264.

22. Quinn N, Critchley P, Marsden CD. Young onset Parkinson's disease. *Mov Disord* 1987; 2(2):73–91.

23. D'Amato RJ, Alexander GM, Schwartzman RJ, et al. Evidence for neuromelanin involvement in MPTP-induced neurotoxicity. *Nature* 1987; 327(6120):324–326.

24. Kurkowska-Jastrzebska I, Wronska A, Kohutnicka M, et al. The inflammatory reaction following 1-methyl-4-phenyl-1,2,3,6-tetrahydropyridine intoxication in mouse. *Exp Neurol* 1999; 156(1):50–61.

25. Burns RS, Markey SP, Phillips JM, et al. The neurotoxicity of 1-methyl-4-phenyl-1,2,3,6-tetrahydropyridine in the monkey and man. *Can J Neurol Sci* 1984; 11(Suppl 1):166–168.

26. Poli A, Gandolfi O, Lucchi R, et al. Spontaneous recovery of MPTP-damaged catecholamine systems in goldfish brain areas. *Brain Res* 1992; 585(1–2):128–134.

27. Heikkila RE, Hess A, Duvoisin RC. Dopaminergic neurotoxicity of 1-methyl-4-phenyl-1,2,3,6-tetrahydropyridine in mice. *Science* 1984; 224(4656):1451–1453.

28. Markey SP, Johannessen JN, Chiueh CC, et al. Intraneuronal generation of a pyridinium metabolite may cause drug-induced parkinsonism. *Nature* 1984; 311(5985):464–467.

29. Boyce S, Kelly E, Reavill C, et al. Repeated administration of N-methyl-4-phenyl 1,2,5,6-tetrahydropyridine to rats is not toxic to striatal dopamine neurones. *Biochem Pharmacol* 1984; 33(11): 1747–1752.

30. DeLong MR. Primate models of movement disorders of basal ganglia origin. *Trends Neurosci* 1990; 13(7):281–285.

31. Bergman H, Wichmann T, DeLong MR. Reversal of experimental parkinsonism by lesions of the subthalamic nucleus. *Science* 1990; 249(4975): 1436–1438.

32. Wichmann T, DeLong MR. Pathophysiology of parkinsonian motor abnormalities. *Adv Neurol* 1993; 60:53–61.

33. Wichmann T, Bergman H, DeLong MR. The primate subthalamic nucleus. I. Functional properties in intact animals. *J Neurophysiol* 1994; 72(2):494–506.

34. Bergman H, Wichmann T, Karmon B, et al. The primate subthalamic nucleus. II. Neuronal activity in the MPTP model of parkinsonism. *J Neurophysiol* 1994; 72(2):507–520.

35. Wichmann T, Bergman H, DeLong MR. The primate subthalamic nucleus. III. Changes in motor behavior and neuronal activity in the internal pallidum induced by subthalamic inactivation in the MPTP model of parkinsonism. *J Neurophysiol* 1994; 72(2):521–530.

36. Benazzouz A, Gross C, Feger J, et al. Reversal of rigidity and improvement in motor performance by subthalamic high-frequency stimulation in MPTP-treated monkeys. *Eur J Neurosci* 1993; 5(4):382–389.

37. Benazzouz A, Boraud T, Feger J, et al. Alleviation of experimental hemiparkinsonism by high-frequency stimulation of the subthalamic nucleus in primates: A comparison with L-Dopa treatment. *Mov Disord* 1996; 11(6):627–632.

38. Bjorklund A. Neural transplantation – an experimental tool with clinical possibilities. *Trends Neurosci* 1991; 14(8):319–322.

39. Bakay RA, Barrow DL, Fiandaca MS, et al. Biochemical and behavioral correction of MPTP Parkinson-like syndrome by fetal cell transplantation. *Ann NY Acad Sci* 1987; 495: 623–640.

40. Bankiewicz KS, Plunkett RJ, Jacobowitz DM, et al. The effect of fetal mesencephalon implants on primate MPTP-induced parkinsonism. Histochemical and behavioral studies. *J Neurosurg* 1990; 72(2):231–244.

41. Elsworth JD, Sladek JR, Jr., Taylor JR, et al. Early gestational mesencephalon grafts, but not later gestational mesencephalon, cerebellum or sham grafts, increase dopamine in caudate nucleus of MPTP-treated monkeys. *Neuroscience* 1996; 72(2):477–484.

42. Sladek JR, Jr., Redmond DE, Jr., Collier TJ, et al. Transplantation of fetal dopamine neurons in primate brain reverses MPTP induced parkinsonism. *Prog Brain Res* 1987; 71:309–323.

43. Nakai M, Itakura T, Kamei I, et al. Autologous transplantation of the superior cervical ganglion into the brain of parkinsonian monkeys. *J Neurosurg* 1990; 72(1):91–95.

44. Freed WJ, Poltorak M, Becker JB. Intracerebral adrenal medulla grafts: A review. *Exp Neurol* 1990; 110(2):139–166.

45. Aebischer P, Goddard M, Signore AP, et al. Functional recovery in hemiparkinsonian primates transplanted with polymer-encapsulated PC12 cells. *Exp Neurol* 1994; 126(2):151–158.

46. Bankiewicz KS, Bringas JR, McLaughlin W, et al. Application of gene therapy for Parkinson's disease: Nonhuman primate experience. *Adv Pharmacol* 1998; 42:801–806.

47. Elsworth JD, Brittan MS, Taylor JR, et al. Upregulation of striatal D2 receptors in the MPTP-treated vervet monkey is reversed by grafts of fetal ventral mesencephalon: An autoradiographic study. *Brain Res* 1998; 795(1–2):55–62.

48. Sortwell CE, Blanchard BC, Collier TJ, et al. Pattern of synaptophysin immunoreactivity within mesencephalic grafts following transplantation in a parkinsonian primate model. *Brain Res* 1998; 791(1–2):117–124.

49. Widner H, Tetrud J, Rehncrona S, et al. Bilateral fetal mesencephalic grafting in two patients with parkinsonism induced by 1-methyl-4-phenyl-1,2,3,6-tetrahydropyridine (MPTP). *N Engl J Med* 1992; 327(22):1556–1563.

50. Falardeau P, Bouchard S, Bedard PJ, Behavioral and biochemical effect of chronic treatment with D-1 and/or D-2 dopamine agonists in MPTP monkeys. *Eur J Pharmacol* 1988; 150(1–2):59–66.

51. Gagnon C, Bedard PJ, Di Paolo T. Effect of chronic treatment of MPTP monkeys with dopamine D-1 and/or D-2 receptor agonists. *Eur J Pharmacol* 1990; 178(1):115–120.

52. Alexander GM, Brainard DL, Gordon SW, et al. Dopamine receptor changes in untreated and (+)-PHNO-treated MPTP parkinsonian primates. *Brain Res* 1991; 547(2):181–189.

53. Alexander GM, Schwartzman RJ, Grothusen JR, et al. Changes in brain dopamine receptors in MPTP parkinsonian monkeys following L-dopa treatment. *Brain Res* 1993; 625(2):276–282.

54. Graham WC, Sambrook MA, Crossman AR. Differential effect of chronic dopaminergic treatment on dopamine D1 and D2 receptors in the monkey brain in MPTP-induced parkinsonism. *Brain Res* 1993; 602(2):290–303.

55. Mierau J, Schingnitz G. Biochemical and pharmacological studies on pramipexole, a potent and selective dopamine D2 receptor agonist. *Eur J Pharmacol* 1992; 215(2–3):161–170.

56. Vermeulen RJ, Drukarch B, Sahadat MC, et al. The dopamine D1 agonist SKF 81297 and the dopamine D2 agonist LY 171555 act synergistically to stimulate motor behavior of 1-methyl-4-phenyl-1,2,3,6-tetrahydropyridine-lesioned parkinsonian rhesus monkeys. *Mov Disord* 1994; 9(6): 664–672.

57. Kebabian JW, Britton DR, DeNinno MP, et al. A-77636: A potent and selective dopamine D1 receptor agonist with anti-parkinsonian activity in marmosets. *Eur J Pharmacol* 1992; 229(2–3):203–209.

58. Blanchet P, Bedard PJ, Britton DR, et al. Differential effect of selective D-1 and D-2 dopamine receptor agonists on levodopa-induced dyskinesia in 1-methyl-4-phenyl-1,2,3,6-tetrahydropyridine-exposed monkeys. *J Pharmacol Exp Ther* 1993; 267(1):275–279.

59. Shiosaki K, Jenner P, Asin KE, et al. ABT-431: The diacetyl prodrug of A-86929, a potent and selective dopamine D1 receptor agonist: in vitro characterization and effects in animal models of Parkinson's disease. *J Pharmacol Exp Ther* 1996; 276(1):150–160.

60. Nomoto M, Jenner P, Marsden CD. The D1 agonist SKF 38393 inhibits the anti-parkinsonian activity of the D2 agonist LY 171555 in the MPTP-treated marmoset. *Neurosci Lett* 1988; 93(2–3):275–280.

61. Close SP, Elliott PJ, Hayes AG, et al. Effects of classical and novel agents in a MPTP-induced reversible model of Parkinson's disease. *Psychopharmacology* 1990; 102(3):295–300.

62. Boyce S, Rupniak NM, Steventon MJ, et al. Differential effects of D1 and D2 agonists in MPTP-treated primates: Functional implications for Parkinson's disease. *Neurology* 1990; 40(6):927–933.

63. Blanchet PJ, Grondin R, Bedard PJ, et al. Dopamine D1 receptor desensitization profile in MPTP-lesioned primates. *Eur J Pharmacol* 1996; 309(1):13–20.

64. Schneider JS, Sun ZQ, Roeltgen DP. Effects of dihydrexidine, a full dopamine D-1 receptor agonist, on delayed response performance in chronic low dose MPTP-treated monkeys. *Brain Res* 1994; 663(1):140–144.

65. Crossman AR, Clarke CE, Boyce S, et al. MPTP-induced parkinsonism in the monkey: Neurochemical pathology, complications of treatment and pathophysiological mechanisms. *Can J Neurol Sci* 1987; 14(Suppl 3):428–435.

66. Clarke CE, Sambrook MA, Mitchell IJ, et al. Levodopa-induced dyskinesia and response fluctuations in primates rendered parkinsonian with 1-methyl-4-phenyl-1,2,3,6-tetrahydropyridine (MPTP). *J Neurol Sci* 1987; 78(3):273–280.

67. Boyce S, Rupniak NM, Steventon MJ, et al. Characterization of dyskinesias induced by L-dopa in MPTP-treated squirrel monkeys. *Psychopharmacology* 1990; 102(1):21–27.

68. Schneider JS. levodopa-induced dyskinesias in parkinsonian monkeys: Relationship to extent of nigrostriatal damage. *Pharmacol Biochem Behav* 1989; 34(1):193–196.

69. Boyce S, Rupniak NM, Steventon MJ, et al. Nigrostriatal damage is required for induction of dyskinesias by L-DOPA in squirrel monkeys. *Clin Neuropharmacol* 1990; 13(5):448–458.

70. Clarke CE, Boyce S, Sambrook MA, et al. Behavioral effects of (+)-4-propyl-9-hydroxynaphthoxazine in primates rendered parkinsonian with 1-methyl-4-phenyl-1,2,3,6-tetrahydropyridine. *Naunyn Schmiedebergs Arch Pharmacol* 1988; 338(1):35–38.

71. Gomez-Mancilla B, Bedard PJ. Effect of D1 and D2 agonists and antagonists on dyskinesia produced by L-dopa in 1-methyl-4-phenyl-1,2,3,6-tetrahydropyridine-treated monkeys. *J Pharmacol Exp Ther* 1991; 259(1):409–413.

72. Nomoto M, Fukuda T. The effects of D1 and D2 dopamine receptor agonist and antagonist on parkinsonism in chronic MPTP-treated monkeys. *Adv Neurol* 1993; 60:119–122.

73. Blanchet PJ, Gomez-Mancilla B, Bedard PJ. DOPA-induced "peak dose" dyskinesia: Clues implicating D2 receptor-mediated mechanisms using dopaminergic agonists in MPTP monkeys. *J Neural Transm Suppl* 1995; 45:103–112.

74. Blanchet PJ, Konitsiotis S, Chase TN. Motor response to a dopamine D3 receptor preferring agonist compared to apomorphine in levodopa-primed 1-methyl-4-phenyl-1,2,3,6-tetrahydropyridine monkeys. *J Pharmacol Exp Ther* 1997; 283(2): 794–799.

75. Pearce RK, Jackson M, Smith L, et al. Chronic L-DOPA administration induces dyskinesias in the 1-methyl-4-phenyl-1,2,3,6-tetrahydropyridine-treated common marmoset (Callithrix Jacchus). *Mov Disord* 1995; 10(6):731–740.

76. Grondin R, Doan VD, Gregoire L, et al. D1 receptor blockade improves L-dopa-induced dyskinesia but worsens parkinsonism in MPTP monkeys. *Neurology* 1999; 52(4):771–776.

77. Akai T, Ozawa M, Yamaguchi M, et al. Combination treatment of the partial D2 agonist terguride with the D1 agonist SKF 82958 in 1-methyl-4-phenyl-1,2,3,6-tetrahydropyridine-lesioned parkinsonian cynomolgus monkeys. *J Pharmacol Exp Ther* 1995; 273(1):309–314.

78. Pearce RK, Banerji T, Jenner P, et al. De novo administration of ropinirole and bromocriptine induces less dyskinesia than L-dopa in the MPTP-treated marmoset. *Mov Disord* 1998; 13(2):234–241.

79. Grondin R, Bedard PJ, Britton DR, et al. Potential therapeutic use of the selective dopamine D1 receptor agonist, A-86929: An acute study in parkinsonian levodopa-primed monkeys. *Neurology* 1997; 49(2):421–426.

80. Filion M, Tremblay L, Bedard PJ. Effects of dopamine agonists on the spontaneous activity of globus pallidus neurons in monkeys with MPTP-induced parkinsonism. *Brain Res* 1991; 547(1):152–161.

81. Blanchet PJ, Calon F, Martel JC, et al. Continuous administration decreases and pulsatile administration increases behavioral sensitivity to a novel dopamine D2 agonist (U-91356A) in MPTP-exposed monkeys. *J Pharmacol Exp Ther* 1995; 272(2):854–859.

82. Goulet M, Morissette M, Calon F, et al. Continuous or pulsatile chronic D2 dopamine receptor agonist (U91356A) treatment of drug-naive 4-phenyl-1,2,3,6-tetrahydropyridine monkeys differentially regulates brain D1 and D2 receptor expression: in situ hybridization histochemical analysis. *Neuroscience* 1997; 79(2):497–507.

83. Blanchet PJ, Grondin R, Bedard PJ. Dyskinesia and wearing-off following dopamine D1 agonist treatment in drug-naive 1-methyl-4-phenyl-1,2,3,6-tetrahydropyridine-lesioned primates. *Mov Disord* 1996; 11(1):91–94.

84. Calon F, Goulet M, Blanchet PJ, et al. levodopa or D2 agonist induced dyskinesia in MPTP monkeys: correlation with changes in dopamine and GABAA receptors in the striatopallidal complex. *Brain Res* 1995; 680(1–2):43–52.

85. Goulet M, Grondin R, Blanchet PJ, et al. Dyskinesias and tolerance induced by chronic treatment with a D1 agonist administered in pulsatile or continuous mode do not correlate with changes of putamenal D1 receptors in drug-naive MPTP monkeys. *Brain Res* 1996; 719(1–2):129–137.

86. Blanchet PJ, Metman LV, Mouradian MM, et al. Acute pharmacologic blockade of dyskinesias in Parkinson's disease. *Mov Disord* 1996; 11(5):580–581.

87. Blanchet PJ, Konitsiotis S, Chase TN. Amantadine reduces levodopa-induced dyskinesias in parkinsonian monkeys. *Mov Disord* 1998; 13(5):798–802.

88. Papa SM BR, Engber TM, Kask AM, et al. Reversal of levodopa-induced motor fluctuations in experimental parkinsonism by NMDA receptor blockade. *Brain Res* 1995; 701:13–18.

89. Papa S, Chase T. levodopa-induced dyskinesias improved by a glutamate antagonist in Parkinsonian monkeys. *Ann Neurol* 1996; 39(5):574–578.

90. Verhagen ML BP, van den Munckhof P, Del Dotto P, et al. A trial of dextromethorphan in parkinsonian patients with motor response complications. *Mov. Disord.* 1998; 13:414–417.

91. Oh JD, Russell DS, Vaughan CL, et al. Enhanced tyrosine phosphorylation of striatal NMDA receptor subunits: effect of dopaminergic denervation and L-DOPA administration [published erratum appears in *Brain Res* 1999 Feb 27; 820(1–2):117]. *Brain Res* 1998; 813(1):150–159.

92. Oh JD, Vaughan CL, Chase TN. Effect of dopamine denervation and dopamine agonist administration on serine phosphorylation of striatal NMDA receptor subunits. *Brain Res* 1999; 821(2):433–442.

93. Normand E, Popovici T, Onteniente B, et al. Dopaminergic neurons of the substantia nigra modulate preproenkephalin A gene expression in rat striatal neurons. *Brain Res* 1988; 439(1–2):39–46.

94. Sivam SP, Krause JE. The adaptation of enkephalin, tachykinin and monoamine neurons of the basal ganglia following neonatal dopaminergic denervation is dependent on the extent of dopamine depletion. *Brain Res* 1990; 536(1–2):169–175.

95. Gudehithlu KP, Duchemin AM, Tejwani GA, et al. Preproenkephalin mRNA and methionine-enkephalin increase in mouse striatum after 1-methyl-4-phenyl-1,2,3,6-tetrahydropyridine treatment. *J Neurochem* 1991; 56(3):1043–1048.

96. Campbell K, Bjorklund A. Prefrontal corticostriatal afferents maintain increased enkephalin gene

expression in the dopamine-denervated rat striatum. *Eur J Neurosci* 1994; 6(8):1371–1383.

97. Henry B, Fox SH, Peggs D, et al. The alpha2-adrenergic receptor antagonist idazoxan reduces dyskinesia and enhances anti-parkinsonian actions of L-dopa in the MPTP-lesioned primate model of Parkinson's disease. *Mov Disord* 1999; 14(5): 744–753.

98. Augood SJ, Emson PC, Mitchell IJ, et al. Cellular localization of enkephalin gene expression in MPTP-treated cynomolgus monkeys. *Brain Res Mol Brain Res* 1989; 6(1):85–92.

99. Herrero MT, Augood SJ, Hirsch EC, et al. Effects of L-DOPA on preproenkephalin and preprotachykinin gene expression in the MPTP-treated monkey striatum. *Neuroscience* 1995; 68(4):1189–1198.

100. Jolkkonen J, Jenner P, Marsden CD. L-DOPA reverses altered gene expression of substance P but not enkephalin in the caudate-putamen of common marmosets treated with MPTP. *Brain Res Mol Brain Res* 1995; 32(2):297–307.

101. Morissette M, Grondin R, Goulet M, et al. Differential regulation of striatal preproenkephalin and preprotachykinin mRNA levels in MPTP-lesioned monkeys chronically treated with dopamine D1 or D2 receptor agonists. *J Neurochem* 1999; 72(2):682–692.

102. Boyce S, Rupniak NM, Steventon M, et al. CCK-8S inhibits L-dopa-induced dyskinesias in parkinsonian squirrel monkeys. *Neurology* 1990; 40(4):717–718.

103. Ekesbo A, Andren PE, Gunne LM, et al. (−)-OSU 6162 inhibits levodopa-induced dyskinesias in a monkey model of Parkinson's disease. *Neuroreport* 1997; 8(11):2567–2570.

104. Gomez-Mancilla B, Bedard PJ. Effect of estrogen and progesterone on L-dopa induced dyskinesia in MPTP-treated monkeys. *Neurosci Lett* 1992; 135(1):129–132.

105. Grondin R, Tahar AH, Doan VD, et al. Noradrenoceptor antagonism with idazoxan improves L-dopa-induced dyskinesias in MPTP monkeys. *Naunyn Schmiedebergs Arch Pharmacol* 2000; 361(2):181–186.

106. Crossman AR, Mitchell IJ, Sambrook MA. Regional brain uptake of 2-deoxyglucose in N-methyl-4-phenyl-1,2,3,6-tetrahydropyridine (MPTP)-induced parkinsonism in the macaque monkey. *Neuropharmacology* 1985; 24(6):587–591.

107. Papa SM, Desimone R, Fiorani M, et al. Internal globus pallidus discharge is nearly suppressed during levodopa-induced dyskinesias. *Ann Neurol* 1999; 46(5):732–738.

108. Alexander GM, Schwartzman RJ, Brainard L, et al. Changes in brain catecholamines and dopamine uptake sites at different stages of MPTP parkinsonism in monkeys. *Brain Res* 1992; 588(2):261–269.

109. Pearce RK, Jackson M, Britton DR, et al. Actions of the D1 agonists A-77636 and A-86929 on locomotion and dyskinesia in MPTP-treated L-dopa-primed common marmosets. *Psychopharmacology* (Berl) 1999; 142(1):51–60.

110. Langston J, Quik M, Petzinger G, et al. Investigating levodopa-induced dyskinesias in the parkinsonian primate. *Ann Neurol* 2000; 47(Suppl 1):S79–S89.

111. Petzinger G, Quik M, Ivashina E, et al. Reliability and validity of a new global dyskinesia rating scale in the MPTP-lesioned non-human primate (Saimiri sciureus). *Mov Disord* 2000; (in press).

112. Mones R. Experimental dyskinesias in normal rhesus monkey. *Adv. Neurol.* 1973; 1:665–669.

113. Bankiewicz KS, Oldfield EH, Chiueh CC, et al. Hemiparkinsonism in monkeys after unilateral internal carotid artery infusion of 1-methyl-4-phenyl-1,2,3,6-tetrahydropyridine (MPTP). *Life Sci* 1986; 39(1):7–16.

114. Smith RD, Zhang Z, Kurlan R, et al. Developing a stable bilateral model of parkinsonism in rhesus monkeys. *Neuroscience* 1993; 52(1):7–16.

115. Bezard E, Imbert C, Deloire X, et al. A chronic MPTP model reproducing the slow evolution of Parkinson's disease: evolution of motor symptoms in the monkey. *Brain Res* 1997; 766(1–2):107–112.

116. Tolwani RJ, Jakowec MW, Petzinger GM, et al. Experimental models of Parkinson's disease: Insights from many models. *Lab Anim Sci* 1999; 49(4):363–371.

117. Lewin R. Brain enzyme is the target of drug toxin [news]. *Science* 1984; 225(4669):1460–1462.

118. Parsons B, Rainbow TC. High-affinity binding sites for [3H]MPTP may correspond to monamine oxidase. *Eur J Pharmacol* 1984; 102(2):375–377.

119. Chiba K, Trevor A, Castagnoli N, Jr. Metabolism of the neurotoxic tertiary amine, MPTP, by brain monoamine oxidase. *Biochem Biophys Res Commun* 1984; 120(2):574–578.

120. Di Monte DA, Wu EY, Irwin I, et al. Production and disposition of 1-methyl-4-phenylpyridinium in primary cultures of mouse astrocytes. *Glia* 1992; 5(1):48–55.

121. Di Monte DA, Wu EY, DeLanney LE, et al. Toxicity of 1-methyl-4-phenyl-1,2,3,6-tetrahydropyridine in primary cultures of mouse astrocytes. *J Pharmacol Exp Ther* 1992; 261(1):44–49.

122. Di Monte DA, Schipper HM, Hetts S, et al. Iron-mediated bioactivation of 1-methyl-4-phenyl-1,2,3,6-tetrahydropyridine (MPTP) in glial cultures. *Glia* 1995; 15(2):203–206.

123. Di Monte DA, Royland JE, Irwin I, et al. Astrocytes as the site for bioactivation of neurotoxins. *Neurotoxicology* 1996; 17(3–4):697–703.

124. Westlund KN, Denney RM, Rose RM, et al. Localization of distinct monoamine oxidase A and monoamine oxidase B cell populations in human brainstem. *Neuroscience* 1988; 25(2):439–456.

125. Tetrud JW, Langston JW. The effect of deprenyl (selegiline) on the natural history of Parkinson's disease. *Science* 1989; 245(4917):519–522.

126. Parkinson's Study Group. Effect of deprenyl on the progression of disability in early Parkinson's disease. *N Eng J Med* 1989; 321:1364–1371.

127. Javitch JA, Snyder SH. Uptake of MPP(+) by dopamine neurons explains selectivity of parkinsonism-inducing neurotoxin, MPTP. *Eur J Pharmacol* 1984; 106(2):455–456.

128. Ricaurte GA, Langston JW, DeLanney LE, et al. Dopamine uptake blockers protect against the dopamine depleting effect of 1-methyl-4-phenyl-1,2,3,6-tetrahydropyridine (MPTP) in the mouse striatum. *Neurosci Lett* 1985; 59(3): 259–264.

129. Mayer RA, Jarvis MF, Wagner GC. Cocaine blocks the dopamine depletion induced by MPTP. *Res Commun Chem Pathol Pharmacol* 1985; 49(1): 145–148.

130. Sundstrom E, Jonsson G. Differential time course of protection by monoamine oxidase inhibition and uptake inhibition against MPTP neurotoxicity on central catecholamine neurons in mice. *Eur J Pharmacol* 1986; 122(2):275–278.

131. Schultz W, Scarnati E, Sundstrom E, et al. The catecholamine uptake blocker nomifensine protects against MPTP-induced parkinsonism in monkeys. *Exp Brain Res* 1986; 63(1):216–220.

132. Bezard E, Gross CE, Fournier MC, et al. Absence of MPTP-induced neuronal death in mice lacking the dopamine transporter. *Exp Neurol* 1999; 155(2):268–273.

133. Ramsay RR, Salach JI, Dadgar J, et al. Inhibition of mitochondrial NADH dehydrogenase by pyridine derivatives and its possible relation to experimental and idiopathic parkinsonism. *Biochem Biophys Res Commun* 1986; 135(1):269–275.

134. Ramsay RR, Salach JI, Singer TP. Uptake of the neurotoxin 1-methyl-4-phenylpyridine (MPP+) by mitochondria and its relation to the inhibition of the mitochondrial oxidation of AND+-linked substrates by MPP+. *Biochem Biophys Res Commun* 1986; 134(2):743–748.

135. Nicklas WJ, Vyas I, Heikkila RE. Inhibition of NADH-linked oxidation in brain mitochondria by 1-methyl-4-phenyl-pyridine, a metabolite of the neurotoxin, 1-methyl-4-phenyl-1,2,5,6-tetrahydropyridine. *Life Sci* 1985; 36(26):2503–2508.

136. Vyas I, Heikkila RE, Nicklas WJ. Studies on the neurotoxicity of 1-methyl-4-phenyl-1,2,3,6-tetrahydropyridine: inhibition of AND-linked substrate oxidation by its metabolite, 1-methyl-4-phenyl-pyridinium. *J Neurochem* 1986; 46(5):1501–1507.

137. Di Monte D, Jewell SA, Ekstrom G, et al. 1-Methyl-4-phenyl-1,2,3,6-tetrahydropyridine (MPTP) and 1-methyl-4-phenylpyridine (MPP+) cause rapid ATP depletion in isolated hepatocytes. *Biochem Biophys Res Commun* 1986; 137(1):310–315.

138. Schapira AH, Cooper JM, Dexter D, et al. Mitochondrial complex I deficiency in Parkinson's disease. *Lancet* 1989; 1(8649):1269.

139. Parker W, Boyson S, Parks J. Abnormalities of the electron transport chain in idiopathic Parkinson's disease. *Ann Neurol* 1989; 26:719–723.

140. Mizuno Y. [Contribution of MPTP to studies on the pathogenesis of Parkinson's disease]. *Rinsho Shinkeigaku* 1989; 29(12):1494–1496.

141. Schapira AH. Human complex I defects in neurodegenerative diseases. *Biochem Biophys Acta* 1998; 1364(2):261–270.

142. Anderson WM, Wood JM, Anderson AC. Inhibition of mitochondrial and Paracoccus denitrificans NADH-ubiquinone reductase by oxacarbocyanine dyes. A structure-activity study. *Biochem Pharmacol* 1993; 45(10):2115–2122.

143. Bindoff LA, Howell N, Poulton J, et al. Abnormal RNA processing associated with a novel tRNA mutation in mitochondrial DNA. A potential disease mechanism. *J Biol Chem* 1993; 268(26):19559–19564.

144. Blin O, Desnuelle C, Rascol O, et al. Mitochondrial respiratory failure in skeletal muscle from patients with Parkinson's disease and multiple system atrophy. *J Neurol Sci* 1994; 125(1):95–101.

145. Mann V, Cooper J, Krige D, et al. Brain, skeletal muscle and platelet homogenate mitochondrial function in Parkinson's disease. *Brain* 1992; 115:333–342.

146. Cardellach F, Marti MJ, Fernandez-Sola J, et al. Mitochondrial respiratory chain activity in skeletal muscle from patients with Parkinson's disease. *Neurology* 1993; 43(11):2258–2262.

147. Di Monte D, Sandy M, Jewell S, et al. Oxidative phosphorylation by intact muscle mitochondria in Parkinson's disease. *Neurodegeneration* 1993; 2(4):275–281.

148. Zweig RM, Singh A, Cardillo JE, et al. The familial occurrence of Parkinson's disease. Lack of evidence for maternal inheritance [published erratum appears in Arch Neurol 1993 Feb;50(2):153]. *Arch Neurol* 1992; 49(11):1205–1207.

149. Gu M, Owen A, Toffa S, et al. Mitochondrial function, GSH and iron in neurodegeneration and Lewy body diseases. *J. Neurol Sci* 1998; 158:24–29.

150. Chan P, DeLanney LE, Irwin I, et al. Rapid ATP loss caused by 1-methyl-4-phenyl-1,2,3,6-tetrahydropyridine in mouse brain. *J Neurochem* 1991; 57(1):348–351.

151. Di Monte D, Sandy MS, Blank L, et al. Fructose prevents 1-methyl-4-phenyl-1,2,3,6-tetrahydropyridine (MPTP)-induced ATP depletion and toxicity in isolated hepatocytes. *Biochem Biophys Res Commun* 1988; 153(2):734–740.

152. Schulz JB, Henshaw DR, Matthews RT, et al. Coenzyme Q10 and nicotinamide and a free radical spin trap protect against MPTP neurotoxicity. *Exp Neurol* 1995; 132(2):279–283.

153. Shults CW, Haas RH, Beal MF. A possible role of coenzyme Q10 in the etiology and treatment of Parkinson's disease. *Biofactors* 1999; 9(2–4):267–272.

154. Frank DM, Arora PK, Blumer JL, et al. Model study on the bioreduction of paraquat, MPP+, and analogs. Evidence against a "redox cycling" mechanism in MPTP neurotoxicity. *Biochem Biophys Res Commun* 1987; 147(3):1095–1104.

155. Di Monte D, Sandy MS, Ekstrom G, et al. Comparative studies on the mechanisms of paraquat and 1-methyl-4-phenylpyridine (MPP+) cytotoxicity. *Biochem Biophys Res Commun* 1986; 137(1):303–309.

156. Adams JD, Jr., Klaidman LK, Leung AC. MPP+ and MPDP+ induced oxygen radical formation with mitochondrial enzymes. *Free Radic Biol Med* 1993; 15(2):181–186.

157. Perry TL, Yong VW, Clavier RM, et al. Partial protection from the dopaminergic neurotoxin N-methyl-4-phenyl-1,2,3,6-tetrahydropyridine by four different antioxidants in the mouse. *Neurosci Lett* 1985; 60(2):109–114.

158. Sershen H, Reith ME, Hashim A, et al. Protection against 1-methyl-4-phenyl-1,2,3,6-tetrahydropyridine neurotoxicity by the antioxidant ascorbic acid. *Neuropharmacology* 1985; 24(12):1257–1259.

159. Baldessarini RJ, Kula NS, Francoeur D, et al. Antioxidants fail to inhibit depletion of striatal dopamine by MPTP. *Neurology* 1986; 36(5):735.

160. Martinovits G, Melamed E, Cohen O, et al. Systemic administration of antioxidants does not protect mice against the dopaminergic neurotoxicity of 1-methyl-4-phenyl-1,2,5,6-tetrahydropyridine (MPTP). *Neurosci Lett* 1986; 69(2):192–197.

161. Perry TL, Yong VW, Hansen S, et al. Alpha-tocopherol and beta-carotene do not protect marmosets against the dopaminergic neurotoxicity of N-methyl-4-phenyl-1,2,3,6-tetrahydropyridine. *J Neurol Sci* 1987; 81(2–3):321–331.

162. Mihatsch W, Russ H, Gerlach M, et al. Treatment with antioxidants does not prevent loss of dopamine in the striatum of MPTP-treated common marmosets: preliminary observations. *J Neural Transm Park Dis Dement Sect* 1991; 3(1):73–78.

163. Blanchet PJ, Konitsiotis S, Hyland K, et al. Chronic exposure to MPTP as a primate model of progressive parkinsonism: a pilot study with a free radical scavenger. *Exp Neurol* 1998; 153(2):214–222.

164. Fredriksson A, Eriksson P, Archer T. MPTP-induced deficits in motor activity: neuroprotective effects of the spintrapping agent, alpha-phenyl-tert-butyl-nitrone (PBN). *J Neural Transm* 1997; 104(6–7):579–592.

165. Klivenyi P, Matthews RT, Wermer M, et al. Azulenyl nitrone spin traps protect against MPTP neurotoxicity. *Exp Neurol* 1998; 152(1):163–166.

166. Matthews RT, Klivenyi P, Mueller G, et al. Novel free radical spin traps protect against malonate and MPTP neurotoxicity. *Exp Neurol* 1999; 157(1):120–126.

167. Ferger B, Teismann P, Earl CD, et al. The Protective Effects of PBN Against MPTP Toxicity Are Independent of Hydroxyl Radical Trapping. *Pharmacol Biochem Behav* 2000; 65(3):425–431.

168. Muralikrishnan D, Mohanakumar KP. Neuroprotection by bromocriptine against 1-methyl-4-phenyl-1,2,3,6-tetrahydropyridine-induced neurotoxicity in mice. *Faseb J* 1998; 12(10):905–912.

169. Acuna-Castroviejo D, Coto-Montes A, Gaia Monti M, et al. Melatonin is protective against MPTP-induced striatal and hippocampal lesions. *Life Sci* 1997; 60(2):L23–L29.

170. Grunblatt E, Mandel S, Gassen M, et al. Potent neuroprotective and antioxidant activity of apomorphine in MPTP and 6-hydroxydopamine induced neurotoxicity. *J Neural Transm Suppl* 1999; 55:57–70.

171. Rojas P, Rios C. Metallothionein inducers protect against 1-methyl-4-phenyl-1,2,3,6-tetrahydropyridine neurotoxicity in mice. *Neurochem Res* 1997; 22(1):17–22.

172. Rojas P, Klaassen CD. Metallothionein-I and -II knock-out mice are not more sensitive than control mice to 1-methyl-4-phenyl-1,2,3,6-tetrahydropyridine neurotoxicity. *Neurosci Lett* 1999; 273(2):113–116.

173. Ferger B, Spratt C, Teismann P, et al. Effects of cytisine on hydroxyl radicals in vitro and MPTP-induced dopamine depletion in vivo. *Eur J Pharmacol* 1998; 360(2–3):155–163.

174. Aubin N, Curet O, Deffois A, et al. Aspirin and salicylate protect against MPTP-induced dopamine depletion in mice. *J Neurochem* 1998; 71(4):1635–1642.

175. Ferger B, Teismann P, Earl CD, et al. Salicylate protects against MPTP-induced impairments in dopaminergic neurotransmission at the striatal and nigral level in mice. *Naunyn Schmiedebergs Arch Pharmacol* 1999; 360(3):256–261.

176. Sriram K, Pai KS, Boyd MR, et al. Evidence for generation of oxidative stress in brain by MPTP: in vitro and in vivo studies in mice. *Brain Res* 1997; 749(1):44–52.

177. Ali SF, David SN, Newport GD, et al. MPTP-induced oxidative stress and neurotoxicity are age-dependent: evidence from measures of reactive oxygen species and striatal dopamine levels. *Synapse* 1994; 18(1):27–34.

178. Chiueh CC, Wu RM, Mohanakumar KP, et al. In vivo generation of hydroxyl radicals and MPTP-induced dopaminergic toxicity in the basal ganglia. *Ann NY Acad Sci* 1994; 738:25–36.

179. Smith TS, Bennett JP, Jr. Mitochondrial toxins in models of neurodegenerative diseases. I: In vivo brain hydroxyl radical production during systemic MPTP treatment or following microdialysis infusion of methylpyridinium or azide ions. *Brain Res* 1997; 765(2):183–188.

180. Thomas B, Muralikrishnan D, Mohanakumar KP. In vivo hydroxyl radical generation in the striatum following systemic administration of 1-methyl-4-phenyl-1,2,3,6-tetrahydropyridine in mice. *Brain Res* 2000; 852(1):221–224.

181. Hussain S, Hass BS, Slikker W, Jr., et al. Reduced levels of catalase activity potentiate MPP+ induced toxicity: comparison between MN9D cells and CHO cells. *Toxicol Lett* 1999; 104(1–2):49–56.

182. Choi WS, Yoon SY, Oh TH, et al. Two distinct mechanisms are involved in 6-hydroxydopamine- and MPP+-induced dopaminergic neuronal cell death: role of caspases, ROS, and JNK. *J Neurosci Res* 1999; 57(1):86–94.

183. Przedborski S, Kostic V, Jackson-Lewis V, et al. Transgenic mice with increased Cu/Zn-superoxide dismutase activity are resistant to N-methyl-4-phenyl-1,2,3,6-tetrahydropyridine-induced neurotoxicity. *J Neurosci* 1992; 12(5):1658–1667.

184. Klivenyi P, St. Clair D, Wermer M, et al. Manganese superoxide dismutase overexpression attenuates MPTP toxicity. *Neurobiol Dis* 1998; 5(4):253–258.

185. Offen D, Beart PM, Cheung NS, et al. Transgenic mice expressing human Bcl-2 in their neurons are resistant to 6-hydroxydopamine and 1-methyl-4-phenyl-1,2,3,6-tetrahydropyridine neurotoxicity. *Proc Natl Acad Sci USA* 1998; 95(10):5789–5794.

186. Yang L, Matthews RT, Schulz JB, et al. 1-Methyl-4-phenyl-1,2,3,6-tetrahydropyride neurotoxicity is attenuated in mice overexpressing Bcl-2. *J Neurosci* 1998; 18(20):8145–8152.

187. Di Monte D, Chan P, Sandy M. Glutathione in Parkinson's disease: A link between oxidative stress and mitochondrial damage? *Ann Neurol* 1992; 32:S111–S115.

188. Graham D. On the origin and significance of neuromelanin. *Arch Pathol Lab Med* 1979; 103:359–362.

189. Chabrier PE, Demerle-Pallardy C, Auguet M. Nitric oxide synthases: targets for therapeutic strategies in neurological diseases. *Cell Mol Life Sci* 1999; 55(8–9):1029–1035.

190. Schulz JB, Matthews RT, Muqit MM, et al. Inhibition of neuronal nitric oxide synthase by 7-nitroindazole protects against MPTP-induced neurotoxicity in mice. *J Neurochem* 1995; 64(2):936–939.

191. Przedborski S, Jackson-Lewis V, Yokoyama R, et al. Role of neuronal nitric oxide in 1-methyl-4-phenyl-1,2,3,6-tetrahydropyridine (MPTP)-induced dopaminergic neurotoxicity. *Proc Natl Acad Sci USA* 1996; 93(10):4565–4571.

192. Hantraye P, Brouillet E, Ferrante R, et al. Inhibition of neuronal nitric oxide synthase prevents MPTP-induced parkinsonism in baboons [see comments]. *Nat Med* 1996; 2(9):1017–1021.

193. Ferrante RJ, Hantraye P, Brouillet E, et al. Increased nitrotyrosine immunoreactivity in substantia nigra neurons in MPTP treated baboons is blocked by inhibition of neuronal nitric oxide synthase. *Brain Res* 1999; 823(1–2):177–182.

194. Liberatore GT, Jackson-Lewis V, Vukosavic S, et al. Inducible nitric oxide synthase stimulates dopaminergic neurodegeneration in the MPTP model of Parkinson disease. *Nat Med* 1999; 5(12):1403–1409.

195. Itzhak Y, Martin JL, Ali SF. Methamphetamine- and 1-methyl-4-phenyl-1,2,3, 6-tetrahydropyridine-induced dopaminergic neurotoxicity in inducible nitric oxide synthase-deficient mice [In Process Citation]. *Synapse* 1999; 34(4):305–312.

196. Castagnoli K, Palmer S, Anderson A, et al. The neuronal nitric oxide synthase inhibitor 7-nitroindazole also inhibits the monoamine oxidase-B-catalyzed oxidation of 1-methyl-4-phenyl-1,2,3,6-tetrahydropyridine. *Chem Res Toxicol* 1997; 10(4):364–368.

197. Di Monte DA, Royland JE, Anderson A, et al. Inhibition of monoamine oxidase contributes to the protective effect of 7-nitroindazole against MPTP neurotoxicity. *J Neurochem* 1997; 69(4):1771–1773.

198. Castagnoli K, Palmer S, Castagnoli N, Jr. Neuroprotection by (R)-deprenyl and 7-nitroindazole in the MPTP C57BL/6 mouse model of neurotoxicity. *Neurobiology* 1999; 7(2):135–149.

199. Matthews RT, Yang L, Beal MF. S-Methylthiocitrulline, a neuronal nitric oxide synthase inhibitor, protects against malonate and MPTP neurotoxicity. *Exp Neurol* 1997; 143(2):282–286.

200. Mackenzie GM, Jackson MJ, Jenner P, et al. Nitric oxide synthase inhibition and MPTP-induced toxicity in the common marmoset. *Synapse* 1997; 26(3):301–316.

201. Tsai MJ, Lee EH. Nitric oxide donors protect cultured rat astrocytes from 1-methyl-4-phenylpyridinium-induced toxicity. *Free Radic Biol Med* 1998; 24(5):705–713.

202. Rose S, Hindmarsh JG, Jenner P. Neuronal nitric oxide synthase inhibition reduces MPP+-evoked hydroxyl radical formation but not dopamine efflux in rat striatum. *J Neural Transm* 1999; 106(5–6):477–486.

203. Youdim MB, Lavie L, Riederer P. Oxygen free radicals and neurodegeneration in Parkinson's disease: a role for nitric oxide. *Ann NY Acad Sci* 1994; 738:64–68.

204. Hunot S, Boissiere F, Faucheux B, et al. Nitric oxide synthase and neuronal vulnerability in Parkinson's disease. *Neuroscience* 1996; 72(2):355–363.

205. Molina JA, Jimenez-Jimenez FJ, Orti-Pareja M, The role of nitric oxide in neurodegeneration. Potential for pharmacological intervention. *Drugs Aging* 1998; 12(4):251–259.

206. Crossman AR, Peggs D, Boyce S, Effect of the NMDA antagonist MK-801 on MPTP-induced parkinsonism in the monkey. *Neuropharmacology* 1989; 28(11):1271–1273.

207. Graham WC, Robertson RG, Sambrook MA, et al. Injection of excitatory amino acid antagonists into the medial pallidal segment of a 1-methyl-4-phenyl-1,2,3,6-tetrahydropyridine (MPTP) treated primate reverses motor symptoms of parkinsonism. *Life Sci* 1990; 47(18):L91–97.

208. Loschmann PA, Lange KW, Kunow M, et al. Synergism of the AMPA-antagonist NBQX and the NMDA-antagonist CPP with L-dopa in models of Parkinson's disease. *J Neural Transm Park Dis Dement Sect* 1991; 3(3):203–213.

209. Turski L, Bressler K, Rettig KJ, et al. Protection of substantia nigra from MPP+ neurotoxicity by

N-methyl-D-aspartate antagonists [see comments]. Nature 1991; 349(6308):414–418.

210. Zuddas A, Oberto G, Vaglini F, et al. MK-801 prevents 1-methyl-4-phenyl-1,2,3,6-tetrahydropyridine-induced parkinsonism in primates. *J Neurochem* 1992; 59(2):733–739.

211. Lange KW, Loschmann PA, Sofic E, et al. The competitive NMDA antagonist CPP protects substantia nigra neurons from MPTP-induced degeneration in primates. *Naunyn Schmiedebergs Arch Pharmacol* 1993; 348(6):586–592.

212. Tabatabaei A, Perry TL, Hansen S, et al. Partial protective effect of MK-801 on MPTP-induced reduction of striatal dopamine in mice. *Neurosci Lett* 1992; 141(2):192–194.

213. Brouillet E, Beal MF. NMDA antagonists partially protect against MPTP induced neurotoxicity in mice. *Neuroreport* 1993; 4(4):387–390.

214. Sonsalla PK, Zeevalk GD, Manzino L, et al. MK-801 fails to protect against the dopaminergic neuropathology produced by systemic 1-methyl-4-phenyl-1,2,3,6-tetrahydropyridine in mice or intranigral 1-methyl-4-phenylpyridinium in rats. *J Neurochem* 1992; 58(5):1979–1982.

215. Kupsch A, Loschmann PA, Sauer H, et al. Do NMDA receptor antagonists protect against MPTP-toxicity? Biochemical and immunocytochemical analyses in black mice. *Brain Res* 1992; 592(1–2): 74–83.

216. Chan P, Di Monte DA, Langston JW, et al. (+)MK-801 does not prevent MPTP-induced loss of nigral neurons in mice. *J Pharmacol Exp Ther* 1997; 280(1):439–446.

217. Michel PP, Agid Y. The glutamate antagonist, MK-801, does not prevent dopaminergic cell death induced by the 1-methyl-4-phenylpyridinium ion (MPP+) in rat dissociated mesencephalic cultures. *Brain Res* 1992; 597(2):233–240.

218. Srivastava R, Brouillet E, Beal MF, et al. Blockade of 1-methyl-4-phenylpyridinium ion (MPP+) nigral toxicity in the rat by prior decortication or MK-801 treatment: a stereological estimate of neuronal loss. *Neurobiol Aging* 1993; 14(4):295–301.

219. Fornai F, Alessandri MG, Fascetti F, et al. Clonidine suppresses 1-methyl-4-phenyl-1,2,3,6-tetrahydropyridine-induced reductions of striatal dopamine and tyrosine hydroxylase activity in mice. *J Neurochem* 1995; 65(2):704–709.

220. Reinhard JF, Jr., Miller DB, O'Callaghan JP. The neurotoxicant MPTP (1-methyl-4-phenyl-1,2,3,6-tetrahydropyridine) increases glial fibrillary acidic protein and decreases dopamine levels of the mouse striatum: evidence for glial response to injury. *Neurosci Lett* 1988; 95(1–3):246–251.

221. Clarke PB, Reuben M. Inhibition by dizocilpine (MK-801) of striatal dopamine release induced by MPTP and MPP+: possible action at the dopamine transporter. *Br J Pharmacol* 1995; 114(2): 315–322.

222. Boireau A, Dubedat P, Bordier F, et al. Riluzole and experimental parkinsonism: antagonism of MPTP-induced decrease in central dopamine levels in mice. *Neuroreport* 1994; 5(18):2657–2660.

223. Benazzouz A, Boraud T, Dubedat P, et al. Riluzole prevents MPTP-induced parkinsonism in the rhesus monkey: a pilot study. *Eur J Pharmacol* 1995; 284(3):299–307.

224. Bezard E, Stutzmann JM, Imbert C, et al. Riluzole delayed appearance of parkinsonian motor abnormalities in a chronic MPTP monkey model. *Eur J Pharmacol* 1998; 356(2–3):101–104.

225. Parkinson's Study Group. A multicenter randomized controlled trial of remacemide hydrochloride as monotherapy for Parkinson's disease. *Neurology* 2000; 54:1583–1588.

226. Otto D, Unsicker K. Basic FGF reverses chemical and morphological deficits in the nigrostriatal system of MPTP-treated mice. *J Neurosci* 1990; 10(6):1912–1921.

227. Date I, Yoshimoto Y, Imaoka T, et al. Enhanced recovery of the nigrostriatal dopaminergic system in MPTP-treated mice following intrastriatal injection of basic fibroblast growth factor in relation to aging. *Brain Res* 1993; 621(1):150–154.

228. Otto D, Unsicker K. FGF-2-mediated protection of cultured mesencephalic dopaminergic neurons against MPTP and MPP+: specificity and impact of culture conditions, non-dopaminergic neurons, and astroglial cells. *J Neurosci Res* 1993; 34(4):382–393.

229. Chadi G, Moller A, Rosen L, et al. Protective actions of human recombinant basic fibroblast growth factor on MPTP-lesioned nigrostriatal dopamine neurons after intraventricular infusion. *Exp Brain Res* 1993; 97(1):145–158.

230. Tomac A, Lindqvist E, Lin LF, et al. Protection and repair of the nigrostriatal dopaminergic system by GDNF in vivo. *Nature* 1995; 373(6512):335–339.

231. Gash DM, Zhang Z, Ovadia A, et al. Functional recovery in parkinsonian monkeys treated with GDNF. *Nature* 1996; 380(6571):252–255.

232. Hadjiconstantinou M, Fitkin JG, Dalia A, Epidermal growth factor enhances striatal dopaminergic parameters in the 1-methyl-4-phenyl-1,2,3,6-tetrahydropyridine-treated mouse. *J Neurochem* 1991; 57(2):479–482.

233. Spina MB, Squinto SP, Miller J, et al. Brain-derived neurotrophic factor protects dopamine neurons against 6-hydroxydopamine and N-methyl-4-phenylpyridinium ion toxicity: involvement of the glutathione system [see comments]. *J Neurochem* 1992; 59(1):99–106.

234. Garcia E, Rios C, Sotelo J. Ventricular injection of nerve growth factor increases dopamine content in the striata of MPTP-treated mice. *Neurochem Res* 1992; 17(10):979–982.

235. Tsukahara T, Takeda M, Shimohama S, et al. Effects of brain-derived neurotrophic factor on 1-methyl-4-phenyl-1,2,3,6-tetrahydropyridine-

induced parkinsonism in monkeys. *Neurosurgery* 1995; 37(4):733–739; discussion 739–741.

236. Hartikka J, Staufenbiel M, Lubbert H. Cyclic AMP, but not basic FGF, increases the in vitro survival of mesencephalic dopaminergic neurons and protects them from MPP(+)-induced degeneration. *J Neurosci Res* 1992; 32(2):190–201.

237. Pearce RK, Collins P, Jenner P, et al. Intraventricular infusion of basic fibroblast growth factor (bFGF) in the MPTP-treated common marmoset. *Synapse* 1996; 23(3):192–200.

238. Date I, Aoi M, Tomita S, et al. GDNF administration induces recovery of the nigrostriatal dopaminergic system both in young and aged parkinsonian mice. *Neuroreport* 1998; 9(10):2365–2369.

239. Gerhardt GA, Cass WA, Huettl P, et al. GDNF improves dopamine function in the substantia nigra but not the putamen of unilateral MPTP-lesioned rhesus monkeys. *Brain Res* 1999; 817(1–2):163–171.

240. Lapchak PA, Araujo DM, et al. Topographical distribution of [125I]-glial cell line-derived neurotrophic factor in unlesioned and MPTP-lesioned rhesus monkey brain following a bolus intraventricular injection. *Brain Res* 1998; 789(1):9–22.

241. Kojima H, Abiru Y, Sakajiri K, et al. Adenovirus-mediated transduction with human glial cell line-derived neurotrophic factor gene prevents 1-methyl-4-phenyl-1,2,3,6-tetrahydropyridine-induced dopamine depletion in striatum of mouse brain. *Biochem Biophys Res Commun* 1997; 238(2):569–573.

242. Steiner JP, Hamilton GS, Ross DT, et al. Neurotrophic immunophilin ligands stimulate structural and functional recovery in neurodegenerative animal models. *Proc Natl Acad Sci USA* 1997; 94(5):2019–2024.

243. Costantini LC, Chaturvedi P, Armistead DM, et al. A novel immunophilin ligand: distinct branching effects on dopaminergic neurons in culture and neurotrophic actions after oral administration in an animal model of Parkinson's disease. *Neurobiol Dis* 1998; 5(2):97–106.

244. Mochizuki H, Nakamura N, Nishi K, et al. Apoptosis is induced by 1-methyl-4-phenylpyridinium ion (MPP+) in ventral mesencephalic-striatal co-culture in rat. *Neurosci Lett* 1994; 170(1):191–194.

245. Jackson-Lewis V, Jakowec M, Burke RE, et al. Time course and morphology of dopaminergic neuronal death caused by the neurotoxin 1-methyl-4-phenyl-1,2,3,6-tetrahydropyridine. *Neurodegeneration* 1995; 4(3):257–269.

246. Desole MS, Sciola L, Delogu MR, et al. Manganese and 1-methyl-4-(2'-ethylpheny1)-1,2,3,6-tetrahydropyridine induce apoptosis in PC12 cells. *Neurosci Lett* 1996; 209(3):193–196.

247. Sheehan JP, Palmer PE, Helm GA, et al. MPP+ induced apoptotic cell death in SH-SY5Y neuroblastoma cells: an electron microscope study. *J Neurosci Res* 1997; 48(3):226–237.

248. Tatton N, Kish S. In situ detection of apoptotic nuclei in the substantia nigra compacta of 1-methyl-4-phenyl-1,2,3,6-tetrahydropyridine-treated mice using terminal deoxynucleotidyl transferase labelling and acridine orange staining. *Neuroscience* 1997; 77(4):1037–1048.

249. Spooren WP, Gentsch C, Wiessner C. TUNEL-positive cells in the substantia nigra of C57BL/6 mice after a single bolus of 1-methyl-4-phenyl-1,2,3,6-tetrahydropyridine. *Neuroscience* 1998; 85(2):649–651; discussion 653.

250. Soldner F, Weller M, Haid S, et al. MPP+ inhibits proliferation of PC12 cells by a p21(WAF1/Cip1)-dependent pathway and induces cell death in cells lacking p21(WAF1/Cip1). *Exp Cell Res* 1999; 250(1):75–85.

251. Hirsch EC, Hunot S, Faucheux B, et al. Dopaminergic neurons degenerate by apoptosis in Parkinson's disease [letter; comment]. *Mov Disord* 1999; 14(2):383–385.

252. Jellinger KA. Is there apoptosis in Lewy body disease? *Acta Neuropathol* (Berl) 1999; 97(4):413–415.

253. Mytilineou C, Cohen G. Deprenyl protects dopamine neurons from the neurotoxic effect of 1-methyl-4-phenylpyridinium ion. *J Neurochem* 1985; 45(6):1951–1953.

254. Le W, Jankovic J, Xie W, et al. (−)-Deprenyl protection of 1-methyl-4 phenylpyridium ion (MPP+)-induced apoptosis independent of MAO-B inhibition [published erratum appears in Neurosci Lett 1997 May 30; 228(1):67]. *Neurosci Lett* 1997; 224(3):197–200.

255. Tatton WG, Greenwood CE. Rescue of dying neurons: a new action for deprenyl in MPTP parkinsonism. *J Neurosci Res* 1991; 30(4):666–672.

256. Wu RM, Chiueh CC, Pert A, et al. Apparent antioxidant effect of l-deprenyl on hydroxyl radical formation and nigral injury elicited by MPP+ in vivo. *Eur J Pharmacol* 1993; 243(3):241–247.

257. Wu RM, Murphy DL, Chiueh CC. Neuronal protective and rescue effects of deprenyl against MPP+ dopaminergic toxicity. *J Neural Transm Gen Sect* 1995; 100(1):53–61.

258. Wu RM, Murphy DL, Chiueh CC. Suppression of hydroxyl radical formation and protection of nigral neurons by l-deprenyl (selegiline). *Ann NY Acad Sci* 1996; 786:379–390.

259. Magyar K, Szende B, Lengyel J, et al. The pharmacology of B-type selective monoamine oxidase inhibitors; milestones in (−)-deprenyl research. *J Neural Transm Suppl* 1996; 48:29–43.

260. Hassouna I, Wickert H, Zimmermann M, et al. Increase in bax expression in substantia nigra following 1-methyl-4-phenyl-1,2,3,6-tetrahydropyridine (MPTP) treatment of mice. *Neurosci Lett* 1996; 204(1–2):85–88.

261. Tatton WG, Wadia JS, Ju WY, et al. (−)-Deprenyl reduces neuronal apoptosis and facilitates neuronal outgrowth by altering protein synthesis without

inhibiting monoamine oxidase. *J Neural Transm Suppl* 1996; 48:45–59.

262. Birkmayer W. (−)-Deprenyl leads to prolongation of L-dopa efficacy in Parkinson's disease. *Mod Probl Pharmacopsychiatry* 1983; 19:170–176.

263. Cosi C, Colpaert F, Koek W, et al. Poly(ADP-ribose) polymerase inhibitors protect against MPTP-induced depletions of striatal dopamine and cortical noradrenaline in C57B1/6 mice. *Brain Res* 1996; 729(2):264–269.

264. Cosi C, Marien M. Decreases in mouse brain AND+ and ATP induced by 1-methyl-4-phenyl-1, 2,3,6-tetrahydropyridine (MPTP): prevention by the poly(ADP-ribose) polymerase inhibitor, benzamide. *Brain Res* 1998; 809(1):58–67.

265. Cosi C, Marien M. Implication of poly (ADP-ribose) polymerase (PARP) in neurodegeneration and brain energy metabolism. Decreases in mouse brain AND+ and ATP caused by MPTP are prevented by the PARP inhibitor benzamide [In Process Citation]. *Ann NY Acad Sci* 1999; 890:227–239.

266. Mandir AS, Przedborski S, Jackson-Lewis V, et al. Poly(ADP-ribose) polymerase activation mediates 1-methyl-4-phenyl-1, 2,3,6-tetrahydropyridine (MPTP)-induced parkinsonism. *Proc Natl Acad Sci USA* 1999; 96(10):5774–5779.

267. Hadjiconstantinou M, Rossetti ZL, Paxton RC, et al. Administration of GM1 ganglioside restores the dopamine content in striatum after chronic treatment with MPTP. *Neuropharmacology* 1986; 25(9): 1075–1077.

268. Hadjiconstantinou M, Mariani AP, Neff NH. GM1 ganglioside-induced recovery of nigrostriatal dopaminergic neurons after MPTP: an immunohistochemical study. *Brain Res* 1989; 484(1–2):297–303.

269. Hadjiconstantinou M, Weihmuller F, Neff NH. Treatment with GM1 ganglioside reverses dopamine D-2 receptor supersensitivity induced by the neurotoxin MPTP. *Eur J Pharmacol* 1989; 168(2):261–264.

270. Saulino MF, Schengrund CL. Differential accumulation of gangliosides by the brains of MPTP-lesioned mice. *J Neurosci Res* 1994; 37(3):384–391.

271. Date I, Felten SY, Felten DL. Exogenous GM1 gangliosides induce partial recovery of the nigrostriatal dopaminergic system in MPTP-treated young mice but not in aging mice. *Neurosci Lett* 1989; 106(3):282–286.

272. Schneider JS. Effects of age on GM1 ganglioside-induced recovery of concentrations of dopamine in the striatum in 1-methyl-4-phenyl-1,2,3,6-tetrahydropyridine-treated mice. *Neuropharmacology* 1992; 31(2):185–192.

273. Fazzini E, Durso R, Davoudi H, et al. GM1 gangliosides alter acute MPTP-induced behavioral and neurochemical toxicity in mice. *J Neurol Sci* 1990; 99(1):59–68.

274. Schneider JS, Yuwiler A. GM1 ganglioside treatment promotes recovery of striatal dopamine concentrations in the mouse model of MPTP-induced parkinsonism. *Exp Neurol* 1989; 105(2):177–183.

275. Rothblat DS, Schneider JS. Effects of GM1 ganglioside treatment on dopamine innervation of the striatum of MPTP-treated mice. *Ann NY Acad Sci* 1998; 845:274–277.

276. Schneider JS, Kean A, DiStefano L. GM1 ganglioside rescues substantia nigra pars compacta neurons and increases dopamine synthesis in residual nigrostriatal dopaminergic neurons in MPTP-treated mice. *J Neurosci Res* 1995; 42(1):117–123.

277. Schneider JS, Distefano L. Response of the damaged dopamine system to GM1 and semisynthetic gangliosides: effects of dose and extent of lesion. *Neuropharmacology* 1995; 34(5):489–493.

278. Schneider JS. MPTP-induced parkinsonism: acceleration of biochemical and behavioral recovery by GM1 ganglioside treatment. *J Neurosci Res* 1992; 31(1):112–119.

279. Schneider JS, Pope A, Simpson K, et al. Recovery from experimental parkinsonism in primates with GM1 ganglioside treatment. *Science* 1992; 256(5058):843–846.

280. Herrero MT, Kastner A, Perez-Otano I, et al. Gangliosides and parkinsonism. *Neurology* 1993; 43(10):2132–2134.

281. Schneider JS, Roeltgen DP, Rothblat DS, GM1 ganglioside treatment of Parkinson's disease: an open pilot study of safety and efficacy. *Neurology* 1995; 45(6):1149–1154.

282. Pai KS, Ravindranath V. Protection and potentiation of MPTP-induced toxicity by cytochrome P-450 inhibitors and inducer: in vitro studies with brain slices. *Brain Res* 1991; 555(2):239–244.

283. Bodis-Wollner I, Chung E, Ghilardi MF, et al. Acetyl-levo-carnitine protects against MPTP-induced parkinsonism in primates. *J Neural Transm Park Dis Dement Sect* 1991; 3(1):63–72.

284. Shahi GS, Das NP, Moochhala SM. 1-Methyl-4-phenyl-1,2,3,6-tetrahydropyridine-induced neurotoxicity: partial protection against striato-nigral dopamine depletion in C57BL/6J mice by cigarette smoke exposure and by beta-naphthoflavone-pretreatment. *Neurosci Lett* 1991; 127(2):247–250.

285. Janson AM, Fuxe K, Goldstein M. Differential effects of acute and chronic nicotine treatment on MPTP-(1-methyl-4-phenyl-1,2,3,6-tetrahydropyridine) induced degeneration of nigrostriatal dopamine neurons in the black mouse. *Clin Investig* 1992; 70(3–4):232–238.

286. Boireau A, Bordier F, Dubedat P, et al. Thalidomide reduces MPTP-induced decrease in striatal dopamine levels in mice. *Neurosci Lett* 1997; 234(2–3):123–126.

287. Marcotte ER, Chugh A, Mishra RK, et al. Protection against MPTP treatment by an analog of Pro-Leu-Gly-NH2 (PLG, MIF-1). *Peptides* 1998; 19(2):403–406.

288. Lau YS, Mouradian MM. Protection against acute MPTP-induced dopamine depletion in mice by adenosine A1 agonist. *J Neurochem* 1993; 60(2):768–771.

289. Aguirre JA, Cintra A, Hillion J, et al. A stereological study on the neuroprotective actions of acute modafinil treatment on 1-methyl-4-phenyl-1,2,3,6-tetrahydropyridine-induced nigral lesions of the male black mouse. *Neurosci Lett* 1999; 275(3):215–218.

290. Corsini GU, Pintus S, Chiueh CC, et al. 1-Methyl-4-phenyl-1,2,3,6-tetrahydropyridine (MPTP) neurotoxicity in mice is enhanced by pretreatment with diethyldithiocarbamate. *Eur J Pharmacol* 1985; 119(1–2):127–128.

291. Irwin I, Wu EY, DeLanney LE, et al. The effect of diethyldithiocarbamate on the biodisposition of MPTP: an explanation for enhanced neurotoxicity. *Eur J Pharmacol* 1987; 141(2):209–217.

292. Miller DB, Reinhard JF, Jr., Daniels AJ, et al. Diethyldithiocarbamate potentiates the neurotoxicity of in vivo 1-methyl-4-phenyl-1,2,3,6-tetrahydropyridine and of in vitro 1-methyl-4-phenylpyridinium. *J Neurochem* 1991; 57(2):541–549.

293. Walters TL, Irwin I, Delfani K, et al. Diethyldithiocarbamate causes nigral cell loss and dopamine depletion with nontoxic doses of MPTP. *Exp Neurol* 1999; 156(1):62–70.

294. Chiba K, Horii H, Kubota E, et al. Effects of N-methylmercaptoimidazole on the disposition of MPTP and its metabolites in mice. *Eur J Pharmacol* 1990; 180(1):59–67.

295. Corsini GU, Zuddas A, Bonuccelli U, et al. 1-Methyl-4-phenyl-1,2,3,6-tetrahydropyridine (MPTP) neurotoxicity in mice is enhanced by ethanol or acetaldehyde. *Life Sci* 1987; 40(9):827–832.

296. Marien M, Briley M, Colpaert F. Noradrenaline depletion exacerbates MPTP-induced striatal dopamine loss in mice. *Eur J Pharmacol* 1993; 236(3):487–489.

297. Hadjiconstantinou M, Hubble JP, Wemlinger TA, et al. Enhanced MPTP neurotoxicity after treatment with isoflurophate or cholinergic agonists. *J Pharmacol Exp Ther* 1994; 270(2):639–644.

298. Tariq M, Khan HA, al Moutaery K, et al. Effect of chronic administration of magnesium sulfate on 1-methyl-4-phenyl-1,2,3,6-tetrahydropyridine-induced neurotoxicity in mice. *Pharmacol Toxicol* 1998; 82(5):218–222.

299. Takahashi RN, Rogerio R, Zanin M. Maneb enhances MPTP neurotoxicity in mice. *Res Commun Chem Pathol Pharmacol* 1989; 66(1):167–170.

300. McGrew D, Irwin I, Langston J. Ethylenebis – but not methyldithiocarbamate enhances MPTP-induced striatal dopamine depletion in mice. *NeuroToxicology* 2000; (in press).

301. Jarvis MF, Wagner GC. Age-dependent effects of 1-methyl-4-phenyl-1,2,5,6-tetrahydropyridine (MPTP). *Neuropharmacology* 1985; 24(6):581–583.

302. Langston JW, Irwin I, DeLanney LE. The biotransformation of MPTP and disposition of MPP+: the effects of aging. *Life Sci* 1987; 40(8):749–754.

303. Gupta M, Gupta BK, Thomas R, et al. Aged mice are more sensitive to 1-methyl-4-phenyl-1,2,3,6-tetra-

304. Ricaurte GA, DeLanney LE, Irwin I, et al. Older dopaminergic neurons do not recover from the effects of MPTP. *Neuropharmacology* 1987; 26(1):97–99.

305. Ricaurte GA, Irwin I, Forno LS, et al. Aging and 1-methyl-4-phenyl-1,2,3,6-tetrahydropyridine-induced degeneration of dopaminergic neurons in the substantia nigra. *Brain Res* 1987; 403(1):43–51.

306. Desole MS, Esposito G, Enrico P, et al. Effects of ageing on 1-methyl-4-phenyl-1,2,3,6-tetrahydropyridine (MPTP) neurotoxic effects on striatum and brainstem in the rat. *Neurosci Lett* 1993; 159(1–2):143–146.

307. Irwin I, Finnegan KT, Delanney LE, et al. The relationships between aging, monoamine oxidase, striatal dopamine and the effects of MPTP in C57BL/6 mice: a critical reassessment. *Brain Res* 1992; 572(1–2):224–231.

308. Saura J, Richards JG, Mahy N. Age-related changes on MAO in Bl/C57 mouse tissues: a quantitative radioautographic study. *J Neural Transm Suppl* 1994; 41:89–94.

309. Finnegan KT, Irwin I, Delanney LE, et al. Age-dependent effects of the 2'-methyl analog of 1-methyl-4-phenyl-1,2,3,6-tetrahydropyridine: prevention by inhibitors of monoamine oxidase B. *J Pharmacol Exp Ther* 1995; 273(2):716–720.

310. Forno LS, Langston JW, DeLanney LE, et al. Locus ceruleus lesions and eosinophilic inclusions in MPTP-treated monkeys. *Ann Neurol* 1986; 20(4):449–455.

311. Rose S, Nomoto M, Jackson EA, et al. Age-related effects of 1-methyl-4-phenyl-1,2,3,6-tetrahydropyridine treatment of common marmosets. *Eur J Pharmacol* 1993; 230(2):177–185.

312. Ovadia A, Zhang Z, Gash DM. Increased susceptibility to MPTP toxicity in middle-aged rhesus monkeys. *Neurobiol Aging* 1995; 16(6):931–937.

313. Irwin I, Delanney L, Chan P, et al. Nigrostriatal monoamine oxidase A and B in aging squirrel monkeys and C57BL/6 mice. *Neurobiol Aging* 1997; 18(2):235–241.

314. Johannessen JN, Chiueh CC, Burns RS, et al. Differences in the metabolism of MPTP in the rodent and primate parallel differences in sensitivity to its neurotoxic effects. *Life Sci* 1985; 36(3):219–224.

315. Hoskins JA, Davis LJ. The acute effect on levels of catecholamines and metabolites in brain, of a single dose of MPTP in 8 strains of mice. *Neuropharmacology* 1989; 28(12):1389–1397.

316. Donnan GA, Kaczmarczyk SJ, Solopotias T, et al. The neurochemical and clinical effects of 1-methyl-4-phenyl-1,2,3,6-tetrahydropyridine in small animals. *Clin Exp Neurol* 1986; 22:155–164.

317. Heikkila RE. Differential neurotoxicity of 1-methyl-4-phenyl-1,2,3,6-tetrahydropyridine (MPTP) in Swiss-Webster mice from different sources. *Eur J Pharmacol* 1985; 117(1):131–134.

318. Hamre K, Tharp R, Poon K, et al. Differential strain susceptibility following 1-methyl-4-phenyl-1,2,3,6-

tetrahydropyridine (MPTP) administration acts in an autosomal dominant fashion: quantitative analysis in seven strains of Mus musculus. *Brain Res* 1999; 828(1–2):91–103.

319. Zimmer J, Geneser FA. Difference in monoamine oxidase B activity between C57 black and albino NMRI mouse strains may explain differential effects of the neurotoxin MPTP. *Neurosci Lett* 1987; 78(3):253–258.

320. Kalaria RN, Harik SI. Blood-brain barrier monoamine oxidase: enzyme characterization in cerebral microvessels and other tissues from six mammalian species, including human. *J Neurochem* 1987; 49(3):856–864.

321. Kalaria RN, Mitchell MJ, Harik SI. Correlation of 1-methyl-4-phenyl-1,2,3,6-tetrahydropyridine neurotoxicity with blood-brain barrier monoamine oxidase activity. *Proc Natl Acad Sci USA* 1987; 84(10):3521–3525.

322. Riachi NJ, Behmand RA, Harik SI. Correlation of MPTP neurotoxicity in vivo with oxidation of MPTP by the brain and blood-brain barrier in vitro in five rat strains. *Brain Res* 1991; 555(1):19–24.

323. Riachi NJ, Harik SI. Strain differences in systemic 1-methyl-4-phenyl-1,2,3,6-tetrahydropyridine neurotoxicity in mice correlate best with monoamine oxidase activity at the blood-brain barrier. *Life Sci* 1988; 42(23):2359–2363.

324. Iacopino A, Christakos S, German D, et al. Calbindin-D28K-containing neurons in animal models of neurodegeneration: possible protection from excitotoxicity. *Brain Res Mol Brain Res* 1992; 13(3):251–261.

325. Lavoie B, Parent A, Bedard PJ. Effects of dopamine denervation on striatal peptide expression in parkinsonian monkeys. *Can J Neurol Sci* 1991; 18(Suppl 3):373–375.

326. German DC, Manaye KF, Sonsalla PK, et al. Midbrain dopaminergic cell loss in Parkinson's disease and MPTP-induced parkinsonism: sparing of calbindin-D28k-containing cells. *Ann NY Acad Sci* 1992; 648:42–62.

327. Parent A, Lavoie B. The heterogeneity of the mesostriatal dopaminergic system as revealed in normal and parkinsonian monkeys. *Adv Neurol* 1993; 60:25–33.

328. Sanghera MK, Manaye KF, Liang CL, et al. Low dopamine transporter mRNA levels in midbrain regions containing calbindin. *Neuroreport* 1994; 5(13):1641–1644.

329. Sanghera MK, Manaye K, McMahon A, et al. Dopamine transporter mRNA levels are high in midbrain neurons vulnerable to MPTP. *Neuroreport* 1997; 8(15):3327–3331.

330. Haber SN, Ryoo H, Cox C, et al. Subsets of midbrain dopaminergic neurons in monkeys are distinguished by different levels of mRNA for the dopamine transporter: comparison with the mRNA for the D2 receptor, tyrosine hydroxylase and calbindin immunoreactivity. *J Comp Neurol* 1995; 362(3):400–410.

331. Airaksinen MS, Thoenen H, Meyer M. Vulnerability of midbrain dopaminergic neurons in calbindin-D28k-deficient mice: lack of evidence for a neuroprotective role of endogenous calbindin in MPTP-treated and weaver mice. *Eur J Neurosci* 1997; 9(1):120–127.

332. Perry TL, Yong VW, Wall RA, et al. Paraquat and two endogenous analogues of the neurotoxic substance N-methyl-4-phenyl-1,2,3,6-tetrahydropyridine do not damage dopaminergic nigrostriatal neurons in the mouse. *Neurosci Lett* 1986; 69(3):285–289.

333. Markey SP, Weisz A, Bacon JP. Reduced paraquat does not exhibit MPTP-like neurotoxicity [letter]. *J Anal Toxicol* 1986; 10(6):257.

334. Brooks AI, Chadwick CA, Gelbard HA, et al. Paraquat elicited neurobehavioral syndrome caused by dopaminergic neuron loss. *Brain Res* 1999; 823(1–2):1–10.

335. Ward C, Duvoisin R, Ince S, et al. Parkinson's disease in 65 pairs of twins and in a set of quadruplets. *Neurology* 1983; 33:815–824.

336. Markopoulou K, Langston JW. Candidate genes and Parkinson's disease: where to next? *Neurology* 1999; 53(7):1382–1383.

337. Tanner CM, Ottman R, Goldman SM, et al. Parkinson disease in twins: an etiologic study. *Jama* 1999; 281(4):341–346.

338. Polymeropoulos MH, Lavedan C, Leroy E, et al. Mutation in the alpha-synuclein gene identified in families with Parkinson's disease. *Science* 1997; 276(5321):2045–2047.

339. Spillantini MG, Schmidt ML, Lee VM, et al. Alpha-synuclein in Lewy bodies [letter]. *Nature* 1997; 388(6645):839–840.

340. Trojanowski JQ, Goedert M, Iwatsubo T, et al. Fatal attractions: abnormal protein aggregation and neuron death in Parkinson's disease and Lewy body dementia [see comments]. *Cell Death Differ* 1998; 5(10):832–837.

341. Vila M, Vukosavic S, Jackson-Lewis V, et al. Alpha-synuclein up-regulation in substantia nigra dopaminergic neurons following administration of the parkinsonian toxin MPTP. *J Neurochem* 2000; 74(2):721–729.

342. Kowall NW, Hantraye P, Brouillet E, et al. MPTP induces alpha-synuclein aggregation in the substantia nigra of baboons. *Neuroreport* 2000; 11(1):211–213.

Hao and colleagues used similar primary mesencephalic (embryonic rat) neuronal culture techniques in amplifying and expanding the initial findings of Yu et al. (5,6). Rather than using cadaveric ventricular CSF, Hao and her collaborators obtained CSF from living patients via lumbar puncture (five with PD; seven controls). Once again CSF from the <10 kDa fraction of PD patients produced an inhibitory effect on cultured neurons, but in Hao's hands this effect was exclusively seen with PD CSF and not with CSF from control patients. Dopaminergic neuronal function, as measured by [³H] DA uptake, was decreased in cultures by 21% following 40 hours incubation with PD CSF, whereas control CSF produced no change. Using tyrosine hydroxylase (TH) immunocytochemistry as a means to identify dopamine neurons, striking and seemingly selective dopaminergic neuronal loss reaching 90% was evident after 90 hours incubation in cultures exposed to PD CSF, compared with no significant cell loss in cultures incubated with control CSF. Because changes in dopamine uptake were evident well before cell loss became apparent, Hao et al. speculated that the toxic element in PD CSF might directly target a specific molecule, such as Complex I, or that it might interact with and impair function of cytoskeletal structures such as neurofilaments. The latter theory was bolstered by their observation, with the aid of high power magnification, that in some surviving TH⁺ neurons TH staining was confined to the cell body, leaving axons and dendrites unstained, which suggests that TH transport was impaired. In either scenario cell function would be impaired first, followed later by cell death.

Much has been written in recent years about the potential for levodopa or DA itself to produce dopaminergic neuronal damage via oxidative stress mechanisms that led to speculation (7,8) (and controversy (9)) that levodopa administration might actually accelerate dopaminergic neuronal loss in PD (see Chapters 28, 32). Because four of the five PD patients, whose CSF was studied in these initial experiments, were receiving levodopa, Hao et al. measured DA levels in three of the five PD CSF samples (and in three additional PD CSF samples) and found DA levels to range from 0.013 μM to 0.026 μM, compared to a range of 0 to 0.013 μM in control CSF. They also observed that DA itself at concentrations of 0.01 to 0.05 μM did not adversely impact either the number or the morphology of DA neurons in culture after 90 hours incubation.

In an effort to further address and clarify this issue Hao and colleagues subsequently studied CSF from 17 untreated PD patients (participants in the DATATOP protocol (10,11). CSF from 14 of the 17 patients was toxic to cultured DA neurons (6), thus exonerating

exogenously administered levodopa as the toxic agent, at least in this paradigm.

Subsequent studies with CSF from the same 17 PD subjects and 5 control CSF samples demonstrated via 2 D-gel electrophoresis the presence of an abnormal protein with a molecular weight of approximately 13,000 in nine of the 17 PD CSF specimens, but in none of the controls (6). The actual identity of the protein, however, was not ascertained.

Colombo and Napp studied the effects of CSF from individuals with PD on primary dissociated cell cultures from not only ventral mesencephalon but also striatum and cerebral cortex (12). Although their techniques differed from those of Yu et al. (4) and Hao et al. (5,6) (they applied CSF to the cultures immediately after seeding, using the CSF as the actual culture medium rather than growing cells in a standard culture medium to which CSF was added) they also demonstrated PD CSF to have a "dystrophic" effect on cultured neurons in that it reduced or abolished cell growth and process formation. Striatal and mesencephalic cultures were more likely to display the dystrophic effect when exposed to PD CSF than were cultures derived from cerebral cortex (60% of striatal and mesencephalic; 40% cortical), whereas control CSF had no dystrophic effect on any cultures.

In contrast to Hao and coworker's experience, the damaging effects of PD CSF did not appear to be confined to DA neurons alone. In contrast to Hao et al., the deleterious effects of PD CSF were primarily evident in CSF from levodopa-treated patients; CSF from the four untreated patients did not show a consistent effect.

Colombo and Napp went on to investigate the effect of glial conditioning on the CSF toxicity by incubating PD CSF with astroglial cells for 24 hours before applying the CSF to striatal or mesencephalic cultures. In the three samples tested in this fashion (all from levodopa-treated patients) glial conditioning abolished the toxic effect of PD CSF on neuronal cultures. This protective effect was specific to astroglial cells in that similar conditioning with fibroblasts did not confer protection. The authors put forward two speculations that could account for the protective effect: glia could either be producing trophic factors that were transferred to the CSF and subsequently protected exposed neurons, or the glia might be sequestering or degrading the toxic substance present in PD CSF. As with earlier investigators, the toxic factor present in CSF from PD patients was not specifically identified.

Le and colleagues published the largest study reported to date on the effects of CSF on cell culture populations (13). They studied CSF from 20 untreated PD patients, 10 levodopa-treated PD patients and 18 controls. Instead of employing primary mesencephalic cell culture, they used two neuronal cell lines for their studies: the hybrid dopaminergic mesencephalic cell line, MES 23.5 (14) and its nondopaminergic parental cell line, N18TG2. As an additional refinement, their studies were performed in a blinded fashion. They found that 50 percent (15/30) of PD CSF samples produced cytotoxicity that was selective for the dopaminergic (MES 23.5) cell line, compared to 11 percent (2/18) of control specimens. No toxicity was evident in the nondopaminergic (N18TG2) cell line. CSF from levodopa-treated patients was more likely to be cytotoxic (70 percent) than was CSF from untreated PD patients (40 percent), but these differences did not achieve statistical significance. Cytotoxicity was not related to either severity or duration of PD, but it was time- and dose-dependent in that cell loss increased with longer exposure to CSF and with increasing CSF concentration.

Staining for DNA fragmentation with the TUNEL technique demonstrated a pattern of nuclear chromatin condensation and nuclear fragmentation in cells exposed to and damaged by PD CSF. This was interpreted by Le et al. as indicative that cell death was occurring via apoptotic mechanisms (see Chapter 29). Tyrosine hydroxylase activity in the cell lines was also inhibited by PD CSF from both treated and untreated individuals.

As with previous investigators, Le and colleagues were not able to specifically identify the toxic agent present in PD CSF. They did not fractionate CSF and could not comment on the possible size of the agent. They did, however, measure levels of the cytokine, tumor necrosis factor α (TNF-α) and found it to be markedly elevated in PD CSF specimens compared to controls. Although the level of TNF-α was not high enough to be cytotoxic, the presence of elevated TNF-α levels in CSF of PD patients raised the possibility of inflammatory or immunologic mechanisms being active in PD.

Thus is the stage set: Cell culture studies from four different laboratories, employing different approaches and methods, uniformly demonstrate that something is present in the CSF of some, though not all, individuals with PD. That something is toxic to dopamine neurons and is a substance that first interferes with function but ultimately is lethal to the neurons. There is disagreement between investigators as to whether the mystery molecule is selectively toxic for DA neurons or whether it also damages other types of neurons. It appears to be relatively small in size, with a molecular weight of approximately 10,000 or less (perhaps up to 13,000), but its exact identity has remained elusive. Cell culture studies have not allowed specific identification of the

toxic agent, but several candidate substances have been identified in studies by other investigators.

CANDIDATE NEUROTOXINS

The discovery that 1-methyl-4-phenyl-1,2,3,6-tetrahydropyridine (MPTP) is capable of producing CNS damage that both clinically and pathologically closely resembles PD (15–20) has led to speculation about, and searches for, possible environmental or endogenously generated neurotoxins that might bear a structural resemblance to MPTP or its active metabolite, 1-methyl-4-phenylpyridinium ion (MPP+) (21–25). Such speculation has received additional impetus from observations that individuals with PD may have a defective ability to catabolize N-methyl compounds, (26) and the realization that certain agricultural chemicals, such as the insecticide rotenone, have a mechanism of action virtually identical to MPP+ (27). Despite these suspicions, the search for MPP+-like substances or MPTP analogs that might be responsible for PD has been inconclusive (28). Nevertheless, information is accumulating that implicates several compounds as potentially playing a role in the pathogenesis of PD.

Tetrahydroisoquinoline and Derivatives

Sandler and colleagues first identified tetrahydroisoquinoline (TIQ) alkaloids in the urine of individuals with PD in 1973 (29), but it was not until the unfolding of the MPTP story that attention was directed toward TIQ or its derivatives as potential etiologic agents in PD. TIQ, which is present in a variety of foods and beverages (including cheese, wine, bananas, milk, and cocoa (30–32), was subsequently found to be present in human brain (33,34), and following chronic subcutaneous injection of up to 104 days in monkeys, to reduce both DA levels and TH activity in substantia nigra (31,35). However, TIQ did not produce actual neuronal death when administered to mice (31,36), and was ultimately judged to be insufficiently noxious to be seriously considered as a candidate toxin for PD. Attention then turned to other, potentially more toxic, TIQ derivatives.

N-Methyl-(R) Salsolinol

Salsolinol (1-methyl-6,7-dihydroxy-1,2,3,4-tetrahydroisoquinoline) was one of the TIQ alkaloids identified in the urine of PD patients by Sandler and colleagues in 1973 (29). It was later also identified in both CSF and brain in studies on non-Parkinsonian subjects (37,38). However, as with TIQ, salsolinol itself does not appear to be sufficiently cytotoxic to be responsible for the neuronal death seen in PD (39,40). Drawing from the knowledge that N-methylation of TIQ increased its cytotoxic potency, Naoi and Maruyama and their colleagues have focused their attention on the N-methylated derivative of salsolinol, N-methylsalsolinol (NMSal), and in particular, its R-enantiomer, NM(R)Sal, in an impressive series of reports that build a case for NM(R)Sal as a potential endogenous toxic agent responsible for the development of PD (39–54).

NM(R)SaL was found in rat striatum in an in vivo microdialysis study (41) and injection of NM(R)SaL into rat striatum produced behavioral changes similar to PD, along with selective depletion of nigral DA neurons (42). In cell culture experiments Maruyama et al. showed that NM(R)Sal was toxic both to PC12 cells (39) and to differentiated human dopaminergic neuroblastoma SH-SY5Y cells. Moreover, the mode of cell death in the SH-SY5Y cells appeared to be via apoptotic mechanisms (43) mediated by caspase 3 (44). It was further demonstrated that NM(R)Sal increased hydroxyl radical formation in rat striatum (45) and that this occurred in the context of oxidation of NM(R)Sal to 1,2-dimethyl-6,7-dihydroxyisoquinolinium ion (DMDHIQ+), which is structurally similar to MPP+ (46).

Although animal and cell culture experiments are interesting, informative, and important, they cannot directly assess the presence and actions of NM(R)Sal in the human and, more specifically, the individual with PD. CSF studies can shed some light in this regard. Maruyama and colleagues studied CSF from 16 patients with newly diagnosed and untreated PD, five patients with multiple system atrophy (MSA), and 29 control subjects (47). All CSF samples were obtained by lumbar puncture. NM(R)Sal was detected in CSF from all three groups, but the mean level in the PD group was significantly higher than both the control and MSA groups (8.32 ± 2.89 nM PD; 4.53 ± 2.08 nM controls; 3.59 ± 1.52 nM MSA). The rate of synthesis of NM(R)Sal was estimated by comparing the ratio of NM(R)Sal to homovanillic acid (HVA), a major metabolite of dopamine. The ratio was significantly higher in the PD group compared to both control and MSA patients. The S-enantiomer of NMSal was undetectable in CSF from all three groups. The elevation of CSF NM(R)Sal in patients with untreated PD was interpreted by Maruyama et al. as indicative of either increased synthesis or reduced catabolism of NM(R)Sal, or both. The stereospecific character of the elevation of NM(R)Sal was felt to be a reflection of enzymatic synthesis of NM(R)Sal in the brains of persons with PD. The authors

suggested that in addition to providing information about the underlying disease process itself, CSF NM(R)Sal levels might be useful as a marker for early or even preclinical PD, although they did not specifically study this issue in any detailed fashion. In a follow-up study, CSF samples were obtained a second time, after an interval that varied from 1.5–2.0 years, from nine of the 16 PD patients (48). By this time all but one of the individuals were taking levodopa. CSF NM(R)Sal levels had decreased in eight of nine subjects and the mean level showed a statistically significant reduction (7.80 ± 2.16 nM vs. 6.15 ± 2.26 nM); the mean CSF NM(R)SaL/HVA ratio also decreased, but the decrease did not achieve statistical significance. Once again the S-enantiomer was not detectable, reinforcing the authors' earlier conclusion that the elevated CSF NM(R)Sal levels reflect in situ biosynthesis of NM(R)Sal in the brain in PD. The reduction in NM(R)Sal levels over time was interpreted as possibly reflecting progressive loss of dopaminergic neurons as part of the disease process.

Maruyama and colleagues then identified NM(R)Sal (and not NM(S)Sal) in the striatum and substantia nigra, but not in the cortex, from brain tissue obtained at autopsy from 10 individuals without neurologic disease (49). Two enzymes were also identified by Naoi and colleagues to explain the stereospecific appearance of NM(R)Sal in the brain and CSF: a primarily cytosolic (R)salsolinol synthase that catalyzed the condensation of dopamine with acetaldehyde into (R)salsolinol (50) and a neutral (R)salsolinol N-methyltransferase, present in both brain and lymphocytes, which converts (R)salsolinol into NM(R)Sal (41,51,52). A third enzyme, an oxidase responsible for the conversion of NM(R)Sal into DMDHIQ+ was also identified in vitro (53).

Naoi and Maruyama have proposed that the following chain of events takes place, which may result in the development of PD: within the brain, (R)salsolinol is formed by enzymatically induced condensation of endogenous dopamine with acetaldehyde and is subsequently converted by a neutral N-methyltransferase, primarily in the striatum into NM(R)Sal, which is then selectively taken up into dopaminergic nerve terminals in the striatum and transported by retrograde axonal flow to the dopaminergic cell bodies in the substantia nigra where it can be oxidized to DMDHIQ+ with associated generation of hydroxyl radicals and subsequent development of dopaminergic cell death via apoptotic mechanisms (54). Individuals who develop PD may have increased N-methyltransferase activity, which propels the chain of events forward.

Although this makes a compelling story, Gerlach and colleagues caution that the evidence implicating NM(R)Sal as the endogenous neurotoxin responsible for PD is still incomplete and that important questions remain to be answered before the scenario described above can be taken as proven fact (55).

CSF investigations have been performed with several other TIQ derivatives, such as salsolinol itself and N-methyl-norsalsolinol (2-methyl-6,7-dihydroxy-1,2,3,4-tetrahydroisoquinoline). Moser and colleagues measured N-methyl-norsalsolinol in 34 PD patients (eight untreated; 26 on levodopa) and in 15 normal control subjects (56). Although N-methyl-norsalsolinol was detected in 53 percent (18/34) of PD CSF samples and in no controls, the authors did not believe that N-methyl-norsalsolinol was responsible for dopamine neuronal toxicity (in other studies it had not been (31)), but rather that the increased levels reflected increased dopamine metabolism in surviving DA neurons in PD. Conflicting results have been reported with CSF salsolinol measurements in PD patients. Muller and colleagues found no increase in salsolinol levels (57,58) while Antiewicz-Michaluk et al. noted an association of increasing CSF salsolinol levels in patients with dementia as a component of their PD (59).

ß-Carbolines

Another family of compounds that has been proposed, on the basis of structural similarities to MPTP and MPP+, as potential neurotoxins responsible for PD are the ß-carbolines. The ß-carbolines are heterocyclic compounds derived from indoleamines such as tryptophan and are found primarily in plants but also occur in fish and beef (60). In addition to these environmental sources ß-carbolines can be manufactured endogenously from condensation of an indoleamine with glyoxylic acid (61). Simple ß-carbolines, such as harman and norharman, are nonpolar compounds and can easily cross the blood–brain barrier (62–63); are probably normal brain constituents and not, themselves, probable neurotoxins (64). Within the brain, however, simple ß-carbolines can undergo N-methylation reactions that result in compounds with more clear neurotoxic potential. Norharman (NH) has received most attention in this regard and 2-methyl-norharman (2-MeNH), most probably as the cation 2-MeNH+, demonstrates definite neurotoxic potential, but at a magnitude 10–20 times less potent than MPP+ (61). Collins and colleagues subsequently found that a second methyl substitution, this time at the 9[indole]-nitrogen, forming 2,9-N, N′-dimethyl-norharman (2,9-Me$_2$NH), resulted in a significantly more potent neurotoxin that also inhibited mitochondrial respiration (66). They noted that 2,9-Me$_2$NH

was toxic to PC12 cells in culture and that guinea pig brain homogenates did possess the ability to manufacture 2,9-Me$_2$NH from NH via 5-adenosylmethionine-dependent N-methylation reactions. Matsubara and colleagues confirmed this and documented that at low doses the cation 2,9-Me$_2$NH+ was relatively selectively toxic for DA neurons in primary mesencephalic cell culture but at higher doses became a non-selective neurotoxin (63). Transient behavioral changes in mice were also noted following subchronic systemic administration of NH and two monomethylated derivatives (2-MeNH and 9-MeNH), presumably due to formation of 2,9-Me$_2$NH+ in the brain (63).

Once again, the question must be asked whether these animal and cell culture experiments have any applicability to humans and CSF studies again provide important information. Matsubara and colleagues obtained CSF samples from 22 PD patients and 11 control subjects (67). Most PD patients were on anti-Parkinson therapy with a variety of agents (exact details were not provided). The simple ß-carboline NH and its monomethylated derivative 2-MeNH+ were detected via HPLC techniques in virtually all CSF samples and tended to be higher in PD CSF, although no statistically significant differences between PD and control groups were discovered. The picture with 2,9-Me$_2$NH+, however, was quite different, in that 12 of the 22 PD patients registered detectable amounts of 2,9-Me$_2$NH+, whereas none of the control CSF samples did. The authors interpreted these results as supporting the contention that endogenously produced ß-carbolines, such as 2,9-Me$_2$NH+, might be involved in the pathogenesis of PD. Further support for this contention comes from Matsubara et al.'s experience with human brain tissue obtained from non-Parkinsonian individuals at autopsy, where 2,9-Me$_2$NH was detected in almost all samples but levels were significantly higher (up to 50-fold) in substantia nigra than in cortex (64).

(E)-4-Hydroxy-2-Nonenal

Much has been written in recent years about the role that oxidative stress mechanisms with free radical generation and lipid peroxidation of cell membranes may play in the development of PD (see Chapter 28) (68–70). This free radical-stimulated cell membrane peroxidation may in itself generate additional toxic products and it is one of these, (E)-4-Hydroxy-2-Nonenal (HNE), that has caught the attention of Selley (71). Malonaldehyde and HNE, along with other aldehydes, are released when membrane-bound arachidonic acid undergoes lipid peroxidation (72). Because HNE is highly lipophilic, it can accumulate in cell membranes and in sufficient concentration become cytotoxic to a variety of cell types, including neurons (71,72,73). This led Selley to measure plasma and CSF HNE concentrations in individuals with PD. Plasma HNE was measured in 20 PD patients, but CSF samples were obtained from only 10 and compared with 10 control subjects. Levels of HNE were significantly elevated in both CSF (1.47 ± 0.76 μM vs 0.38 ± 0.14 μM) and plasma (0.68 ± 0.15 μM vs 0.47 ± 0.12 μM) of patients with PD compared to controls. Furthermore, HNE concentrations in the range of those found in PD CSF were found to be toxic to DA neurons in rat mesencephalic primary cultures (71), which led Selley to suggest that HNE might be the toxic agent noted in earlier CSF studies (4,5,12,13). Further studies on HNE are clearly warranted.

CONCLUSION

This chapter focused on the apparent presence and possible identity of a factor or factors present in the CSF of individuals with PD that might be toxic for DA neurons and, thus, an etiologic agent for PD. It must also be acknowledged that CSF has been studied in PD in many additional fashions, such as measuring DA metabolites or other substances, that have nothing directly to do with CSF neurotoxicity and are beyond the scope of this chapter.

Although the total number of studies (and investigators) pursuing the issue of CSF toxicity in PD is quite small, potentially important information has emerged. Cell culture studies seem to clearly and consistently indicate the presence of some toxic factor or factors in the CSF of many patients with PD. Investigation for the responsible agent have largely focused on substances, such as TIQ derivatives and ß-carbolines, that bear structural similarity to the known DA neurotoxin, MPTP. This is a natural area on which to initially focus, but it is also important to recognize that this could be the equivalent of looking for lost keys under the street lamp because that is where the light is best and investigative minds should not be closed to considering and pursuing other clues in the effort to solve the riddle of PD. For now, studies of CSF toxicity and related searches for neurotoxins in PD have provided provocative food for thought.

REFERENCES

1. Rowland LP, Fink ME, Rubin L. Cerebrospinal fluid: Blood-brain barrier, brain edema, and hydrocephalus. In: Kandel ER, Schwartz JH, Jessell TM (eds). *Principles of Neuroscience.* Third Edition. New York: Elsevier Science Publishing 1991:1050–1060.

2. Carvey PM, Ptak LR, Lo ES, et al. Homogenates of parkinsonian striatum enhance DA-uptake in rat mesencephalic cultures relative to control striatum. *Neurology* 1990; 40(Suppl 1):402.

3. Carvey PM, Ptak LR, Nath ST, et al. Striatal extracts from patients with Parkinson's disease promote dopamine neuron growth in mesencephalic cultures. *Exp Neurol* 1993; 120:149–152.

4. Yu SJ, Lo ES, Cochran EJ, et al. Cerebrospinal fluid from patients with Parkinson's disease alters the survival of dopamine neurons in mesencephalic culture. *Exp Neurol* 1994; 125:15–24.

5. Hao R, Norgren RB, Lau Y-S, et al. Cerebrospinal fluid of Parkinson's disease patients inhibits the growth and function of dopaminergic neurons in culture. *Neurology* 1995; 45:138–142.

6. Hao R, Fu L, Pfeiffer RF. Abnormal protein found in CSF from PD patients by 2D-gel electrophoresis. *Neurology* 1998; 50(Suppl 4):A386.

7. Melamed E, Offen D, Shirvan A, et al. Levodopa toxicity and apoptosis. *Ann Neurol* 1998; 44(Suppl 1): S149–S154.

8. Tanaka M, Sotomatsu A, Kanai H, et al. Dopa and dopamine cause cultured neuronal death in the presence of iron. *J Neurol Sci* 1991; 101:198–203.

9. Agid Y, Ahlskog E, Albanese A, et al. Levodopa in the treatment of Parkinson's disease: A consensus meeting. *Mov Disord* 1999; 14:911–913.

10. The Parkinson Study Group. Effect of deprenyl on the progression of disability in early Parkinson's disease. *N Eng J Med* 1989; 321:1364–1371.

11. Parkinson Study Group. Cerebrospinal fluid homovanillic acid in the DATATOP study on Parkinson's disease. *Arch Neurol* 1995; 52:237–245.

12. Colombo JA, Napp MI. Cerebrospinal fluid from L-Dopa-treated Parkinson's disease patients is dystrophic for various neural cell types ex vivo: Effects of astroglia. *Exp Neurol* 1998; 154:452–463.

13. Le W-D, Rowe DB, Jankovic J, et al. Effects of cerebrospinal fluid from patients with Parkinson's disease on dopaminergic cells. *Arch Neurol* 1999; 56:194–200.

14. Crawford GD Jr, Le W-D, Smith RG, et al. A novel N18TG2 x mesencephalon cell hybrid expresses properties that suggest a dopaminergic cell line of substantia nigra origin. *J Neurosci* 1992; 12:3392–3398.

15. Langston JW, Ballard P, Tetrud JW, et al. Chronic parkinsonism in humans due to a product of meperidine-analog synthesis. *Science* 1983; 219: 979–980.

16. Ballard PA, Tetrud JW, Langston JW. Permanent human parkinsonism due to 1-methyl-4-phenyl-1,2,3,6-tetrahydropyridine (MPTP): seven cases. *Neurology* 1985; 35:949–956.

17. Langston JW, Forno LS, Rebert CS, et al. Selective nigral toxicity after systemic administration of 1-methyl-4-phenyl-1,2,3,6-tetrahydropyridine (MPTP) in the squirrel monkey. *Brain Res* 1984; 292:390–394.

18. Markey SP, Johannessen JN, Chiueh CC, et al. Intraneuronal generation of a pyridinium metabolite may cause drug-induced parkinsonism. *Nature* 1984; 311:464–467.

19. Burns RS, Chiueh CC, Markey SP, et al. A primate model of parkinsonism: Selective destruction of dopaminergic neurons in the pars compacta of the substantia nigra by N-methyl-4-phenyl-1,2,3,6-tetrahydropyridine. *Proc Natl Acad Sci USA* 1983; 80:4546–4550.

20. Heikkila RE, Hess A, Duvoisin RC. Dopaminergic neurotoxicity of 1-methyl-4-phenyl-1,2,3,6-tetrahydropyridine in mice. *Science* 1984; 224:1451–1453.

21. Koller W, Vetere-Overfield B, Gray C, et al. Environmental risk factors in Parkinson's disease. *Neurology* 1990; 40: 1218–1221.

22. Kopin IJ. Toxins and Parkinson's disease: MPTP parkinsonism in humans and animals. In: Yahr MD, Bergmann KJ (eds). *Parkinson's Disease (Advances in Neurology, Vol. 45)*. New York: Raven Press. 1986; 137–144.

23. Langston JW. MPTP: Insights into the etiology of Parkinson's disease. *Eur Neurol* 1987; 1:2–10.

24. Markey SP, Schmuff NR. The pharmacology of the parkinsonian syndrome producing neurotoxin MPTP (1-methyl-4-phenyl-1,2,3,6-tetrahydropyridine) and structurally related compounds. *Med Res Rev* 1986; 6:389–429.

25. Tanner CM, Langston JW. Do environmental toxins cause Parkinson's disease? A critical review. *Neurology* 1990; 40(Suppl 3):17–30.

26. Williams AC, Pall HS, Steventon GB, et al. N-methylation of pyridines and Parkinson's disease. In: Narabayashi H, Nagatsu T, Yanagisawa N, Mizuno Y (eds). *Parkinson's Disease from Basic Research to Treatment (Advances in Neurology, Vol. 60)*. New York: Raven Press. 1993:194–196.

27. Heikkila RE, Nicklas WJ, Vyas I, et al. Dopaminergic toxicity of rotenone and the 1-methyl-4-phenylpyridinium ion after their stereotaxic administration to rats: Implication for the mechanism of 1-methyl-4-phenyl-1,2,3,6-tetrahydropyridine toxicity. *Neurosci Lett* 1985; 62:389–394.

28. Ikeda H, Markey CJ, Markey SP. Search for neurotoxins structurally related to 1-methyl-4-phenylpyridine (MPP+) in the pathogenesis of Parkinson's disease. *Brain Res* 1992; 575:285–298.

29. Sandler M, Bonham Carter S, Hunter KR, et al. Tetrahydroisoquinoline alkaloids: In vivo metabolites of L-dopa in man. *Nature* 1973; 241:439–443.

30. Niwa T, Yoshizumi H, Tatematsu A, et al. Presence of tetrahydroisoquinoline, a parkinsonism-related compound, in foods. *J Chromatogr* 1989; 493:345–352.

31. Yoshida M, Ogawa M, Suzuki K, et al. Parkinsonism produced by tetrahydroisoquinoline (TIQ) or the analogs. In: Narabayashi H, Nagatsu T, Yanagisawa N, Mizuno Y (eds). *Parkinson's Disease from Basic Research to Treatment (Advances in Neurology, Vol. 60)*. New York: Raven Press. 1993:207–211.

32. Makino Y, Ohta S, Tachikawa O, et al. Presence of tetrahydroisoquinoline and 1-methyl-tetrahydroisoquinoline in foods: Compounds related to Parkinson's disease. *Life Sci* 1988; 43:373–378.

33. Ohta S, Kohno K, Makino Y, et al. Tetrahydroisoquinoline and 1-methyl-tetrahydroisoquinoline are present in the human brain: Relation to Parkinson's disease. *Biomed Res* 1987; 8:453–456.

34. Niwa T, Takeda N, Kaneda N, et al. Presence of tetrahydroisoquinoline and 2-methyl-tetrahydroisoquinoline in parkinsonian and normal human brains. *Biochem Biophys Res Commun* 1987; 144: 1084–1089.

35. Nagatsu T, Yoshida M. An endogenous substance of the brain, tetrahydroisoquinoline, produces parkinsonism in primates with decreased dopamine, tyrosine hydroxylase and biopterine in the nigrostriatal regions. *Neurosci Lett* 1988; 87:178–182.

36. Ogawa M, Araki M, Nagatsu I, et al. The effect of 1,2,3,4-tetrahydroisoquinoline (TIQ) on mesencephalic dopaminergic neurons in C57BL/6J mice: Immunohistochemical studies – tyrosine hydroxylase. *Biogenic Amines* 1989; 6:427–436.

37. Sjoequist B, Eriksson A, Winblad B. Salsolinol and catecholamines in human brain and their relation to alcoholism. *Prog Clin Biol Res* 1982; 90:57–67.

38. Sjoequist B, Borg S, Kvande H. Salsolinol and methylated salsolinol in urine and cerebrospinal fluid from healthy volunteers. *Subst Alcohol Actions Misuse.* 1981; 2:73–77.

39. Maruyama W, Takahashi T, Minami M, et al. Cytotoxicity of dopamine-derived 6,7-dihydroxy-1,2,3,4-tetrahydroisoquinolines. In: Narabayashi H, Nagatsu T, Yanagisawa N, Mizuno Y (eds). *Parkinson's Disease from Basic Research to Treatment (Advances in Neurology, Vol. 60)* New York: Raven Press. 1993:224–230.

40. Naoi M, Dostert P, Yoshida M, et al. N-methylated tetrahydroisoquinolines as dopaminergic neurotoxins. In: Narabayashi H, Nagatsu T, Yanagisawa N, Mizuno Y (eds). *Parkinson's Disease from Basic Research to Treatment (Advances in Neurology, Vol. 60)*. New York: Raven Press. 1993:212–217.

41. Maruyama W, Nakahara D, Ota M, et al. N-methylation of dopamine-derived 6,7-dihydroxy-1,2,3,4-tetrahydroisoquinoline, (R)salsolinol, in rat brains: In vivo microdialysis study. *J Neurochem* 1992; 59:395–400.

42. Naoi M, Maruyama W, Dostert P, et al. Dopamine-derived endogenous 1(R), 2(N)-dimethyl-6,7-dihydroxy-1,2,3,4-tetrahydroisoquinoline, N-methyl-(R)-salsolinol, induced parkinsonism in rat: Biochemical, pathological and behavioral studies. *Brain Res* 1996; 709:285–295.

43. Maruyama W, Strolin Benedetti M, Takahashi T, et al. A neurotoxin N-methyl(R)salsolinol induces apoptotic cell death in differentiated human dopaminergic neuroblastoma SH-SY5Y cells. *Neurosci Lett* 1997; 232:147–150.

44. Akao Y, Nakagawa Y, Maruyama W, et al. Apoptosis induced by an endogenous neurotoxin, N-methyl(R) salsolinol, is mediated by activation of caspase 3. *Neurosci Lett* 1999; 267:153–156.

45. Maruyama W, Nakahara D, Dostert P, et al. Dopamine-derived isoquinolines as dopaminergic neurotoxins and oxidative stress. In: Hanin I, Yoshida M, Fisher A (eds). *Alzheimer's and Parkinson's Disease: Recent Development*. New York: Plenum Press. 1995:575–581.

46. Maruyama W, Dostert P, Matsubara K, et al. N-methyl(R)salsolinol produces hydroxyl radicals: involvement to neurotoxicity. *Free Rad Biol Med* 1995; 19:67–75.

47. Maruyama W, Abe T, Tohgi H, et al. A dopaminergic neurotoxin, (R)-N-methylsalsolinol, increases in parkinsonian cerebrospinal fluid. *Ann Neurol* 1996; 40:119–122.

48. Maruyama W, Abe T, Tohgi H, et al. An endogenous MPTP-like dopaminergic neurotoxin, N-methyl(R)salsolinol, in the cerebrospinal fluid decreases with progression of Parkinson's disease. *Neurosci Lett* 1999; 262:13–16.

49. Maruyama W, Sobue G, Matsubara K, et al. A dopaminergic neurotoxin, 1(R),2(N)-dimethyl-6,7-dihydroxy-1,2,3,4-tetrahydroisoquinoline, N-methyl(R) salsolinol, and its oxidation product, 1,2(N)-dimethyl-6,7-dihydroxyisoquinolinium ion, accumulate in the nigrostriatal system of the human brain. *Neurosci Lett* 1997; 223:61–64.

50. Naoi M, Maruyama W, Dostert P, et al. A novel enzyme enantio-selectively synthesizes (R)salsolinol, a precursor of a dopaminergic neurotoxin, N-methyl(R)salsolinol. *Neurosci Lett* 1996; 212:183–186.

51. Naoi M, Maruyama W, Matsubara K, et al. A neutral N-methyltransferase activity in the striatum determines the level of an endogenous MPP+-like neurotoxin, 1,2-dimethyl-6,7-dihydroxyisoquinolinium ion, in the substantia nigra of human brains. *Neurosci Lett* 1997; 235:81–84.

52. Naoi M, Maruyama W, Nakao N, et al. (R)Salsolinol n-methyltransferase activity increases in parkinsonian lymphocytes. *Ann Neurol* 1998; 43:212–216.

53. Naoi M, Maruyama W, Zhang JH, et al. Enzymatic oxidation of the dopaminergic neurotoxin, 1(R),2(N)-dimethyl-6,7-dihydroxy-1,2,3,4-tetrahydroisoquinoline, into 1,2(N)-dimethyl-6,7-dihydroxyisoquinolinium ion. *Life Sci* 1995; 57:1061–1066.

54. Naoi M, Maruyama W. N-methyl(R)salsolinol, a dopamine neurotoxin, in Parkinson's disease. In: Stern GM (ed). *Parkinson's Disease (Advances in Neurology, Vol. 80)*. Philadelphia: Lippincott Williams & Wilkins. 1999:259–264.

55. Gerlach M, Koutsilieri E, Riederer P. N-methyl-(R)-salsolinol and its relevance to Parkinson's disease. *Lancet* 1998; 351:850–851.

56. Moser A, Scholz J, Nobbe F, et al. Presence of N-methyl-norsalsolinol in the CSF: Correlations with dopamine metabolites of patients with Parkinson's disease. *J Neurol Sci* 1995; 131:183–189.

57. Müller T, Przuntek H, Kuhn W, et al. No increase of synthesis of (R)salsolinol in Parkinson's disease. *Mov Disord* 1999; 14:514–515.

58. Müller T, Sällström Baum S, Häussermann P, et al. R- and S-salsolinol are not increased in cerebrospinal fluid of parkinsonian patients. *J Neurol Sci* 1999; 164:158–162.

59. Antkiewicz-Michaluk L, Krygowska-Wajs A, Szczudlik A, et al. Increase in salsolinol level in the cerebrospinal fluid of parkinsonian patients is related to dementia: Advantage of a new high-performance liquid chromatography methodology. *Biol Psychiatr* 1997; 42:514–518.

60. Gross GA, Turesky RJ, Fay L, et al. Heterocyclic aromatic amine formation in grilled bacon, beef and fish in grill scrapings. *Carcinogenesis* 1993; 14:2313–2318.

61. Neafsey EJ, Drucker G, Raikoff K, et al. Striatal dopaminergic toxicity following intranigral injection in rats of 2-methyl-norharman, a ß-carbolinium analog of N-methyl-4-phenylpyridinium ion (MPP+). *Neurosci Lett* 1989; 105:344–349.

62. Rommelspacher H, Damm H, Strauss S, et al. Ethanol induces an increase of harman in the brain and urine of rats. *Naunyn Schmiedebergs Arch Pharmacol* 1984; 327:107–113.

63. Matsubara K, Gonda T, Sawada H, et al. Endogenously occurring ß-carboline induces parkinsonism in nonprimate animals: A possible causative protoxin in idiopathic Parkinson's disease. *J Neurochem* 1998; 70:727–735.

64. Matsubara K, Collins MA, Akane A, et al. Potential bioactivated neurotoxicants, N-methylated ß-carbolinium ions, are present in human brain. *Brain Res* 1993; 610:90–96.

65. Rollema H, Booth RG, Castagnoli N Jr. In vivo dopaminergic neurotoxicity of the 2-ß-methylcarbolinium ion, a potential endogenous MPP+ analog. *Eur J Pharmacol* 1988; 153:131–134.

66. Collins MA, Neafsey EJ, Matsubara K, et al. Indole-N-methylated ß-carbolinium ions as potential brain-bioactivated neurotoxins. *Brain Res* 1992; 570:154–160.

67. Matsubara K, Kobayashi S, Kobayashi Y, et al. ß-carbolinium cations, endogenous MPP+ analogs, in the lumbar cerebrospinal fluid of patients with Parkinson's disease. *Neurology* 1995; 45:2240–2245.

68. Jenner P, Olanow CW. Understanding cell death in Parkinson's disease. *Ann Neurol* 1998; 44(Suppl 1):S72–S84.

69. Münch G, Gerlach M, Sian J, et al. Advanced glycation end products in neurodegeneration: More than early markers of oxidative stress? *Ann Neurol* 1998; 44(Suppl 1):S85–S88.

70. Schapira AHV, Gu M, Taanman J-W, et al. Mitochondria in the etiology and pathogenesis of Parkinson's disease. *Ann Neurol* 1998; 44(Suppl 1):S89–S98.

71. Selley ML. (E)-4-Hydroxy-2-nonenal may be involved in the pathogenesis of Parkinson's disease. *Free Radic Biol Med* 1998; 25:169–174.

72. Esterbauer H, Schaur RJ, Zollner H. Chemistry and biochemistry of 4-hydroxynonenal, malonaldehyde and related aldehydes. *Free Radic Biol Med* 1991; 11:81–128.

73. Mark RJ, Lovell MA, Markesbery WR, et al. A role for 4-hydroxynonenal, an aldehydic product of lipid peroxidation, in disruption of ion homeostasis and neuronal death induced by amyloid beta-peptide. *J Neurochem* 1997; 68:255–264.

32

Levodopa: 30 Years of Progress

Tanya Simuni, M.D., and Howard Hurtig, M.D.

University of Pennsylvania Health System, Philadelphia, Pennsylvania

INTRODUCTION

Levodopa was first used to treat Parkinson's disease (PD) in the early 1960s, and by the time it was approved by the U.S. FDA in 1967, it was hailed as one of the most important advances in the pharmacotherapy of neurologic diseases of the twentieth century. Its development was based on a series of major advances in the understanding of the neurochemical mechanisms underlying the disease. Now, more than 30 years later and despite significant advances in the pharmacotherapy of PD, levodopa remains the gold standard of treatment. The gold, however, has been tarnished by a variety of intrinsic problems and complications of long-term use, such as motor fluctuations (on-off phenomenon) and dyskinesias, which can be no less disabling than the Parkinsonian symptoms it suppresses. Moreover, the early and unrealistic belief that levodopa could actually cure the disease by simply replacing a missing neurotransmitter or slow the inevitable progression of the underlying degeneration in the substantia nigra (SN) was quickly undercut by the harsh truth of practical experience. In fact, one of the most active controversies swirling around levodopa today centers on whether it might *increase* the pace of neurodegeneration of neurons in the SN by promoting oxidative neurotoxicity.

In this chapter the history of levodopa's development and the major milestones that punctuate its maturation as the mainstay of treatment for PD are reviewed. This chapter also covers the impact of levodopa on the mortality and morbidity of PD, the proposed mechanism of levodopa- induced complications (fluctuations and dyskinesias), and the evidence that levodopa is toxic to neurons.

HISTORICAL REVIEW

In his classic 1817 monograph *"An Essay on the Shaking Palsy,"* James Parkinson (1) first described a series of six patients afflicted by the highly visible malady that now bears his name. The precision of much of the description is remarkable considering that Parkinson examined only three of the patients directly, whereas the others were observed by him as a vigilant spectator on the streets of London. His language has forever captured the cardinal manifestations of the disease, although the accuracy of some of his observations (i.e., the bold and italicized segments) have been refuted by modern experience: "Involuntary tremulous motion, with *lessened muscular power*, in parts not in action and even when supported: with the propensity to bend the trunk forward and to pass from a walking to a running pace: the senses and the *intellect being unimpaired*." Parkinson himself did not comment on how to treat this new condition. Instead, he concluded his essay with an appeal "to those who humanely employ anatomical examination in detecting the courses and nature of diseases" to study the brain and find the cause. Later in the nineteenth century Jean-Martin Charcot described a "pill rolling" tremor and masked face as particular features of PD (2). As a corrective revision, he commented on the absence of weakness and the occasional impairment of intellect. By the beginning of the twentieth century, the clinical picture of the disease was well defined but the pathologic substrate remained unknown. In 1913 Lewy (3) first described the characteristic eosinophilic intracytoplasmic inclusion bodies in various regions of the brain stem but mistakenly reported that the SN was not affected. It was only a few years later in 1919 that Tretiakoff (4) discovered that the neuronal degeneration of the SN was a consistent pathologic signature in the brains of patients with clinical Parkinsonism.

The first pharmacotherapy for PD was introduced over a century ago by Ordenstein in 1867 (5). Belladonna alkaloids, which were administered to PD patients to control drooling, were incidentally found to improve stiffness and tremor. In the early 1950s synthetic anticholinergic drugs, such as benztropine mesylate (Cogentin) and trihexyphenidyl (Artane) had been introduced. Although benefit was modest and inconsistent, anticholinergics remained the cornerstone of therapy for nearly a hundred years. The reason anticholinergics ameliorate symptoms in PD is not clear. It is believed that they block muscarinic receptors in the striatum and thereby restore balance to the polarity that normally characterizes the relationship between dopamine and acetylcholine.

Because pharmacologic therapy was largely ineffective (except in dampening tremor), neurosurgical ablation of a variety of sites in the brain and spinal cord became a popular alternative. The clinical observations that parkinsonian tremor arrested after cerebrovascular accident on the side of the paralysis led to the conclusion that well-placed surgical lesions in particular motor centers might be useful in suppressing symptoms (6). Early surgical trials showed that lesions in the cortex or descending pyramidal tracts could truly arrest tremor but often at the expense of paralysis. In 1952 Cooper (7) serendipitously discovered that accidental ligation of the anterior choroidal artery abolished parkinsonian tremor and rigidity without causing paralysis by producing a lesion in the globus pallidus. A variety of approaches were subsequently used with the major targets being globus pallidus (8) and later thalamus (9), specifically for tremor suppression. Surgical treatment was almost totally eclipsed by the immediate and widespread efficacy of levodopa only to rise again 30 years later as a select method of controlling levodopa-related complications (dyskinesias), as computerized imaging, refined stereotactic techniques, and advances in understanding the circuitry of the basal ganglia brought remarkable sophistication to the process of targeting appropriate regions of the brain for surgical manipulation.

Dopamine and the Rational Treatment of Parkinson's Disease

The development of levodopa as effective pharmacotherapy for PD was a logical outcome of advances in understanding the pathophysiology of Parkinsonism. In the early 1950s, Brodie et al. (10) discovered that reserpine depleted serotonin in the brains of rats by altering storage in synaptic vesicles, following which, Carlsson et al. (11) demonstrated that reserpine had the same effect on dopamine. He further showed that the motor slowing or bradykinesia induced by administration of reserpine to rabbits could be reversed by administration of levodopa, an inert precursor of dopamine. Subsequent investigations by Carlsson et al. (12) and by Bertler and Rosengren showed that dopamine was highly concentrated in the caudate and

putamen of the basal ganglia (13) (the striatum), compared with other biogenic amines such as noradrenaline that accumulated in the brainstem. By the end of the 1950s, these findings had led to the hypothesis that dopamine deficiency was the biochemical link to the patholophysiology of PD. Hornykiewiecz (14), whose seminal work and landmark publication in 1960 proved the hypothesis correct, subsequently wrote, "On the basis of these findings (in animals), it was to my mind a very simple and very logical step to go from animal to human brain to see whether it was possible to discover any abnormalities of dopamine metabolism in certain neurological disorders involving the basal ganglia." Ehringer and Hornykiewicz (15) studied the brains of patients dying of PD and consistently demonstrated a 90% reduction in the concentration of dopamine in the striatum and substantia nigra. They also showed that the content of striatal homovanillic acid (HVA), a stable byproduct of dopamine metabolism, directly correlated with the degree of dopamine deficiency and of cell loss in the SN (16). They further observed that parkinsonism associated with chronic manganese poisoning was also characterized by degeneration of nigral neurons and a decrease in dopamine and HVA in the striatum and SN (17). Therefore nigral cell death was the common pathologic denominator in all syndromes of parkinsonism, irrespective of etiology.

By the mid-1960s sophisticated histofluorescence techniques had been developed and new knowledge quickly accumulated. Anden et al. (18), using this new methodology, demonstrated that dopamine was concentrated in neurons of the SN pars compacta (pc) and that axonal terminals projected cephalad to the striatum. Poirier and Sourkes (19), by showing that a unilateral nigral lesion in the monkey could cause ipsilateral depletion of striatal dopamine, mapped the previously unknown nigrostriatal pathway and thus explained the relationship between neuronal loss in the SNpc and dopamine depletion in the striatum.

These pivotal discoveries provided the foundation for the logical next step: treatment of PD by replacing the depleted neurotransmitter dopamine. The simplicity of the concept had to be a siren signal that implementation would not be easy.

Levodopa Therapy

Among the early findings of research into the pharmacologic properties of dopamine was that it did not penetrate the blood–brain barrier (BBB). Its immediate amino acid precursor dihydroxyphenylalanine (dopa) could, however, cross the barrier and enter the brain, where it was enzymatically converted to dopamine. Proof of access lay in levodopa's ability to reverse the behavioral effects of reserpine in experimental animals and elevate brain dopamine levels when administered systemically. In 1961 two independent research groups launched clinical trials of dopa in patients with advanced PD. Birkmayer and Hornykiewicz (20) administered dopa intravenously to parkinsonian patients in doses up to 150 mg. They observed "complete abolition or substantial reduction" of parkinsonian akinesia. Barbeau (21) et al. reported similar results following oral doses up to 300 mg of dopa daily (21). These early therapeutic experiments were soon repeated by many other investigators with conflicting and frequently unimpressive results. Birkmayer and Hornykiewicz (22) later reported positive response to dopa in only half of the patients and saw no recognizable effect if the patient's previous anticholinergic medication had been withdrawn. In 1964 McGeer and Zeldowitz (23) treated 10 patients with an oral dose of dopa ranging from 1 to 3 gm daily. Only two of ten patients improved at the highest dose, and they concluded that dopa was not useful. In their experiment, dopa was combined with pyridoxine because of the erroneous belief that pyridoxine, a cofactor for dopa decarboxylase in the dopa-to-dopamine-conversion reaction, would enhance the therapeutic impact. The fact that pyridoxine actually diminishes the effect of dopa by potentiating peripheral decarboxylation was not appreciated until five years later when it was described by Duvoisin and coworkers (24).

Challenged by the inconsistent and even disappointing early experience with dopa therapy, George Cotzias achieved what others could not by bringing dedication and an unswerving vision to the goal of proving that dopa really works. After years of patient trial and error he and his colleagues reported in 1967 (25) that high doses (4–16 grams) of oral racemic (D, L) dopa brought about "either complete, sustained disappearance or marked amelioration of Parkinsonism" in 8 of 16 patients. There was a clear dose–response relationship; only the patients on the highest dose responded. However, 25% of the patients developed granulocytopenia attributable to the drug and withdrew from the trial. In the same study the patients were exposed to melanocyte-stimulating hormone and phenylalanine, a dopa precursor, both of which aggravated the Parkinsonian symptoms. The authors concluded that D, L dopa was effective in certain cases of parkinsonism, but the significant risk of granulocytopenia nullified its potential as a useful anti-parkinson drug.

Two years later Cotzias et al. (26) published the results of a study of levodopa (L-dopa) in 28 patients with PD. Twenty experienced marked and sustained improvement for up to two years. The daily dose of levodopa ranged from 4.5 to 8 gm. None of the patients experienced the granulocytopenia observed with the use of D, L-dopa. Nausea and vomiting, adverse drug effects common to other studies of dopa in PD, were overcome by initiation of low-dose treatment, followed by slow-dose escalation. In the same study, the authors observed choreiform involuntary movements in 14 of 28 patients, ranging from mild to severe and correlating in severity with duration of the disease. Within the next few years similar studies using large oral doses of levodopa were reported by Yahr et al. (27), McDowell et al. (28), Markham (29), Godwin-Austen (30) and others, confirming the dramatic findings reported by Cotzias. A major breakthrough in the treatment of PD was duly recognized – Cotzias received the Lasker award in 1970 – but just as important was the idea that replacement pharmacotherapy could be successful and might be applicable to other neurodegenerative disorders with specific biochemical defects.

The next five years were marked by a number of studies that supported pronounced and sustained response of all Parkinsonian symptoms to treatment with levodopa. Markham (29) demonstrated that the overall response to medication achieved at one year was sustained at two and a half years. Similar results were published by Yahr (31), Cotzias et al. (32), as well as Godwin-Austen. At the same time, clinicians pointed to differential response of symptoms of parkinsonism to medication with tremor responding less predictably (33).

The complete or near complete reversal of the physical signs and symptoms of a chronic progressive neurodegenerative disorder had not been previously seen. The spectacle of patients being able to get out of bed and wheelchair to resume long lost daily and athletic activities was truly incredible to professional and lay witnesses alike. Furthermore, the evidence that levodopa was having a long-term impact on the natural history of PD began to accumulate. When progression of Parkinsonian disability was compared in 182 patients receiving levodopa treatment with a cohort of patients from the prelevodopa era, Hoehn (34,35) found that patients on levodopa remained stable in each Hoehn and Yahr stage of the disease three to five years longer than was the case in the prelevodopa era. Also, the number of patients classified as disabled or dead in each stage was reduced by 30 to 50%. Yet there was no detectable difference in the severity of the Parkinsonian symptoms between treated and untreated patients evaluated in the setting of withdrawal from levodopa, suggesting that the benefit derived from using levodopa was purely nigral degeneration or decrease in the density of striatal dopamine terminals (114). However, intrastriatal administration of high doses of levodopa to rats did produce degeneration of presynaptic dopaminergic terminals (115). High concentrations of levodopa are potentially toxic to normal dopaminergic neurons, in some species and not in others. No study has shown that systemic administration of levodopa in human equivalent doses causes degeneration of dopaminergic cells in normal animals.

Is Levodopa Toxic in Animals with a Lesioned Nigrostriatal System?

Two pivotal studies evaluated the effect of exposure to levodopa on the 6-hydroxy dopamine (6-OHDA) animal model of PD. Blunt et al. (116) lesioned the nigrostriatal pathway in rats and investigated the effect of chronic levodopa exposure on dopaminergic cell survival. Animals were assigned to a control group (lesion but no levodopa) and a treated group (lesion plus levodopa/carbidopa feedings for 27 weeks). The experiment demonstrated that the animals fed with levodopa/carbidopa had greater loss of dopaminergic cells on the lesioned side than control animals, especially in the ventral segmental area. The number of dopaminergic cells on the nonlesioned contralateral side was not affected in either group. Blunt et al. concluded that a damaged dopaminergic system is susceptible to further damage from levodopa-induced oxidative stress, and it translates into an increased risk of treatment-related, accelerated neurodegeneration.

A more recent study by Murer and colleagues (117) used a similar design but expanded it considerably. Animals exposed to levodopa or placebo for 26 weeks had either a sham or actual unilateral 6-hydroxy dopamine lesion that caused moderate or severe damage. The various groups were compared. There was no significant difference in the number of surviving dopaminergic neurons between rats treated with levodopa versus rats treated with placebo. In contrast, surviving cells in the SN of the moderately lesioned rats treated with levodopa had a higher concentration of dopaminergic neurons compared with placebo-treated animals. The authors concluded that chronic levodopa exposure is not toxic to dopaminergic neurons of either healthy or 6-OHDA-lesioned rats. On the contrary, the authors postulated that levodopa can actually promote dopamine function and recovery in the rats with moderate degrees of 6-OHDA-induced damage. The authors attributed the difference between their results and the ones obtained by Blunt et al. to the variable degree of the 6-OHDA-induced lesion, which was more extensive in the Blunt study. The key determinant of a neurotrophic levodopa effect was considered to be the number of surviving dopaminergic cells before levodopa exposure.

Is Levodopa Toxic in Humans?

There is no convincing data from human studies to support the hypothesis that levodopa promotes nigral cell death in PD. Normal individuals treated with chronic levodopa as a result of a mistaken diagnosis of PD do not develop Parkinsonism or changes in striatal metabolism on positron emission tomography (PET) scans (118,119), and nigral degeneration is not present at autopsy in these cases (118,120). However, it can be argued that the normal brain is more resistant to oxidative stress than the parkinsonian brain. Autopsy data from patients with PD has not demonstrated any difference in the number of surviving nigral cells between levodopa-treated and levodopa-untreated patients (121), notwithstanding the difficulty of making quantitative comparisons in SN severely depleted of neurons by end-stage PD. Moreover, active axonal outgrowth has been demonstrated in a fetal mesencephalic transplant performed on a levodopa-treated patient with PD who subsequently died of unrelated causes (122). Such active fetal tissue proliferation despite continuous levodopa treatment argues against drug toxicity in vivo.

Enhanced survival of PD patients in the post-levodopa era is used as another argument against levodopa-induced neurotoxicity. The landmark study of the natural history of PD in the pre-levodopa era by Hoehn and Yahr (c. 1967) (35) reported a mortality rate 2.9 times greater than the age-matched population. Studies performed soon after the introduction of levodopa revealed a favorable but variable effect on mortality rates. Yahr (123) reexamined 597 of the patients who were treated with levodopa between 1967 and 1973 and showed that the mortality had decreased from 2.9 to 1.46 times the expected rate. Hoehn (124) reported a similar mortality ratio of 1.5 in 182 patients who were followed since the advent of levodopa therapy and concluded that life expectancy in the treated patients was close to that of the general population. Diamond and colleagues (125) demonstrated a positive correlation between early initiation of levodopa and improved mortality. Other studies showed less optimistic results, and the mortality ratios ranged from 1.85 to 2.4 (126–128). One of the explanations for the discrepancy in mortality ratios between the early and later studies is that reduced mortality is a somewhat transitory benefit experienced during the first years of levodopa therapy but partly reversed by the progressive nature of PD even in the face of optimal and sustained levodopa therapy (129). Lees and Stern observed that the mortality ratio was 1.46 in

- Levodopa remains the most effective drug for treating the symptoms of PD, notwithstanding the problems related to chronic use. Maximal levodopa efficacy is achieved by the concomitant use of an inhibitor of peripheral dopa decarboxylase.
- There is no evidence that levodopa is toxic to human beings, notwithstanding the experimental findings supporting toxicity in vitro.
- Motor complications associated with chronic oral levodopa therapy occur inevitably from the interaction between progressive nigrostriatal degeneration and the unique pharmacodynamic properties of levodopa.
- The question of whether treatment with levodopa should be initiated early or later in the course of illness remains unanswered. That debate may continue into the twenty-second century.
- Combination pharmacotherapy is a major advance in the management of PD. The evolution of this practice is the result of major achievements in drug development and the emergence of the randomized clinical trial as the most rigorous measure of drug efficacy.
- The fashion of treating "young" Parkinsonians with dopamine agonists as a levodopa-sparing strategy has a sound theoretical and empirical basis. It is not yet clear that the strategy makes a difference over the long course of PD.
- The Achilles heel of levodopa therapy is the drug's short half-life and erratic intestinal absorption. A simple and effective system of continuous parenteral delivery of levodopa has been pursued but not realized. The goal may yet be within reach.

REFERENCES

1. Parkinson J. *An Essay on the Shaking Palsy.* London: Sherwood, Neely, and Jones, 1817.
2. Charcot JM. *Lecons sur les Malades de Systeme Nerveux: Faltes a la Salpetriere.* Paris, Delahaye et Lacrosmier,1871: 155–188.
3. Lewy FH. Zue pathologischen Anatomie der Parlysis agitans. *Deutsche Z Nervenheilkunde* 1913; 50:50–55.
4. Tretiakoff C. Contribution a l'etude de l'anatomie pathologiqaue du Locus Niger de Soemmering. Paris: Thesis, 1919.
5. Ordenstein I. *Sur la paralysie agitante* Paris, Martinet. 1867.
6. Putman TJ. Treatment of unilateral paralysis agitans by section of the lateral pyramidal tract. *Arch Neurol Psychiatry* 1940; 44:950–976.
7. Cooper IS. Ligation of the anterior choroidal artery for involuntary movements of parkinsonism. *Arch Neurol* 1952; 75:36–48.
8. Svennilson E, Torvik A, Lowe R, et al. Treatment of parkinsonism by stereotactic thermolesions in the pallidal region: A clinical evaluation of 81 cases. *Acta Psychiatric Neurol Scand* 1960; 35:358–377.
9. Webster DD. Dynamic evaluation of thalamotomy in Parkinson's disease: Analysis of 75 consecutive cases. In: Gillingham FJ, Donaldson IML (eds.). *Third Symposium on Parkinson's Disease.* Edinburgh: E&S Livingstone, 1969:266–271.
10. Brodie BB, Comer MS, Costa E, et al. The role of brain serotonin in the mechanism of the central action of reserpine. *J Pharmacol Exp Ther* 1966; 152(2):340–349.
11. Carlsson A, Lindquist M, Magnusson T. 3, 4-dihydroxyphenylalaninen and 5-hydroxytryptophan as reserpine antagonists. *Nature* 1957; 180:200.
12. Carlsson A, Lindquist M, Magnusson T, et al. On the presence of 3 hydroxytyramine in brain. *Science* 1958; 127:471–472.
13. Bertler A, Rosengren E. Occurrence and distribution of catecholamines in brain. *Acta Physiol Scand* 1959; 47:350–361.
14. Hornykiewicz O. Physiologic, biochemical and pathological backgrounds of levodopa and possibilities for the future. *Neurology* 1970; 20:1–5.
15. Ehringer H, Hornykiewicz O. Verteilung von Noradrenalin und Dopamin (3- Hydroxytyramin) im Gehirn des Menschen und ihr Verhalten bei Erkrankungen des extrapyramidalen Systems. *Wein Klin Wochenschr* 1960; 38:1236–1239.
16. Bernheimer H, Birkmayer W, Hornykiewicz O, et al. Zur Differenzie-rung des Parkinson-Syndrome: Biochemisch-neurohistologische Vergleichsuntersuchungen. *Proc 8th Int Conf Neurol* (Vienna); 1965:145.
17. Hornykiewicz O. Parkinson's disease. From brain homogenates to treatment. *Fed Proc Fed Am Soc Exp Biol* 1973; 32:183–190.
18. Anden NE, Carlsson A, Dahlstrom A, et al. Demonstration and mapping of nigroneostriatal dopamine neurons. *Life Sci* 1964; 3:523–530.
19. Poirier LJ, Sourkes TL. Influence of the substantia nigra on the catecholamine content of the striatum. *Brain* 1965; 88:181–192.
20. Birkmayer W, Hornykiewicz O. Der 1–3,4 Dioxyphenylalanin (= DOPA)- Effekt bei der Parkinson-Akinese. *Wien Jklin Wochenschr* 1961; 73:787–788.
21. Barbeau A, Sourkes TL, Murphy CF. Les catecholamines dans la maladie de Parkinson, In: J de Ajuriaguerra (ed.). *Monoamines et Systeme Nerveaux Central.* Geneva: Georg, 1962; 247–262.
22. Birkmayer W, Hornykiewicz O. Weitere experimentelle untersuchungen uber beim Parkinson-syndrom und reserpine-parkinsonismus. *Arch Psychiatry Zeitschr Neurol* 1964; 206:367–381.

23. McGeer PL, Zeldowitz LR. Administration of dihydroxyphenylalanine to Parkinsonian patients. *Can Med Assoc J* 1964; 90:463–466.

24. Duvoisin RC, Yahr MD, Cote L. Pyridoxine reversal of L-dopa effect in Parkinsonism. *Trans Am Neurol Assoc* 1969; 94:81–84.

25. Cotzias GC, Van Woert MH, Schiffer LM. Aromatic amino acids and modifications of Parkinsonism. *N Eng J Med* 1967; 276:374–379.

26. Cotzias GC, Papavasiliou PS, Gellene R. Modification of Parkinsonism: Chronic treatment with L-dopa. *N Eng J Med* 1969; 280:337–345.

27. Yahr MD, Duvoisin RC, Schear MJ, et al. Treatment of Parkinsonism with levodopa. *Arch Neurol* 1969; 21:343–354.

28. McDowell FH, Lee JE, Sweet R, et al. The treatment of Parkinson's disease with dihydroxyphenylalanine. *Ann Intern Med* 1970; 72:19–25.

29. Markham CH. Thirty months trial of levodopa in Parkinson's disease. *Neurology* 1972; 22:17–22.

30. Godwin-Austen RB, Tomlinson EB, Frears CC, et al. Effects of L-DOPA in Parkinson's disease. *Lancet* 1969; 2:165–168.

31. Yahr MD, Duvoisin RC, Hoehn MM, et al. L-Dopa (L-3,4-dihydroxyphenylanine) – its clinical effects in Parkinsonism. *Trans Am Neurol Assoc* 1968; 93:56–63.

32. Cotzias GC, Papavsiliou PS, Steck A, et al. Parkinsonism and levodopa. *Clin Pharm Ther* 1970; 12:319–322.

33. Yahr MD, Duvoisin RC. Drug therapy of Parkinsonism. *N Eng J Med* 1972; 287:20–24.

34. Hoehn MM. Parkinson's disease: Progression and mortality. *Adv Neurol* 1987; 457–461.

35. Hoehn MM, Yahr MD: Parkinsonism: Onset, progression and mortality. *Neurology* 1967; 17:427–442.

36. Barbeau A, McDowell FH (eds.). L-Dopa and Parkinsonism. Philadelphia: FA Davis, 1970.

37. Godwin-Austen RB. The long term therapeutic effect of levodopa in the treatment of Parkinsonism. *Adv Neurol* 1973; 3:23–27.

38. Wade DN, Mearrick PT, Morris JL. Active transport of L-DOPA in the intestine. *Nature* 1973; 242:463–465.

39. Hardie RJ, Malcom SL, Lees AJ, et al. The pharmacokinetics of intravenous and oral levodopa in patients with Parkinson's disease who exhibit on-off fluctuations. *Br J Pharmacol* 1986; 22:429–436.

40. Nutt JG, Feldman JH. Pharmacokinetics of levodopa. *Clin Neuropharm* 1984; 7:35–49.

41. Nutt JG, Woodward WR, Hammerstad JP, et al. The "on-off" phenomenon in Parkinson's disease: Relation to levodopa absorption and transport. *N Engl J Med* 1984; 310:483–488.

42. Nutt JG, Woodward WR, Anderson JL. Effect of carbidopa on pharmacokinetics of intravenously administered levodopa: Implications for mechanism of action of carbidopa in the treatment of Parkinsonism. *Ann Neurol* 1985; 13:537–544.

43. Wade LA, Katzman R. 3-O-Methyldopa uptake and inhibition of L-dopa at the blood- brain barrier. *Life Sci* 1975; 17:131–136.

44. Hefti F, Melamed E, Wurtman RJ. The site of dopamine formation in rat striatum after L-dopa administration. *J Pharmacol Exp Ther* 1980; 217:189–197.

45. Poewe W: L-dopa in Parkinson's disease: Mechanisms of action and pathophysiology of late failure. In: Jankovic J, Tolosa E (eds.). Parkinson's disease and Movement Disorders. Baltimore: Williams & Wilkins, 1993:103–113.

46. Bunny BS, Walter JR, Roth RH, et al. Dopaminergic neurons: Effects of antipsychotic drugs and amphetamine on single cell activity. *J Pharmacol Exp Ther* 1973; 85:560–571.

47. Schwartz J-C, Giros B, Martres M-P, et al. The dopamine receptor family: Molecular biology and pharmacology. *Sem Neurosci* 1992; 4:99–108.

48. Obeso JA, Luquin MR, Grandas F, et al. Motor response to repeated dopaminergic stimulation in Parkinson's disease. *Clin Neuropharm* 1992; 15:75–79.

49. Oreland L. Monoamine oxidase, dopamine and Parkinson's disease. *Acta Neurol Scand* 1991; 81(Suppl 136):60–65.

50. Marsden CD, Parkes JD, Quinn N. Fluctuations of disability in Parkinson's disease: Clinical aspects. In: Marsden CD, Fahn S (eds.). *Movement Disorders*. London: Butterworths, 1982:96–119.

51. Quinn N, Critchley P, Marsden CD. Young onset Parkinson's disease. *Mov Disord* 1987; 2:73–91.

52. The Parkinson Study Group. Impact of deprenyl and tocopherol treatment on Parkinson's disease in DATATOP patients requiring levodopa. *Ann Neurol* 1996; 39:37–45.

53. Block G, Liss C, Reines S, et al. Comparison of immediate-release and controlled-release carbidopa/levodopa in Parkinson's disease: A multicenter 5 year study. The CR FIRST Study Group. *Eur Neurol* 1997; 37:23–27.

54. De Jong GJ, Meerwaldt JD, Schmitz PI. Factors that influence the occurrence of response variations in Parkinson's disease. *Ann Neurol* 1987; 22: 4–7.

55. Bedard PJ, Blanchet PJ, Levesque D, et al. Pathophysiology of L-dopa induced dyskinesias. *Mov Disord* 1999; 14(Suppl 1):4–8.

56. Obeso JA, Lingzaroso G, Gorospe, et al. Complications associated with chronic levodopa therapy in Parkinson's disease. In: Olanow CW, Obeso JA (eds.). *Beyond the decade of the brain*. Kent: Wells Medical Limited, 1997:11–35.

57. Rascol O. L-Dopa-induced peak-dose dyskinesias in patients with Parkinson's disease. A clinical pharmacologic approach. *Mov Disord* 1999; 14(Suppl 1):19–32.

58. Caraceni T, Scigliano G, Mussico M. The occurrence of motor fluctuations in parkinsonian patients treated

long-term with levodopa: Role of early treatment and disease progression. *Neurology* 1991; 41:380–384.

59. Wooten GF. Progress in understanding the pathophysiology of treatment-related fluctuations in Parkinson's disease. *Ann Neurol* 1988; 24:366–371.

60. Fabbrini G, Mouradian MM, Juncos JL, et al. Motor fluctuations in Parkinson's disease: Central pathophysiological mechanisms. Part I. *Ann Neurol* 1988; 24:366–371.

61. Mouradian MM, Juncos JL, Fabbrini G, et al. Motor fluctuations in Parkinson's disease: Pathogenetic and therapeutic studies. *Ann Neurol* 1987; 22:475–479.

62. Leenders KL, Palmer AJ, Quinn N, et al. Brain dopamine metabolism in patients with Parkinson's disease measured with positron emission tomography. *J Neurol Neurosurg Psychiatry* 1986; 49:853–860.

63. Colosimo, Merello M, Hughes AJ, et al. Motor response to acute dopaminergic chalenge with apomorphine and levodopa in Parkinson's disease: Implications for the pathogenesis of the "on-off" phenomenon. *J Neurol Neurosurg Psychiatry* 1996; 60:634–637.

64. Rodriguez M, Lera G, Vaamonde J, et al. Motor response to apomorphine in asymmetric Parkinson's disease. *J Neurol Neurosurg Psychiatry* 1994; 57:562–566.

65. Vaamonde J, Luquin MR, Obeso JA. Subcutaneous lisuride infusion in Parkinson's disease: Response to chronic administration in 34 patients. *Brain* 1991; 114:601–614.

66. Kempster PA, Frankel JP, Stern JM, et al. Comparison of motor response to apomorphine and levodopa in Parkinson's disease. *J Neurol Neurosurg Psychiatry* 1990; 53:1004–1007.

67. Mouradian MM, Heuser IJE, Baronti F, et al. Modification of central dopaminergic mechanisms by continuous levodopa therapy for advanced Parkinson's disease. *Ann Neurol* 1990; 27:18–23.

68. Juncos JL, Engber TM, Raisman R, et al. Continuous and intermittent levodopa differentially affect basal ganglia function. *Ann Neurol* 1989; 25:437–478.

69. Grace AA. Phasic versus tonic dopamine release and the modulation of dopamine system responsivity: A hypothesis for the etiology of schizophrenia. *Neuroscience* 1991; 41:1–24.

70. Jenner P. The rational for use of dopamine agonists in Parkinson's disease. *Neurology* 1995; 45(Suppl 3):S6–S12.

71. Rinne UK. Early combination of bromocriptine and levodopa in the treatment of Parkinson's disease: A 5-year follow-up. *Neurology* 1987; 37:826–828.

72. Factor SA, Weiner WJ. Early combination therapy with bromocriptine and levodopa in Parkinson's disease. *Mov Disord* 1993; 8:257–262.

73. Metman LV, Del Doto P, Van den Munckhof P, et al. Amantadine as treatment for dyskinesias and motor fluctuations in Parkinson's disease. *Neurology* 1998; 50:1323–1326.

74. Metman VL, Del Doto P, Blanchet PJ, et al. Blockade of glutaminergic transmission as treatment of dyskinesias and motor fluctuations in Parkinson's disease. *Amino Acids* 1998; 14:75–82.

75. Fahn S. Is levodopa toxic? *Neurology* 1996; 47(Suppl 3):S184–S195.

76. Agid Y. Levodopa. Is toxicity a myth? *Neurology* 1998; 50:858–863.

77. Jenner P, Shapira AHV, Marsden CD. New insights into the cause of Parkinson's disease. *Neurology* 1992; 42:2241–2250.

78. Cross CE. Oxygen radicals and human disease. *Ann Intern Med* 1987; 107:526–545.

79. Southorn PA, Powis G. Free radicals in medicine: Chemical nature and biological reactions. *Mayo Clin Proc* 1988; 63:381–389.

80. Fahn S, Cohen G. The oxidant stress hypothesis in Parkinson's disease: Evidence supporting it. *Ann Neuro* 1992; 32:804–811.

81. Olanow CW, Youdim MHB. Iron and neurodegeneration: Prospects for neuroprotection. In: Olanow CW, Jenner P, Youdim MHB (eds.). *Neurodegeneration and Neuroprotection in Parkinson's Disease*. London: Academic Press, 1996:55–67.

82. Cohen G. The pathobiology of Parkinson's disease: Biochemical aspects of dopamine neuron senescence. *J Neural Transm* 1983; (Suppl 19):89–103.

83. Oreland L. Monoamine oxidase, dopamine and Parkinson's disease. *Acta Neurol Scand* 1991; 81(Suppl 136):60–65.

84. Graham DG. Oxidative pathways for catecholamines in the genesis of neuromelanin and cytotoxic quinones. *Mol Pharmacol* 1978; 14:633–643.

85. Graham DG. On the origin and significance of neuromelanin. *Arch Pathol Lab Med* 1979; 103:359–362.

86. Youdim MBH, Ben-Schachar D, Riederer P. Is Parkinson's disease a progressive siderosis of substantia nigra resulting in iron and melanin induced neurodegeneration? *Acta Neurol Scand* 1989; 80(Suppl 126):47–54.

87. Perry TL, Godin DV, Hansen S. Parkinson's disease: A disorder due to nigral glutathione deficiency. *Neurosci Lett* 1982; 33:305–310.

88. Sofic E, Lange KW, Jellinger K, et al. Reduced and oxidized glutathione in the substantia nigra of patients with Parkinson's disease. *Neurosci Lett* 1992; 142:128–130.

89. Sian J, Dexter DT, Lees AJ, et al. Alterations in glutathione levels in Parkinson's disease and other neurodegenerative disorders affecting basal ganglia. *Ann Neurol* 1994; 36:348–355.

90. Dexter DT, Sian J, Rose S, et al. Indices of oxidative stress and mitrochondrial function in individuals with incidental Lewy body disease. *Ann Neurol* 1994; 35:38–44.

91. Pardo B, Mena MA, de Yebenes JG. L-DOPA inhibits complex IV of the electron transport chain in catecholamine-rich human neuroblastoma NB69 cells. *J Neurochem* 1995; 64:576–582.

155. Olanow CW, Jenner P, Brooks S. Dopamine agonists and neuroprotection in Parkinson's disease. *Ann Neurol* 1998; 44:S167–S174.

156. Factor SA. Dopamine agonists. *Med Clin North Am* 1999; 83(2):415–443.

157. Rascol O, Brooks DJ, Korczyn AD, et al. A five year study of the incidence of dyskinesia in patients with early Parkinson's disease who were treated with ropinirole or levodopa. *N Engl J Med* 2000; 342(20):1484–1491.

158. Barone P, Bravi D, Bermejo-Pareja F, et al. Pergolide monotherapy in the treatment of early PD. *Neurol* 1999; 53:573–579.

159. Carrion A, Weiner WJ, Shulman LM. A three and a half year experience with pramipexole monotherapy in patients with early Parkinson's disease. *Neurol* 1998; 50:A330.

160. Montastruc JL, Rascol O, Senard JM. Treatment of Parkinson's disease should begin with a dopamine agonist. *Mov Disord* 1999; 14:725–730.

161. Bunny BS, Walter JR, Roth RH, et al. Dopaminergic neurons:Effect of antipsychotic drugs and amphetamine on single cell activity. *J Pharm Exp Ther* 1973; 85:560–571.

162. Marion MH, Stocchi F, Quinn NP, et al. Repeated levodopa infusion in fluctuating Parkinson's disease: Clinical and pharmacokinetic data. *Adv Neurol* 1986; 9:165–181.

163. Shoulson I, Glaubiger GA, Chase TN. On-off response: Clinical and biochemical correlations during oral and intravenous levodopa administration in Parkinsonian patients. *Neurology* 1975; 25:1144–1148.

164. Nutt JG, Carter JH, Woodward W, et al. Does tolerance develop to levodopa? Comparison of 2- and 21-H levodopa infusion. *Mov Disord* 1993; 8:139–143.

165. Kurlan R, Rubin AJ, Miller CH, et al. Duodenal delivery of levodopa for on-off fluctuations in parkinsonism: Preliminary results. *Ann Neurol* 1986; 20:262–266.

166. Sage JL, Trooskin S, Sonsalla PK. Long-term duodenal infusion of levodopa for motor fluctuations in Parkinsonism. *Ann Neurol* 1988; 24:87–89.

167. Kurth MC, Tetrud JW, Tanner CM, et al. Double-blind, placebo-controlled, cross-over study of duodenal infusion of levodopa/carbidopa in Parkinson's disease patients with "on-off" fluctuations. *Neurology* 1993; 43:1698–1703.

168. Pappert EJ, Goetz CG, Niederman F, et al. Liquid levodopa/carbidopa produces significant improvement in motor function without dyskinesia exacerbation. *Neurology* 1996; 47:1493–1495.

169. Steiger MJ, Stocchi F, Bramante L, et al. The clinical efficacy of single morning doses of levodopa methyl ester: Dispersible Madopar and Sinemet Plus in Parkinson's disease. *Clin Neuropharm* 1992; 15:501–504.

170. Djaldetti R, Ziv I, Melamed E. Impaired absorption of oral levodopa: A major cause for response fluctuations in Parkinson's disease. *Isr J Med* 1996; 32:1224.

171. Lindvall O. Update on fetal transplantation: The Swedish experience. *Mov Disord* 1998; 13(Suppl 1):83–87.

172. Lapchak PA. A preclinical development strategy designed to optimize the use of glial cell line-derived neurotrophic factor in the treatment of Parkinson's disease. *Mov Disord* 1998; 13(Suppl 1):49–54.

173. Kang UJ. Potential of gene therapy for Parkinson's disease: Neurobiologic issues and new developments in gene transfer methodologies. *Mov Disord* 1998; 13(Suppl 1):59–72.

33

Amantadine and Anticholinergics

Charles H. Adler, M.D., Ph.D.

Mayo Clinic, Department of Neurology, Scottsdale, Arizona

AMANTADINE AND ANTICHOLINERGICS

Before the discovery of levodopa for the treatment of Parkinson's disease (PD) the treatment of choice was trihexyphenidyl (Artane) or other anticholinergic medications. At about the same time that levodopa trials demonstrated its efficacy, the serendipitous finding that amantadine was beneficial in PD was published (1). Both groups of drugs continue to play important roles in the treatment of PD today, and they are the topic of this chapter.

AMANTADINE

The serendipitous discovery that amantadine (Symmetrel) had antiparkinsonian effects improving rest tremor, rigidity, and akinesia was made by Schwab et al. (1) in 1968 when a PD patient took this drug as influenza A prophylaxis. This woman improved during the six weeks she took amantadine and deteriorated when it was discontinued. Since that time there have been numerous reports of amantadine's beneficial effects as monotherapy in early, untreated PD, (1–6) and in stable, treated PD, (4,7) and as adjunct treatment to levodopa in more advanced, fluctuating patients (8–11). Although the mechanism of action is not completely clear, its clinical role is well established.

Pharmacology

Amantadine hydrochloride, 1-adamantanamine, is a tricyclic amine that is minimally metabolized and is excreted in the urine (dosing should be reduced in patients with decreased creatinine clearance) (12,13). It is well absorbed when given orally. Maximum blood levels occur between one and four hours, and the half-life is approximately 15 hours in healthy patients but increases with age (14.7 hours in young, 28.9 hours in elderly) (12,13). Amantadine sulfate can be administered orally or intravenously (IV) with equivalent motor effects in PD at a dose of 200 mg/d (14). The maximum concentration and area under the curve are greater when the drug is given IV, however, clinical efficacy of the orally administered formulation was equivalent (14). Unfortunately, amantadine sulfate is not available in the United States, but in countries where it is available, it can be useful for patients who are unable to take medications orally.

The mechanism of action of amantadine in PD is not clear. Much evidence suggests that amantadine's effect is mediated through the dopamine system: (*1*) It causes stereotypy and amphetamine-like turning behavior in rats (15). (*2*) It stimulates locomotor activity (16,17) and reverses catalepsy (15) in catecholamine-depleted animals, suggesting a direct dopamine agonist effect. (*3*) Its behavioral effect is not influenced by pretreatment with the presynaptic dopamine depleting agents, reserpine and tetrabenzine, both of which disrupt catecholamine storage vesicles. Therefore, amantadine may promote the release of extravesicular intraneuronal dopamine (18,19). (*4*) Several studies have suggested that amantadine is a weak inhibitor of dopamine uptake (15,20,19). While synthesizing the data regarding amantadine's effect on dopaminergic systems, it appears that its ability to release dopamine from extravesicular stores may be the most crucial effect, then its dopamine receptor agonist activity, and the least likely effect is the inhibition of dopamine reuptake (15). There is also some evidence to suggest a possible anticholinergic effect of amantadine (21).

The excitatory neurotransmitter, glutamate, may play a role in PD, and inhibition of the N-methyl-D-aspartate (NMDA) receptor subtype of glutamate receptors may be beneficial in treating PD patients (see Chapter 38). Amantadine has been shown to have NMDA antagonist activity that may also provide some of its antiparkinsonian effect. NMDA antagonists block subthalamic nucleus overactivity, enhance striatal dopamine release and turnover, and protect nigral neurons from death in certain animal models (22). Further support for the benefits of a NMDA receptor antagonist in PD is found in the work of Klockgether and Turski (23) and Greenamyre et al. (24) with animals. It was shown that in monoamine-depleted rats, NMDA antagonists potentiate the effects of levodopa even when levodopa is given in subtherapeutic doses (24,23). Greenamyre et al. also demonstrated potentiation of levodopa's effect in Parkinsonian monkeys while comparing remacemide hydrochloride (a glutamate antagonist) to placebo with a duration of action of more than five hours (24). There was no effect of NMDA receptor antagonist monotherapy in either the rat or the monkey models (23,22). Additionally, Engber et al. (25) have shown that NMDA receptor antagonists can reverse levodopa-induced motor fluctuations in a rat model, and Papa and Chase (26) have shown that levodopa-induced dyskinesias improve with glutamate antagonist treatment in MPTP-induced Parkinsonian monkeys.

A placebo-controlled trial of dextromethorphan in six advanced PD patients showed reduced levodopa-induced dyskinesias without a change in levodopa's motor effects (27). However, dextromethorphan is not completely selective for the NMDA receptor (27). Results from placebo-controlled treatment trials suggest that the more specific NMDA receptor antagonist remacemide is beneficial when it is added to levodopa in PD (28). Whether amantadine's mechanism of action relates to NMDA receptor antagonist activity is not clearly established but is theoretically possible.

Clinical Use in Early Parkinson's Disease

The clinical benefit of amantadine in PD was first established by Schwab et al. in 1969 (1). They found, in an open-label study of 163 PD patients, that 66% had improvement in bradykinesia and rigidity on 200 mg/d with some tremor benefit as well (1). Although there was a decline in benefit after four to eight weeks of treatment, patients continued to be improved when compared to baseline at eight months. However, when amantadine was discontinued patients that had lost the benefit over time had rebound worsening of symptoms (1). The same group then reviewed their two-year experience with amantadine in 351 patients on 200 mg/d for ≥60 days (5). Maximum benefit was between two to three weeks with 64% improving at 60 days. They found no correlation between the

severity of PD and the effectiveness of amantadine, and found that patients on no medication or those already on levodopa, could benefit (5).

Placebo-controlled trials have also documented benefit with amantadine. Barbeau et al. (2) compared amantadine 100 mg bid with placebo in a crossover design and found statistically significant improvement with amantadine in the 54 patients studied. When they compared their amantadine data with that of levodopa, from a previous study, only 44% had "moderate or better improvement" with amantadine as compared with 88% of those having received levodopa (2). Dallos et al. (4) studied 62 patients, already on anticholinergic therapy, with a diagnosis of either idiopathic PD, postencephalitic or arteriosclerotic parkinsonism. Some patients had prior thalamotomies. There was improvement in akinesia > rigidity and no change in tremor. The maximum benefit was between two to three weeks with some lessening of benefit at four weeks (4). Butzer et al. (3) found 20 of 26 PD patients preferred amantadine over placebo in a crossover study.

Zeldowicz and Huberman (6) found that 19 of 77 patients on amantadine alone improved for a mean duration of 21 months, and 46 patients had significant improvement with combined use of amantadine and levodopa as opposed to monotherapy with either drug (6). In a placebo-controlled crossover study, Savery (7) found that in 42 patients (Hoehn and Yahr stage II–IV) already taking levodopa, 95% had improvement on 100–200 mg/d of amantadine. Comparing amantadine with the anticholinergic benzhexol, Parkes et al. (29) found that each drug produced a 15% reduction in disability as monotherapy and a 40% reduction when the drugs were combined. Koller (30) found that amantadine reduced tremor 23% compared with the anticholinergic trihexyphenidyl's 59% benefit and levodopa's 55% benefit.

In contrast to its symptomatic effects, another potential reason to treat early PD patients with amantadine is the possibility that it may be "neuroprotective." Uitti et al. (31) reviewed the charts of all patients diagnosed with Parkinsonism in their clinic from 1968 to 1990. A total of 836 parkinsonism cases were reviewed, 92% of which had PD. Amantadine treatment (for a minimum of two months) was found to be an independent predictor of improved survival. Of the 836 parkinsonism patients, 250 had been on amantadine 100 mg bid, and mean duration of treatment was 37 months (median = 24 months). The mechanism by which this effect occurred is not clear, although the authors speculate that it is the NMDA antagonist activity of amantadine that may be critical (31). No controlled study of amantadine as a "neuroprotective" agent has been undertaken to date.

Clinical Use in Advanced Parkinson's Disease

Long considered as a drug for early PD it has recently become apparent that amantadine has a role in the treatment of patients with advanced PD. Amantadine was first reported to benefit PD patients with postprandial motor fluctuations by DeDevitiis et al. (9). They studied 19 patients, 16 of whom benefited from the addition of amantadine. In an open-label study of 20 patients with motor fluctuations (19 – predictable wearing-off, 1 – unpredictable on-off), Shannon et al. (11) added amantadine 100 mg 1-2x/d to levodopa ± bromocriptine or pergolide. Eleven (55%) of the patients had subjective improvement in the severity of motor fluctuations at two months and a 30% improvement in their disability scores. Those who responded were initially more disabled and had more severe fluctuations than those that did not respond. The patient with unpredictable on-off fluctuations did not respond. The mean duration of improvement was 5.7 months (range = 2–12 months) (11).

Adler et al. (8) reported that amantadine's benefit in four patients with advanced PD can last up to two years. They were the first to present patients who not only demonstrated benefit for predictable wearing off but also a reduction in dyskinesias and dystonia. They also found that even if a patient had failed amantadine early in the course of the disease, it may be effective later in the disease (8). One study of MPTP-induced parkinsonism in monkeys demonstrated that levodopa-induced dyskinesias improved when treated with an NMDA antagonist (26).

Metman et al. (32) studied amantadine in 18 patients with advanced PD using a placebo-controlled crossover design. Treatment was for three weeks and 14 patients completed the study (four terminated because of side effects). Amantadine reduced dyskinesia severity by 60% compared to placebo with no change in Parkinsonian motor scores. The degree of dyskinesia reduction was directly correlated to plasma amantadine concentration. A reduction in motor fluctuations and improvement in activities of daily living scores were statistically significant. The average dose of amantadine was 350 mg/d (higher than normally used in clinic practice). Following the controlled trial, patients were placed on open-label amantadine and most patients had sustained benefit for 12 months (32). Thus a potential advantage of adding amantadine to levodopa for dyskinesias is that there is no reduction in the motor effects of levodopa, a problem that often occurs using other dyskinesia reducing strategies (32).

Side Effects

GI discomfort, nausea, sleep disturbance, and nervousness are frequent acute side effects of amantadine (3,7,6,15,33). Chronic treatment with amantadine may result in livedo reticularis of the legs, characterized by reddish-purple skin discoloration, especially when the legs are dependent (6,7,15). Shealy et al. (34) first reported this in 10 of 18 women treated with 100–200 mg/d. Ankle edema was also found, both with and without livedo reticularis (34). In most cases symptoms resolve within two to four weeks of discontinuing the drug. The livedo reticularis is generally not associated with serious consequences. However, Shulman et al. reported a patient with amantadine-induced neuropathy, which was associated with severe livedo reticularis (35).

In more advanced cases of PD, especially in patients with an underlying dementia or those already taking other antiparkinsonian drugs, hallucinations may be a significant problem with the addition of amantadine (15).

Neuroleptic malignant syndrome has been reported after withdrawal of amantadine in PD (36). Patients developed confusion, autonomic dysfunction, hyperthermia, leucocytosis, and elevation of creatinine kinase. Additionally, Factor et al. (37) reported the development of acute delirium in three patients on long-term (4–18 years) amantadine therapy who discontinued the drug. All three patients developed confusion, agitation, disorientation, and paranoia, and all required reinstitution of therapy with amantadine for resolution (37). All three patients had advanced PD with dementia and a history of hallucinations, however, none had neuroleptic malignant syndrome.

Amantadine is contraindicated in patients with glaucoma, hepatic or renal disease, prostate hypertrophy, and in women who are pregnant or lactating (33). Because the drug is excreted unmetabolized in the urine, dosage must be reduced in patients with reduced creatinine clearance (12,13).

Summary

Despite our incomplete knowledge of its mechanism of action in PD, amantadine is an effective treatment for early and advanced patients. Monotherapy in early patients and adjunctive therapy to levodopa in patients with motor fluctuations or dyskinesias should be considered. Contrary to what has often been stated amantadine may have prolonged benefit in both early and advanced patients (38). Dosing should start at 100 mg/d and can be increased to 100 mg tid, with most patients improving on 100 mg bid. Nausea, vomiting, livedo reticularis, and hallucinations may occur.

ANTICHOLINERGICS

Anticholinergic agents are compounds originally derived from plants of the *Solanaceae* family. The effects of belladona alkaloids were noted in the nineteenth century by Charcot, and its effects on PD were described by Ordenstein (39,40). In the mid- to late-1920s studies of cholinergic and anticholinergic agents in postencephalitic parkinsonism (41,42) followed by Milhorat's studies in PD (43) supported the role of the cholinergic system in parkinsonism (44).

Pharmacology

Anticholinergic agents can be divided into those occurring in nature and those that are synthetically derived. Before an understanding of the pharmacology of PD, all naturally occurring "medications" were tested in patients with parkinsonism, but only those agents containing the belladonna alkaloids were effective. Feldberg (44–46) is credited with first postulating that atropine and scopolamine, both naturally occurring belladonna alkaloids, had their effect by central atropine-acetylcholine antagonism. Before the 1950s atropine and scopolamine (the natural belladonna alkaloids.) were primarily used in PD. In the 1950s synthetic anticholinergic agents were introduced which included benztropine (Cogentin), trihexyphenidyl (Artane), procyclidine (Kemadrin), biperiden (Akineton), and ethopropazine (Parsidol) (44).

Anticholinergic drugs act by blocking acetylcholine receptors. There are two types of acetylcholine receptors, the muscarinic and the nicotinic. Distribution is quite different with the muscarinic receptors being located in the central nervous system (CNS), smooth muscle, cardiac muscle, and parasympathetically innervated glands, such as the salivary glands. Nicotinic receptors are located on striated muscle and in the autonomic ganglia. The beneficial effect of agents in PD is mediated by CNS muscarinic receptor blockade (39).

The clinical effectiveness of anticholinergic agents has been correlated with multiple different in vitro effects, which include (1) antagonism of the central toxic effects in mice of the cholinomimetic agent oxotremorine (44,47), (2) antagonism of drug-induced circling movements (48), and (3) antagonism of physostigmines tremorigenic effect (49).

However, as often happens, patient trials appear to have preceded much of the traditional animal experimentation. In 1959, Nashold published a series of 11 PD patients demonstrating that direct infusion of acetylcholine into the globus pallidus caused an increase in contralateral tremor while infusion of an anticholinergic agent, oxypheninium

bromide, reduced contralateral tremor, and rigidity (50). This led to Barbeau's hypothesis that PD was secondary to a deficit in dopamine, leading to a relative overactivity of cholinergic function in the CNS (51).

This was followed by in vivo studies in monkeys which demonstrated that carbachol (a muscarinic cholinergic agonist) injections into the caudate nucleus induced contralateral rest tremor that was inhibited by anticholinergic agents (52,53). Further human studies demonstrated that the centrally active cholinergic agent physostigmine exacerbated existing PD signs although centrally active anticholinergic agents (scopolamine or benztropine) reversed this effect (45,44). Central and not peripheral anticholinergic action was crucial to the antiparkinsonian effect (45). The effects of the cholinergic agents only occurred in preexisting symptoms, thus a cholinergic mechanism was not likely the underlying etiology of PD (45,44).

The only pharmacokinetic data available for an anticholinergic agent is for trihexyphenidyl. The reported half-life is 1.7 hours in patients with dystonia (54). Studies of levodopa absorption in the presence or absence of chronic treatment with an anticholinergic, orphenadrine, revealed no significant difference for maximal levodopa concentration, time to maximal concentration, or area under the curve in six patients. One patient did have an increase in plasma concentration of levodopa and two had a decrease (55). The pharmacokinetics of orphenadrine was not studied.

Clinical Use

The actual scientific literature regarding the use of anticholinergics in PD is limited. Techniques used to study tremor and other symptoms, the type of anticholinergic that was used, daily dose, duration of treatment, and variable patient population, all make the earlier studies difficult to interpret. Doshay and Constable (56) found that 77% of 117 patients with various forms of Parkinsonism, treated with open-label trihexyphenidyl, had improvement, with rigidity being more responsive than tremor, little effect akinesia was reported. Doshay et al. (57) then reported the results for benztropine (Cogentin) in 20 patients with Parkinsonism (six – idiopathic, eight – arteriosclerotic, six – postencephalitic). They found some benefit alone or with trihexyphenidyl but no quantification is provided (57). The five-year summary of treatment in 302 patients found that 52% had improvement mostly in tremor and rigidity (58).

In 1965 Strang (59) reported the effects of open-label benztropine in 94 patients with parkinsonism (11 – postencephalitic and 24 – arteriosclerotic). Sixty patients were on benztropine alone, although 34 were on other medications including other anticholinergics. Less than 50% of those treated had benefit for tremor, rigidity, akinesia, or gait. Maximum benefit required dosing three to four times a day and a total dose of 3–6 mg/d (59).

Tourtellotte et al. (54) reported a double-blind, placebo-controlled crossover study of benztropine in 29 idiopathic PD patients. All patients were on levodopa and global assessments by the patient and physician showed significant improvement on benztropine. Rigidity, finger-tapping speed, and activity of daily living scores improved by 10% (54). Another double-blind study, procyclidine versus levodopa in 46 parkinsonian patients, revealed that levodopa was much more effective than procyclidine for rigidity and other clinical measures (60).

Koller (30) found, in nine idiopathic PD patients on no medications, that trihexyphenidyl reduced tremor amplitude by 59% compared to 23% for amantadine and 55% for levodopa. Five patients preferred trihexyphenidyl although four preferred levodopa. Other studies of tremor using quantitative measures found benefit with anticholinergics (61), although some other studies have not supported this effect (62).

Comparing benzhexol with amantadine, Parkes et al. (29) reported that each drug produced a 15% reduction in disability as monotherapy with a 40% reduction, when the drugs were combined. This combination had an equivalent effect when compared to giving levodopa, which caused a 36% reduction in disability scores (29). The anticholinergic, procyclidine, can be useful in PD patients with foot dystonia (63).

Individual Agents

Trihexyphenidyl (Artane)

Trihexyphenidyl is a synthetic piperidine anticholinergic agent with efficacy in PD (64). Because of potential side effects all anticholinergics should be started at a low dose and gradually titrated upward (65). The starting dose for trihexyphenidyl is 0.5–1 mg/d and the dose should be increased no faster than every 7–14 days. Dose increases of one mg/d is reasonable and a dose of 2 mg three to four times per day is the usual goal.

Procyclidine (Kemadrin)

Procyclidine is another piperidine agent that has similar efficacy to trihexyphenidyl. Some find fewer side effects with this agent. The dose is begun at 2.5 mg/d and

increased gradually to a maximum of approximately 30 mg/d.

Benztropine (Cogentin)

Benztropine is a synthetic agent that has both the benzhydryl group found in diphenhydramine and the tropine group found in atropine (57). It is more potent than trihexyphenidyl and less sedating than diphenhydramine. This drug is effective in PD and requires dosing two to three times per day (59). The dose is begun at 0.5 mg/d and can be raised to 4–8 mg/d.

Antihistamines

This class of drugs also have anticholinergic activity and are mildly effective in patients with PD (39). Diphenhydramine (Benadryl) and orphenadrine (Disipal, Norflex) have been most commonly used. However, both are sedating, and are best used to help induce sleep. The starting dose is 25 mg/d and it can be titrated to 150–200 mg/d in divided doses. No data regarding the nonsedating antihistamines, such as astemizole (Hismanil) and loratadine (Claritin) exist for the treatment of PD.

Phenothiazines

Phenothiazines primarily act as dopamine receptor antagonists with some anticholinergic activity. Thus most drugs in this family result in worsening of motor symptoms. The only agent in this class that is effective in treating PD is ethopropazine hydrochloride (Parsidol Parsitan) (39). This drug is not available in the United States but can be purchased in Canada.

Side Effects

The use of anticholinergic drugs in the treatment of PD is often difficult because of the multitude of side effects that occur. In young patients this is less of an issue than in the elderly. Drug dose must be titrated very slowly and patients must be informed of the many side effects.

Anticholinergic agents block muscarinic acetylcholine receptors throughout the body. At low doses, blockade of these receptors in the salivary glands results in dry mouth, often the first side effect described (57,59). Parenthetically, low dose anticholinergics can be helpful in treating the profound sialorrhea some patients experience. As the dose is increased muscarinic receptor blockade in the smooth muscle of the GI tract results in constipation that can progress to intestinal pseudo-obstruction and bowel dilation requiring aggressive intervention (57,45,59). Effects on the bladder can result in urinary retention, especially in male patients. Nausea, drowsiness, abdominal cramps, and mild tachycardia can also occur (45). Dry skin and impaired sweating may lead to heat stroke. Anticholinergics are contraindicated in patients with closed-angle glaucoma (39,65). Some of these peripheral anticholinergic side effects may be counteracted by a low dose (30–60 mg/d) of pyridostigmine (Mestinon), an acetylcholinesterase inhibitor used in patients with myasthenia gravis.

The central side effects of the anticholinergic agents can be quite problematic. These drugs can cause confusion and memory loss at any stage of the disease (66,67), and in the more advanced and demented patients hallucinations and disorientation can occur (68). In a study of 27 hospitalized parkinsonian patients with dementia 6 of 13 (46%) not receiving an anticholinergic suffered confusional states, whereas 13 of 14 (93%) on an anticholinergic had confusional states (69). Neuropsychologic testing revealed that trihexyphenidyl 2 mg tid given as monotherapy (six patients) or added to levodopa (two patients) or amantadine (four patients) did not effect digit span, however, recall and learning tasks were worse after trihexyphenidyl treatment (66). Ataxia and dizziness may occur (59). These agents can also cause orobuccal dyskinesias in PD patients (70).

Side effects can only be treated by lowering or discontinuing the drug. Withdrawal of anticholinergics should never occur quickly given the potential for rebound worsening of symptoms (71). As with other drugs, side effects with one anticholinergic does not predict side effect with all of them (72).

Summary

Anticholinergics may be useful as monotherapy in early, untreated PD and as adjunct therapy to patients already on levodopa. Although somewhat unclear from the actual data published, anticholinergics appear to most benefit rigidity and tremor. PD patients with dystonia may respond to anticholinergics. Peripheral side effects include dry mouth, blurred vision, and constipation, whereas central side effects include dizziness, confusion, memory loss, hallucinations and dyskinesia. All anticholinergic agents should be started at a very low dose and gradually titrated, with elderly and more debilitated patients tolerating much lower doses than younger patients. Clearly, the use of these drugs in patients over 65 requires vigilance and caution.

REFERENCES

1. Schwab RS, England AC, Poskanzer DC, et al. Amantadine in the treatment of Parkinson's disease. *JAMA* 1969; 208:1168–1170.
2. Barbeau A, Mars H, Botez MI, et al. Amantadine-HCL (Symmetrel) in the management of Parkinson's disease: A double-blind cross-over study. *Can Med Assoc J* 1971; 105:42–62.
3. Butzer JF, Silver DE, Sahs AL. Amantadine in Parkinson's disease: A double-blind, placebo-controlled, crossover study with long-term follow-up. *Neurology* 1975; 25:603–606.
4. Dallos V, Heathfield K, Stone P, et al. Use of amantadine in Parkinson's disease: Results of a double-blind trial. *Br Med J* 1970; 4:24–26.
5. Schwab RS, Poskanzer DC, England AC, et al. Amantadine in Parkinson's disease. Review of more than two years experience. *JAMA* 1972; 222:792–795.
6. Zeldowicz LR, Huberman J. Long-term treatment of Parkinson's disease with amantadine, alone and combined with levodopa. *Can Med Assoc J* 1973; 109:588.
7. Savery F. Amantadine and a fixed combination of levodopa and carbidopa in the treatment of Parkinson's disease. *Dis Nervous System* 1977; 38:605–608.
8. Adler CH, Stern MB, Vernon G, et al. Amantadine in advanced Parkinson's disease: Good use of an old drug. *J Neurol* 1997; 244:336–337.
9. DeDevitiis E, D'Andrea F, Signorelli CD, et al. L'amantadina nel trattamento dell'ipokinesia transitoria di pazienti parkinsoniani in corso di terapia con L-DOPA. *Minerva Med* 1972; 409:4007–4008.
10. Fahn S, Isgreen WP. Long-term evaluation of amantadine and levodopa combination in parkinsonism by double-blind cross-over analyses. *Neurology* 1975; 25:695–700.
11. Shannon KM, Goetz CG, Carroll VS, et al. Amantadine and motor fluctuations in chronic Parkinson's disease. *Clin Neuropharmacol* 1987; 10:522–526.
12. Aoki FY, Sitar DS. Clinical pharmacokinetics of amantadine hydrochloride. *Clin Pharmacokinet* 1988; 14:5135–5151.
13. Bleidner WE, Harmon JB, Hewes WE, et al. Absorption, distribution and excretion of amantadine hydrochloride. *J Pharmacol Exp Ther* 1965; 150:484–490.
14. Muller T, Kuhn W, Quack G, et al. Intravenous application of amantadine and anti-parkinsonian efficacy in parkinsonian patients. *J Neural Transm* 1995; 46(Suppl):407–413.
15. Bailey EV, Stone TW. The mechanism of action of amantadine in parkinsonism: A review. *Arch Int Pharmacoldyn* 1975; 216:246–262.
16. Heikkila RE, Cohen G. Evaluation of amantadine as a releasing agent or uptake blocker for H3-dopamine in rat brain slices. *Eur J Pharmacol* 1972; 20:156–160.
17. Lassen JB. The effect of amantadine and (+)-amphetamine on motility in rats wafter inhibition of

monoamine synthesis and storage. *Psychopharmacology (Berlin)* 1973; 29:55–64.

18. Farnebo LO, Fuxe K, Goldstein M, et al. Dopamine and nonadrenaline releasing action of amantadine in the central and peripheral nervous system: A possible mode of action in Parkinson's disease. *Eur J Pharmacol* 1971; 16:3827–38.

19. Stromberg U, Svensson TH, Waldeck B. The effect of amantadine on the uptake of dopamine and nonadrenaline by rat brain homogenates. *J Pharm Pharmacol* 1970; 22:957–962.

20. Heimans RLH, Rand M, Fennessy MR. Effects of amantadine on uptake and release of dopamine by a particulate fraction of rat basal ganglia. *J Pharm Pharmacol* 1972; 24:875–879.

21. Nastuck WC, Su PC, Doubilet P. Anticholinergic and membrane activities of amantadine in neuromuscular transmission. *Nature* 1976; 264:76–79.

22. Greenamyre JT, O'Brien CF. N-methyl-D-aspartate antagonists in the treatment of Parkinson's disease. *Arch Neurol* 1991; 48:977–981.

23. Klockgether T, Turski L. NMDA antagonists potentiate anti-Parkinsonian actions of levodopa in monoamine-depleted rats. *Ann Neurol* 1990; 28:539–546.

24. Greenamyre JT, Eller RV, Zhany Z, et al. Anti-Parkinsonian effects of remacemide hydrochloride, a glutamate antagonist in rodent and primate models of Parkinson's disease. *Ann Neurol* 1994; 35:655–661.

25. Engber TM, Papa SM, Boldry RC, et al. NMDA receptor blockade reverses motor response alterations induced by levodopa. *Neuroreport* 1994; 5:2586–2588.

26. Papa SM, Chase TN. Levodopa-induced dyskinesias improved by a glutamate antagonist in parkinsonian monkeys. *Ann Neurol* 1996; 39:574–578.

27. Metman LV, Del Dotto P, Natte R, et al. Dextromethorphan improves levodopa-induce dyskinesias in Parkinson's disease. *Neurology* 1998; 51:203–206.

28. Parkinson Study Group. The glutamate antagonist remacemide improves motor performance in levodopa-treated Parkinson's disease. *Neurology* 1999; 52(Suppl 2):A262(Abstract).

29. Parkes JD, Baxter RC, Marsden CD, et al. Comparative trial of benzhexol, amantadine and levodopa in the treatment of Parkinson's disease. *J Neurol Neurosurg Psychiatry* 1974; 37:422–426.

30. Koller WC. Pharmacologic treatment of parkinsonian tremor. *Arch Neurol* 1986; 43:126–127.

31. Uitti RJ, Rajput AH, Ahlskog JE, et al. Amantadine treatment is an independent predictor of improved survival in Parkinson's disease. *Neurology* 1996; 46:1551–1556.

32. Metman LV, Del Dotto P, van den Munckhof P, et al. Amantadine as treatment for dyskinesias and motor fluctuations in Parkinson's disease. *Neurology* 1998; 50:1323–1326.

33. Danielczyk W. Twenty-five years of amantadine therapy in Parkinson's disease. *J Neural Transm* 1995; 46:399–405.

34. Shealy CN, Weeth JB, Mercier D. Livedo reticularis in patients with parkinsonism receiving amantadine. *JAMA* 1970; 212:1522–1523.

35. Shulman LM, Minegar A, Weiner WJ. Amantadine induced neuropathy. *Neurology* 1999; 53:1862–1865.

36. Factor SA, Singer C. Neuroleptic malignant syndrome. In: Lang AE, Weiner WJ (eds). *Drug-Induced Movement Disorders*. Mount Kisco: Futura Publishing, 1992:199–230.

37. Factor SA, Molho ES, Brown DL. Acute delirium after withdrawal of amantadine in Parkinson's disease. *Neurology* 1998; 50:1456–1458.

38. Factor SA, Molho ES. Transient benefits of amantadine in Parkinson's disease: The facts about the myth. *Mov Disord* 1999;

39. Comella CL, Tanner CM. Anticholinergic drugs in the treatment of Parkinson's disease. In: Koller WC, Paulson G (eds). *Therapy of Parkinson's Disease*. 2nd ed. New York: Marcel Dekker, 1995:109–122.

40. Ordenstein L. *Sur la Paralysie et la Sclerose in Plaque Generalise*. Paris:Martinet, 1867.

41. Marinesco G, Bourguignon G. Variations de la chronaxie et de l'attitude des membres sous l'influence de la scopolamine et de l'eserine dans deux cas de syndromes Parkinsoniens postencephalitiques. *C R Soc Biol (Paris)* 1927; 97:207.

42. Zucker K. Uber die Wirkung der physostigmine bei erkrankungen des extrapyramidalen systems. *M Psych Neurol* 1925; 58:11.

43. Milhorat AT. Studies in diseases of muscle: IX. Effect of quinine and prostigmine methyl sulfate on muscular rigidity in paralysis agitans. *Arch Neurol Psychiatry* 1941; 45:74.

44. Duvoisin RC. Cholinergic-anticholinergic antagonism in Parkinsonism. *Arch Neurol* 1967; 17:124–136.

45. Duvoisin RC. The mutual antagonism of cholinergic and anticholinergic agents in Parkinsonism. *Trans Am Neurol Assoc* 1966; 91:73–79.

46. Feldberg W. Present views on the mode of action of acetylcholine in the central nervous system. *Physiol Rev* 1945; 25:596.

47. Everett GM, Blockus LE, Sheppard IM. Tremor induced by tremorine and its antagonism by antiparkinson drugs. *Science* 1956; 124:79.

48. Dejong MC, Funcke ABH. Sinistrotorsion in guinea pigs as a method of screening anti-parkinsonian drugs. *Arch Int Pharmacodyn* 1962; 137:375.

49. Faucon G, Lavarenne J, Collard M. Mis en evidence de l'activite anti-Parkinonienne au moyen du tremblement eserinique. *Therapie* 1965; 20:137.

50. Nashold BS. Cholinergic stimulation of globus pallidus in man. *Proc Soc Exp Biol Med* 1959; 101:68–69.

51. Barbeau A. The pathogenesis of Parkinson's disease: A new hypothesis. *Can Med Assoc J* 1962; 87:802–807.

52. Connor JD, Rossi GV, Baker WW. Antagonism of intracaudate carbachol tremor by local injections

of catecholamines. *J Pharmacol Exp Ther* 1967; 155:545–551.

53. Velasco F, Velasco M, Romo R. Effect of carbachol and atropine perfusions in the mesencephalic tegmentum and caudate nucleus of experimental tremor in monkeys. *Exp Neurol* 1982; 78:450–460.

54. Burke R, Fahn S. Pharmacokinetics of trihexyphenidyl after acute and chronic administration. *Ann Neurol* 1982; 12:94.

55. Contin M, Riva R, Martinelli P, et al. Combined levo-dopa-anticholinergic therapy in the treatment of Parkinson's disease. *Clin Neuropharm* 1991; 14:148–155.

56. Doshay LJ, Constable K. Artane therapy for parkinsonism: Preliminary study of results of 117 cases. *JAMA* 1949; 140:1317–1322.

57. Doshay LJ, Constable K, Fromer S. Preliminary study of a new anti-parkinsonian agent. *Neurology* 1952; 2:233–243.

58. Doshay LJ. Five-year study of benztropine (Cogentin) methanesulfate. *JAMA* 1956; 162:1031–1034.

59. Strang RR. Experiences with Cogentin in the treatment of parkinsonism. *Acta Neurol Scand* 1965; 145:413–418.

60. Timberlake WH. Double-blind comparison of levodopa and procyclidine in parkinsonism, with illustrations of levodopa-induced movement disorders. *Neurology* 1970; 20:31–35.

61. Agate FJ, Doshay LJ, Curtis FK. Quantitative measurement of therapy in paralysis agitans. *JAMA* 1956; 160:353–354.

62. Norris JW, Vas CJ. Mehixene hydrochloride and parkinsonian tremor. *Acta Neurol Scand* 1967; 43:535–538.

63. Poewe WH, Lees AJ. Pharmacology of foot dystonia in parkinsonism. *Clin Neuropharmacol* 1987; 10:47–56.

64. Rix A, Fischer RG. Comparison of trihexyphenidyl and dihydromorphanthridine derivative in control of tremor of parkinsonism. *South Med J* 1972; 65:1305–1389.

65. Olanow CW, Koller WC. An algorithm (decision tree) for the management of Parkinson's disease: Treatment guidelines. *Neurol* 1998; 50(Suppl 3):S1–S57.

66. Koller WC. Disturbance of recent memory function in parkinsonian patients on anticholinergic therapy. *Cortex* 1984; 20:307–311.

67. Sadeh M, Braham J, Modan M. Effects of anticholinergic drugs on memory in Parkinson's disease. *Arch Neurol* 1982; 39:666–667.

68. Goetz CG, Tanner CM, Klawans HL. Pharmacology of hallucinations induced by long-term drug therapy. *Am J Psychiatry* 1982; 139:494–497.

69. de Smet Y, Ruberg M, Serdaru M, et al. Confusion, dementia and anticholinergics in Parkinson's disease. *J Neurol Neurosurg Psychiatry* 1982; 45:1161–1164.

70. Hauser RA, Olanow CW. Orobuccal dyskinesia associated with trihexyphenidyl therapy in a patient with Parkinson's disease. *Mov Disord* 1993; 8:512–514.

71. Hurtig HI. Advanced Parkinson's disease and complications of treatment. In: Stern MB, Hurtig HI (eds). *The Comprehensive Management of Parkinson's Disease.* New York: PMA Publishing Corp, 1988:119–158.

72. Hurtig HI. Anticholinergics for Parkinson's disease. *Ann Neurol* 1980; 7:495.

34

Monoamine Oxidase Inhibitors

Theresa A. Zesiewicz, M.D., and Robert A. Hauser, M.D.
University of South Florida, Tampa, Florida

INTRODUCTION AND HISTORY

Amines are weakly basic organic compounds that contain a nitrogen group (1,2). They are described as primary, secondary, or tertiary depending on whether one, two, or three carbon atoms are attached to the nitrogen atom (1). Primary amines are also called "monoamines," and include the catecholamines dopamine, norepinephrine, and 5-hydroxytryptamine (Figure 34-1). These chemicals play an integral role in neurotransmission. Many neuropsychiatric pharmaceutical agents act by inhibiting or promoting their formation, release, metabolism, or reuptake (3,4).

Monoamine oxidases (MAOs) are intracellular enzymes that play a role in the catabolism of neuroactive amines (3). They are located in the outer mitochondrial membrane and comprise isozymes A and B. MAOs catalyze the oxidative deamination of monoamines (5,6) via a reaction between dioxygen and $R-CH_2-NH_2$ to form $R-CHO$, NH_3, and H_2O_2 (7). Monoamine oxidase inhibitors (MAOIs) inhibit the action of monoamine oxidases. However, oxidation via MAO is not the rate-limiting step in the catabolism of monoamines. Because of the ubiquitous nature of the enzyme, considerable inhibition must occur before any changes in monoamine concentrations are observed.

Research into the nature and function of monoamines and their oxidases began at the turn of the century. In the late 1800s, Schmiedeberg et al. (8) discovered that almost all monoamines containing the atomic grouping $-CH_2-NH_2$ are metabolized to ammonia (NH_3). The first monoamine oxidase identified was tyramine oxidase in 1928 (9). Zeller later proposed the term *monoamine oxidase* for the group of enzymes whose main function is the oxidative deamination of monoamines (10–12).

In the 1950s and 1960s, several drugs used to treat tuberculosis were noted to be mood elevators (13–15). Some patients experienced euphoria and were noted to

"dance in the hall" during treatment (16). One anti-tuberculosis medication, isonicotinic acid hydrazide, or iproniazid, was found to be a potent MAO inhibitor (17). Kline et al. (18) conducted an open-label trial of iproniazid in depressed, institutionalized patients and found that approximately 70% experienced significant improvement in mood. Iproniazid was later introduced as the first antidepressant medication (19).

The mood elevating properties of iproniazid suggested that MAOIs could function as "psychic energizers." Knoll and Ecseri, seeking a compound with amphetamine-like stimulating effects and potent MAO inhibition, synthesized phenylisopropyl-N-methylpropinylamine or E-250 (20,21). E-250 was found to be a strong, irreversible inhibitor of the MAO that metabolized benzylamine (21) and phenylethylamine (22). It also inhibited the effects of tyramine (22). The compound was separated into two isomers, and the L-form was named "deprenyl."

In 1968 Johnston synthesized 2,3-dichlorophenoxypropyl-N-methylpropinylamine, or clorgyline, and found it to be similar in structure to deprenyl (23). He designated the form of MAO with greater affinity for clorgyline, "MAO A," and the type with lower affinity for clorgyline and greater affinity for deprenyl, "MAO B."

MONOAMINE OXIDASE: BIOCHEMISTRY AND MECHANISM OF ACTION

MAOs are a family of flavin-containing enzymes that catalyze the oxidative deamination of norepinepherine, epinephrine, dopamine, serotonin, and a variety of other monoamines to their corresponding aldehydes (24,25) by the reaction:

$$R-CH_2-NH_2 + O_2 + H_2O$$
$$\rightarrow R-CHO + NH_3 + H_2O_2 \ (27).$$

365

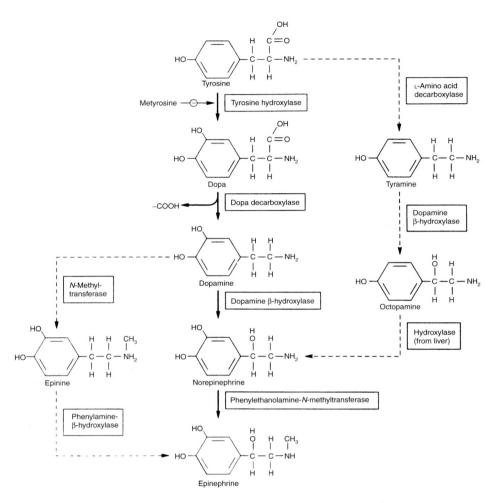

FIGURE 34-1. Biosynthesis of catecholamines. The rate-limiting step is the conversion of tyrosine to DOPA. (Reproduced with permission from Greenspan FS, Sterewler FJ: *Basic and Clinical Endocrinology*, 5th edition, Appleton and Lange, 1996).

The amine is oxidized to an iminium ion, and the flavin (FAD) is reduced (26). The iminium ion is then hydrolyzed to an aldehyde (27), and the reduced flavin is reoxidized with molecular oxygen (27).

MAO A and B show 71 percent sequence homology. The flavin sites on both forms of MAO are identical (28), thereby accounting for overlapping substrate specificities and inhibitor sensitivities (29). Although often described as selective, most MAO inhibitors are truly selective only at low concentrations (30).

MAO A primarily catabolizes serotonin and octopamine, whereas MAO B metabolizes benzylamine, phenylethylamine, milacemide, and N-methylhistamine. MAO B also deaminates long-chain diamines and tertiary cyclic amines such as 1-methyl-4-phenyl-1,2,3,6-tetrahydropyridine (MPTP) (31). Both enzymes catabolize dopamine, epinephrine, norepinephrine, tyramine, tryptamine, 3-methoxytryamine, and kynuramine (common substrates) (31).

MONOAMINE OXIDASE: ANATOMY AND LOCALIZATION

MAO A and B are intracellular enzymes in the CNS and peripheral tissues (32). Most MAO is tightly bound to the outer mitochondrial membrane (33,34), although a small portion can be found in the microsomal fraction of the cell. MAO can exist as part of a membrane unit containing A and B forms embedded in a phospholipid structure. MAO A activity is thought to be phospholipid-dependent, whereas MAO B activity is not (35).

MAO is present in most peripheral organs, blood vessel walls, and ventricular surfaces, but is absent in red blood cells and blood plasma (36–39). MAO A constitutes a large portion of the enzyme in the pancreas, intestine, and spleen and is the sole form in the human placenta (40–42). In contrast,

MAO B predominates in skin and skeletal muscle, and is the sole form in platelets. The human liver contains both forms (43). The human brain contains predominantly MAO B (about 70–80%) (44–47), whereas the rodent brain contains predominantly MAO A (48).

In the brain, MAO A is primarily located in catecholamine cells, and is usually situated intraneuronally in synaptosomes (49). MAO A containing neurons include those in the locus ceruleus, nucleus subceruleus, periventricular regions of the hypothalamus, and dopaminergic neurons in the striatum (50,51). Using specific antibodies to determine the immunocytochemical localization of MAO A, Westlund found that the MAO A content of the substantia nigra is low relative to the number of cells that are tyrosine hydroxylase–positive (51).

MAO B is the predominant extraneuronal form of the enzyme (51). It is located in the central nervous system astrocytes and in serotonergic neurons, including the raphe dorsalis in the midbrain. More than 80% of deamination in the frontal cortex is due to glial MAO B (52). Both protoplasmic and fibrillary astroctyes in the brain contain MAO B, whereas oligodendrocytes do not contain the enzyme. MAO B is also found in brain regions lacking a blood-brain barrier. It is found on either side of the midline in the medulla and pons, which includes cells in the raphe pallidus, raphe obscureus, raphe magnus, raphe pontis (61), and nucleus centralis superior.

Both MAO A and B activity are present in adrenergic nerve terminals in the hypothalamus, in the cortical projections from the posterior hypothalamus to the hippocampus, and paraventricular and supraoptic nuclei of the hypothalamus, medulla, and spinal cord (53).

In both rat and human brain (54), dopamine can be metabolized by either MAO A or Yang and Neff demonstrated that dopamine is metabolized by both in vitro, while Green and coworkers observed similar findings in rat brain in vivo. Glial cells in the human substantia nigra contain both forms of the enzyme (55), and may be responsible for MAO activity in this area. Using dopamine as a substrate, the highest MAO activity is in the nucleus accumbens (56).

The half-life for turnover of MAO B in experimental animals is approximately 6 to 30 days. The half-life of MAO B in pig brain is approximately 6.5 days (57). Using ^{11}Cl-deprenyl positron emission tomgraphy (PET), Arnett et al. (57) determined the half-life for turnover of MAO B in baboons to be 30 days.

MONOAMINE OXIDASE INHIBITORS: REVERSIBLE AND IRREVERSIBLE

MAO inhibitors may be reversible or irreversible. Reversible inhibitors are competitive, mixed (noncompetitive) or uncompetitive (58). MAO B inhibitors are not sterically hindered from binding to MAO A and are therefore less selective than MAO A inhibitors (59,60).

Selective MAO A inhibitors are formed by the substitution of the α-hydrogen by a methyl group on a monoamine (61,62). Harmaline, mexiletine, procaine, debrisoquine, $(\pm)\alpha$-methyltryptamine, and pirlindole are examples of reversible MAO A inhibitors (63). Other reversible MAO A inhibitors include amiflamine (64) and tolaxtone (65), which inhibit MAO A in vitro and in vivo. Many substances with other biologic functions also act as reversible MAO A inhibitors including amphetamine (1-methyl-2-phenylethylamine) (48), tetracaine, procainamide, propranolol, many formanilides (48), proflavine (66), salsolinol (67), and some xanthones (68). CGP 11305 (69) behaves as a short-acting MAO A inhibitor in vitro, and befloxatone is a newer, reversible MAO A inhibitor (70). Potent irreversible MAO A inhibitors include clorgyline, cyclopropylamines, and the hydrazines (71). Moclobemide is also a reversible MAO A inhibitor (72).

There are far fewer MAO B inhibitors than MAO A inhibitors. Some examples of reversible MAO-B inhibitors are benzyl alcohol, benzyl cyanide, and cyanophenol in vitro. The tricyclic antidepressants amitriptyline and imipramine (73) are MAO B inhibitors at lower concentrations than are needed for MAO A inhibition (74–76). MD 240928 and caroxazome are also reversible MAO B inhibitors (77). Lazabemide (Ro 19-6327) is a selective, rapidly reversible MAO B inhibitor (78). Irreversible MAO B inhibitors include the acetylenic compounds selegiline (deprenyl) and pargyline, the cyclopropylamines, and the hydrazines that include phenylhydrazine and benzylhydrazine. Rasagiline [R(+)−N−propargyl-1-aminoindane] is a newer selective irreversible MAO B inhibitor (79).

MONOAMINE OXIDASE INHIBITORS: HYPERTENSIVE CRISIS

Patients treated with early, nonselective MAO inhibitors including iproniazid, phenelzine, and tranylcypromine occasionally experienced dangerous hypertensive episodes when they ate foods rich in tyramine such as cheese, yeast, chicken liver, snails, pickled herring, red wines, and broad beans, or other indirectly-acting amines (80). This phenomenon is known as "the cheese effect." Tyramine is a sympathomimetic amine that is normally metabolized by MAO A in the intestine, but when absorbed results in the release of intraneuronal norepinephrine, leading to hypertensive crisis. Levodopa can also cause hypertensive crisis when MAO A is inhibited. Therefore, patients receiving nonspecific MAO or MAO A inhibitor medications must restrict tyramine in the diet and cannot take levodopa.

Selegiline (deprenyl), a relatively specific MAO B inhibitor, is free from the "cheese effect" when used in oral doses up to 10 mg/day. Knoll et al. (81) selected the levorotatory isomer of E-250 for further development because it inhibited the release of biogenic amines and acted in vivo and in vitro as a potent tyramine antagonist. It was later discovered that the cheese effect was generally not induced by this isomer even when administered with large amounts of tyramine. Elsworth et al. (82) found that individuals taking oral selegiline at a dose of 10 mg/day could tolerate 150 to 200 mg of tyramine without cardiovascular effects. However, there is increased sensitivity to tyramine with oral selegiline at a dose of 30 mg/day (55), and transient increases in blood pressure have been reported with selegiline at a dose of 20 mg/day. Thus oral selegiline 10 mg/day or less does not necessitate a tyramine-restricted diet and can be given safely with levodopa. Significant MAO A inhibition may occur with oral selegiline doses of 20 mg per day or more and should ordinarily be avoided.

Selegiline: Pharmacology

Pharmacokinetics of Selegiline

Selegiline is a relatively selective, irreversible MAO B inhibitor. It is considered a "suicide inhibitor" because it forms a covalent bond with MAO, and loss of MAO inhibition is dependent on generation of new enzyme. Selegiline is lipophilic and readily absorbed from the gastrointestinal tract. The absolute bioavailability of selegiline is roughly 10% (83). Ninety-four percent is bound to plasma proteins, with strong binding to macroglobulins (84,85). Maximal concentrations are achieved approximately 1/2 to 2 hours after oral administration (86). Studies of platelets in PD patients have shown that within two to four hours after a single 5 mg dose of selegiline, MAO B activity is inhibited by 86%, whereas within 24 hours of a 10 mg dose MAO B activity is inhibited by almost 98% (87). Selegiline readily crosses the blood–brain barrier and accumulates in brain regions rich in MAO B, including the striatum, thalamus, cortex, and brain stem (88).

Selegiline is metabolized in the liver by the microsomal cytochrome P-450 system to (-)-desmethylselegiline (DES), and l-(-)-methamphetamine (1-MA) (89); the latter compound is further metabolized to amphetamine and p-hydroxylated metabolites (55) (Figure 34-2). These metabolites are conjugated with glucuronic acid to form inactive metabolites (55). Selegiline may also be metabolized outside the liver. Three metabolites have been identified in serum and urine: l-(-)-methamphetamine, l-(-)-amphetamine, and (-)-desmethylselegiline (DES) (90). Desmethylselegiline has activity as an irreversible MAO B inhibitor, but it is much less potent than selegiline in vitro (55,91,92).

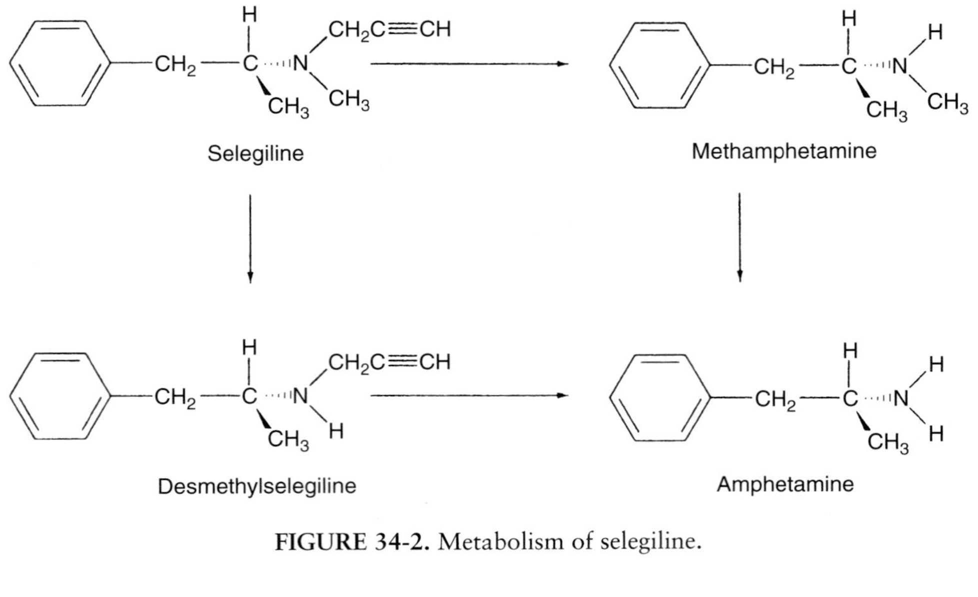

FIGURE 34-2. Metabolism of selegiline.

Mechanisms of Action

Selegiline may provide symptomatic antiparkinsonian benefit through a number of mechanisms. Chronic administration of selegiline increases striatal dopamine concentration in rats (93,94). This is thought to be due to MAO B inhibition in striatal glia as MAO B is essentially absent from nigrostriatal nerve terminals (95). Selegiline may also act by inhibiting dopamine reuptake (92) and by blocking presynaptic dopamine receptors (96). In rats, intraperitoneal selegiline increases 2-phenylethylamine concentration (97), which may increase dopamine release. Metabolites of selegiline, including amphetamine, may also promote dopamine release although the concentrations of these metabolites are probably too small to provide significant clinical benefit.

In addition to symptomatic antiparkinsonian effects, selegiline is thought by some to provide neuroprotective effects. The evidence for these effects and their mechanisms are discussed in Chapter 43.

Side Effects

Selegiline is usually well tolerated. The most frequent side effect is an increase in dyskinesia when it is added to a levodopa regimen in patients who have already developed dyskinesia. In some patients the increase in dyskinesia may occur without improvement in motor features. Additional side effects include nausea, dizziness, dryness of the mouth, sleep disturbances, confusion, anxiety, hallucinations, and orthostatic hypotension. When combined with levodopa therapy orthostatic hypotension may be marked and unassociated with compensatory tachycardia. It is reversible within days after stopping selegiline. Related to this is supine hypertension. The causes of these phenomenon are unknown (97a). Dopaminergic adverse reactions can typically be managed by lowering the levodopa dose (98). Gastric ulcer activation and urinary disturbances (99) have been reported (100,101), and some patients may have an elevation of liver function tests (102). Psychiatric abnormalities with selegiline use, which include hypomania and paranoia are rare (103–105).

Drug Interactions

Selegiline can interact with other drugs resulting in a variety of complications. The constellation of stupor, muscular rigidity, severe agitation, and elevated temperature has been reported in some patients receiving the combination of selegiline and meperidine (106). This is typical of the interaction of meperidine and MAOIs. Selegiline is therefore contraindicated for use with meperidine and this contraindication is usually extended to other opioids. The combined use of selegiline and other MAO inhibitors may result in hypotension, and their concomitant use is not recommended (107).

The combined use of selective serotonin reuptake inhibitor (SSRI) antidepressants and selegiline can cause the "serotonin syndrome," which result in some combination of: mental status changes, myoclonus, diaphoresis, hyperreflexia, tremor, diarrhea, shivering, incoordination, and fever (108). The syndrome may, on rare occasions, progress to seizures, coma, or death (109). Treatment of the serotonin syndrome consists of discontinuation of the offending agent, and supportive measures. The pathophysiology of the serotonin syndrome may be related to enhanced stimulation of 5-HT receptors in the brainstem and spinal cord (110).

Serotonin syndrome due to the combination of selegiline and an SSRI antidepressant is rare. Two chart reviews of patients taking the combination of an SSRI and selegiline failed to detect side effects which had not already been reported with each respective medication (110,111). The Parkinson Study Group found that of 4,568 PD patients treated with an antidepressant and selegiline, only 0.24% reported symptoms that were thought to be consistent with the serotonin syndrome (112). There were no fatalities. In routine clinical practice, selegiline and SSRI antidepressants are commonly used together, but clinical monitoring appears warranted.

Selegiline Clinical Trials

Selegiline in Early Parkinson's Disease

Selegiline monotherapy provides modest symptomatic benefit in early PD. In the DATATOP study, 800 patients were randomized to receive selegiline 10 mg/day or placebo. Total and motor UPDRS scores improved significantly at one and three months. Total UPDRS scores improved 2.07 ± 6.36 at one month in selegiline-treated patients compared to 0.11 ± 5.98 in placebo-treated patients (p < 0.001) and 1.56 ± 7.04 in selegiline-treated patients at three months compared to a worsening of 1.34 ± 6.70 in placebo-treated patients (p < 0.001) (113). In a more recent study of 157 patients, Palhagen et al. (114) noted significant improvement in total and motor UPDRS scores at six weeks and three months following the introduction of selegiline. At three months, total UPDRS scores improved 1.1 ± 4.3 in the selegiline group compared with a worsening of 0.4 ± 4.0 in the placebo group (p < 0.05). Similarly, the French Selegiline Multicenter

Trial of 93 patients identified significant improvements in total and motor UPDRS scores at one and three months.

Several smaller studies were unable to identify early symptomatic effects, probably due to power limitations (115). In a study of 54 patients, Tetrud and Langston did not identify symptomatic benefit at one month (116) and in a Finnish study of 52 patients, symptomatic benefit was not identified at three weeks or two months (117). It can be concluded that selegiline monotherapy in early PD provides minor symptomatic effects that is evident in larger studies by four to six weeks of therapy.

Withdrawal of selegiline results in a loss of symptomatic benefit. Loss of benefit depends on generation of new MAO B and may take several months. The half-life for human MAO B synthesis has been estimated to be as long as 40 days (114). In the DATATOP study, there was no significant loss of symptomatic benefit one month following selegiline withdrawal. However, at two months, total UPDRS scores had worsened 2.34 ± 4.95 points in selegiline-treated patients compared to 0.48 ± 5.72 in placebo-treated patients ($p < 0.001$) (113). Several smaller studies were unable to detect this effect. Tetrud and Langston did not find significant clinical changes during a one-month washout in 54 patients (116), and Palhagen et al. (114) found no evidence of clinical deterioration during a two-month washout in 157 patients.

Selegiline delays the need for (additional) symptomatic therapy in early PD. In the DATATOP study, selegiline significantly delayed the need for levodopa. The probability of reaching end point (need for levodopa) was significantly reduced in patients assigned to selegiline (hazard ratio, 0.50; 95% confidence interval, 0.41–0.62; $p < 0.001$). Subjects assigned to selegiline reached end point at a projected median of 719 days compared to 454 days for subjects assigned to placebo, representing a difference of nine months (113). Tetrud and Langston (116) found that patients taking selegiline required levodopa at a mean of 548.9 days compared to 312.1 days for placebo-treated patients ($p < 0.002$). Palhagen et al. (114) noted that the median time for levodopa was 12.7 months in their selegiline group, compared to 8.6 months in the placebo group ($p = 0.028$). Myllyla et al. (117) found a mean of 545 ± 90 days in their selegiline group compared to 372 ± 28 days in the placebo group ($p = 0.03$), a difference of almost six months. It can therefore be concluded that selegiline monotherapy delays the need for symptomatic therapy by six to nine months.

The mechanism by which selegiline delays the need for symptomatic therapy is not clearly defined. It is possible that the delay is entirely due to selegiline's symptomatic effect. However, it is not known whether this small symptomatic effect is sufficient to account for all of the delay in need for levodopa that was observed in these studies. The delay is potentially consistent with a neuroprotective effect but this remains to be proven. It is not possible to separate symptomatic and possible neuroprotective effects of selegiline in these studies.

During selegiline monotherapy a slowing of progression of measures of parkinsonian disability is observed. Tetrud and Langston (116) identified a 50% decrease in the rate of progression in UPDRS motor scores in their selegiline group compared to placebo ($p = 0.002$). In the DATATOP trial, there was a significantly slower rate of decline in UPDRS scores in patients taking selegiline compared to those taking placebo through six months of follow-up (113). Palhagen et al. (114) reported a progression in total UPDRS score of 7.5 ± 8.4 points from baseline to start of washout (median time = 12.7 months) in the selegiline group compared to 10.6 ± 9.6 points (median time = 8.6 months) in the placebo group ($p = 0.042$). Myllyla et al. (117) also noted significantly less progression of disability in parkinsonian symptoms as measured by the Columbia University Rating Scale in their selegiline group up to one year. Again, the mechanism(s) underlying these observations are not clearly defined. A decline in the rate of progression of disability as measured from an untreated baseline to a point during treatment may be due, wholly or in part, to symptomatic effects regardless of whether significant symptomatic benefit was observed in that study.

Olanow and coworkers (118) reported significantly less progression in UPDRS scores from an untreated baseline to an untreated endpoint following medication wash-out. Patients were randomized to selegiline or placebo and to symptomatic treatment with bromocriptine or levodopa. Endpoint evaluation at 14 months was completed after a two-month wash-out of selegiline and a one-week wash-out of bromocriptine and levodopa. The change in total UPDRS scores from baseline to final visit was 0.4 ± 1.3 in the selegiline group compared to 5.8 ± 1.4 in the placebo group ($p < 0.001$). Palhagen et al. (114) also assessed progression of UPDRS scores from an untreated baseline to an untreated endpoint following an eight-week wash-out of selegiline. Total UPDRS scores worsened significantly less in the selegiline group (11.3 ± 9.1) than in the placebo group (14.2 ± 10.9), when the length of time to reach the endpoint of need for levodopa was used as the covariate ($p = 0.033$). These observations are potentially consistent with a neuroprotective effect from selegiline, but it cannot be determined if the wash-outs were of sufficient duration to allow resolution of all symptomatic effects.

Once patients require levodopa therapy, selegiline allows symptomatic control with lower levodopa doses. Myllyla et al. (117) randomized patients to selegiline 10 mg/day or placebo until initiation of levodopa, and then followed them for at least two years. Required doses of levodopa were significantly lower in the selegiline group compared to the placebo group (p < 0.001). In selegiline-treated patients, the levodopa dose increased from 272 ± 75 mg/day to 358 ± 117 mg/day over 24 months, whereas in the placebo group the dose of levodopa almost doubled, from 293 ± 117 mg/day to 543 ± 150 mg/day. Selegiline-treated patients also required significantly fewer levodopa doses per day (3.5 vs. 4.5, p = 0.01). DATATOP subjects who reached endpoint and required levodopa were invited to join an open-label extension in which they received selegiline 10 mg/day and levodopa as needed and were followed for an additional 18 months. Patients who had originally been assigned to selegiline took levodopa for a significantly shorter period of time (p < 0.0001) and received significantly lower total cumulative levodopa doses (p < 0.02). However, the total daily levodopa dose at final evaluation was similar between groups. These observations are consistent with the fact that selegiline delays the need for levodopa and patients on levodopa can be controlled with lower levodopa doses (113). In the DATATOP extension, levodopa dose requirements were equal once patients in both groups were taking selegiline (119). This suggests that the differences observed may be due to symptomatic rather than neuroprotective effects. Other findings by the PSG (119a), in patients reaching end point (requiring levodopa), also support the idea that the effects were symptomatic. In this report they found that complications of levodopa therapy that include motor fluctuations, dyskinesia, and freezing occurred at the same time and in the same proportion of patients treated with deprenyl as those not originally treated with deprenyl.

Selegiline in Advanced Parkinson's Disease Patients

Selegiline affords mild to moderate symptomatic benefit as an adjunct to levodopa in advanced patients. It is for this indication that selegiline was approved by the FDA in the United States. In an early open-label trial, Rinne et al. (120) found that the addition of selegiline 10 mg/day in advanced patients on stable doses of levodopa significantly improved tremor, rigidity, and bradykinesia. In double-blind controlled studies, Siversten et al. (121) noted

significant improvement in tremor (p = 0.02) and Heinonen et al. (122) noted significant improvement in tremor (p = 0.010), rigidity (p = 0.027), and hypokinesia (p = 0.004) (122).

In patients with motor fluctuations, selegiline prolongs the short duration levodopa response and reduces "off" time. In an open-label trial, Rinne et al. (120) found that 68% of patients showed significant improvement in on–off phenomena. Motor fluctuations were less frequent and less severe. In double-blind crossover trials, Heinonen et al. (122) and Lees et al. (123) identified significantly less end-of-dose akinesia in patients taking selegiline. In a larger, double-blind placebo-controlled, parallel group trial of 96 fluctuating PD patients, Golbe et al. (124) observed better mean hourly symptom control in 58% of patients randomized to selegiline compared to 26.1% of patients randomized to placebo (p < .01). Improvement was also noted in dressing, dysarthria, hypomimia, sialorrhea, and tremor (p < 0.05).

When used as an adjunct to levodopa, selegiline allows a reduction in daily levodopa dose of about 10 to 25% (121–123). For example, Golbe et al. (124) found that mean daily levodopa dosages were decreased by 17% in the selegiline group compared to 7% in the placebo group.

Selegiline may worsen dyskinesia when initially added to levodopa, thereby necessitating levodopa dose reductions. Once the levodopa dose is reduced, dyskinesia is usually no worse than at baseline. Golbe et al. (124) found that approximately 60 percent of patients taking selegiline and 30% of patients taking placebo reported a worsening of dyskinesia two or three days after starting treatment. In most cases symptoms resolved after several days when the levodopa dosage was reduced.

Thus selegiline is useful as an adjunct to levodopa in patients with advanced disease to improve symptoms and reduce off-time. If dyskinesia emerges or worsens, the levodopa dose should be reduced. Patients are often controlled on 10 to 25 percent less levodopa.

Selegiline and Mortality

The Parkinson's Disease Research Group of the United Kingdom (125) reported a 60 percent increase in mortality rate in PD patients who were randomized to levodopa and selegiline compared to levodopa alone. A total of 624 patients were randomized to one of three groups: levodopa, levodopa plus selegiline, or bromocriptine. After a mean duration of 5.6 years, 44 (17.7%) deaths were observed in the levodopa group, compared with 76 (28%) deaths in the levodopa plus selegiline group (p = 0.05). The number in the bromocriptine group was not given. The increase in mortality became apparent after 2.5 to 3.5 years of treatment.

Questions have been raised regarding methodologic issues in this study and the validity of its conclusions. Multiple interim analyses were performed without apparent statistical adjustment in regard to mortality (126). In addition, the on-treatment analysis did not confirm the findings of the intention-to-treat analysis. Further, both treatment arms (levodopa and levodopa plus selegiline) experienced surprisingly high mortality rates. Mortality rates of 50.7 and 32.1/1,000 were observed in the levodopa/selegiline and levodopa groups, respectively, while a meta-analysis of five long-term trials yielded mortality rates of 12.5 and 16.7/1,000 (125).

Other long-term trials have not identified the same increase in mortality with selegiline. In the DATATOP trial and a subsequent open-label extension, the overall death rate was 17.1% (137 of 800), or 2.1% per year through a mean of 8.2 years of observation (127). Mortality rate was unaffected by any of the treatments. In another study, three (6%) deaths occurred in the selegiline group through a mean follow-up of 4.5 years with no significant difference in mortality rate between groups, and no trend toward increased mortality with selegiline use (118). Thus, although the U.K. study raises concerns, no firm conclusions can be drawn. Experience from other studies suggests mortality is not increased and the drug can be considered safe.

Selegiline Use by Alternate Routes

Selegiline administration via a transdermal patch or a sublingual wafer may provide clinical benefits that cannot be achieved with oral selegiline administration. The selegiline transdermal system provides relatively stable selegiline blood concentrations through the day and minimizes the formation of metabolites. Oral selegiline undergoes first pass metabolism, and has an elimination half-life of about two hours. The transdermal system avoids the first pass effect, thereby increasing bioavailability and decreasing metabolite production. Higher blood and brain selegiline concentrations may be achieved before MAO A in the gut is inhibited to the extent that creates a risk of hypertensive crisis. Higher selegiline brain concentrations might provide greater symptomatic benefit by completely inhibiting brain MAO B and possibly some MAO A. Inhibition of MAO A within the substantia nigra might increase intraneuronal dopamine pools and facilitate dopamine release.

Rohatagi et al. (79) administered selegiline transdermal system (STS) to six healthy male volunteers using 1–4 1.83 mg/cm^2-patches daily for five days and observed higher blood concentrations of selegiline compared with oral tablets. Selegiline delivery increased proportionally from 7.7 ± 0.9 mg using one STS/day to 29.2 ± 5.2 mg following four STS/day. AUC also increased linearly with dose.

Hauser et al. (128) evaluated the tolerability and safety of transdermal selegiline monotherapy in mild to moderate PD. Patients who were well controlled on levodopa underwent baseline evaluation following a two-week levodopa washout. One selegiline transdermal system (delivering 8.5 mg/24 hours) was then applied each day for eight weeks. The most common adverse events were dizziness (28%), headache (16%), and pruritis (16%). For patients completing eight weeks on study medication, UPDRS total and motor scores improved significantly (-2.53 ± 4.37, p < 0.05; -1.80 ± 3.32, p = 0.05).

Sublingual selegiline preparations also avoid first pass metabolism and may also allow greater brain MAO inhibition. The sublingual form of selegiline is a fast dissolving tablet that disintegrates in the mouth and is absorbed. This formulation is referred to as Zydis-selegiline. There is no need for water and the resulting plasma level of selegiline is higher than that of the standard oral form. Both sublingual and transdermal selegiline are presently being evaluated as adjuncts to levodopa in patients who experience motor fluctuations.

OTHER MAO INHIBITORS

Rasagiline

Rasagiline [R(+)−N−propargyl-1-aminoindane] is a selective irreversible MAO B inhibitor. Unlike selegiline, the racemic form (AGN-1135) is not metabolized to amphetamine-like derivatives (129). Rasagiline is well absorbed orally and effectively passes the blood-brain barrier. It is a potent MAO B inhibitor, and 1 mg daily causes more than 90% inhibition of platelet MAO B after seven days. Rasagiline effects a high degree of MAO inhibition in rat brain, and enhanced dopamine release is observed with chronic administration. Phase I clinical trials have found it safe in human volunteers. As with selegiline, there is interest in possible neuroprotective effects (129).

In a phase II placebo-controlled, double-blind study, this drug was found safe and well tolerated in 56 previously untreated patients (129a). In addition, symptomatic improvement was seen in UPDRS scores. A phase III trial is in progress.

Lazabemide

Lazabemide (Ro 19-6327) is a selective, rapidly reversible MAO B inhibitor, chemically unrelated to selegiline (130). Lazabemide has a high degree of MAO B selectivity, and is not metabolized to amphetamine or its derivatives. Even at high doses, lazabemide is devoid of any tyramine potentiation ("cheese effect") (131). Lazabemide does not cause dopamine release nor induce ipsilateral turning in 6-hydroxydopamine-lesioned rats (132).

In a six-week double-blind trial, 201 early untreated PD patients were randomized to receive lazabemide 100 to 400 mg/day or placebo. Lazabemide treatment was associated with significant improvement in the activities of daily living component of the UPDRS, but other scores were unchanged (130). A higher incidence of insomnia, decreased hematocrit, and elevated serum alanine aminotransferase levels were associated with lazabemide at doses of 400 mg/day.

In another double-blind, placebo-controlled trial, 321 otherwise untreated patients were randomized to receive lazabemide 25 to 200 mg/day or placebo, and were followed for up to one year (133). The primary endpoint was the time to reach functional disability severe enough to warrant levodopa therapy. The risk of reaching endpoint was reduced by 51% for patients receiving lazabemide compared to placebo (p = 0.008). No symptomatic effects were noted.

The Parkinson Study Group (134) conducted a tolerability study of lazabemide in 137 patients who experienced a stable response to levodopa. Subjects were randomized to receive lazabemide 100 to 400 mg/day, or placebo for eight weeks. Lazabemide was as well tolerated as placebo, but there was an increased frequency of dopaminergic side effects including dyskinesia, nausea, and dystonia in lazabemide-treated groups.

Thus, lazabemide and rasagiline could provide other alternatives to selegiline in the treatment of PD in the future. Rasagiline is currently being tested in phase III trails. Both drugs lack the side effects related to amphetamine metabolites of selegiline.

CONCLUSION

Monoamine oxidase plays an integral role in the metabolism of intracerebral dopamine, and inhibitors of the enzyme provide benefit in PD. The most widely used MAOI is selegiline, a selective, irreversible MAO-B inhibitor. Unlike early nonselective MAOIs, selegiline is free from the "cheese effect" when used in oral doses up to 10 mg/day. In addition to inhibiting dopamine metabolism, it may also block dopamine reuptake and augment dopamine release. Selegiline monotherapy provides modest symptomatic benefit in early PD, and significantly delays the need for dopamine-replacement therapy. Whether this confers a long-term benefit is not known. Once levodopa is required, selegiline allows symptomatic control with lower levodopa doses. In advanced disease, selegiline provides mild to moderate symptomatic benefit as an adjunct to levodopa. Off time is reduced and symptom control is improved. If dopaminergic side effects emerge with the introduction of selegiline, the levodopa dose should be reduced. Mortality associated with selegiline use remains controversial. Although one study found a higher mortality rate in patients randomized to selegiline (125), other studies have not identified an increase in mortality.

Transdermal and sublingual selegiline delivery systems are currently under investigation. It is hoped that these alternate delivery systems will allow greater brain MAO inhibition and provide more symptomatic benefit without making patients susceptible to the "cheese effect." Rasagiline and lazabemide are investigational oral MAO-B inhibitors. Future research efforts will seek to determine how to increase the magnitude of clinical benefit provided by MAO inhibitors. Combination therapies to further enhance dopamine release, inhibit dopamine metabolism and block dopamine reuptake and may provide greater symptomatic effects.

Several MAO inhibitors provide neuroprotective actions in cell culture and animal model systems. Although clinical trials have yielded results that are consistent with a neuroprotective effect, it has not yet been possible to conclusively prove such an effect. New long-term studies that include positron emission tomography (PET) or single photon emission computed tomography (SPECT) to assess the rate of loss of dopamine neurons may be of value to evaluate possible neuroprotective effects in PD patients. The usefulness of MAO inhibitors in the treatment of PD in the future may well depend on finding ways to provide greater symptomatic benefit (such as alternate delivery systems or combination therapies) or in conclusively demonstrating neuroprotective benefit.

ACKNOWLEDGMENT

The authors wish to thank Albert Azzaro, Ph.D. for his kind review of the manuscript and his helpful suggestions.

REFERENCES

1. Hardman JG, Limbird LE, eds. Goodman & Gilman's *The Pharmacological Basis of Therapeutics*.

Ninth edition. New York: McGraw-Hill, 1996; 209–212.

2. Smith AD, Datta SP, Howard Smith G, et al. eds. *Oxford Dictionary of Biochemistry and Molecular Biology*. Oxford, New York, Tokyo: Oxford University Press, 1997;31.

3. Nicoll. Introduction to the pharmacology of CNS drugs. In: Katzung BG, ed. *Basic and Clinical Pharmacology*. Stamford: Appleton and Lange, 1998:352.

4. Clark WG, Brater DC, Johnson AR. General aspects of neuropharmacology. In: *Goth's Medical Pharmacology*. Twelfth edition. St. Louis: Mosby, 1988:83.

5. Westlund KN. The distribution of monoamine oxidases A and B in normal human brain. In: Lieberman A, Olanow CW, Youdim MBH, et al. eds. *Monoamine Oxidase Inhibitors in Neurological Diseases*. New York, Basel, Hong Kong: Marcel Dekker, 1994:1

6. Lefkowitz RJ, Hoffman BB, Taylor P. Neurotransmission. The autonomic and somatic motor nervous systems. In: Hardman JG, Limbird LE, Molinoff PB, et al. eds. Goodman & Gilman's *The Pharmacological Basis of Therapeutics*. Ninth Edition. New York: McGraw-Hill, 1996:123.

7. Davison AN. Physiological role of monoamine oxidase. *Physiol Rev* 1958; 38:729–747.

8. Schmiedeberg O. Uber das verbaltnis des ammoniaks und der primaren monoaminbasen zur harnstoffbildung im thierkorper. *Naunyn Schmiedebergs Arch Pharmacol* 1977; 8:1–14.

9. Hare. Tyramine oxidase – I. A new enzyme system in liver. *Biochem J* 1928; 22:968–979.

10. Zeller EA. Uber den enzymatischen abbau von histamin und diaminen. *Helv Chim Acta* 1938; 21:881–890.

11. O'Brien EM, Tipton K. Biochemistry and mechanism of action of monoamine oxidases A and B. In: Lieberman A, Olanow CW, Youdim MBH, et al. eds. *Monamine Oxidase Inhibitors in Neurological Disease*. New York, Basel, Hong Kong: Marcel Dekker, 1994:31–77.

12. Blaschko H. The natural history of amine oxidases. *Rev Physiol Biochem Pharmacol* 1974; 70:84–148.

13. Pletcher A. Monoamine oxidase inhibitors: effects related to psychostimulation. In: Efron DH, ed. *Psychopharmacology. A Review of Progress 1957–1967*. Washington: US Government Printing Office.

14. Schiele BC. Antidepressants: Comparison of clinical effect in anergic schizophrenia and the depressed states. *Ann NY Acad Sci* 1963; 107:1131–1138.

15. Bryant JM, Schvartz N, Torosdag S, et al. Long-term antihypertensive effect of pargyline HCL with and without diuretic sulfonamides. *Ann NY Acad Sci* 1963; 107:1023–1032.

16. Pletcher A. The discovery of antidepressants: A winding path. *Experientia* 1991; 47:4–8.

17. Zeller EA, Barsky J. In vivo inhibition of liver and brain monoamine oxidase by 1-isonicotinyl-2-isopropyl hydrazine. *Proc Soc Exp Biol Med* 1952; 81:459–461.

18. Loomer HP, Saunders JC, Kline NS. A clinical and pharamcodynamic evaluation of iproniazid as a pyschic energizer. *Psychiat Res Rep Am Psychiat Associa* 1958; 8:129–141.

19. Loomer HP, Sauncers JC, Kline NS. Iproniazid, an amine oxidase inhibitor, as an example of a psychic energizer. *Congres Rec* 1957; 1382–1390.

20. Knoll J, Magyar K. Some puzzling pharmacological effects of monoamine oxidase inhbitors. *Adv Biochem Psychopharmacol* 1972; 5:393–408.

21. Knoll H, Ecseri Z, Kelemen K, et al. Phenylisopropyl-methylpropinylamine (E-250), a new spectrum psychic energizer. *Arch Int Pharmacodyn* 1965; 155:154–164.

22. Yang HYT, Neff NH. The monoamine oxidases of brain: Selective inhibition with drugs and the consequences for the metabolism of the biogenic amines. *J Pharmacol Exp Ther* 1974; 189:733–740.

23. Johnston JP. Some observations upon a new inhibitor of monoamine oxidase in brain tissue. *Biochem Pharmacol* 1968; 17:1285–1297.

24. Kearney EB, Salach JI, Walker WH, et al. Structure of the covalently bound flavin of monoamine oxidase. *Biochem Biophys Res Commun* 1971; 42:490–496.

25. Neff NH, Goridis C. Neuronal monoamine oxidase: Specific enzyme types and their rates of formation. *Adv Biochem Psychopharmacol* 1972; 5:307–323.

26. Yasunobu KT, Gomes B. Mitochondrial amine oxidase (MAO) (beef liver). *Meth Enzymol* 1971; 17:709.

27. Yasunobu KI, Oi S. Mechanistic aspects of the bovine hepatic monoamine oxidase reaction. *Adv Biochem Psychopharmacol* 1972; 5:91–105.

28. Nagy J, Salach JI. Identity of the active site flavin-peptide fragments from the human "A"-form and the bovine "B"-form of monoamine oxidase. *Arch Biochem Biophys* 1981; 208:388–394.

29. Ramsay RR, Singer TP. The kinetic mechanisms of monoamine oxidases A and B. *Biochem Soc Trans* 1991:219–223.

30. Dahlstrom A, Fuxe K. Evidence for the existence of monoamine-containing neurons in the central nervous system. I. Demonstration of monoamines in the cell bodies of brainstem neurons. *Acta Physiol Scand* 1965; 62(Suppl 232):1–55.

31. May T, Strauss S, Rommelspacher H. [3H] Harman labels selectively and with high affinity the active site of monoamine oxidase (EC1.4.3.4) subtype A (MAO-A) in rat, marmoset, and pig. *J Neural Transm* (suppl)1990; 32:93–102.

32. Lewinsohn R, Glover V, Sandler M. Development of benzylamine oxidase and monoamine oxidase A and B in man. *Biochem Pharmacol* 1980; 29:1221–1230.

33. Pugh CEM, Quastel JH. Oxidation of aliphatic amines by brain and other tissues. *Biochem J* 1937; 31:2306–2321.

34. Quastel JH. Amine oxidases. In: Lajta A. ed. *Handbook of Neurochemistry*. New York: Plenum, 1970:285–312.

35. White HL, Stine DK. Monoamine oxidases A and B as components of a membrane complex. *J Neurochem* 1982; 38:1429–1436.

36. Blaschko H. Amine oxidase and amine metabolism. *Pharmacol Rev* 1952; 4:415–458.

37. Arai R, Kimura H, Maeda T. Topographic atlas of monoamine oxidase-containing neurons in the rat brain studies by an improved histochemical method. *Neurology* 1986; 19:905–925.

38. Kithama K, Denney Rm, Maeda T, Jouvet M. Distribution of type B monoamine oxidase immunoreactivity in the cat brain with reference to enzyme histochemistry. *Neuroscience* 1991; 44:185–204.

39. Willoughby J, Glover V, Sandler M. Histochemical localization of monoamine oxidases A and B in rat brain. *J Neural Transm* 1988; 74:29–42.

40. Lewinsohn R, Glover V, Sandler M. Development of benzylamine oxidase and MAO-A and -B in man. *Biochem Pharmacol* 1980; 29:1220–1230.

41. Riederer P, Reynolds GP, Yodim MBH. Selectivity of MAO inhibitors in human brain and their clinical consequences. In: Youdim MBH, Paykel ES. eds. *Monoamine Oxidase Inhibitors – The State of the Art*. Chichester: Wiley & Sons, 1981:63–76.

42. White HL, Tansik RL. Characterization of multiple substrate binding sites of MAO. In: Singer TP, von Korff RW, Murphy DL. eds. *Monoamine Oxidase: Structure, Function, Altered Functions*. New York: Academic Press, 1979:129–144.

43. Callingham BA. Substrate selective inhibition of monoamine oxidase by mexiletine. *Br J Pharmacol* 1977; 61:118.

44. Glover V, Sandler M, Owen F, et al. Dopamine is a monoamine oxidase B substrate. *Nature* 1979; 265:80–81.

45. Fowler CJ, Tipton KF. On the substrate specificities of the two forms of monoamine oxidase. *J Pharm Pharmacol* 1984; 36:111–115.

46. Reynolds GP, Riederer P, Rausch WD. Dopamine metabolism is human brain: effects of monoamine oxidase inhibition in vitro by (−)deprenyl and (+) and (−) tranylcypromine. *J Neural Transm* 1980; 16:173–178.

47. Murphy DL, Redmond D, Garrick N, et al. Brain region differences and some characteristics of monoamine oxidase type A and B activities in the vervet monkey. *Neurochem Res* 1979; 4:53–62.

48. Fowler CJ, Callingham BA, Mantle TJ, et al. Monoamine oxidase A and B: a useful concept? *Biochem Pharmacol* 1978; 27:97–101.

49. Oreland L. Monoamine oxidase, dopamine and Parkinson's disease. *Acta Neurol Scand* 1991; 84:60–65.

50. Levitt P, Pintar JE, Breakefield XO. Immunocytochemical demonstration of monoamine oxidase B in brain astrocytes and serotonergic neurons. *Proc Natl Acad Sci USA* 1982; 79:6385–6389.

51. Westlund KN, Kenney RM, Kochersperger LM, et al. Distinct monoamine oxidase A and B populations in primate brain. *Science* 1985; 230:181–183.

52. Oreland L, Arai Y, Stenstrom A, et al. Monoamine oxidase activity and localization in the brain and the activity in relation to psychiatric disorders. *Mod Probl Pharmacopsychiat* 1982; 19:246–254.

53. Wouterlood FG, Gaykema RPA. Innervation of histaminergic neurons in the posterior hypothalamic region by medial preoptic neurons. Anterograde tracing with *Phaselous vulgaris* leucoagglutinin combined with immunocytochemistry of histidine decarboxylase in the rat. *Brain Res* 1988; 455:170–176.

54. Youdim MBH, Green AR. Biogenic monoamine metabolism and functional activity in iron-deficient rats: behavioural correlates. *Ciba Found Symp* 1976; 51:201–225.

55. Heinonen EH, Lammintausta. A review of the pharamcology of selegiline. *Acta Neurol Scand* 1991; 84:44–59.

56. Kalaria RN, Mitchell MJ, Harik SI. Monoamine oxidases of the human brain and liver. *Brain* 1988; 111:1441–1451.

57. Arnett CD, Fowler JS, Macgregor RR, et al. Turnover of brain monoamine oxidase measure in vivo by positron emission tomography using L-(11C)deprenyl. *J Neurochem* 1987; 49:522–527.

58. Tipton KF, Fowlert CJ. In: Tipton KF, Dosteret P, Strolini Benedetti M, eds. *Monoamine Oxdiase and Disease*. London: Academic Press, 1984:27.

59. Zeller EA, Arora KL, Gurne DH, et al. In: Singer TP, Von Korff RW, Murphy DL, eds. *Monoamine Oxidase: Structure, Function, and Altered Functions*. New York: Academic, 1979:335.

60. Fowler CJ, Ross SB. Selective inhibitors of monoamine oxidase A and B: biochemical, pharmacological, and clinical properties. *Med Res Rev* 1984; 4:323–358.

61. Tipton KF, McCRodden JM, Kalir AS, et al. Inihibition of rat liver monoamine oxidase by alpha-methyl- and N-propargyl-amine derivatives. *Biochem Pharmacol* 1982; 31:1251–1255.

62. Ask AL, Hellstrom W, Norrman S, et al. Selective inhibition of the A form of monoamine oxidase by 4-dimethylamino-alpha-methylphenylalkylamine derivatives in the rat. *Neuropharmacology* 1982; 21:299–308

63. Fowler CJ, Strolin Benedetti M. Cimoxatone is a reversible tight-binding inhibitor of the A form of rat brain monoamine oxidase. *J Neurochem* 1983; 40:510–513.

64. Ogren SO, Ask AL, Holm AC, et al. In: Youdim MBH, Paykel ES, eds. Monoamine oxidase

inhibitors. The state of the art. Chichester: Wiley & Sons, 1981:103–112.

65. Keane PE, Kan JP, Sontag N, et al. Monoamine oxidase inhibition and brain amine metabolism after oral treatment with toloxatone in the rat. *J Pharm Pharmacol* 1979; 31:752–754.

66. Urbaneja M, Knowles CO. Formanilide inhibition of rat brain monoanmine oxidase. *Gen Pharmacol* 1979; 10:309–314.

67. Meyerson LR, McMurtrey KD, Davis VE. Neuro-amine-derived alkaloids: substrate-preferred inhibitors of rat brain monoamine oxidase in vitro. *Biochem Pharmacol* 1976; 25:1013–1020.

68. Suzuki O, Katsumata Y, Oya M, et al. Inhibition of type A and type B monoamine oxidase by naturally occurring xanthones. *Planta Med* 1981; 42:17–21.

69. Rovei V, Caille D, Curet O, et al. Biochemical pharmacology of befloxatone (MD 370503), a new potent reversible MAO-A inhibitor. *J Neural Transm* 1994; 339–347.

70. Waldmeier PC, Felner AE, Tipton KF. The mono-amine oxidase inhibiting properties of CGP 11305 A. *Eur J Pharmacol* 1983; 94:73–83.

71. Johnston JP. Some observations upon a new inhibitor of monoamine oxidase in brain tissue. *Biochem Pharmacol* 1968; 17:1285–1297.

72. Da Prada M, Keller HH, Schaffner R, et al. In: Kamijo K, Usdin E, Nagatsu T, eds. *Monoamine Oxidase: Basic and Clinical Frontiers.* Amsterdam: Excerpta Medica,1981:183.

73. Strolin Benedetti M, Destert P. Stereochemical aspects of MAO interactions: reversible and selective inhibitors of monoamine oxidase. *TIPS* 1985; 246–251.

74. Roth JA, Gillis CN. Deamination of beta-phenylethylamine by monoamine oxidase-inhibition by imipramine. *Biochem Pharmacol* 1974; 23:2537–2545.

75. Roth JA, Gillis CN. Some structural requirements for inhibition of type A and B forms of rabbit monoamine oxidase by tricyclic psychoactive drugs. *Mol Pharmacol* 1975; 11:28–35.

76. Edwards DJ, Change SS. Multiple forms of monoamine oxidase in rabbit platelets. *Life Sci* 1975; 17:1127–1134.

77. Dostert P, Strolin Benedetti M, Guffroy C. Different stereoselective inhibition of monoamine oxidase-B by the R- and S-enantiomers of MD 780236. *J Pharm Pharmacol* 1983; 335:161–165.

78. Henriot S, Kuhn C, Kettler R, et al. Lazabemide (Ro-19-6327), a reversible and highly sensitive MAO-B inhibitor: preclinical and clinical findings. *J Neural Transm Supp* 1994; 41:321–325.

79. Rohatagi S, Barrett JS, DeWitt KE, et al. Integrated pharamacokinetics and metabolic modeling of selegiline and metabolites after transdermal administration. *Biopharm Drug Dispos* 1997; 18:567–584.

80. Marley E, Blackwell B. Interactions of monoamine oxidase inhibitors, amines, and foodstuffs. *Adv Pharmacol Chemother* 1970; 8:186–239.

81. Knoll J, Vizi ES, Somogyi G. A phenyl-isopropyl-methylpropinylamine (E-250) tyraminantagonists hatasa. MTA V. *Oszt Kozl* 1967; 18:33–37.

82. Elsworth JD, Glover V, Reynolds GP. Deprenyl administration in man: A selective monoamine oxidase B inhibitor without the "cheese effect." *Psychopharmacology* 1978; 57:33–38.

83. Mahmood I, Marinac JS, Wilsie S, et al. Pharmacokinetics and relative bioavailability of selegiline in healthy volunteers. *Biopharm Drug Dispos* 1995; 16:535–545.

84. Szoko E, Kalasz H, Kerecsen L, et al. Binding of (-)-deprenyl to serum proteins. *Pol J Pharmacol Pharm* 1984; 36:413–421.

85. Kalasz H, Herescen L, Knoll J, Pucsok J. Chromatographic studies on the binding action and metabolism of (-)-deprenyl. *J Chromatogr* 1990; 499:589–599.

86. Benakis A. *Pharmacokinetic Study in Man of 14 C Jumex.* Study report, data on file, Framos Group Ltd Research Center, 1981.

87. Ahola R, Haapalinna A, Heinonen E, et al. Protection by L-deprenyl of intact peripheral sympathetic neurons exposed to neurotoxin 6-hydroxy-dopamine (6-OHDA). 11th Symposium of Parkinson's Disease, Rome, March 26–30, 1994. *New Trends Clin Neuropharamcol* 1994; 7:287.

88. Fowler JS, MacGregor RR, Wolf AP, et al. Mapping human brain monoamine oxidase A and B with 11C-labeled suicide inactivators and PET. *Science* 1987; 23:481–485.

89. Yoshida T, Yamada Y, Yamamoto T, et al. Metabolism of deprenyl, a selective monoamine oxidase (MAO) B inhibitor in rat: relationship of metabolism to MAO-B inhibitory potency. *Xenobiotica* 1986; 16:129–136.

90. Knoll J. R-(-)-deprenyl (selegiline, MoverganR) facilitates the activity of the nigrostriatal dopaminertic neuron. *J Neural Transm* 1987(Suppl 25):44–66.

91. Borbe HO, Neibich G, Nickel B. Kinetic evaluation of MAO-B activity following oral administration of selegiline and desmethyl-selegiline in rat. *J Neural Transm* 1990; 32:131–137.

92. Knoll J. The possible mechanism of action of (-)-deprenyl in Parkinson's disease. *J Neural Transm* 1978; 43:177–193.

93. Tipton KF. What is it that l-deprenyl (selegiline) might do? *Clin Pharmacol Ther* 1994; 56:781–796.

94. Zsilla G, Foldi P, Held G, et al. The effect of repeated doses of (-) deprenyl on the dynamics of monoaminergic transmission. Comparison with clorgyline. *Pol J Pharmacol Pharm* 1986; 38:57–67.

95. Salo PT, Tatton WG. Deprenyl reduces the death of motoneurons caused by axotomy. *J Neurosci Res* 1992; 31:394–400.

96. Bronzetti E, Felici L, Ferrante F, et al. Effect of ethylcholine mustard axiridium (AF64A) and of the

monoamine oxidase-B-inhibitor L-deprenyl on the morphology of rat hippocampus. *Int J Tissue React* 1992; 14:175–182.

97. Tatton WG, Seniuk NA. "Trophic-like" actions of (-)-deprenyl on neurons and astroglia. *Acad Biomed Drug Res* 1994; 7:238–248.

97a. Churchyard A, Mathias CJ, Lees AJ. Selegiline-induced postural hypotension in Parkinson's disease: A longitudinal study on the effects of drug withdrawal. *Mov Disord* 1999; 14:246–251.

98. Myllyla W, Sotaniemi K, Make-Ikola O, et al. Role of selegiline in combination therapy of Parkinson's disease. *Neurology* 1996; 47:200–209.

99. Waters CH. Side effects of selegiline (Eldepryl). *J Geriatr Psychiatry Neurol* 1992; 5:31–34.

100. Yahr MD, Mendoza MR, Moros D, et al. Treatment of Parkinson's disease in early and late phases: Use of pharmacological agents with special reference to deprenyl (selegiline). *Acta Neurol Scand* 1983; 95:95–102.

101. Elizan TS, Moros DA, Yahr MD. Early combination of selegiline and low-dose levodopa as initial symptomatic therapy in Parkinson's disease. *Arch Neurol* 1991; 48:31–34.

102. Golbe LI. Long-term efficacy and safety of deprenyl (selegiline) in advanced Parkinson's disease. *Neurology* 1989; 39:1109–1111.

103. Boyson SJ. Psychiatric effects of selegiline [letter]. *Arch Neurol* 1991; 48:902.

104. Menza MA, Golbe LI. Hypomania in a patient receiving deprenyl (selegiline) after adrenal-striatal implantation for Parkinson's disease. *Clin Neuropharmacol* 1988; 1:549–551.

105. Kurlan R, Dimitsopulos R. Selegiline and manic behavior in Parkinson's disease. *Arch Neurol* 1991; 48:31–34.

106. Zornberg GL, Bodkin JA, Cohen BM. Severe adverse interaction between pethidine and selegiline. *Lancet* 1991; 337:246.

107. Pare CMB, Mousawi MA, Sandler M, et al. Attempts to attenuate the "cheese effect." *J Affect Disord* 1989; 9:137–141.

108. Sternbach H. The serotonin syndrome. *Am J Psychiatry* 1991; 148:705–713.

109. Feigher JP, Boyer WF, Tyler DL, et al. Adverse consequences of fluoxetine-MAOI combination therapy. *J Clin Psychiatry* 1990; 51:222–225.

110. Waters CH. Fluoxetine and selegiline. *Can J Neurol Sci* 1994; 21:259–261.

111. Toyama SC, Iacono RP. Is it safe to combine a selective serotonin reuptake inhibitor with selegiline? *Ann Pharmacother* 1994; 28:405–406.

112. Richard I, Kurlan R, Tanner C et al. Serotonin syndrome and the combined use of deprenyl and an antidepressant in Parkinson's disease. Parkinson Study Group. *Neurology* 1997; 48:1070–1077.

113. Parkinson Study Group. Effects of tocopherol and deprenyl on the progression of disability on early Parkinson's disease. *N Engl J Med* 1993; 328:176–183.

114. Palhagen S, Heinonen EH, Hagglund J, et al. Selegiline delays the onset of disability in de novo parkinsonian patients. *Neurology* 1998; 51:520–525.

115. Allain H, Cougnard J, Neukirch HC. Selegiline in de novo parkinsonian patients: The French Selegiline Multicenter Trial. *Acta Neurol Scand Suppl* 1991; 136:73–78.

116. Tetrud JW, Langston JW. The effect of deprenyl (selegiline) on the natural history of Parkinson's disease. *Science* 1989; 245:519–522.

117. Myllyla VV, Sotaniemi KA, Vuorinen JA, et al. Selegiline in de novo parkinsonian patients: The Finnish study. *Mov Disord* 1993; 8(Suppl 1):41–44.

118. Olanow CW, Hauser RA, Gauger L, et al. The effect of deprenyl and levodopa on the progression of signs and symptoms in Parkinson's disease. *Ann Neurol* 1995; 38:771–777.

119. Parkinson Study Group. Impact of deprenyl and tocopherol treatment on Parkinson's disease in DATATOP subjects not requiring levodopa. *Ann Neurol* 1996; 39:29–36.

119a. Parkinson Study Group. Impact of deprenyl and tocopherol treatment on Parkinson's disease in DATATOP patients requiring levodopa. *Ann Neurol* 1996; 39:37–45.

120. Rinne UK, Siirtola T. Sonninen V. L-deprenyl treatment on 'on-off' phenomena in Parkinson's disease. *J Neural Transm* 1978; 43:253–262.

121. Sivertsen B, Dupont E, Mikkelsen B, et al. Selegiline and levodopa in early or moderately advanced Parkinson's disease: A double-blind controlled short- and long-term study. *Acta Neurol Scand Suppl* 1989; 126:147–152.

122. Heinonen EH, Rinne UK. Selegiline in the treatment of Parkinson's disease. *Acta Neurol Scand* 1989; 126:103–111.

123. Lees AJ. Current controversies in the use of selegiline hydrochloride. *J Neural Transm* 1987; 25:157–162.

124. Golbe LI, Lieberman AN, Muenter MD, et al. Deprenyl in the treatment of symptom fluctuations in advanced Parkinson's disease. *Clin Neuropharmacol* 1988; 11:45–55.

125. Lees AJ. Parkinson's Disease Research Group of the United Kingdom. Comparison of therapeutic effects and mortality data of levodopa and levodopa combined with selegiline in patients with early, mild Parkinson's disease. *BMJ* 1995; 311:1602–1607.

126. Olanow CW, Fahn S, Langston JW, et al. Selegiline and mortality: A point of view. *Ann Neurol* 1996; 40:841–845.

127. The Parkinson Study Group. Mortality in DATATOP: A multicenter trial in early Parkinson's disease. *Ann Neurol* 1998; 43:318–325.

128. Hauser RA, Stern MC, Olanow CW, et al. Tolerability and safety of transdermal selegiline monotherapy in mild to moderate Parkinson's disease. *Mov Disord* 1998; 13:256.

129. Finberg JP, Takeshima T, Johnston JM, et al. Increased survival of dopaminergic neurons by rasagiline, a monoamine oxidase B inhibitor. *Neuroreport* 1998; 9:703–707.

129a. Marek K, Friedman J, Hauser R, et al. Phase II evaluation of rasagiline mesylate (TVP-1012), a novel anti-parkinsonian drug in parkinsonian patients not using levodopa/carbidopa. *Mov Disord* 1997; 12:838–839.

130. The Parkinson Study Group. A controlled trial of lazabemide (Ro 19–6327) in untreated Parkinson's disease. *Ann Neurol* 1993; 33:350–356.

131. Dingemanse J, Wood N, Jorga K et al. Pharmacokinetics and pharmacodynamics of single and multiple doses of the MAO-B inhibitor lazabemide in healthy subjects. *Brit J Clin Pharmacol* 1997; 43:41–47.

132. Carruba MO, Picotti GB, Miodini JP, et al. Blood sampling by chronic cannulation technique for reliable measurements of catecholamines and other hormones in plasma of conscious rats. *J Pharmacol Meth* 1981; 5:292–303.

133. The Parkinson Study Group. Effect of lazabemide on the progression of disability in early Parkinson's disease. *Ann Neurol* 1996; 40:99–107.

134. The Parkinson Study Group. A controlled trial of lazabemide (Ro19–6327) in levodopa-treated Parkinson's disease. *Arch Neurol* 1994; 51:342–347.

35

Dopamine Agonists

Puiu F. Nisipeanu

Department of Neurology, Hill Yaffe Hospital, Hadera

and

Amos D. Korczyn

Sackler Faculty of Medicine, Tel-Aviv University Medical School, Ramat-Aviv, Israel

Although levodopa affords considerable symptomatic benefit in Parkinson's disease (PD), it obviously does not prevent the continuous progression of the disease, and its long-term use is associated with complex motor and psychiatric complications. Additionally, the unresolved debate concerning levodopa neurotoxicity (see Chapter 32) helped to generate a variety of therapeutic strategies devoted to manage these complications including delaying or reducing the use of levodopa (1,2).

During the last few years a number of drugs, belonging to different classes and operating through different mechanisms, have been shown to be useful in PD. New dopaminergic agonists, selegiline, and catechol-O-methyltransferase (COMT) inhibitors were found to be effective as monotherapy or as an adjunct to levodopa offering more nuanced choices. Therapeutic decisions need to be correlated with disease severity, patient age, concurrent morbidity and concomitant medication, expectations, and individual needs.

Two important facts emerged during the last decades that contributed to the understanding of the role of dopamine in motor behavior and in parkinsonism:

1. Dopamine interacts with different receptors, grouped into 2 families, D_{1A}, D_{1B}, and D_{1C} (the D_1 family) and D_2, D_3, D_4 (the D_2 family), on the basis of their molecular homology and relation to the common second messenger cAMP (3).
2. The anti-parkinsonian efficacy is principally derived from stimulation of D_2 receptors and perhaps D_3 and D_4 receptors.

Unlike dopamine itself, which is a full agonist of both D_1 and D_2 receptors, most dopamine agonists (DAA) are not fully effective in activating even D_2 receptors, (Table 35-1). These drugs demonstrate their maximal efficacy in vitro, or on denervated receptors. However, in situations of greater clinical relevance, they will compete with endogenous dopamine and may prevent it from exhibiting its full effect. Because of their cumbersome structure they may attach themselves to the receptors for longer periods than dopamine, thus possibly manifesting functional antagonistic properties. The functional outcome depends on the amount of dopamine (either endogenous or derived from levodopa) compared to that of the specific DAA and its relative potency. Theoretically, a higher dose of DAA may be required to achieve its full effect in the presence of endogenous dopamine.

The distribution of dopamine receptors in the CNS extends well beyond the basal ganglia, and also includes the nucleus accumbens, hypothalamus, pituitary, hippocampus, frontal cortex, olfactory tubercle, the brain stem and the spinal cord (4). Administration of DAA may activate these receptors as well, thus accounting for some of the frequent side effects of the drugs, including psychiatric manifestations, somnolence, nausea, and hormonal changes. In addition, effects on dopamine receptors outside the CNS may contribute to some cardiovascular effects (mainly hypotension) and nausea. Finally, older DAA are not selective to dopamine receptors and some of the side effects can perhaps be accounted for by interaction with other receptors, particularly serotonergic.

DAA represent the most efficacious therapy for PD after levodopa. It is remarkable to note that the first studies with DAA, using apomorphine (5,6) and bromocriptine (7) despite small patient numbers and

Table 35-1 Selected Pharmacodynamic Characteristics of Dopamine Agonists

Drug	Class	Dopamine Receptors Activity		Other Receptors Activity	
		D_1 (D_1, D_5)	D_2 (D_2, D_3, D_4)	$5HT_{1/2}$	$\alpha_{1/2}$
Bromocriptine	Ergot	Antagonist	Moderate–marked agonist	Agonist	Agonist
Pergolide	Ergot	Agonist	Marked agonist	Agonist	Agonist
Lisuride	Ergot	Variable	Marked agonist	Agonist	None
Cabergoline	Ergot	Very weak agonist	Marked agonist	None	None
Ropinirole	Non-Ergot	None	Marked agonist (D_3>D_2)	None	None
Pramipexole	Non-Ergot	None	Marked agonist (D_3>D_2)	None	Moderate agonist
Apomorphine	Non-Ergot	Weak agonist	Marked agonist	None	None

short treatment durations established their efficacy and potential usefulness. These results were to be confirmed later in larger trials. Numerous dopaminergic agents have been examined in the treatment of patients with parkinsonism. Their development follows a classic sequence: (1) capability to elicit dopaminomimetic effects on the neuroendocrine system; (2) ability to bind to different dopamine receptors in vitro; (3) to show dopamine-like action on animals and to reverse parkinsonism in experimental models; (4) human studies in PD.

DAA possess pharmacokinetic and pharmacodynamic qualities, which at least in theory are advantageous over levodopa. First, they act directly on dopamine receptors and thus bypass the need for conversion and storage in nigrostriatal neurons. Also, they do not depend (as does levodopa) on amino acid transporters for absorption across the gastrointestinal tract and the blood-brain barrier and consequently may be taken with meals. Their metabolism in the liver is much more limited than that of levodopa and thus the hepatic first pass effect is minimal. Consequently, most of them have much longer half-lives than levodopa and provide more continuous dopaminergic stimulation. Some exhibit low protein-binding, thus limiting the possibility of pharmacokinetic interactions with other drugs, and none adversely interferes with levodopa pharmacokinetics. Because of the diverse dopaminergic receptor specificity of DAA, some may act more selectively on one subtype, which possibly offers a higher therapeutic index, and possibly diminishes some side effects (Table 35-1). Finally, the expense of DAA treatment may be higher than that of levodopa at equivalent dosages, although, interestingly, the newer DAA are not necessarily the most expensive.

However, with the possible exception of apomorphine, even the newest DAA are less efficacious than levodopa, particularly in patients with more severe disease. Moreover, as the treatment is usually initiated at low dosage and the titration period may be prolonged for weeks or months to improve compliance until tolerance to the peripheral side effects develops, improvement is usually delayed. It may take longer to discover the responding patients and the adequate daily dose. In addition to having lower potency, DAA are less well tolerated than levodopa, with a higher occurrence of adverse events, mainly hallucinations and confusion, which together contribute to higher dropout rates among DAA treated patients.

A substantial proportion of patients initially treated with DAA will need levodopa supplementation within a few months or years. This is partly because of poor tolerability to higher DAA doses, but may also reflect the belief that DAA are less efficacious. However, some patients can benefit from DAA monotherapy for considerably longer periods. Even if levodopa is added, the reduced dose requirement may decrease the incidence of side effects, particularly dyskinesias.

The fact that levodopa requires activation by metabolic conversion to dopamine can explain its limitations in advanced disease, when dopaminergic terminals have largely degenerated. It could then be expected that DAA, which act directly at dopamine receptors, would be particularly useful in advanced disease. Unfortunately, this is not the case, and patients with advanced PD still require levodopa and cannot be treated with DAA monotherapy. The reason for this is not clear, but it has been speculated that to achieve maximal efficacy, D_2 and D_1 receptors need to be activated (8). Most DAA are not able to provide this stimulation, and endogenous dopamine may be required. As the disease progresses, endogenous dopamine is depleted but can be replaced by dopamine derived from conversion of exogenous levodopa by nondopaminergic cells.

PROTECTIVE EFFECTS OF DOPAMINE AGONISTS

Over the years, a notion has emerged that DAA may provide "neuroprotection" (9), that is, slow the progression of the neuronal degeneration in PD (10). Although this assumption has only limited experimental support and no clinical support, it may still be useful to review its theoretical basis.

Although the pathogenesis of PD is not clear, a neurotoxic theory has gained acceptance, implying damage to dopaminergic neurons by oxidative species generated in the breakdown of dopamine (see Chapter 28). According to this theory, excessive turnover of dopamine may lead to neurodegeneration (presumably by metabolism by intraneuronal MAO to toxic oxygen species). DAA may decrease this turnover by two mechanisms. First, stimulation of presynaptic DA receptors on dopaminergic cell bodies and terminals may inhibit the firing and release of dopamine, and thus indirectly reduce its turnover. Second, the use of DAA in parkinsonism will decrease levodopa consumption (levodopa sparing effect) and thus prevent oxidation of the drug within dopaminergic neurons.

Clinical evidence for a neuroprotective influence of DAA is meager. The development of novel sensitive tests to assess the amount of disease progression such as striatal fluorodopa uptake on PET or SPECT scans in conjunction with clinical findings may provide the opportunity to verify putative neuroprotection. In an ongoing five-year, double-blind study 45 early PD patients, started on either ropinirole or levodopa, were scanned (PET) at baseline approximately two years later (11). Preliminary results, available from a small number of these patients, showed a trend (nonsignificant) toward relative sparing of dopamine terminals in the ropinirole group. This trend became significant in the subgroup of patients with less than two years disease duration. It is premature to make any definitive conclusions from this study at this time. Other trials evaluating other DAA and their putative neuroprotection are under way.

ADVERSE EFFECTS OF DOPAMINE AGONISTS

Because DAA differ from each other in structure and in some pharmacologic properties, which include effects on nondopaminergic receptors (Table 35-1), it is reasonable to assume that they will have distinctive adverse effects profile. However, ergot and nonergot

DAA share a variety of peripheral and central adverse effects (12).

The most common "peripheral" dopaminergic adverse effects are nausea, vomiting, and orthostatic hypotension, each having a mixed peripheral and central component. These adverse effects are dose- and time-dependent, being particularly prevalent during therapy initiation, and tend to diminish or disappear over weeks as peripheral tolerance develops. Nausea and vomiting result from direct dopamine stimulation of chemoreceptors in the area postrema, which lacks a blood-brain barrier (BBB). Orthostatic hypotension is probably due to both central and peripheral dopaminergic effects. Both effects can potentially be blocked by dopamine antagonists, but these may cause parkinsonism to become more severe. Domperidone, a D_2-receptor antagonist, which does not cross the BBB is very helpful in this situation (13).

Central dopaminergic adverse effects are dominated by psychiatric symptomatology, with a spectrum similar to that seen with levodopa (14). However, DAA induce psychiatric side effects more commonly than levodopa does, particularly in patients with advanced disease. The variety of psychiatric manifestations include mood disturbances (depression, irritability, euphoria, hypomania), vivid dreams, nightmares, sleep difficulties, inappropriate sexual behavior, benign hallucinations (i.e., with retained insight), hallucinations (visual, rarely auditory or tactile), delusions, agitation, confusion, and paranoid psychosis. Their occurrence varies in different studies, but is generally dose-dependent and is more common following longer treatment. The higher potential of DAA to induce serious psychiatric adverse effects in patients with a psychiatric history (usually not included in therapeutic trials), in the elderly or in cognitively impaired patients imposes a particular problem. Notably, the early presence of visual hallucinations, especially when associated with fluctuations in mental status and cognitive dysfunction, in older patients with mild parkinsonian symptoms and lack of tremor, suggests a diagnosis of dementia with Lewy bodies (15). See Chapter 16.

These psychiatric side effects usually occur in the context of treatment of PD patients; interestingly, when used for galactorrhea they are rarely seen, either because of the dose and duration of treatment or the age of the patients. It is possible that the pathology of PD predisposes patients to develop psychotic manifestations.

Psychotic symptoms occur with DAA monotherapy and when combined with levodopa. The psychotic manifestations may occur on the background of clear consciousness (i.e., be "schizophreniform"), or on a background of confusion (i.e., fulfilling diagnostic criteria for drug-induced delirium).

The psychotic manifestations will sometimes disappear following lowering of the DAA or of levodopa (if given concurrently) (16), although it is not uncommon for antipsychotic therapy to be required for years. However, drug withdrawal is frequently impractical because the patients' motor condition usually deteriorates. The same objection applies to treatment with typical neuroleptic drugs such as trifluoperazine (17) or haloperidol. Newer, so-called "atypical" antipsychotics are superior because these will not jeopardize the parkinsonian state of the patient (see Chapters 37, 42). Low-dose clozapine treatment has been demonstrated to be the most effective of these drugs so far (18,19).

Bromocriptine and other ergot derivative–induced psychotic manifestations were initially attributed to serotonergic effects because of their similarity to the effects of LSD. The fact that levodopa could induce similar reactions has been explained by the assumption that levodopa was taken up by serotonergic terminals, converted to dopamine and released. However, the fact that identical manifestations occur with selective D_2 agonists such as pramipexole and ropinirole substantiates the dopaminergic nature of these effects (also supported by the fact that they can be antagonized with selective dopamine blockers). It is customary to associate bromocriptine psychosis with action on limbic dopamine receptors. However, the demonstration that the striatum also subserves mental functions suggests an alternative hypothesis.

Ergot derivatives were associated with pleuropulmonary, pericardial, and retroperitoneal inflammatory-fibrotic pathology (12,20,21). As bromocriptine was the first DAA and the most widely used, most cases with these reactions were described in bromocriptine-treated patients and only occasionally as a result of treatment with pergolide, lisuride, cabergoline, and mesulergine (22,23). Pleuropulmonary fibrosis is the most frequent, with a reported prevalence of 2 to 5% at five years (24). Whether this complication is specific to ergot derivatives is a matter of debate as there has been one case reported with the nonergot ropinirole (25).

Other uncommon but potentially serious side effects related to the ergot vasoconstrictive properties are Raynaud's phenomenon, livedo reticularis, erythromelalgia, and possibly exacerbation of angina pectoris.

Peripheral edema, which is common in PD, has also been observed in patients treated with DAA more frequently than in parallel groups treated with placebo. The mechanism is not clear but the phenomenon is not limited to ergot derivatives.

Other reactions, which are common to all DAA, consist of reduction of anterior pituitary hormone secretion, particularly prolactin. This effect is used therapeutically in the treatment of hyperprolactinemia and prolactinomas.

Data on the safety of DAA are largely derived from controlled drug studies. These usually included well over 1,000 patients and are likely to have identified the most common adverse events but not necessarily those with a frequency of 0.1% or less, such as idiosyncratic events. More importantly, these studies excluded patients with severe comorbidity, and therefore data on the safety of DAA are limited for patients with such disorders as severe coronary artery disease, active peptic ulcer, or a history of psychotic events or epilepsy, and data on possible interactions with drugs commonly used in these conditions are also meager. By the same token, data on teratogenicity are limited. Nevertheless, it should be stressed that except for fibrosis, life-threatening reactions have not been reported by any of the DAA.

DRUG INTERACTIONS

The most obvious drug interactions are those with other drugs acting on dopamine receptors, either as agonists or as antagonists. Antihypertensive drugs could potentially enhance the tendency to hypotension and syncope. Paradoxically, severe hypertension has been reported to occur in women taking ergot derivatives during pregnancy or in the puerperium.

Macrolide antibiotics, such as erythromycin, may increase the bioavailability of ergot derivatives.

Ropinirole is metabolized by the cytochrome P450 enzyme, CYP1A2, thus allowing a potential interaction with other drugs using this enzyme. Indeed, ciprofloxacin, which inhibits the enzyme, was found to increase serum levels of ropinirole. There is no pharmacokinetic interaction at steady state between levodopa and ropinirole (26).

APOMORPHINE

Apomorphine hydrochloride, a nonaddictive derivative of morphine, was the first DAA ever used in PD (5). It has a unique structure and had been employed for several decades in medicine because of its emetic properties. This effect is shared by all DAA, but because apomorphine can be injected, this effect is fast, short-lived, and more pronounced. Presently apomorphine is being used together with the peripheral dopamine receptor antagonists domperidone and, in the United States, trimethobenzamide, which prevents many of these reactions.

Because of its sedative properties, apomorphine was first used in Sydenham's chorea by Weill (27), who suggested that it may be of value in PD. This was ultimately demonstrated by Schwab and coworkers (5), who, by injecting apomorphine, produced a short but striking improvement of tremor and rigidity. These findings lay dormant for over 20 years, until Cotzias and coworkers (6) showed in a double-blind, placebo-controlled study that apomorphine injected subcutaneously improved extrapyramidal features in parkinsonian patients chronically treated with levodopa. This improvement started shortly after the injection, became maximal at 30'–60' and dissipated after approximately two hours. Unfortunately, patients experienced disturbing side effects including drowsiness, nausea, vomiting, hypotension, bradycardia, and syncope. The capability of apomorphine to reverse akinetic "off" periods in fluctuating patients, observed by Cotzias and coworkers was amply confirmed later in double-blind and open-label studies (28,29). The efficacy of apomorphine in reducing time spent "off" is usually maintained for many years. Patients with biphasic dyskinesias may be helped by using intermittent injections.

Another suggested use of apomorphine is in differentiating PD from other Parkinsonian syndromes. PD is essentially a "presynaptic" disorder, whereas "Parkinson plus" syndromes (PSP, MSA, CBGD,) include a significant postsynaptic component. The clinical diagnosis of these disorders is not always easy (30). Of course, the loss of a large number of postsynaptic elements (striatal neurons and/or dopamine receptors) does not preclude the possibility that DAA will have an effect (e.g., the efficacy of cholinesterase inhibitors in myasthenia gravis), but this efficacy will decrease as the postsynaptic changes advance. Therefore, DAA could theoretically be used as a diagnostic aid. In particular, apomorphine injection has been proposed as an ideal agent for this purpose (31).

The first attempt to answer this question was to test patients with a clear diagnosis (PD or other parkinsonian syndromes), but the more relevant information will come from patients with parkinsonism of unclear etiology who would be followed up until the diagnosis is clear. Although this has not yet been performed, even the preliminary data from those whose diagnosis is clear have not been promising. The apomorphine test was positive in nearly 20 percent of patients with "parkinsonism plus" syndromes, which indicates that it represents a test of dopaminergic responsiveness rather than one specific for PD (32).

Apomorphine is rapidly and completely absorbed following subcutaneous administration, reaching rapid equilibrium between plasma and brain (33). The onset of action is also rapid (<20') and the duration is variable correlated with the apomorphine dose, but typically quite shorter than that of levodopa. This duration is shortened with disease progression and a steepening of the dose–response relation may also occur (34). Special prefilled "penject" syringes for intermittent bolus injection or minipumps for continuous subcutaneous infusion are available, but the quality of response was almost identical (35). The primary use in advanced PD patients is as "rescue" therapy from "off" periods that are intractable. The bolus injections are easier and better tolerated than the continuous infusion. Some studies suggested that intermittent injection be used up to 10 times per day. If more than that is required, they should be switched to continuous infusion (25).

Another indication for apomorphine is replacing oral levodopa in the preoperative management of parkinsonian patients undergoing abdominal surgery (36). In addition, timely injection of apomorphine may ameliorate swallowing problems, off-period belching, off-pain and painful dystonia, and perhaps constipation, anismus, adynamic bowel, and neurogenic hyperreflexic bladder (37).

Other routes of administration are currently being evaluated for apomorphine. The sublingual use of apomorphine tablets is followed by a motor response of a magnitude identical to the subcutaneous route, although with a longer latency (20'–40'). Intranasally administered apomorphine is also effective, with a latency of effect and duration almost identical to those obtained by injecting apomorphine (38). Rectal administration of apomorphine suppositories, however, produces poor effects.

Side Effects

The most common side effects of apomorphine, similar to those of other DAA, consist of nausea, vomiting, and hypotension, which can be prevented by earlier and concomitant administration of domperidone. Many patients will be able to discontinue domperidone after weeks or months because of the development of tolerance to the peripheral side effects. Neuropsychiatric complications increasingly occur with long-term apomorphine treatment, but they may be less common than with other DAA, perhaps related to its short duration of action. A stereotyped pattern consisting of unjustified increase of daily injections, severely disturbed sexual behavior, and finally, acute psychomotor agitation was recently reported, suggesting that a psychologic dependence may occur (39).

Other rare or exceptional complications included transient Coombs' positive autoimmune hemolytic anemia, leg edema, transient atrial fibrillation, cardiac arrest, penile erections, and precipitation of migraine attacks in migrainous parkinsonians. The onset of yawning often heralds the effect of the drug. The benefit of apomorphine is marred in most patients by the development of local reactions: small nodules at injection sites, severe stomatitis, nasal vestibulitis, a disagreeable burning feeling, or transient nasal obstruction after intranasal administration. Ulcerations and necrosis with subsequent abdominal wall scarring at injection sites are often attributed to poor hygiene practice (37,28,29). The cutaneous reactions are more common with continuous infusion than with intermitted injection.

BROMOCRIPTINE

Bromocriptine (2-Br-α-ergocryptine) was the first dopamine receptor agonist licensed for the treatment of PD. The mean dosage in the original paper of Calne and coworkers (7) was 18.8 mg/day. Shortly thereafter, much higher doses (mean daily dose 79 mg) were employed (40), which led to a significant reduction in levodopa ("dopa sparing effect") and improvement of many parkinsonian features (40).

Starting with a low dose (1 mg/day) a slow escalation allows increased tolerability (41). Again, the association with a peripheral dopaminergic blocking drug, domperidone, prevents many undesirable side effects (13).

Clinical Studies in Early Parkinson's Disease

Few trials rigorously evaluated bromocriptine use in levodopa-naive patients. However, several trials have been reported in this situation. Some of the studies were open-label, some were double-blind, placebo-controlled trials that were of short duration, and some were open-label or double-blind evaluations of bromocriptine monotherapy versus low-dose levodopa monotherapy (42–47). The results of these studies demonstrated that bromocriptine was superior to placebo in improving early symptoms but was inferior to levodopa, providing modest effects in milder patients. A substantial proportion of patients on bromocriptine monotherapy (approximately 30%) had lack of efficacy with treatment, and a larger proportion of patients had to drop out because of acute side effects such as nausea, orthostatic hypotension, and confusion. In one particular parallel group trial, levodopa was more effective than bromocriptine (48). One important conclusion derived from this trial and supported by Montastruc and coworkers was that bromocriptine induced less dyskinesia or wearing off (44,49). However, since relatively few patients were

able to tolerate high doses for long periods [some studies even suggested that it was only three to six months (50)], the use of bromocriptine as a first-line drug was abandoned. These conclusions were supported by more recent studies (42,51,52).

Based on these findings related to diminished fluctuations, Rinne performed an uncontrolled, nonrandomized study involving 76 patients treated with bromocriptine monotherapy (50). Those patients who tolerated this therapy continued while the majority added levodopa and both groups were compared with a historical control group of 217 patients receiving levodopa monotherapy. Results of this study showed that combined therapy of bromocriptine and low-dose levodopa had an efficacy equal to that achieved by higher doses of levodopa and induced substantially fewer motor fluctuations and dyskinesias after a five-year follow-up (50). Early combination therapy became the recommended therapy by many for early disease. His work, however, was criticized (53,54) because of its open-label, nonrandomized design. Several studies were initiated in an attempt to verify the results of Rinne. One supportive study was reported by Rascol and coworkers (55) in an abstract. These authors presented the results of a prospective open-label trial in which 240 PD patients were randomized to receive either levodopa monotherapy or levodopa plus bromocriptine. After five years of follow-up there was no significant levodopa-sparing effect. However, they did find that there was a 208-day (15%) delay in the onset of fluctuations in the combination group which was statistically significant and that the total number of late motor complications was reduced by one-third in the combination group. A large number of dropouts may have affected the outcome. One other small study, which supported early combination therapy, randomized in an open fashion 31 patients to receive high-dose bromocriptine therapy to which levodopa was later added (approximately three years later) and 29 patients to receive levodopa alone (49). There was no difference in efficacy between the two groups, and at the end of five years there was no difference in the incidence of wearing-off phenomenon in the two groups, although in the combination group wearing-off may have been delayed. However, there was a difference in peak dose dyskinesias which occurred later and less frequently in the combination group than in the levodopa group. The authors concluded that high doses of bromocriptine monotherapy for the first three years delayed the occurrence of motor fluctuations and dyskinesia when compared with levodopa monotherapy from the start. Several other trials did not demonstrate superior efficacy with this treatment strategy (42,45–47,56,57). Of interest is that three of these were double-blind studies. Most of these trials were unable to confirm Rinne's results, but it must be emphasized that both the supportive studies and the majority of the negative studies were performed with evident methodological flaws, such as an unblinded treatment or a small number of patients, making firm conclusion difficult.

Bromocriptine in Advanced Parkinson's Disease

Numerous open and double-blind trials (58) confirmed the results of the pioneering study of Calne and coworkers (7). This improvement occurred in 60 percent of patients and was expressed by improvement in all manifestations of "off" phenomenon – frequency, severity, duration, and diminished dyskinesias subsequent to reduction of levodopa dosage. Bromocriptine was found to prolong the duration of levodopa action in patients with motor fluctuations. There were a significant number of withdrawals usually related to adverse events. Most of these studies were carried out before 1985 in over 500 patients. As the result of methodological differences, these studies are difficult to compare with studies of newer agents. There has been one recent study using modern methods that is worth further discussion. Guttman and coworkers (59) compared bromocriptine to placebo as adjunctive therapy in advanced PD patients with motor fluctuations. In this multicenter, double-blind, parallel-group study, patients were randomized to receive pramipexole, bromocriptine, or placebo. The study was powered to compare each agonist with placebo, not with each other. There were 84 patients randomized to bromocriptine, and an average dose of 22.6 mg/day was used after nine months of therapy. There was a 14 percent improvement in the activities of daily living score and 23.8 percent improvement in motor score (Parts II and III in the UPDRS score) and both were significantly better than placebo. In addition, there was a 29.7 percent improvement in percent off time per day. This study confirmed the results of the earlier trials.

PERGOLIDE

Pergolide mesylate (8-beta-methyl-thiomethyl-6-N-propylegoline), a semisynthetic ergoline compound, is a dopaminergic agonist with dose-dependent D_2/D_1 activities: selective D_2 agonist stimulation at low dose, mixed with D_1 agonism at higher doses (60). Pergolide has a high affinity for the presynaptic D_2 autoreceptor at low doses. It was approved for use in 1989. On a mg basis, this drug is approximately 10 percent more potent than bromocriptine. It has a much longer half-life, up to 27 hours.

Clinical Studies in Early PD

A few trials investigated the efficacy of pergolide in de novo PD patients (61–63), and these included relatively small numbers of patients, most of whom could not be maintained on monotherapy for more than one year, partly because of the frequent gastrointestinal and psychiatric side effects. Also, levodopa was required in approximately half because of inadequate symptom control. In those who tolerated the drug, however, dyskinesias, wearing off, or motor fluctuations were rarely recorded and motor examination improved. The first well-controlled trial in early patients was reported in 1999. Barone and coworkers (64) reported the results of a multicenter, placebo-controlled, parallel-group, randomized 12-week trial. Of the 105 patients enrolled, 53 patients received pergolide and 52 patients received placebo. Twelve patients had previously received levodopa. Patients were initiated on 0.05 mg per day and over the first three weeks followed a fixed titration to 0.25 three times a day. Thereafter increases in dosage were at the discretion of the investigators. Forty-six placebo subjects and 44 pergolide subjects completed the full study. The mean pergolide dose at final visit was 2.06 mg per day. The primary end point was the percentage of patients who fulfilled criteria for responder status, defined as more than 30 percent improvement in the motor portion of the UPDRS. This was seen in 56.6 percent of the pergolide subjects and only 17.3 percent of those receiving placebo (p < 0.001). There were also significant differences between groups with regard to decrease in UPDRS total, Part II (ADL) and Part III (motor exam scores). The most prominent adverse events were nausea (32.1%), somnolence (15.1%; not significantly different from placebo, which was 5.8%), dizziness (13.2%), and insomnia and vomiting (both 9.4%).

Pergolide in Advanced Disease

A multicenter, double-blind, placebo-controlled pivotal trial demonstrated the effectiveness of pergolide as add-on to levodopa in advanced PD and demonstrated a significant levodopa-sparing effect (65). The efficacy of pergolide was significant in almost all clinical measures of these patients with advanced disease. That study involved 16 centers and was of 24 weeks duration. One hundred and eighty-nine patients were randomized to pergolide, 187 to placebo and approximately 30 subjects dropped out in each group. The mean final dose was 2.94 mg per day and patients reduced their mean levodopa dose by approximately 25 percent (235 mg/day) versus only 5 percent in control group. There was a decrease in percent "off" time per day of 32 percent, which translated to approximately two hours decrease in "off" time per day. With the Columbia PD scale there was a 35 percent decrease in the motor portion and a 30 percent decrease in activities of daily living. Total PD score was decreased by greater than 25 percent in 56 percent of the pergolide treated patients and 25 percent of the controls. The most common adverse events reported in this study were an increase in dyskinesia (62% vs. 25% in placebo group); nausea (24%); hallucinations (14%), which were the most troubling of all adverse events; drowsiness (10%); and insomnia (8%). With regard to the dyskinesia, the lowering of levodopa dose led to a decrease of dyskinesia, and in the end there was no significant difference between the treatment group and controls. This study demonstrated clear efficacy of pergolide as an adjunct to levodopa in the treatment of advanced PD. There had been seven other smaller double-blind trials published between 1985 and 1988 which examined 162 patients with a usual duration of treatment was 24 to 26 weeks and several open-label trials examining over 100 patients. Short-term trials demonstrated results that were similar to those seen in the double-blind studies, and long-term effects of pergolide in advanced PD patients have also been examined in trials lasting up to seven years. The results were similar to the work of Olanow and coworkers (65), with improvement being maintained in some studies for at least four years. For more detailed review, see Factor (25).

Side Effects

In addition to the usual reactions to DAA, the use of pergolide in older patients with advanced PD was suspected to be associated with cardiotoxicity and led to a temporary suspension of clinical trials. Subsequent studies did not support a deleterious cardiac effect of pergolide (66,67). Nevertheless, it is frequently suggested that patients prone to cardiac dysrhythmias may need closer monitoring. Those with unstable or serious cardiac disease were excluded from recent trials, so safety data on these patients are meager. Other rare side effects were erythematous swelling of legs, leukopenia, and elevation of aspartate aminotransferase.

LISURIDE

Lisuride, 3-(9,10-didehydro 6 methyl -8α-ergolinyl)-1,1-diethyl urea) hydrogen maleate is a semisynthetic ergot derivative, unique because it is effective at such low doses that efficacious concentrations of lisuride can be dissolved in water and used in intravenous (i.v) or subcutaneous (s.c) administration (68). Lisuride is

a full agonist with high affinity to the D_2 receptors but also has high affinity for serotonin receptors and a duration of action of 1 to 3 hours. An increase in body weight and reduced recurrence rates of migraine attacks were attributed to its serotoninergic activity (69).

Clinical Studies in Early Parkinson's Disease

Rinne (70) conducted an open label, randomized, parallel group trial in 90 de novo PD patients never treated with levodopa. Patients were allocated to receive lisuride, levodopa, or lisuride and levodopa from the beginning. A follow-up at four years demonstrated that lisuride had a long-term benefit for a small proportion of patients, with only 17 percent of patients maintained on monotherapy and that its antiparkinsonian efficacy was significantly lower than that of levodopa. Nevertheless, none of the five patients maintained on lisuride for four years exhibited wearing-off or dyskinesias, and those with early combination of lisuride and levodopa had significantly fewer motor fluctuations and dyskinesias than patients on levodopa monotherapy.

Lisuride as Add-on to Levodopa

Studies performed in the early 1980s, some of them double-blind versus placebo or in comparison to bromocriptine, demonstrated a significant clinical improvement and a levodopa-sparing effect by lisuride (71). It was found to be superior to bromocriptine. Comparison of oral lisuride in combination with levodopa versus only levodopa in patients with increased motor disability and marked fluctuations showed antiparkinsonian efficacy, as well as statistically significant reduction in "off" time and less dyskinesias (72).

Lisuride was used in parenteral administration, subcutaneous injections, and especially subcutaneous infusions to counteract disabling motor fluctuations and dyskinesias. The round-the-clock infusion of lisuride dramatically prolonged the antiparkinsonian effect of levodopa and widened its therapeutic window, supporting the view that continuous dopamine replacement greatly eliminates motor fluctuations and peak-dose dyskinesias. Marked reduction of "off" hours was achieved and sustained for many months. This effect occurred at doses of 0.5 to 8 mg/day. However, this improvement was later followed in most patients by dyskinesias and "off" periods difficult to control. A major disadvantage was the frequent occurrence of psychiatric side effects, especially severe psychosis in up to one-third of patients. Injection site nodules developed in every patient (73,74).

The manufacturer opted to terminate the development of lisuride pumps, and presently only apomorphine is widely available for parenteral administration in severely fluctuating patients.

CABERGOLINE

Cabergoline, 1-[(6-alleylergolin-8β-yl) carbonyl]-1-[3-dimethylamino) propyl]-3- ethylurea is a long-acting orally administered D_2 agonist that, because of its very long elimination half-life (65 to 110 hours), may be given once a day (75) or even on alternate days. However, the overall benefit of this property is still uncertain (60), although it may be useful to patients with nocturnal fluctuations, especially dystonic pain, nocturnal awakenings, and early morning dystonia.

Cabergoline was one of the most widely investigated antiparkinsonian dopaminergic agonists as approximately 4,000 patients were exposed to it before marketing (76).

Clinical Studies in Early Parkinson's Disease

Cabergoline alone or in early combination with levodopa decreases significantly the risk of motor complications. Approximately one-third of patients remained on monotherapy for almost four years (77).

Cabergoline as Adjunct to Levodopa

The efficacy of carbergoline as adjunct to levodopa has been suggested in numerous open and controlled studies in the last decade (78–82) demonstrating a levodopa sparing effect of cabergoline (decreased levodopa dose of 20%) improvement on ADL and motor examination scores (decreased by 20% and 15%, respectively) and reduction in "off"-time using a median daily dose of 3.5 mg. Improvement was maintained for two years in one-third of the patients. The effectiveness was similar to that found with bromocriptine.

Tolerability

Cabergoline-associated adverse events did not differ essentially from those of other dopaminergic agonists (67). Pleuropulmonary changes occurred in 3.4 percent after at least one year. Although this figure is considerably higher than reported for other DAA, it was based on chest skiagrams that were performed at baseline and every six months. Recently, constrictive pericarditis and later pleuropulmonary fibrosis were reported in a former smoker, receiving 10 mg cabergoline daily for more than one year (18). The drug has been marketed in Europe for PD but not in the United States. It is marketed in the United States for hyperprolactinemia, but is extremely expensive.

OTHER DOPAMINE AGONISTS

Lergotrile, a synthetic ergoline, was discarded because of its severe adverse effects, especially hepatotoxicity (41). Mesulergine (CU 32-085), an ergoline derivative with variable antiparkinsonian efficacy, was investigated mostly in open studies but later withdrawn because of a high occurrence of testicular Leydig's cell tumors in long-term exposed rats. Another novel ergoline derivative, **CQA206-291** with potent D_1 and D_2 agonist activity that showed significant antiparkinsonian qualities and acceptable tolerability, was also abandoned from future development because of laboratory-demonstrated toxicity (83). **Terguride** (9,10-transdihydrolisuride) possesses mixed agonist and antagonist properties at striatal D_2 receptors, depending on the dopamine receptor status: full agonist activity can be demonstrated at denervated, supersensitive sites and inhibition of full agonists at normal receptors. This partial D_2 dopamine agonist showed antiparkinsonian activity in animal models and it was suggested that it may be helpful in reducing dyskinesias. However, less impressive results were obtained in a double-blind controlled trial (84). **Almirid** (α-dihydroergocryptine) is to date the last ergot compound licensed for use in PD, available in some European countries (85).

NONERGOT DRUGS

Other D_2 agonists are aminotetralines structurally unrelated to the ergolines. Two of them, **N-0437** and its (−) enantiomer **N-0923**, were effective in rat and monkey models of PD. Other candidate drugs tested in parkinsonian patients, also unrelated to the ergolines, were **PHNO** [(+)-4-propyl-9-hydroxynaphthoxazine) and its controlled-release formulation **MK-458**, the most potent D_2 receptor agonist known to date. In addition to its oral absorption, PHNO is easily absorbed when given transdermally or injected subcutaneously, has a three to four hour therapeutic effect, which may be extended up to 10 hours with a controlled-release formulation. However, its effects as add-on therapy were less than expected based on the experimental models. Also, **MK-458** was significantly less effective than pergolide, to which it had been compared (86). **Piribedil**, another nonergoline derivative with D_2 agonist activity and an active metabolite (active at D_1 receptors), was introduced as add-on therapy in some European countries in the early 1970s. It induced more nausea and vomiting than ergot derivatives without additional clinical benefit (87).

Finally, two new nonergoline drugs were recently introduced and made widely available in 1997: **ropinirole** and **pramipexole**. Both are synthetic D_2 receptor agonists with a similar pharmacodynamic spectrum. They will be described in more detail.

ROPINIROLE

Ropinirole (4-{2- (dipropylamino) ethyl] 1 3 dihydro 2H indol 2 one HCl) is a potent, nonergoline dopaminergic D_2 agonist. Its affinity order for D_2 receptor subtypes is $D_3 > D_2 > D_4$, similar to dopamine, with ropinirole being 20-fold more selective for the human D_3 than D_2 receptors (21,88–90). Ropinirole has no affinity for D_1 receptors and negligible or no affinity for 5HT, GABA, benzodiazepine, muscarinic acetylcholine, and central adrenoreceptors. Its elimination half-life is five to seven hrs.

Clinical Studies in Early Parkinson's Disease

Several large prospective, double-blind, multicenter studies entered patients with early (stage I to III Hoehn and Yahr) PD (91–95). They were respectively placebo-controlled, (six-month duration, 241 patients), levodopa-controlled (five-year duration, 268 patients), and bromocriptine-controlled (three-year duration, 335 patients). Patients were enrolled if they had not been treated with levodopa (or had been treated for less than six weeks) and required symptomatic therapy. Patients receiving selegiline were also enrolled. In all trials, ropinirole and the controller drug were titrated, reaching a maximum dose of 24 mg per day ropinirole, 1200 mg per day of levodopa, and 40 mg per day of bromocriptine.

The results of these trials support the efficacy of ropinirole. In the study by Adler and coworkers (91), 241 patients were randomized to receive ropinirole (n = 116) or placebo (n = 125) in a prospective, multicenter, double-blind, randomized, parallel-group trial lasting 24 weeks. Patients were stratified by use of or non-use of selegiline. The primary outcome measure was percent reduction in the motor examination portion and total score of the UPDRS. In addition, a responder was defined as a patient with a greater than 30 percent reduction in UPDRS motor scale. Secondary end points included the number of patients requiring levodopa, time to initiation of levodopa therapy, number with insufficient response, and clinical global impression score. An average dose of 15.7 mg per day for ropinirole patients resulted in an average 24 percent decrease in UPDRS motor score versus an increase

of 3 percent in the placebo group. This difference was significant. Forty-seven percent of ropinirole patients were responders compared with 20 percent in the placebo group, and 11 percent of ropinirole patients required levodopa because of insufficient response compared with 29 percent in the placebo group. A statistically significant improvement in the motor examination score (24–32%) was observed in ropinirole-treated patients compared with a worsening in placebo-treated patients.

In the comparison with bromocriptine (94), early PD patients not treated with levodopa were randomized in a double-blind trial involving 37 centers. The study enrolled 335 patients, 168 randomized to ropinirole and 167 to bromocriptine. Patients were allowed to use levodopa in an open-label fashion as a rescue therapy if they were inadequately treated. At six months, 86 percent of the patients continued, with only 14 percent in each group dropping out. Patients were stratified with regard to treatment or non-treatment with selegiline. Total UPDRS motor score improved significantly in both groups, but ropinirole provided a significantly more robust change than bromocriptine. In the responder group (patients with a 30% or more drop in UPDRS motor score), ropinirole again was significantly better than bromocriptine. An interesting finding in this study was that when only the groups with no selegiline therapy were compared, ropinirole demonstrated an even more robust difference in response compared to bromocriptine. However, when comparing the groups with selegiline, there was no difference between the two agonists. The authors suggested that selegiline in some way augmented the efficacy of bromocriptine but not the efficacy of ropinirole. The percentage of patients with dyskinesias was low in both groups and adverse events occurred in 80 percent of both groups, although most of them were minor and there were no significant differences. Ropinirole at a mean dose of 8.3 mg per day demonstrated a superior effect on early parkinsonian symptoms than a mean dose of 16.8 mg of bromocriptine per day. A three-year follow-up (93) showed that DAA monotherapy was maintained in 60 percent (of patients remaining in the study) of ropinirole-treated patients (mean dose 12 ± 6) and 53% of bromocriptine-treated group (mean dose 24 ± 8 mg). The UPDRS scores showed definite improvement for both groups, although the ADL score was significantly better for ropinirole.

These trials provided strong support for the effectiveness of DAA for at least several years in PD patients. It also suggested but did not clearly demonstrate that ropinirole may be superior to bromocriptine unless selegiline is coadministered.

Ropinirole in Advanced Parkinson's Disease

Ropinirole was also used as adjunctive therapy in the treatment of patients with levodopa-induced motor fluctuations. The principal study for this population was reported by Lieberman and coworkers (96). It was a six-month, double-blind, placebo-controlled, randomized, parallel-group trial comparing ropinirole to placebo in PD patients with wearing-off effect and dyskinesia. The randomization design provided that of every three patients, two were randomized to ropinirole and one to placebo. Patients were stratified according to whether they received selegiline or not. The dosage of ropinirole was increased to a minimum of 7.5 mg per day, and at that time a planned decrease in levodopa dose was implemented. The primary end point of the study measured the number of responders in each group defined as patients who could achieve a 20 percent or greater decrease in levodopa dose and a 20 percent or greater reduction in percent "off" time between baseline and final visit. Secondary variables included levodopa dose change and change in "off" time from baseline. UPDRS scores were not used. One hundred and forty-nine patients were randomized to ropinirole (n = 95) or placebo (n = 54). Seventy-three percent completed the study. Results demonstrated that 28 percent of ropinirole-treated patients were considered responders while the same was true for 11 percent of placebo patients. Reduction in levodopa dose in the ropinirole group was 31 percent compared with only 6 percent in the placebo group. Hours "off" per day were reduced by approximately 12 percent (1.9 hours) in the ropinirole group and 5 percent (0.8 hours) in the placebo group. Dyskinesia was the only side effect that was significantly more common in the ropinirole group (33.7%). Other smaller studies in advanced patients have demonstrated similar results (97–99). One can conclude that ropinirole is effective in treating advanced disease as a partial substitute for and as an adjunct to levodopa. Like the other agonists, it cannot replace levodopa completely.

Compared with bromocriptine, both drugs showed efficacy, although ropinirole was significantly better in patients already receiving a high dose of levodopa and in patients who had motor fluctuations (100,101).

Tolerability and Adverse Events

The nonergoline structure of ropinirole and its selective D_2 agonist action suggested a possibly different profile of adverse reactions as compared with ergoline dopaminergic agents, particularly with regard to psychiatric manifestations such as hallucinations and confusion, but this has not been confirmed.

Schrag and coworkers (102) reviewed safety and tolerability data on a total of 1,364 parkinsonian patients exposed to ropinirole, over 70 percent for more than six months and 44 percent for more than one year. As the majority of patients were treated in double-blind randomized studies, the comparison of ropinirole with bromocriptine or levodopa was also possible.

In early PD monotherapy studies, nausea (47.6%), dizziness (24.1%), and somnolence (22.3%) were the most frequent reported side effects. A similar percentage (21.8%) of patients reported dizziness in the placebo group and in bromocriptine groups (19.2%), which suggests that dizziness is not a particularly common adverse experience with DAA. Hallucinations were rare in early-therapy trials, but occurred more commonly with ropinirole and bromocriptine than with levodopa.

The adverse experiences recorded in add-on studies showed a similar proportion of central dopaminergic side effects (dyskinesias, hallucinations, insomnia) for ropinirole and bromocriptine. Only somnolence occurred clearly more frequently among ropinirole-treated patients – 11.4 percent versus 6.4 percent bromocriptine, 7.9 percent placebo (90). A patient who experienced a "sleep attack" at 16 mg ropinirole dose was recently reported (103).

The occurrence of orthostatic hypotension in monotherapy was similar for ropinirole (7.0%) and levodopa (7.9%), whereas it was 10.8% in bromocriptine group and 4.8% in placebo-receiving patients. In adjunct-therapy studies it occurred more in placebo (13.2%) than in DAA-treated groups (ropinirole 10.8%, bromocriptine 7.4%). Domperidone pretreatment may prevent postural symptoms at the initiation of treatment, as tolerance to the hypotensive effect of ropinirole will develop later. Surprisingly, leg edema, which has been traditionally attributed to nondopaminergic peripheral effects of ergot derivatives, appeared in 6.4 percent of ropinirole-treated patients.

The time frame of adverse effects revealed the high incidence of gastrointestinal symptoms at the initiation of therapy with ropinirole (this may be reduced by prophylactic or on demand use of domperidone) and the increasing incidence of hallucinations with prolonged duration and higher doses. Hallucinations are the leading reason for withdrawal in add-on studies (3.2%).

One case of pleural inflammation and sclerosis has been reported but has no other fibrolic complications. No significant changes were revealed in laboratory tests.

It may be concluded that the adverse experiences profile of ropinirole is quite similar to that of bromocriptine, both in early and add-on therapy of PD, with the exception of pleuropulmonary, pericardial or retroperitoneal reactions, which probably occur less frequently with ropinirole.

PRAMIPEXOLE

Pramipexole (PPX), a synthetic amino benzathiazole derivative, is another nonergot full dopamine D_2 receptor agonist, acting preferentially at presynaptic D_2 autoreceptors (in nondenervated striatum) with even stronger affinity for the D_3 subtype than ropinirole (104,105). It has a half-life of 8 to 12 hours and typical doses are 3 to 4.5 mg/day.

Clinical Studies in Early Parkinson's Disease

Three double-blind, placebo-controlled studies evaluated the efficacy and tolerability of PPX in early PD (106–108) using a titration reaching a maximum (if required) of 4.5 to 6.0 mg per day. All demonstrated a significant therapeutic advantage over placebo. Shannon and coworkers (107) reported the results of an 18-center, six-month trial in 335 patients who were randomized to receive pramipexole (n = 164) or placebo (n = 171). More than 80 percent of patients completed the trial. The primary efficacy end points were the ADL and motor portions of the UPDRS. They found a 22 to 29 percent improvement in the ADL score and a 25 to 31 percent improvement in the motor score, both of which were statistically significant and maintained for the entire six months. The most common adverse events – and ones that were significantly more common with active therapy when compared to placebo – included nausea (39%), insomnia (25.6%), constipation (17.7%), and somnolence (18.3%). Symptomatic orthostasis was absent. Visual hallucinations occurred in 9.7 percent, which was also significantly greater than placebo. A similar result was reported in a smaller early phase trial (106). The Parkinson Study Group (108) reported on a dose-ranging study that involved 20 sites and evaluated four doses of pramipexole and placebo in a double-blind, parallel group, randomized trial. 264 patients were randomized to receive 1.5 mg (n = 54), 3 mg (n = 50), 4.5 mg (n = 54), 6 mg (n = 55), or placebo (n = 51). There was a six-week dose escalation followed by a four-week maintenance period. The primary outcome measure for efficacy was total UPDRS score, and tolerability was measured by the ability of patients to complete the study. There was a linear trend between mean response and dosage and this was highly significant; however, it was found that the magnitude of the mean response was similar across all active groups (20% improvement in UPDRS) and in all cases significantly different from placebo. Pramipexole seemed to be more effective in patients who were more severely impaired. They were unable to find a minimally effective dose since 1.5 mg per day was also significantly effective. With regard to tolerability, 98 percent of placebo patients completed the study, 81 percent in the 1.5-mg group, 92 percent in the 3-mg group, 78 percent in the 4.5-mg group, and 67 percent in the 6-mg group. These numbers were significantly smaller in all active groups with the exception of 3 mg per day, compared with placebo. The major side effects of the drug were somnolence, dizziness, nausea, and hallucinations, and all of these increased with increasing doses. The dose between 4.5 mg per day and 6 mg per day caused the most side effects. Based on this trial, it was thought that the optimum dosage of pramipexole monotherapy in early PD patients is between 1.5 mg per day and 4.5 mg per day. Thus, pramipexole demonstrated clear efficacy in early patients, and long-term follow-up has demonstrated prolonged efficacy without the need for levodopa in a notable percentage of these patients.

Pramipexole in Advanced Parkinson's Disease

Two large double-blind, placebo-controlled, multicenter studies performed in advanced PD patients with motor fluctuations (59,109) showed marked and statistically significant improvement for PPX over placebo in motor disability and decrease in "off" time. Levodopa dose was also significantly reduced. Lieberman and coworkers (109) reported the results of an eight-month trial with a seven-week ascending dose phase followed by a six-month maintenance phase. The pramipexole group escalated the dose to a maximum of 4.5 mg divided into three doses. The primary efficacy end points included improvement in the ADL subscore of UPDRS (averaging "on" and "off" scores) and the motor exam score while "on." There were numerous secondary end points, including measures from fluctuation diaries. Three hundred and sixty patients were enrolled with 179 randomized to placebo and 181 to pramipexole. The averaged ADL score was significantly improved, by 22 percent, and that was maintained over the entire duration of the study. The motor exam score also was significantly improved when compared to placebo, with a decrease of about 25 percent. The percent "off" time when comparing the last visit (after 8 months) to baseline significantly decreased by 31 percent. A measure of severity of "off" times also demonstrated significant improvements. Levodopa dose was reduced in the pramipexole group by 27 percent as compared to 5 percent in the placebo group.

The major adverse events reported included dyskinesia (61.3%), asymptomatic orthostatic hypotension (48.1%), dizziness (36.5%), insomnia (22.7%), hallucinations (19.3%), nausea (17.7%), and symptomatic orthostatic hypotension (16%). All of these were more common in the active treatment group than in the placebo group. Guttman and coworkers (59) reported another large nine-month trial with three treatment groups: placebo, pramipexole with escalating dose up to 4.5 mg per day, and bromocriptine with an escalating dose up to 30 mg per day (discussed earlier). The study was not powered for a comparison of the two agonists, but the purpose of adding a bromocriptine treatment arm was to evaluate whether the methodology was appropriate for demonstrating efficacy of an agonist over placebo. All patients were required to have wearing-off phenomenon, and there was a three-month ascending dose phase followed by a six-month maintenance phase. The primary efficacy end point measures were the ADL and motor exam scores for the UPDRS (during "on" time) and the difference they demonstrated from baseline. There were a large number of secondary end point measures similar to that studied by Lieberman and coworkers (109), but additionally there were evaluations of quality of life measures. Two hundred and forty-six subjects were randomized in the trial. At an average dose of 3.36 mg per day, pramipexole resulted in a significant improvement in ADL score (26.7 percent lower than baseline) and in motor exam score during "on" time (34.9 percent when compared to baseline). There was also a reduction in average percent "off" time compared to controls (15%), which translated to an increase in 2.5 hours "on" per day. The percent decrease in "off" time in the pramipexole group was 45.6 percent compared with 5.5 percent for placebo. Significant improvement in one particular quality of life measure (Euro QOL) was seen in the pramipexole group compared with placebo. The most common adverse events that occurred in the pramipexole group included dyskinesia (40%), dizziness (33%), insomnia (28%), headache (20%), hallucinations (14%), confusion (14%), orthostatic hypotension (40%), and nausea (36%). All these percentages were greater than those seen in placebo. Overall, the results of this trial were quite similar to those seen by Lieberman and coworkers (109).

Safety and Tolerability

Pramipexole was well tolerated. The usual dopaminergic side effects were observed, namely, somnolence, insomnia, nausea, hallucinations, confusion, and orthostatic hypotension. Long-term data confirm the safety of PPX (110). However, a serious side effect was recently reported by Frucht and coworkers (103). Eight patients receiving PPX fell asleep during driving. The sleep attacks disappeared after discontinuing PPX or reducing the dose. This possibility of sudden impairment of alertness must be made known to driving patients. Further observations have suggested that this is a class problem.

COMPARISON OF DOPAMINE AGONISTS

Apart from apomorphine, which is reserved as a rescue option to a small category of problematic patients, the present selection of DAA includes at least four ergot derivatives – some of them used for approximately 25 years – and two nonergoline compounds, ropinirole and pramipexole. Bromocriptine, pergolide, lisuride, cabergoline, ropinirole, and pramipexole have different potencies and affinities at dopamine receptors (Table 36-1). Although all are highly potent at D_2 and D_3 receptors, ropinirole and pramipexole are 10 times more potent at the D_3 than at the D_2 receptor, bromocriptine is 10 times more potent at D_2 than at D_3 and only pergolide acts as a D_1 agonist. DAA were tried and reported to be effective as levodopa adjuncts, as monotherapy in early PD and in early combination with levodopa.

It is clear that the DAA are more alike than different. Nevertheless, particular differences exist (Table 35-2). However, few head-to-head comparisons between DAA were reported, making comparisons difficult because of differences in design and patient populations in the various studies. Perhaps not surprisingly, the few head-to-head comparisons between DAA which have been published show superiority of the newer agents over bromocriptine (For review see Factor 1999).

COMPARISON OF DOPAMINE AGONISTS WITH LEVODOPA

Several prospective, randomized, double-blind studies have recently been completed in which dopamine agonists or levodopa were used as monotherapy in early PD. The aim of these studies was not only to evaluate efficacy and safety of agonists compared with levodopa in previously untreated patients but also to determine if long-term outcomes differ with regard to motor complications. These studies used ropinirole, pramipexole, and pergolide. The pergolide study is unpublished at this time. The first study was a five-year

Table 35-2 Clinical Use of Dopamine Agonists.

Drug	Initial Dose (mg)	Titration	Usual Daily Dose (mg)	Maximal Dose in Drug Studies (mg)
Bromocriptine	1.25 × 2	1–2 weeks	10–40	120
Pergolide	0.05	3 days	3	10
Lisuride	0.2	weekly	1.5–5	10
Cabergoline	0.5	weekly	3–6	8
Ropinirole	0.25 × 3	weekly	9	24
Pramipexole	0.125 × 3	weekly	1.5–4.5	6

All drugs are usually given tid, except for cabergoline, which is given only once daily.

comparison of ropinirole and levodopa in 268 patients (111). For every subject randomized to levodopa, two patients were randomized to ropinirole. Open-label rescue levodopa supplementation was allowed. Approximately half of the patients withdrew by the end of five years. The study showed that ropinirole, at a mean dose of 16.5 mg per day, was well tolerated and could be maintained as monotherapy in some patients. The primary end point was the appearance of dyskinesias as measured by item 32 on the UPDRS. Dyskinesias were shown to occur earlier and more frequently in patients treated with levodopa than in those treated with ropinirole. Regardless of levodopa supplementation, 20 percent of ropinirole subjects experienced dyskinesias by the end of five years versus 45 percent of levodopa subjects. Before the addition of rescue levodopa, 5 percent of the ropinirole group and 36 percent of the levodopa group developed dyskinesias. The differences were statistically significant. There were no differences between the two groups with regard to the occurrences of wearing off or freezing gait, although the latter was more common in the ropinirole group. The change from baseline of the UPDRS ADL subscore was similar between the two groups, but there was a significant difference in favor of the levodopa group for the change from baseline of the UPDRS motor subscore, which improved approximately four times greater in the levodopa group. This difference in efficacy was reported in the six-month interim report published earlier (85). This indicates that patients receiving ropinirole had less motor improvement than those in the levodopa arm. As the dose of ropinirole used was considered to be submaximal in most patients, it is possible that further gains could have been made with more aggressive therapy. A post hoc analysis of this study showed that the increased risk for dyskinesias occurred mostly in those patients who were younger than 70 years old when recruited (112).

The CALM-PD study was a 23.5-month prospective, randomized, double-blind study comparing pramipexole with levodopa in 301 early PD patients (104). It was carried out by 22 sites in the Parkinson Study Group. The primary end point was the time of first occurrence of motor complications: wearing off, on-off, or dyskinesias. Open-label (rescue) levodopa was allowed is this study also when patients needed supplementation to their experimental therapy. Patients were randomized so that 151 patients were treated with pramipexole and 150 received levodopa. Motor complications occurred in 28 percent of the pramipexole group and 51 percent of the levodopa group at 23.5 months. Dyskinesias occurred in 10 percent of the pramipexole patients and 31 percent of the levodopa patients by the end of study, and wearing off occurred in 24 percent of the pramipexole patients and 38 percent of those treated with levodopa. Both differences were significant. However, a significantly greater number of pramipexole patients required levodopa supplementation, and the mean improvement in the total UPDRS scores were significantly better in the levodopa group (9.2 vs. 4.5 points). Levodopa dose requirement was significantly higher in the levodopa group. The PELMOPET study (pergolide vs. l-dopa in early PD) has been completed, and although a detailed analysis has not been published, the results presented at conferences seem to be qualitatively similar to the results of these other two studies.

These trials included neuroimaging substudies to analyze for possible neuroprotection from dopamine agonists. The CALM-PD study used B-CIT SPECT scanning techniques at baseline and month 23 in 82 patients (78 returned for the month 23 scan) (113,114). The mean change per year of CIT uptake was similar for both treatment groups (20% decline in the pramipexole group vs. 24.5% in the levodopa group). Fluoro-dopa PET studies were done in the ropinirole and pergolide trials (11). In the ropinirole study 28 ropinirole-treated patients and 9 levodopa-treated patients were evaluated. A trend was seen toward preservation of dopaminergic function in the striatum in the ropinirole group, especially in those who had the disease for less than two years. These results are difficult to interpret because of the small patient numbers. The pergolide study also used PET studies. Although as yet unpublished, the results demonstrated no significant differences between treatment groups (presented at the 6th International Congress of Parkinson's Disease and Movement Disorders).

It appears that dopamine agonists, when used in early PD patients, cause less dyskinesia and wearing off effect but at the cost of less robust motor control. It is not clear what the mechanism is that leads to fewer complications with the dopamine agonists. Follow-up studies should determine whether the precipitation of dyskinesias by levodopa is irreversible or whether they could be eliminated (or at least reduced) through partial replacement of levodopa by dopamine agonists. The imaging studies suggest that agonists are not neuroprotective and that levodopa is not toxic, but longer follow-up is needed. While these studies have addressed many issues, still more unanswered ones have arisen. This leaves the question as to what is appropriate first-line therapy for the symptomatic treatmnent of PD an ongoing controversy. Obviously, as no direct comparisons between the three DAA agents have been attempted, conclusions as to their relative efficacy and safety cannot be made. At this time, using a DAA or levodopa would be appropriate. Therapy should be individualized according to the patient's needs.

CONCLUSIONS

The accumulated clinical experience has led to two important conclusions regarding the advantages and clinical roles of DAA. The first is that, although all DAA (with the notable exception of apomorphine) have lower potency than levodopa, they have other properties that make them potentially helpful in ameliorating motor fluctuations which can be incapacitating in advanced PD. Thus, DAA in combination with levodopa became a mainstay therapy in this situation. More excitingly, accumulating evidence with several DAA suggests that monotherapy in de novo patients can be maintained for at least one year in many patients, and that when additional levodopa is required, this will be at a relatively low dose. This strategy seems to decrease and delay the development of dyskinesias and perhaps wearing off effect. It is not clear whether this is due to the levodopa-sparing effect of DAA (preventing the formation of oxidative products), the activation of presynaptic D_2 receptors, the putative neuroprotective effects of DAA, the low D_1 activation, or the longer duration of action.

The limitations of DAA are due to their low efficacy, relative to dopamine itself at postsynaptic receptors, and their side effect profile. The "peripheral" adverse actions, such as nausea and hypotension, can be antagonized by dopamine blocking drugs, particularly domperidone, which does not cross the blood-brain barrier (115). However, this agent is not available worldwide and it would be advantageous if DAA existed with a higher central : peripheral activity ratio. The development of such agents might also allow for a more rapid dose escalation in new patients, without the need to wait for tolerance to develop. The major psychiatric side effects – hallucinations, delusions, and confusion – may be caused by the action of DAA on D_4 rather than D_2 receptors. Thus, there is a potential to develop D_2 superselective agonists, devoid of action at D_4 sites, the use of which should not be limited by psychiatric manifestations.

Other major questions, such as what to do in case of failure of a first DAA as add-on therapy, to switch to another DAA (116) or to another drug class, such as catechol-O-methyl transferase inhibitors, and whether the use of DAA may impact mortality rate (117,118) are still unanswered.

REFERENCES

1. Jenner P. The rationale for the use of dopamine agonists in Parkinson's disease. *Neurology* 1995; 45:S6–S12.
2. Watts RL. The role of dopamine agonists in early Parkinson's disease. *Neurology* 1997; 49:S34–S48.
3. Sibley DR, Monsma FJJ. Molecular biology of dopamine receptors. *Trends Pharmacol Sci* 1992; 13:61–69.
4. Missale C, Russel SN, Robinson SW, et al. Dopamine receptors: from structure to function. *Physiol Rev* 1998; 78:189–225.
5. Schwab RS, Amador LV, Lettvin JY. Apomorphine in Parkinson's disease. *Trans Amer Neurol Assoc* 1951; 76:251–253.
6. Cotzias GC, Papavasiliou PS, Fehling C, et al. Similarities between neurologic effects of L-dopa and of apomorphine. *N Engl J Med* 1970; 282:31–33.
7. Calne DB, Techenne PF, Leigh PN, et al. Treatment of parkinsonism with bromocriptine. *Lancet* 1974; 2:1355–1356.
8. Carlson JH, Bergstrom DA, and Walters JG. Stimulation of both D_1 and D_2 dopamine receptors appears necessary for full expression of postsynaptic effects of dopamine agonists: A neurophysiological study. *Brain Res* 1987; 400:205–218.
9. Koller WC. Neuroprotection for Parkinson's disease. *Ann Neurol* 1998; 44:S155–S159.
10. Olanow CW. Dopamine agonists and neuroprotection in Parkinson's disease. *Ann Neurol* 1998; 44:S167–S174.

11. Rakshi JS, Bailey DL, Uema T, et al. Is ropinirole a selective D$_2$ receptor agonist, neuroprotective in early Parkinson's disease? An [^{18}F)dopa PET study. *Neurology* 1998; 50:A330.

12. Rajput AH. Adverse effects of ergot derivative dopamine agonists. In Olanow CW, Obeso JA, (eds.), *Dopamine Agonists in Early Parkinson's Disease* Kent, U.K.: Wells Medical Limited, 1997; 209–216.

13. Agid Y, Pollak P, Bonnet AM, et al. Bromocriptine associated with a peripheral dopamine blocking agent in treatment of Parkinson's disease. *Lancet* 1979; 1:570–572.

14. Saint-Cyr JA, Taylor AE, Lang AE. Neuropsychological and psychiatric side effects in the treatment of Parkinson's disease. *Neurology* 1993; 43:S47–S52.

15. Goetz CG, Vogel C, Tanner CM, et al. Early dopaminergic drug-induced hallucinations in parkinsonian patients. *Neurology* 1998; 51:811–814.

16. Boyd A. Bromocriptine and psychosis: A literature review. *Psych Quarterly* 1995; 66:87–95.

17. Klawans HL, Weiner WJ. Attempted use of haloperidol in the treatment of L-dopa-induced dyskinesias. *J Neurol Neurosurg Psychiatry* 1974; 37:427–430.

18. Parkinson Study Group. Low-dose clozapine for the treatment of drug-induced psychosis n Parkinson's disease. *N Engl J Med* 1999; 340:757–763.

19. Rabey JM, Treves TA, Neufeld MY, et al. Low-dose clozapine in the treatment of levodopa induced mental disturbances in Parkinson's disease. *Neurology* 1995; 45:432–434.

20. Ling LH, Ahlskog JE, Munger TM, et al. Constrictive pericarditis and pleuropulmonary disease linked to ergot dopamine agonist therapy (cabergoline) for Parkinson's disease. *Mayo Clin Proc* 1999; 74:371–375.

21. Hillerdal G, Lee J, Blonkvist A, et al. Pleural disease during treatment with bromocriptine in patients previously exposed to asbestos. *Eur Respir* 1997; 10:2711–2715.

22. Frans E, Dom R, and Demedts M. Pleuropulmonary changes during treatment of Parkinson's disease with a long-acting ergot derivative, cabergoline. *Eur Respir J* 1992; 5:263–265.

23. Shaunak S, Wilkins A, Pilling JB, et al. Pericardial, retroperitoneal, and pleural fibrosis induced by pergolide. *J Neurol Neurosurg Psychiatry* 1999; 66:79–81.

24. Rinne UK. Pleuropulmonary changes during long-term bromocriptine treatment for Parkinson's disease. *Lancet* 1981; i:44.

25. Factors. Dopamine agonists. *Med Clin North Am* 1999; 83:415–443.

26. Taylor AC, Beerahee A, Citerone DR, et al. Lack of a pharmacokinetic interaction at steady state between ropinirole and L-dopa in patients with Parkinson's disease. *Pharmacotherapy* 1999; 19:150–156.

27. Weill E. De l'apomorphine dans certains troubles nerveux. *Lyon Med* 1884; 48:411–419.

28. Colzi A, Turner K, and Lees AJ. Continuous waking-day subcutaneous apomorphine therapy in the treatment of levodopa-induced dyskinesias and "on-off" phenomena in Parkinson's disease. *Mov Disord* 1997; 12:428.

29. Frankel JP, Lees AJ, Kempster PA, et al. Subcutaneous apomorphine in the treatment of Parkinson's disease. *J Neurol Neurosurg Psychiatry* 1990; 53:96–101.

30. Korczyn AD. Parkinson's disease: One disease entity or many? *J. Neural Transm* 1999; 56:107–111.

31. Hughes AJ, Lees AJ, and Stern GM. Apomorphine test to predict dopaminergic responsiveness in parkinsonism syndromes. *Lancet* 1990; 336:32–34.

32. Hughes AJ, Colosimo C, Kleendorfer B, et al. The dopaminergic response in multiple system atrophy. *J Neurol Neurosurg Psychiatry* 1992; 55:1009–1013.

33. Gancher ST, Woodward WR, Boucher RB, et al. Peripheral pharmacokinetics of apomorphine in humans. *Ann Neurol*, 1989; 26:232–238.

34. Metman LV, Locatelli MD, Bravi D, et al. Apomorphine responses in Parkinson's disease and the pathogenesis of motor complications. *Neurology* 1997; 48:369–372.

35. Kempster PA, Frankel JP, Stern GM, et al. Comparison of motor response to apomorphine and levodopa in Parkinson's disease. *J Neurol Neurosurg Psychiatry* 1990; 53:1004–1005.

36. Broussolle E, Marion MH, and Pollak P. Continuous subcutaneous apomorphine as replacement for levodopa in severe parkinsonian patients after surgery. *Lancet* 1992; 340:859–860.

37. Chaudhuri KR, and Clough C. Subcutaneous apomorphine in Parkinson's disease. *Br Med J* 1998; 316:641.

38. Dewey RB, Maraganore DM, Ahlskog JE, et al. A controlled clinical trial of intranasal epomorphine as rescue therapy for "off" periods in fluctuating Parkinson's disease. *Ann Neurol* 1995; 38:329(A).

39. Courty E, Durif F, Zenut M, et al. Psychiatric and sexual disorders induced by apomorphine in Parkinson's disease. *Clin Neuropharmacol* 1997; 20:140–47.

40. Kartzinel R, and Calne DB. Studies with bromocriptine – Part 1. "on-off" phenomena. *Neurology* 1976; 26:508–570.

41. Teychenne PF, Bergsrud D, Racy A, et al. Bromocriptine: Low-dose therapy in Parkinson disease. *Neurology* 1982; 32:577–583.

42. Hely MA, Morris JG, Reid WG, et al. The Sydney multicenter study of Parkinson's disease: A randomized, prospective five year study comparing low dose bromocriptine with low-dose levodopa-carbidopa. *J Neurol Neurosurg Psychiatry* 1994; 57:903–910.

43. Herskovits E, Yorio A, Herrera E, et al. Use of bromocriptine in "de novo" parkinsonian patients. *Adv Therapy* 1986; 3:29–38.

44. Montastruc JL, Rascol O, and Rascol A. A randomized controlled study of bromocriptine versus levodopa in previously untreated Parkinsonian patients: A 3-year follow-up. *J Neurol Neurosurg Psychiatry* 1989; 52:773–775.

45. Nakanishi T, Mizuno Y, Goto I, et al. A nationwide collaborative study on the long-term effects of bromocriptine in patients with Parkinson's disease: First interim report in Japan. *Eur Neurol* 1988; 28 (Suppl 1):3–8.

46. Nakanishi T, Iwata M, Goto I, et al. Nationwide collaborative study on the long-term effects of bromocriptine in the treatment of Parkinsonian patients: final report. *Eur Neurol* 1992; 32(Suppl 1):9–22.

47. Weiner WJ, Factor SA, Sanchez-Ramos JR, et al. Early combination therapy (bromocriptine and levodopa) does not prevent motor fluctuations in Parkinson's disease. *Neurology* 1993; 43:21–27.

48. Lees AJ, and Stern GM. Sustained bromocriptine therapy in previously untreated patients with Parkinson's disease. *J Neurol Neurosurg Psychiatry* 1981; 44:1020–1023.

49. Montastruc JL, Rascol O, Senard JM, et al. A randomised controlled study comparing bromocriptine to which levodopa was later added, with levodopa alone in previously untreated patients with Parkinson's disease: A five year follow up. *J Neurol Neurosurg Psychiatry* 1994; 57:1034–1038.

50. Rinne UK. Early combination of bromocriptine and levodopa in the treatment of Parkinson's disease: A 5-year follow-up. *Neurology* 1987; 37:826–828.

51. Bergamasco B, Benna P, and Scarzella L. Long-term bromocriptine treatment of de novo patients with Parkinson's disease: A seven-year follow-up. *Acta Neurol Scand*, 1990; 81:383–387.

52. Ogawa N, Kanazawa I, Kowa H, et al. Nationwide multicenter prospective study on the long-term effects of bromocriptine for Parkinson's disease: Final report of a ten-year follow-up. *Eur Neurol* 1997; 38:37–49.

53. Factor SA, Weiner WJ. Early combination therapy with bromocriptine and levodopa in Parkinson's disease. *Mov Disord* 1993; 8:257–262.

54. Goetz CG. Dopaminergic agonists in the treatment of Parkinson's disease. *Neurology* 1990; 40(Suppl 3):50–54.

55. Rascol A, Olsson JE, Worm-Petersen J, et al. Early combination of bromocriptine with levodopa in the treatment of Parkinson's disease: A five-year multicentric study. *Mov Disord* 1994; 9(Suppl 1):102.

56. Fischer PA, Przuntek H, Majer M, et al. Combined treatment of early stages of Parkinson's syndrome with bromocriptine and levodopa: A multi-center evaluation. *Deutsch Med Wscher* 1984; 109:1279–1283.

57. Moore AP, Bakheit M, Henderson L, et al. Early combination of bromocriptine with levodopa in the treatment of Parkinson's disease: A five year double blind study. *Ann Neurol* 1994; 36:281.

58. Lieberman AN, Goldstein M. Bromocriptine in Parkinson's disease. *Pharmacol Rev* 1985; 37:217–227.

59. Guttman M. International Pramipexole-Bromocriptine Study Group. Double-blind comparison of pramipexole and bromocriptine treatment with placebo in advanced Parkinson's disease. *Neurology* 1997; 49:1060–1065.

60. Langtry HD, and Clissold SP. Pergolide: A review of its pharmacological properties and therapeutic potential in Parkinson's disease. *Drugs* 1990; 39:491–506.

61. Mizuno Y, Kondon T, and Narabayashi H. Pergolide in the treatment of Parkinson's disease. *Neurology* 1997; 45:S12–S21.

62. Wolters E, Tissingh G, Bergmans P, et al. Dopamine agonists in Parkinson's disease. *Neurology* 1995; 45:S28–S34.

63. Rinne UK. Early dopamine agonist therapy in Parkinson's disease. *Mov Disord* 1989; 4(Suppl 1):S86–S94.

64. Barone P, Bravi D, Bermejo-Pareja F, et al. Pergolide monotherapy in the treatment of early Parkinson's disease: A randomized controlled study. *Neurology* 1999; 53:573–579.

65. Olanow CW, Fahn S, Muenter M, et al. A multicenter, double-blind placebo-controlled trial of pergolide as an adjunct to treatment in Parkinson's disease. *Mov Disord* 1994; 9:40–42.

66. Kurlan R, Millar C, Knapp R, et al. Double-blind assessment of potential pergolide-induced cardiotoxicity. *Neurology* 1986; 36:993–995.

67. Sayler ME, Street JS, Bosoworth JC, et al. Analysis of mortality in pergolide-treated patients with Parkinson's disease. *Neuroepidemiology* 1996; 15:26–32.

68. Horowski R, Dorow R, Loschmann P, et al. Oral and parenteral use of lisuride in Parkinson's disease: Clinical pharmacology and implications for therapy in parkinsonism and aging. In Calne DB, Comi G, Crippa R, et al. (eds.). *Parkinsonism and Aging*. New York: Raven Press, 1989; 269–286.

69. Uitti RJ, Ahlskog JE. Comparative review of dopamine receptor agonists in Parkinson's disease. *Drugs* 1996; 5:369–388.

70. Rinne UK. Lisuride, a dopamine agonist in the treatment of early Parkinson's disease. *Neurology* 1989; 39:336–339.

71. McDonald RJ, and Horowski R. Lisuride in the treatment of parkinsonism. *Eur Neurol* 1983; 22:240–255.

72. Rabey JM, Streifler U, Treves T, and Korczyn AD. A long-term comparative study of lisuride and levodopa in Parkinson's disease, in Parkinsonism and Aging. In Calne DB, Crippa D, Comi G, et al. (eds.), New York: Raven Press, 1989; 261–268.

73. Vaamonde J, Luquin MR, Obeso JA. Subcutaneous lisuride infusion in Parkinson's disease. *Brain* 1991; 114:601–614.

74. Baronti F, Mouradian MM, Davis TL, et al. Continuous lisuride effects on central dopaminergic mechanisms in Parkinson's disease. *Ann Neurol* 1992; 32:776–781.

75. Fariello RG. Pharmacodynamic and pharmacokinetic features of cabergoline: Rationale for use in Parkinson's disease. *Drugs* 1998; 55:10–16.

76. Marsden CD. Clinical experience with cabergoline in patients with advanced Parkinson's disease treated with levodopa. *Drugs* 1998; 55:17–22.

77. Rinne UK, Bracco F, Chouza C, et al. Early treatment of Parkinson's disease with cabergoline delays the onset of motor complications: Results of a double-blind levodopa controlled trial. *Drugs* 1998; 55:23–30.

78. Jori MC, Franceschi MN, Giusti MC, et al. Clinical experience with cabergoline, a new ergoline derivative, in the treatment of Parkinson's disease. *Adv Neurol* 1990; 53:539–543.

79. Ahlskog JE, Muenter MD, Maraganore DM, et al. Fluctuating Parkinson's disease: Treatment with the long-acting dopamine agonist cabergoline. *Arch Neurol* 1994; 51:1236–1241.

80. Lieberman A, Imke S, Muenter M, et al. Multicenter study of cabergoline, a long-acting dopamine receptor agonist, in Parkinson's disease patients with fluctuating responses to levodopa-carbidopa. *Neurology* 1993; 43:1981–1984.

81. Inzelberg R, Nisipeanu P, Rabey JM, et al. Double-blind comparison of cabergoline and bromocriptine in Parkinson's disease with motor fluctuations. *Neurology* 1996; 47:785–788.

82. Inzelberg R, Nisipeanu P, Rabey JM, et al. Long-term tolerability and efficacy of cabergoline, a new long-acting dopamine agonist, in Parkinson's disease. *Mov Disord* 1995; 10:604–607.

83. Tolosa E, Marti M, Valldeoriola F, et al. History of levodopa and dopamine agonists in Parkinson's disease treatment. *Neurology* 1998; 50:S2–S10.

84. Pacchetti C, and Martignoni E. Terguride in fluctuating parkinsonian patients: A double-blind study versus placebo. *Mov Disord* 1993; 8:463–465.

85. Battistin L, Bardin PG, Ferro-Milone F, et al. Alpha-dihydroergocryptine in Parkinson's disease: A multicentre randomized double blind parallel group study. *Acta Neurol Scand*, 1999; 99:36–42.

86. Ahlskog JE, Muenter MD, Bailey PA, et al. Dopamine agonist treatment of fluctuating parkinsonism: D-2 (controlled-release MK-458) vs combined D-1 and D-2 (Pergolide). *Arch Neurol* 1992; 49:560–569.

87. Rondot P, and Ziegler M. Activity and acceptability of piribedil in Parkinson's disease: A multicenter study. *J Neurol* 1992; 239:528–534.

88. Eden RY, Costall B, Domeney AH, et al. Preclinical pharmacology of ropinirole (SK&F 101468-A) a novel dopamine D_2 agonist. *Pharmacol Biochem Behav* 1991; 38:147–154.

89. Tulloch IF. Pharmacologic profile of ropinirole: A nonergoline dopamine agonist. *Neurology* 1997; 49:558–562.

90. Dechant KL, and Plosker GI. Ropinirole. *CNS Drugs* 1997; 8:335–341.

91. Adler CH, Sethi KD, Hauser RA, et al. Ropinirole for the treatment of early Parkinson's disease. *Neurology* 1997; 49:393–399.

92. Korczyn AD, Brooks DJ, Brunt ER, et al. Ropinirole versus bromocriptine in the treatment of early Parkinson's disease: A 6-month interim report of a 3-year study. *Mov Disord* 1998; 13:46–51.

93. Korczyn AD, Brunt ER, Larsen JP, et al. A 3-year randomized trial of ropinirole and bromocriptine in early Parkinson's disease. *Neurology* 1999; 53:364–370.

94. Rascol O, Brooks DJ, Brunt ER, et al. Ropinirole in the treatment of early Parkinson's disease: A 6-month interim report of a 5-year levodopa controlled study. *Mov Disord* 1998; 13:39–45.

95. Rascol O, Group, a t S Ropinirole reduces risk of dyskinesia when used in early PD. AAN 51st Annual Meeting, Toronto, 1999.

96. Lieberman A, Olanow CW, Sethi K, et al. A multicenter trial of ropinirole as adjunct treatment for Parkinson's disease. *Neurology* 1998; 51:1057–1062.

97. Rascol O, Lees AJ, Senard JM, et al. Ropinirole in the treatment of levodopa-induced motor fluctuations in patients with Parkinson's disease. *Clin Neuropharmacol* 1996; 19:234–245.

98. Brooks DJ, Torjanski N, Burn DJ. Ropinirole in the symptomatic treatment of Parkinson's disease. *J Neural Transm* 1995; 45(Suppl):231–238.

99. Vidailhet MJ, Bonnet AM, Belal S, et al. Ropinirole without levodopa in Parkinson's disease. *Lancet* 1990; 336:316.

100. Group RS. A double-blind comparative study of ropinirole versus bromocriptine in the treatment of parkinsonian patients not optimally controlled on L-dopa. *Mov Disord* 1996; 11:188.

101. Brunt ER, Korczyn AD, Lieberman A, et al. The long-term efficacy of ropinirole as an adjunct to L-dopa. AAN 51st Annual Meeting, Toronto (1999).

102. Schrag AE, Brooks DJ, Brunt E, et al. The safety of ropinirole, a selective nonergoline dopamine agonist, in patients with Parkinson's disease. *Clin Neuropharmacol* 1998; 21:169–175.

103. Frucht S, Rogers JD, Greene PE, et al. Falling asleep at the wheel: Motor vehicle mishaps in persons taking pramipexole and ropinirole. *Neurology* 1999; 52:1908–1910.

104. Mierau J, and Schingnitz G. Biochemical and pharmacological studies on pramipexole, a potent and selective dopamine D_2 receptor agonist. *Eur J Pharmacol* 1992; 215:161–170.

105. Piercey MF. Pharmacology of pramipexole, a dopamine D_3-preferring agonist useful in treating Parkinson's disease. *Clin Neuropharmacol* 1998; 21:141–151.

106. Hubble JP, Koller WC, Cutler NR, et al. Pramipexole in patients with early Parkinson's disease. *Clin Neuropharmacol* 1995; 18:338–347.

107. Shannon KM, Bennett Jr, JP, Friedman JH. Efficacy of pramipexole, a novel dopamine agonist, as monotherapy in mild to moderate Parkinson's disease. *Neurology* 1997; 49:724–728.

108. Parkinson Study Group. Safety and efficacy of pramipexole in early Parkinson disease: A randomized dose-ranging study. *JAMA* 1997; 278:125–130.

109. Lieberman A, Ranhosky A, and Korts D. Clinical evaluation of pramipexole in advanced Parkinson's disease: Results of a double-blind, placebo-controlled, parallel-group study. *Neurology* 1997; 49:162–168.

110. Factor SA, Weiner WY, Jankovic J, et al. Four year safety and adverse events in an open-label experience of 306 patients on pramipexole for Parkinson's disease. *Neurology* 1999; 52:A407–408.

111. Rascol O, Brooks DJ, Korczyn AD, De Deyn PP, Clarke CE, Lang AE. A five-year study of the incidence of dyskinesia in patients with early Parkinson's disease who were treated with ropinirole or levodopa. 056 Study Group. *N Engl J Med* 2000; 342(20):1484–91.

112. Korczyn AD, Keens J, Oldham M, and Macrae S. The safety and efficacy of ropinirole as early therapy in elderly patients with Parkinson's disease. *Neurology* 2000; 54(Suppl 3): A89.

113. Parkinson Study Group. Pramipexole vs. levodopa as initial treatment for Parkinson's disease: A randomized controlled trial. *JAMA* 2000; 284:1931–1938.

114. Marek K and the Parkinson Study Group. B-CIT/SPECT assessment of progression of Parkinson's disease in subjects participating in the CALM-PD study. *Neurology* 2000; 54(Suppl 3):A90.

115. Korczyn AD. Autonomic nervous system disturbances in Parkinson's disease. In Streifler MB, Korczyn AD, Melamed E, et al. (eds.), *Advances in Neurology: Parkinson's Disease: Anatomy, Pathology, Therapy* New York: Raven Press, 1990; 463–468.

116. Goetz CG, Blasucci L, and Stebbins GT. Switching dopamine agonists in advanced Parkinson's disease: Is rapid titration preferable to slow? *Neurology* 1999; 52:1227–1229.

117. Przuntek H, Welzel D, Blummer E, et al. Bromocriptine lessens the incidence of mortality in L-dopa treated parkinsonian patients: Prado-study discontinued. *Eur J Clin Pharmacol* 1992; 43:357–363.

118. Hely MA, Morris JGL, Traficante R, et al. The Sydney multicenter study of Parkinson's disease: Progression and mortality at 10 years. *J Neurol Neurosurg Psychiatry* 1999; 67:300–307.

36

Catechol-O-Methyltransferase (COMT) Inhibitors

Cheryl Waters, M.D., F.R.C.P.(C)
Columbia University, New York, New York

LIMITATIONS OF LEVODOPA

To appreciate the rationale for the use of catechol-*O*-methyltransferase (COMT) inhibitors, it is important to understand the metabolism of levodopa. The majority (70%) of oral levodopa is rapidly metabolized in the liver and intestinal mucosa to dopamine via dopa decarboxylase. Even while levodopa is being absorbed, it is undergoing decarboxylation. A second pathway of metabolism occurs via COMT to produce 3-*O*-methyldopa (3-OMD). Less than 1% of administered oral levodopa penetrates the brain. The peripheral production of dopamine results in side effects such as nausea, hypotension, and cardiac arrhythmias. With the use of peripheral dopa decarboxylase inhibitors (e.g., carbidopa and benserazide), the dose of levodopa is substantially reduced (about 70%) and peripheral side effects markedly attenuated (1).

In spite of this advance, only 5 to 10% of oral levodopa reaches the brain. With the inhibition of dopa decarboxylase, other pathways are activated. In particular, COMT metabolizes levodopa to 3-OMD. The half-life of 3-OMD is about 15 hours compared with about one hour for levodopa. It has been suggested that 3-OMD may compete with levodopa for the energy dependant transport mechanism used for penetration into the brain. Large amounts of 3-OMD may decrease the efficacy of levodopa in animals and patients with Parkinson's disease (PD). 3-OMD is of no benefit to the Parkinsonian brain: whether it has deleterious properties is under speculation. COMT is one of the main enzymes responsible for metabolism of levodopa and other catecholamines. It is located in the liver, kidney and gut wall as well as in the central nervous system (CNS) neurons and glia (2).

RATIONALE FOR COMT INHIBITORS

COMT inhibitors are used in conjunction with levodopa/carbidopa in PD patients to lengthen levodopa's duration of action. Peripheral metabolism of levodopa is reduced by carbidopa and COMT inhibitors. This allows for a greater portion of the dose of levodopa to remain in the circulation for transport to the brain (Figure 36-1). In this way, COMT inhibitors lengthen levodopa's duration of action by prolonging its half-life in plasma and increasing the amount of levodopa that is available to enter the brain (2). This is an important development because the shortening of the duration of response to levodopa has been associated with the onset of motor fluctuations (3). A recent study by Block and colleagues observed a low (20%) but definite prevalence of response fluctuations after five years of treatment with levodopa–carbidopa therapy (immediate release [IR] or controlled release [CR]) (4).

In addition, preclinical and clinical studies suggest that current therapeutic regimens provide only intermittent stimulation of dopamine receptors (5). This intermittent stimulation may lead to neuronal changes downstream that contribute further to the development of motor complications. Dopamine replacement regimens that provide continuous stimulation of dopamine receptors may prevent or ameliorate the motor complications of PD. Therefore patients should obtain significant advantages from adjunctive therapy with a COMT inhibitor, which may result in the stabilizing or "smoothing out" of dopamine levels.

After a number of years many patients treated with levodopa develop motor fluctuations (6). Motor fluctuations of the "wearing off" type are the most common. Because these fluctuations result from a shortening of levodopa's duration of action, they are also the known as end-of-dose deterioration. Eventually, progression

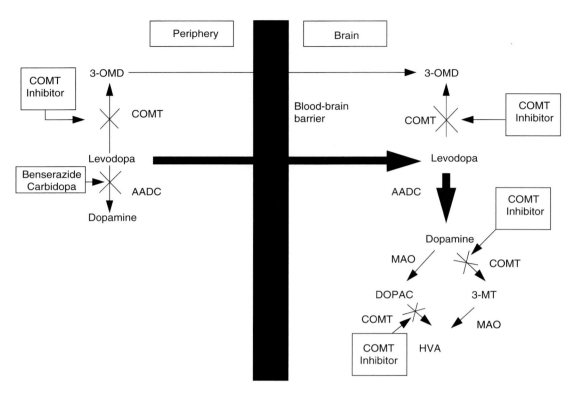

FIGURE 36-1. Metabolism of levodopa: Effects of peripheral and central COMT inhibition AADC, aromatic amino acid decarboxylase; COMT, catechol-*O*-methyltransferase, DOPAC, 3,4-dihydroxyphenylacetic acid; HVA, homovanillic acid; MAO, monoamine oxidase; 3-MT, 3-methoxytyramine; 3-OMD, 3-*O*-methyldopa.

of PD results in loss of terminals and the inability of the remaining neurons to store dopamine; both contribute to the increasing severity and unpredictability of the motor fluctuations. As this occurs, motor function fluctuates between two states: the "on" state, when plasma levodopa concentrations remain within the therapeutic range and optimally control bradykinesia, tremor, and rigidity; and the "off" state, when plasma levels decline, the medication's effect diminishes, and mobility is compromised.

As the disease advances, and with long-term levodopa use, many patients show an enhanced sensitivity to even small fluctuations in blood concentrations of levodopa (1). They also may experience peak-dose dyskinesias (choreic or dystonic movements) that occur when plasma concentrations of levodopa are at their highest (6,7). Furthermore, disease progression can bring complications in motor response that may be unrelated to the dosing interval. These abrupt and often unpredictable fluctuations, also called random fluctuations or the "on-off" phenomena, can become the most disabling symptoms of PD and are generally not amenable to therapeutic intervention.

Patients in the early stages who have not developed fluctuations are categorized as having nonfluctuating,

or stable, PD. As a rule, in these early stages, bid or tid administration of levodopa/carbidopa in patients provides constant control of Parkinsonian symptoms. Eventually, most patients experience some degree of "on" and "off" states as the disease progresses. The goals of drug development in PD are symptomatic relief; delay or prevention of disease progression; avoidance of "wearing off" fluctuations; amelioration of "wearing off" fluctuations when they do develop; and management of other associated problems of PD such as psychosis, cognitive impairment, and depression (6). The challenge for the clinician is to use the range of pharmacologic interventions appropriately to achieve maximum benefit for the patient.

Patients with nonfluctuating disease seem to have sufficient presynaptic dopaminergic neurons to store and release dopamine, thus avoiding fluctuations in intrasynaptic dopamine levels and facilitating long-duration responses. In patients with advanced disease, residual neurons are thought to have a diminished capacity to take up levodopa and to store and release dopamine, thus shortening the duration of response. Intrasynaptic dopamine concentrations begin to reflect the fluctuating plasma levels of levodopa that correspond to periodic administration of levodopa.

Table 36-1   Strategies for Extending Levodopa Effect
• Increase amount of levodopa administered per dose • Increase frequency of levodopa doses • Switch to controlled-release preparations of levodopa • Provide direct intraduodenal infusion of levodopa • Inhibit peripheral catechol-*O*-methyltransferase (decreasing metabolism of levodopa to 3-*O*-methyldopa)

Although controversial, clinical evidence suggests that fluctuating levels of levodopa are associated with motor complications, and continuous levels of levodopa ameliorate these problems, researchers are focusing on extending the duration of each dose of levodopa to sustain a more consistent plasma level. This may be achieved by administering levodopa infusions, substituting CR formulations for IR formulations, and adding COMT inhibitors (Table 36-1).

Some believe that increasing the dose of levodopa or the frequency of dosing can lead to the patient's development or worsening of dyskinesias. Either strategy steepens the dose-response curve for levodopa, narrowing the therapeutic index and heightening sensitivity to minute changes in drug availability (3).

CLINICAL STUDIES WITH COMT INHIBITORS

Tolcapone

Pharmacokinetics of Tolcapone

Tolcapone is a COMT inhibitor that acts both peripherally and centrally (animal data only) although clinical response seems to be primarily related to its peripheral effects. Tolcapone, like entacapone, was shown in several studies to increase the half-life of levodopa (2). Tolcapone increases the area under the curve (AUC) for levodopa. This occurs without a concomitant increase in peak plasma concentration. At a 200 mg dose of tolcapone, the AUC increases by 94%. Inhibition of 3-OMD formation is substantial and dose-dependent (8). The overall clearance of tolcapone is low, which translates to good bioavailability. The elimination half-life is 2.1 hours. The inhibition of erythrocyte COMT is stronger and considerably longer with tolcapone than with entacapone.

Studies in Patients with Fluctuating Parkinson's Disease

In a study conducted by Kurth and colleagues (9), tolcapone prolonged the time that patients received clinical benefits from levodopa. In addition, patients were able to reduce their total levodopa dose requirements. This multicenter, double-blind, placebo-controlled study included patients (n = 151) who initially required at least three doses of IR levodopa/carbidopa daily. All patients had idiopathic PD and were experiencing a predictable "on" time in response to the first morning dose of levodopa/carbidopa and at least two predictable end-of-dose "off" time episodes (with a combined "off" time >2 hours). Primary efficacy measures were the investigators' 10-hour evaluation of "off" time and the Unified Parkinson's disease rating scale (UPDRS) motor subscale (part 3) AUC. Clinical evaluations were made just before and after six weeks of treatment with tolcapone (50 mg, 200 mg, or 400 mg three times a day [tid]). At both evaluations, UPDRS motor subscale scores as well as "on-off" and dyskinesia assessments were made at 30-minute intervals over a 10-hour period. Compared with placebo the difference between baseline and week six for all three doses of tolcapone significantly reduced "off" time by an average of 40%; ($-0.4\% \pm 2.7\%$ [placebo]; $-16.6\% \pm 2.7\%$ [50-mg tid group]; $-16.1\% \pm 2.8\%$ [200-mg tid group]; and $-18.1\% \pm 3.0\%$ [400-mg tid group]; $P < 0.01$). The change in AUC was statistically and significantly different from placebo for all tolcapone dosages from baseline to week six (-11.4 ± 8.6 [placebo]; -44.8 ± 8.9 [50-mg tid group]; -37 ± 8.9 [200-mg tid group]; and -49.1 ± 10.1 [400-mg tid group]; $P < 0.05$). Both the total daily dose of levodopa/carbidopa and the dosing frequency were significantly reduced in patients receiving tolcapone either 200 mg or 400 mg tid.

Although generally well tolerated, tolcapone was associated with typical dose-related dopaminergic side effects in some patients. Dopamine-related adverse events increased during the first two weeks of treatment in all tolcapone groups but diminished as levodopa dosages were adjusted downward. The most frequently reported adverse event was dyskinesias; 21.4% of the placebo group and approximately 50% of the tolcapone-treated patients reported this event at least once during the six-week study. Nausea was reported in approximately 12% of the placebo group and in 25% of the tolcapone-treated group. Postural hypotension was reported by 12% of the placebo group and between 7.5% and 18.4% of the tolcapone-treated patients. These side effects could be either ameliorated or eliminated by reducing the dosage of levodopa/carbidopa. Dizziness (5.3% to 10%

of tolcapone-treated patients versus 0% of placebo patients) and urine discoloration (4.9% to 23.7% of tolcapone-treated patients versus 0% of placebo patients) were also noted. No significant changes in the mean values of vital sign parameters were observed, and no significant differences were observed between the tolcapone and placebo patients in any vital sign parameters. Additionally, no abnormal laboratory tests results were reported that were related to tolcapone.

Welsh and colleagues recently assessed the effect of tolcapone (50 mg, 200 mg, or 400 mg tid) versus placebo on quality of life (QOL) in patients who were receiving levodopa/carbidopa therapy over a 6-week period (10). This study was conducted in parallel with the double-blind, placebo-controlled, dose-response study previously described. (10) QOL was measured by the Sickness Impact Profile (SIP) and adjustment to illness was measured by the Psychosocial adjustment to Illness scale – Self-report. Objective assessment of the impact of PD was measured by the UPDRS. Patient ratings of total illness impact $(P = 0.003)$, physical impact $(P = 0.002)$, and psychosocial impact $(P = 0.007)$ improved significantly when subjects in the three tolcapone-treated groups were compared with those receiving placebo (9).

In a double-blind, parallel group trial involving 11 centers, Rajput and colleagues studied (202) patients who were experiencing "wearing off" phenomenon on levodopa therapy; patients were at least 30 years old and had been treated with levodopa for at least one year (11). At the start of the study, patients were taking at least four doses daily of levodopa/carbidopa (or three doses daily if two were a CR formulation). Patients were experiencing predictable motor fluctuations at the end of a dosing interval that could not be eliminated by adjusting their existing therapy.

The principal efficacy measurement was "off" and "on" time assessed by patient diaries. Investigators' global assessment (IGA) was used to evaluate change in "wearing off" phenomenon and severity of PD symptoms. UPDRS scale was used to assess Parkinsonian symptoms and impact on QOL was measured. After baseline assessments, patients were randomized to receive either tolcapone (100 mg or 200 mg tid) or placebo in addition to levodopa/carbidopa. After three months of treatment with tolcapone, data from the patients' daily diaries were analyzed. The patients experienced statistically significant reduction in the duration of "off" time – a mean reduction of 3.2 hours – compared with baseline when treated with tolcapone 200 mg tid $(P < 0.01)$ (Table 36-2) (11). A subgroup of these patients received tolcapone for

Table 36-2 Efficacy Data: Change from Baseline to Month 3. Reprinted with permission from Rajput A, et al. *Neurology* 1997; 49:1066–1071 (16).

	Placebo	100 mg	200 mg
Daily "off" time	−1.4	−2.3	−3.2*
% baseline	−20	−32	−48

*$P < 0.01$

12 months, during which further reductions in total daily levodopa dose were achieved and reduced "off" time was maintained. The dosage of levodopa was significantly reduced in patients receiving either dosage of tolcapone compared with those receiving placebo $(P < 0.01)$ and the number of daily doses was also significantly reduced $(P < 0.01)$ (11).

Over the long term, tolcapone therapy was well tolerated, and the most frequent dopaminergic adverse events were dyskinesias and nausea, both of which occurred early in the study and were generally transient. Dyskinesias were satisfactorily controlled by adjusting levodopa dose. Diarrhea and constipation were the most frequent nondopaminergic events and accounted for the majority of withdrawals from the trial (4% and 8% withdrew from the 100-mg tid and 200-mg tid groups, respectively, and 3% withdrew from the placebo group) (11). Tolcapone treatment was associated with elevated liver enzymes in three patients in the 100-mg tid group versus two patients in the 200-mg tid group.

In European study, Baas and colleagues demonstrated that tolcapone reduces "off" time and levodopa requirements in patients (n = 177) experiencing predictable fluctuations, thereby improving the efficacy of long-term levodopa therapy (12). During the study, in addition to levodopa/benserazide, patients received either tolcapone (100 mg or 200 mg tid) or placebo for three months. At three months, changes in the frequency of "wearing off" fluctuations were assessed, along with other efficacy parameters. Compared with placebo, adding tolcapone 100 mg tid to the regimen produced statistically significant reductions in "off" time (31.5% decrease; $P < 0.05$); statistically significant increases in "on" time (21.3% increase, $P < 0.01$); and statistically significant reductions in the mean daily levodopa dose (decrease of 109 mg, $P < 0.05$). "On" time was increased by 20.6% $(P < 0.01)$ and "off" time was decreased by 26.2% (NS) with tolcapone 200 mg tid. Diarrhea resulted in withdrawals in seven percent of the 100-mg tid group and 10% of the 200-mg tid group.

The latest study of tolcapone in patients with fluctuating disease was reported by Adler et al. (12a) in 1998. This study was a placebo-controlled, double-blind, randomized trial involving 15 centers. Patients were on levodopa at least for one year and had to be using a minimum of four doses of standard formulation levodopa or three doses if two were of the controlled-release type. They had to have end-of-dose failure but not unpredictable "on–off" and be on a stable dose of levodopa for at least four weeks. Patients were randomized to receive placebo, and tolcapone 100 mg tid or 200 mg tid. Primary efficacy measures were changes in "on" and "off" time measured by diaries. Secondary efficacy measures were UPDRS, IGA, dyskinesia scale, and SIP. A total of 215 patients enrolled: mean duration of PD was 10.5 years, mean duration of levodopa therapy was 8.5 years, and 76% had dyskinesias. A six-week study showed significant increase in "on" time for both tolcapone groups (2.1 hours for 100 mg tid, 2.3 hours for 200 mg tid) versus placebo (0.3 hours) ($P < .001$). "Off" time decreased by two hours in the 100-mg tid group, 2.5 hours in the 200-mg tid group and 0.3 hours in the placebo group ($P < .005$). Levodopa dose significantly decreased by 23% in 100-mg tid group, 29% in 200-mg tid group compared to placebo ($P < .001$), and the number of doses per day also decreased in active treatment groups. Adverse events were similar to previous studies.

Comparison to Dopamine Agonists

The relative effectiveness and tolerability of a COMT inhibitor versus a dopamine agonist as adjunctive therapy to levodopa have been compared recently in a randomized, single-blind study conducted in Europe (13). Over an eight-week period, investigators compared the effects of adjunctive therapy with tolcapone (200 mg tid) versus bromocriptine (mean final dose, 22.4 mg/d) in 146 levodopa-treated patients with fluctuating disease. Tolcapone was shown to be more effective than bromocriptine for increasing the mean "on" time and decreasing the mean "off" time, and was also better tolerated (Table 36-3). Patients treated with tolcapone required less levodopa and experienced fewer CNS adverse effects (psychosis and hallucinations) than patients treated with bromocriptine.

These results demonstrate that when used as an adjunct to levodopa therapy in patients with fluctuating disease, tolcapone is as effective or more so than the dopamine agonist bromocriptine. In addition, tolcapone has the advantage of not requiring titration at the start of treatment. Tolcapone also leads to significant reductions in the total daily dose of levodopa

Table 36-3 Efficacy and Tolerability of Bromocriptine Compared with Tolcapone as Adjunctive Therapies to Levodopa. Adapted with permission from Agid Y et al. *Lancet* 1997; 350:712–713 (30).

Clinical Effect	Bromocriptine (n = 74)	Tolcapone (n = 72)
Levodopa		
Reduction in total daily dose (mg)	-30.0 ± 20.3	$-124.0 \pm 21.5^*$
Patients reduced dosage/d	11%	-33%
"On-Off" Time		
Change in mean "off" time (hours)	-2.4 ± 0.4	-3.0 ± 0.5
Mean change in "off" time/mean baseline "off" time	-37.9%	-43.7%
Change in "on" time (hours)	$+2.1 \pm 0.5$	$+2.8 \pm 0.5$
Mean change in "on" time/mean baseline "on" time	27.5%	36.6%
Investigators' Global Assessment		
Efficacy: patients improved	69%	82%[†]
Tolerability: patients improved	9%	16%
UPDRS Subscale II Score		
Change in ADL	-0.1 ± 0.4	-0.9 ± 0.5
UPDRS Subscale III Score		
Change in motor function	-3.3 ± 1.0	-3.1 ± 1.05

In this open-label study, either tolcapone (200 mg tid) or bromocriptine (mean final dose, 22.4 mg/d) was administered to patients also receiving levodopa. Data are mean ± standard error of the mean (SEM) between baseline and week eight or percentages of patients at week eight. UPDRS, Unified Parkinson's Disease Rating Scale; ADL, activities of daily living.
*$P < 0.01$
†$P < 0.05$

and to improvements in "wearing off" fluctuations. Tolcapone was associated with a much lower incidence of peripheral dopaminergic events (e.g., nausea) than was bromocriptine.

In Phase III tolcapone studies for patients with fluctuating disease, in which about one-third of them received a dopamine agonist concomitantly with tolcapone as an adjunct to levodopa and a dopa decarboxylase inhibitor, no serious safety concerns were identified. However, the incidence of orthostatic complaints and hallucinations was found to be higher among those receiving dopamine agonists with tolcapone than among those receiving only tolcapone (11). The incidence of dyskinesias was approximately 8–10% higher in the dopamine agonist group.

Patients with Nonfluctuating Parkinson's Disease

For patients who have not developed motor fluctuations (the "stable" patient), tolcapone has been studied to assess its ability to delay their development and improve activities of daily living (ADL) scores. Researchers have hypothesized that providing smooth and continued delivery of levodopa in patients with nonfluctuating disease, by using adjunctive therapy, may positively influence the development of motor fluctuations.

The major outcome variable was the percent change in the ability to perform ADL as measured by UPDRS subscale II. After six months of therapy, the patients receiving tolcapone 100 mg or 200 mg tid showed statistically significant improvement on the ADL (subscale II) and motor function (subscale III) sections of the UPDRS, compared with patients who received placebo (14). For example, there was an 18% (-1.4 ± 0.3) and a 20% (-1.6 ± 0.3) improvement in ADL scores in patients receiving tolcapone 100 mg tid ($P < 0.05$) or tolcapone 200 mg tid ($P < 0.01$). In contrast, there were no significant changes in the ADL or motor scores of patients receiving placebo over the same six-month period ($+0.1 \pm 0.6$ change on subscales II and III).

Along with the improvements in motor function, patients receiving tolcapone 100 mg and 200 mg tid were able to reduce their total daily levodopa dose by 6% and 9%, respectively ($P < 0.001$ for both groups). In contrast, patients in the placebo group required an additional 47 mg of levodopa over the same six-month period, which was not accompanied by a decrease in impairment.

Compared with placebo-treated patients, a significantly lower proportion of patients treated with 200 mg tid tolcapone developed evidence of motor fluctuations at six months as measured by the UPDRS (subscale IV).

In this study, patients treated with tolcapone 100 mg tid ($P < 0.01$ vs placebo) or 200 mg tid ($P < 0.05$ vs placebo) also experienced statistically significant improvements in the physical subscale of the Sickness impact profile (SIP), the QOL measure used in this trial.

Dupont and colleagues assessed the effect of tolcapone on levodopa dose in patients with stable PD whose "wearing off" phenomena had been controlled with more frequent levodopa dosing (15). In this double-blind, placebo-controlled study, 97 patients were randomly assigned to receive placebo or tolcapone (200 mg or 400 mg tid) for six weeks. On the morning of the first day of the treatment period, the levodopa dose was reduced by 35% and subsequently titrated as needed. In case of dyskinesias, increasing the dose interval, mainly in the afternoon, was preferred to decreasing the size of a single dose (except when the first daily dose was not tolerated) (15). After six weeks of treatment, patients in the 200-mg tid group crossed over to the 400-mg tid group and vice versa for another three weeks. Patients receiving placebo remained on placebo until the end of the nine-week study. The primary efficacy parameter was change in levodopa dosage from baseline to week six. Other efficacy parameters were IGA, UPDRS subscales I (mentation, behavior, mood), II (ADL), III (motor functions), and IVb (clinical fluctuations). Safety assessments included levodopa-induced symptoms, dyskinesia-rating scale, UPDRS subscales IVa (dyskinesias) and IVc (other complications), IGA of tolerability, vital signs, electrocardiograms (ECG), and laboratory analyses. Efficacy was analyzed via hypothesis testing for the first six-week treatment period.

At the end of the six-week treatment period, both tolcapone groups evidenced a greater reduction in total daily dose (27% for 200-mg tid group and 25% for 400-mg tid group) and number of doses of levodopa (-1.3 for 200 mg tid group and -1.5 for 400 mg tid group) compared with the placebo group (19% decrease in dose and -1.1 doses per day), but these differences did not reach statistical significance. The tolcapone 200-mg tid group demonstrated the greatest improvement in estimated mean scores for all efficacy parameters ($P < 0.05$ vs placebo only for a change in UPDRS subscale II). The changes seen in the tolcapone 400-mg tid group were nearly indistinguishable from those in the placebo group. However, the results indicate that levodopa dosage reduction in the tolcapone treatment groups did not occur at the expense of other efficacy parameters.

As in previous studies, nausea and dyskinesias were the most frequently reported dopaminergic adverse events. The most unexpected nondopaminergic event frequently reported was diarrhea, which was reported by three patients (nine percent) in the tolcapone 200-mg tid treatment group and six patients (19%) in the 400-mg tid treatment group. The majority of the adverse events reported were mild and reversible.

Entacapone

Pharmacokinetics of Entacapone

Entacapone is rapidly absorbed and exhibits linear pharmacokinetics up to a dose of 200 mg (8). The bioavailability of entacapone is low at 35%. It is rapidly metabolized in the liver. Entacapone has a greater volume of distribution than tolcapone and is metabolized rapidly, whereas tolcapone becomes protein-bound. Therefore, entacapone is cleared more rapidly from the body than tolcapone.

Early Studies of Entacapone

In a four-week, open-label trial, entacapone was shown to improve "on" time from 2.3–3.4 hours per dose of levodopa (16). Dyskinesias were seen as a side effect. These results were validated in a crossover trial of entacapone and placebo (17). In this study, entacapone prolonged the duration of a motor response to an individual dose of levodopa by 34 minutes. Dyskinesia duration was similarly prolonged. From home diaries, "on" time was found to be prolonged by 2.1 hours per day.

Entacapone has been studied pharmacologically and was found to increase the area under the curve (AUC) for levodopa without enhancing T_{max} or C_{max} (18). It prolongs the elimination half-life of levodopa, thus extending its action. This was true when tested with either orally or intravenously administered levodopa (19). Entacapone increased the duration of action of single doses of levodopa by 56%. Plasma 3-OMD concentrations were reduced by 60%. During chronic administration of this drug for eight weeks, the daily requirements for levodopa were reduced by 27%. Patients reported that the percentage of day "on" time was 77% during treatment with entacapone, dropping to 44% when this drug was withdrawn.

Parkinson Study Group and Nordic Study Group

A large, multicenter, placebo-controlled, double-blind, randomized, 24-week study of entacapone was conducted by the Parkinson Study Group (20). Two hundred and five patients were randomized to receive either entacapone 200 mg or placebo with each dose of levodopa. The primary efficacy endpoint was the change in "on" time while awake. Entacapone treatment increased "on" time by 5 percent (approximately one hour) per day consistently throughout all 24 weeks of the study (20). The effect of entacapone treatment was especially dramatic in patients with the lowest amount of "on" time (<55%) at baseline (i.e., patients who were most impaired). The total UPDRS score improved in 10% of patients treated with entacapone at week 24. Entacapone reduced patients' levodopa requirements by 100 mg/d on average. The investigators' global evaluations of the patients revealed a shift in the positive direction in those patients treated with entacapone compared with the placebo group, who shifted in a negative direction ($P = 0.002$) (Table 36-4). When entacapone was withdrawn, in a blinded staggered drug withdrawal period, the beneficial effects were rapidly lost.

Table 36-4 Distribution of Responses on the Investigators' Global Evaluation of the Patient at Baseline and at Week 24. Reprinted with permission from Parkinson Study Group. *Ann Neurol* 1997; 42:747–755 (18).

	Very Poorly	Poorly	Rather Poorly	Not Well, Not Poorly	Rather Well	Well	Very Well
Baseline							
Placebo	1	2	11	42	32	13	1
Entacapone	0	3	14	35	29	18	4
Week 24							
Placebo	1	7	28	30	26	7	3
Entacapone	1	4	9	30	33	24	2

The investigator was asked to rate how the patient had been doing in terms of his or her Parkinson's disease during the week preceding the visit.

The most frequently reported adverse events in the entacapone group were dyskinesias, urine discoloration, dizziness, nausea, and constipation. Dyskinesias were reported most frequently during the first eight weeks of the trial (30 of 33 patients in the placebo group; 53 of 55 patients in the entacapone group) (20). However, after the levodopa dosage was adjusted, dyskinesias resolved in approximately one-third of the patients within the eight weeks. No differences were observed between entacapone and placebo groups in vital signs, laboratory tests, or ECG results.

Similar results with entacapone have been reported by the Nordic Study Group (n = 171) (21). This was also a six month double-blind, placebo-controlled trial using patient diaries as the primary outcome measure. Treatment with entacapone increased daily "on" time. Baseline daily "on" time was 9–10 hours, which was increased by 1.3 hours after entacapone treatment. Treatment with entacapone also reduced the mean total UPDRS scores when "on" by approximately 10% compared to scores for patients receiving placebo. The benefits of treatment with entacapone were lost within 2–3 hours of the last dose administered and before the beginning of the next scheduled dose cycle (20,21).

Patients with Nonfluctuating Parkinson's Disease

There are no data available on the use of entacapone on stable patients. However, at the time of this writing, a multicenter, double-blind study is in progress.

SAFETY OF COMT INHIBITORS

Management of Dopaminergic Adverse Events

Both tolcapone and entacapone have the potential to increase dopaminergic adverse events in patients receiving levodopa. The most frequent adverse events associated with COMT inhibitors (those occurring in >5% of treated patients) have been dopaminergic in nature, for example, peak-dose dyskinesias, nausea, or hallucinations. These have been mild, and reducing the levodopa dose when tolcapone or entacapone is administered tends to minimize their occurrence (9,11,12,21). The short-term studies conducted to date have shown that administration of COMT inhibitors is safe and well tolerated in patients with PD (9,22). In clinical trials of tolcapone, the majority of patients required a decrease in their daily levodopa dose if their daily levodopa dose initially was >600 mg or if they had moderate or severe dyskinesias before beginning tolcapone treatment (11). In those patients

who required a levodopa dose reduction, the average reduction in daily dosage was 30%.

Management of Nondopaminergic Adverse Events

Nondopaminergic adverse events such as diarrhea, headache, increased sweating, and abdominal pain have been observed. Diarrhea is the most frequent reason given for patients' withdrawing from the long-term tolcapone trials (11,14). However, Waters and colleagues reported that in 92 to 95% of patients diarrhea abated or was mild enough that patients continued tolcapone on a long-term basis (14). With tolcapone, severe diarrhea affects approximately 5 to 10% of patients. Furthermore, almost all cases of severe diarrhea developed during the first three months of treatment. Approximately one half of patients who experienced diarrhea elected to discontinue treatment with tolcapone. After three months, the incidence of diarrhea was equivalent to that in the placebo-treated patients. Thereafter, all patients tolerated tolcapone extremely well (12). If a patient does not develop diarrhea in the first six months, it is unlikely to occur.

Entacapone has also been associated with hypotension and constipation, but the incidence of diarrhea (5%) and gastrointestinal cramping has been relatively low (19).

Between 6 and 12 weeks after the start of tolcapone treatment, some patients had increased levels of alanine aminotransferase (ALT) and aspartate aminotransferase (AST) (>3 times the upper limit of normal); 3% receiving 200 mg tid and 1% receiving 100 mg tid. Within two to four weeks of discontinuing treatment, both AST and ALT levels tended to return to normal without any other hepatic adverse effects observed (12,14). In patients who continued treatment, liver enzyme abnormalities resolved spontaneously without sequelae (14). Six patients were withdrawn from the studies because of elevated transaminases (11,12,14).

As of October 1998, three deaths from acute fulminant hepatic failure have been reported in association with the use of tolcapone. Thus new prescribing information is being adopted. Tolcapone is recommended for patients experiencing symptom fluctuations and who are no longer being satisfactorily treated with other medications for PD. Tolcapone's benefit is quickly apparent. If after three weeks no clinical benefit is seen, tolcapone should be stopped. Liver function should be tested before starting the compound, and monitoring of liver function is required every two weeks for one year, every four weeks for an additional six months, and then every two months for the lifetime of the patient. Since the introduction of liver monitoring, no new deaths have been reported with tolcapone. Patients should also be advised of the need for self-monitoring for the signs of liver failure. In the United States informed written consent must be obtained. As the dose is increased from 100 mg tid to 200 mg tid the monitoring should be repeated as if the patient had just been initiated. Because of the potential for rhabdomyolysis, it is recommended that this drug is not used in patients with severe dyskinesia. If it is necessary to discontinue tolcapone, it should be done with care as sudden withdrawal of any dopaminergic drug may lead to worsening of PD or a hyperpyrexia, confusion (neuroleptic malignant-like) syndrome. (2) Entacapone has not been associated with liver toxicity. It has been approved by the FDA for use in fluctuating PD patients without the requirement of liver function monitoring. COMT inhibitors can change the color of the patients urine to bright yellow or orange. This is not a cause for alarm and has no toxicity associated with it, but patients should be informed of this possibility.

Safety When Used with Selegiline

Tolcapone has been shown to be effective and tolerable when used with selegiline and levodopa (22,24).

DIFFERENCES BETWEEN TOLCAPONE AND ENTACAPONE

Both tolcapone and entacapone are peripheral inhibitors of COMT; however, several important distinctions need to be made between the two drugs.

Pharmacokinetics

Differences between the two drugs can be mostly attributed to differences in their pharmacokinetic profiles (Table 36-5) (8). Both are rapidly absorbed and exhibit linear pharmacokinetics up to a dose of 200 mg (8). Since only a small amount of tolcapone is lost during first-pass metabolism in the liver, the absolute bioavailability of tolcapone after oral administration is 70%. This is significantly higher than the bioavailability of entacapone (35%), which is rapidly metabolized in the liver. Entacapone has a greater volume of distribution than tolcapone and is metabolized rapidly, whereas tolcapone becomes protein-bound. Therefore entacapone is cleared more rapidly from the body than tolcapone (8).

Tolcapone and entacapone have similar half-lives (2.1 ± 0.6 hours vs 3.4 ± 2.7 hours). Tolcapone is active in both the periphery and, in animal studies, in the brain, whereas entacapone inhibits only peripheral

Table 36-5 Pharmacokinetic Parameters of Entacapone and Tolcapone after Administration of 200 mg. Adapted with permission from Jorga KA, *Clin Neuropharmacol* 1998; 21(Supp1):S9–S16 (18).

	Tolcapone	Entacapone
Cmax (ug/mL)	6.3 ± 2.9	1.8 ± 0.8
Tmax (h)	1.8 ± 1.3	0.7 ± 0.2
AUC (h*ug/mL)	18.5 ± 5.2	1.6 ± 0.3
Half-life (h)	2.1 ± 0.6	3.4 ± 2.7

Values are mean ±SD.

COMT activity. However, central COMT inhibition with tolcapone has not been proven conclusively to occur in humans (23), and any possible clinical advantage of central activity is not known.

Dosing Regimens

The recommended dosing regimens are significantly different for tolcapone and entacapone. The schedule for tolcapone is 100 mg or 200 mg tid at six-hour intervals. Entacapone 200 mg is administered simultaneously with each dose of levodopa (18).

Use with Different Formulations of Levodopa

Jorga and colleagues have demonstrated that adjunctive treatment with tolcapone potentiates the clinical effects of levodopa, irrespective of the levodopa–carbidopa formulation (25). The results were obtained for all of the following formulations of levodopa/carbidopa after coadministration with tolcapone 200 mg: 100 mg/10 mg; 100 mg/25 mg; 200 mg/20 mg; 200 mg/50 mg; 250 mg/25 mg (IR); and 200 mg/50 mg (CR) (25). Comparable effects have been observed when tolcapone was administered with both single-dose and multiple-dose regimens (26).

The effects of entacapone combined with levodopa/carbidopa differ from those of tolcapone in combination with levodopa/carbidopa. In a study by Ahtila and colleagues, normal volunteers were treated simultaneously with entacapone (200 mg) and CR levodopa/carbidopa (27). Even though entacapone extended the time that levodopa remained within the therapeutic range, the effect on levodopa bioavailability was less with the CR formulation than had been demonstrated previously with standard levodopa.

PATIENT SELECTION CRITERIA

COMT inhibitors are likely to play an important role in the long-term management of patients with PD.

Therefore it is important to identify those patients who will be most responsive to this therapy.

Patients Residing Alone or in Nursing Homes

Because they may reduce or eliminate the need for other adjunctive therapies such as selegiline, amantadine, anticholinergic agents, and dopamine agonists, COMT inhibitors should also be very beneficial not only to those elderly PD patients living alone but also to PD patients living in nursing homes. COMT inhibitors, by extending the duration of action of each dose of levodopa, have been shown to reduce the total number of daily levodopa doses that need to be administered to each patient (11,20).

In many elderly patients, there are concerns about cognitive dysfunction with the dopamine agonists (6,28). Hallucinations and delusions are commonly assumed to complicate the advanced PD when dopaminergic drug treatment has been given for an extended period and a high dosage is required to control motor symptoms. However, Graham and colleagues found that these behavioral problems were more prevalent among idiopathic PD patients when a direct-acting dopamine receptor agonist was prescribed concomitantly with levodopa therapy regardless of age at onset of PD, stage of the disease, "on" motor disability, cognitive function, or dosage of levodopa (28).

If problems arise with cognition, physicians can reduce and/or eliminate anticholinergic agents, amantadine, selegiline, and dopamine agonists. The COMT inhibitors can be substituted if the motor fluctuations become troublesome.

COMPARISONS OF COMT INHIBITORS WITH OTHER THERAPIES FOR PARKINSON'S DISEASE

Dopamine Agonists (see previous section)

Sinemet® CR

There has been no study directly comparing the ability of Sinemet® CR to extend levodopa's benefit versus a COMT inhibitor. CR preparations are effective for the management of simple "wearing off" phenomena (6). However, by virtue of their slow-release property, there is a delay in the onset of effect. CR preparations can augment or worsen end of day dyskinesias. COMT inhibitors offer the advantage of ameliorating "wearing off" fluctuations without a delay in onset. In addition, the levodopa dose can be adjusted downward if dyskinesias appear.

CONCLUSION

Unique among the adjunctive therapies for PD, COMT inhibitors effectively extend and enhance the duration and action of levodopa. COMT inhibitors effectively increase "on" time, reduce "off" time, improve the patient's ability to perform ADL, increase motor function scores on UPDRS subscales, and may reduce the dosage of levodopa needed.

Unlike dopamine agonists, COMT inhibitors have an effect on levodopa pharmacokinetics after the first dose. If dopaminergic side effects occur with COMT inhibitors, the dose of levodopa can be reduced. COMT inhibitors do not require titration for optimal effect.

COMT inhibitors are an option in the treatment of Parkinson's disease in patients with fluctuating motor responses. Patients and physicians need to be aware of the new requirements for liver function monitoring with the recently released tolcapone.

FDA requests that all cases of serious liver injury occurring in Parkinson's patients whether on TASMAR or any other drug, be reported to the Agency via the MEDWATCH by phone at 1-800-FDA-1088, by fax at 1-800-FDA-0178, by mail at MEDWATCH HF-2, FDA 5600 Fishers Lane, Rockville, MD 20857, or on the MEDWATCH web site at *www.FDA.gov/medwatch*.

REFERENCES

1. LeWitt PA. Treatment strategies for extension of levodopa effect. *Neurol Clin* 1992; 10:511–527.
2. Kurth MC, Adler CH. COMT inhibition: A new treatment strategy for Parkinson's disease. *Neurology* 1998; 50:S3–S14.
3. Mouradian MM, Heuser IJ, Baronti F, et al. Modification of central dopaminergic mechanisms by continuous levodopa therapy for advanced Parkinson's disease. *Ann Neurol* 1990; 27:18–23.
4. Block G, Liss C, Reines S, et al. Comparison of immediate-release and controlled-release carbidopa/levodopa in Parkinson's disease. *Eur Neurol* 1997; 37:23–27.
5. Chase TN. Levodopa therapy: Consequences of the nonphysiologic replacement of dopamine. *Neurology* 1998; 50(Suppl):S17–S25.
6. Waters CH. Managing the late complications of Parkinson's disease. *Neurology* 1997; 49(Suppl 1):S49–S57.
7. Juncos JL. Levodopa: Pharmacology, pharmacokinetics, and pharmacodynamics. *Neurol Clin* 1992; 10:487–509.
8. Jorga KM. COMT inhibitors: Pharmacokinetics and pharmacodynamic comparisons. *Clin Neuropharmacol* 1998; 21:S9–S16.

9. Kurth MC, Adler CH, Saint Hilaire M-H, et al. Tolcapone improves motor function and reduces levodopa requirement in patients with Parkinson's disease experiencing motor fluctuations: A multicenter, double-blind, randomized, placebo-controlled trial. *Neurology* 1997; 48:81–87.

10. Welsh MD, Ved N, Waters CH. Psychosocial adjustment and illness impact in Parkinson's disease patients before and after treatment with tolcapone (Tasmar). *Neurology* 1996; 46:A322. Abstract.

11. Rajput AH, Martin W, Saint Hilaire M-H, et al. Tolcapone improves motor function in Parkinsonian patients with the "wearing-off" phenomenon: A double-blind, placebo-controlled, multicenter trial. *Neurology* 1997; 49:1066–1071.

12. Baas H, Beiske AG, Ghika J, et al. COMT inhibition with tolcapone reduces "wearing-off" phenomenon and levodopa requirements in fluctuating Parkinsonian patients. *J Neurol Neurosurg Psychiatry* 1997; 63:421–428.

12a. Adler CH, Singer C, O'Brien C et al. Randomized, placebo-controlled study of tolcapone in patients with fluctuating parkinson's disease treated with levodopa carbidopa. *Arch Neurol* 1998; 55:1089–1095.

13. Agid Y, Destee A, Durif F, et al. Tolcapone, bromocriptine, and Parkinson's disease. *Lancet* 1997; 350:712–713.

14. Waters CH, Kurth M, Bailey P, et al. Tolcapone in stable Parkinson's disease: Efficacy and safety of long-term treatment. *Neurology* 1997; 49:665–671.

15. Dupont E, Burgunder J-M, Findley L, et al. Tolcapone added to levodopa in stable Parkinsonian patients: A double-blind, placebo-controlled study. *Mov Disord* 1997; 12:928–934.

16. Ruottinen HM, Rinne UK. A double-blind pharmacokinetic and clinical dose-response study of entacapone as an adjuvant to levodopa therapy in advanced Parkinson's disease. *Clin Neuropharmacol* 1996; 19:283–296.

17. Ruottinen HM, Rinne UK. Entacapone prolongs levodopa response in a one-month double-blind study in Parkinsonian patients with levodopa-related fluctuations. *J Neurol Neurosurg Psychiatry* 1996; 6:36–40.

18. Kaakkola S, Teravainen H, Ahtila S, et al. Effect of entacapone, a COMT inhibitor, on clinical disability and levodopa metabolism in Parkinsonian patients. *Neurology* 1994; 44:77–80.

19. Nutt JG, Woodward WR, Beckner RM, et al. Effect of peripheral catechol-*O*-methyltransferase inhibition on the pharmacokinetics and pharmacodynamics of levodopa in Parkinsonian patients. *Neurology* 1994; 44:913–919.

20. Parkinson Study Group. Entacapone improves motor fluctuations in levodopa-treated Parkinson's disease patients. *Ann Neurol* 1997; 42:747–755.

21. Rinne UK, Larsen JP, Siden A, et al. Entacapone enhances the response to levodopa in Parkinsonian patients with motor fluctuations. *Neurology* 1998; 51:1309–1314.

22. Davis TL, Roznoski M, Burns RS. Acute effects of COMT inhibition on L-DOPA pharmacokinetics in Patients treated with carbidopa and selegiline. *Clin Neuropharm* 1995; 18:333–337.

23. Roberts JW, Cora-Locatelli G, Bravi D, et al. Catechol-*O*-methyltransferase inhibitor tolcapone prolongs levodopa/carbidopa action in Parkinsonian patients. *Neurology* 1994; 44:2685–2688.

24. Hauser R, Molho E, Shale H, et al. A pilot evaluation of the tolerability, safety, and efficacy of tolcapone alone and in combination with oral selegiline in untreated Parkinson's disease patients: Tolcapone De Novo Study Group. *Mov Disord* 1998; 13:643–647.

25. Jorga K, Fotteler B, Sedek G, et al. The effect of tolcapone on levodopa pharmacokinetics is independent of levodopa/carbidopa formulation. *J Neurol* 1998; 245:223–230.

26. Jorga K, Dingemanase J, Fotteler B, et al. Pharmacokinetics-pharmacodynamics of a novel COMT inhibitor during multiple dosing regimens. *Clin Pharmacol Ther* 1993; 53(Suppl 2):II–40. Abstract.

27. Ahtila S, Kaakkola S, Gordin A, et al. Effect of entacapone, a COMT inhibitor, on the pharmacokinetics and metabolism of levodopa after administration of controlled-release levodopa-carbidopa in volunteers. *Clin Neuropharmacol* 1995; 18:46–57.

28. Graham J, Grünewald R, Sagar H. Hallucinosis in idiopathic Parkinson's disease. *J Neurol Neurosurg Psychiatry* 1997; 63:434–441.

37

Atypical Antipsychotics

Joseph H. Friedman, M.D.

Memorial Hospital of Rhode Island, Pawtucket, Rhode Island

and

Herbert Y. Meltzer, M.D.

Vanderbitt University Medical Center, Nashville, Tennessee

INTRODUCTION

Soon after levodopa was introduced in the late 1960s a plethora of mental side effects was observed. These included euphoria, depression, mania, hypersexuality, hallucinations, delusions, confusional states, and sleep disturbances (1–5). Most of these truly represented the effects of levodopa on patients with idiopathic Parkinson's disease (PD). An unknown, but significant percentage of these treated patients had postencephalitic Parkinsonism, which itself caused behavior abnormalities (6). In addition, some patients who had been "locked in" for years were able to communicate once started on the drug. Because their baseline mental state was not known, the levodopa may simply have allowed its expression. Regardless of the underlying state, some Parkinsonian patients clearly developed psychotic symptoms when placed on levodopa, posing the dilemma of which problem to treat: the motor dysfunction or the mental dysfunction. Either levodopa had to be reduced or a neuroleptic antipsychotic needed to be added. Both choices resulted in worsened Parkinsonism.

When clozapine was first being tested as an antipsychotic for schizophrenia in the early 1970s, it was characterized as "atypical." The definition of "atypical" antipsychotic has remained elusive. A variety of pharmacologic characteristics have been sited as possible standards from which to measure the atypicality of these agents (6a,6b). Before listing these it is important to realize that, whatever the definition, clozapine remains the prototype of this class of drugs and that to which all others are compared. The search for newer agents is directed at finding drugs with similar efficacy but no risk for agranulocytosis and hence no need for blood monitoring. In earlier times, before use in patients, these drugs were classified as atypical if they failed to induce catalepsy (an unresponsive state with waxy flexibility) or antagonize amphetamine-induced stereotypy in rodents. Also, receptor-binding profiles were considered important (Table 37-1), especially with regard to an increase in 5HT and decrease in D2 binding (an increase in the 5HT/D-2 binding ratio) being more prominent in atypical vs typical agents. In patients, a drug is atypical if it has no effect on elevating prolactin levels and has increased efficacy on negative symptoms of schizophrenia compared with typical antipsychotics. Finally, perhaps most important, is the relatively low incidence of extrapyramidal side effects in psychiatric patients. Table 37-2 summarizes the behavior of the four currently available atypical antipsychotics with regard to these pharmacologic characteristics. What is seen is a lack of uniformity between them. As is discussed later, not all of these drugs behave clinically in an atypical manner. So the definition remains a moving target. We believe that the litmus test for a neuroleptic being "atypical" is the ability to treat PD patients without worsening motor features of the disease (6c).

The potential benefit that antipsychotic drugs, which did not cause parkinsonism, provided for patients with PD was recognized early as 1978 (7). Moskovitz et al. wondered whether clozapine might be such a drug. It is therefore somewhat surprising that clozapine was not tried in psychotic PD patients until 1985 (8) and it was not until the 1990s that the number of published reports describing its efficacy mushroomed, documenting its effectiveness and tolerability in PD patients.

Since clozapine was introduced, other antipsychotic drugs considered "atypical" have been commercially

Table 37-1   Receptor Binding of Atypical Antipsychotics

Drug	D-1	D-2	5HT-2A	α1	α2	H-1	M-1
Clozapine	++	++	+++	+++	+++	+++	++++
Risperidone	+	+++	++++	++	+++	++	0
Olanzapine	++	++	++++	+++	0	++++	++++
Quetiapine	+	+	+	+++	+	++++	+

D = Dopamine, 5HT = Serotonin, Alpha = alpha adrenergic, H = Histaminic, M = Muscarinic.

Table 37-2   Summary of Atypical Characteristics of Atypical Antipsychotics

Characteristics	Clozapine	Risperidone	Olanzapine	Quetiapine
Fails to induce catalepsy or antagonize amphetamine stereotypys	+	−	−	+
5HT/D-2 ratio	+	+	+	+
No Prolactin elevation	+	−	±	+
Improves negative symptoms	+	+	+	+
Decreased EPS	+	−	?	?

released, and others have been close behind. However, not all atypicals have comparable ability to spare extrapyramidal function, making some more useful than others in treating various aspects of PD (9,10). In addition, clozapine has been shown to have properties making it useful in treating certain motor symptoms of PD as well (11).

We would first like to point out some of the difficulties in interpreting the effects of antipsychotic drugs on parkinsonism as measured in clinical trials of schizophrenic patients. Most studies enrolled subjects who had received typical neuroleptics until shortly before the study drug was begun (12–14). "Washout" periods, if any, range from zero to seven days for patients receiving oral neuroleptics. Thus a subject may have been taking large doses of a high-potency neuroleptic, and then taken off the drug for less than a week before starting the study drug. This short period of time may be adequate for the antipsychotic effect to wear off, but the parkinsonian effects may last for months. Low concentrations of neuroleptic drugs have been shown to persist in animal brain (15) and human PET (positron emission tomography) studies (16). If a study drug has a lower parkinson-inducing potency than the neuroleptic previously used, the Parkinsonism will improve during the study, even if the drug itself causes Parkinsonism. The second problem is the much younger age of schizophrenics than PD patients (mean 35–40 years) in drug trials. This makes them less sensitive to extrapyramidal side effects. The third problem with neuroleptic studies is the universal use of the Simpson–Angus scale (17) for Parkinsonism that is heavily biased towards assessment of rigidity and measured in a manner most neurologists would not consider reliable (i.e., arm rigidity is measured by having the psychotic patient passively drop his arms to his side and rating the velocity of the arms falling). How well the Simpson-Angus Scale correlates with the Unified Parkinson's disease rating scale (UPDRS) (18), the generally accepted instrument used in studies on PD, is not known. It is therefore difficult to extrapolate results concerning motor function from psychiatric drug trials on relatively young schizophrenics to older PD patients.

PSYCHOSIS

All of the drugs used to treat PD may induce psychosis (see Chapter 42). How the patterns of psychopathology induced by anticholinergics, amantadine, dopamine agonists, or levodopa differ has not been well studied (19). More often than not, patients take more than one anti-PD medication, and they frequently take anxiolytics or antidepressants as well. The so-called "dopaminomimetic psychosis" is relatively stereotypic, however (20,21). Visual hallucinations are the most common symptoms (22). Typically these hallucination are of people, less commonly animals or objects such as tractors or statues. These images are not usually threatening, although they may be. The single most common hallucination is of strangers who silently watch the patient. These are more common in the evening but also occur during the day. The images do not interact with the patient and do not make any sounds. They disappear when touched. Most patients have insight and realize that these are not real. Auditory hallucinations that are very common in schizophrenia occur much less frequently than visual hallucinations in Parkinson's patients. The next most common psychotic symptoms are delusional. Jealous delusions, of spouse infidelity, no matter how bizarre the notion, and paranoid delusions of people stealing things, peddling drugs in the basement, and so forth, are the most typical. Symptoms common in schizophrenia, such as thought broadcasting, ideas of reference, pressured speech, grandiosity, and negative symptoms (anhedonia, apathy, emotional withdrawal, thought blocking) are not encountered.

Psychosis, defined as a major psychiatric illness in which reality testing is impaired, usually causing severe communication and social problems (23), may arise abruptly or insidiously. It is usual for patients to have suffered with this problem for months without discussing it for fear of being labeled as "crazy." In addition, both patient and spouse are frequently embarrassed by allegations of infidelity. Although psychosis may develop after a new drug has been added or an old drug increased, it may occur without any apparent precipitant. Pre-PD psychiatric history does not appear to play any role, as a risk factor, except in patients who develop hallucinations very early (24). Concurrent medical illnesses such as infections or thyroid dysfunction, must be considered possible precipitants.

A standard approach to treating this problem has been developed. Drugs with the greatest risk to benefit ratio are either reduced or stopped first (20). The anticholinergics are decreased or stopped followed by selegiline, amantadine, dopamine agonists, catechol-o-methyl transferase (COMT) inhibitors, and finally levodopa. If at some point, motor dysfunction caused by drug reduction becomes intolerable, an atypical antipsychotic is begun.

The prevalence of hallucinations is about 20 to 30% of drug-treated patients (22), whereas frank psychosis is seen in about 5 to 8% (20,21). Psychosis is more common in the elderly and the demented but may occur in younger, nondemented patients without an earlier psychiatric history.

It should be noted that psychosis is a major problem that is more important in triggering nursing home placement than the inability to walk (25). In addition, the psychic stress on a patient who is completely dependant on a spouse believed to be deceitful must be extraordinarily high (26). Psychosis in PD also appears to be associated with a markedly increased mortality rate (27,28).

When commencing treatment, it must be clear what the target symptoms are. Visual hallucinations, for example, may not merit treatment other than a medication reduction, whereas paranoid or jealous delusions should be treated.

As of this writing there are four drugs classified as atypical antipsychotics: clozapine, risperidone, olanzapine, and quetiapine. Others are forthcoming.

CLOZAPINE

Clozapine has been the subject of over 30 publications describing its use in drug-induced psychosis (DIP) in PD (8,29–53). However, all but one was supportive (54). Over 400 patients have been reported, with a consistent success rate greater than 80%, both in the meta-analysis and in the larger studies themselves. The one dissenting study (54) was the first double-blind, placebo-controlled trial. It included only six subjects. In this study clozapine was initiated at and escalated to an excessively high dose. The other reports are primarily single case reports or small series but also include many prospective open-label studies and a double-blind, placebo-controlled trial. In the prospective and retrospective studies, the rate of a "good" or "excellent" response has generally been over 80%. Side effects were generally limited to sedation or orthostatic hypotension but occasionally confusion was seen and rare cases of granulocytopenia, which has always reversed on stopping clozapine, were reported. On high doses, weight gain has occurred.

Clozapine is effective, at low doses, in improving psychosis without exacerbating parkinsonism in a four-week, multisite, double-blind, placebo-controlled trial involving 60 subjects (28). Whereas the typical dose range for treating psychosis is 300–900 mg/d, clozapine was used in doses ranging from 6.25 to 50 mg/d. Subjects were eligible for the study if they had psychotic symptoms for four weeks or more, were able to maintain stable doses of all their medications, and were deemed "safe" to manage for four weeks on placebo. Patients with possible medical or primary psychiatric causes for their psychosis were excluded. The minimum degree of psychosis was determined by the clinical question, "If this patient did not have PD, would treatment with a typical neuroleptic be indicated?" Patients could be demented as long as they were able to be assessed on the measures of mental and psychiatric function employed in the study: the Mini-Mental State Exam; the Brief Psychiatric Rating Scale (BPRS); the Survey Assessment of Positive Symptoms (SAPS); and the Clinical Global Impression Scale (CGIS). PD was rated using the UPDRS, the Hoehn and Yahr Staging, the Schwab and England activities of daily living scale, and the Step–Seconds test of gait speed. It should be noted that no validated scale had been published for assessing psychosis in PD, so that the BPRS, a widely used scale in schizophrenia trials was employed, along with the global scale, which provided a general "gestalt" rating psychosis on a one to seven scale.

The results of this study supported the open-label reports. At a mean dose of 28 mg/d, clozapine improved psychosis by clinically and statistically significant amounts. Parkinson tremor improved by 1.5 units on the UPDRS, but other items on the UPDRS were not changed, and the overall UPDRS and other measures of Parkinsonism were unchanged or improved but not by significant amounts. The degree of improvement of the psychosis was greater than that typically seen in schizophrenia trials. One patient was dropped because of transient leukopenia, one because of sedation, and a third because of myocardial infarction. Three subjects in the placebo group also dropped out – two for psychiatric reasons and one for pneumonia.

In a three-month open-label extension of the four-week study, in which all subjects were treated with clozapine, without knowledge of the treatment assignment in the double-blind portion of the study, the beneficial results were similar (28a). The mean dose used was approximately 28 mg/d (range 6.25 to 50 mg/d) and the improvement on scales measuring both parkinsonism and psychosis were about equal to those found in part one. A second subject dropped out because of reversible leukopenia. Most unexpected, however, was the death of five subjects during the extension phase and a sixth who died shortly after completing the study. Three of these deaths occurred in nursing home patients who had advance directives not to be treated for life-threatening illnesses. The other three deaths occurred in patients who lived at home. In no case did the local investigator believe that clozapine was implicated in anyway with the death. It should be noted that this high death rate has not been described before in DIP in PD or with clozapine but that increased mortality in PD has been associated with psychosis (27). The high death rate may reflect the special characteristics of patients who agreed to participate in the study.

The usual side effects of anticholinergics – dry mouth, constipation, urinary retention, and blurred vision – were not found with clozapine, although clozapine has potent central nervous system (CNS) antimuscarinic effects. Clozapine also increases the release of acetylcholine in the prefrontal cortex (55) that may counteract some of its antimuscarinic effects. Clozapine is to be a partial muscarinic M1 receptor agonist in vivo (56). There is also evidence that clozapine is an agonist at the cloned muscarinic M4 receptor expressed in transfected cells (57,58).

Olanzapine is also an M4 agonist but not risperidone or quetiapine (58).

Prescribing clozapine in the United States is cumbersome because of a requirement for weekly monitoring of the white blood count (WBC) for six months followed by biweekly WBC checks. In other countries, monitoring is either optional or monthly after six months. To guarantee compliance, each patient must be registered in a central registry maintained by the drug company. The results of the weekly WBC must be provided, in writing, to the pharmacist who can dispense only enough clozapine to last until the next WBC check. When many patients are on clozapine and each uses a different laboratory and pharmacy, the amount of administrative time required is large and not reimbursed, making clozapine use onerous for the prescribing physician. However, clinics with large numbers of patients can organize programs with nurse assistants to efficiently manage its use.

RISPERIDONE

Risperidone was the second drug released as an atypical antipsychotic in the United States. Only a small number of publications have appeared addressing its efficacy in PD (59–64). The first report described improved psychosis in PD patients without worsening parkinsonism in six patients. This was countered by other reports in which marked worsening of motor features occurred even at low doses (61,62). Three further reports were published; The first study was a long-term study of ten subjects by the author of the first positive report, (60) in which only three of ten subjects remained on risperidone. The second study was a retrospective study (63) in which parkinsonism was not measured but was thought to have not worsened. The third was a retrospective study in 39 patients with akinetic rigid syndromes, (64) 32 of whom had PD. Twenty-three of the 39 had complete or near complete remission of psychiatric symptoms and four others were much better. UPDRS scores were stable at six months. Only six patients did poorly either for psychiatric or for motor reasons.

Risperidone causes significant prolactin elevations at all clinical doses. Its ability to cause Parkinsonism in patients with schizophrenia is very dose-dependent. At the low end of the dose range for treating schizophrenia, 1 to 4 mg/d, it produces less parkinsonism than typical neuroleptics at comparable doses. However, at higher doses it loses some of its atypical features. It has recently been reported to produce a lower rate of tardive dyskinesia in elderly demented patients compared with typical neuroleptics (M. Brecker, personal communication). Rosebush et al. (64a) studied the frequency of EPS in neuroleptic naive patients admitted to an acute psychiatric service and treated with either halperidol or risperidone. The frequency of akathisia, parkinsonism, and dyskinesia were comparable. Thus risperidone behaves more like a typical than an atypical antipsychotic.

We believe that enough experience exists in the literature and PD research community to conclude that risperidone is less likely to be tolerated by patients with PD than other atypical agents and should be reserved for use after other drugs have failed.

OLANZAPINE

Olanzapine is closer to clozapine in its effects on animal behavior than risperidone. In animals and humans it induces transient and minor prolactin secretion (12). It induces catalepsy and inhibits apomorphine-induced stereotypy only at high doses. Clozapine does not cause either. These are animal behaviors predictive of low extrapyramidal effects in patients. No patient has so far been reported to have had any acute dystonic reaction when on olanzapine, but at least one patient has been described who developed tardive dyskinesia with olanzapine (65).

The first report of olanzapine's effect on DIP in PD was an open-label prospective trial involving 15 non-demented patients (66). All improved, including two who had previously failed to respond to clozapine. After two months no patient's parkinsonism became worse. Anti-PD medications were fixed for the first 50 days and then altered as needed. When anti-PD medications were increased, Parkinsonism improved but psychosis did not recur. The mean olanzapine dose in this study was 6.5 mg, in comparison to the usual dose required in schizophrenia of 5 to 20 mg/d. This contrasts with the clozapine dose required in DIP, which is less than 1/10 of that required in schizophrenia.

Unfortunately, as with risperidone, the next publications reported that some PD patients suffered worsening of their parkinsonism. Jimenez-Jimenez reported (67) two patients whose Parkinsonism worsened. Friedman and Jacques (68) reported that only eight of nineteen patients with akinetic-rigid syndromes, not all PD, including some with dementia, were able to stay on olanzapine. Parkinsonism worsened in the others, including one who required hospitalization for increased parkinsonian features. Friedman et al. (69) also found that only 3 of 12 PD patients who were psychiatrically stable on clozapine for DIP,

were able to make a transition from clozapine to olanzapine without worsening parkinsonism. Again, one required hospitalization for worsening motor function. Molho and Factor reported (70) that 10 of 12 PD patients treated with low-dose olanzapine suffered worsening Parkinsonism. In six of these the worsening was described as "dramatic". One required hospitalization.

Churchyard and Isanek followed 23 patients prospectively (71) and described marked improvement in psychosis without significant worsening of Parkinsonism. However, the only measure used for Parkinsonism was the Hoehn-Yahr stage and no measure was made of psychosis. In addition, 12 patients had been treated with neuroleptics (not described) before starting olanzapine. The mean dose of olanzapine was 4.3 mg/d with a range of 2.5 to 7.5 mg/d Paranoia resolved in all eight patients who had this symptom, and hallucinations improved in 20. Nursing home placement was avoided in 11 of 14 considered "at risk". Weiner et al. (72) in a retrospective review of 21 patients treated with a mean dose of 5 mg/d found that 12 had a good psychiatric response without a decline in parkinsonism, one had a good psychiatric response but worsened parkinsonism, and eight had worsened parkinsonism without psychiatric benefit. Unfortunately, there were no standardized measures of either psychiatric function or Parkinsonism. Graham et al. reported (73) that two of five PD patients could not tolerate olanzapine because of worsened Parkinsonism.

Overall, olanzapine was an effective antipsychotic in DIP but in five of seven reports it caused worsening Parkinsonism in a substantial percentage of patients. Some patients required hospitalization. We cannot easily explain the discrepancy in the results of these reported studies. The populations may have varied. Wolters et al. suggested that the difference may relate to the presence of dementia, which leads to poor tolerability (73a). In addition the measures used, differed. These differences alone may not fully explain the different outcomes.

A multicenter, double-blind, placebo-controlled trial is currently in progress to assess olanzapine's efficacy on psychosis and motor function in Parkinson's disease. Until this study is reported, we believe that olanzapine should be used cautiously. Obviously, low doses (2.5–5 mg/d) should be the goal.

QUETIAPINE

Quetiapine is the most recently released atypical antipsychotic drug, and less information exists regarding its effect on DIP. Quetiapine most closely resembles clozapine in animal models. It does not induce catalepsy or block amphetamine-induced stereotypy. (74) It also does not increase serum prolactin levels. (75) In schizophrenia trials, no acute dystonic reactions occurred. Juncos et al. (76) followed 15 akinetic-rigid patients, including patients with progressive supranuclear palsy, PD, and other neurodegenerative disorders for one year. Psychosis improved and, although anti-PD medications were not altered, motor functions, except for tremor, improved as well. A mean dose of 70 mg/d was used, in contrast to the usual 150–750 mg/d required in schizophrenia. Juncos et al. (77) treated 40 patients with PD and psychosis (as part of larger trial using quetiapine to treat psychosis in the elderly) at a mean dose of 75 mg/d and followed then for 12 months. Twenty patients dropped out because of a variety of side effects or lack of efficacy but not worsening parkinson. The other 20 patients showed benefit in both psychiatric and motor scores and, in general, no worsening Parkinsonism was seen. The improved motor scores were transient and may have related to the discontinuation of earlier psychiatric drugs.

Samanta and Stacy (78) treated 10 PD patents in an open-label study at a mean dose of 37.5 mg/d and found that six had significant improvement in psychosis without a significant change in motor function, although seven had mild worsening in their UPDRS score. Rosenfeld et al. (79) prospectively followed 24 patients with DIP in PD. Ten had baseline and four-week follow-up measures of psychosis and parkinsonism using the BPRS and UPDRS with clinically and statistically significant improvement on the BPRS with a slight but insignificant decline in the UPDRS motor section (2.7 points). The other 14 had no BPRS baseline measure. UPDRS motor scores obtained at the last visit, before quetiapine was prescribed over the telephone, compared with scores repeated after starting quetiapine showed minimal change in parkinsonism. Twenty of the 24 did well enough to remain on quetiapine for more than eight weeks. One patient died of causes considered unrelated to the drug. Three subjects were intolerant of quetiapine because of orthostatic hypotension, headache, nausea or persistent hallucinations. The same authors attempted to convert psychiatrically stable PD patients on clozapine or olanzapine to quetiapine but were able to do this successfully only in 5 of 11. (80) Six (five on clozapine and one on olanzapine) were unable to make the crossover because of confusion, erratic behavior, or increased hallucinations. No patient had worsening of akinesia or rigidity although one clozapine-treated patient's tremor worsened. A later review (81), including the same subjects as Rosenfeld et al. extended treatment to 34 neuroleptic naive PD patients (demented and nondemented) plus 25 attempted crossovers from clozapine (22) or olanzapine (3). Twenty-eight of the 34 (82%) neuroleptic naive patients had marked improvement or complete amelioration of psychosis. In 12 patients with pre-and post-treatment BPRS scores, a clinically and statistically significant improvement was seen. Seven of the 34 had worsened parkinsonism, and overall there was a mild but statistically significant worsening of the UPDRS. Six were unable to tolerate quetiapine because of orthostasis, nausea confusion, or lack of response. The mean dose used was 44.6 mg/d. Seventeen of the 25 (68%) psychiatrically stable PD patients successfully crossed over to quetiapine without change in psychosis or Parkinsonism (BPRS and UPDRS motor scale, respectively). Eight switched back to clozapine or olanzapine. No distinguishing features could be determined between those successfully converted to quetiapine and the others. Crossover failures were due to increased Parkinsonism, recurrent hallucinations, agitation, and dyskinesia.

OTHER DRUGS FOR TREATING LEVODOPA PSYCHOSIS

Other agents related to clozapine, risperidone, olanzapine, and quetiapine that have been reported to be effective in the treatment of levodopa psychosis and to be tolerable include zotepine (82), melperone (83), and mianserin (84). The former are both proven antipsychotic drugs in the treatment of schizophrenia, although mianserin, generally thought of as an antidepressant, has also been found to be useful in the treatment of negative symptoms of schizophrenia as an adjunct to neuroleptic drugs. All three agents are relatively more potent $5HT_2$ than D2 antagonists. The results reported by Barbato et al. (83) for melperone were dramatic. Twenty-eight of 30 patients with psychotic symptoms were found to respond to melperone with improvement in psychosis and no worsening of Parkinsonian symptoms. The mean dose was about 20% of that used to treat schizophrenia. Melperone is available primarily in Europe. Ondansetron, a $5HT_3$ antagonist, is also reported to be effective in 15 of 16 patients in an open-label, short-term study (84a) but it works better for hallucinations than delusions. There were no major side effects. Ondansetron has not been found to be effective in the treatment of schizophrenia but may not have been adequately studied.

TREMOR

Clozapine is the only atypical antipsychotic reported to improve tremor in PD (51,85–90). Risperidone and olanzapine may worsen or induce tremor, whereas quetiapine appears to be less likely to do this. However, patients switched from clozapine to quetiapine may experience an increase in tremors, which may be due to the loss of clozapine's antitremor effect rather than quetiapine-induced worsening.

The first report of clozapine improving tremor did not state the rationale for using the drug (89). It reported improvement in the tremor of PD, essential tremor, alcohol-induced tremor, and the tremor of multiple sclerosis, as well as combined tremors. This paper further describes a reduction in both amplitude and frequency. No other publication has reported altered frequency as a medication effect.

Four open-label trials of clozapine reported improvement in tremor in primarily nonpsychotic but also some psychotic patients with PD (85,86,88,89). In most of these cases, the tremors had been refractory to other medications, including anticholinergic drugs. Thus the antitremor effect of clozapine was thought to be either unrelated or in addition to its anticholinergic effect. Friedman et al. (87) attempted to prove this hypothesis by performing a double-blind, crossover trial comparing benztropine with clozapine for 20 PD patients with tremor. Their subjects, however, did not necessarily have tremors refractory to other drugs, or even severe tremors, as had been the case in earlier reports. They found that clozapine, at doses up to 100 mg, was about as effective as doses of benztropine considered to have equal CNS antimuscarinic activity. However, clozapine and benztropine were not equally effective in each individual, suggesting that an antimuscarinic effect was not the explanation.

Two double-blind trials reported similar benefit. The PSYCLOPS study (28), a double-blind trial comparing clozapine with placebo in 60 psychotic PD patients also examined tremor, in isolation from the other manifestations of PD, using the single tremor item on the UPDRS motor scale. Although not all subjects had tremor, the mean improvement on clozapine was 1.5 (on a zero to four scale) on a mean dose of 27 mg/d, which was both clinically and statistically significant. Bonnucelli et al. treated (90), in a double-blind manner, 17 PD patients with tremor unresponsive to levodopa, with a single dose of clozapine 12.5 mg/d and reported that 15 improved by 50% or more. This improvement was maintained in an open label extension for move than a year. The mean daily dose was 45 mg/d in the open-label study. One multicenter retrospective review of clozapine's effects on 172 PD patients also reported benefit on tremors (51).

The authors believe that there is convincing data obtained from different sites, using different methods (including three double-blind trials), that clozapine is effective in treating PD tremor. The authors urge the reader to review the videotape that accompanies the report by Friedman and Lannon (86) to see how impressive this response can be. The mechanism of clozapine's antitremor activity is not known. Although one study found a benefit similar to that of benztropine, we note that three publications specifically reported clozapine's benefit in patients who had failed anticholinergics (85,86,88). Olanzapine, whose anticholinergic activity is similar to clozapine's does not have this effect. Olanzapine is also an M4 agonist. Clozapine, although a potent CNS anticholinergic agent, generally lacks peripheral anticholinergic effects such as dry mouth, constipation, and urinary retention (91). It has been reported to increase acetylcholine release (55). Finally, it is not possible to truly compare anticholinergics because they each have their own pattern of effects on the various muscarinic receptors, of which at least five have been identified (92).

Although not universally accepted, we recommend a trial of clozapine in PD patients with refractory tremors before referring a patient for a thalamic deep brain stimulation or thalamotomy. The initial dose should be 12.5 mg in the evening, as clozapine is very sedating. The dose is increased slowly to a ceiling of 50 mg twice daily. However, few PD patients can tolerate this high dose. In addition to the sedation, high doses act as appetite enhancers, causing weight gain. Obviously, one aims for the lowest dose that helps, without inducing bothersome side effects.

OTHER MOTOR ASPECTS OF PARKINSON'S DISEASE

Risperidone has been reported to be helpful in reducing dyskinesias induced by levodopa (93) in eight advanced cases. However, aside from this one report, none of the other atypical antipsychotics, with the exception of clozapine, have been reported as useful in controlling motor aspects of PD. Clozapine has been shown, in very careful experiments by Bennett et al. (94) to reduce dyskinesias without altering the "on" response to levodopa. Unfortunately, the dose required was more 200 mg/d, causing the subjects to increase their sleep time by two hours each day. Clozapine has also been reported to reduce dyskinesias at a much lower dose (35). It has also been reported to reduce nocturnal akathisia and dystonia associated with PD (11).

CONCLUSION

Robust and reliable data support the use of low-dose clozapine for treating DIP in PD when the offending drugs cannot be reduced without impairing motor function. Clozapine not only spares motor function but actually improves tremor. It is the only atypical proven to have this effect in controlled double blind studies. Less strong data suggests that quetiapine also improves psychosis without worsening motor function but appears not to improve any aspect of motor function. So far, this effect is only supported by open-label trials. Like clozapine, quetiapine must be used at a much lower dose than what is used in schizophrenia. Quetiapine does not cause granulocytopenia; therefore, blood monitoring is not required. It is therefore much easier to prescribe than clozapine. Olanzapine is helpful to some PD patients but clearly causes worsening parkinsonism in a substantial number. Risperidone is the least well tolerated agent but may be effective and tolerable at very low doses in some patients.

We recommend that either quetiapine or clozapine be used as the first line drug (6c). We start with quetiapine 12.5 mg QHS and increase as tolerated and as needed, in which sedation is the usual limiting side effect. We start clozapine at 6.25 mg or 12.5 mg qhs depending on the age and frailty of the patient and titrate, as with quetiapine, giving all or most of the dose at bedtime. Most patients probably require treatment with one of there agents for life but attempts to wean them should be considered if the psychosis is well controlled for several months. Our experience has been that relapses induced by lowering the dose can easily be controlled by increasing it again.

ADDENDUM

We have not considered the issue of cognitive impairment in PD and the potential benefit derived from atypical antipsychotic drugs in this regard. There is strong evidence that clozapine improves some types of memory in schizophrenia. The evidence that olanzapine and risperidone also improve cognition is increasing. Research is needed to determine if any of these agents improve cognition in patients with PD as well.

Acknowledgments

Mary Eddy for manuscript preparation; Jorge Juncos, M.D. for sharing data.

REFERENCES

1. Celesia GC, Barr AN. Psychosis and psychiatric manifestations of levodopa therapy. *Arch Neurol* 1970; 23:193–200.
2. Cotzias GC, Papavasilou PS, Ginos JZ, et al. Metabolic modification of Parkinson's disease and of chronic manganese poisoning. *Ann Rev Med* 1971; 22:205–326.
3. Goodwin FK. Psychiatric side effects of levodopa in men. *JAMA* 1971; 218:1915–1921.
4. Jenkins RB, Groh RH. Mental symptoms in parkinsonian patients treated with L-Dopa. *Lancet* 1970; 2:177–180.
5. Mindham RHS. Psychiatric symptoms in parkinsonism. *J Neurol Neurosurg, Psychiatry* 1970; 33:188–191.
6. Friedman JH. Post encephalitic parkinsonism. In: Stern MB, Koller WC (ed). *Parkinsonian Syndromes*. New York: Marcel Dekker, 1993:203–226.
6a. Richelson E. Preclinical pharmacology of neuroleptics: Focus on new generation compounds. *J Clin Psychiatry* 1996; 57(Suppl 11):4–11.
6b. Casey DE. The relationship of pharmacology to side effects. *J Clin Psychiatry* 1997; 58(Suppl 10):55–62.
6c. Friedman JH, Factor SA. Atypical neuroleptics in the treatment of drug-induced psychosis in Parkinson's disease. *Mov Disord* 2000; 15:201–211.
7. Moskovitz C, Moses H III, Klawans HL. Levodopa-induced psychosis: A kindling phenomenon. *Am J Psychiatry* 1978; 135:669–675.
8. Scholz E, Dichgans J. Treatment of drug-induced exogenous psychosis in parkinsonism with clozapine and fluperlapine. *Eur Arch Psychy Neurol Sci* 1985; 235:60–64.
9. Arndt J, Skarsfeld T. Do novel antipsychotics have similar pharmacologic characteristics? A review of the evidence. *Neuropsychopharm acology* 1998; 18:63–101.
10. Meltzer HY, Matsubara S, Lee J-C. Classification of typical and atypical antipsychotic drugs on the basis of dopamine D1, D2 and serotonin$_2$ pKi values. *J Pharmacol Exp Ther* 1989; 251:238–246.
11. Factor SA, Friedman JH. The Emerging role of Clozapine in the treatment of movement disorders. *Mov Disord* 1997; 12:483–496.
12. Beasley CM jr, Sanger T, Satterlee W, et al. Olanzapine versus Placebo: Results of a double blind, fixed dose olanzapine trial. *Psychopharmacol* 1996; 124:159–167.
13. Small JG, Hirsch SR, Arvanitis LA, et al. Quetiapine in Patients with Schizophrenia. A high and low-dose double-blind comparision with placebo. *Arch Gen Psychiatry* 1997; 54:549–557.
14. Zimbroff DL, Kane JM, Tamminga CA, et al. Controlled, dose-response study of sertindol and Haloperidol in the treatment of schizophrenia. *Am J Psychiatry* 1997; 154:782–791.

15. Cohen BM, Tsumeizumi T, Baldessarini RJ, et al. Differences between antipsychotic drugs in persistence of brain levels and behavioral effects. *Psychopharmacology* 1992; 108:338–344.

16. Nyberg S, Farde L, Halldin C. Delayed normalization of central D2 dopamine receptor availability after discontinuation of haloperidol decanoate: Preliminary findings. *Arch Gen Psychiatry* 1997; 54:953–958.

17. Simpson GM, Amuso D, Blair JH, et al. Phenothiazine produced extrapyramidal disturbance. *Arch Gen Psychiatry* 1964; 10:127–136.

18. Lang AE, Fahn S. Assessment of Parkinson's disease. In: Munsat TL (ed.). *Quantification of neurologic deficit.* Boston: Butterworths, 1989:285–309.

19. Goetz CG, Tanner CM, Klawans HL. Pharmacology of hallucinations induced by long-term drug therapy. *Am J Psychiatry* 1982; 139:494–497.

20. Factor SA, Molho ES, Podskalny GD, et al. Parkinson's disease: Drug-induced psychiatric states. In: Weiner WJ, Lang AE (eds). *Behavioral Neurology of Movement Disorders*: Advances in Neurology, vol 65. New York, Raven Press, 1995:115–138.

21. Friedman JH. Management of levodopa psychosis. *Clin Neuropharmacol* 1991; 14(4):283–295.

22. Sanchez-Ramos JR, Ortoll R, Paulson GW. Visual hallucinations associated with Parkinson's disease. *Arch Neurol* 1996; 53:1265–1268.

23. Kaplan HI, Saddock BJ. Synopsis of psychiatry. 7th ed. Baltimore: Williams and Wilkins, 1996.

24. Goetz CG, Vogel C, Tanner LM, et al. Early versus late hallucinations in Parkinson's disease. *Neurology* 1998; 51:811–814.

25. Goetz CG, Stebbins GT. Risk factors for nursing home placement in advanced Parkinson's disease. *Neurology* 1993; 43:2227–2229.

26. Carter JH, Stewart BJ, Archold PG. The Parkinson's Study Group. Living with a person who has Parkinson's disease: The spouse's perspective by stage of the disease. *Mov Disord* 1998; 33:20–28.

27. Goetz CG, Stebbins G. Mortality and hallucinations in nursing home patients with advanced Parkinson's disease. *Neurology* 1995; 45:669–671.

28. Parkinson Study Group. Low dose clozapine for the treatment of drug-induced psychosis in idiopathic parkinson's disease: Results of the double blind, placebo controlled PSYCLOPS trial. *N Eng J Med* 1999; 340:757–763.

28a. Factor SA, Friedman JH, Lannon MC, et al. Clozapine for the treatment of drug-induced psychosis in Parkinson's disease: Results of the 12 week open label extension in the PSYCLOPS trial. *Mov Disord* 2001; 16:135–139.

29. Bear D, Lawson W, Burns S, et al. Clozapine in idiopathic Parkinson's. *Biol Psychiatry* 1989; 25:160A–165A.

30. Bernardi F, Del Zompa M. Clozapine in idiopathic Parkinson's disease (letter). *Neurology* 1990; 40:1151.

31. Brewer MA, Kurth MC, Imke SC, et al. Safety and effectiveness of clozapine for Parkisonian patients with psychosis. *Neurology* 1995; 45(Suppl 4):A252.

32. Chacko RC, Hurley RA, Harper RG, et al. Clozapine for acute and maintenance treatment of psychosis in Parkinson's disease. *J Neuropsychiatry Clin Neurosci* 1995; 7:471–475.

33. Diederich N, Keipes M, Graas M, et al. Clozapine in the treatment of mental manifestations of Parkinson's disease. *Rev Neurol (Paris)* 1995; 151:251–257.

34. Factor SA, Brown D, Molho ES, et al. Clozapine: A two-year open trial in Parkinson's disease patients with psychosis. *Neurology* 1994; 44:544–546.

35. Factor SA, Brown D. Clozapine prevents recurrence of psychosis in Parkinson's disease. *Mov Disord* 1992; 7:125–131.

36. Friedman JH, Max J, Swift R. Idiopathic Parkinson's disease in a chronic schizophrenic patient: Long-term treatment with clozapine and L-Dopa. *Clin Neuropharmacol* 1987; 10:470–475.

37. Friedman JH, Lannon MC, Caley C. Clozapine for movement disorder patients: A retrospective analysis of 38 patients. *Ann Neurol* 1992; 32:277.

38. Gonski PN. The use of clozapine in Parkinson's disease. *Aust NZ J Med* 1994; 24:585.

39. Greene P, Cote L, Fahn S. Treatment of drug-induced psychosis in Parkinson's disease with clozapine. *Adv Neurol* 1993; 60:703–706.

40. Kahn N, Freeman A, Juncos JL, et al. Clozapine is beneficial for psychosis in Parkinson's disease. *Mov Disord* 1992; 41:1699–1700.

41. Lanazasoro G, Suerez JA, Marti Masso JF. Clozapine in Parkinson's disease: Three years experience. *Mov Disord* 1992; 7(Suppl):100.

42. Lew MF, Waters CF. Clozapine treatment of Parkinsonism with psychosis. *J Am Geriatr Soc* 1993; 41:669–671.

43. Ostergaard K, Dupont E. Clozapine treatment of drug-induced psychotic symptoms in late stages of Parkinson's disease. *Act Neurol Scand* 1988; 78:349–350.

44. Pfeiffer RF, Kang J, Graber B, et al. Clozapine for psychosis in Parkinson's disease. *Mov Disord* 1990; 5:239–242.

45. Pinter MM, Helscher RJ. Therapeutic effect of clozapine in psychotic decompensation in idiopathic Parkinson's disease. *J Neurol Transm Park Dis Dement Sect* 1993; 5:135–146.

46. Rabey JM, Treves TA, Neufeld MY, et al. Low-dose clozapine in the treatment of levodopa-induced mental disturbances in Parkinson's disease. *Neurology* 1995; 45:432–434.

47. Roberts HE, Dean RC, Stoudemire A. Clozapine treatment of psychosis in Parkinson's disease. *J Neuropsychiatry* 1989; 1:190–192.

48. Rosenthal SH, Fenton ML, Harnett DS. Clozapine for the treatment of levodopa-induced psychosis in Parkinson's disease. *Gen Hosp Psychiatry* 1992; 14:285–286.

49. Ruggieri S, De Pandis MF, Bonamartini A, et al. Low dose of clozapine in the treatment of dopaminergic psychosis in Parkinson's disease. *Clin Neuropharmacol* 1997; 20:204–209.

50. Rui-Silva M, Magalhaes M, Viseu M, et al. Clozapine in the treatment of psychosis in Parkinsonism. *J Neurol* 1995; 242(Suppl 2):138.

51. Trosch RM, Friedman JH, Lannon MC, et al. Clozapine use in Parkinson's disease: A retrospective analysis of a large multicentered clinical experience. *Mov Disord* 1998; 13:377–382.

52. Wagner ML, Defilippi JL, Menza A, et al. Clozapine for the treatment of psychosis in Parkinson's disease. *J Neuropsychiatry Clin Neurosci* 1996; 8:276–280.

53. Wolk SI, Douglas CJ. Clozapine treatment of psychosis in Parkinson's disease: A report of 5 consecutive cases. J Clin Psychiatry 1992; 53:373–376.

54. Wolters ECh, Hurwitz TA, Mak E, et al. Clozapine in the treatment of Parkinsonian patients with dopaminomimetic psychosis. *Neurology* 1990; 40:832–834.

55. Parada MA, Hernandez L, Puig de Parada M, et al. Selective action of acute systemic clozapine on acetylcholine release in rat prefrontal cortex by reference to the nucleus accumbens and striatum. *J Pharmacol Exp Ther* 1997; 281(1):582–8.

56. Ogren SO. Pharmacology of atypical neuroleptic drugs: Relevance for muscarinic mechanisms in schizophrenia. Presented at annual meeting of the American College of Neuropsychopharmacology, San Juan, Puerto Rico, 1992.

57. Zorn SH, Jones SB, Ward KM, et al. Clozapine is a potent and selective muscarinic M4 receptor agonist. *Eur J Pharmacol Mol Pharmacol.* 1994; Sect 269 R1.

58. Zeng XP, Le F, Richelson E. Muscarnic M4 receptor activation by some atypical antipsychotic drugs. *Eur J Pharmacol* 1997; 321:349–354.

59. Meco G, Allesandri A, Bonifati V, et al. Risperidone for hallucinations in levodopa treated Parkinson's disease patients. *Lancet* 1994; 343:1370–1371.

60. Meco G, Alessandri A, Guistini P, et al. Risperidone in levodopa-induced psychosis in advanced Parkinson's disease: An open label long term study. *Mov Disord* 1997; 12:610–612.

61. Ford B, Lynch T, Greene P. Risperidone in Parkinson's disease. *Lancet* 1994; 344:681.

62. Rich SS, Friedman JH, Ott BR. Risperidone versus clozapine in the treatment of psychosis in six patients with Parkinson's disease and other akinetic-rigid syndromes. *J Clin Psychiatry* 1995; 56:556–559.

63. Workman RJ Jr, Orengo CA, Bakey AA, et al. The use of risperidone for psychosis and agitation in demented patients with Parkinson's disease. *J Neuropsychiatry Clin Neurosci* 1997; 9:594–597.

64. Leopold NA. Risperidone treatment of drug-related psychosis in patients with parkinsonism. *Mov Disord* 2000; 15:301–304.

64a. Rosebush PI, Mazurek MF. Neurologic side effects in neuroleptic naive patients treated with haloperidol or risperidone, *Neurology* 1999; 52:782–785.

65. Meco G, Fabrizio E, Alessandi A, et al. Risperidone in levodopa-induced dyskinesia. *J Neurol Neurosurg Psychiatry* 1998; 64:135–142.

66. Wolters EC, Jansen EN, Tuynman-Qua HG, et al. Olanzapine in the treatment of dopaminomimetic psychosis in patients with Parkinson's disease. *Neurology* 1996; 47:1085–1087.

67. Jimenez-Jimenez FJ, Talon-Barranco A, Orti-Pareja, et al. Olanzapine can worsen Parkinsonism. *Neurology* 1998; 50:1183–1184.

68. Friedman JH, Goldstein SM, Jacques C. Substituting clozapine for olanzapine in psychiatrically stable Parkinson's disease patients: Results of an open-label pilot trial. *Clin Neuropharmacol* (In press).

69. Friedman JH, Goldstein SM. Olanzapine in the treatment of dopaminomimetic psychosis in patients with Parkinson's disease. *Neurology* 1998; 50:1195–1196.

70. Molho ES, Factor SA. Worsening of motor features of parkinsonism with olanzapine. *Mov Disord* 1999; 14:1014–1016.

71. Churchyard A, Iansek R. Olanzapine as treatment of the neuropsychiatric complications of Parkinson's disease: An open-label study. *Mov Disord* 1998; 13(Suppl 2):188.

72. Weiner WJ, Minagar A, Shulman L. Olanzapine for the treatment of hallucinations/delusions in Parkinson's disease. *Mov Disord* 1998; 13(Suppl 2):62.

73. Graham JM, Sussmen JP, Ford KS, et al. Olanzapine in the treatment of hallucinosis in idiopathic Parkinson's disease: A cautionary note. *J Neurol Neurosurg Psychiatry* 1998; 65:774–777.

73a. Wolters EC, Jansen ENH, Tuynman-Qua HG, Bermans PLM. Olanzapine in the treatment of dopaminomimetic psychosis in patients with Parkinson's disease. *Neurology* 1998; 50:1196.

74. Moore NA, Tye NC, Axton MS, et al. The behavioral pharmacology of olanzapine: A novel "atypical" antipsychotic agent. *J Pharmacol Exp Ther* 1992; 262:545–551.

75. Moore NA, Coligaro DO, Wong DT, et al. The pharmacology of olanzapine and other new.antipsychotic agents. *Curr Opin Invest Drug* 1993; 2:281–293.

76. Juncos JL, Evatt ML, Jewert D. Long-term effects of quetiapine fumarate in Parkinsonism complicated by psychosis. *Neurology* 1998; 50(Suppl 4):A70–A71.

77. Juncos JL, Young P, Sweitzer D, et al. Quetiapine improves psychotic symptoms associated with Parkinson's disease. *Neurology* 1999; 52(Suppl 2):A262.

78. Samanta J, Stacy M. Quetiapine in the treatment of hallucinations in advanced Parkinson's disease. *Mov Disord* 1998; 13(Suppl 2):274.

79. Rosenfeld M, Friedman JH, Jacques C. Quetiapine pilot trial in dopamimetic psychosis (DP) in

Parkinson's disease (PD). Presented at the 5th International Congress of Parkinson's Disease and Movement Disorders, October 10–14, 1998.

80. Friedman JH, Jacques CJ, Fernandez HH, Quetiapine for drug-induced psychosis in Parkinson's disease. Fifth International Congress of Parkinson's disease and Movement Disorders. New York, Oct 1998.

81. Fernandez HH, Friedman JH, Jacques CJ. Quetiapine for the treatment of dopamimetic psychosis in PD.

82. Arnold G, Trenkwalker C, Schwartz JL, et al. Zotepine reversibly induces akinesia and rigidity in Parkinson's disease patients with resting tremor or drug-induced psychosis. *Mov Disord* 1994; 9:238–240.

83. Barbato L, Monge A, Stocchi F, et al. Melperone in the treatment of iatrogenic psychosis in Parkinson's disease. *Func Neurol* 1996; 11:201–207.

84. Ikeguchi K, Kuroda A. Mianserin treatment of patients with psychosis induced by anti parkinsonian drugs. *Eur Arch Psychiatry Clin Neurosci* 1995; 244:320–324.

84a. Zoldan J, Friedberg G, Livneh M, et al. Psychosis in advanced Parkinson's disease: Treatment with ondansetron, a 5-HT3 receptor antagonist. *Neurology* 1995; 47:1608–1609.

85. Fischer PA, Baas H, Hefner R. Treatment of Parkinsonian tremor with clozapine. *J Neural Transm Park Dis Dement Sect* 1990; 2:233–238.

86. Friedman JH, Lannon MC, Clozapine-responsive tremor in Parkinson's disease. *Mov Disord* 1990; 5:225–229.

87. Friedman JH, Lannon MC. Benztropine versus clozapine for the treatment of tremor in Parkinson's disease. *Neurology* 1997; 4(48):1077–1081.

88. Jansen ENH. Clozapine in the treatment of tremor in Parkinson's disease. *Acta Neurol Scand* 1994; 89:262–265.

89. Pakkenberg H, Pakkenberg B. Clozapine in the treatment of tremor. *Acta Neurol Scand* 1986; 73:295–297.

90. Bonuccelli U, Ceravolo R, Salvetti S, et al. Clozapine in Parkinson's disease tremor: Effects of acute and chronic administration. *Neurology* 1997; 49:1587–1590.

91. Baldessarini RJ, Frankenburg FR. Clozapine: A Novel Antipsychotic Agent. *N Eng J Med* 1991; 324: 746–754.

92. Bolden C, Cusack B, Richelson E. Clozapine is a potent and selective muscarinic antagonist at the five cloned human muscarinic acetylcholine receptors expressed in the CHO-K1 cell. *Eur J Pharmacol* 1991; 192:205–206.

93. Raja M. Tardive dyskinesia induced by olanzapine. *Mov Disord* 1998; 13(Suppl 2):276.

94. Bennett JP jr, Landon ER, Dietrich S, et al. Suppression of dyskinesias in advanced Parkinson's disease: Moderate daily clozapine doses provide long-term dyskinesia reduction. *Mov Disord* 1994; 9:409–414.

38

Excitatory Amino Acid Receptor Antagonists

Fabio Blandini

Neurological Institute "C. Mondino", Pavia, Italy

and

J. Timothy Greenamyre

Emory University, Atlanta, Georgia

INTRODUCTION

Almost 40 years ago, Ehringer and Hornykiewicz identified the loss of melanized, dopaminergic neurons of the substantia nigra pars compacta (SNc) as the pathologic marker of Parkinson's disease (PD) (1). Since SNc neurons project primarily to the caudate-putamen, it became apparent that the motor symptoms of PD – rigidity, bradykinesia, and tremor – were directly related to the dopaminergic depletion of the nigrostriatal pathway. This led to the adoption of dihydroxyphenylalanine (levodopa), the direct precursor of dopamine, as the first-choice therapy for PD. In the four decades since the original description of PD-related pathobiochemical changes, significant progress has been made in the understanding of PD pathophysiology.

Therapy with levodopa has significant shortcomings. After a variable period of time, usually between five and seven years, most patients begin to experience fluctuations in the motor response to the drug ("on-off" and "wearing off" phenomena). Long-term therapy with levodopa can also induce a number of side effects, including dyskinesias and hallucinations (2), which are extremely troublesome for the patient and caregiver. These considerations have stimulated a profound interest in alternative therapeutic strategies for PD. The recognition of the central role that the excitatory amino acid, glutamate, plays in the pathophysiology of the disease has suggested the possibility that glutamate antagonists may be new therapeutic tools for PD.

EXCITATORY NEUROTRANSMISSION IN THE CENTRAL NERVOUS SYSTEM

Excitatory neurotransmission in the brain and spinal cord is mediated mainly by the acidic amino acid, L-glutamate. Glutamate is the most abundant free amino acid in the central nervous system (CNS) and is capable of inducing an excitatory response in almost all CNS neurons. Besides its role in excitatory neurotransmission, glutamate is involved in the molecular mechanisms underlying learning processes and synaptic plasticity. Glutamate is stored in synaptic vesicles within nerve terminals, from which it is released in a Ca^{++}-dependent manner upon depolarization (3). Glutamate's action is terminated mainly by high-affinity, Na^+-dependent uptake into neurons and glia (4). Once in the glial cell, glutamate is converted to glutamine, which diffuses into nerve terminals. Within the terminal, glutamine is converted to glutamate (5) (Figure 38-1).

Glutamate activates several types of receptors that have been grouped into two distinct classes: *ionotropic* and *metabotropic* receptors. The family of ionotropic receptors includes three subgroups: NMDA (N-methyl-D-aspartate), AMPA (α-amino-3-hydroxy-5-methylisoxazole propionic acid), and KA (kainic acid) receptors, according to their preferred agonist (6). Activation of ionotropic receptors leads to opening of associated ion channels and subsequent cellular influx of ions. In contrast, activation of metabotropic receptors, which are linked to G proteins, produces

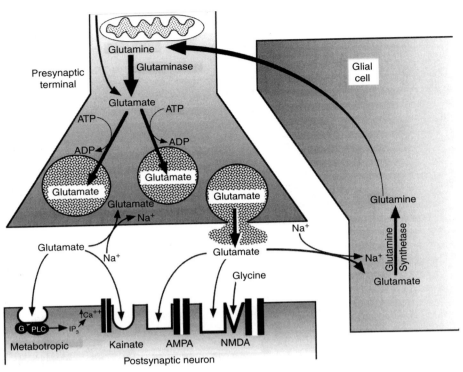

FIGURE 38-1. The glutamatergic synapse. Glutamate in the synaptic cleft can act on ionotropic receptors (NMDA, AMPA, and kainate) or metabotropic receptors. Glutamate is transported into glia where it is converted to glutamine, which can diffuse back to neurons.

changes in cyclic nucleotides or phosphoinositol metabolism (6,7).

This original classification has been updated with the application of molecular cloning technology, which has led to a more detailed understanding of the characteristics of glutamate receptor features. It has been demonstrated, for example, that NMDA, AMPA, and KA receptors are composed of subunits encoded by different gene families and that their pharmacologic specificities and ionic conductances depend on subunit composition. So far, 14 cDNAs encoding glutamate receptor subunits – five for the NMDA receptor, four for the AMPA receptor and five for the KA receptor – have been identified. As for metabotropic receptors, eight cDNAs encoding different subtypes have been cloned. The existence of numerous variants deriving from alternative splicing and editing of RNA further increases the molecular diversity of glutamate receptors (8). In addition, cDNAs for two other subunits, called $\delta 1$ and $\delta 2$, have been cloned (9). At present, however, the function of these subunits is poorly understood.

NMDA Receptors

Two families of subunits, NMDAR1 (or NR1) and NMDAR2 (or NR2), have been identified for the NMDA receptor. There are eight alternative splice variants of the NR1 subunit, whereas the second family consists of four members, NR2A through NR2D, sharing only an 18 to 20% amino acid sequence homology to NMDAR1 (10). The NR1 subunit serves as the fundamental subunit to form heteromeric NMDA receptors, whereas NR2 subunits alone do not form functional receptors. Incorporation of an NR2 subunit, however, induces massive increases in the functional response of the NMDA receptor. In addition, heteromeric NMDA receptors display different properties, depending on what NR2 subunit is present. Therefore NR2 subunits can be considered as modulatory components of the NMDA receptor (8).

The main characteristic of the NMDA receptor is that its activation causes massive influx of Ca^{++} and Na^+ to the intracellular compartment. In addition to glutamate and certain analogs (NMDA, ibotenic acid, quinolinic acid), different substances can bind to other specific sites on the receptor and affect its function. There is a glycine binding site on the NMDA receptor, which differs from the glycine receptor in that it is strychnine-insensitive. Both the glycine and glutamate sites must be occupied by ligands for receptor activation to occur (10). For this reason, glutamate and glycine are termed *coagonists*.

Other potential coagonists are D-alanine and D-serine, which bind to the same site as glycine (11). NMDA receptor activation is also modulated by the binding of polyamines, such as spermine and spermidine (12), which increase the ability of glutamate and glycine to open the NMDA receptor ion channel. Extracellular Zn^{++} and pH levels also influence NMDA receptor function. Zn^{++} acts as an antagonist (13), whereas reduction in extracellular pH decreases activation of the receptor (14).

An essential feature of the NMDA receptor is that, at normal resting membrane potential, the associated ion channel is blocked by physiologic concentrations of extracellular Mg^{++} (15). Because this Mg^{++} blockade is voltage-dependent, occupation of the glutamate and glycine sites cannot activate a Ca^{++} current if a neuron is kept in a highly polarized or hyperpolarized state. On the other hand, if a neuron is depolarized, Mg^{++} is extruded from the channel and glutamate and glycine cause Ca^{++} (and Na^+) influx (Figure 38-2).

Specific compounds acting at several distinct sites on the receptor-channel complex can antagonize activation of the NMDA receptor. Competitive antagonists, such as D-2-amino-5-phosphovalerate (D-AP5) or 3-((±)-2-carboxypiperazin-4-yl) propyl-1-phosphonic acid (CPP), block the glutamate

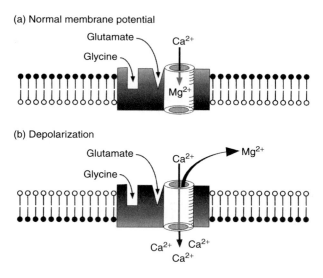

FIGURE 38-2. The NMDA receptor is a ligand-gated ion channel that is permeable to calcium (and sodium). (**A**) At normal resting membrane potential, magnesium blocks the ion channel and prevents calcium influx. The magnesium block of the NMDA receptor is voltage-dependent (**B**) In the setting of membrane depolarization, magnesium is extruded from the channel, and calcium can flow inward. Maintenance of membrane potential requires a constant source of energy. As a result, impaired mitochondrial function can cause depolarization and facilitate NMDA receptor activation.

binding site. Glycine site antagonists, such as 7-chlorokynurenate, prevent glycine from binding. Drugs like MK-801, phencyclidine, and remacemide prevent current flow by binding to the activated (open) state of the ion channel, whereas ifenprodil antagonize the effect of glutamate, possibly by binding to the polyamine site (6). Interestingly, the subunit composition of the NMDA receptor affects its pharmacologic profile. For example, it has been shown that NR1–NR2A receptors are more sensitive than NR1–NR2C and NR1–NR2D receptors to the effect of MK-801 (16), and drugs such as ifenprodil are selective antagonists of receptors containing the NR2B subunit.

AMPA Receptors

Four subunits, GluR1–GluR4, have been cloned for the AMPA receptor. Like the NMDA receptor, the AMPA receptor is a ligand-gated ion channel. A major functional difference between AMPA and NMDA receptors is the permeability to Ca^{++}. Binding of glutamate, or analogs like AMPA and quisqualic acid, to the AMPA receptor is associated primarily with an influx of Na^+ into the neuron. However, some native AMPA receptors are highly permeable to Ca^{++} (17,18). The four subunits that have been described for this receptor can assemble in various combinations that determine the functional characteristics of the receptor. For example, although GluR1 and GluR3 can form homomeric or heteromeric ion channels permeable to Ca^{++}, the inclusion of a GluR2 subunit prevents Ca^{++} permeability (19). Further complexity derives from the fact that slightly different mRNA splice variants (called "flip" and "flop") exist for each subunit (20). In terms of physiologic and pharmacologic profiles, as well as anatomical distribution, this gives rise to a wide spectrum of AMPA receptors. Agonists or antagonists of the AMPA receptor can act at three distinct binding sites: a glutamate binding site, a desensitization site, and a site located within the ion channel. Competitive antagonists, such as 2,3-dihydroxy-6-nitro-7-sulphamoyl-benzo (F) quinoxaline (NBQX) and 6-(1H-imidazol-1-yl)-7-nitro-2,3(1H,4H)-quinoxalinedione (YM90K), bind to the glutamate binding site. Compounds such as cyclothiazide, aniracetam, or GYKI 52466 affect the receptor desensitization site. Another group of substances, including the joro spider toxin and its analogs, block the ion flow by binding to a site within the ion channel (8).

KA Receptors

Five subunits – GluR5, GluR6, GluR7, KA1, and KA2 – have been identified for the KA receptor. The GluR5–GluR7 subunits represent low-affinity binding sites for kainate, whereas KA1 and KA2 subunits are high-affinity binding sites. Functional receptors can only be formed by GluR5 or GluR6 homomers. GluR7, KA1, or KA2 subunits do not form functional channels (21). However, it is likely that both functioning and nonfunctioning subunits combine in native KA receptors. As far as ion permeability is concerned, homomeric GluR6 receptors show substantial permeability to Ca^{++} (22).

The substantial lack of specific antagonists for the KA receptor has limited the understanding of the pharmacology and functions of this receptor type. In fact, at high concentrations, classical AMPA antagonists, such as CNQX, generally antagonize KA receptors as well. Among the putative selective inhibitors of the KA receptor, 5-nitro-6,7,8,9-tetrahydrobenzo[g]indole-2,3-dione-3-oxime (NS-102) has shown selective displacement of low-affinity [^{3}H]kainate binding (23). In cultured hippocampal neurons, NS-102 blocks the responses mediated by activation of the KA receptor, without affecting AMPA receptors (24). Notwithstanding the widespread distribution of KA receptors in the CNS, their physiologic role remains poorly understood.

Metabotropic Receptors

Metabotropic receptors (mGluRs) differ from ionotropic receptors in that, rather than being linked to ion channels, they are coupled to G proteins and cytoplasmic enzymes. The mGluRs, while retaining the transmembrane domains that characterize G-protein-coupled receptors, possess a large N-terminal extracellular domain in which the glutamate binding site is located (25).

Eight genes and several splice variants coding for mGluRs have been isolated. The mGluRs have been divided into three groups, based on sequence similarity and transduction pathways. Group I includes mGluR1 (splice variants: a,b,c,d,e) and mGluR5 (splice variants: a,b). Group II includes mGluR2 and mGluR3. Group III includes mGluR4a, mGluR4b, mGluR6, mGluR7a, mGluR7b, and mGluR8. The primary structure of the eight subtypes of mGluR is closely related, and the amino acid sequence shows more than 40% homology. Within the same subgroup, the homology increases up to 70% (26). Activation of group I mGluRs stimulates phospholipase C, which results in the formation of inositol-1,4,5-triphosphate (IP_3) and subsequent release of Ca^{++} from intracellular storage compartments. Stimulation of mGluR1 results also in adenosine cyclic 3',5'-phosphate cAMP formation and release of arachidonic acid. Members of the other two subgroups of mGluRs are negatively coupled to adenylate cyclase (7,27).

Certain agonists of the ionotropic receptors, such as glutamate, quisqualate, and ibotenate, are also active on mGluRs. Conversely, glutamate analogs like 1-aminocyclopentane-1,3-dicarboxylic acid (ACPD) and L-2-amino-4-phosphobutanoate (L-AP4) are specific for mGluRs. The prototypic agonist for group I mGluRs is 3,5-dihydrophenylglycine (DHPG), whereas DCG-IV activates group II mGluRs selectively. Sensitivity to L-AP4 characterizes group III mGluRs. The lack of selective antagonists has been recently overcome by the synthesis of new compounds that show high selectivity for the different subgroups of mGluRs. For example, (RS)-1-aminoindan-1,5-dicarboxylic acid (AIDA) has been shown to act as a potent competitive antagonist for group I mGluRs (28). Analogously, (2S,1'S,2'S)-2-methyl-2-(2'-carboxycyclopropyl)glycine (MCCG) and α-methyl-L-AP4 (MAP4) are selective antagonists for group II and III mGluRs, respectively (29,30).

Group I mGluRs show a postsynaptic localization, although a preferential presynaptic localization has been reported for some members of group II and III. Group I mGluRs seem to show synergistic interactions with the NMDA receptor. Indeed, activation of group I mGluRs enhances NMDA currents and NMDA-mediated toxicity. These effects may be because of the activation of phosphokinase C – resulting from the intracellular Ca^{++} mobilization – that relieves the Mg^{++} blockade within the NMDA-gated ion channel. Conversely, group II and III mGluRs show a negative modulatory effect on glutamatergic transmission, and their activation causes a reduction in the release of glutamate (7).

GLUTAMATE-MEDIATED TRANSMISSION IN THE BASAL GANGLIA: RELEVANCE TO PD PATHOPHYSIOLOGY

The functional architecture of the basal ganglia has attracted the interest of numerous researchers. This has led to the formulation of a model in which the basal ganglia contribute, with sensory-motor cortex and motor thalamus, to form a functional loop that regulates the execution of voluntary movements (31,32) (see Chapter 22). According to the model, excitatory, glutamatergic, inputs from the cortex are funneled, through the striatum, to the basal ganglia output nuclei substantia nigra pars reticulata (SNr) and medial globus pallidus (MGP). SNr and MGP, in turn, project to the ventral lateral and ventral anterior nuclei of the thalamus, which project back to the cortex, thus closing the loop.

According to this model, striatal projections reach the output nuclei through a direct and an indirect pathway. A subset of striatal GABAergic neurons, containing dynorphin and substance P as co-transmitters and expressing D_1 dopamine receptors, project directly to SNr and MGP. A different subset of GABAergic neurons, containing enkephalin and expressing D_2 receptors, project to the lateral globus pallidus (LGP), which sends GABAergic projections to the subthalamic nucleus (STN). The STN, in turn, sends glutamatergic efferents to SNr and MGP, both of which send GABAergic fibers to the motor thalamus (33,34) (Figure 38-3).

In this model glutamate mediates excitatory transmission at crucial points of the circuit. Indeed, glutamate receptors are expressed abundantly in basal ganglia. Binding studies suggest a differential distribution for glutamate receptors across the circuit. It has been shown that NMDA receptors have a higher density than AMPA receptors in the striatum, where they are particularly enriched in the projection neurons. The

opposite seems to occur in the other nuclei (35,36). Subsequent studies, using in situ hybridization and immunocytochemistry techniques for the investigation of single subunits have provided further insights and partially modified the picture. It has been shown that subunits of the same receptor subtype are expressed differentially in the basal ganglia nuclei or even within the same nucleus. Kosinski et al. (37) have recently shown a preferential expression of NR1, NR2B, and NR2C subunits in the human striatum, compared with the globus pallidus. Conversely, the NR2D subunit appears to be expressed preferentially in the globus pallidus, whereas NR2A is present equally in both regions (37). In the striatum of rat, projection neurons differ from interneurons in terms of the specific NR subunit mRNAs they express (38). AMPA receptor subunits also show a differential expression in projection neurons and interneurons; in particular, the GluR1 subunit does not appear to be expressed on projection neurons in rats (39). On the other hand, GluR1 appears to be expressed abundantly in striatal projections neurons in the primate brain (Greenamyre et al., unpublished data).

It has been suggested that, at least in rats, AMPA receptors have a higher relative density than NMDA receptors in STN, SNr, globus pallidus (GP, the rodent homolog of LGP), and entopeduncular nucleus (EP, the homolog of MGP) (36). In keeping with this view, intrapallidal infusion of the AMPA–kainate receptor antagonist NBQX reduces the firing rate of GP neurons significantly, whereas no effect is observed when the NMDA antagonist MK-801 is injected (40). However, Bernard and Bolam have recently shown that 80% of spiny projection neurons in the striatum express both the NMDA NR1 and the AMPA GluR2/3 subunits in rats (41). Analogously, in the globus pallidus, the rodent homolog of LGP, most NR1-positive synapses are also positive for GluR2/3. In addition, GluR 1, 2/3, 4 and NR1 subunits appear to be evenly distributed in both the entopeduncular nucleus, the rodent homolog of MGP, and STN (42). Therefore it is likely that glutamatergic transmission is mediated by variable combinations of NMDA and AMPA receptors, the relative contribution of each receptor changing from region to region.

In the striatum functional interactions occur between dopaminergic and glutamatergic pathways. Endogenous dopamine modulates the cortical input to the striatum, possibly acting at presynaptic D_2 receptors located on corticostriatal terminals (43). Dopamine depletion of the striatum, or blockade of striatal D_2 receptors, causes increases in the striatal release of glutamate (44,45) and downregulation of NMDA receptors (46). In addition, recent evidence shows that

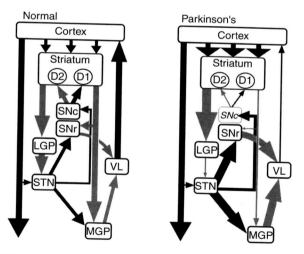

FIGURE 38-3. Schematic diagram of basal ganglia functional anatomy. In this scheme, black arrows represent excitatory pathways and gray arrows represent inhibitory pathways; the relative thickness of the arrows denotes firing pattern or signal strength. In PD, excitatory glutamatergic pathways from cortex to striatum, and from subthalamus (STN) to medial globus pallidus (MGP), substantia nigra pars reticulata (SNr) and substantia nigra pars compacta (SNc) become overactive. Blockade of glutamate receptors in striatum, SNr or MGP improves the symptoms of PD. Blockade of glutamate receptors in SNc may be neuroprotective.

dopamine influences the expression of single NMDA and AMPA receptor subunits. D_1 and D_2 receptors seem to play opposite roles in this phenomenon. Indeed, expression of NR1 and GluR1 subunits is reduced in the striatum of transgenic mice with a selective deficiency of D_{1A} dopamine receptors (47). On the other hand, chronic administration of haloperidol, a dopamine D_2 blocker, causes induction of GluR2 mRNA in the rat striatum (48). The strong relationship between dopamine and glutamate receptors is further supported by the observation that mRNA transcripts for D_1 and D_2 receptors, and for NR1, GluR1 and GluR2/3 subunits are coexpressed in striatal neurons (49).

The importance of glutamate in the functional organization of basal ganglia is further emphasized by the fact that a fundamental component of basal ganglia circuitry, the STN, is glutamatergic. Subthalamic neurons show selective glutamate-like immunoreactivity but do not stain for other transmitters (50,51). STN activity plays a major role in modulating basal ganglia output. Electrical stimulation of STN, which mimics subthalamic hyperactivity, induces metabolic activation in SNr as well as GP and EP (52). Conversely, STN ablation reduces oxidative metabolism in the same nuclei (53,54).

PD-Related Changes in the Functional Organization of Basal Ganglia

The degenerative process that characterizes PD causes a functional rearrangement of basal ganglia circuitry. According to the current model, the impairment of the nigrostriatal pathway leads to increased activity of the basal ganglia output nuclei, as a result of enhanced glutamatergic drive from the subthalamic nucleus (Figure 38-3). Indeed, a number of experimental studies have reported increases in neuronal firing rate (55,56), glucose metabolism (57), and activity of mitochondrial enzymes (46) in the subthalamic nucleus, or its targets, following nigrostriatal lesion. In rats, lesion of the nigrostriatal pathway also causes down-regulation of glutamate receptors in STN targets, which is in keeping with the hypothesized hyperactivity of subthalamic glutamatergic projections (46). Human studies also support the view that STN hyperactivity plays a central role in PD pathophysiology. For example, disappearance of PD symptoms has been reported in a patient after the occurrence of a subthalamic hematoma (58). Furthermore, Lange et al. have reported downregulation of NMDA receptors in the medial globus pallidus of PD patients, which has been interpreted to be a consequence of increased activity of subthalamic projections to the medial globus pallidus (59).

The model, which still maintains substantial validity, has nevertheless been recently criticized and is currently being revised (60,61). In particular, the mechanism proposed to explain the functional changes of the STN associated with the striatal dopamine denervation is not entirely satisfactory. For example, according to the model, STN hyperactivity results from reduction of the inhibitory control exerted by LGP (31). In fact complete removal of the pallidal influence causes only a slight increase in the firing rate of subthalamic neurons, far less pronounced than the increase observed in animal models of Parkinson's disease (62). Thus alternative explanations for STN hyperactivity are being taken into consideration. Dopamine is likely to play an important role at the subthalamic level. STN receives dopaminergic projections from the SNc (63) and has dopamine receptors (64), which mediate the functional response of the nucleus to a variety of dopaminergic drugs (56,65,66). In addition, recent evidence shows that, in the rat, unilateral subthalamic lesion followed by administration of the dopamine agonist apomorphine causes selective increases of glucose utilization in contralateral STN targets (67). Therefore, the nigral degeneration may cause a dopaminergic "denervation" of the STN, contributing to the pathologic hyperactivity of the nucleus.

THE ROLE OF GLUTAMATE-MEDIATED TOXICITY IN THE ETIOPATHOGENESIS OF PD

No single causative agent has been identified for idiopathic PD. The recent hypothesis that genetic factors might underlie PD seems to apply to a small percentage of PD cases. In fact, mutations in the α-synuclein gene, on chromosome 4, have been found in a restricted number of families in Greece, Italy, and Germany (68). Other studies have failed to find such mutations in other cases of familial PD or, more importantly, in any case of sporadic PD (69–70).

PD pathogenesis is most likely multifactorial, and different, concomitant events contribute to the neuronal damage. Among the mechanisms proposed, mitochondrial defects and oxidative stress may play primary roles (see Chapter 28). Selective deficiency of mitochondrial complex I (NADH:ubiquinone oxidoreductase) has been repeatedly found in parkinsonian patients (71,72). The role of oxidative stress in PD pathogenesis has also been demonstrated. Various markers of lipid peroxidation and oxidative damage to DNA are increased in the SNc of Parkinsonian patients, with respect to normal subjects (73–75). These phenomena may be the consequence of the altered efficiency of endogenous anti-oxidants, such as glutathione or the enzyme superoxide dismutase, which may render PD patients more vulnerable to the cytotoxic effects of reactive oxygen species (ROS) forming in the SNc. Indeed, glutathione is deficient in the substantia nigra of these patients (76,77), whereas the activity of superoxide dismutase is increased (78) to compensate the increased formation of ROS.

Oxidative stress may also account for the nigral defect of complex I, which is highly vulnerable to oxidative damage (79). On the other hand, the impairment of mitochondrial respiration is associated with increased ROS formation (80). Thus oxidative stress and mitochondrial defects are intimately connected, and it is difficult to identify the initiating factor.

Glutamate may play an additional role in the etiopathogenesis of PD. Besides its central role in excitatory neurotransmission, glutamate can also act as a neurotoxin. Glutamate neurotoxicity or "excitotoxicity" (81) is caused primarily by a massive influx of extracellular Ca^{++}, secondary to activation of the NMDA receptor (82). The increase in cytoplasmic Ca^{++} activates a number of Ca^{++}-dependent enzymes involved in the catabolism of proteins, phospholipids, and nucleic acid, as well as in the synthesis of nitric oxide (NO). This leads to necrotic cell death through different pathways, including membrane breakdown, cytoskeletal alterations, and NO-derived free radicals (83).

Mitochondria represent one of the main intracellular targets of excitotoxicity. It is at the mitochondrial level that NMDA receptor-induced ROS formation takes place (84). The susceptibility of mitochondria to NMDA-mediated toxicity is due to the role that these organelles play in buffering intracellular Ca^{++}. They sequester Ca^{++} when cytoplasmic levels rise abnormally, as following NMDA receptor activation, in a rapid and reversible fashion (85). Laser scanning confocal microscopy reveals that the NMDA-mediated increase in cytosolic Ca^{++} concentrations is coupled with privileged access of Ca^{++} to mitochondria, compared with nonNMDA receptor or voltage-dependent Ca^{++} channel activation (86). The NMDA-induced accumulation of Ca^{++} into mitochondria is reversible. However, with prolonged receptor activation, the reversibility of mitochondrial Ca^{++} sequestration appears to be impaired (85). This mechanism may contribute to the mitochondrial dysfunction associated with excitotoxicity. Glutamate can also trigger apoptosis (see Chapter 29), a gradual

process of cell elimination resulting from the activation of cell death programs, both in vitro (87) and in vivo (88). The glutamate-induced mitochondrial impairment may contribute to this phenomenon, as a decrease in the mitochondrial membrane potential seems to be a critical effector of apoptosis (89).

An alternative form of toxicity is based on the ability of glutamate to induce ROS formation in neuronal cells, with a mechanism that does not involve the activation of glutamate receptors. In this case, glutamate inhibits the uptake of cystine, which is required for the intracellular synthesis of glutathione. Reduced availability of cystine causes reduction of glutathione levels, increased formation of ROS, and, ultimately, cell death (90). Interestingly, cell death induced by glutamate with this mechanism shows the morphologic characteristics of both apoptosis and necrosis (91).

Indirect Glutamate Toxicity

Excessive stimulation of the NMDA receptor, because of increased levels of glutamate or to decreased removal from the synaptic cleft of the transmitter, results in *direct* excitotoxicity. However, glutamate can be toxic *indirectly* also.

The ion channel associated with the NMDA receptor is blocked by extracellular Mg^{++}. This blockade, which prevents influx of Ca^{++} in the presence of physiologic concentrations of glutamate, is voltage-dependent. Therefore if a neuron is depolarized, the Mg^{++} blockade is relieved and binding of glutamate leads to a large Ca^{++} influx (Figure 39-2). Maintenance of membrane polarity is a process that requires a continuous energy supply. Consequently, impaired mitochondrial function causes depolarization (92). The result is that, if a cell is depolarized because of a bioenergetic deficit, even nontoxic levels of glutamate become lethal (93). This has led to formulation of the "indirect excitotoxic hypothesis" (94,95), according to which any process that impairs a neuron's ability to maintain normal membrane potential enhances its vulnerability to the toxic effects of glutamate. Substantial experimental evidence has supported this hypothesis, showing that the inhibition of mitochondrial respiration, both in vitro and in vivo, causes "excitotoxic" lesions. The excitotoxic nature of these lesions is confirmed by the fact that they are prevented by NMDA antagonists (96). Therefore, it is likely that in PD, glutamate synergizes with a preexisting metabolic defect (complex I deficiency) to induce or worsen the neurodegenerative damage in the SNc.

PROSPECTS OF GLUTAMATE ANTAGONISTS FOR PD THERAPY

Glutamate plays a crucial role in the functional organization of basal ganglia nuclei. Glutamate mediates the excitatory transmission from the cortex to the striatum. More importantly, glutamatergic projections from the STN modulate the activity of the output nuclei of the circuit. Furthermore, as a neurotoxin, glutamate might play a role in the degenerative process affecting the SNc neurons. Drugs that are capable of antagonizing the effects of glutamate might have beneficial effects in PD therapy, as both *symptomatic* and *neuroprotective* agents.

The hyperactivity and altered firing patterns of SNr and MGP that follow lesions of the nigrostriatal pathway are due, in large part, to the enhanced glutamatergic drive from the STN. Lesion or functional inactivation of the STN ameliorates parkinsonian symptoms in MPTP-treated monkeys (97,98). In rats, nigrostriatal lesion increases the firing rate and metabolic activity of SNr and EP (the rodent homolog of MGP), and these changes are abolished by selective lesion of the STN (99,100). These experimental findings have led to the introduction of surgical procedures that improve PD motor symptoms by abolishing the activity of STN (101) (see Chapter 49). These procedures are performed in a limited number of patients who present with profound motor impairment, which cannot be medically managed. Pharmacologic manipulation of glutamatergic neurotransmission, at the level of either the STN or its target nuclei, may also improve PD symptoms. In parkinsonian monkeys, stereotactic administration of the nonselective glutamate antagonist, kynurenate, into the MGP reverses parkinsonian signs in a reversible, dose-dependent fashion (102). Similarly, microinjections of glutamate antagonists into the EP, SNr, or STN have shown anti-Parkinsonian effects in dopamine-depleted rats (103,104). Systemic administration of glutamate antagonists, particularly in combination with levodopa, has also proved highly effective. Coadministration of the AMPA antagonist, NBQX, or the competitive NMDA antagonist, CPP, with threshold doses of levodopa ameliorates parkinsonian symptoms in animal models of PD (103,105). Similarly, the clinical response to coadministration of levodopa and remacemide, a low-affinity NMDA receptor channel blocker with anticonvulsant properties, has been shown to be better than levodopa alone (106). Remacemide can also potentiate threshold doses of selective D_2 receptor agonists and, when added to a maximally effective dose of agonist, can further improve motor function without apparent side effects

or worsening of dyskinesias (Greenamyre et al., unpublished data). Glutamate antagonists are also effective in counteracting the motor response complications induced by long-term treatment with levodopa. Papa and Chase (107) have recently demonstrated that LY 235959, a competitive NMDA antagonist, suppresses oral dyskinesias and attenuates choreic movements in MPTP-lesioned monkeys.

Indirect excitotoxicity might be involved in the degenerative process affecting SNc neurons in PD. This view is supported by the fact that NMDA antagonists protect the substantia nigra against MPPT toxicity (108). Analogously, the noncompetitive NMDA antagonist MK-801, the competitive antagonist LY274614, and the glycine site antagonist 7-chlorokynurenate block the toxicity of a mitochondrial poison in vivo (109). In addition, J. Zhang et al. have recently shown that the apoptosis induced by dopamine in dopaminergic cell cultures is partially attributable to increased vulnerability to nontoxic levels of glutamate (110). In the setting of excitotoxic damage to SNc neurons, it is likely that STN hyperactivity plays a major role. There is anatomic evidence of a glutamatergic pathway connecting the STN to the SNc (111). There is also evidence that the STN affects the activity of nigral neurons (112). Therefore STN disinhibition would result in glutamatergic overstimulation of SNc residual neurons. This may result in a self-sustaining vicious circle, and the nigrostriatal damage may cause STN hyperactivity, which in turn would worsen the nigrostriatal damage (113). This seems conceivable, in particular, if one considers that the deficit of complex I affecting the SNc of Parkinsonian patients renders nigral neurons more vulnerable to the toxic effects of glutamate. Indeed, in rats, STN lesion protects SNc neurons against the toxicity of 6-hydroxydopamine (114) and prevents transneuronal degeneration of the substantia nigra pars reticulata (115). Therefore inhibition of STN hyperactivity, particularly in the early phase of the disease, may protect residual SNc neurons against glutamate-mediated toxicity and slow the progression of the disease.

Human Studies

These experimental data have promoted interest in the potential effectiveness of glutamate antagonists in the clinical management of PD. It has been recognized, for example, that three drugs used for treatment of PD patients – amantadine (see Chapter 33), memantine, and budipine – are NMDA receptor antagonists (116–119). Recently, it has been reported that coadministration of levodopa with amantadine reduced severity of levodopa-induced dyskinesias by 60%, without altering the anti-parkinsonian effects (120). A number of other drugs with apparent antiglutamatergic effects have also been examined. Zipp et al. showed that lamotrigine, a glutamate-release inhibitor, had anti-Parkinsonian activity when coadministered with levodopa (121). However, a subsequent, controlled clinical trial did not confirm the efficacy of this drug (122). Ifenprodil, a noncompetitive antagonist of the NMDA receptor at the polyamine modulatory site, did not improve PD symptoms when used as an add-on therapy to levodopa (123). Conflicting results have been obtained with dextromethorphan, a dextrorotatory analog of codeine that modulates the ion channel linked to the NMDA receptor by acting at the phencyclidine site. Although Bonuccelli's group reported that dextromethorphan can improve, at high doses, some PD features (124), other authors failed to show any significant amelioration with this drug (125). Virtually all these studies have been severely limited by uncertainties of drug dosing and very small sample sizes.

In contrast, promising results have been obtained with remacemide (an NMDA channel blocker), which has already shown significant anti-Parkinsonian activity in MPTP-treated monkeys (106). Recent studies conducted by the Parkinson Study Group have demonstrated that the addition of remacemide in fluctuating PD patients treated optimally with conventional drugs reduced "off" time and improved motor function without worsening any "dopaminergic" side effects, such as dyskinesias or hallucinations (126). The magnitude of the effect on "off" time was similar to a COMT inhibitor and the improvement in motor function was similar to a dopamine receptor agonist. This combination of effects, which has not been seen with any conventional therapy, is particularly encouraging since it was not associated with any significant deleterious events.

There have been no prospective clinical trials of glutamate antagonists as neuroprotective drugs in PD. However, it has been reported that the use of the NMDA antagonist, amantadine, by patients with PD is an independent predictor of improved survival (127). Although this was a retrospective study, it indicates that future examination of this important issue is warranted.

CONCLUSION

Current therapeutic strategies for PD rely on replacement of dopamine, inhibition of its metabolism, or direct stimulation of dopamine receptors. An increasing body of evidence suggests that the excitatory amino acid, glutamate, is likely to play a primary role in PD pathogenesis. Enhanced activity of glutamatergic projections from the STN is probably responsible for PD motor symptoms. STN hyperactivity may also sustain the progression of the degenerative process affecting the SNc. Therefore drugs capable of antagonizing the effects of glutamate might represent a valuable tool for the development of new symptomatic and neuroprotective strategies for therapy of PD.

REFERENCES

1. Ehringer H, Hornykiewicz O. Verteilung von noradrenalin und dopamin (3-hydroxytyramin) im gehirn des menschen und ihr verhalten bei erkrankungen des extrapyramidalen systems. *Klinische Wochenschrift* 1960; 1236–1239.
2. Koller WC, Hubble JP. Levodopa therapy in Parkinson's disease. *Neurology* 1990; 40(Suppl 3): 40–47.
3. McMahon HT, Nicholls DG. Transmitter glutamate release from isolated nerve terminals: Evidence for biphasic release and triggering by localized Ca^{++}. *J Neurochem* 1991; 56:86–94.
4. Kanai Y, Smith CP, Hediger MA. The elusive transporters with a high affinity for glutamate. *Trends Neurosci* 1993; 16:359–365.
5. Nicklas WJ. Glial-neuronal inter-relationships in the metabolism of excitatory amino acids. In: Roberts PJ, Storm-Mathisen J, Bradford HF (eds). *Excitatory Amino Acids*. London: Macmillan, 1986:57–66.
6. Greenamyre JT, Porter RHP. Anatomy and physiology of glutamate in the CNS. *Neurology* 1994; 44(Suppl 8):S7–S13.
7. Nicoletti F, Bruno V, Copani A, et al. Metabotropic glutamate receptors: A new target for the therapy of neurodegenerative disorders? *Trends Neurosci* 1996; 19:267–271.
8. Ozawa S, Kamiya H, Tsuzuki K. Glutamate receptors in the mammalian central nervous system. *Prog Neurobiol* 1998; 54:581–618.
9. Hollmann M, Heinemann S. Cloned glutamate receptors. *Ann Rev Neurosci* 1994; 17:31–108.
10. McBain CJ, Mayer L. N-methyl-D-aspartic acid receptor structure and function. *Physiol Rev* 1994; 74:723–760.
11. Kemp JA, Leeson PD. The glycine site of the NMDA receptor – five years on. *Trends Pharmacol Sci* 1993; 14:20–25.
12. Willias K, Romano C, Dichter MA, et al. Modulation of the NMDA receptor by polyamines. *Life Sci* 1991; 48:469–498.
13. Christne CW, Choi DW. Effect of zinc on NMDA-receptor-mediated channel currents in cortical neurons. *J Neurosci* 1990; 10:108–116.

14. Traynelis SF, Cull-Candy SG. Proton inhibition of N-methyl-D-aspartate receptors in cerebellar neurons. *Nature* 1990; 345:347–350.

15. Mayer ML, Westbrook GL, Guthrie PB. Voltage-dependent block by Mg of NMDA responses in spinal cord neurons. *Nature* 1984; 309:261–263.

16. Mori H, Mishina M. Review: Neurotransmitter receptors VIII, Structure and functions of the NMDA receptor channel. *Neuropharmacology* 1995; 34:1219–1237.

17. Hollman M, O'Shea-Greenfield A, Rodgers SW, et al. Cloning by functional expression of a member of the glutamate receptor family. *Nature* 1989; 342:643–648.

18. Keinanen K, Wisden W, Sommer B, et al. A family of AMPA-selective glutamate receptors. *Science* 1990; 249:556–560.

19. Hollman M, Hartley M, Heinemann S. Ca^{2+} permeability of KA-AMPA-gated glutamate receptor channels depends on subunit association. *Science* 1991; 252:851–853.

20. Sommer B, Keinanen K, Verdoon TA, et al. Flip and flop: A cell-specific functional switch in glutamate-operated channels of the CNS. *Science* 1990; 249:1580–1585.

21. Bettler B, Mulle C. Review: Neurotransmitter receptors II. AMPA and kainate receptors. *Neuropharmacology* 1995; 34:123–139.

22. Köhler M, Burnashev N, Sakmann B, et al. Determination of Ca^{2+} permeability in both TM1 and TM2 of high-affinity kainate receptor channels: Diversity by RNA editing. *Neuron* 1993; 10:491–500.

23. Johansen TH, Drejer J, Nielsen EO. A novel non-NMDA receptor antagonist shows selective displacement of the low-affinity [³H]kainate binding. *Eur J Pharmacol* 1993; 246:195–204.

24. Lerma J, Paternain AV, Naranjo JR, et al. Functional kainate selective glutamate receptors in cultured hippocampal neurons. *Proc Natl Acad Sci USA* 1993; 90:11688–11692.

25. O'Hara PJ, Sheppard PO, Thogersen H, et al. The ligand-binding domain in metabotropic glutamate receptor is related to bacterial periplasmic binding proteins. *Neuron* 1993; 11:41–52.

26. Pin JP, Duvoisin R. Review: Neurotransmitter receptors I. The metabotropic glutamate receptors: Structure and functions. *Neuropharmacology* 1995; 34:1–26.

27. Aramori I, Nakanishi S. Signal transduction and pharmacologic characteristics of a metabotropic receptor, mGluR1, in transfected CHO cells. *Neuron* 1992; 8:757–765.

28. Pellicciari R, Marinozzi M, Natalini B, et al. Synthesis and pharmacologic characterization of all sixteen stereoisomers of 2-(2'-carboxy-3'-phenylcyclopropyl) glycine. Focus on (2S,1'S,2'S,3'R)-2-(2'-carboxy-3'-phenylcyclopropyl)glycine, a novel and selective group II metabotropic glutamate receptors antagonist. *J Med Chem* 1996; 39:2259–2269.

29. Knopfel T, Lukic S, Leonard T, et al. Pharmacologic characterization of MCCG and MAP4 at the mGluR1b, mGluR2, and mGluR4a human metabotropic glutamate receptor subtypes. *Neuropharmacology* 1995; 34:1099–1102.

30. Jane DE, Jones PL, Pook PC, et al. Actions of two new antagonists showing selectivity for different subtypes of metabotropic glutamate receptor in the neonatal rat spinal cord. *Br J Pharmacol* 1994; 112:809–816.

31. Albin RL, Young AB, Penney JB. The functional anatomy of basal ganglia disorders. *Trends Neurosci* 1989; 12:366–375.

32. Green CR. The neostriatal mosaic: Multiple levels of compartmental organization. *Trends Neurosci* 1992; 15:133–139.

33. Graybiel AM. Neurotransmitters and neuromodulators in the basal ganglia. *Trends Neurosci* 1990; 13:244–254.

34. Kita H, Kitai ST. Efferent projections of the subthalamic nucleus in the rat: Light and electron microscopic analysis with the PHA-L method. *J Comp Neurol* 1987; 260:435–452.

35. Tallaksen-Greene SJ, Wiley RG, Albin RL. Localization of striatal excitatory amino acid binding site subtypes to striatonigral projection neurons. *Brain Res* 1992; 594:165–170.

36. Albin RL, Makowiec RL, Hollingsworth ZR, et al. Excitatory amino acid binding sites in the basal ganglia of the rat: A quantitative autoradiographic study. *Neuroscience* 1992; 46:35–48.

37. Kosinski CM, Standaert DG, Counihan TJ, et al. Expression of N-methyl-D-aspartate receptor subunit mRNAs in the human brain: Striatum and globus pallidus. *J Comp Neurol* 1998; 390:63–74.

38. Landwehrmeyer GB, Standaert DG, Testa CM, et al. NMDA receptor subunit mRNA expression by projection neurons and interneurons in rat striatum. *J Neurosci* 1995; 15:5297–5307.

39. Tallaksen-Greene SJ, Albin RL. Localization of AMPA-selective excitatory amino acid receptor subunits in identified populations of striatal neurons. *Neuroscience* 1994; 61:509–519.

40. Soltis RP, Anderson LA, Walters JR, et al. A role for non-NMDA excitatory amino acid receptors in regulating the basal activity of rat globus pallidus neurons and their activation by subthalamic nucleus. *Brain Res* 1994; 666:21–30.

41. Bernard V, Bolam, JP. Subcellular and subsynaptic distribution of the NR1 subunit of the NMDA receptor in the neostriatum and globus pallidus of the rat: Colocalization at synapses with the GluR2/3 subunit of the AMPA receptor. *Eur J Neurosci* 1998; 10:3721–3736.

42. Clarke NP, Bolam JP. Distribution of glutamate receptor subunits at neurochemically characterized synapses in the entopeduncular nucleus and subthalamic nucleus of the rat. *J Comp Neurol* 1998; 397:403–420.

43. Calabresi P, Pisani A, Mercuri NB, et al. The corticostriatal projection: From synaptic plasticity to dysfunctions of the basal ganglia. *Trends Neurosci* 1996; 19:19–24.

44. Calabresi P, Mercuri NB, Sancessario G, et al. Electrophysiology of dopaminedenervated striatal neurons. Implications for Parkinson's disease. *Brain* 1993; 116:433–452.

45. Yamamoto BK, Cooperman MA. Differential effects of chronic antipsychotic treatment on extracellular glutamate and dopamine concentrations. *J Neurosci* 1994; 14:4159–4166.

46. Porter RH, Greene JG, Higgins DS, et al. Polysynaptic regulation of glutamate receptors and mitochondrial enzyme activities in the basal ganglia of rats with unilateral dopamine depletion. *J Neurosci* 1994; 14:7192–7199.

47. Ariano MA, Drago J, Sibley DR, et al. Striatal excitatory amino acid receptor subunit expression in the D_{1A}-dopamine receptor-deficient mouse. *Dev Neurosci* 1998; 20:237–241.

48. Brene S, Messer C, Nestler EJ. Expression of messenger RNAs encoding ionotropic glutamate receptors in rat brain: Regulation by haloperidol. *Neuroscience* 1998; 84:818–823.

49. Ariano MA, Larson ER, Noblett KL, et al. Coexpression of striatal dopamine receptor subtypes and excitatory amino acid subunits. *Synapse* 1997; 26:400–414.

50. Robledo P, Feger J. Excitatory influence of rat subthalamic nucleus to substantia nigra pars reticulata and the pallidal complex: Electrophysiologic data. *Brain Res* 1990; 518:47–54.

51. Brotchie JM, Crossman AR. D-[^{3}H]aspartate and [^{14}C]GABA uptake in the basal ganglia of rats following lesions in the subthalamic region suggest a role for excitatory amino acid but not GABA-mediated transmission in subthalamic nucleus efferents. *Exp Neurol* 1991; 113:171–181.

52. Tzagournissakis M, Dermon CR, Savaki HE. Functional metabolic mapping of the rat brain during unilateral electrical stimulation of the subthalamic nucleus. *J Cereb Blood Flow Metab* 1994; 14:132–144.

53. Blandini F, Greenamyre JT. Effect of subthalamic nucleus lesion on mitochondrial enzyme activity in rat basal ganglia. *Brain Res* 1995; 669:59–66.

54. Blandini F, Porter RHP, Greenamyre JT. Autoradiographic study of mitochondrial complex I and glutamate receptors in the basal ganglia of rats after unilateral subthalamic lesion. *Neurosci Lett* 1995; 186:99–102.

55. Bergman H, Wichmann T, Karmon B, et al. The primate subthalamic nucleus. II. Neuronal activity in the MPTP model of Parkinsonism. *J Neurophysiol* 1994; 72:507–520.

56. Kreiss DS, Mastropietro CW, Rawji SS, et al. The response of subthalamic nucleus neurons to dopamine receptor stimulation in a rodent model of Parkinson's disease. *J Neurosci* 1997; 17:6807–6819.

57. Mitchell IJ, Clarke CE, Boyce S, et al. Neural mechanisms underlying Parkinsonian symptoms based upon regional uptake of 2-deoxyglucose in monkeys exposed to 1-methyl-1,2,3,6-tetrahydropyridine. *Neuroscience* 1989; 32:231–226.

58. Sellal F, Hirsh E, Lisovoski F, et al. Contralateral disappearance of Parkinsonian signs after subthalamotomic hematoma. *Neurology* 1992; 42:255–256.

59. Lange KW, Kornhuber J, Riederer P. Dopamine–glutamate interactions in Parkinson's disease. *Neurosci Biobehav Rev* 1997; 21:393–400.

60. Albin RL, Young AB, Penney JB. The functional anatomy of disorders of the basal ganglia. *Trends Neurosci* 1995; 18:63–64.

61. Chesselet MF, Delfs JM. Basal ganglia and movement disorders: An update. *Trends Neurosci* 1996; 19:417–422.

62. Hassani OK, Mouroux M, Feger J. Increased subthalamic neuronal activity after nigral dopaminergic lesion independent of disinhibition via the globus pallidus. *Neuroscience* 1996; 72:105–115.

63. Hassani OK, Feger J, Yelnik J, et al. Evidence for a dopaminergic innervation of the subthalamic nucleus in the rat. *Brain Res* 1997; 749:88–94.

64. Dawson TM, Barone P, Sidhu A, et al. The D_1 dopamine receptor in the rat brain: Quantitative autoradiographic localization using an iodinated ligand. *Neuroscience* 1988; 26:83–100.

65. Kreiss DS, Anderson LA, Walters JR. Apomorphine and dopamine D1 receptor agonists increase the firing rate of subthalamic nucleus neurons. *Neuroscience* 1996; 72:863–876.

66. Ruskin DN, Marshall JF. D_1 dopamine receptors influence Fos immunoreactivity in the globus pallidus and subthalamic nucleus of intact and nigrostriatal-lesioned rats. *Brain Res* 1995; 703:156–164.

67. Blandini F, Conti G, Martignoni E, et al. Modifications of local cerebral metabolic rates for glucose and motor behavior in rats with unilateral lesion of the subthalamic nucleus. *J Cereb Blood Flow Metab* 1999; 19:149–154.

68. Polymeropoulos MH, Lavedan C, Leroy E, et al. Mutation in the *α-synuclein* gene indentified in families with Parkinson's disease. *Science* 1997; 276:2045–2047.

69. Krüger R, Kuhn W, Müller T, et al. Ala30Pro mutation in the gene encoding *α*-synuclein in Parkinson's disease. *Nat Genet* 1998; 18:106–108.

70. Gasser T, Muller-Myhsok B, Wszolek ZK, et al. Genetic complexity and Parkinson's disease. *Science* 1997; 277:388–389.

71. Parker WD, Boyson SJ, Parks JK. Abnormalities of the electron transport chain in idiopathic Parkinson's disease. *Ann Neurol* 1989; 26:719–723.

72. Schapira AHV, Cooper JM, Dexter D, et al. Mitochondrial complex I deficiency in Parkinson's disease. *J Neurochem* 1990; 54:823–827.

39

Other Therapies

Eric Siemers, M.D.

Lilly Research Laboratories, Indianapolis, Indiana

and

Allison Brashear, M.D.

Indiana University School of Medicine, Indianapolis, Indiana

INTRODUCTION

Although the use of dopaminergic drugs continues to be the mainstay for the treatment of motor disability in Parkinson's disease (PD), other symptoms and signs of the disorder do not appear to be mediated by loss of dopaminergic cells. Given improvements in dopaminergic therapies, many patients now survive into the later stages of PD when nondopaminergic symptoms and signs may become of primary importance. Given the more widespread degeneration that is presumed to occur in later stages of the disease, treatment of these symptoms remains difficult. Clearly, the most effective treatment of these symptoms would be the development of agents that slow the progression of PD so that patients never develop these disabilities; however we are not at that point yet. Symptomatic therapy for these difficulties with a variety of agents can be attempted.

Symptoms of PD that are not felt to be related to dopaminergic deficiency include dementia, autonomic failure, and freezing of gait with postural imbalance. Dystonia may be seen in PD either when dopaminergic agents are likely to be subtherapeutic (i.e., early morning or off-period dystonia) or when the combined effect of dopaminergic agents is above the therapeutic window (i.e., dystonia seen in the context of dyskinetic movements; on-period dystonia). Thus for patients with marked response fluctuations and a small therapeutic window, dystonia may be problematic. Tremor, either resting or postural, may be resistant to dopaminergic therapies. This is also true for off periods and dyskinesia that sometimes require a different approach. This chapter will review other types of medications that have to be used in the treatment of PD patients.

TREATMENT OF DEMENTIA ASSOCIATED WITH PARKINSON'S DISEASE

Past studies regarding dementia in patients with preexisting PD suggest the frequency of PD–associated dementia ranges from 8 to 81% (1,2); a rise in prevalence has been noted over the last three decades. More recent studies suggest that a mean of approximately 40% of patients with PD may also have dementia (3) (see Chapter 15). In addition, the recent interest in diffuse lewy body disease (DLBD) and suggestions that some patients with PD may also develop concomitant Alzheimer's disease (AD) makes the true estimate of dementia associated with PD difficult to determine (4) (see Chapter 16).

The neuropsychiatric symptoms associated with PD may manifest as memory loss, confusion, inappropriate behavior, poor attention span (5) or psychosis. Symptoms may be attributable to medications used to treat motoric manifestations, particularly anticholinergic medications (6). Persistence of cognitive or behavioral problems will dramatically alter the treatment of the symptoms of PD as medications often need to be substantially decreased or discontinued. Psychosis associated with medications or dementia may improve with conventional therapies, including neuroleptic medications, although these drugs tend to worsen motor features. Use of new agents such as, clozapine (7), olanzapine (8), risperidone (9), and quetiapine (10) as well as electroconvulsive therapy (11) have been shown to be effective in small studies of patients with PD and severe behavioral problems. Although these agents have revolutionized treatment of psychosis, some controversy exists (see Chapter 37 for details).

Advances in the treatment of AD, including the introduction of tacrine (12) and later donapezil, have heightened interest in the treatment of PD-associated dementia. The dementia associated with PD is defined by occurrence one year or more after the onset of PD and in the absence of drugs capable of inducing PD-like symptoms. Although tacrine has been studied in several multicenter, double-blind, clinical trials for treatment of AD, no similar studies of dementia associated with PD exist. A small pilot study of the use of tacrine 20 mg tid in seven patients with dementia occurring after a long-standing diagnosis of PD has been reported (13). Improvement in dementia scores of these patients was reported, and it included improved mini-mental state and hallucinations. There was no worsening of parkinsonism. Donepezil has shown modest improvement in neuropsychologic test results and clinician's global impressions in several double-blind randomized clinical trials in the treatment of AD (14,15). No studies of donepezil in patients with dementia associated with PD have been performed. In the United States several small clinical trials to assess the safety and efficacy of donepezil in these subjects are underway. Concerns about the increased cholinergic action and subsequent worsening of PD motoric symptoms will need to be addressed. One case of tacrine-induced Parkinsonism has been reported (16). Although donepezil does not have the significant risk of hepatic toxicity associated with tacrine, the issues of cost and limited potential benefits must be addressed with patients and their families. It has been suggested that dementia with lewy bodies may have the potential of being more responsive to cholinergic inhibitors than AD.

Dietary supplements, such as vitamin E (17) (α-tocopherol) and estrogen (18) have been suggested to be effective in postponing clinical decline in patients with AD. The DATATOP Study did examine vitamin E as a neuroprotective agent in PD, but the results were negative (19). With regard to estrogen, several studies have shown that it could possibly reduce the risk for AD (with a dose–response effect) and perhaps delay its onset in postmenopausal women, although these findings have not been consistent (20). One recent study demonstrated a lack of symptomatic efficacy of estrogens for this disease although the treatment was short term (21). In PD the work is preliminary but certainly of interest. Estrogens have not only been studied in relation to dementia of PD patients but also relating to PD risk and symptomatic effects. Marder et al. (20) examined the effect of estrogen use on the risk of developing PD in women and dementia in

female PD patients. This was a retrospective survey of participants of a community-based study of PD from Washington Heights–Inwood, New York. There were 87 nondemented PD patients, 80 demented PD patients, and 989 healthy controls. Estrogen-replacement therapy was associated with a lower risk of dementia in women with PD (consistent with some studies in Alzheimer's) but was not associated with the presence of PD; thus it did not protect against the occurrence of PD. One other study looked at the effect of estrogen therapy on risk of PD. Benedetti et al. (22) used a case-control study and found 75 postmenopausal female PD patients. They were matched with 75 non-PD controls. There was a slight but nonsignificant difference regarding estrogen use in the two groups.

The clinical effect of estrogen on movement disorders has been confusing. Estrogen has been shown to have both prodopaminergic and antidopaminergic effects. Should this compound be found to decrease the risk of PD or dementia associated with PD the question of effect on clinical symptoms remains a pertinent one. Saunders-Pullman (23) reported the results of a retrospective chart review in women with early (<5 years) PD who were not yet treated with levodopa to examine effect on disease disability. Thirty-four patients were found to have received treatment with estrogens whereas 104 were not. The estrogen-treated group had a significantly lower UPDRS score indicating less disability; however, these patients had a earlier onset of disease. Blanchet et al. (24) examined the short-term use of high-dose estrogen (17B-estradiol) in a prospective, double-blind, placebo-controlled, crossover trial involving eight female PD patients. Each portion of the trial was two weeks in duration with a two-week washout between phases. Diaries and response to a levodopa challenge test were used to evaluate the effect of estrogen on the clinical symptoms. The threshold dose of levodopa needed to produce an anti-PD effect was decreased significantly. No other changes were noted. Three patients had worsening of dyskinesias. This would suggest a prodopaminergic effect.

The effect of estrogens on PD may relate to several possible mechanisms. It may have trophic influences on dopaminergic cells (25) and alter number or sensitivity of dopamine receptors (23) or inhibition of COMT (26). Whatever the mechanism, the effect of estrogen on PD has generated quite a bit of enthusiasm and will be a fertile area of research in the coming decade.

Many practitioners and patients will take herbal remedies (i.e., gingko biloba, ginseng, melatonin), which are currently available over-the-counter. The safety of long-term use, the effect of these agents on the symptoms of PD, and any interactions between many over-the-counter treatments and medication used to treat PD remains unknown.

TREATMENT OF DYSTONIA ASSOCIATED WITH PARKINSON'S DISEASE

Dystonia is an involuntary muscle spasm leading to twisting of the limb, neck, or trunk. It may be a symptom associated with PD or may be caused by levodopa. Dystonia before the morning dose of levodopa may be relieved by treating the motor symptoms of PD, whereas dystonic posturing associated with the onset of peak-dose dyskinesia may be treated by reducing dopaminergic drugs. Decreasing each dose of levodopa may improve the dystonia but can worsen the rigidity and bradykinesia. In cases of refractory dystonia, especially in cranio-cervical distribution, localized injections of the involved muscles with botulinum toxin is accepted as temporary therapy (27–31). Standard doses used in idiopathic dystonia is a good starting point. With repeated injections of botulinum toxin type A (BTX), some patients may develop antibodies to the toxin and no longer benefit from treatments (32). In addition to BTX, other serotypes of botulinum toxin – type B (33), type F (34,35), and type C (36) – are being investigated for clinical use. Recently, botulinum toxin has been used also to treat drooling in PD. Doses of 7.5–15 units per parotid gland provides substantial improvement (37).

A number of drugs have been used to treat dystonia in PD. Nauseida et al. (38) recommended baclofen to treat foot dystonia in PD. At doses up to 40 mg per day they described prompt reduction or complete relief of the problem. Quinn and Marsden (39) successfully used lithium to treat off-period dystonia in patients failing other more standard approaches. It was the result of a seven patient double-blind crossover study using daily doses of 600 to 1400 mg. Dystonia was reduced or abolished within 2 weeks.

TREATMENT OF AUTONOMIC FAILURE

Although autonomic failure is more prominently seen in association with multiple system atrophy, it can also be seen in idiopathic PD, albeit usually to a lesser degree. A number of modalities have been used in the treatment of orthostatic hypotension (40–42). Non-pharmacologic therapy includes sleeping with the head elevated to increase activity of the renin–angiotensin system at night and the use of caffeine-containing beverages after meals. Patients should be reminded to liberalize their intake of salt and water. Support stockings can also be of benefit but are not always tolerated by patients. Pharmacologic treatments include prostaglandin synthesis inhibitors such as indomethacin that may provide a modest benefit (40). Octreotide, a somatostatin analog, inhibits release of vasodilator peptides and may be useful (41), although it must be given subcutaneously. Intravascular volume may be maintained with the use of fludrocortisone acetate taken at bedtime (40–42). Desmopressin (DDAVP) nasal spray may be taken at night both to reduce nocturnal polyuria and to improve intrasvascular volume and blood pressure in the morning (41,43). Patients should be watched carefully for heart failure and pedal edema when using these agents. A number of vasoconstrictors can also be used. These include midodrine, a peripherally acting α_1 agonist as well as ephedrine and phenylpropanolamine (40–42).

Genitourinary problems may occur in PD, although they are more commonly seen with multiple system atrophy. Urinary incontinence due to detrusor hyper-reflexia can be treated with anticholinergic agents such as oxybutinin, but their use may precipitate urinary retention (43) and may be accompanied by other typical anticholinergic adverse effects including memory loss. Tolterodine does not cross the blood–brain barrier and may induce less central anticholinergic problems. In the case of urinary retention, bethanechol chloride, a cholinergic muscarinic agonist, can be used (40). Intermittent catheterization or a chronic indwelling catheter are rarely necessary in idiopathic PD. Impotence may be treated with intracavernosal injections of papaverine or implantation of a penile prosthesis (41,43). The use of sildenafil in PD has also been recently reported (44,45). Zesiewicz et al. (44) treated ten men with PD (mean 7.5 years) and erectile dysfunction with sildenafil citrate 50 to 100 mg and evaluated them after eight sexual encounters. This was an open-label trial. There was a significant improvement in the sexual health inventory scores with no worsening of PD (measured by UPDRS scores) and no change in Beck depression inventory. It was concluded that sildenafil was safe and effective for erectile dysfunction in PD. Brewer and Stacy (45) evaluated this drug in 22 patients with PD in a less formal manner. They found the sildenafil citrate to be safe and effective for erectile dysfunction in men with PD. In the two studies side effects included headache and flushing.

disease, age of onset of Parkinsonism, and levodopa dose may influence the time of onset of these problems.

DEVELOPMENT OF MOTOR FLUCTUATIONS

The manner in which motor fluctuations develop is important for understanding the pathogenesis and for designing therapies for the problem. The clinical impressions of how the response to levodopa changes differ somewhat from the measured changes in motor function that occur during long-term levodopa therapy. Accurately defining the natural history of how the response to levodopa changes during long-term therapy is important, as the time course of changes may implicate and exclude various pathogenetic mechanisms for fluctuations and dyskinesia.

Motor fluctuations are commonly envisioned to be because of a single effect of levodopa on motor function. However, there is evidence that the motor performance of a levodopa-treated PD patient is the summation of several different responses to levodopa plus contributions from endogenous dopamine (9,10). There are at least three different motor responses to levodopa. The *short-duration response* is a motor improvement that roughly parallels the elevation of plasma levodopa after a dose of drug and is measured in minutes to hours. The short-duration response is responsible for the peak motor response – the response that has been the focus of attention in the clinic and in basic and clinical research. The *long-duration response*, first described by Cotzias (11) and Muenter (12), is a motor improvement that builds up over days and, likewise, decays over days. It has received relatively little attention. A *negative or inhibitory response* is a worsening of motor function that follows (and may precede) a short-duration response (13–15). The negative response worsens the "off" condition for minutes up to an hour and is therefore sometimes termed the *super off*. These three responses to levodopa are superimposed on a diurnal pattern of motor function that is evident in levodopa-untreated and levodopa-treated PD patients. The diurnal motor pattern is characterized by better motor performance in the morning (sleep benefit (16–18) and worse function in the evenings. Finally, there is the residual endogenous dopaminergic function that presumably accounts for what motor function remains when a patient has been taken off levodopa for several weeks. This endogenous dopamine production may be virtually

nil as indicated by the virtual immobility of severely affected, untreated PD patients. The endogenous dopamine plus the long-duration response are the main determinants of the "off" motor function. Currently, there is no method to dissociate the contributions of the long-duration levodopa response and the endogenous dopamine production to motor function without prolonged withdrawal from levodopa, which is usually precluded for ethical, medical, and logistical reasons.

The clinical definition of the stable response is a levodopa-induced improvement of motor function in the absence of motor fluctuations in a patient taking four or less doses of levodopa/carbidopa per day. The stable response is characteristically observed in patients early in the course of the disease and early in long-term levodopa therapy, the so-called "honeymoon" period that lasts several years. It is commonly envisioned that the stable response is because the short-duration response to each dose of levodopa/carbidopa is sufficiently long that the effects of each dose overlap with the previous dose to produce a sustained response. However, measurement of motor performance in patients with a stable response suggests that the sustained improvement appears to be largely because of the long-duration response. If patients' motor function is measured in the morning after 12 hours without levodopa, or even several days without medication, it can be seen that their motor function is still appreciably better than that before they began levodopa (9). Stable responding subjects do have motor fluctuations related to the short-duration response that is superimposed on the long-duration response, but the patients are unaware and untroubled by them (9). The negative response and diurnal variation are usually not important at this stage.

Motor fluctuations first appear clinically as "wearing off" when bradykinesia emerges at the end of dose cycles or in the morning after being without levodopa overnight. This is commonly attributed to shortening of the short-duration response. Motor effects no longer seem to last the four to six hours between doses. The short-duration response is briefer in "wearing-off" patients (19–22), but there is neither a direct correlation with duration of action and presence of fluctuations nor are the differences between stable and fluctuating patients very great (20,22). The often ignored characteristic of fluctuating patients is that there is a large, clinically appreciable difference in motor function between the "on" and 'off" motor states (20,22,23). Thus another change between fluctuating and stable patients is that the short-duration response, generally measurable from the beginning of therapy, becomes larger and clinically more significant. The peak levodopa response does not increase; rather deterioration in the "off" motor function makes the magnitude of the short-duration response larger. Precisely how much of this deterioration in the "off" motor function is related to changes in the long-duration response and how much is related to further loss of endogenous dopaminergic function is not known. It is, however, known that a long-duration response is still present in severely affected PD patients (24,25) and is approximately the magnitude of the long-duration response in less-severe PD patients. Thus loss of endogenous dopamine production seems more likely to explain the increasing "off" motor disability. The negative response may also appear at this time and further augment "off" disability. Finally, diurnal patterns of response become apparent with better function in the morning and poorer response to medications in the afternoon (26,27).

The more marked motor fluctuations, termed *on-off*, are clinically characterized by rapid switches between "on" and "off," which is seemingly unrelated to oral dosing with levodopa. It occurs in severely affected patients with large differences in "on" and "off" motor function and who are on complex, frequent dosing regimens. The unpredictable response to oral levodopa is in contrast to the predictable, dose-responsive responses to intravenous boluses or brief infusions in these patients (23,28). This observation indicates that the unpredictable "on-off" response is largely pharmacokinetic in origin. Unpredictability is enhanced by administering frequent, small doses of levodopa in the vain hope that this strategy will yield relatively constant plasma levodopa concentrations.

DEVELOPMENT OF LEVODOPA-INDUCED DYSKINESIA

Dyskinesia is almost an invariable component of motor fluctuations and a consideration in treating fluctuations. Dyskinesia occurring when the patient is "on" is frequently termed *peak-dose* dyskinesia. This term is misleading in that dyskinesia is generally present throughout the time the patient is "on" and is physically, emotionally, or cognitively active (i.e., dyskinesia is brought out by motor activity and any form of stress and, conversely, is reduced by relaxation and inactivity). Furthermore, many patients have an increase in dyskinesia at the beginning and end of a dose cycle – a mild form of the so-called diphasic dyskinesia (29).

How the dyskinesia dose–response relationship is altered during long-term levodopa therapy should offer clues to the pathogenesis of dyskinesia. The thresholds and time course for dyskinesia and anti-Parkinsonian effects are reported to be similar in patients with motor fluctuations (28,30). The important question is what happens during the first months of treatment as dyskinesia first appears. There are three hypotheses.

One hypothesis is that the threshold for dyskinesia is initially much higher than that for an anti-Parkinsonian effect and that the dyskinesia threshold is lowered by repeated dosing of levodopa until it approximates the anti-Parkinsonian effect threshold (28,30). The threshold is a marker for the initial inflection of the dose-response curve or the equivalent of an "effective dose 05" (dose producing 5% of the maximum response). Thus lowering of the dyskinesia threshold would be equivalent to shifting the dose–response curve to the left. The slope of the dyskinesia dose-response curve and the maximum response (Emax) could also change, but the essential feature is the leftward shift and reduction of dose required to produce dyskinesia (often expressed as the reduction in ED50, the dose producing 1/2 of the maximum response). The problem with this hypothesis is that there have been few (28) or no (30) subjects described with newly developed dyskinesia that fall between the subjects who have no dyskinesia at all (and in whom no threshold can be determined because they do not have dyskinesia) and the fluctuating subjects with dyskinesia thresholds that are similar to anti-Parkinsonian thresholds. Thus there are no subjects with dyskinesia in whom the initial high threshold postulated by this model can be demonstrated. In conclusion, although intuitively attractive, the leftward shift of the dose-response curve is an unproven model of how dyskinesia develops.

A second model is that rather than a leftward shift of the dose–response curve, an increase in Emax from clinically undetectable to clinically apparent explains the development of dyskinesia (31). This hypothesis is also based on scanty data: three stable patients exhibited mild dyskinesia at doses of levodopa that were as low or lower than those inducing an anti-Parkinsonian action in the subjects or those inducing dyskinesia in fluctuating subjects (23). The Emax hypothesis would explain the increase in severity of levodopa-induced dyskinesia during long-term levodopa therapy.

The third model contradicts both of the above models and suggests that neither the ED50 nor the Emax of the dose (concentration)–response curve for dyskinesia change during levodopa therapy (32). These conclusions are based on longitudinal studies in 11 PD subjects who had received levodopa for an average of four years and had dyskinesia for one year upon entry into the study. Concentration (as opposed to dose)–response curves were derived from pharmacokinetic–pharmacodynamic modeling. Instead of the dyskinesia concentration–response curve shifting, the anti-Parkinsonian concentration–response curve shifted to the right. That is, the threshold for the anti-Parkinsonian action increased during long-term therapy, whereas that for dyskinesia did not change. The severity of dyskinesia (Emax) also did not change over the three years of the study although the scale used (33) was relatively insensitive to changes in severity of dyskinesia.

It is obvious that more careful observations, as dyskinesia initially appears, are critical to deciding between these different models of development of dyskinesia. Understanding the clinical course of events will indicate the type and time course of biochemical events that might underlie development of dyskinesia.

Two unproven concepts guide treatment of dyskinesia. The first concept is that there are different thresholds for dyskinesia and for anti-Parkinsonian actions of levodopa. Most studies using single parenteral doses of levodopa find that the thresholds for dyskinesia and anti-Parkinsonian actions are similar in "wearing-off" and "on-off" patients (23,28). Thus the concept of dosing to exceed the anti-Parkinsonian threshold and not the dyskinesia threshold is problematic, particularly, when the short half-life of levodopa is considered.

The second unproven concept is that severity of dyskinesia is dose-related. However, several studies have indicated that severity of dyskinesia is not very dose-related and more of an all-or-nothing phenomenon (23,30,34). The duration of dyskinesia is, nonetheless, dose-related (23,30,34). Thus small doses of levodopa will not necessarily reduce the severity of dyskinesia although they will shorten the time dyskinesia is present. By patient history, dyskinesia tends to have a diurnal pattern; if present, it tends to be more severe in the evening.

TREATMENT OF FLUCTUATIONS AND DYSKINESIA

Aims

The strategies for managing PD patients with motor fluctuations are dictated by the physician's clinical experience and his or her weighing of clinical studies and their interpretations. What follows is admittedly a personal algorithm and is a mixture of science and style.

Several principles guide treating patients with fluctuations. First, educate the patient that fluctuations generally cannot be eliminated but may be made more bearable. Second, determine what fluctuates and what causes disability. Third, make responses predictable by controlling pharmacokinetic factors and administering adequate doses. Fourth, make the response to each dose sufficiently long such that it is useful to the patient. Fifth, reduce "off" disability. Sixth, avoid drug toxicity and tolerance by limiting cumulative doses of anti-Parkinsonian agents. Seventh, treat "on" dyskinesia and "off" dystonia. These will be considered in the following sections.

Determining What Fluctuates

To effectively treat fluctuations, it is important to have a clear picture of what is fluctuating and in what pattern. A careful history in the clinic may be sufficient; If not, having the patient come to the clinic for several hours may allow the clinician to see the "on" and "off" states. The clinician should be aware that the response to the first dose cycle may be different from the response to dose cycles later in the day. Home videos are another manner in which the "on" and "off" manifestations can be seen. Home diaries, with the patient, care giver, and physician agreeing on what constitutes "off" and what constitutes "on" before the diary is filled out may yield diurnal patterns of response. It is important to recognize that the motor fluctuations are often accompanied by fluctuations in anxiety level, mood, autonomic function, and sensation. Anxiety, as part of the "off" experience, is frequently a major contributor to distress. It may be that therapy needs to be directed to these phenomena rather than to motor fluctuations.

Making Responses Predictable

Unpredictable levodopa responses are generally related to pharmacokinetic causes. The most important pharmacokinetic characteristic of levodopa is the short plasma half-life. This in turn makes the variable absorption and distribution of levodopa very important. The most common cause of unpredictable responses is frequent small doses of levodopa. The duration of response to each dose of levodopa is, like other drugs, proportional to the size of the dose; larger doses give longer responses (35). Small levodopa doses will give brief periods of motor improvement, and thereby increase the motor fluctuations. Furthermore, because small doses will produce plasma concentrations that are closer to the threshold for anti-Parkinsonian effects, delays or reductions in absorption may cause individual doses to fail to reach threshold. Controlled-release levodopa preparations are associated with lower plasma concentrations, more erratic absorption, and, consequently, erratic responses in many subjects. Because of these considerations, when faced with a patient with seemingly unpredictable response to levodopa, a good strategy is to switch the patient to regular levodopa given at three- to four-hour intervals without altering the total daily dose of levodopa. The schedule for administration of other anti-Parkinsonian agents should be adjusted so that they are given with levodopa. This will almost always convert the unpredictable response into a predictable response and provide a starting point for adjusting medications. There is another benefit of this regimen; a simpler regimen will increase compliance and reduce the variability caused by patients' efforts to titrate their medications with self-developed, complex formulas based on response.

The short half-life of levodopa (one to two hours) makes it impossible to maintain relatively constant plasma concentrations of levodopa. Further, the absorption of levodopa is largely in the small bowel so that variations in gastric emptying or bowel transit time may alter absorption. Avoiding giving levodopa with meals (36–38) or ferrous sulfate (39), reconsidering the need for anticholinergics that may slow gastric emptying (40), and possibly adding antacids or domperidone to enhance gastric emptying (41,42) are methods to enhance absorption. Levodopa enters the brain via a saturable large neutral amino acid (LNAA) transporter, and their entry may be influenced by plasma concentrations of LNAAs. Increases in LNAA concentrations after meals and the tendency for these concentrations to increase during the day underlie some unpredictable motor fluctuations (36) and the diurnal pattern of declining response to levodopa during the day (27). The standard American diet contains about twice the recommended daily amount of protein. Low-protein diets will enhance levodopa effects (43) but are difficult to implement. Rather than a low-protein diet, avoiding meals with very high protein may be the best compromise. A dietician may be very helpful to patients in implementing such diets and also in helping them to avoid protein malnutrition.

Making Responses Usable

A predictable response that only lasts for a few minutes is of little use to the patient. The response must be of sufficient duration such that the patient can accomplish various activities. Methods to prolong the response to each dose of the drug include giving larger doses of levodopa (23,34), using controlled-release preparations in patients who do not have complicated fluctuations, adding dopamine agonists, selegiline,

amantadine or COMT inhibitors. Amantadine, which is generally thought of as a drug to use in early PD, may be dramatically helpful in some fluctuating patients. There is a tendency to continue to escalate doses of anti-Parkinsonian agents to lengthen "on" time, but the clinician should be aware that this is a strategy with diminishing returns. The most striking example of this phenomenon in the author's clinic was a 50-year-old man who had been maintained on carbidopa/levodopa 25/250 every three hours and who, to cope with wearing-off at the end of each dose cycle, progressively increased his carbidopa/levodopa to 25/250 every 45 minutes around the clock and still had wearing-off. This case and some studies suggest that tolerance develops with continuous therapy (44–48). For this reason, it is worthwhile to try to limit the total drug intake and to provide some drug-free periods, generally overnight. Another limitation to increasing anti-Parkinsonian medications is an exacerbation of dyskinesia that is considered later.

Reducing "Off" Disability

Dopamine agonists are often considered to reduce "off" disability, although what has been measured in trials is a reduction in "off" time and "off" ADLs (49). Pallidotomy reduces "off" severity in some investigator's hands but not in others (50,51), and it is best to consider an improvement in "off" disability a bonus and not the indication for pallidotomy. Deep brain stimulation of the pallidum or subthalamic nucleus can reduce "off" severity (52–54), but it is an experimental procedure at this point. Similarly, fetal mesencephalic grafting into the putamen may reduce "off" disability (55). Anxiety, panic attacks, and depression as "off" phenomena may be amenable to conventional therapy and thereby reduce the "off" distress.

Reducing Cumulative Drug Intake

There is a tendency to increase anti-Parkinsonian drugs during long-term treatment because an increase in levodopa will temporarily reduce "off" time. However, this benefit wanes over weeks to months necessitating a further increase in levodopa. The author tries to keep his patients on 1,200 mg or less of levodopa per day. Some times, it is possible to get as good, if not better, control of fluctuations with lower doses of levodopa and with less-adverse effects (56). One strategy is to try to minimize levodopa use during the night and to focus on other methods to give the patient a comfortable night's sleep. Trazadone or benzodiazepines may help with sleep and therapy for restless legs, and "off" dystonia and nocturia may improve sleep.

Controlling "On" Dyskinesia

The first strategy for reducing dyskinesia is to reduce anti-Parkinsonian medications that are adjunctive therapy and may contribute to dyskinesia. Selegiline can promote dyskinesia and is the first drug to consider tapering and discontinuing, if possible. Controlled-release levodopa preparations may increase dyskinesia, and switching to immediate release may reduce dyskinesia and increase the predictability of a motor response. Dopamine agonists rarely cause dyskinesia by themselves but added to levodopa they may augment dyskinesia. Therefore stopping agonists may reduce dyskinesia. Levodopa itself may be reduced. As discussed earlier, trying to prevent dyskinesia by frequent, small doses is generally ineffective and leads to short, unpredictable motor responses. A second strategy is to add drugs. Amantadine may have antidyskinetic effects and, paradoxically, may reduce dyskinesia while increasing "on" time. Buspirone has been reported to reduce dyskinesia (57) but is not dramatic in the author's experience. Fluoxetine and propranolol have also been used to treat dyskinesia (57a,b). Adding dopamine agonists and reducing levodopa may be very effective, particularly if levodopa can be markedly reduced or stopped (58). A third strategy for severe disabling dyskinesia is pallidotomy contralateral to the most affected side (59,60). Bilateral pallidotomy is effective at reducing dyskinesia bilaterally but with an unacceptable rate of speech, swallowing, and balance problems. Unilateral pallidotomy combined with contralateral pallidal stimulation may, in the future, be a manner to prevent adverse effects of bilateral procedures.

Reducing "Off" Dystonia

"Off" period dystonia is a painful posture or cramp, generally occurring in the foot or leg, that appears when plasma levodopa concentrations are low. For this reason, "off" period dystonia is particularly common in the morning before the first dose of levodopa. It is also frequently brought on by movement, typically, walking to the bathroom upon arising. There are several methods to cope with this problem. The easiest is to have the patient take the first dose of levodopa while in bed, perhaps dissolving the tablet in water to hasten absorption, and waiting 15 to 30 minutes before arising. A second method is to use a controlled-release levodopa preparation at bedtime that will sometimes carry over to the next morning. A third method is to add a dopamine agonist to the anti-Parkinsonian drug regimen. Antispasticity drugs such as baclofen have been of little use in the author's experience. Finally, although "off" period dystonia

is rarely an indication for pallidotomy by itself, this phenomenon, like "on" dyskinesia, is generally relieved by contralateral pallidotomy.

Prevention of Motor Complications

The knowledge that levodopa-induced fluctuations and dyskinesia will ultimately complicate the management of a majority of patients with Parkinsonism is dictating treatment of patients early in the course of the disease. As these complications are clearly related to levodopa and are rare to nonexistent with other drugs including the dopamine agonists, one strategy is to delay levodopa use until absolutely necessary. This could preserve the patient's function and may subsequently reduce levodopa use by combining it with other anti-Parkinsonian drugs. There is no doubt that initiating dopaminergic treatment with dopamine agonists will delay the need for levodopa by one to three years and that the incidence of motor complications during that time will be very low (61). However, when levodopa is added, motor complications will emerge with the same or shortened latency as when levodopa is the first dopaminergic treatment (61). This may be related to the observation that delaying initiation of levodopa shortens the interval to appearance of motor fluctuations (62), probably because emergence of motor complications is related to disease severity (63). Another strategy for early treatment of Parkinsonism is based on the theoretical importance of pulsatile administration of levodopa to the development of motor complications (64). Attempts to test this theory by comparing immediate release carbidopa/levodopa and controlled-release preparations has not shown any difference in motor complications after five years of treatment (8). Controlled-release carbidopa/levodopa does not produce constant dopaminergic stimulation, and so it may be argued that the failure to show differences is not a test of the theory. However, it is also important to realize that the animal studies supporting this theory are using levodopa doses that could be difficult to extrapolate to the clinic situation (65). In conclusion, there are strong feelings about the proper manner to manage early PD patients, but they are based more on interpretation of basic studies rather than proven clinical tenets (66,67).

Because motor fluctuations and dyskinesia are related to disease severity, another method of minimizing fluctuations is to reduce the "off" disability. This means either increasing or at least maintaining the long-duration response and preventing or reversing the further loss of the endogenous nigrostriatal dopaminergic system. Neuroprotective strategies arguably are largely theoretical at this point (68). Deep brain stimulation of pallidum (52,53) and subthalamic nucleus (54,69), fetal mesencephalic grafting (55,70), and perhaps pallidotomy may reduce "off" disability and thereby fluctuations. The mechanism underlying the long-duration response is completely mysterious and, when understood, may offer other strategies to improve function and reduce motor complications.

Acknowledgments

Preparation of this manuscript is supported in part by the National Parkinson's Foundation and by NIH grant 5 R01 NS21062-14.

REFERENCES

1. Sweet RD, McDowell FH. Five years treatment of Parkinson's disease with levodopa: Therapeutic results and survival of 100 patients. *Ann Intern Med* 1975; 83:456–463.

2. Barbeau A. High-level levodopa therapy in severely akinetic Parkinsonian patients: Twelve years later. In: Rinne UK, Klinger M, Stamm G (eds.). *Parkinson's Disease: Current Progress, Problems and Management.* Amsterdam/New York: Elsevier, 1980:229–239.

3. Poewe WH, Lees AJ, Stern GM. Low-dose L-DOPA therapy in Parkinson's disease: A 6-year follow-up study. *Neurology* 1986; 36:1528–1530.

4. Hely MA, Morris JGL, Reid WGJ, et al. The Sidney multicentre study of Parkinson's disease: A randomized, prospective five year study comparing low dose bromocriptine with low dose levodopa-carbidopa. *J Neurol Neurosurg Psychiatry* 1994; 57:903–910.

5. Kostic V, Przedborski S, Flaster E, et al. Early development of levodopa-induced dyskinesias and response fluctuations in young-onset Parkinson's disease. *Neurology* 1991; 41:202–205.

6. Quinn N, Critchley P, Marsden CD. Young onset Parkinson's disease. *Mov Disord* 1987; 2, No. 2:73–91.

7. Schrag A, Ben-Shlomo Y, Brown R, et al. Young-onset Parkinson's disease revisited – Clinical features, natural history and mortality. *Mov Disord* 1998; 13:885–894.

8. Block GA, Liss CL, Reines S, et al. Comparison of immediate-release and controlled release carbidopa/levodopa in Parkinson's disease. *Eur Neurol* 1997; 37:23–27.

9. Nutt JG, Carter JH, Van Houten L, et al. Short- and long-duration responses to levodopa during the first year of levodopa therapy. *Ann Neurol* 1997; 42:349–355.

10. Nutt JG, Holford NHG. The response to levodopa in Parkinson's disease: Imposing pharmacological law and order. *Ann Neurol* 1996; 39:561–573.

11. Cotzias GC, Van Woert MH, Schiffer LM. Aromatic amino acids and modification of Parkinsonism. *N Engl J Med* 1967; 276:374–379.

12. Muenter MD, Tyce GM. L-DOPA therapy of Parkinson's disease: Plasma L-DOPA concentration, therapeutic response, and side effects. *Mayo Clin Proc* 1971; 46:231–239.

13. Nutt JG, Gancher ST, Woodward WR. Does an inhibitory action of levodopa contribute to motor fluctuations? *Neurology* 1988; 38:1553–1557.

14. Kempster PA, Frankel JP, Stern GM, et al. Comparison of motor response to apomorphine and levodopa in Parkinson's disease. *J Neurol Neurosurg Psychiatry* 1990; 53:1004–1007.

15. Contin M, Riva R, Martinelli P, et al. Response to a standard oral levodopa test in Parkinsonian patients with and without motor fluctuations. *Clin Neuropharmacol* 1990; 13:19–28.

16. Marsden CD. "On-Off" Phenomena in Parkinson's Disease. In: Rinne UK, Klinger M, Stamm G (eds.). *Parkinson's Disease: Current progress, problems and management.* Amsterdam New York: Elsevier/North-Holland Biomedical Press, 1980:241–254.

17. Currie LJ, Bennett JP, Harrison MB, et al. Clinical correlates of sleep benefit in Parkinson's disease. *Neurology* 1997; 48:1115–1117.

18. Merello M, Hughes A, Colosimo C, et al. Sleep benefit in Parkinson's disease. *Mov Disord* 1997; 12:506–508.

19. Fabbrini G, Mouradian MM, Juncos JL, et al. Motor fluctuations in Parkinson's disease: Central pathophysiological mechanisms, Part I. *Ann Neurol* 1988; 24:366–371.

20. Gancher ST, Nutt JG, Woodward WR. Response to brief levodopa infusions in parkinsonian patients with and without motor fluctuations. *Neurology* 1988; 38:712–716.

21. Contin M, Riva R, Martinelli P, et al. Longitudinal monitoring of the levodopa concentration–effect relationship in Parkinson's disease. *Neurology* 1994; 44:1287–1292.

22. Colosimo C, Merello M, Hughes AJ, et al. Motor response to acute dopaminergic challenge with apomorphine and levodopa in Parkinson's disease: Implications for the pathogenesis of the on-off phenomenon. *J Neurol Neurosurg Psychiatry* 1996; 61:634–637.

23. Nutt JG, Woodward WR, Carter JH, et al. Effect of long-term therapy on the pharmacodynamics of levodopa: Relation to on-off phenomenon. *Arch Neurol* 1992; 49:1123–1130.

24. Kaye JA, Feldman RG. The role of L-DOPA holiday in the long-term management of Parkinson's disease. *Clin Neuropharmacol* 1986; 9:1–13.

25. Nutt JG, Carter JH, Woodward WR. Long duration response to levodopa. *Neurology* 1995; 45:1613–1616.

26. Rusk GD, Siemers ER. Diurnal variation in motor ability in Parkinson's disease. *Ann Neurol* 1993; 34:266–267. (Abstract)

27. Nutt JG, Carter JH, Lea ES, et al. Motor fluctuations during continuous levodopa infusions in patients with Parkinson's disease. *Mov Disord* 1997; 12:285–292.

28. Mouradian MM, Juncos JL, Fabbrini G, et al. Motor fluctuations in Parkinson's disease: Central pathophysiological mechanisms, Part II. *Ann Neurol* 1988; 24:372–378.

29. Marconi R, Lefebvre-Caparros D, Bonnet A, et al. Levodopa-induced dyskinesia in Parkinson's disease: Phenomenology and pathophysiology. *Mov Disord* 1994; 9:2–12.

30. Metman LV, van den Mundkhof P, Klaassen AAG, et al. Effects of supra-threshold levodopa doses on dyskinesia in advanced Parkinson's disease. *Neurology* 1997; 49:711–713.

31. Nutt JG, Gancher ST, Woodward WR. Motor fluctuations in Parkinson's disease. *Ann Neurol* 1987; 25:633.

32. Contin M, Riva R, Martinelli P, et al. Relationship between levodopa concentration, dyskinesias, and motor effect in Parkinsonian patients: A 3-year follow-up. *Clin Neuropharmacol* 1997; 20:409–418.

33. Goetz CG, Stebbins GT, Shale HM, et al. Utility of an objective dyskinesia rating scale for Parkinson's disease: Inter- and intrarater reliability assessment. *Mov Disord* 1994; 9:390–394.

34. Nutt JG, Woodward WR. Levodopa pharmacokinetics and pharmacodynamics in fluctuating Parkinsonian patients. *Neurology* 1986; 36:739–744.

35. Levy G. Kinetics of pharmacologic effects. *Clin Pharmacol Ther* 1966; 7:362–372.

36. Nutt JG, Woodward WR, Hammerstad JP, et al. The "On-off" phenomenon in Parkinson's disease: Relation to levodopa absorption and transport. *N Engl J Med* 1984; 310:483–488.

37. Baruzzi A, Contin M, Riva R, et al. Influence of meal ingestion time on pharmacokinetics of orally administered levodopa in Parkinsonian patients. *Clin Neuropharmacol* 1987; 10:527–537.

38. Contin M, Riva R, Martinelli P, et al. Effect of meal timing on the kinetic-dynamic profile of levodopa/carbidopa controlled release in Parkinsonian patients. *Eur J Clin Pharmacol* 1998; 54:303–308.

39. Campbell NRC, Rankine D, Goodridge AE, et al. Sinemet–ferrous sulphate interaction in patients with Parkinson's disease. *Br J Clin Pharmacol* 1990; 30:599–605.

40. Algeri S, Cerletti C, Curcio M, et al. Effect of anticholinergic drugs on gastrointestinal absorption of L-DOPA in rats and in man. *Eur J Pharmacol* 1976; 35:293–299.

41. Rivera-Calimlim L, Dujovne CA, Morgan JP, et al. L-Dopa treatment failure: Explanation and correction. *BMJ* 1970; 4:93–94.

42. Soykan I, Sarosiek K, Shifflett J, et al. Effect of chronic domperidone therapy on gastrointestinal symptoms and gastric emptying in patients with Parkinson's disease. *Mov Disord* 1997; 12:952–957.

43. Pincus JH, Barry KM. Protein redistribution diet restores motor function in patients with dopa-resistant "off" periods. *Neurology* 1988; 38:481–483.

44. Coleman RJ, Quinn NP, Traub M, et al. Nasogastric and intravenous infusions of (+)-4-propyl-9-hydroxynaphthoxazine (PHNO) in Parkinson's disease. *J Neurol Neurosurg Psychiatry* 1990; 53:102–105.

45. Cedarbaum JM, Silvestri M, Kutt H. Sustained enteral administration of levodopa increases and interrupted infusion decreases levodopa dose requirements. *Neurology* 1990; 40:995–997.

46. Cedarbaum JM, Clark M, Toy LH, et al. Sustained-release of (+)-PHNO [MK-458 (HPMC)] in the treatment of Parkinson's disease: Evidence for tolerance to a selective D2-receptor agonist administered as a long-acting formulation. *Mov Disord* 1990; 5:298–303.

47. Gancher ST, Nutt JG, Woodward WR. Time-course of tolerance to apomorphine in Parkinsonism. *Clin Pharmacol Ther* 1992; 52:504–510.

48. Nutt JG, Carter JC, Woodward WR. Effect of brief levodopa holidays on the short-duration response to levodopa: Evidence for tolerance to the anti-Parkinsonian effects. *Neurology* 1994; 44:1617–1622.

49. Lieberman A, Ranhosky A, Korts D. Clinical evaluation of pramipexole in advanced Parkinson's disease: Results of a double-blind, placebo-controlled, parallel-group study. *Neurology* 1997; 49:162–168.

50. Lozano AM, Lang AE, Galvez-Jimenez N, et al. Effect of GPi pallidotomy on motor function in Parkinson's disease. *Lancet* 1995; 346:1383–1387.

51. Johansson F, Malm J, Nordh E, et al. Usefulness of pallidotomy in advanced Parkinson's disease. *J Neurol Neurosurg Psychiatry* 1997; 62:125–132.

52. Gross C, Rougier A, Guehl D, et al. High-frequency stimulation of the globus pallidus internalis in Parkinson's disease: A study of seven cases. *J Neurosurg* 1997; 87:491–498.

53. Pahwa R, Wilkinson S, Smith D, et al. High-frequency stimulation of the globus pallidus for the treatment of Parkinson's disease. *Neurology* 1997; 49:249–253.

54. Limousin P, Pollak P, Benazzouz A, et al. Effect on Parkinsonian signs and symptoms of bilateral subthalamic nucleus stimulation. *Lancet* 1995; 345:91–95.

55. Lindvall O, Widner H, Rehncrona S, et al. Transplantation of fetal dopamine neurons in Parkinson's disease: One-year clinical and neurophysiological observations in two patients with putaminal implants. *Ann Neurol* 1992; 31:155–165.

56. Barbeau A. The clinical physiology of side effects in long-term L-DOPA therapy. *Adv Neurol* 1974; 5:347–365.

57. Bonifati V, Fabrizio E, Cipriani R, et al. Buspirone in levodopa-induced dyskinesia. *Clin Neuropharmacol* 1994; 17:73–82.

57a. Durif F, Vidailhet M, Bonnet AM, et al. Levodopa-induced dyskinesias are improved by flouxetine. *Neurology* 1995; 45:1855–1858.

57b. Carpentier AF, Bonnet AM, Vidailhet M, et al. Improvement of levodopa-induced dyskinesia by propranolol in Parkinson's disease. *Neurology* 1996; 46:1548–1551.

58. Facca A, Sanchez-Ramos J. High-dose pergolide monotherapy in the treatment of severe levodopa-induced dyskinesia. *Mov Disord* 1996; 11:327–341.

59. Lang AE, Lozano AM, Montgomery E, et al. Posteroventral medial pallidotomy in advanced Parkinson's disease. *N Engl J Med* 1997; 337:1036–1042.

60. Samuel M, Caputo E, Brooks DJ, et al. A study of medial pallidotomy for Parkinson's disease: Clinical outcome, MRI localization and complications. *Brain* 1998; 121:59–75.

61. Montastruc JL, Rascol O, Senard JM, et al. A randomized controlled study comparing bromocriptine to which levodopa was later added, with levodopa alone in previously untreated patients with Parkinson's disease: A five year follow up. *J Neurol Neurosurg Psychiatry* 1994; 1034–1038.

62. Cedarbaum JM, Gandy SE, McDowell FH. "Early" initiation of levodopa treatment does not promote the development of motor response fluctuations, dyskinesias, or dementia in Parkinson's disease. *Neurology* 1991; 41:622–629.

63. Langston WJ, Ballard P. Parkinsonism induced by 1-methyl-4-phenyl-1,2,3,6-tetrahydropyridine (MPTP): Implications for treatment and the pathogenesis of Parkinson's disease. *Can J Neurol Sci* 1984; 11:160–165.

64. Chase TN, Engber TM, Mouradian MM. Palliative and prophylactic benefits of continuously administered dopaminomimetics in Parkinson's disease. *Neurology* 1994; 44(Suppl 6):S15–18.

65. Trugman JM, Hubbard CA, Bennett JP. Dose-related effects of continuous levodopa infusion in rats with unilateral lesions of the substantia nigra. *Brain Res* 1996; 725:177–183.

66. Ahlskog JE. Treatment of early Parkinson's disease: Are complicated strategies justified? *Mayo Clin Proc* 1996; 71:659–670.

67. Watts RL. The role of dopamine agonists in early Parkinson's disease. *Neurology* 1997; 49(Suppl 1):S34–S48.

68. Olanow CW. Attempts to obtain neuroprotection in Parkinson's disease. *Neurology* 1997; 49(Suppl):S26–S33.

69. Limousin P, Krack P, Pollak P, et al. Electrical stimulation of the subthalamic nucleus in advanced Parkinson's disease. *N Engl J Med* 1998; 339:1105–1111.

70. Defer G, Geny C, Ricolfi F, et al. Long-term outcome of unilaterally transplanted Parkinsonian patients. *Brain* 1996; 119:41–50.

41

Fluctuations of Nonmotor Symptoms

Jacob I. Sage, M.D.

Robert Wood Johnson Medical School, New Brunswick, New Jersey

GENERAL PRINCIPLES

The majority of patients with Parkinson's disease (PD) begin to experience a fluctuating response to levodopa (LD) within five years of initiating treatment (1). The most common fluctuations consist of changes in motor function presumably associated with alterations in the concentration and efficacy of striatal dopamine (2). High-concentration motor effects usually consist of dyskinesias (peak dose dyskinesias chorea or dystonia) and are associated with the "on" state. Low concentration or reduced efficacy of striatal dopamine is associated with the reemergence of Parkinsonian motor symptoms ("off" state, end-of-dose wearing off) and frequently with chorea (diphasic) and dystonia (early morning dystonia, diphasic dystonia (3,4).

Although the treatment of patients with advanced PD places major emphasis on controlling or reducing motor fluctuations, it has become increasingly clear that nonmotor fluctuations may be equally or even more incapacitating and common (5). Riley and Lang have suggested that most nonmotor fluctuations can be classified into three groups: sensory, autonomic, and cognitive/psychiatric (6). One hundred and thirty patients with motor fluctuations had been studied and it was shown that at least 17% had nonmotor fluctuations as well (5). In a significant number of patients, these nonmotor phenomena were a major, if not the major, cause of discomfort or disability.

It is important to note that many of the nonmotor phenomena to be discussed are present in PD patients as a constant complaint and not as a fluctuating problem. Paresthesias, pain, drooling, orthostatic hypotension, urinary frequency, hallucinations, depression, anxiety, and dementia, just to name the most obvious ones, are difficulties that some patients face all the time. A number of these complaints, most commonly pain and depression, can even be seen as an initial or early symptom of PD.

The focus of this chapter, however, will be on situations in which these nonmotor problems appear in temporal patterns that are closely associated with fluctuating concentrations of dopaminergic medications and of resultant changes in motor function. We will apply the Riley and Lang classification to nonmotor phenomena that occur both in the "on" state and in the "off" state. Nonmotor complications occurring in association with the "on" state are better known and therefore more frequently diagnosed than those occurring in the "off" state. Recognizing all nonmotor fluctuations depends on knowledge of the phenomena that can occur and relating the individual event with either a hypodopaminergic or hyperdopaminergic state. Nonmotor symptoms and signs must be related carefully to motor signs and symptoms and to the timing of medications to make an accurate judgement about whether the patient is experiencing an "on" or "off" problem. Appropriate therapeutic adjustments can then be made (7).

NONMOTOR PHENOMENA ASSOCIATED WITH THE "ON" STATE (TABLE 41-1)

Akathisia

Akathisia is a feeling of inner restlessness associated with a sense of the need to move. Patients describe an experience in which there is an inability to remain at rest. They find relief of this uncomfortable sensation only when they move about, either by walking or sometimes, when seated or recumbant, by moving the trunk or limbs. Some patients experience this sensation in one limb or one half of the body, usually the side with worse Parkinsonism. About half of the patients experiencing akathisia find that there is no relationship

Table 41-1 Nonmotor phenomena associated with the "on" state

Sensory
Akathisia
Pain associated with dystonia
Internal tremor
Autonomic
Sweating
Flushing
Nausea
Hypotension
Cognitive/Psychiatric
Confusion
Hallucinations
Anxiety
Cognitive dysfunction
Hypomania
Sexual deviance
Hypersexuality
Others
Dyspnea

to the timing of medications or Parkinsonian state while the remainder of patients are evenly divided between those with akathisia in the "on" state and those with this sensation in the "off" state (8).

Akathisia, when it occurs as a peak dose phenomenon, generally starts from 30 minutes to one hour after a patient's "on" period has begun and may last until that patient goes "off". It begins with peak plasma levodopa (and presumably brain dopamine) concentration and abates as these levels go down. Ten percent of patients experience akathisia in the beginning of dose pattern, starting about 10 minutes after levodopa ingestion and lasting only for 15 to 30 minutes. Some of these patients have diphasic akathisia associated with suboptimal levodopa concentrations or an inhibitory effect of levodopa, which is discussed later.

The sense of a need to move, which is true akathisia, probably should be distinguished from mild chorea. Many patients with mild chorea do not even realize they are moving and have no sensation of a need to move. In some fluctuators, however, akathisia is a prelude to chorea or dystonia. In such patients, slight increases in the dose of levodopa or other dopaminergic agents will produce obvious chorea, suggesting that the perception of akathisia may occasionally mark the beginning of choreiform movements. Anxiety, depression, or even claustrophobia may be expressed by a perceived need to move about during an "on" phase in a fluctuating patient. As with other types of fluctuations,

akathisia can begin shortly after the onset of levodopa treatment or many years after initiation of therapy.

Pain Associated with Dystonia

Only ten percent of PD patients with pain have it during the "on" state. Virtually all of these patients have pain associated with dystonia and only a few have it with chorea (9). Patients with "on" type pain usually have cramps or tightness, most commonly in the neck, face, or paraspinal muscles of the upper trunk. Face and neck pain associated with dystonia is obvious on inspection. Paraspinal dystonic pain may be mistaken for nonspecific back pain and needs to be looked for with careful inspection of the involved body parts during an "on" period. Foot and leg pain can sometimes be seen with "on" periods but is generally seen at times of maximal Parkinsonism ("off" periods).

Sweating and Flushing

Profuse sweating and flushing during the "on" state is almost always associated with severe chorea (10). Since sweating during periods of choreiform movement is related more to excessive physical activity than to poor heat dissipation, the entire body sweats, although head and neck areas may be somewhat more involved than the limbs or lower trunk (11).

Nausea

Although nausea is not an uncommon problem with the initiation of dopaminergic therapy, it usually disappears or is minimized as treatment continues (12). Patients with advanced disease on long-term levodopa therapy rarely begin to experience nausea. Such patients are usually on high doses of levodopa and have nausea shortly after each dose in association with the peak plasma concentration. Nausea often occurs in these patients only with the first dose of the day but it can also occur with every dose or can get worse with each successive dose throughout the day.

Hypotension

Both the supine and standing blood pressures in fluctuating PD patients are significantly lower in the "on" state than in the "off" state (13). Since many patients with advanced PD have low blood pressure, further reduction in standing BP during an "on" can lead to symptomatic orthostatic hypotension (OH) and syncope. Although the majority of patients with measured OH on routine office examination (drop in BP greater than 15 mm Hg) are asymptomatic, a major cause of unexplained dizziness during the "on" state in fluctuating Parkinsonian patients is OH (14). These patients do not experience dizziness every time the BP drops or every time they are "on" but are only intermittently symptomatic, which makes the diagnosis difficult. Furthermore, such complaints of "dizziness" due to OH must be distinguished from those related to postural instability. Multiple BP measurements or even continuous ambulatory BP monitoring may be necessary to make a diagnosis in equivocal cases.

Cognitive or Psychiatric

In general, fluctuating PD patients do not have more psychopathology or increased cognitive deficits during the "on" state than patients without motor fluctuations. Most PD patients have more psychopathology during "off" states when compared to "on" periods. One should always be careful in assuming that a psychiatric or cognitive deficit in any given patient is an "on" phenomenon only. Despite this caveat, in rare patients, hallucinations, delusions, and even mania and punding may be seen as a manifestation of the "on" state only or may be worsened during an "on" period.

Some patients with severe nighttime akinesia require bedtime levodopa to sleep comfortably. These patients are at increased risk for nighttime hallucinations. Night-time hallucinations are relatively frequent and it is difficult to say if this situation (taking bedtime levodopa) should be classified as a psychosis associated with the "on" state or is more accurately considered a levodopa associated psychosis occurring during the night.

Hypomania may occur in the "on" state (15). We have seen patients who went on buying sprees, gambled excessively, or were hypersexual during such "on" periods. Others have reported sexually deviant behavior such as masochism, exhibitionism, and bondage associated only with "on" states (16). Most of these patients become more rational and even repentant as the "on" state wears off.

Depression that occurs mainly with the "on" state is almost always associated with severe choreiform dyskinesias (17). Many patients whose mood fluctuates with their motor state also have depression when "off", but they feel normal during an "on" state without dyskinesias. This pattern of mood fluctuations argues for a reactive depression due to increased disability in such patients.

Punding is a stereotyped behavior characterized by repeated cleaning, polishing, taking things apart, putting things together, to name a few. Fernandez et al. described several patients with this type of behavior during "on" time (17a).

NONMOTOR FLUCTUATIONS ASSOCIATED WITH THE "OFF" STATE

Abnormalities of Sensation

Pain Without Dystonia

About 25% of patients with "off" state, nonmotor phenomena have sensory symptoms, most of these are being complaints of pain (18–21). Commonly, these pains mimic a radicular or neuropathic distribution. Patients describe a shooting sensation from proximal leg or arm locations traveling distally to the fingers or toes. The sensation is usually constant (although it may be paroxysmal), beginning as the levodopa dose is wearing off and continuing until the next dose "kicks in". Other common types of pain include deep, boring pain perceived to be in the bones of the legs, usually distally but sometimes felt above the knee. This feeling has been likened to "ripping the flesh from the bone." Patients also describe superficial, burning dysesthesias that can be compared to a raw sunburn but more often is a tingling or a feeling of numbness in the distal leg or toes. Patients with pain from other cases, such as low back arthritis, also notice fluctuations in pain. Their pain though present continuously, is worse in "off" state than in the "on" state. In some, approaching the treatment of pain from this angle may be more successful than using pain relievers.

There are a number of syndromes which are distinguished by the location of pain and are seen more rarely than those enumerated. Pain in the proximal arm and pectoral area (21), "whole body" pain, proximal limb burning, burning of the nipples and pain similar to trigeminal neuralgia have all been seen as "off" phenomena (5). Abdominal pain is perhaps the most dramatic of these less common presentations. It occurs just as the "off" period begins, often doubling the patient over with an excruciating intra abdominal cramplike feeling. The patient reports the symptoms as if he was experiencing an acute abdomen without a sense of external cramping of the abdominal musculature. Inspection of the abdominal muscles reveals nothing unusual and there is no visible bloating.

Pain with Dystonia

Pain may be associated with obvious dystonia (22). Since "off" dystonia commonly involves the leg and foot, this type of pain is usually associated with a severe cramp in the dorsiflexors of the great toe, the gastrocnemius, anterior tibial or posterior tibial, although any muscles of the leg or foot may be involved. Some patients experience off dystonia in other parts of the body and report pain in the back,

Table 41-2   Nonmotor phenomena associated with the "off" state

Sensory
Limb pain
Abdominal pain
Facial pain
Dysesthesias
Akathisia
Dyspnea
Internal tremor

Autonomic
Malignant hyperthermia
Dysphagia
Belching
Drooling
Anismus
Facial flushing
Limb edema
Drenching sweats
Urinary frequency and urgency
Nausea
Abdominal bloating
Cough
Hunger
Stridor
Pupillary dilation

Cognitive psychiatric
Cognitive dysfunction
Depression
Panic
Anxiety
Hallucinations
Moaning/screaming

abdominal muscles, an arm, or even the head and neck. This is far less common than foot or leg involvement.

Akathisia

Two other sensory phenomena that occur with "off" periods are akathisia and sensory dyspnea. Akathisia has already been discussed as a peak-dose phenomenon but is more commonly seen in the "off" state. Off akathisia can be so severe that bradykinetic patients may require passive movement of the extremities to keep the discomfort levels tolerable. Akathisia should not be related to immobility alone. One must also exclude other causes of a need to move such as severe rigidity, positive sensory phenomena like itching, burning or paresthesias, restless leg syndrome, claustrophobia, anxiety, or depression and diphasic dyskinesias, or end-of-dose dyskinesias all of which can mimic akathisia.

Sensory Dyspnea

Sensory dyspnea is the distressing feeling that one cannot take another breath (5). During such periods there is no observable abnormality of breathing, which is in sharp contrast to dyspnea associated with peak dose chorea in which the respirations appear visibly chaotic (22A). Because breathing patterns and rates are normal during these episodes, it is unlikely that chest muscle rigidity is responsible for the complaints. Despite the discomfort, most patients are not anxious. There is no evidence of autonomic or motor dysfunction during each episode other than the usual "off" phenomena characteristic of each patient. In particular, there is no stridor or other evidence of upper airway obstruction and no dystonia or chorea. It is a sensation of dyspnea and therefore the symptoms have been classified as sensory in nature. The dyspneic feeling usually disappears within minutes after a levodopa dose begins to take effect.

Internal Tremor

The term *internal tremor* describes an often encountered subjective complaint that patients with Parkinson's disease experience. This is a sensation of a tremor that is felt inside the limbs or axial regions with no observable tremor at the same time. A sensation of internal tremor has been reported in up to 44% of patients with PD. Internal tremor can be episodic most often lasting between 5 and 30 minutes. It may occur on a daily basis or it may occur one to four times per week. Eighty percent of patients who experience internal tremor report no predictable schedule to its occurrence. More than half of the patients report the sensation of internal tremor when they are feeling anxious. Internal tremor is described by patients as being unpleasant, uncomfortable, or painful. Internal tremor is most often experienced in the extremities. More than half of the patients are unaware of any association between the sensation of internal tremor and whether they are "on" or "off". Those patients who note an association of internal tremor and fluctuations, usually experience it during an "off" period. Internal tremor is not terribly responsive to anti-Parkinsonian medications. Internal tremor is often relieved by axiolytic agents (12a).

Autonomic Dysfunction

Drenching Sweats

Sweating abnormalities have been noted in PD patients since the early descriptions of Gowers and Charcot (23,24). Excessive intermittent head and neck sweating and patchy impairment of thermoregulatory sweating suggests that abnormal sweating patterns are primarily disease-related. After the introduction of levodopa therapy in 1967, it also became clear that episodes of profuse sweating occurred in a fluctuating pattern similar to motor dysfunction (10). Excessive whole body sweating can accompany severe peak dose chorea and probably represents an impairment of thermoregulation during hard exercise. The most severe drenching sweats, however, occur as part of the spectrum of "off" period levodopa-related fluctuations (25).

Profuse sweating during periods of subtherapeutic plasma levodopa concentrations suggests that this phenomenon results from inadequate central dopaminergic stimulation. The sweating, usually involving the head and neck, begins as plasma levels of levodopa fall below the threshold necessary to maintain the "on" state and may last for an hour or more if the patient does not take another dose of levodopa. Most often these episodes occur during the night, several hours after the last evening dose of levodopa. Patients may drench their clothing and the bedsheets often necessitating a change of bed clothes and bed linen. Sweating, like diphasic dyskinesias, does not necessarily occur each time the levodopa level falls or even every night. Patients may experience night sweats for many months only to have them disappear for no apparent reason.

The most likely reason that abnormal sweating is seen most often as an end-of-dose or night-time only pattern is related to the fact that most methods of levodopa administration produce rapid rises to peak levodopa concentrations followed by a gradual return to baseline. The concentration window at which sweating occurs may be achieved briefly as levodopa levels rise just before the dose becomes effective. Diphasic events such as profuse sweats are usually too fleeting to notice or may not occur at all before most "on" states and only develop as the patient is wearing off.

Urinary Frequency and Urgency

Patients with PD often have detrusor hyperactivity that leads to urinary frequency, urgency, and nocturia (12,26). Nocturia is the most common urinary complaint, followed by daytime symptoms. If daytime frequency or urgency occur early, causes such as mechanical obstruction from prostatism should be considered. Significant problems with daytime frequency can be seen in the "off" state. Such patients are usually on a schedule of frequent levodopa doses and exhibit "wearing off" less than three hours after each dose. As a dose of medication wears off, patients develop urinary frequency and urgency that lasts until the next dose takes effect. The sense of urgency in these patients

may be severe enough that they need to return to the bathroom every few minutes during an "off" period. In some patients, this sense of urgency recurs each time the levodopa wears off. This type of urgency and frequency may be seen in patients whose "off" symptoms are severe (marked bradykinesia, tremor, rigidity, and gait disturbance) but is also seen in patients with less severe "off" states.

Malignant Hyperthermia

Most reported cases of hyperthermia, tachycardia, tachypnea, sweating, and mental status deterioration occur in dopaminergic medication withdrawal and are thought to represent an abnormality of central dopaminergic thermoregulatory systems. The signs and symptoms occur within several days after discontinuation of therapy and may or may not be accompanied by elevations in serum creatine kinase. In rare patients, stupor, hyperthermia and to a variable extent the other signs noted previously, may occur repeatedly in association with "off" episodes in the context of severe motor fluctuations. In at least one reported case, this syndrome led to the death of a patient (27).

Gastrointestinal Tract Dysmotility

Autonomic pathology and dysfunction in patients with PD is widespread and responsible for a number of problems related to different parts of the gastrointestinal tract, some of which are exacerbated during "off" periods (28–32). Lewy bodies have been found within degenerating colonic neurons (myenteric plexus), and the primary clinical correlate is slowed stool transit time and constipation is related to impaired colonic muscle contraction. Some patients may even develop sigmoid volvulus and megacolon (33). Vagal dysfunction may delay gastric emptying, especially of solids. Esophageal peristalsis, mediated by the dorsal motor nucleus of the vagus, is probably abnormal with resultant segmental esophageal spasm and reflux in many cases. One observation is that infusion of dopamine relaxes the gastroesophageal sphincter. Both parasympathetic and sympathetic inputs mediate small bowel motility, whereas salivation is primarily a parasympathetic phenomenon controlled by the cholinergic superior and inferior salivatory nuclei.

Dysphagia, in patients who do not normally complain of swallowing difficulty, or exacerbation of existing dysphagia during "off" periods has several causes (34,35). The most common cause of dysphagia during "offs" is a slowing down of the musculature that propels food from the mouth backward into the pharynx. This neural control system involves voluntary buccolingual striated muscle and is therefore a motor rather than a nonmotor phenomenon. Once food enters the esophagus, it is rapidly propelled via a complex reflex mechanism culminating in food entering the stomach. During "offs", patients may complain of a lump in the throat as food becomes lodged in the esophagus. This can be something that occurs only during an "off" or as an exacerbation of a complaint present to a lesser degree at other times as well. Transit of food is often slowed in the lower third of the esophagus where peristalsis is most impaired. Some patients complain more of heartburn secondary to esophageal reflux during "off" periods. Two patients have been reported with paroxysmal belching that is associated with esophageal dysmotility and involuntary aerophagia during the "off" state. Subcutaneous apomorphine improved esophageal motility in these patients (as shown by radiologic evaluation) with resolution of belching and aerophagia for the duration of dopamine agonist-induced "on" time.

Drooling is a common complaint in patients with PD. Some patients with drooling find that they appear to have a marked overproduction of saliva during their "off" periods. A few patients with little or no drooling all during "on" experience a sudden onset of drooling with each "off". These periodic increases in drooling often seem so excessive that it is hard not to infer a significant increase in saliva production as a dose of levodopa is wearing off, although no such increased production has ever been adequately documented. An alternative explanation is that increased drooling during "offs" reflects a decrease in the automatic, unconscious swallowing of saliva with subsequent pooling in the mouth and drooling. The author has witnessed several such episodes and it seems reasonable to him that there is some role for excessive saliva production.

Abdominal pain during "off" is usually associated with dystonia. A number of patients with abdominal complaints associated with the "off" state have disturbances related to the sudden onset of "intestinal gas pain" (36). These symptoms can occur as each levodopa dose wears off or they may sometimes develop during the night after the last daytime dose of medication has been given, often after awakening the patient from sleep. Some rare patients have visible abdominal bloating during such episodes. Anismus has even been reported as a wearing off phenomenon (37,38).

There are a host of other infrequently reported symptoms and signs of autonomic dysfunction that can be seen during "off" periods (5), which include pupillary dilation, tachycardia, pallor, facial flushing, cough, hunger, stridor, and body temperature changes. Although nausea is usually related to the effect of peak levodopa concentrations on the central vomiting mechanism, the author has seen at least one patient with "off" state nausea presumably associated with gastointestinal hypomotility and increased intestinal gas. Limb edema, although usually due to poor mobility, can be seen as an "off" phenomenon. In one case, hand swelling occurred as a dose of levodopa wore off and disappeared within an hour after the next dose took effect. In this patient, poor mobility of the limb is an unlikely explanation of the rapid onset and clearing of "off" period edema that was probably a result of autonomic dysfunction.

Cognitive or Psychiatric

Panic or Anxiety

Panic attacks are the most debilitating nonmotor "off" period symptoms. One study reported a frequency of 24% in PD patients (38a). It usually occurs when wearing off has been present for a few years. Panic begins abruptly with many patients describing an uncontrolled feeling that death or some other terrible event is imminent. It is often associated with other symptoms including shortness of breath, palpitations, trembling, sweating, abdominal distress, and chest pain. This frightening sensation disappears just as suddenly with the onset of the next "on" state. Reports suggest that panic always occurs in the setting of generalized anxiety (39,40). This is not necessarily true in all cases since some personally observed patients with panic attacks were anxious only during "off" states.

Since these panic episodes can occur in the setting of severe bradykinesia, it is conceivable that the feeling of panic might be merely a consequence of the motor problem with its associated fear and discomfort. This is probably not an adequate explanation for most patients. Many patients with end-of-dose panic have been seen whose "off" bradykinesia, rigidity, or other signs of Parkinsonism were not that much more severe than in their "on" condition.

The distinction between panic and anxiety in these patients is somewhat arbitrary. Some patients for whom the word panic is not quite appropriate have severe anxiety as an end-of-dose phenomenon. There is probably a continuum from mild "off" period anxiety to severe panic.

Depression

Depression is common in patients with PD occurring in as many as 50% (41,42). Some PD patients experience mood swings of a large amplitude, which go in tandem with their motor fluctuations (43). The symptoms of depression in these patients are often out of proportion to their motor dysfunction and can be the most disabling part of the disease. In one survey study, as many as two-thirds of fluctuating patients reported some mood swings (44).

Depressive symptoms and signs are usually linked to "off" periods, appearing abruptly as a dose of medication wears off and ceasing just as quickly as the next dose takes effect. In some patients, depression has been associated both with "off" state bradykinesia and during "on" periods with severe dyskinesias, suggesting a reactive process linked to motor impairment rather than a biochemical state of the brain (17). In the majority of patients with mood swings related to motor fluctuations, significant depression is seen in "off" states only. A study comparing fluctuating Parkinsonian patients and those similarly immobile from rheumatoid arthritis showed increased "off" period depression in the PD patients (45). This suggests that the depressive symptoms are related to the underlying biochemical, molecular, and structural causes of fluctuations and are not a psychologic reaction to immobility.

Hallucinosis

The abrupt onset of hallucinations and confusion can occur in "off" periods (46). In some personally observed cases, hallucinations began 30–60 minutes after levodopa wore off. The psychosis was accompanied by marked exacerbations of Parkinsonism both of which improved when the next dose began to take effect. A few cases of "off" period moaning and screaming accompanying hallucinosis and pain have been reported (47). One case of "off" state moaning alone has been seen without confusion, hallucinations, or screaming.

Cognitive Changes

Cognitive function is difficult to assess accurately in fluctuating patients, a fact that may account for differing opinions by various authors (48–52). One study finds that verbal recall ability is state-dependent, that is, it is better if patients are in the same motor state as they were the previous day when asked to recall a verbal task the next day, regardless of whether they were "on" or "off". Some investigations report diminished mental ability in the "off" state. However, tests of high cortical function that depend on the integrity of motor systems skew results toward findings that suggests worsening mental ability during "off" states. At least one report demonstrates a deterioration

in intellectual functioning during "off" states that was related to deterioration in affect and arousal scores. Another study suggests that some aspects of frontal lobe cognitive function may be improved in "off" states while others are better during "on" periods. Most of the evidence and our own experience suggests that significant numbers of patients do have selective deficits in cognitive function during "off" states. These problems vary from patient to patient and are certainly not present in all patients with complaints of cognitive dysfunction during "off" periods. Delayed memory function, particularly for names, and perseveration or festination of speech are two problems that are most frequently seen in these patients. Many complain of increased difficulty in concentrating, although this is difficult to measure. When there is a difference in cognitive functioning between "on" and "off" states, it is usually mild, and not often troublesome.

TREATMENT

Treatment of nonmotor fluctuations is not always possible but should be aimed at diminishing "off" time or peak dose effects whichever is appropriate. (see Chapter 40). There are a few special points worth noting. In several patients with severe "off" pain," the benefit derived from tolcapone, a catechol-o-methyl transferase (COMT) inhibitor has been particularly impressive. Some of the patients with "off" state depression who were not depressed during "on" periods and did not benefit from antidepressants were helped by pramipexole. Not much benefit has been found from botulinum toxin in patients with painful dystonia related to either "on" or "off". Anismus seems to be helped in a number of patients by injections of apomorphine. Drenching sweats in many patients appears to have a limited time course, lasting for several months and diminishing in intensity or even disappearing for long periods of time for seemingly no reason at all. Recognition of the symptoms and signs of nonmotor fluctuations will prevent unnecessary investigations and useless treatments.

REFERENCES

1. Wooten GF. Progress in understanding the pathophysiology of treatment-related fluctuations in Parkinson's disease. *Ann Neurol* 1988; 24:363–365.
2. Sage JI, Mark MH. Basic mechanisms of motor fluctuations. *Neurology* 1994; 44(Suppl 6):S10–S14.
3. Muenter MD, Sharpless NS, Tyce GM, et al. Patterns of dystonia ("I-D-I" and "D-I-D") in response to

l-dopa therapy for Parkinson's disease. *Mayo Clin Proc* 1977; 52:163–174.

4. McHale DM, Sage JI, Sonsalla PK, et al. Complex dystonia of Parkinson's disease: Clinical features and relation to plasma levodopa profile. *Clin Neuropharmacol* 1990; 13:164–170.

5. Hillen ME, Sage JI. Nonmotor fluctuations in patients with Parkinson's disease. *Neurology* 1996; 47:1180–1183.

6. Riley DE, Lang AE. The spectrum of levodopa-related fluctuations in Parkinson's disease. *Neurology* 1993; 43:1459–1464.

7. Sage JI, Mark MH, McHale DM, et al. Benefits of monitoring plasma levodopa in Parkinson's disease patients with drug-induced chorea. *Ann Neurol* 1991; 29:623–628.

8. Lang AE, Johnson K. Akathisia in idiopathic Parkinson's disease. *Neurology* 1987; 37:477–481.

9. Sage JI, Kortis HI, Sommer W. Evidence for the role of spinal cord systems in Parkinson's disease-associated pain. *Clin Neuropharmacol* 1990; 13:171–174.

10. Barbeau A. The clinical physiology of side effects of long-term l-DOPA therapy. *Adv Neurol* 1974; 5:347–364.

11. Appenzeller O, Goss JE. Autonomic deficits in Parkinson's syndrome. *Arch Neurol* 1971; 24:50–57.

12. Tanner CM, Goetz CG, Klawans HL. Autonomic nervous system disorders in Parkinson's disease. In: Koller WC (ed.). *Handbook of Parkinson's disease.* New York: Marcel Dekker, 1992: 185–215.

12a. Shulman LM, Singer C, Bean JA, et al. Internal tremor in patients with Parkinson's disease. *Mov Disord* 1996: 11:3–7.

13. Weiner WJ, Bergen D. Prevention and management of the side effects of levodopa. In: Klawans HL (ed.). *Clinical neuropharmacology*, vol 2. New York: Raven Press, 1977.

14. Hillen ME, Wagner ML, Sage JI. "Subclinical" orthostatic hypotension is associated with dizziness in elderly patients with Parkinson's disease. *Arch Phys Med Rehabil* 1996; 77:710–712.

15. Hardie RT, Lees AJ, Stern GM. On-off fluctuations in Parkinson's disease. *Brain* 1984; 107:487–506.

16. Quinn NP, Toone B, Lang AE, et al. Dopa dose-dependent sexual deviation. *Br J Psychiatry* 1983; 142:296–298.

17. Menza MA, Sage JI, Marshall E, et al. Mood changes and "on-off" phenomena in Parkinson's disease. *Mov Disord* 1990; 5:148–151.

17a. Fernandez HH, Friedman JH. Punding on L-dopa. *Mov Disord* 1999; 14:836–838.

18. Snider SR, Fahn S, Isgreen WP, et al. Primary sensory symptoms in Parkinsonism. *Neurology* 1976; 26:423–429.

19. Koller WC. Sensory symptoms in Parkinson's disease. *Neurology* 1984; 34:957–959.

20. Goetz CG, Tanner CM, Levy M, et al. Pain in Parkinson's disease. *Mov Disord* 1986; 1:45–49.

21. Quinn NP, Lang AE, Koller WC, et al. Painful Parkinson's disease. *Lancet* 1986; 1:957–959.

22. Sage JI, McHale DM, Sonsalla PK, et al. Continuous levodopa infusions to treat complex dystonia in Parkinson's disease. *Neurology* 1989; 39:888–891.

22a. Weiner WI, Goetz C, Nausieda PA, et al. Respiratory dyskinesias: Extrapyramidal dysfunction presenting as dyspnea. *Ann Int Med* 1978; 3:134–140.

23. Gowers WR. A manual of disease of the nervous system. Philadelphia:Blakiston, 1888.

24. Charcot JM. *Maladies du syteme nerveux*, vol 1. Paris: Battaille, 1892.

25. Sage JI, Mark MH. Drenching sweats as an off phenomenon in Parkinson's disease: Treatment and relation to plasma levodopa profile. *Ann Neurol* 1995; 37:120–122.

26. Fitzmaurice H, Fowler CJ, Rickards D, et al. Micturition disturbance in Parkinson's disease. *Br J Urol* 1985; 57:652–656.

27. Pfeiffer RF, Sucha EL. "On-off"-induced lethal hyperthermia. *Mov Disord* 1989; 4:338–341.

28. Koller WC, Silver DE, Lieberman A (eds). An algorithm for the management of Parkinson's disease. *Neurology* 1994; 44(Suppl 10):S19–S27.

29. Edwards LL, Quigley EMM, Hofman R, et al. Gastrointestinal symptoms in Parkinson's disease: 18, month follow-up study. *Mov Disord* 1993; 8:83–86.

30. Edwards LL, Pfeiffer RF, Quigley EMM, et al. Gastrointestinal symptoms in Parkinson's disease. *Mov Disord* 1991; 6:151–156.

31. Edwards LL, Quigley EMM, Pfeiffer RF. Gastrointestinal dysfunction in Parkinson's disease: Frequency and pathophysiology. *Neurology* 1992; 42:726–732.

32. Edwards LL, Quigley EMM, Harned RK, et al. Defacatory function in Parkinson's disease: Response to apomorphine. *Ann Neurol* 1993; 33:490–493.

33. Caplan LH, Jacobson HG, Rubinstein BM, et al. Megacolon and volvulus in Parkinson's disease. *Radiology* 1965; 85:73–79.

34. Bushmann M, Dobmeyer SM, Leeker L, et al. Swallowing abnormalities and their response to treatment in Parkinson's disease. *Neurology* 1989; 39:1309–1314.

35. Edwards LL, Quigley EMM, Harned RK, et al. Characterization of swallowing and defecation in Parkinson's disease. *Am J Gastroenterology* 1994; 89:15–25.

36. Kempster PA, Lees AJ, Crichton P, et al. Off-period belching due to a reversible disturbance of oesophageal motility in Parkinson's disease and its treatment with apomorphine. Mov Disord 1989; 4:47–52.

37. Mathers SE, Kempster PA, Law PJ, et al. Anal sphincter dysfunction in Parkinson's disease. Arch Neurol 1989; 46:1061–1064.

38. Mathers SE, Kempster PA, Swash M, et al. Constipation and parodoxical puborectalis contraction in anismus and Parkinson's disease: A dystonic

phenomenon? *J Neurol Neurosurg Psychiatry* 1988; 51:1503–1507.

38a. Vasfuez A, Jiminez-Jiminez FJ, Garcia-Rviz P, et al. "Panic attacks" in Parkinson's disease: A long-term complication of levodopa therapy. *Acta Neurol Scand* 1993; 87:14–18.

39. Stein MB, Heuser IJ, Juncos JL, et al. Anxiety disorders in patients with Parkinson's disease. *Am J Psychiatry* 1990; 147:217–220.

40. Routh LC, Black JL, Ahlskog JE. Parkinson's disease complicated by anxiety. *Mayo Clin Proc* 1987; 62:733–735.

41. Marsden CD, Parkes JD. "On and off" variability and response swings in Parkinson's disease. In: Rose FC, Capildeo R, (eds). *Research Progress in Parkinson's disease*. Kent England:Pitman Medical; 1981: 265–264.

42. Menza M, Forman N, Sage J, et al. Psychiatric symptoms in Parkinson's disease: A comparison between patients with and without "On-off" symptoms. *Biol Psychiatry* 1993; 33:682–684.

43. Keshavan MS, David AS, Narayanen HS, et al. "On-off" phenomena and manic depressive mood shifts: Case report. *J Clin Psychiatry* 1986; 47:93–94.

44. Nissenbaum H, Quinn NP, Brown RG, et al. Mood swings associated with the "On-off" phenomenon in Parkinson's disease. *Psychol Med* 1987; 17:899–904.

45. Cantello R, Gilli M, Riccio A, et al. Mood changes associated with "end of dose deterioration" in Parkinson's disease: A controlled study. *J Neurol Neurosurg Psychiatry* 1986; 49:1182–1190.

46. Sage JI, Duvoisin RC. Sudden onset of confusion with severe exacerbation of Parkinsonism during levodopa therapy. *Mov disord* 1986; 1:267–270.

47. Steiger MJ, Quinn NP, Toone B, et al. Off-period screaming accompanying motor fluctuations in Parkinson's disease. *Mov Disord* 1991; 6:89–90.

48. Huber SJ, Shulman HG, Paulson GW, et al. Dose-dependent memory impairment in Parkinson's disease. *Neurology* 1989; 39:438–440.

49. Delis D, Direnfeld L, Alexander MP, et al. Cognitive fluctuations associated with on-off phenomenon in Parkinson's disease. *Neurology* 1982; 32:1049–1052.

50. Girotti E, Carella F, Grassi MP, et al. Motor and cognitive performance of Parkinsonian patients in the on and off phases of the disease. *J Neurol Neurosurg Psychiatry* 1986; 49:657–660.

51. Gotham AM, Brown RG, Marsden CD. "Frontal" cognitive function in patients with Parkinson's disease "on" and "off" levodopa. *Brain* 1988; 11:299–321.

52. Poewe W, Berger W, Benke T, et al. High speed memory scanning in Parkinson's disease: Adverse effects of levodopa. *Ann Neurol* 1991; 29:670–673.

42

Psychosis and Related Problems

Eric S. Molho, M.D.

The Parkinson's Disease and Movement Disorder Center of Albany Medical Center, Albany, New York

INTRODUCTION

The early years of levodopa therapy for Parkinson's disease (PD) was accompanied by great optimism that dopamine replacement therapy might provide a cure or, at least, a lasting reversal of symptoms. It was soon realized that levodopa therapy was not a cure for PD and that there were a number of long-term complications associated with its use. Among the problems were several drug-induced psychiatric states. The one that may be considered the most disabling and frustrating is drug-induced psychosis (DIP)(1). In fact, recent studies have indicated that hallucinations are a major risk factor for nursing home placement in PD patients (2) and that such placement is often permanent and may be associated with a high mortality rate (3). Recently, psychosis in PD has received increased attention because of the clearly demonstrated efficacy of clozapine in treating this problem (4). This chapter will review the history, clinical features, and mechanisms of DIP in PD and outline a practical approach to its treatment. Mania and hypersexuality will also be addressed, but other psychiatric disorders such as depression (Chapter 17) and anxiety (Chapter 18) are discussed elsewhere in this text.

DRUG-INDUCED PSYCHOSIS: TERMINOLOGY, HISTORY, AND FREQUENCY

In the past, the terms *levodopa psychosis*, *drug-induced psychosis* and *dopaminomimetic psychosis* were used indiscriminately to describe several different psychiatric syndromes occurring in PD. The broad application of these terms has hindered understanding of the frequency, pathophysiology and treatment of these disorders. It is now clear that there are several

distinct psychiatric syndromes with psychotic features that occur in PD. These syndromes will be divided into two broad categories; those associated with a clear sensorium and those occurring on a background of confusion (5). Patients with a clear sensorium may suffer from hallucinations, delusions or both. By DSM-III-R criteria these correspond to an organic delusional syndrome or an organic hallucinosis (6). The organic confusional psychosis is seen in patients with a clouded sensorium and can vary in intensity from a mild confusional state to a frank delirium. These have been redefined in DSM-IV as delusional disorder, psychotic disorder, or delirium secondary to general medical condition, with PD being the medical condition. There seems to be general agreement that all these syndromes can be induced by dopaminergic medications but they are distinct in their epidemiology, pathophysiology, and response to treatment (5,7–10).

A review of psychosis in PD from the prelevodopa era indicates that not all psychotic symptoms are drug-related. Coexistent and premorbid psychiatric disease can occur, including schizophrenia (5). There is also little question that psychiatric symptoms, including psychosis, can be a prominent feature of secondary parkinsonism, particularly, the postencephalitic form (11) and diffuse Lewy body disease (12). However, the occurrence of hallucinations, delusions and other psychotic symptoms as a primary feature of PD is controversial.

In James Parkinson's original description of the disease he concluded, "... *by the absence of any injury to the senses and to the intellect, we are taught that the morbid state does not extend to the encephalon*" (13). This view of PD as a process that spares the intellect and psychologic functioning was held for almost a century. In 1903, E. Regis (14) categorized the mental disorders associated with parkinsonism, and specifically mentioned depression as an early phenomenon and hallucinations as a symptom associated with advanced disease. In 1922, 140 patients with PD were reviewed, and postencephalitic parkinsonism patients were specifically excluded (15). Depression was found in these patients and was thought to be reactive in nature, but no mention of psychotic symptoms was made. Another review in 1923 presented several patients with "paralysis agitans" and prominent symptoms of psychosis (16). Early features, such as sleep disturbance, withdrawal from social situations, and suspiciousness were mentioned. Also discussed were more dramatic symptoms such as paranoid delusions and hallucinations that were "...generally limited to the organic sensations and tactile sense..." (16). In 1950, Schwab et al. (17) described a number of psychiatric symptoms in "PD" including paroxysmal depression, paranoia, and schizoid reactions. However, it is clear from a review of the case histories in this paper that all the patients described had a history of encephalitis or oculogyric crisis, or both, and probably had postencephalitic parkinsonism rather than PD. Thus it appears that psychosis occurred in PD before the levodopa era. However, it must have been rare and a number of these cases might have had secondary forms of parkinsonism, especially postencephalitic.

During the initial levodopa trials in PD, it became apparent that various psychiatric syndromes were occurring with a much higher frequency in treated patients than in untreated patients. Unfortunately, it is difficult to determine the incidence with which these problems occurred because the early studies varied with regard to the inclusion criteria, the dosages of levodopa employed, and the classification of the psychiatric side effects reported. Studies that included patients with postencephalitic Parkinsonism reported incidences of psychiatric symptoms as high as 55% (18). Most of the studies reporting a significant incidence of psychosis used levodopa dosages in excess of 4 gm per day or did not specify the specific dosages used (19–26). On the other hand, Cheifetz et al. (27) reported no incidence of psychosis in 34 patients treated with 4 gm per day or less. In addition, some authors included patients with preexisting psychiatric symptoms in their data although others excluded these patients. While reporting side effects, confusional states were sometimes lumped with other forms of psychosis, although other studies attempted to be more specific in their definitions.

In 1971, Goodwin reviewed the psychiatric side effects of levodopa that occurred in 908 patients who were previously treated in major studies (28). He found an overall incidence of 20% (range 10–50%). Confusional states including delirium were most common with an overall incidence of 4.4%. Psychosis,

including delusions and hallucinations, occurred with a frequency of 3.6%.

In these early reviews, there is little question that psychiatric side effects were much more likely to occur in patients with certain predisposing characteristics. Dementia was mentioned by a number of authors as a risk factor (23,26,28,29). A confusional psychosis was particularly common in these patients. Other significant risk factors were advanced age (25), premorbid psychiatric illness (23,27,28), and exposure to high daily doses of levodopa (27). More recent reviews have confirmed advanced age and cognitive decline as strong risk factors for the development of hallucinations (7,30,31) and have added depression (30,31), sleep disorder (30), altered dream phenomena (32), and visual loss (33) as significant clinical accompaniments to visual hallucinations in PD. Goetz et al. (34) suggested that early onset hallucinations (within three months of starting levodopa therapy) are not typical of idiopathic PD. Rather, the occurrence of hallucinations early in the course of levodopa treatment suggests the presence of premorbid psychiatric illness or an atypical Parkinsonian syndrome, such as diffuse Lewy body disease or Alzheimer's disease with extrapyramidal signs.

Recent reviews have also confirmed the high incidence of various forms of psychosis in patients treated with levodopa and implicating each of the other anti-Parkinsonian drugs in current use (1,5,7,10). Graham et al. (35) found an overall incidence of hallucinations of 25% in a hospital-based outpatient population of PD patients. In the first extensive community-based survey of patients with PD, Aarsland et al. (31) found an overall frequency of DIP in 15.8%, whereas 9.8% had specific hallucinations. Individual reports on bromocriptine and pergolide have shown these agents to cause hallucinations, delusions, and confusional states with a frequency comparable to that of levodopa (7,36–42). The newest available dopamine agonists, pramipexole and ropinirole, which are currently in widespread use have shown a similar tendency (43). DIP has also been reported with experimental and less-available dopamine agonists, such as cabergoline (44), lisuride (45), apomorphine (46), lergotrile, and mesulergine (47). The frequency of DIP with various agonists in trials has varied depending on the stage of PD being evaluated. Selegiline may be particularly prone to causing psychotic symptoms in susceptible individuals. This is most common when it is given concurrently with other anti-Parkinsonian medications (7,48,49). Even propranolol that is occasionally used in PD to treat tremor, has been reported to cause hallucinations (50).

Amantadine and anticholinergic medications, have also been associated with confusional and nonconfusional psychotic states in PD patients. When given in isolation, the frequency of these problems is low (8,51). However, when given in combination with other PD medications they are much more likely to cause an acute, confusional psychosis (1,7,8,10,52). The acute confusional syndromes seen with anticholinergic medications are more common in older or demented patients and in some cases can result in a frank delirium (10). Paradoxically, acute delirium has also been described with amantadine withdrawal in patients who had been treated chronically with this agent (53).

The COMT (catechol-O-methyltransferase) inhibitors are a novel class of anti-Parkinsonian medication whose beneficial effect is achieved through increasing the bioavailability of concomitantly administered levodopa. Tolcapone was the first of these agents to be approved for use in PD. In clinical trials, tolcapone was shown to dramatically increase the duration of action and potency of levodopa which resulted in improvement of motor fluctuations (54,55 and (see Chapter 36)). Not surprisingly, patients treated with tolcapone also experienced an increase in dopaminergic side effects, including hallucinations. Sometimes dramatic reductions in the levodopa dose was required to treat this complication of tolcapone treatment (54,55). Clinical practice has confirmed that tolcapone must be used with caution in patients prone to cognitive side effects from levodopa, and that some patients will experience DIP for the first time when started on this medication.

Entacapone is another COMT inhibitor that was approved by the U.S. Food and Drug Administration (FDA) in October 1999. Hallucinations and other dopaminergic side effects have been encountered with a similar frequency to tolcapone (56), and it is expected that susceptible individuals will have to be treated cautiously to avoid this complication of therapy.

CLINICAL FEATURES

The clinical characteristics of DIP in PD are now well defined. Visual hallucinations are the most common of these disorders (7) with recent estimates approximating 30% in treated individuals (7,9,30,35,51,57). Hallucinations can be defined as *spontaneously fabricated perceptions occurring although awake*. In PD, hallucinations usually occur on a background of a clear sensorium, however, a concomitant confusional state is common in older or demented patients (7,9). Hallucinations are usually fully formed, nonthreatening images of people or animals, and tend to be nocturnal, recurrent, and stereotyped for each patient (7,9). For most, the imagined figures seem familiar and friendly, although in others, they appear to be innocuous strangers. Some patients will typically see adults sitting around their home as if they belong there. Others may describe children wandering around the house. In some cases, the visions are solitary whereas in others there may be a crowded room full of figures. Another common scenario occurs when patients peer outside through a window and see children playing in the yard or men working. One patient of the author reported seeing a parade passing in front of her home on several occasions, whereas another saw elaborate construction scenarios being played out. Visions of animals are common. Cats, dogs, and other benign furry creatures are typical as is the occurrence of insects. Occasionally, there will be an erotic overtone to the visions (30), and about 28% of the time hallucinations will have a threatening or frightening quality (51).

Oddly, many patients will claim to realize the fabricated nature of these images, and describe them to family members and physicians in such neutral terms that they seem to be no more extraordinary than a visit from a neighbor. In most patients, these hallucinations are fleeting and may disappear if they look directly at the image, move toward it or even blink their eyes (30). According to Klawans (9) the phenomena "... *usually conform to boundaries imposed by actual concurrent sensory input and often concern individuals and experiences that were significant in the patient's life*."

Pure auditory hallucinations are extremely rare in patients with PD but a secondary auditory component has been reported in 26%–40% of patients with visual hallucinations (35,51). In a more recent review, auditory hallucinations accompanied visions in 8% of patients (58) and were described as human voices, which were "... *nonimperative, nonparanoid, and often incomprehensible*." The author has seen two patients who, in addition to benign visual hallucinations, also reported hearing music periodically unconnected to their other hallucinations. Both claimed that the music was of a particular style but could not identify a specific tune. One of these patients heard the music along with muffled voices that seemed to emanate from the air-conditioning ducts in her house. She actually attempted to tape record the sounds and play them back for her husband, who could not hear them.

Tactile hallucinations are also extremely rare (51). In a recent report, a patient was described as "... *feeling as if her bowels and bladder extruded from the distal parts of her upper limbs*" (59). This was interpreted by the authors, as a somatic hallucination of visceral origin (cenesthetic hallucination).

True illusions, which are distortions of actual visual stimuli, are also uncommon but do occur in some patients (35,51). Typically, patients will report seeing faces in patterned fabric, misinterpret a curtain blown by the wind as a person moving or mistake crumbs on a tablecloth for small bugs. One of our patients has reported intermittently that other people's faces appear to be distorted in grotesque ways. Although difficult to classify as either a true hallucination or illusion, some patients will report the "sensation" that someone is standing beside or behind them (30). As true illusions, this phenomenon may herald the onset of more typical hallucinations.

Hallucinations in PD are quite different from the more common hallucinatory syndromes seen with mind-altering drugs or schizophrenia. Absent are the flashing lights, elaborate shifting patterns, and bizarre distortions of time and space that are otherwise seen with illicit hallucinogenic drugs (60). Synesthesias, such as seeing sounds as colors also do not occur in PD. Although auditory hallucinations can occur, verbal commands and ego-dystonic critical commentaries typical of paranoid schizophrenia do not occur (30).

Abnormal dreaming and sleep disturbances seem to be closely related to the presence of hallucinations and other drug-induced psychiatric phenomena in PD patients. In fact, Nausieda et al. (61) showed that 98% of patients with psychiatric side effects from their medications also experienced sleep disturbance in the form of sleep fragmentation, excessive day time sleepiness, altered dreams or parasomnias, such as sleep talking, sleep walking, and nocturnal myoclonus. They also found that hallucinations occurred in 39% of patients with sleep disturbance and only 4% of patients with normal sleep patterns. It is the combination of sleep disorders and nocturnal psychiatric phenomenon that make the patients so difficult to manage by caregivers. It is usual for hallucinations to blend indistinguishably with dream phenomena possessing similar themes (9). On some occasions they are difficult to separate by patient and physician.

Abnormal dreaming and sleep disruption, in general, seem to be specific for dopaminergic therapy and become more common as the duration of therapy increases (61,62). Scharf et al. (62) found three types of abnormal dream phenomena in a population of 88 patients with PD. Vivid dreams were most common, occurring in 20 of the 88 patients interviewed (27%). These were described as "... *qualitatively vivid, seemingly real, temporally condensed, internally organized and coherent, often affectively neutral, with a frequent theme of persons and events from the*

dreamer's remote past." Night terrors were the next most common occurring in 6.8% of these patients. The family must report these occurrences because the patient is always amnestic for the event. Typically, the patient is said to shout and thrash about in their sleep as if in a terrible fight, and awaken the next morning without any recollection of the event. Nightmares were seen in only 5.7% of the 88 patients interviewed. They were much like classic, frightening nightmares but can be paranoid in nature and are usually described by the patients as distinctly different from their usual dreams.

It is clear that sleep disruption, altered dreaming and hallucinations tend to coexist in PD patients. However, it is still unknown if these clinical phenomena occur independently of one another or if there is a causal relationship. A recent review of the subject found no statistical interaction between sleep disruption and hallucinations, (32) but they did find that altered dream phenomena was independently related to both sleep disruption and hallucinations. They postulated that altered dreaming was pivotal and perhaps causally related to the other two clinical problems.

Delusions are not as common as hallucinations in PD but they usually constitute a more serious problem for the patient and physician. Delusions are false beliefs that are based on incorrect inference, are held despite evidence to the contrary, and are not ordinarily accepted by other members of one's culture (6). In PD, delusions are usually paranoid in nature. They most often occur on a background of a clear sensorium without other elements of a thought disorder, as that seen in schizophrenia (9). They can occur as a side effect of any of the currently used anti-Parkinsonian medications (7) including the COMT inhibitors (personal observation). Klawans (9) indicated that about 3% of patients treated with levodopa for two or more years would experience this type of organic delusional syndrome. More common estimates are 7 to 8% (92) but they go as high as 17% (7). Specific examples mentioned in the literature include fears of being injured, poisoned, filmed (63) and even delusions of grandeur (25). In the authors' experience, delusions of spousal infidelity and elaborate conspiracies on the part of family members and even physicians are particularly common. The belief that family members or friends have been replaced by identical appearing emposteres (the capgras phenomenon) has also been reported (36,64). This syndrome and others such as it are classified as delusional mistaken identification syndromes. Related to this are syndromes of reduplication, where persons or places are duplicated or replaced (64). The entity, which is reduplicated or replaced is stereotyped and of a personal nature. One patient, who was an artist, thought his paintings were being replaced by reproductions.

When hallucinations or delusions occur on a background of a clouded sensorium, disorientation, impaired concentration or other cognitive impairment, the term organic confusional psychosis can be used. This complication of therapy is much more likely to occur in patients with dementia or in those treated with anticholinergic medications (7,29). Dopamine agonists have also been prone to cause this syndrome (7).

Klawans et al. (9,51) have suggested that this confusional syndrome rarely arises de novo in PD patients. They found that organic confusional psychosis is usually associated with a pre-existing nonconfusional psychotic state. In fact, they indicated that the various levodopa psychoses generally do not occur in isolation in a given patient. Rather, there is a continuum or progression in most patients from altered dreaming to dreams plus hallucinations, to a nonconfusional organic delusional syndrome, and ultimately to a confusional state superimposed on the other symptoms. This phenomenon may be due to a dopaminergic "kindling phenomenon" (51). This phenomenon of symptoms does not occur in all patients, and DIP with hallucinations can begin without any previous sleep disturbance.

MECHANISMS OF PSYCHOSIS

The mechanisms responsible for producing DIP in PD are poorly understood. In some patients, anti-Parkinsonian medications precipitate acute psychiatric symptoms by unmasking a premorbid psychiatric state. This had occurred in schizophrenics (65) and patients with manic-depressive illness (28) who were exposed to levodopa. For the majority of PD patients, however, there is no premorbid psychiatric disorder. Thus other characteristics peculiar to PD patients, anti-Parkinsonian medications or both must be important.

It has been known for many years that drugs that are structurally similar to dopamine, such as lysergic acid diethylamide (LSD), mescaline and amphetamines, can cause elaborate hallucinations and other psychotic symptoms in otherwise healthy individuals (65). The discovery that levodopa could also precipitate psychiatric symptoms, coupled with the dramatic efficacy of dopamine receptor blockers (neuroleptics) in treating endogenous psychosis, formed the basis for the dopamine theory of psychosis (65). Clinical evidence that supports this hypothesis includes the de novo, dose-related appearance of hallucinations in PD patients treated with levodopa, the reliable disappearance of these symptoms with dose reduction

and the efficacy of traditional neuroleptics (dopamine antagonists) in treating this problem.

Several specific mechanisms have been proposed to explain how exogenously administered levodopa can cause psychosis. Early theories were based on the effects of dopamine on other monoamine systems in the brain, such as the serotonergic and noradrenergic systems (19,28). It was also suggested that as part of the metabolism of dopamine, certain patients might form a greater proportion of toxic metabolites, such as methylated derivatives, which could precipitate these symptoms (28).

More recent theories have been based on the unique dopamine receptor physiology associated with PD, and the varied effects of dopamine and other dopamine receptor agonists on different dopamine systems. It is well known that dysfunction of the nigrostriatal dopamine system and the resulting denervation of otherwise normal striatal neurons is responsible for the motor symptoms of PD. This process may result in hypersensitivity of striatal dopamine receptors. The early appearance of psychotic symptoms in patients treated with dopaminergic medications has been attributed to stimulation of these hypersensitive receptors (51). In support of this, Rinne has found increased striatal dopamine receptor numbers in postmortem specimens of PD patients with psychosis (66). Although dopamine receptor hypersensitivity may be a plausible explanation for psychotic symptoms occurring in PD patients initially treated with levodopa, the more common problem of psychotic symptoms emerging after several years of dopaminergic therapy is not likely to be due to this phenomenon. It should be noted that early psychosis is unusual and atypical for PD (34). In addition, work with the atypical neuroleptic clozapine has shown that the mesolimbic dopamine pathway may be more significant in the genesis of schizophrenia and dopaminomimetic psychosis than the nigrostriatal pathway (67).

To explain the late appearance of psychosis in PD, Klawans et al. (68) introduced a concept of levodopa-induced dopamine receptor hypersensitivity. They have shown in animal models that chronic stimulation of dopamine receptors can cause dopaminergic induced stereotyped behavior to appear at subthreshold doses and with a shorter latency, than in animal not chronically exposed to dopaminergic stimulation. Thus chronic exposure to dopamine agonists causes hypersensitivity of dopamine receptors rather than the expected result of down regulation. In applying this model to levodopa-induced psychosis, Moskovitz et al. (51) proposed that two populations of dopamine sensitive neurons exist in the striatum and limbic cortex. They suggested that a dopamine-facilitated, neuronal population might predominate in limbic cortex and thus be responsible for the psychotic symptoms observed with chronic levodopa treatment. On the basis of this theory, one might imagine it as an ideal agent for treating dopaminomimetic psychosis that preferentially blocks dopamine facilitated neurons in the mesolimbic cortex and spares the striatal neuronal population. Such a drug could be used in Parkinsonian patients with DIP without worsening the motor symptoms of PD.

Clinical experience suggests that hallucinations are generally linked primarily to the size and frequency of levodopa doses in susceptible individuals. However, recent experiments by Goetz et al. (69) question this link. They administered high-dose intravenous levodopa to nondemented PD patients already experiencing daily hallucinations. Neither steady nor pulse infusions of levodopa precipitated hallucinations in these patients. Clearly, other factors, such as environment, must be important in acutely triggering hallucinations and other symptoms of psychosis.

Dysfunction of central serotonergic pathways has also been explored as a cause of DIP. Postmortem studies have shown that patients with this complication have low brain stem levels of serotonin (61). In addition, acute administration of levodopa reduces brain serotonin levels by several possible mechanisms including; (1) interfering with the transport of L-tryptophan across the gut and blood-brain barrier, and (2) inhibiting tryptophan hydroxylase and replacing serotonin in presynaptic storage sites (8,28,61). Dysfunction of serotonergic systems is also suggested by the frequent association of dopaminergic psychosis with sleep disturbance and altered dreaming, both of which seem to have a serotonergic basis (30,61).

Recently, E. Melamed et al. (70) showed that administration of levodopa causes an increased turnover of serotonin in rat brain. They proposed that overstimulation of central serotonergic (5HT3) receptors results from levodopa-induced elevations in serotonin release and concluded that this mechanism is partially responsible for levodopa-induced hallucinosis.

TREATMENT OF PSYCHOSIS: GENERAL CONSIDERATIONS

There are some patients with psychotic symptoms secondary to dopaminergic medications that do not require antipsychotic therapy. Those patients with hallucinosis on the background of a clear sensorium may not need or want therapeutic intervention, especially when the hallucinations are intermittent, brief, nonthreatening and the patients have preserved insight. In fact, some patients actually claim to gain pleasure from the symptoms. These patients should be watched carefully because escalation of psychotic symptoms may occur without provocation (71).

In patients with a sudden onset of psychotic symptoms, it is important to investigate for triggering events, such as urinary and pulmonary infections, metabolic disturbance, cerebrovascular events, or traumatic brain injury. Treatment of these underlying conditions is paramount and may be sufficient. Postoperative psychosis is another situation that may not require specific therapy. In one study (72), psychosis occurred in nearly 60% of PD patients who had surgical intervention. It was found to be 2.8 to 8.1 times more frequent in PD than in the general geriatric population under these circumstances. The authors (72) attributed the psychotic symptoms to the underlying condition and not dopaminergic medications. The study did not discuss treatment in general, except to indicate that lowering anti-Parkinsonian medication doses may result in a worsening of the patient's overall condition. The authors' own experience with this situation suggests that once patients are allowed to increase activity and, more frequently, when they are discharged home, the psychosis will improve spontaneously. This has not been formally studied. Other possible causes of postoperative psychosis include anesthetics, pain medications, alteration in environment, metabolic encephalopathy or infection.

The first step in treating DIP when treatment is necessary is to decrease anti-Parkinsonian medications. An extreme of this therapeutic plan would be a "drug holiday" or the transient cessation of dopaminergic therapy. However, Weiner et al. (73) distinguished between the two. They indicated that lowering medication doses usually leads to a worsening of motor status in PD with some improvement of psychosis, although the "drug holiday" may clear psychotic symptoms completely, and ultimately, improve PD motor symptoms. It is clear from experience, that lowering medications can be helpful and is usually well tolerated (19,25). Marsden and Fahn (74) suggested decreasing and then removing adjunctive medications first, before lowering levodopa. It may take days for the symptoms to improve (5) and psychosis may persist in some patients. As medications are discontinued, the patient will eventually experience intolerable worsening of motor symptoms. This would lead to the unenviable decision of choosing between having a patient who is immobile and free of psychotic symptoms or one who is mobile and psychotic (74).

In the 1970s and early 1980s many physicians used the "drug holiday" to treat PD patients with various late complications, including psychosis. Medications were typically withdrawn for 5–14 days and this invariably led to significant physical disability. Many patients became bedridden, unable to move or even swallow. As Friedman noted (75) this was "... *not a holiday in the usual sense*". These holidays were performed, for the most part, in patients with complications, limiting dose and efficacy of levodopa. Sweet et al. (76) initially demonstrated an enhanced motor response to levodopa immediately after a "drug holiday". Other studies have supported this finding (73,77,78) by observing a preholiday level response with approximately half the required levodopa dosage. Weiner et al. (73) showed that all six patients with psychosis improved dramatically with a drug holiday. In general, one-year follow-up revealed loss of efficacy and return to preholiday disability in most patients (75,77), with increasing requirements of levodopa. Four of the initial six patients with psychosis were still psychosis-free at 12 months (73,77) and the investigators indicated that this was a realistic means of managing this late complication. Ultimately, however, the holiday has no effect on the overall course of the disease (78).

It is now well recognized that there are major drawbacks to the "drug holiday". First, it requires long-term hospitalization, which is costly. The patients have the terrifying experience of becoming completely immobile. In addition, approximately 30% do not improve and some patients never return to their baseline level of functioning (W.J. Weiner; personal communication). Nursing care must be meticulous to prevent complications that include decubitus ulcer, compression neuropathy (79), joint contracture, aspiration pneumonia, deep venous thrombosis, pulmonary embolism (77,80), and depression (75,77). In addition, the sudden cessation of dopaminergic medications can lead to a potentially lethal syndrome similar to the neuroleptic malignant syndrome (75,77,81). In this situation patients will have hyperthermia, mental status change, autonomic dysfunction, along with extreme rigidity and worsening of all other features of PD. There is usually an increase in serum creatine kinase, elevation in white blood count (WBC) and a drop in serum iron levels. Patients may die from respiratory failure, aspiration pneumonia, pulmonary embolism, cardiovascular complications or renal failure. Considering the gravity of these complications "drug holiday" should not be promoted as a routine, therapeutic measure and, in fact, has been abandoned in most major medical centers (75). It should only be used as last resort in patients who have extreme toxic side effects (usually psychosis) and when patients cannot tolerate lower doses of dopaminergic medications or other medications that are used to treat DIP (77). If a "drug holiday" is carried out, a movement disorder specialist should be involved in the patient's care.

In the past, drug therapy for dopaminomimetic psychosis included standard neuroleptics, particularly low potency agents. Marsden and Fahn (74) indicated that although the use of these agents was "illogical", the addition of a small dose of thioridazine could allow a compromise between the relative disability imposed by psychosis or the immobility. Other investigators (82,83) have also indicated that low doses of typical antipsychotics need not exacerbate PD. However, it is clear that in most cases neuroleptics, including thioridazine, caused marked exacerbation of PD symptoms (36,84–88). In addition to the risk of worsening PD disability, PD patients are elderly and therefore at great risk for tardive dyskinesia. In conclusion, these drugs should simply be avoided especially now when other options are available. Other medications used unsuccessfully, in the past, for treatment of psychosis in PD include L-tryptophan (89), methylsergide, and physostigmine (5).

Clozapine

Clozapine is a unique drug that has now become the "gold standard" for treating DIP in PD patients. Clozapine is considered to be an "atypical" antipsychotic because it does not cause catalepsy in laboratory animals (i.e., increase in muscle tone and postural abnormalities) (67) and is associated with minimal risk of drug-induced Parkinsonism, dystonia and akathisia (67,85,90,91). It is this unique ability to be able to effectively treat psychosis without causing parkinsonism that led to the initial attempts to use this drug in PD a decade ago. Since then its safety and efficacy, in this setting, has been demonstrated in numerous open-label studies (92) and in two major multicenter, double-blind, placebo-controlled trials (4,93) (see Chapter 37). This accumulated experience with clozapine has shown that it can be used in small doses to rapidly reverse symptoms of psychosis. Patients should be started on a dose of 6.25 to 12.5 mg at bedtime and then increased by 12.5 mg increments every 4–7 days until there is adequate control of symptoms or until the occurrence of adverse effects.

Sedation is the most common side effect but its occurrence should be used to therapeutic advantage. Frequently, patients with DIP also have sleep disruption and some degree of reversal of their normal sleep–wake cycle. These patients often spend nights awake, agitated, hallucinating, and engaged in paranoid behaviors such as looking through their house for intruders. During the day they are sleepy and more disoriented. Caregivers become sleep-deprived, emotionally stressed and physically exhausted. When clozapine therapy is started as a bedtime dose the most dramatic initial benefit is usually restored restful sleep. This is a result that is greatly appreciated by all involved. It is also a sign that the clozapine dose is at, or very near, an effective antipsychotic dose. Most patients will obtain these benefits with 50 mg or less at bedtime. Occasionally, acutely psychotic patients will need to be given doses as high as 150–200 mg per day until their symptoms are under control. Later, a smaller maintenance dose can be used to prevent recurrence. Some patients on a single bedtime dose will experience breakthrough symptoms the next day, in the late afternoon or early evening. In this situation, a small additional daytime dose (usually less than 25 mg) is sufficient. If sedation is a problem in the morning, the bedtime dose can be lowered or moved one to two hours earlier in the evening.

Once psychotic symptoms are adequately controlled and the patient is sleeping through the night, it is usually possible to carefully increase anti-Parkinsonian medication doses to improve motor functioning. Small increases in daytime levodopa doses are possible but it is best to keep nighttime doses to the absolute minimum. Adjunctive medications such as dopamine agonists, selegiline or COMT inhibitors will have usually been dramatically reduced in dose or eliminated before starting clozapine. These medications need to be used with caution in patients requiring antipsychotic therapy, and in patients with a significant dementia they should be avoided.

Clozapine is associated with other adverse effects in PD patients. Sialorrhea and delirium are the most frequent adverse effects other than sedation (67,85). These appear to be dose-related adverse events and are a common cause of dose limitation. Orthostatic hypertension can also be a problem with PD patients, because many already have this problem caused either by anti-Parkinsonian medications or autonomic dysfunction. Seizures are of concern in schizophrenics, occurring in up to 4% of these patients (67,94,95), and this is related to EEG changes that have been well described. Both seizures and EEG changes are dose-related phenomena. This would explain why no seizures have been reported in PD. The incidence of seizures is less than 1% at doses under 300 mg per day, 2.7% at daily doses of 300–600 mg per day and 4.4% at doses greater than 600 mg per day (94). We have examined EEGs in three PD patients before initiating clozapine and then during therapy at a mean daily dose of 54 mg per day with no changes observed.

The adverse effect of most concern with clozapine is agranulocytosis (Agran). The 1975 occurrence of eight deaths from septicemia out of 16 patients with Agran in Europe (84,85) delayed the marketing of this drug in the United States. The estimated risk of Agran in schizophrenic patients treated with clozapine is 1–2% (95,96), which is higher than standard psychotropic medications. An analysis of data from February 1990 to April 1991 examined the risk in schizophrenic patients, in the United States (96). Agran was defined as a neutrophil count of less than $500/mm^3$. Out of 11,555 patients treated, 73 had Agran and two died from secondary septicemia. Cumulative incidence at one year was 0.8% and at 18 months was 0.91%. The peak hazard ratio was at three months (both deaths occurred within 1.5 months). This adverse effect is an idiosyncratic response to clozapine and is not dose related. An apparent prodrome of 29 days that was characterized by a gradual decrease in WBC, was observed. Precipitous drops in the granulocyte count have been seen. The relative risk of this complication increased with age and was also higher in women than in men.

Current guidelines in the United States require weekly monitoring of the white blood cell count for the first six months of clozapine therapy and every other week thereafter. It is recommended that therapy should be interrupted when WBC drops to less than $3,000/mm^3$ or absolute neutrophil count drops to less than $1,500/mm^3$. Permanent discontinuation is recommended if the WBC is less than $2,000/mm^3$ or neutrophil count becomes less than $1,000/mm^3$. Also, patients with a baseline WBC of less than $3,500/mm^3$ or a neutrophil count of less than $1,500/mm^3$ or a history of immune deficiency should not be treated. Apparently, these guidelines have been effective in reducing the risk of Agran associated with clozapine treatment. Honigfeld et al. (97) reviewed the incidence of Agran in 99,502 patients treated with clozapine according to these guidelines between 1990 and 1994. They found that 382 cases of Agran (0.38%) and 12 deaths had occurred, and that this was dramatically reduced from the 995 cases of Agran and 149 deaths that would have been predicted based on the preguideline incidence of 1–2%. Only one patient with PD has been reported to have true Agran (88). This patient had a protracted course but survived. However, in one of the double-blind studies, two patients had to discontinue over a four-month period because of WBC drop. (4)

Other hematologic side effects that may occur with clozapine include mild asymptomatic eosinophilia, chronic leukocytosis that may be associated with a low-grade fever, and lymphopenia (less than 600 lymphocytes/mm^3), which is usually asymptomatic or may be associated with diarrhea and fever (67). The etiology of these problems is not known (98). One other adverse event of concern is neuroleptic malignant syndrome. One case was described in a patient with clozapine and carbamazepine therapy and the other in a patient with clozapine combined with lithium therapy (81).

The main obstacle to long-term success with clozapine therapy in PD is progression of underlying disease, particularly dementia. Greene et al. (88) demonstrated that of four patients with marked dementia treated with clozapine, only one improved and the rest experienced adverse events. Factor et al. (99) in a long-term trial showed that as dementia progressed (illustrated by a decrease in mini-mental status score) psychosis began to reemerge and adverse effects became more of a dose-limiting problem. It is believed that nondemented patients can tolerate long-term therapy. In those patients with significant dementia, efficacy and tolerance will decline.

Other Atypical Antipsychotics

Safe and effective alternatives for the treatment of DIP in PD have been sought because of the small but significant risk of agranulocytosis associated with clozapine, and the need for frequent blood testing. Three additional antipsychotic medications are now available that have been considered to have an "atypical" pharmacologic profile – risperidone, olanzapine, and quetiapine (see Chapter 37).

Risperidone was the second "atypical" antipsychotic approved in the United States. An initial open-label report suggested that it could be used successfully to treat DIP in PD without worsening of motor symptoms (100). However, since then there have been several reports of less-favorable results (101–103). Significant worsening of motor features was encountered in many patients. It is now clear that risperidone can cause intolerable motor deterioration in PD patients even at low doses (<6 mg per day). Risperidone is no longer considered an option in PD patients, and its designation as an "atypical" antipsychotic has been questioned (104,105).

The next "atypical" antipsychotic medication that became available for use in PD patients was olanzapine. This drug was actually developed to specifically imitate the unique pharmacologic profile of clozapine without the associated risk of agranulocytosis (106). As with risperidone, the initial report on the use of olanzapine for DIP in PD was very encouraging. Wolters et al. (107) found that olanzapine was effective in treating DIP in 15 nondemented PD patients. No worsening of motor functioning was seen in this open-label prospective study. Unfortunately, the subsequent literature concerning the use of olanzapine in this setting has, once again, been less impressive. Several open-label studies have found that significant motor deterioration can be seen in some PD patients treated with this medication (108–112). In the author's own clinic the experience with olanzapine has also been disappointing. In a retrospective analysis of 12 patients they treated with olanzapine, symptoms of psychosis were improved in nine patients (75%) but nine patients (75%) also experienced significant motor deterioration (113). Only one of the original 12 subjects was still using olanzapine successfully at the time of the analysis.

The reason for the disparity between the initial favorable results and the subsequent studies is unclear but may relate to the differences in patient populations and the methods of dose titration. Wolters et al. (114) pointed out that the poor results reported in subsequent studies were in some instances observed in patients with atypical parkinsonian syndromes and included patients with dementia. In addition, the starting dose of olanzapine in Wolters' report was 1 mg per day, which is less than half the initial dose of 2.5–5.0 mg per day used in subsequent studies (the lowest dose currently available in the United States is a 2.5 mg pill). Whether more stringent patient selection and gentler dose titration will prevent motor complications is unclear, but a multicenter, double-blind, placebo-controlled trial is currently underway and should help resolve these issues.

An additional concern about the safety of olanzapine has been raised recently by three single-case reports linking this medication to neutropenia. In the first report, a patient experienced prolongation of neutropenia associated with clozapine therapy after being switched to olanzapine (115). In the second case, there was recurrence of neutropenia on olanzapine after recovery from clozapine associated neutropenia (116). In the third report, true agranulocytosis occurred in a patient treated with olanzapine, five months after the discontinuation of clozapine (117). Despite the extreme rarity of these cases, greater vigilance for this potential complication is warranted, particularly in patients who have experienced neutropenia with clozapine.

The most recent and, perhaps, most promising "atypical" antipsychotic medication introduced as an alternative to clozapine, is quetiapine. It appears to be effective in treating DIP in PD at doses of 50 to 100 mg per day, but in some patients, doses as high as 400 mg per day have been required (118–122). Although minimal worsening of motor symptoms has been observed, judging from this preliminary literature and the author's own experience, it seems unlikely that this will constitute a significant clinical problem. Controlled, clinical trials are needed to further clarify the benefits and side effects associated with the use of quetiapine in this setting.

Nonneuroleptic Therapies

Approaches to the treatment of DIP, other than atypical antipsychotic medications, have been used with some success. Ondansetron is a serotonin (5HT3) receptor antagonist that was approved by the FDA in 1991 for chemotherapy-induced emesis (123). This drug has been used successfully in the treatment of schizophrenia (124) and has only rarely caused dystonia or akathisia (123). It does not have significant dopamine receptor blocking properties and there have been no apparent cases of ondansetron-induced parkinsonism. Zoldan et al. (125) treated, 16 PD patients with psychosis, with ondansetron in open-label fashion. Doses ranged from 12–24 mg per day. All but one patient experienced a moderate to marked improvement in psychiatric symptoms and the drug was well tolerated. In one additional study these optimistic findings were not fully reproduced (126). Results of these studies add credence to the serotonin hypothesis regarding pathogenic mechanism of DIP. Further studies of this drug are needed. However, a major obstacle to more widespread testing and use of this medication is its extremely high cost.

It has also been suggested that electroconvulsive therapy (ECT) may be useful in the treatment of dopaminomimetic psychosis (5,127). Hurwitz et al. (127) treated two PD patients suffering from chronic nonconfusional psychosis with bilateral ECT (one received six treatments and the other three). It not only cleared the psychosis but also allowed for the use of higher doses of dopaminergic medications. After five months one patient had no recurrence and the other patient, six month later, had only occasional visual illusions. It is probable that patients with confusional states will not achieve the same benefit, and confusion is considered a contraindication for ECT (5,128).

There also seems to be interest in using ECT to treat PD patients because of its ability to improve motor symptoms (129–131). It is believed that this improvement is because of an enhancement of dopamine transmission caused by ECT (132). It is hard to explain the antipsychotic effect of ECT on the background of increased responsiveness of dopamine receptors and Hurwitz et al. (127) suggest that improvement in psychosis may be due to an effect via nondopaminergic mechanisms.

The improvement of motor features of PD by ECT is most likely transient (129,130). In addition, the antidepressant effects of ECT are also unsustained and patients should be treated with antidepressant agents for long-term maintenance. Although the two patients with psychosis (127) were without recurrence after 5 to 6 months, the author's experience indicates that this effect may also be transient and may only last weeks to months. In general, this would not make ECT a logical choice as a primary agent in the treatment of DIP in PD. The adverse effects of memory loss and delirium are also of concern. However, in those situations where clozapine does not improve psychosis or when significant side effects occur at dose levels that do not improve psychosis, ECT can be used as an adjunct (133).

TREATMENT: SUMMARY

The treatment of DIP in PD can be approached in a stepwise fashion. First, it is necessary to search for and treat any triggering factors, such as infection that may have precipitated decompensation in an otherwise stable patient. Even a minor urinary tract infection can cause dramatic deterioration in patients prone to this problem. If no such triggers are present and the symptoms are mild, a modest reduction in anti-Parkinsonian medication dose will usually be sufficient. Because mild symptoms are commonly limited to the nighttime hours, a reduction or discontinuation of the patient's bedtime dose of medication may be all that is necessary. In more severely affected patients, the next step is to decrease or stop adjunctive medications. This should be done one drug at a time and in the order of decreasing risk to benefit ratio. Anticholinergic medications should be stopped first. Then selegiline, dopamine agonists, and finally, amantadine are eliminated. Tolcapone is poorly tolerated in PD patients prone to DIP and should be avoided. If psychosis continues, an attempt should be made to decrease the dose of levodopa. If this leads to a significant increase in disability, an antipsychotic medication will be required.

Clozapine is the only antipsychotic medication that has been proven in controlled, clinical trials to effectively control DIP without worsening parkinsonism. However, based on promising preliminary data and the author's own experience and ease of use (no need for blood monitoring) the author feels that quetiapine is a reasonable alternative as a first-line medication for treating DIP. If quetiapine is not effective or side effects prevent further increases in dose, clozapine is recommended as the antipsychotic of choice. It is important to remember that PD patients are particularly prone to sedation with these medications and therapy should be initiated with a low dose and increased in small increments. Frequent communication between the physician and the patient's caretaker is essential during this difficult period. Once DIP is controlled, a smaller maintenance dose is usually possible and a careful optimization of anti-Parkinsonian medications can be attempted.

In the rare patient who does not respond to either of these medications, a trial of olanzapine is justified, but the patient should be carefully monitored for worsening of parkinsonism. Risperidone and other typical antipsychotics are not appropriate choices for treating DIP in PD and should be avoided. Occasional patients will not respond to the earlier measures and more drastic reductions in levodopa will be necessary. This will usually be associated with severe worsening of parkinsonism and should be done in a hospital setting under the supervision of a movement disorder specialist. In a patient with resistant psychosis and a clear sensorium, psychiatric consultation should be obtained and ECT can be used as a measure of last resort.

MANIA

Mania (41,48,134–138), hypomania (22,28,139), and euphoria (19,41) have all been reported as side effects of dopaminergic medications. Symptoms of hypomania and mania have ranged from extreme optimism to uncontrollable spending sprees. Goodwin (28) reported that the incidence of hypomania was 1.5% in 908 patients treated with levodopa. Goodwin and associates (140) in 1972 treated 11 depressed, non-PD patients with levodopa to evaluate its possible effects on depression. Six patients, all with a history of previous manic or cyclothymic behavior, developed acute mania or hypomania when treated with 4–10 gm per day. O'Brien and colleagues (141) reported an interesting case of a man who developed episodes of inappropriate laughter and grandiosity that occurred in cycles, approximately 90 minutes after each 6 gm dose of levodopa. Jouvent et al. (142) reported 2 of 10 patients with PD who developed hypomania on high doses of bromocriptine. Mania has also occurred in two non-PD patients treated with bromocriptine for postpartum suppression of lactation (136,137). Both patients were taking bromocriptine for approximately one week before developing manic symptoms. After the withdrawal of bromocriptine and with the treatment of haloperidol for three to seven days, all signs of mania was resolved. Euphoria developed in a single patient after pergolide was added to their previous medication regimen (41). Recently, acute mania was reported in PD patients taking selegiline (48,138). Boyson (48) described five women with PD who

developed acute mania when selegiline was added to their anti-PD medications. Two of these patients had previous symptoms of cyclothymia but had not been diagnosed with this disorder. Mendez (143) described a single patient who became hypomanic on selegiline after adrenal cell transplantation. Other authors (138,144) warned against the concomitant use of selegiline and antidepressants (especially fluoxetine) because of the possibility of precipitating acute mania. Recently, pramipexole has been noted to result in mood elevation in PD patients (145). Although we are unaware of any formal reports of mania with this drug, the potential certainly exists.

Mania, hypomania, and euphoria do not occur in untreated PD (10). These are rare, treatment-related adverse effects and have occurred in PD and non-PD patients treated with dopaminergic agents. Patients with previous signs of mania or hypomania may experience an acute exacerbation if given these medications.

HYPERSEXUALITY

Increased libido and return of penile erection, after years of impotence, have been reported in PD patients treated in early levodopa trials (20,141). However, these cases were not associated with aberrant sexual behavior. Subsequently, other investigators confirmed a renewed interest in sex among patients treated with levodopa, and in rare cases, this led to sexual desires out of proportion to their premorbid sexual profile and sexual activities outside personal and society norms (146). Some were reported to become more voyeuristic or experience a disinhibition of long-suppressed erotic fantasies involving public indecent exposure or sadomasochism (147). Unfortunately, some of these patients acted to fulfill their desires causing great embarrassment to themselves and their families. In many of these patients, the increased sexual desire and preoccupation is not accompanied by a return of sexual function. Impotence remains common among these individuals (146). In the author's experience, this led to compulsive self-stimulation in some patients, although in others constant requests were made of the spouse for genital stimulation even if orgasm cannot be achieved.

Hypersexuality seems to be a rare complication of anti-Parkinsonian therapy and is estimated to occur in 0.9 to 3% of patients (28,148). It is more common in men and has been reported to occur with all dopaminergic medications (7,146) including recent reports on apomorphine (149), pramipexole, and ropinirole (150). Uitti et al. (146) reported two cases of hypersexuality occurring in PD patients after thalamotomy. Some authors have reported an association between hypersexuality and psychosis or hypomania (28). However, patients without signs of either disorder have developed this problem (147). In addition, premorbid sexual behavior does not always predict the presence or absence of drug-induced hypersexuality (146).

Although preoccupation with sex and erotic fantasy usually resolves when PD medications are reduced, they are likely to resume if rechallenged with similar doses (146,147). Low-potency neuroleptics have been helpful in treating some PD patients with this complication, however, as expected, their use has been limited by worsening of motor functioning (147). The author has had good success using clozapine in patients with problematic sexual behavior, many of whom also have some degree of DIP. Fernandez et al. have reported a case of zoophilia (sexual contact with the family dog) precipitated by dopaminergic medications that responded to clozapine therapy (151). Cyproterone, an antitestosterone agent, was mildly beneficial in one male patient but additional medications were required to ultimately control the uncharacteristic behavior (147).

The exact mechanism of how anti-Parkinsonian medications cause hypersexuality is still not known. It would be reasonable to think that dopaminergic mechanisms are responsible, but there is no direct evidence for this. One recent report found fluctuating penile erection corresponding to peak dose effects of levodopa (152), but this does not directly relate to aberrant sexual behavior particularly in patients who remain impotent. Uitti and colleagues (146) have speculated that prolactin may play a role. They based this opinion on the clinical observation that patients with prolactin secreting tumors, who suffer a decline in sexual drive, can experience a reversal of this problem when given bromocriptine. Although hypersexuality remains a rare psychiatric complication of the treatment of PD, it can potentially limit therapy.

Impotence is reported in 40–60% of male PD patients. Sildenafil (Viagra) is being used more frequently by male PD patients with sexual dysfunction. There has been one report of 22 PD patients treated effectively with sildenafil without significant side effects (153). However, the author believes that this medication needs to be prescribed with caution in PD because of the possibility that patients with impotence may also have some degree of DIP, hypersexuality or deviant sexual behavior. The patient is unlikely to volunteer this information when asking for sildenafil. The author recommends that any PD patient considering treatment with sildenafil be carefully screened for the presence of DIP or hypersexuality. Further the patients sexual partner should be interviewed separately to be sure they are also in favor of this treatment.

Acknowledgment

This work was supported by the Albany Medical Center Parkinson's Research Fund.

REFERENCES

1. Fischer P, Danielczyk W, Simanyi M, et al. Dopaminergic psychosis in advanced Parkinson's disease. In: Streifler MB, Korczyn AD, Melamed E, et al. (eds.). *Advances in Neurology*, Vol. 53: *PD: Anatomy, Pathology, and Therapy*. New York: Raven Press, 1990; 391–397.
2. Goetz CG, Stebbins GT. Risk factors for nursing home placement in advanced Parkinson's disease. *Neurology* 1993; 43:2227–2229.
3. Goetz CG, Stebbins GT. Mortality and hallucinations in nursing home patients with advanced Parkinson's disease. *Neurology* 1995; 45:669–671.
4. The Parkinson Study Group. Low-dose clozapine for the treatment of drug-induced psychosis in Parkinson's disease. *N Engl J Med* 1999; 340:757–763.
5. Friedman JH. The management of the levodopa psychoses. *Clin Neuropharmacol* 1991; 14:283–295.
6. American Psychiatric Association. *Diagnostic and statistical manual of mental disorders*. 3rd edn., revised. Washington, D.C. American Psychiatric Association, 1987.
7. Cummings JL. Behavioral complications of drug treatment of Parkinson's disease. *J Am Geriatr Soc* 1991; 33:708–716.
8. Weiner WJ, Bergen D. Prevention and management of the side effects of levodopa. In: Klawans HL (ed.). *Clinical Neuropharmacology*. Vol. 2. New York: Raven Press, 1977; 1–23.
9. Klawans HL. Levodopa-induced psychosis. *Psychiatric Ann* 1978; 8:447–451.
10. Mayeux R. PD: A review of cognitive and psychiatric disorders. *Neuropsych, Neuropsycho Behav Neurol* 1990; 3:3–14.
11. Hoehn MM, Yahr MD. Parkinsonism: Onset, progression and mortality. *Neurology* 1967; 17:427–442.
12. Mckeith IG, Galasko D, Kosaka K, et al. Consensus guidelines for the clinical and pathological diagnosis of dementia with Lewy bodies (DLB): Report of the consortium on DLB international workshop. *Neurology* 1996; 47:1113–1124.
13. Parkinson J. *An Essay on the Shaking Palsy*. London: Neely and Jones, 1817.
14. Regis E. *Precis de Psychiatrie*. Paris: Gaston Doiz, 1906.
15. Patrick HT, Levy DM. PD: A clinical study of one hundred and forty-six cases. *Arch Neurol Psychiatry* 1922; 7:711–720.

16. Jackson JA, Free GBM, Pike HV. The psychic manifestations in paralysis agitans. *Arch Neurol Psychiatry* 1923; 10:680–684.

17. Schwab RS, Fabing HD, Prichard JS. Psychiatric symptoms and syndromes in Parkinson's disease. *Am J Psychiatry* 1950; 107:901–907.

18. Calne DB, Stern GM, Laurence DR, et al. L-dopa in post-encephalitic Parkinsonism. *Lancet* 1969; 1:744–746.

19. Celesia GG, Barr AN. Psychosis and other psychiatric manifestations of levodopa therapy. *Arch Neurol* 1970; 23:193–200.

20. Yahr MD, Duvoisin RC, Schear MJ, et al. Treatment of Parkinsonism with levodopa. *Arch Neurol* 1969; 21:343–354.

21. Cotzias GC, Papavasilou PS, Gellene R. Modification of Parkinsonism: Chronic treatment with L-dopa. *N Engl J Med* 1969; 280:337–345.

22. McDowell F, Lee JE, Swift T, et al. Treatment of Parkinson's syndrome with L-dihydroxyphenylalanine (levodopa). *Ann Intern Med* 1970; 72:29–35.

23. Damasio AR, Lobo-Antunes J, Macedo C. Psychiatric aspects in Parkinsonism treated with L-dopa. *J Neurol Neurosurg Psychiatry* 1971; 34:502–507.

24. Mawdsley C. Treatment of Parkinsonism with levodopa. *Brit Med J* 1970; 1:331–337.

25. Jenkins RB, Groh RH. Mental symptoms in Parkinsonian patients with L-dopa. *Lancet* 1970; 2:177–180.

26. Celesia GG, Wanamaker WM. Psychiatric disturbances in Parkinson's disease. *Dis Nerv Syst* 1972; 33:577–583.

27. Cheifetz DI, Garron DC, Leavitt F, et al. Emotional disturbance accompanying the treatment of Parkinsonism with L-dopa. *Clin Pharmacol Ther* 1970; 12:56–61.

28. Goodwin FK. Psychiatric side effects of levodopa in man. *JAMA* 1971; 218:1915–1920.

29. Sacks OW, Kohl MS, Messeloff CR, et al. Effects of levodopa in parkinsonian patients with dementia. *Neurology* 1972; 22:516–519.

30. Sanchez-Ramos JR, Ortoll R, Paulson GW. Visual hallucinations associated with Parkinson's disease. *Arch Neurol* 1996; 53:1265–1268.

31. Aarsland D, Larsen JP, Cummings JL, et al. Prevalence and clinical correlates of psychotic symptoms in Parkinson's disease. *Arch Neurol* 1999; 56; 595–601.

32. Pappert EJ, Goetz CG, Niederman FG, et al. Hallucinations, sleep fragmentation, and altered dream phenomena in Parkinson's disease. *Mov Disord* 1999; 14:117–121.

33. Lepore FE. Visual loss as a causative factor in visual hallucinations associated with Parkinson's disease. *Arch Neurol* 1997; 54:799.

34. Goetz CG, Vogel C, Tanner CM, et al. Early dopaminergic drug-induced hallucinations in Parkinsonian patients. *Neurology* 1998; 51:811–814.

35. Graham JM, Grunewald RA, Sagar HJ. Hallucinosis in idiopathic Parkinson's disease. *J Neurol Neurosurg Psychiatry* 1997; 63:434–440.

36. Lipper S. Psychosis in patients on bromocriptine and levodopa with carbidopa. *Lancet* 1976; 2:571–572.

37. Calne DB, Williams AC, Neophytides A, et al. Long-term treatment of Parkinsonism with bromocriptine. *Lancet* 1978; 1:735–738.

38. White AC, Murphy TJC. Hallucinations caused by bromocriptine. *Brit J Psychiatry* 1977; 130:104.

39. Olanow WC, Alberts MJ. Double-blind controlled study of pergolide mesylate as an adjunct to Sinemet in the treatment of Parkinson's disease. In: Yahr MD, Bergmann KJ (eds.). *Advances in Neurology*, Vol. 45. New York: Raven Press,1986; 555–560.

40. Kurlan R, Miller C, Levy R, et al. Long-term experience with pergolide therapy of advanced Parkinsonism. *Neurology* 1985; 35:738–742.

41. Lang AE, Quinn N, Brincat S, et al. Pergolide in late-stage Parkinson's disease. *Ann Neurol* 1982; 12:243–247.

42. Stern Y, Mayeux R, Ilson J, et al. Pergolide therapy for Parkinson's disease: Neurobehavioral changes. *Neurology* 1984; 34:201–204.

43. Factor SA. Dopamine agonists. *Med Clin N Am* 1999; 83:415–443.

44. Hutton JJ, Morris JL, Brewer MA. Controlled study of the anti-Parkinsonian activity and tolerability of cabergoline. *Neurology* 1993; 43:613–616.

45. Rinne UK. Lisuride, a dopamine agonist in the treatment of early Parkinson's disease. *Neurology* 1989; 39:336–339.

46. Frankel JP, Lees AJ, Kempster PA, et al. Subcutaneous apomorphine in the treatment of Parkinson's disease. *J Neurol Neurosurg Psychiatry* 1990; 53:96–101.

47. Lieberman AN, Goldstein M, Gopinathan G, et al. D-1 and D-2 agonists in Parkinson's disease. *Can J Neurol Sci* 1987; 14:466–473.

48. Boyson SJ. Psychiatric effects of selegiline [Letter]. *Arch Neurol* 1991; 48:902.

49. Venezia P, Mohr E, Grimes D. Deprenyl in Parkinson's disease: Mechanisms, neuroprotective effect, indications and adverse effects. *Can J Neurol Sci* 1992; 19:142–146.

50. Fleminger R. Visual hallucinations and illusions with propranolol. *Brit Med J* 1978; 1:1182.

51. Moskovitz C, Moses H, Klawans HL. Levodopa-induced psychosis: A kindling phenomenon. *Am J Psychiatry* 1978; 135:669–675.

52. Schwab RS, England AC, Poskanzer DC, et al. Amantadine in the treatment of Parkinson's disease. *JAMA* 1969; 208:1168–1170.

53. Factor SA, Molho ES, Brown DL. Acute delirium after withdrawal of amantadine in Parkinson's disease. *Neurology* 1998; 50:1456–1458.

54. Adler CH, Singer C, O'Brien C, et al. Randomized, placebo-controlled study of tolcapone in patients with fluctuating Parkinson's disease treated with levodopa-carbidopa. *Arch Neurol* 1998; 55:1089–1095.

55. Rajput AH, Martin W, Saint-Hilaire MH, et al. Tolcapone improves motor function in Parkinsonian

patients with the "wearing-off" phenomenon: A double-blind, placebo-controlled, multicenter trial. *Neurology* 1997; 49:1066–1071.

56. Parkinson Study Group. Entacapone improves motor fluctuations in levodopa-treated Parkinson's disease patients. *Ann Neurol* 1997; 42:747–755.

57. Tanner CM, Vogel C, Goetz CG, et al. Hallucinations in Parkinson's disease: A population study (abstract). *Ann Neurol* 1983; 14:136.

58. Inzelberg R, Kipervasser S, Korczyn AD. Auditory hallucinations in Parkinson's disease. *J Neurol Neurosurg Psychiatry* 1998; 64:533–535.

59. Jimenez-Jimenez FJ, Orti-Pareja M, Gasalla T, et al. Cenesthetic hallucinations in a patient with Parkinson's disease. *J Neurol Neurosurg Psychiatry* 1997; 63:120.

60. Kluver H. Neurobiology of normal and abnormal perception. In: Hoch P, Zubin J (eds.). *Psychopathology of Perceptions*. New York:Grune & Stratton; 1965.

61. Nausieda PA, Weiner WJ, Kaplan LR, et al. Sleep disruption in the course of chronic levodopa therapy: An early feature of the levodopa psychosis. *Clin Neuropharmacol* 1982; 5:183–194.

62. Sharf B, Moskovitz C, Lupton MD, et al. Dream phenomena induced by chronic levodopa therapy. *J Neurol Trans* 1978; 43:143–151.

63. Serby M, Angrist B, Lieberman A. Mental disturbances during bromocriptine and lergotrile treatment of Parkinson's disease. *Am J Psychiatry* 1978; 135:1227–1229.

64. Roane DM, Rogers JD, Robinson JH, et al. Delusional misidentification in association with Parkinsonism. *J Neuropsy Clin Neurosci* 1998; 10:194–198.

65. Yaryura-Tobias JA, Diamond B, Merlis S. Psychiatric manifestations of levodopa. *Dis Nerv System* 1970; 31:60–63.

66. Rinne UK. Brain neurotransmitter receptors in Parkinson's disease. In: Marsden CD, Fahn S (eds.). *Movement Disorders*. Boston: Butterworth Scientific, 1982; 59–74.

67. Baldesserini RJ, Frankenburg FR. Clozapine: A novel antipsychotic agent. *N Engl J Med* 1991; 324:740–754.

68. Klawans HL, Goetz CG, Nausieda PA, et al. Levodopa-induced dopamine receptor hypersensitivity. *Ann Neurol* 1977; 2:125–129.

69. Goetz CG, Pappert EJ, Blasucci LM, et al. Intravenous levodopa in hallucinating Parkinson's disease patients: High-dose challenge does not precipitate hallucinations. *Neurology* 1998; 50:515–517

70. Melamed E, Zoldan J, Friedberg G, et al. Is hallucinosis in Parkinson's disease due to central serotonergic hyperactivity? *Mov Disord* 1993; 8:406–407.

71. Goetz CG, Tanner CM, Klawans HL. Pharmacotherapy of hallucinations induced by long-term drug therapy. *Am J Psychiatry* 1982; 139:494–497.

72. Golden WE, Lavender RC, Metzer WS. Acute postoperative confusion and hallucinations in Parkinson's disease. *Ann Int Med* 1989; 111:218–222.

73. Weiner WJ, Koller WC, Perlik S, et al. Drug holiday and management of Parkinson's disease. *Neurology* 1980; 30:1257–1261.

74. Marsden CD, Fahn S. Problems in PD. In: Marsden CD and Fahn S eds. *Movement Disorders*. London: Butterworth Scientific, 1981:1–7.

75. Friedman JH. "Drug holidays" in the treatment of Parkinson's disease: A brief review. *Arch Intern Med* 1985; 145:913–915.

76. Sweet RD, Lee JE, Spiegel H, et al. Enhanced response to low doses of levodopa after withdrawal from chronic treatment. *Neurology* 1972; 22:520–525.

77. Klawans HL, Goetz CG, Tanner CM, et al. Levodopa-free periods ("drug holidays") in the management of Parkinsonism. *Adv Neurol* 1983; 37:33–43.

78. Mayeux R, Stern Y, Mulvey K, et al. Reappraisal of temporary levodopa withdrawal ("drug holiday") in Parkinson's disease. *N Engl J Med* 1985; 313:724–728.

79. Kurlan R, Baker P, Miller C, et al. Severe compression neuropathy following sudden onset of Parkinsonian immobility. *Arch Neurol* 1985; 42:720.

80. Direnfield L, Spero L, Marotta J, et al. The L-dopa on-off effect in Parkinson's disease: Treatment by transient drug withdrawal and dopamine receptor sensitization. *Ann Neurol* 1978; 4:473–475.

81. Factor SA and Singer C. Neuroleptic malignant syndrome. In: Lang AE and Weiner WJ (eds.). *Drug-induced movement disorders*. Mount Kisco, N.Y. Futura Publishing Co, Inc., 1992:199–230.

82. Hale MS, Bellizzi J. Low dose perphenazine and levodopa/carbidopa therapy in a patient with Parkinsonism and a psychotic illness. *J Nerv Ment Dis* 1980; 168:312–314.

83. Crow TJ, Johnstone EC, McClelland HA. The coincidence of schizophrenia and Parkinsonism: Some neurochemical implications. *Psychol Med* 1976; 6:227–233.

84. Scholz E, Dichgans J. Treatment of drug-induced exogenous psychosis in parkinsonism with clozapine and fluperlapine. *Eur Arch Psychiatr Neurol Sci* 1985; 235:60–64.

85. Friedman JH, Lannon MC. Clozapine in the treatment of psychosis in Parkinson's disease. *Neurology* 1989; 39:1219–1221.

86. Wolk SI, Douglas CJ. Clozapine treatment of psychosis in Parkinson's disease: A report of five consecutive cases. *J Clin Psychiatry* 1992; 53:373–376.

87. Lew MF, Waters CH. Clozapine treatment of Parkinsonism with psychosis. *JAGS* 1993; 41:669–671.

88. Greene P, Cote L, Fahn S. Treatment of drug-induced psychosis in Parkinson's disease with clozapine. *Adv Neurol* 1993; 60:703–706.

89. Beasley BL, Nutt JG, Davenport RW, et al. Treatment with tryptophan of levodopa-associated psychiatric disturbances. *Arch Neurol* 1980; 37:155–156.

90. Wolters EC, Hurwitz TA, Peppard RF, et al. Clozapine: An antipsychotic agent for Parkinson's disease? *Clin Neuropharmacol* 1989; 12:83–90.

91. Casey DE. Clozapine: Neuroleptic-induced EPS and tardive dyskinesia. *Psychopharmacology* 1989; 99:S47-S53.

92. Factor SA, Friedman JH. The emerging role of clozapine in the treatment of movement disorders. *Mov Disord* 1997; 12:483-496.

93. French Clozapine Parkinson Study Group. Clozapine in drug-induced psychosis in Parkinson's disease. *Lancet* 1999; 353:2041-2042.

94. Devinsky O, Honigfeld G, Patin J. Clozapine-related seizures. *Neurology* 1991; 41:369-371.

95. Alphs LD, Meltzer HY, Bastani B, et al. Side effects of clozapine and their management. *Pharmacol Psychiat* 1991; 24:46.

96. Alvir JMJ, Lieberman JA, Safferman AZ, et al. Clozapine-induced agranulocytosis: incidence and risk factors in the United States. *N Engl J Med* 1993; 329:162-167.

97. Honigfeld G, Arellano F, Sethi J, et al. Reducing clozapine-related morbidity and mortality: 5 years experience with the Clozaril National Registry. *J Clin Psychiatry* 1998; 59[Suppl 3]:3-9.

98. Gerson SL. Clozapine-deciphering the risks. *N Engl J Med* 1993; 329:204-205.

99. Factor SA, Brown D, Molho ES, et al. Clozapine: A two year open trial in Parkinson's disease patients with psychosis. *Neurology* 1994; 44:544-546.

100. Meco G, Alessandria A, Bonifati V, et al. Risperidone for hallucinations in levodopa-treated Parkinson's disease patients. *Lancet* 1994; 343:1370-1371.

101. Meco G, Alessandria A, Giustini P, et al. Risperidone in levodopa-induced psychosis in advanced Parkinson's disease: An open-label, long-term study. *Mov Disord* 1997; 12:610-611.

102. Ford B, Lynch T, Greene P. Risperidone in Parkinson's disease. *Lancet* 1994; 344:681.

103. Rich SS, Friedman JH, Ott BR. Risperidone versus clozapine in the treatment of psychosis in six patients with Parkinson's disease and other akinetic-rigid syndromes. *J Clin Psychiatry* 1995; 56:556-559.

104. Rosebush PJ, Mazurek MF. Neurologic side effects in neuroleptic-naive patients treated with haloperidol or risperidone. *Neurology* 1999; 52:782-785.

105. Friedman JH, Factor SA. Atypical antipsychotics in the treatment of drug-induced psychosis in Parkinson's disease. *Mov Disord* 2000; 15:201-211.

106. Bymaster FP, Rasmussen K, Calligaro DO, et al. In vitro and in vivo biochemistry of olanzapine: A novel, atypical antipsychotic drug. *J Clin Psychiatry* 1997; 58[Suppl 10]:28-36.

107. Wolters EC, Jansen ENH, Tuynman-Qua HG, et al. Olanzapine in the treatment of dopaminomimetic psychosis in patients with Parkinson's disease. *Neurology* 1996; 47:1085-1087.

108. Friedman JH. Olanzapine in the treatment of dopaminomimetic psychosis in patients with Parkinson's disease. *Neurology* 1998; 50[Letter]:1195-1196.

109. Friedman JH, Goldstein SM, Jacques C. Substituting clozapine for olanzapine in psychiatrically stabe

Parkinsons disease patients: Results of an open-label pilot trial. *Clin Neuropharmacol* 1998; 21:285-288.

110. Jimenez-Jimenez FJ, Tallon-Barranco A, Orti-Pareja M, et al. Olanzapine can worsen Parkinsonism. *Neurology* 1998; 50:1183-1184.

111. Graham JM, Sussman JD, Ford KS, et al. Olanzapine in the treatment of hallucinosis in idiopathic Parkinson's disease: A cautionary note. *J Neurol Neurosurg Psychiatry* 1998; 65:774-777.

112. Weiner WJ, Minagar A, Shulman LM. Olanzapine for the treatment of hallucinations/delusions in Parkinson's disease. *Mov Disord* 1998; 13[Suppl 2]:62.

113. Molho ES, Factor SA. Worsening of motor features of Parkinsonism with olanzapine. *Mov Disord* 1999; 14:1014-1016.

114. Wolters EC, Jansen ENH, Tuynman-Qua HG, et al. Olanzapine in the treatment of dopaminomimetic psychosis in patients with Parkinson's disease. *Neurology* 1998; 50[Letter]:1196.

115. Flynn SW, Altman S, MacEwan GW, et al. Prolongation of clozapine-induced granulocytopenia associated with olanzapine. *J Clin Psychopharmacol* 1997; 17:494-495.

116. Benedetti F, Cavallaro R, Smeraldi E. Olanzapine-induced neutropenia after clozapine-induced neutropenia. *Lancet* 1999; 354:567.

117. Naumann R, Felber W. Heilmann H, Reuster T. Olanzapine-induced agranulocytosis. *Lancet* 1999; 354:566-567.

118. Fernandez HH, Friedman JH, Jacques C, et al. Quetiapine for the treatment of drug-induced psychosis in Parkinson's disease. *Mov Disord* 1999; 14:484-487.

119. Parsa MA, Bastani B. Quetiapine (Seroquel) in the treatment of psychosis in patients with Parkinson's disease. *J Neuropsychiatry Clin Neurosci* 1998; 10:1-4.

120. Juncos JL, Arvanitis L, Sweitzer D, et al. Quetiapine improves psychotic symptoms associated with Parkinson's disease. *Neurology* 1999; 52[Suppl 2]:A262.

121. Targum SD, Criden MR, Rubin A, et al. Efficacy of seroquel (quetiapine) in Parkinson's patients with psychosis. *Mov Disord* 1997; 12:842.

122. Samanta J, Stacy M. Quetiapine in the treatment of hallucination in advanced Parkinson's disease. *Mov Disord* 1998; 13[Suppl 2]:274.

123. Halperin JR, Murphy B. Extrapyramidal reaction to ondansetron. *Cancer* 1992; 69:1275.

124. White A, Corn TH, Feetham C, et al. Ondansetron in treatment of schizophrenia. *Lancet* 1991; 337:1173.

125. Zoldan J, Friedberg G, Livneh M, et al. Psychosis in advanced Parkinson's disease: Treatment with ondansetron, a 5-HT3 receptor antagonist. *Neurology* 1995; 45:1305-1308.

126. Eichhorn TE, Brunt E, Oertel WH. Ondansetron treatment of L-dopa-induced psychosis. *Neurology* 1996; 47:1608-1609.

127. Hurwitz TA, Calne DB, Waterman K. Treatment of dopaminomimetic psychosis in Parkinson's disease with electroconvulsive therapy. *Can J Neurol Sci* 1988; 15:32-34.

128. Brown GI. Parkinsonism depression and ECT. *Am J Psychiatry* 1975; 132:1084.

129. Stern MB. Electroconvulsive therapy in untreated Parkinson's disease. *Mov Disord* 1991; 6:265.

130. Douyon R, Serby M, Klutchko B, et al. ECT and Parkinson's disease revisited: A "naturalistic" study. *Am J Psychiatry* 1989; 146:1451–1455.

131. Abrams R. ECT for Parkinson's disease. *Am J Psychiatry* 1989; 146:1391–1393.

132. Fochtmann L. A mechanism for the efficacy of ECT in Parkinson's disease. *Convulsive Ther* 1988; 4:321–327.

133. Factor SA, Molho ES, Brown DL. Combined clozapine and electroconvulsive therapy for the treatment of drug-induced psychosis in Parkinson's disease. *J Neuropsychiatry Clin Neurosci* 1995; 7:304–307.

134. Ryback RS, Schwab RS. Manic response to levodopa therapy: Report of a case [Letter]. *N Engl J Med* 1971; 285:788–789.

135. Pearlman C. Manic behavior and levodopa [Letter]. *N Engl J Med* 1971; 285:1326–1327.

136. Vlissides D, Gill D, Castelow J. Bromocriptine-induced mania [Letter]? *Br Med J* 1978; 1:510.

137. Brook NM, Cookson IB. Bromocriptine-induced mania [Letter]? *Br Med J* 1978; 1:790.

138. Kurlan R, Dimitsopulos T. Selegiline and manic behavior in Parkinson's disease. *Arch Neurol* 1992; 49:1231.

139. Barbeau A, Mars H, Gill-Joffroy L. Adverse clinical side effects of levodopa therapy. In: McDowell FH, Markham CM (eds.). *Contemporary Neurology-Recent Advances in Parkinson's Disease.* Philadelphia: F.A. Davis Company, 1971:204–237.

140. Goodwin F, Murphy D, Brodie K, et al. Levodopa: Alterations in behavior. Clin Pharmacol Ther 1971; 12:383–396.

141. O'Brien CP, DiGiacomo JN, Fahn S, et al. Mental effects of high-dosage levodopa. *Arch Gen Psychiatry* 1971; 24:61–64.

142. Jouvent R, Abensour P, Bonnet A, et al. Anti-Parkinsonian and antidepressant effects of high doses of bromocriptine; An independent comparison. *J Affect Disord* 1983; 5:141–145.

143. Mendez MA, Golbe LI. Hypomania in a patient receiving deprenyl (selegiline) after adrenal-striatal implantation for Parkinson's disease. *Clin Neuropharmacol* 1988; 11:549–551.

144. Suchowersky O, deVries J. Possible interaction between deprenyl and Prozac [Letter]. *Can J Neurol Sci* 1990; 17:352–353.

145. Pogarell O, Kunig G, Oertel WH. A non-ergot dopamine agonist, pramipexole, in the therapy of advanced Parkinson's disease: Improvement of Parkinsonian symptoms and treatment-associated complications. A review of three studies. *Clin Neuropharmacol* 1997; 20[Suppl 1]:S28–S35.

146. Uitti RJ, Tanner CM, Rajput AH, et al. Hypersexuality with anti-Parkinsonian therapy. *Clin Neuropharmacol* 1989; 12:375–383.

147. Quinn NP, Toone B, Lang AE, et al. Dopa dose-dependent sexual deviation. *Brit J Psychiatry* 1983; 142:296–298.

148. Lesser RP, Fahn S, Snider SR, et al. Analysis of the clinical problems in Parkinsonism and the complications of long-term levodopa therapy. *Neurology* 1979; 29:1253–1260.

149. Courty E, Durif F, Zenut M, et al. Psychiatric and sexual disorders induced by apomorphine in Parkinson's disease. *Clin Neuropharmacol* 1997; 2:140–147.

150. Colcher A, Simuni T, Stern M, et al. Dopamine agonists produce hypersexuality. *Mov Disord* 1998; 13[Abstract]:122.

151. Fernandez HH, Durso R. Clozapine for dopaminergic-induced paraphilias in Parkinson's disease. *Mov Disord* 1998; 13:597–598.

152. Jimenez-Jimenez FJ, Tallon-Barranco A, Cabrera-Valdivia F, et al. Fluctuating penile erection related with levodopa therapy. *Neurology* 1999; 52:210.

153. Brewer M, Stacy M. Sildenafil citrate therapy in men with Parkinson's disease. *Mov Disord* 1998; 13[Abstract]:860.

43

Status of Protective Therapies

Andrew D. Siderowf, M.D., and Matthew B. Stern, M.D.
University of Pennsylvania, Philadelphia, Pennsylvania

Therapy for Parkinson's disease (PD) can be divided into three main categories: (1) symptomatic, (2) restorative and (3) neuroprotective. Effective symptomatic therapy for PD has existed since the demonstration by Cotzias (1) that dopamine replacement with exogenous levodopa could reverse most of the clinical manifestations of PD. More recently, therapies such as neural transplantation (2) have shown the potential to restore the capacity to produce dopamine in PD patients. However, therapy that actually alters the underlying process of neurodegeneration in PD remains a largely unattained goal in spite of a number of areas of active research. This chapter will review the status of currently available and emerging therapies with potential neuroprotective activity (Tables 43-1, 43-2) and address some of the issues related to evaluating these agents in clinical trials.

DEFINITION OF NEUROPROTECTION AND RELEVANCE TO PARKINSON'S DISEASE

Neuroprotection is a therapeutic strategy intended to slow or halt the progression of neuronal loss (3) and thereby alter the natural history of disease. As contrasted with symptomatic therapy, neuroprotective therapies act on the pathogenic mechanisms underlying the clinical manifestations of the disease. A partially neuroprotective therapy slows the course of disease, although a therapy that is fully neuroprotective completely arrests disease progression.

The term *neurorescue* has recently been used to describe a distinct type of neuroprotection. Neurorescue is based on the concept that a population of cells is dysfunctional but not irreversibly injured, and may be restored to normal function (4). In contrast to traditional neuroprotective therapies that would be expected to have no immediate effect on

symptoms, neurorescue therapies may improve clinical manifestations of the disease and slow or stop disease progression.

The concept of neuroprotection obviously has great relevance to PD. Because the rate of disease progression in PD is relatively slow, and little disability is associated with the early stages of disease (5), therapies that slow but do not entirely arrest disease progression would result in significant reduction in the burdens of PD.

MECHANISMS OF NEURONAL INJURY IN PARKINSON'S DISEASE

Development of rational neuroprotective therapies is predicated on understanding the underlying causes of neuronal injury in PD. The mechanisms are reviewed in detail in Chapter 28, and will be covered briefly here. Among the pathologic processes that have been implicated in PD, the mechanisms of oxidative stress and excitotoxicity have received the most attention. Perhaps the strongest evidence for oxidative stress comes from experiments showing impaired mitochondrial electron transport chain function, particularly in complex I, resulting in increased free radical production and cellular injury (6–8). Excitotoxicity, is closely related to oxidative stress and results from a cascade of events initiated by pathologically high levels of excitatory neurotransmitters, particularly glutamate or increased cellular responsiveness to normal levels (9). Stimulation of the ionotropic N-methyl D-aspartate (NMDA) glutamate receptor allows the intracellular entry of large amounts of calcium that in turn may trigger the production of reactive oxygen species and a variety of other pathologic processes (10).

Other potential mechanisms of cellular injury in PD include inflammation and glial cell dysfunction. A possible role of inflammation in the pathogenesis of PD has been suggested by the finding that the substantia nigra

Table 43-1 Current Status of Agents with Possible Neuroprotective Activity in PD

Compound	Stage of Development
MAO-B inhibitors	
Selegiline	Approved by FDA
Lazabemide	Finished phase III trials*
Rasagiline	Phase III trials under way
Dopamine Agonists	
Bromocriptine	Approved by FDA
Pergolide	Approved by FDA
Pramipexole	Approved by FDA
Ropinirole	Approved by FDA
Glutamate antagonists	
Remacemide	Phase II–III trials under way
Amantadine	Approved by FDA
Dextromethorphan	Approved by FDA
Riluzole	Approved by FDA for ALS, trial in PD under way
Antioxidative therapy	
CoenzymeQ10	Pilot study completed
Vitamin C (ascorbic acid)	Available
Vitamin E (alpha tocopherol)	Available
Emerging therapies	
Immunophilins	Clinical trials under way
GDNF	Phase I clinical trials under way**

* not currently marketed in the United States.
** recent trials have been discontinued because of poor tolerability and minimal efficacy.

Table 43-2 Status of Evidence for Classes of Neuroprotective Therapies

Class of Compound	Evidence for Rationale*	Preclinical Evidence**	Clinical Evidence***
MAO-B inhibitors	++	+++	+/−
Dopamine agonists	++	+++	+/−
Anti-glutamate agents	++	++	N/A
Anti-oxidant vitamins	++	++	−
CoenzymeQ	+++	++	N/A
Neurotrophic factors	++	+++	N/A
Immunophilins	++	++	N/A

* two plus (++) indicates evidence for rationale from nonhuman primate models, three plus (+++) indicates evidence for rationale from human studies (e.g., pathological studies or studies using tissue samples from PD patients).
** two plus (++) indicates supportive evidence in animal models other than nonhuman primate. Three plus (+++) indicates supportive evidence in nonhuman primates.
*** evidence for protective effect of MAO-B inhibitors (specifically selegiline) is controversial in spite of large scale trials designed to detect neuroprotective effect. Preliminary evidence suggests dopamine agonists may delay emergence motor complications (dyskinesia and motor fluctuations). A large-scale trial (25) showed no effect of vitamin E on the progression of PD. N/A indicates that no evidence is currently available.

pars compacta (SNpc) from Parkinsonian patients contains increased levels of inflammatory mediators, such as interluken-1 β, interferon-γ, and tumor-necrosis factor-α (11). Glial involvement in PD has been suggested by studies showing both that the concentration of reduced glutathione (GSH) and mitochondrial complex I activity are decreased to about 30 percent of normal in substantia nigra homogenates from patients. This result cannot be explained by neuronal loss alone because dopaminergic neurons probably account for no more than about 2 percent of tissue in such samples (12). These mechanisms are additional rational targets for neuroprotective therapies.

NEUROPROTECTIVE THERAPY FOR PARKINSON'S DISEASE

Selegiline

Selegiline is the only monoamine oxidase type B (MAO-B) inhibitor that is commercially available in the United States. At doses of 5 to 10 mg per day, it is a selective MAO-B inhibitor, and is devoid of the hypertensive "cheese effect" associated with nonselective MAO inhibition (13). Selegiline has been the subject of more intense study than any other potentially neuroprotective compound for PD. However, a great deal of controversy remains regarding whether it possesses neuroprotective properties, and, if present, the mechanism of action.

A substantial body of research suggests several possible mechanisms by which selegiline may protect degenerating neurons from oxidative injury, and thus alter the underlying course of PD. First, it may protect against the effects of oxidative environmental toxins that act via a mechanism similar to the neurotoxin 1-methyl-4 phenyl-1,2,3,6-tetrahydropyridine (MPTP) (14). The conversion of MPTP, which is a pro-toxin, to the active toxin 1-methyl-4-phenylpyridium (MPP+) is catalyzed by MAO-B, and treatment with selegiline can block the conversion, protecting dopaminergic neurons from MPTP-mediated injury (15,16). Second, it can decrease the formation of endogenous free radicals by inhibiting the MAO-B mediated metabolism of dopamine, which results in the formation of H_2O_2. In addition, animal experiments (17–19) have shown that selegiline induces the expression of the free radical scavenger superoxide dismutase (SOD), and may thus improve the ability of cells to buffer against reactive oxygen species.

It has been proposed that the protective effects of selegiline could result from novel actions including inhibition of apoptosis. Tatton and Greenwood (20)

reported that selegiline protects dopaminergic neurons against the neurotoxic action of MPTP even when it is given three days after MPTP administration. Furthermore, these investigators showed that the drug can rescue dopaminergic neurons from MPP+ induced cell death when the active toxin is administered directly (20). These findings suggest that the mechanism of protection is independent of MAO-B inhibition. Subsequently, Tatton and colleagues demonstrated that treatment with selegiline promotes the expression of genes known to prevent apoptosis (21). These findings suggest an alternative neuroprotective mechanism for selegiline.

Two large-scale, prospective, monotherapy studies have attempted specifically to assess the neuroprotective effect of selegiline in PD patients. Tetrud and Langston (22) studied 54 subjects with early PD who were randomized to receive either selegiline 10 mg per day or placebo and then followed until they either required additional symptomatic therapy (levodopa) or had been in the study three years. In this study, there was a delay in reaching endpoint of approximately nine months and clinical disease progression was apparently slowed by 40 to 83% per year in the selegiline treated group.

The DATATOP (Deprenyl and tocopherol antioxidative therapy of Parkinsonism) study (23) randomized 800 subjects to receive selegiline, tocopherol (vitamin E), a combination of the two, or placebo in a 2×2 factorial design. During interim analysis of this study, a substantially reduced likelihood of reaching endpoint in the selegiline but not in the tocopherol treated group was found, and the selegiline randomization was terminated prematurely. The hazard ratio for reaching endpoint was 0.43, and because of the large sample size, the "p value" for this result was 10^{-10}. The initial conclusion from both Tetrud and Langston and DATATOP study was of an apparent protective effect of selegiline on the progression of PD.

However, validity of the results of both studies has been questioned over concern that the delay in need for additional therapy was due to a symptomatic effect rather than a neuroprotective effect (24). Tetrud and Langston noted no symptomatic wash-in or washout effect in their relatively small group of patients, suggesting no meaningful symptomatic effect of selegiline. The DATATOP investigators found a small but statistically significant wash-in effect after one and three months of treatment. Similarly, a small washout effect was noted in the final staggered blinded washout in DATATOP (25), raising the possibility that symptomatic effects were at least partly responsible for the differences in reaching endpoint. In addition, several short-term studies have noted a symptomatic effect of selegiline (26,27). Given the long pharmacodynamic effect of selegiline, it has been suggested that a longer washout would have shown an even greater symptomatic effect (28) in the DATATOP study. Thus the question of whether selegiline is indeed protective has not been adequately resolved.

More recently, Palhagen and coworkers (29) studied the effect of selegiline in 157 patients with early, untreated PD in a design that included an eight-week washout period. These investigators found a significant delay in the progression of Unified Parkinson's disease rating scale (UPDRS) scores and delay in the time until the emergence of disability significant enough to require levodopa therapy. Selegiline was noted to have a small initial symptomatic effect. However, after the eight-week washout period, no significant differences in the deterioration of disability between the groups was noted in any of the clinical rating scales. The authors interpreted their results, which suggested that, beside having a slight symptomatic effect, selegiline may also have a neuroprotective effect.

Olanow and coworkers (30) used a different study design to address the issue of neuroprotection with selegiline. They carried out a 14-month prospective randomized double-blind, placebo-controlled study of 100 patients with early PD. Subjects were randomized to one of four groups: selegiline plus carbidopa/levodopa, placebo plus carbidopa/levodopa, selegiline plus bromocriptine or placebo plus bromocriptine. To avoid confounding effects of treatment, at the end of the study, subjects were washed out from selegiline for two months and from levodopa or bromocriptine for one week. The final evaluation, performed off all treatments, showed a statistically significant increase in the rate of progression of disease in the patients that had not received selegiline. Because of the long washout from selegiline, these results are more likely due to a neuroprotective rather than a symptomatic effect. However, because of the adjunct treatment design, it is difficult to compare results from this trial to the monotherapy trials, and the proposed neuroprotective effect of selegiline remains controversial.

More controversial are the findings of the Parkinson's Disease Research Group of the United Kingdom (PDRG-UK) (31). This group found that patients randomized to receive levodopa plus selegiline in their long-term open study had a 60% *increase* in mortality in comparison to those receiving levodopa alone. This is the only report of increased mortality with selegiline and it is not consistent with previous studies in animals (32) and PD patients (33), which suggest that selegiline may prolong life expectancy. Analysis of other long-term studies of early PD and a meta-analysis have not

shown a similar increase in mortality in association with selegiline (28,34,35). Several concerns have been raised (24) regarding the design of the PDRG-UK study. One concern is that mortality in the PDRG-UK study was unusually high in both the group receiving selegiline (28%) and in the nonselegiline group (18%). Other problems include a large proportion of subjects who failed to complete the study in their original treatment assignment, and relatively poor documentation of the causes of death. In spite of these concerns, the data from the PDRG-UK must not be entirely dismissed and further information regarding potentially increased mortality during selegiline therapy should be sought.

Other MAO-B Inhibitors

Lazabemide is a selective, reversible, inhibitor of MAO-B(36) that is not currently available for use in the United States. It has approximately 100-fold greater selectivity in inhibiting MAO-B compared with MAO-A, making the possibility of a cheese reaction very unlikely. Unlike selegiline, it is not metabolized to potentially active compounds such as methamphetamine and amphetamine (these metabolites may have been the cause of symptomatic improvement of selegiline (37). Lazabemide has been the subject of three placebo-controlled clinical trials in patients with early PD (38–40). These studies showed that lazabemide has barely detectable symptomatic effects and also has the ability to delay the need for levodopa by about 50% when compared to placebo. These effects are very similar to those obtained in clinical trials of selegiline.

Rasagiline (R(+)-N-propargyl-1-aminoindane) is a selective, irreversible, inhibitor of MAO-B that is also not metabolized into amphetamine derivatives (41). It has been shown to have neuroprotective effects in a variety of experimental systems (42). In a pilot study of untreated PD patients, it was well tolerated, and appeared to have symptomatic effects similar to those of selegiline (43). Rasagiline is currently the subject of a large-scale, placebo-controlled clinical trial.

Dopamine Agonists

Dopamine agonists have been used to treat PD since the early 1970s. Initially, they were used as an adjunct to levodopa in patients who developed motor fluctuations (44–46). More recently, dopamine agonists have been used as monotherapy in the early stages of PD (47,48) based on the idea that delaying the introduction of levodopa may delay the emergence of levodopa-related complications, including motor fluctuations and dyskinesias. Attention has also been focused on the possibility that dopamine agonists may have neuroprotective and symptomatic effects in PD. Several potential neuroprotective mechanisms have been proposed including: (1) reduction of the need for exogenous levodopa resulting in reduced free radical production; (2) stimulation of auto-receptors resulting in reduced dopamine turnover and catabolism; (3) direct anti-oxidant or neuroprotective properties; and (4) reduction of glutamatergic subthalamic nucleus output, resulting in reduced excitotoxicity.

Studies of dopamine agonists as adjunctive therapy to levodopa have consistently demonstrated that combined therapy produces a comparable level of anti-Parkinsonian control with a reduced levodopa dose requirement (49,50). Initiating therapy with a dopamine agonist in patients with mild symptoms permits a delay before the introduction of levodopa (48). If it is true that higher cumulative exposure to levodopa accelerates the degenerative process in PD, these levodopa sparing effects may be neuroprotective. Dopamine agonists may also reduce the rate of dopamine metabolism. Carter (51) has shown that addition of the dopamine agonist pramipexole to a cell culture of dopaminergic neurons reduces the concentration of dopamine in the medium. Similarly, in vivo studies have shown that several dopamine agonists may reduce firing rates of dopaminergic neurons (52). Slowed dopaminergic metabolism may translate into reduced production of reactive oxygen species.

Evidence for direct neuroprotective effects has been reported with many dopamine agonists in excitotoxic and oxidative stress models of neurodegeneration. For example, bromocriptine has been shown to mitigate excitotoxic injury by enhancing the ability of cells to buffer extracellular glutamate (53,54), by reducing the susceptibility of cultured neurons to MPTP mediated toxicity (55), and by acting as a free radical scavenger (56). Pramipexole has been shown to reduce cell loss in toxic and ischemic models of neuronal injury (57). In addition, pramipexole has been shown to attenuate oxygen radical generation and inhibit mitochondrial transition pore opening in a dose-dependent fashion (58). Felten (59) showed that low doses of pergolide protected against age-related loss of dopaminergic neurons in Fisher rats.

Some clinical studies have suggested that initial treatment with dopamine agonists rather than levodopa may be associated with reduced frequency of motor complications (60,61) (see Chapter 35). For example, Montastruc and coworkers (61) showed in a randomized, unblinded study that motor complications may be less frequent in patients receiving the combination of bromocriptine and levodopa than in those receiving levodopa alone. It is worth noting that the rate of motor complications in the levodopa treated group in this study was unusually high. Nonetheless, these findings are consistent with preclinical data from Pearce and coworkers (62) showing that MPTP-treated nonhuman primates are less likely to develop dyskinesias when treated with dopamine agonists, such as ropinirole or bromocriptine, than when treated with levodopa. It has been hypothesized that reduction in motor complications observed with dopamine agonists may be related to constant rather than pulsatile stimulation of dopamine receptors (63), however, the delay in the development of motor complications may also be evidence of a neuroprotective effect.

Few clinical studies have directly addressed the neuroprotective effects of dopamine agonists. Olanow and coworkers (30) evaluated the rate of deterioration in UPDRS over a period of 14 months in patients randomized to receive either levodopa or bromocriptine, with or without selegiline. At the end of the study, there was no significant difference in the degree of deterioration in UPDRS scores between the levodopa and bromocriptine treated groups, suggesting no substantial protective effect. In another prospective, double-blind study, Przuntek and coworkers (64) randomized patients to receive treatment with bromocriptine plus levodopa, when necessary, versus levodopa monotherapy. This trial was suspended prematurely due to the observation of lower mortality in the bromocriptine treated group. These results had not been observed previously, and remain to be confirmed in other trials.

In summary, several lines of reasoning suggest that dopamine agonists may have neuroprotective properties. A substantial body of preclinical evidence from studies in animal models of Parkinsonism and in vitro systems shows that dopamine agonists have neuroprotective potential. Preliminary clinical studies show that early use of dopamine agonists may delay the emergence of motor complications. However, this remains controversial. Definitive studies of the effect of the early use of dopamine agonists on the emergence of motor complications, and studies to assess the effect of these agents on disease progression, are in progress.

Stereotactic Surgery

It has been suggested (65) that stereotactic surgical procedures which reduce outflow from the subthalamic nucleus (STN) may have neuroprotective and symptomatic effects. The STN is the principal source of glutamatergic output in the basal ganglia. In pathophysiologic models of PD, loss of dopaminergic input to the striatum results in loss of inhibition of the STN. The result of this disinhibition may be excessive excitatory outflow with the potential for glutamate-mediated excitotoxic injury. There is preclinical evidence to support this line of reasoning. In rat and primate models, STN ablation induces reductions in mitochondrial enzyme activity, glutamic acid decarboxylase (GAD) mRNA expression, and 2-deoxyglucose uptake in the ipsilateral SNr and globus pallidus (66–69). These metabolic changes may reflect a reduction in the potential for excitotoxic injury.

More direct experimental evidence for a protective effect of STN ablation remains elusive. In a rodent model, STN ablation protected dopaminergic neurons from 6-OHDA toxicity (70). In a primate model, however, no such protective effect of STN lesioning was observed. In this experiment, lesions were created in the STN before administration of MPTP. Postmortem counting of dopaminergic neurons did not show differences in cell loss between the lesioned and unlesioned sides (68). However, large doses of MPTP were employed, and neuroprotection was not the primary aim of this study. Studies of nonhuman primates designed to evaluate the protective effects of STN ablation, and clinical evaluation of Parkinsonian patients who have undergone stereotactic ablation or stimulation of the STN, may clarify the potential neuroprotective effects of these procedures.

Glutamatergic Agents

On the basis of "weak excitotoxicity" hypothesis indicating that a slight excess of glutamatergic activity may be neurotoxic (10), a number of agents that inhibit glutamatergic transmission are being examined. These agents antagonize the action of glutamate at NMDA receptors or interfere with glutamate transmission. These drugs include dextromethorphan, amantadine, remacemide, and riluzole. Because glutamatergic transmission is an important part of basal ganglia physiology, these agents may have symptomatic and neuroprotective effects.

Remacemide hydrochloride is a noncompetitive inhibitor of glutamate at NMDA receptors. It was initially developed as an antiepileptic drug, and human trials have demonstrated that it is an effective and well-tolerated anticonvulsant (71). In vitro studies have shown that remacemide and its desglycine metabolite prevent NMDA-induced depolarization in rat hippocampal slices (71). Remacemide has been shown to have neuroprotective effects in several animal models of ischemic injury (71). Remacemide has no anti-Parkinsonian effects on monoamine-depleted rats when administered alone (72), however, when combined with a threshold dose of levodopa, remacemide increased motor activity in monoamine-depleted rats and in MPTP-treated rhesus monkeys (73). On the basis of its ability to antagonize glutamate, and thus prevent excitotoxic injury, there is reason

to believe that remacemide may have neuroprotective and symptomatic effects in PD. Human trials of remacemide in PD for symptomatic treatment and as potential neuroprotection are ongoing. Early phase trials on PD patients have demonstrated symptomatic effects similar to those seen in animal models. More importantly, the drug has been proven safe and well tolerated in PD patients (73a).

Amantadine is a tricyclic amine that has been used as a treatment for PD, for decades. Its mechanism of action is not certain, but anticholinergic and dopamine reuptake inhibition have been suggested (74). Amantadine has recently been shown to be a weak NMDA antagonist (75), and has been demonstrated to reduce levodopa-induced involuntary movements in advanced PD (76). In a retrospective study, Uitti and coworkers (77) found that treatment with amantadine was an independent predictor of survival in patients with PD.

The commonly available ingredient in cough medication, dextromethorphan, is also a weak NMDA antagonist. It has effects similar to those of amantadine on levodopa-induced dyskinesia (78). Because of their antiglutamatergic activity, their benign or beneficial clinical profile in PD, and history of safe use, both amantadine and dextromethorphan are logical candidates to be tested as neuroprotective agents.

Riluzole is a novel glutamate antagonist that was originally developed as an anticonvulsant. Although the mechanism of action of riluzole is not certain, it has been suggested that it interferes with glutamate release (79). Riluzole does not appear to compete for binding with either NMDA or non-NMDA receptors (80,81). It has been shown to slightly delay the progression of amyotrophic lateral sclerosis (ALS), in two placebo-controlled clinical trials. In one study (82), 155 ALS patients were randomized to receive either 100 mg of riluzole or placebo. After 18 months of treatment, there was approximately a 35% decrease in risk of tracheostomy or death in the riluzole-treated group. A second randomized, controlled trial of 959 patients receiving riluzole (83) also showed statistically significant improvements in tracheostomy-free survival. Because of proposed overlap in the pathophysiology of PD and ALS (6), riluzole has been considered to be a potentially neuroprotective agent for PD. It has been shown to exert neuroprotective effects in animal models of Parkinsonism including MPTP-mediated neurotoxicity in mice and marmosets and 6-OHDA-mediated injury in rats (84–86). Clinical trials to test the neuroprotective effects of riluzole in PD are underway.

Antioxidants: Vitamin C and Vitamin E

Vitamin E (alpha-tocopherol) has long been viewed as a potential neuroprotective agent, particularly in view of the oxidative stress hypothesis of PD. It acts as an antioxidant by blocking lipid peroxidation and trapping peroxyl radicals (87). Vitamin E has been shown to have neuroprotective effects in several experimental systems (88). A case-controlled, community-based study (89) suggested that high dietary intake of vitamin E may protect against the development of PD. However, other epidemologic studies (90,91) have failed to find an association between vitamin E intake and PD. The effect of vitamin E at a dose of 2,000 IU per day was evaluated in the DATATOP trial. After a mean of 14 months of treatment, no effect was observed in patients receiving vitamin E compared to placebo (25). This adequately powered negative trial suggests that vitamin E is not a potent neuroprotective agent at the dosage used in DATATOP. Nonetheless, proponents of vitamin E suggest that the negative results of the DATATOP trial can be explained by the poor penetration of vitamin E into the CNS. One study (56) found no increase in CSF vitamin E levels in spite of dosing of 4,000 IU per day. Therefore, the possibility that it may have a mild effect cannot be entirely excluded, especially at high doses or over sustained periods of time.

Vitamin C (ascorbic acid) is another compound with antioxidant properties that has been considered as a neuroprotective agent in PD. Vitamin C protects against dopamine autooxidation in cell culture (92), and may act synergistically with selegiline (93) to protect against oxidative injury. Several epidemiologic studies have failed to find a relationship between intake of vitamin C and the risk of PD (91,94). However, in an open trial, Fahn (95) found that the need to introduce levodopa therapy was delayed up to 2.5 years in patients treated with high-dose combination therapy with vitamins C and E compared to controls not treated with antioxidants. This result has not been confirmed in a randomized, placebo-controlled trial. On the basis of current evidence, the neuroprotective effects of vitamin C, as those of vitamin E, are probably quite modest.

Co-Enzyme Q10

Co-Enzyme Q10 (CoQ), also known as ubiquinone, is a lipid soluble compound that acts as an electron acceptor in complex I and complex II of mitochondria (96). CoQ has antioxidant properties, and has been shown to scavenge free radicals generated within microsomal membranes more effectively than vitamin E (97). Brain levels of CoQ decline with age, being about 50 percent greater in young adults compared to the elderly (98,99) and have been shown to be lower in PD patients compared to age-matched controls (100,101). Favit and coworkers (102) found

that CoQ protected against neuronal death in two in vitro models. Treatment with CoQ has also been shown to be neuroprotective in rodent models (103).

CoQ has been studied in a number of human diseases where mitochondrial defects are considered to be present. It has been shown to improve myocardial function and exercise duration in congestive heart failure (104). It is also safe in pilot studies in Huntington's disease (105) and mitochondrial encephalopathies (106). In a pilot study, PD (107) patients treated with CoQ showed normalization of mitochondrial complex I activity. However, because of the small sample size, the results did not reach statistical significance. A larger clinical study in PD patients designed to assess the effects of CoQ on mitochondrial function and potential neuroprotective actions is currently under way.

FUTURE STRATEGIES

Immunophilins

Immunophilins are a group of molecules related to CyclosporineA (CyA) including FK 506 GPi 1046, and rapamycin. The principal clinical role of immunophilins is as immunosuppressive agents in patients who have undergone organ transplantation (108). Many immunophilins are small, orally-active molecules that have the ability to cross the blood-brain barrier (109). Nonimmunosuppressive derivatives of immunophilins have been developed that retain their effects on neurons. The notion that immunophilins may be neuroprotective came from studies showing that they could inhibit nitric oxide synthase (NOS), and thus prevent excitotoxic injury. Subsequently, FK 506 was shown to reduce neuronal injury in animal models of cerebral ischemia (110). Nonimmunosuppressive derivatives have been shown to protect against MPTP and 6-OHDA mediated injury to dopaminergic neurons (111). On the basis of this preclinical data, these agents appear to hold promise as potential neuroprotective agents. Clinical trials in PD patients are under way.

Neurotrophic Factors

Neurotrophic factors are another class of compounds that have the potential to be highly effective neuroprotective therapies. They are a group of naturally occurring molecules, many of which are not structurally related to each other, that are required for the survival and development of neurons (112). In theory, these molecules may possess both neuroprotective and restorative properties. The neurotrophic factor that has been of greatest interest in PD is glial cell line–derived neurotrophic factor (GDNF). It belongs to a distinct family of trophic factors distantly related to the transforming growth factor-β superfamily (113). GDNF has been shown to protect from 6-OHDA-mediated injury in rodents, (114) and to mediate recovery from such injury (115). In nonhuman primates, Gash and coworkers (116) demonstrated marked increase in tyrosine hydroxylase staining and increased numbers of dopaminergic fibers in MPTP-treated rhesus monkeys, following GDNF administration. These primates also showed marked behavioral improvement as a result of the treatment.

A major disadvantage to GNDF as therapy for CNS disease is that it must be given by intra-ventricular infusion. However, several studies have explored other novel delivery systems for neurotrophic factors. Tseng and colleagues (117) implanted genetically engineered hamster kidney cells adjacent to the midbrain of Wistar rats, and demonstrated preservation of tyrosine hydroxylase positive neurons following mid-brain transsection. Choi-Lundberg and colleagues (118) used adenovirus vectors to transfect cells in adult rats to produce GDNF. These genetically engineered animals showed markedly reduced susceptibility to 6-OHDA toxicity compared to nontransfected animals. This study illustrates the potential to apply gene therapy techniques in PD. Other gene therapy strategies that have been explored include engineering cells to express anti-apoptosis gene products or free radical scavengers, such as superoxide dismutase (SOD) (119). Strategies such as these in which both the therapeutic agent and the delivery system are products of advances in molecular biology may be an important paradigm for the future (Table 43-2). For detailed discussion of gene therapy see Chapter 45.

Issues in Design of Neuroprotective Trials

Achieving a convincing demonstration of neuroprotection in clinical trials has proved to be as challenging and as crucial as identifying neuroprotective compounds in the laboratory. Because of the slow rate of disease progression, neuroprotective trials are necessarily of long duration, involve large numbers of subjects and are costly. Identifying methods for testing promising compounds in more efficient trials has been a major challenge for clinical investigators. A second major challenge has been to separate symptomatic from neuroprotective effects. Suggested approaches to this problem have included novel experimental designs, and the use of functional imaging as a biologic marker for disease progression.

Although the DATATOP study established many of the standard procedures for neuroprotective trials in PD, it is unlikely that resources will be available to carry out similar trials for more than a few very promising compounds. To evaluate the relatively large number of potential compounds, more efficient clinical trial methods must be found. One response (120) to this challenge is to identify subsets of patients who may be more likely to respond to a given intervention, and carry out small trials in these populations. It is possible to take advantage of recent advances in genetics, molecular biology, and imaging to identify such populations. For example, the discovery of a mutation in the α-synuclein gene on chromosome 4 that is responsible for autosomally dominant inherited parkinsonism (121) in several Mediterranean kindreds, and investigations with positron emission tomography (PET) (122), and single photon emission computerized tomography (SPECT) (43) have suggested that it is possible to identify asymptomatic at-risk individuals for trials of neuroprotective agents. Trials in such individuals offer the possibility of preventing the emergence of parkinsonian symptoms. In addition, using PET techniques, Morrish and coworkers (123) have suggested that the rate of neuronal loss may be more rapid in early PD than later in the course of the disease. Therefore, it may be easier to detect a neuroprotective effect in asymptomatic at-risk individuals, or in patients with very early rather than well-established disease.

Certain interventions may be more likely to be neuroprotective in distinct subpopulations of PD patients. For example, the mechanism of action of CoQ appears to be to normalize mitochondrial complex I and II activity (107). Using platelet-mitochondrial cybrids (124), patients with defects in mitochondrial function can be identified. It may be reasonable to preferentially select patients with clearly defined defects in complex I and II activity for early clinical trials. The limitation of using enriched subgroups is that such studies do not necessarily generalize to all patients with clinically defined PD. Nonetheless, studies in subgroups could be used to screen potential agents before embarking on long and costly trials.

Separating neuroprotective effects from symptomatic effects has proved to be a very difficult methodologic issue in designing neuroprotective trials. Clearly, the DATATOP experience is the most prominent example of this challenge. However, many other potentially neuroprotective compounds including dopamine agonists, glutamate antagonists, and surgical interventions have established effects on parkinsonian symptoms that may interfere with the detection of small but clinically meaningful changes in the natural history of disease.

One approach to this problem has been to discontinue or "washout" the study drug for a period of time before the final clinical evaluation. The rationale for this strategy is that protective effects are likely to remain after washout, although symptomatic effects should dissipate. Several washout strategies have already been employed. Olanow and coworkers (30) combined a long-term washout of selegiline with a short-term washout of levodopa and bromocriptine symptomatic therapy in an effort to improve patient compliance with the long duration of withdrawal of selegiline required by that compound's long pharmacodynamic half-life. In another study, a blinded, staggered washout strategy was devised (25) to prevent unblinding or reverse-placebo effect during washout.

A second proposed option to distinguish between symptomatic and neuroprotective effects is the "randomized start" trial (see Figure 43-1) (125). In this design, patients are randomized to begin active treatment either right away or after a specified time interval. Symptomatic effects will lead to the group that started later "catching up" in clinical performance to the first group, and no difference between the groups will be detectable. However, if there is a true neuroprotective effect and the separation in starting time is sufficient, the performance of the two groups will remain distinct, even if a symptomatic effect is present. Because all patients receive treatment at some time in this trial design, there is probably a good patient acceptance, although the essential elements of randomization, placebo-control, and blinding are retained. The randomized start design has been employed in neuroprotective trials of Alzheimer's disease (126), but has not yet been used in PD.

The use of biologic markers including PET and SPECT imaging, represent another approach to demonstrating neuroprotection with compounds that may also have symptomatic effects. PET and SPECT have been refined to the point that they possess sufficient precision to be used as markers of nigral cell degeneration in clinical trials. Fluorodopa PET was the first functional imaging modality used to assess the integrity of dopamine terminal function in vivo. The loss of uptake observed with this technique appears to reflect dopaminergic terminal density, correlates with nigral cell counts obtained at autopsy (127), and is related to disease progression as measured by the UPDRS and Hoehn-Yahr Staging (128). Morrish and coworkers (122) estimated the rate of striatal dopamine loss at about 9 to 12% per year. Control patients showed no loss of dopaminergic uptake for over three years.

SPECT imaging of the dopamine transporter may provide a more convenient and less expensive alternative to PET imaging. The dopamine transporter is located on the presynaptic membrane of dopaminergic terminals, and provides a marker of dopaminergic innervation of the striatum (129). Imaging with radio-labeled compounds that bind to the dopamine transporter protein including (123I-β)CIT have demonstrated dopamine transporter loss in patients with early PD compared to controls (130), and that transporter loss in PD patients is correlated with disease severity (131). One disadvantage to β-CIT imaging is that the ligand must be administered 24 hours before imaging. As a result, other SPECT tracers with similar affinities for the dopamine transporter are being developed (132).

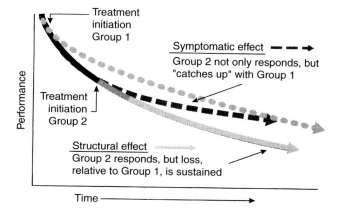

FIGURE 43-1. Schematic representation of randomized-start trial showing effects of symptomatic and neuroprotective therapies. Note that protective effects can be detected even in the presence of symptomatic effects. (From Koller, *Annals of Neurology* 1998, with permission).

CONCLUSION

Neuroprotection remains a highly desirable and elusive goal in the treatment of PD. A number of potentially neuroprotective compounds are available, but none have been convincingly demonstrated to confer neuroprotection for PD. Significant advances in understanding the pathophysiologic processes underlying PD, and a body of preclinical evidence demonstrating neuroprotection in model systems for a number of candidate compounds, raise the hope that neuroprotective therapy for PD is achievable. The challenges for the twenty-first century will continue to be to develop promising compounds, to select the compounds that should be brought from the bench to the clinic, and to develop a sound and standardized clinical method to evaluate these compounds in PD.

REFERENCES

1. Cotzias GC, Papavasilioou PS, Gellene R. Modification of parkinsonism – chronic treatment with L-dopa. *N Engl J Med* 1969; 280:337–345.

2. Kordower JH, Goetz CG, Freeman TB, et al. Dopaminergic transplants in patients with Parkinson's disease: Neuroanatomical correlates of clinical recovery. *Exp Neurol* 1997; 144:41–46.

3. Shoulson I. Neuroprotective clinical strategies for Parkinson's disease. *Ann Neurol* 1992; 32(Suppl): S143–S145.

4. Shults CW. Neurotrophic factors. In: Watts RL, Koller WC (eds). *Movement Disorders, Neurologic Principles and Practice*. New York: McGraw-Hill, 1997:117–123.

5. Poewe WH, Wenning GK. The natural history of Parkinson's disease. *Ann Neurol* 1998; 44:S1–S9.

6. Bowling AC, Beal MF. Bioenergetic and oxidative stress in neurodegenerative diseases. *Life Sciences* 1995; 56:1151–1171.

7. Olanow CW. Oxidative reactions in Parkinson's disease. *Neurology* 1990; 40:22–29.

8. Inzelberg R, Shapira T, Korczyn AD. Effects of atropine on learning and memory functions in dementia. *Clin Neuropharm* 1990; 13:241–247.

9. Lipton SA, Rosenberg PA. Excitatory amino acids as a final common pathway for neurological disorders. *N Engl J Med* 1994; 330:613–622.

10. Albin RL, Greenamyre JT. Alternative excitotoxic hypotheses. *Neurology* 1992; 42:733–738.

11. Hirsch HC, Hunot S, Damier P, et al. Glial cells and inflammation in Parkinson's disease: A role in neurodegeneration? *Ann Neurol* 1998; 44(Suppl 1): S115–S120.

12. Jenner P, Olanow CW. Understanding cell death in Parkinson's disease. *Ann Neurol* 1998; 44:S72–84.

13. Knoll J. Deprenyl (selegiline): The history of its development and pharmacological action. *Acta Neurol Scand* 1983; 68(Suppl 95):57–80.

14. Langston JW, Ballard PA, Tetrud JW, et al. Chronic parkinsonism in humans due to a product of meperidine analog synthesis. *Science* 1983; 219:979–980.

15. Heikkila RE, Manzino L, Duvoisin RC, et al. Protection against the dopaminergic neurotoxicity of 1-methyl-4- phenyl-1,2,3,6-tetrahydropyridine (MPTP) by monoamine oxidase inhibitors. *Nature* 1984; 311:467–469.

16. Singer TP, Castagnoli NJ, Ramsay RR, et al. Biochemical events in the development of parkinsonism induced by 1-methyl-4-phenyl-1,2,3,6-tetrahydropyridine. *J Neurochem* 1987; 49:1–8.

17. Knoll J. Extension of life span of rats by long-term (-)deprenyl treatment. *Mt Sinai J Med* 1988; 55:67–74.

18. Carrillo M-C, Kanai S, Nokubo M. (-)Deprenyl induces activities of both superoxide dismutase and catalase but not of glutathione peroxidase in the striatum of young male rats. *Life Sci* 1991; 48:517–521.

19. Clow A, Hussain T, Glover V. (-)-Deprenyl can induce soluble superoxide dismutase in rat striata. *J Neural Transm Gen Sect* 1991; 86:77–80.

20. Tatton WG, Greenwood CE. Rescue of dying neurons: A new action for deprenyl in MPTP Parkinsonism. *J Neurosci Res* 1991; 30:666–677.

21. Tatton WG, Chalmers-Redman RME. Modulation of gene expression rather than monoamine oxidase inhibition: (-)-deprenyl-related compounds in controlling neurodegeneration. *Neurology* 1996; 47:S171–S183.

22. Tetrud JW, Langston JW. The effect of deprenyl (selegiline) in the natural history of Parkinson's disease. *Science* 1989; 245:519–522.

23. Parkinson Study Group. Effect of deprenyl on the progression of disability in early Parkinson's disease. *N Engl J Med* 1989; 321:1364–1371.

24. Olanow CW, Fahn S, Langston JW, et al. Selegiline and mortality in Parkinson's disease. *Ann Neurol* 1996; 40:841–845.

25. Parkinson Study Group. Effects of tocopherol and deprenyl on the progression of disability in early Parkinson's disease. *N Engl J Med* 1993; 328:176–183.

26. Allain H, Pollak P, Neukirch HC, et al. Symptomatic effect of selegiline in de novo parkinsonian patients. *Mov Disord* 1993; 8:536–540.

27. Myllyla VV, Sontaniemi KA, Vuorinen JA, et al. Selegiline as initial treatment in de novo parkinsonian patients. *Neurology* 1992; 42:339–343.

28. Olanow CW. Selegiline: Current perspectives on issues related to neuroprotection and mortality. *Neurology* 1996; 47:S210–S216.

29. Palhagen S, Heinonen EH, Hagglund J, et al. Selegiline delays the onset of disability in de novo parkinsonian patients. Swedish Parkinson Study Group. *Neurology* 1998; 51:520–525.

30. Olanow CW, Hauser RA, Gauger L, et al. The effect of deprenyl and levodopa on the progression of Parkinson's disease. *Ann Neurol* 1995; 38:833–834.

31. Lees AJ, on behalf of the Parkinson's Disease Research Group of the UK. Comparison of therapeutic effects and mortality data of levodopa and levodopa combined with selegiline in patients with early mild Parkinson's disease. *BMJ* 1995; 311:1602–1607.

32. Knoll J. The striatal dopamine dependency of life span in male rats: Longevity study with (-)deprenyl. *Mech Ageing Dev* 1988; 46:237–262.

33. Birkmayer W, Knoll J, Riederer P. Increased life expectancy resulting from addition of L-deprenyl to Modopar treatment of Parkinson's disease: A long-term study. *J Neural Transm* 1985; 64:113–127.

34. Parkinson Study Group. Mortality in DATATOP: A multicenter trial in early Parkinson's disease. *Ann Neurol* 1998; 43: 318–325.

35. Maki-Ikola O, Kilkku O, Heinonen E. Other studies have not shown increased mortality. *BMJ* 1996; 312:702–702.

36. Da-Prada M, Kettler R, Keller HH, et al. From moclobemide to Ro 19-6327 and Ro 41-1049: The

development of a new class of reversible selective MAO-A and MAO-B inhibitors. *J Neural Transm* 1990; 29(Suppl):279–292.

37. Da-Prada M, Kettler R, Keller HH, et al. Ro 19-6327, a reversible, highly selective inhibitor of type B monoamine oxidase, completely devoid of tyramine-potentiating effects: Comparisons with selegiline. In: Dahlstrom A (ed.). *Progress in Catecholamine Research.* New York: Alan R Liss, 1988:359–363.

38. Parkinson Study Group. Effect of lazabemide on the progression of disability in early Parkinson's disease. *Ann Neurol* 1996; 40:99–107.

39. Parkinson Study Group. A controlled trial of lazabemide (Ro 19-6327) in levodopa-treated Parkinson's disease. *Arch Neurol* 1994; 51:427–442.

40. Parkinson Study Group. A controlled trial of lazabemide (Ro 19-6327) in untreated Parkinson's disease. *Ann Neurol* 33, 350–356.

41. Finberg JP, Lamensdorf I, Commissiong JW, et al. Pharmacology and neuroprotective properties of rasagiline. *J Neural Transm* 1996; Suppl 48:95–101.

42. Finberg JP, Takeshima T, Johnston JM, et al. Increased survival of dopaminergic neurons by rasagiline, a monoamine oxidase B inhibitor. *Neuroreport* 1998; 9:703–707.

43. Marek KL, Friedman J, Hauser R, et al. A phase II evaluation of rasagiline mesylate (TVP-1012), a novel anti-parkinsonian drug, in parkinsonian patients not using levodopa/carbidopa. *Mov Disord* 1997; 12:838.

44. Kartzinel R, Teychenne P, Gillespie MM, et al. Bromocriptine and levodopa (with or without carbidopa) in Parkinsonism. *Lancet* 1976; 2:272–275.

45. Calne DB, Burton K, Beckman J, et al. Dopamine agonists in Parkinson's Disease. *Can J Neurol Sci* 1984; 11:221–224.

46. Olanow CW, Fahn S, Muenter MD, et al. A multicenter, double-blind, placebo-controlled trial of pergolide as an adjunct to Sinemet in Parkinson's disease. *Mov Disord* 1994; 9:40–47.

47. Shannon KM, Bennett JPJ, Friedman JH. Efficacy of pramipexole, a novel dopamine agonist, as monotherapy in mild to moderate Parkinson's disease. The Pramipexole Study. *Neurology* 1997; 49:724–728.

48. Adler CH, Sethi KD, Hauser RA, et al. Ropinirole for the treatment of early Parkinson's disease. The Ropinirole Study. *Neurology* 1997; 49:393–399.

49. Lieberman A, Ranhosky A, Korts D. Clinical evaluation of pramipexole in advanced Parkinson's disease: Results of a double-blind, placebo-controlled, parallel group study. *Neurology* 1997; 49:162–168.

50. Rascol O, Lees AJ, Senard JM, et al. Ropinirole in the treatment of levodopa-induced motor fluctuations in patients with Parkinson's disease. *Clin Neuropharm* 1996; 19:234–245.

51. Carter AJ, Muller RE. Pramipexole, a dopamine D2 antagonist receptor antagonist, decrease the extracellular concentration of dopamine in vivo. *Eur J Pharmacol* 1991; 200:65–72.

52. Piercey MF, Camacho-Ochoa M, Smith MW. Functional roles for dopamine-receptor subtypes. *Clin Neuropharmacol* 1995; 18:34–42.

53. Yamashita H, Kawakami H, Zhang YX, et al. Neuroprotective mechanism of bromocriptine. *Lancet* 1995; 346:1305.

54. Sawada H, Ibi M, Kihara T, et al. Dopamine D2-type agonists protect mesencephalic neurons from glutamate neurotoxicity: Mechanisms of neuroprotective treatment against oxidative stress. *Ann Neurol* 1998; 44:110–119.

55. Muralikrishnan D, Mohanakumar KP. Neuroprotection by bromocriptine against 1-methyl-4-phenyl-1,2,3,6-tetrahydropyridine-induced neurotoxicity in mice. *FASEB* 1998; 12:905–912.

56. Pappert EJ, Tangney CC, Goetz CG, et al. Alpha-tocopherol in the ventricular cerebrospinal fluid of Parkinson's disease patients: Dose-response study and correlations with plasma levels. *Neurology* 1996; 47:1037–1042.

57. Sethi VH, Wu H, Oostveen JA, et al. Neuroprotective effects of the dopamine agonists pramipexole and bromocriptine in 3-acetylpyridine-treated rats. *Brain Res* 1997; 754:181–186.

58. Cassarino DS, Fall CP, Smith TS, et al. Pramipexole reduces reactive oxygen species production in vivo and in vitro and inhibits the mitochondrial permeability transition produced by the parkinsonian neurotoxin methylpyridium ion. *J Neurochem* 1998; 71:295–301.

59. Felten DL, Felten SY, Fuller RW, et al. Chronic dietary pergolide preserves nigrostriatal neuronal integrity in aged Fischer 344 rats. *Neurobiol of Aging* 1992; 13:339-351.

60. Rinne UK. Early combination of bromocriptine and levodopa in the treatment of Parkinson's disease: A 5 year follow-up. *Neurology* 1987; 37:826–828.

61. Montastruc JL, Rascol O, Senard JM, et al. A randomized controlled study comparing bromocriptine to which levodopa was later added, with levodopa alone in previously untreated patients with Parkinson's disease: A five year follow-up. *J Neurol Neurosurg Psychiatry* 1994; 57:1034–1038.

62. Pearce RKB, Banerji T, Jenner P, et al. Effects of repeated treatment with L-dopa, bromocriptine and ropinirole in drug-naive MPTP-treated common marmosets. *Brit J Pharmacol* 1996; 118:37.

63. Olanow CW, Jenner P, Brooks D. Dopamine agonists and neuroprotection in Parkinson's disease. *Ann Neurol* 1998; 44:S167–S174.

64. Przuntek H, Welzel D, Blumner E, et al. Bromocriptine lessens the incidence of mortality in L-dopa-treated Parkinsonian patients: Prado-study discontinued. *Eur J Clin Pharmacol* 1992; 43:357–363.

65. Rodriguez MC, Obeso JA, Olanow CW. Subthalamic nucleus-mediated excitotoxicity in Parkinson's disease: A target for neuroprotection. *Ann Neurol* 1998; 44:S175–S188.

66. Blandini F, Greenamyre JT. Prospects of glutamate antagonists in the therapy of Parkinson's disease. *Fund Clin Pharmacol* 1998; 12:4–12.

67. Delfs JM, Ciaramitaro VM, Parry TJ, et al. Subthalamic nucleus lesions: Widespread effects on changes in gene expression induced by nigrostriatal dopamine depletion in rats. *J Neurosci* 1995; 15:6562–6575.

68. Guridi J, Herrero MT, Luquin MR, et al. Subthalamotomy in parkinsonian monkeys. Behavioral and biochemical analysis. *Brain* 1996; 119:1717–1727.

69. Mitchell IJ, Sambrook MA, Crossman AR. Subcortical changes in the regional uptake of [3H]-2-deoxyglucose in the brain of the monkey during experimental choreiform dyskinesia elicited by injection of a gamma-aminobutryric acid antagonist into the subthalamic nucleus. *Brain* 1985; 108:405–422.

70. Piallat B, Benazzouz A, Benabid AL. Subthalamic nucleus lesions on rats prevents dopaminergic nigral neuron degeneration after striatal 6-OHDA injection: behavioral and immunohistochemical studies. *Eur J Neurosci* 1996; 8:1408–1414.

71. Palmer GC, Cregan EF, Borrelli AR, et al. Neuroprotective properties of the uncompetitive NMDA receptor antagonist remacemide hydrochloride. *Ann NY Acad Sci* 1995; 765:236–247.

72. Klockgether T, Turski L. NMDA antagonists potentiate antiparkinsonian effects of L-dopa in monoamine-depleted rats. *Ann Neurol* 1990; 28:536–539.

73. Greenamyre JT, Eller RV, Zhang Z, et al. Antiparkinsonian effects of remacemide, a glutamate antagonist, in rodent and primate models of Parkinson's disease. *Ann Neurol* 1994; 35:655–661.

73a. Parkinson Study Group. A randomized, controlled trial of remacemide for motor fluctuations in Parkinson's disease. *Neurology* 2001; 56:455–462.

74. Goetz CG. New lessons from old drugs: Amantadine and Parkinson's disease. *Neurology* 1998; 50:1211–1212.

75. Stoof JC, Booij J, Drukalrch B. Amantadine as N-methyl-D-aspartaic acid receptor antagonist. *Clin Neurol Neurosur* 1992; 94:S4–S6.

76. Verhagen ML, Del Dotto P, van den Munckhof P, et al. Amantadine as treatment for dyskinesias and motor fluctuations in Parkinson's disease. *Neurology* 1998; 50:1323–1326.

77. Uitti RJ, Rajput AH, Ahlskog JE, et al. Amantadine treatment is an independent predictor of improved survival in Parkinson's disease. *Neurology* 1996; 46:1551–1556.

78. Verhagen ML, Blanchet PJ, van den Munckhof P, et al. A trial of dextromethorphan in parkinsonian patients with motor response complications. *Mov Disord* 1998; 13:414–417.

79. Doble A, Hubert JP, Blanchard JC. Pertussis toxin pretreatment abolishes the inhibitory effect of riluzole and carbechol on D-3H-aspartate release from cultured cerebellar granule cells. *Neurosci Lett* 1992; 140:254.

80. Malgouris C, Bardot F, Daniel M, et al. Riluzole, a novel antiglutamate, prevents memory loss and hippocampal damage in ischemic gerbils. *J Neurosci* 1989; 9:3720–3727.

81. Cheramy A, Barbieto L, Godeheu G, et al. Riluzole inhibits the release of glutamate in the caudate nucleus of the cat in vivo. *Neurosci Lett* 1992; 147:209–212.

82. Bensimon G, Lacomblez L, Meininger V. A controlled trial of riluzole in amyotrophic lateral sclerosis. ALS/Riluzole Study Group. *N Engl J Med* 1994; 330:585–591.

83. Lacomblez L, Bensimon G, Leigh PN, et al. Dose-ranging study of riluzole in amyotrophic lateral sclerosis. Amyotrophic Lateral Sclerosis/Riluzole Study Group II. *Lancet* 1996; 347:1425–1431.

84. Barneoud P, Mazadier M, Miquet JM, et al. Neuroprotective effects of riluzole on a model of Parkinson's disease in the rat. *Neuroscience* 1996; 74:971–983.

85. Benazzouz A, Boraud T, Dubedat P, et al. Riluzole prevents MPTP-induced parkinsonism in the rhesus monkey: A pilot study. *Eur J Pharmacol* 1995; 284:299–307.

86. Boireau A, Miquet JM, Dubedat P, et al. Riluzole and experimental Parkinsonism: Partial antagonism of MPP(+)-induced increase in striatal extracellular dopamine in rats in vivo. *Neuroreport* 1994; 5:2157–2160.

87. Halliwell B, Gutteridge JMC. Oxygen radicals and the nervous system. *TINS* 1985; 8:22–26.

88. Gerlach M, Riederer P, Youdim MB. Neuroprotective therapeutic strategies. Comparison of experimental and clinical results. *Biochem Pharmacol* 1995; 50:1–16.

89. De Rijk MC, Breteler MM, den Breeijen JH, et al. Dietary antioxidants and Parkinson disease. The Rotterdam Study. *Arch Neurol* 1997; 54:762–765.

90. Scheider WL, Hershey LA, Vena JE, et al. Dietary antioxidants and other dietary factors in the etiology of Parkinson's disease. *Mov Disord* 1997; 12:190–196.

91. Logroscino G, Marder K, Cote L, et al. Dietary lipids and antioxidants in Parkinson's disease: A population-based, case-control study. *Ann Neurol* 1996; 39:89–94.

92. Offen D, Ziv I, Sternin H, et al. Prevention of dopamine-induced cell death by thiol antioxidants: Possible implications for treatment of Parkinson's disease. *Exp Neurol* 1996; 141:32–39.

93. Pardo B, Mena MA, Fahn S, et al. Ascorbic acid protects against levodopa-induced neurotoxicity on a catecholamine-rich human neuroblastoma cell line. *Mov Disord* 1993; 8:278–284.

94. Fernandez-Calle P, Jimenez-Jimenez FJ, Molina JA, et al. Serum levels of ascorbic acid (vitamin C) in patients with Parkinson's disease [see comments]. *J Neurol Sci* 1993; 118:25–28.

95. Fahn S. A pilot trial of high-dose alpha-tocopherol and ascorbate in early Parkinson's disease. *Ann Neurol* 1992; 32:S128–S132.

96. Frei B, Kim MC, Ames BN. Ubiquinol-10 is an effective lipid-soluable antioxidant at physiological concentrations. *Proc Natl Acad Sci* 1990; 87:4879–4883.

97. Stocker R, Bowry VW, Frei B. Ubiquinol-10 protects human low density lipoprotein more efficiently against lipid peroxidation than does alpha-tocopherol. *Proc Natl Acad Sci* 1991; 88:1646–1650.

98. Soderberg M, Edlund C, Kristensson K, et al. Lipid composition in different regions of the human brain during aging. *J Neurochem* 1990; 54:415–423.

99. Erstner L, Dallner G. Biochemical, physiological and medical aspects of ubiquinone function. *Biochem Biophys Acta* 1995; 1271:195–204.

100. Matsubara T, Azuma T, Yoshida S, et al. Serum coenzyme Q-10 level in Parkinson syndrome. In: Folkers K, Littarru GP, Yamagami T (eds). *Biomedical and Clinical Aspects of Coenzyme Q*. New York: Elsevier Science, 1991:159–166.

101. Shults CW, Haas RH, Passov D, et al. Coenzyme Q10 levels correlate with the activities of complexes I and II/III in mitochondria from parkinsonian and non-parkinsonian subjects. *Ann Neurol* 1997; 42:261–264.

102. Favit A, Nicoletti F, Scapagnini U, et al. Ubiquinone protects cultured neurons against spontaneous and excitotoxin-induced degeneration. *J Cerebral Blood Flow Metab* 1992; 12:638–645.

103. Beal MF, Henshaw DR, Jenkins BH, et al. Coenzyme Q10 and nicotinamide block striatal lesions produced by the mitochondrial toxin malonate. *Ann Neurol* 1994; 36:882–888.

104. Wilson MF, Frishman WH, Giles T, et al. Coenzyme Q10 therapy and exercise duration in stable angina. In: Folkers K, Littarru GP, Yamagami T (eds). *Biomedical and Clinical Aspects of Coenzymeq*. New York: Elsevier Science, 1991:339–348.

105. Kieburtz K, Feigin A, McDermott M, et al. A controlled trial of remacemide hydrochloride in Huntington's disease. *Mov Disord* 1996; 11:273–277.

106. Peterson PL. The treatment of mitochondrial myopathies and encephalomyopathies. *Biochem Biophys Acta* 1995; 1271:275–280.

107. Shults CW, Beal MF, Fontaine D, et al. Absorption, tolerability, and effects on mitochondrial activity of oral coenzyme Q10 in parkinsonian patients. *Neurology* 1998; 50:793–795.

108. Morris PJ. Cyclosporine, FK-506 and other drugs in organ transplantation. *Curr Opin Immunol* 1991; 3:748–751.

109. Snyder SH, Lai MM, Burnett PE. Immunophilins in the nervous system. *Neuron* 1998; 21:283–294.

110. Sharkey J. Butcher SP. Immunophilins mediate the neuroprotective effects of FK 506 in focal cerebral ischemia. *Nature* 1994; 371:336–339.

111. Steiner JP, Connolly MA, Valentine HL, et al. Neurotrophic actions of nonimmunosuppressive analogues of immunosuppressive drugs FK506, rapamycin and cyclosporin A. *Nat Med* 1997; 3:421–428.

112. Tuszynski MH. Gage FH. Neurotrophic factors and diseases of the nervous system. *Ann Neurol* 1994; 35:S9–S12.

113. Gash DM, Zhang Z, Gerhardt G. Neuroprotective and neurorestorative properties of GDNF. *Ann Neurol* 1998; 44:S121–S125.

114. Kearns CM, Cass WA, Smoot K, et al. GDNF protection against 6-OHDA: Time dependence and requirement for protein synthesis. *J Neurosci* 1997; 17:7111–7118.

115. Hoffer BJ, Hoffmann A, Bowenkamp K, et al. Glial cell line-derived neurotrophic factor reverses toxin-induced injury to midbrain dopaminergic neurons in vivo. *Neurosci Lett* 1994; 182:107–111.

116. Lapchak PA, Gash DM, Jiao S, et al. Glial cell line-derived neurotrophic factor: A novel therapeutic approach to treat motor dysfunction in Parkinson's disease. *Exp Neurol* 1997; 144:29–34.

117. Tseng JL, Baetge EE, Zurn AD, et al. GDNF reduces drug-induced rotational behavior after medial forebrain bundle transection by a mechanism not involving striatal dopamine. *J Neurosci* 1997; 17:325–333.

118. Choi-Lundberg DL, Lin Q, Chang Y-N, et al. Dopaminergic neurons protected from degeneration by GDNF gene therapy. *Science* 1997; 275:838–841.

119. Kang UJ. Potential of gene therapy for Parkinson's disease: Neurobiologic issues and new developments in gene transfer methodologies. *Mov Disord* 1998; 13(Suppl 1):59–72.

120. Marsden CD, Olanow CW. The causes of Parkinson's disease are being unraveled and rational neuroprotective therapy is close to reality. *Ann Neurol* 1998; 44:S189–S196.

121. Polymeropoulos MH, Lavedan C, Leroy E, et al. Mutation in the alpha-synuclein gene identified in families with Parkinson's disease. *Science* 1997; 276:2045–2047.

122. Morrish PK, Sawle GV, Brooks DJ. Clinical and [18F] dopa PET findings in early Parkinson's disease. *J Neurol Neurosurg Psychiatry* 1995; 59:597–600.

123. Morrish PK, Rakshi JS, Bailey DL, et al. Measuring the rate of progression and estimating the preclinical period of Parkinson's disease with [18F]dopa PET. *J Neurol Neurosurg Psychiatry* 1998; 64:314–319.

124. Swerdlow RH, Parks JK, Miller SW, et al. Origin and functional consequences of the complex I defect in Parkinson's disease. *Ann Neurol* 1996; 40:663–671.

125. Leber P. Slowing the progression of Alzheimer disease: Methodologic issues. *Alz Dis Assoc Dis* 1997; 11(Suppl 5):S10–S21.

126. Whitehouse PJ, Kittner BJ, Roessner M, et al. Clinical trial designs for demonstrating disease-course-altering effects in dementia. *Alz Dis Assoc Dis* 1998; 12:281–294.

127. Snow BJ, Tooyama I, McGeer EG, et al. Human positron emission tomographic [18-F]fluorodopa studies correlate with dopamine cell counts and levels. *Ann Neurol* 1993; 34:324–330.

128. Piccini P, Morrish PK, Turjanski N, et al. Dopaminergic function in familial Parkinson's disease: A clinical and 18F-dopa positron emission tomography study. *Ann Neurol* 1997; 41:222–229.

129. Kaufman MJ, Madras BK. Severe depletion of cocaine recognition sites associated with the dopamine transporter in Parkinson's-diseased striatum. *Synapse* 1991; 9:43–49.

130. Seibyl JP, Marek KL, Quinlan D, et al. Decreased single-photon emission computed tomographic [123I]β-CIT striatal uptake correlates with symptom severity in Parkinson's disease. *Ann Neurol* 1995; 38:589–598.

131. Marek KL, Seibyl JP, Zoghbi SS, et al. [123I] beta-CIT/SPECT imaging demonstrates bilateral loss of dopamine transporters in hemi-Parkinson's disease. *Neurology* 1996; 46:231–237.

132. Meegalla SK, Plossl K, Kung MP, et al. Specificity of diastereomers of [99mTc]TRODAT-1 as dopamine transporter imaging agents. *J Med Chem* 1998; 41:428–436.

44

Treatment Approaches for Early Parkinson's Disease

J. Eric Ahlskog, Ph.D., M.D.

Mayo Clinic, Rochester, Minnesota

INTRODUCTION

The subject of the medical treatment of early Parkinson's disease (PD) continues to trigger controversy and philosophic differences. There has been increasing focus on a means of slowing PD progression and possible long-term consequences of early therapy. Much has been written, and some therapeutic recommendations are based on hypothetical constructs and animal models far removed from clinical practice. In this discussion, the focus is on therapeutic strategies primarily based on clinical evidence in humans.

GENERAL NEUROPROTECTIVE STRATEGIES

Background

Parkinson's disease is a progressive disorder. There are two areas of therapeutic concern and interest regarding this progression: (1) levodopa therapy may contribute to the progression; (2) certain other medications may slow disease progression. Most of the therapeutic recommendations relating to these issues have been based on two theoretical constructs, the oxidant stress hypothesis of PD and the MPTP (1-methyl-4-phenyl-1,2,3,6-tetrahydropyridine) model of parkinsonism.

The oxidant stress hypothesis of PD (see Chapter 28) (1,2) is based on the recognition that the dopaminergic substantia nigra is a major focus of the pathology. Dopamine is oxidatively metabolized via monoamine oxidase (MAO), potentially yielding oxyradical metabolites, which can also be generated by dopamine auto-oxidation. Within the substantia nigra, the high iron and neuromelanin concentrations and perhaps reduced scavenger enzyme levels may facilitate these oxyradical reactions. There is evidence of oxyradical damage in postmortem substantia nigra (3–5), although it is uncertain whether this is an epiphenomenon. A final common pathway of cell destruction may involve oxidative processes. A critical implication of the oxidant stress hypothesis is that increased substantia nigra dopamine levels resulting from levodopa treatment may fuel the oxidative fire and result in increased toxic metabolities.

The MPTP model of PD resulted from the discovery that this meperidine analog destroys the substantia nigra and was the cause of levodopa-responsive parkinsonism in humans who self-injected this substance (see Chapter 30) (6). Studies in animals revealed that biologic conversion to the metabolite, MPP+, via MAO-B, is necessary for the substantia nigra toxicity. This can be blocked by pretreatment with MAO-B inhibitors, most notably selegiline (7). An obvious implication from these studies is that selegiline might have a neuroprotective effect in idiopathic PD, assuming that there might be some shared pathophysiologic similarities.

Limiting Levodopa Therapy Because of Concerns About Toxicity

The oxidant stress hypothesis predicts that levodopa treatment should be toxic and this concern has gained much publicity. This concern has been heightened by multiple studies that have shown levodopa to be toxic when added to pure neuronal cell cultures (8). This is problematic for clinicians because levodopa therapy is the most potent and effective treatment available for PD. Numerous lines of evidence, however, argue against substantial levodopa toxicity.

1. Coincident with the introduction of levodopa therapy 30 years ago a significant improvement

in PD mortality rates was observed (9–14) even when potential confounding variables were statistically controlled (15). Parenthetically, a more recent study (16), suggesting increased mortality associated with levodopa therapy (compared to bromocriptine), is uninterpretable because of confounding factors (17).

2. The neuropathologic appearance of PD did not change with the introduction of levodopa therapy (18).

3. PD pathology is not simply confined to dopaminergic or catecholaminergic cells and involves such nuclei as the cholinergic nucleus basalis (19).

4. PD patients from the 1960s, whose levodopa therapy was delayed because of unavailability, gained no advantage over post-levodopa era patients starting levodopa therapy early, (matched for symptom duration) (20).

5. In a one-year treatment trial followed by medication washout, the rates of symptom progression were the same among patients randomized to levodopa versus bromocriptine monotherapy (21).

6. Levodopa treatment of other conditions has not been associated with evidence of clinical deterioration, the development of parkinsonism, or neuropathologic findings of substantia nigra toxicity (22–25).

7. Mice that were administered huge doses of levodopa daily for up to 18 months did not develop substantia nigra pathology (26–28).

8. Lipid peroxidation products (malondialdehyde) don't increase in the circulation with levodopa therapy, in contrast to diabetes mellitus, which is known to be associated with oxidant stress (29).

9. Interpretation of the in vitro evidence of levodopa toxicity is problematic. Cell cultures are devoid of the normal homeostatic and protective mechanisms such as glia, physiologic barriers, and cytoprotective enzymes. Recent studies demonstrated that levodopa is not toxic in vitro when glial cells are present in the culture medium (30,31); in fact, levodopa is neuroprotective in that setting (32).

Thus, despite theoretical concerns about levodopa toxicity, there is little convincing evidence for this.

Selegiline as Neuroprotective Therapy

The MPTP model raised the hypothetical possibility that MAO-B inhibition with selegiline might slow the progression of PD. Theoretically, nigrostriatal

oxidative stress should be reduced by selegiline inhibition of dopamine oxidative metabolism by MAO-B. The large, multi-center DATATOP (Deprenyl and Tocopherol Antioxidative Therapy of Parkinsonism) trial was designed to assess whether selegiline has a neuroprotective effect (33). Although selegiline benefited patients in this study, it was not possible to separate a simple symptomatic effect from an effect on disease progression. Two extensions of this study followed (34,35), with the premise that patients who had received selegiline in the earlier DATATOP trial should have less-advanced disease than the group who had been randomized to placebo. It was expected that these selegiline-treated patients would reach subsequent progression milestones later than placebo-treated patients. However this was not the case. The frequency of progression sufficient to require levodopa initiation (34), and the frequency of developing levodopa motor complications (35) were similar in the two groups. One retrospective study also failed to identify an advantage of early selegiline treatment in reducing the frequency of PD motor progression or levodopa motor complications (36).

A subsequent Swedish multi-center study (37) was modeled after the DATATOP trial, but with a longer (two month) washout phase (i.e., the end-of-study phase when patients were withdrawn from study drugs and then retested). The earlier DATATOP investigation had been criticized because the known 40-day half-life of brain MAO-B inhibition by selegiline (38) exceeded the one-month washout phase. This Swedish study demonstrated that selegiline treatment delayed the need for levodopa initiation, although the delay was modest (four months) and could be explained on the basis of a symptomatic effect. Symptomatic effects were illustrated by significant improvement at six weeks of treatment (wash-in phase) and deterioration during the two-month washout phase. There was a small, but statistically significant beneficial effect of selegiline on the rate of clinical motor progression from baseline to the end of the washout phase. Whether this translates into a true neuroprotective effect is open to speculation.

A significant increase in the mortality rate was associated with chronic selegiline administration in one multi-center investigation (39). However, this potentially worrisome report has been criticized on the basis of methodologic shortcomings (17) and runs contrary to substantial other experience (40).

There is very limited clinical support for selegiline as neuroprotective therapy and it's symptomatic effect confounds interpretation of the clinical trials. Many neurologists who previously prescribed this as the initial treatment for PD patients no longer subscribe to this practice. Despite the paucity of supporting data, some still advocate early selegiline administration, as evidenced by this quote from a recent publication: "Selegiline, because of its putative neuroprotective effect, should therefore be considered as initial treatment for PD" (41).

Dopamine Agonists as Neuroprotective Therapy

Animal models have suggested that pergolide (42), bromocriptine (43), pramipexole (44,45) and ropinirole (45a) may have neuroprotective effects. Similar conclusions have been drawn from in vitro studies of pramipexole (46–48). Neuroprotection by these drugs has not been directly assessed in any clinical trial. Thus, there is currently no good clinical basis for use of dopamine agonist drugs as neuroprotective treatment.

STRATEGIES FOR REDUCING MOTOR COMPLICATIONS: DYSKINESIAS, FLUCTUATIONS

Background

With the passage of several years and progression of PD in that time, levodopa treatment often results in less consistent effects. Early in the course, levodopa therapy produces a long-duration response (55); the effect is not dependent on the timing of the levodopa dose and these patients do not experience a clinical decline for several days if they discontinue levodopa. Later in the course, many patients experience a short-duration levodopa effect as their primary response; following each levodopa dose, motor improvement lasts several hours or less and then the effect "wears off." Sometimes the effects change rapidly ("on-off") and occasional doses don't kick-in ("skipped dose effects" or "no-on"). These phenomena are the basis for so-called clinical fluctuations. Superimposed on these clinical problems are levodopa-induced dyskinesias, which can be severe and disabling in their own right (see Chapter 40). Much has been written about early treatment strategies that might delay, present, or reduce the subsequent frequency of these motor complications of levodopa therapy.

Pathophysiology of Levodopa-Related Motor Fluctuations and Dyskinesias

Both pre and postsynaptic mechanisms appear to contribute to these motor problems. Prominent clinical fluctuations do not occur early in this progressive disease and presumably do not appear until the loss of striatal dopaminergic presynaptic terminals becomes marked and reaches a threshold (56). Both animal

models (57,58), and experience with MPTP-induced Parkinsonism in humans (59), indicate that severe dopaminergic nigrostriatal loss is a necessary prerequisite for levodopa motor complications. When depletion of dopaminergic terminals is nearly complete, (at least within restricted regions of the striatum), synaptic dopamine concentrations presumably can no longer be regulated. There is no steady presynaptic release to maintain continuous dopamine concentrations or reuptake to prevent excessive levels.

Postsynaptic mechanisms also appear to play a role in the development of levodopa motor complications. In the normal state, dopaminergic stimulation of striatal receptors is primarily tonic, which contrasts with the intermittent stimulation of oral levodopa therapy. Ongoing pulsatile stimulation may induce downstream receptor effects that promote motor fluctuations and dyskinesias (60,61). Evidence in favor includes the following:

1. Monkeys with severe MPTP-induced nigrostriatal neuronal loss, do not develop dyskinesias immediately after oral levodopa administration; these occur after a minimum of a few days to several of weeks of therapy (58,62), consistent with an effect induced downstream from the receptor.
2. Switching to continuous intravenous levodopa infusion for 1–2 weeks reduces motor swings and elevates the dyskinesia threshold in fluctuating PD patients (63); on reinstitution of oral therapy, reversion to the baseline state develops over about a week (63).
3. After chronic, continuous dopamine agonist infusion, the thresholds for levodopa fluctuations improve substantially (64).

This evidence has raised concern that routine levodopa administration may predispose to subsequent motor fluctuations and dyskinesias (65). These concerns have generated a variety of alternative treatment strategies, and each of these based on their clinical merits will be considered.

Delaying Levodopa Therapy to Delay Fluctuations

An often-cited retrospective study of PD patients seen in a movement disorder clinic suggested that early levodopa initiation predisposes to wearing-off and on–off phenomena (66); a subsequent study found similar results (67). These studies were criticized because of substantial patient selection bias; patients presenting with more severe and more progressive disease were more likely to have been started early on levodopa therapy (68). Four subsequent retrospective

Dopamine Agonist Medication Dosing
(See Chapter 35)

If a dopamine agonist is chosen as early therapy, the North American physician has four choices: bromocriptine (Parlodel), pergolide (Permax), pramipexole (Mirapex), and ropinirole (Requip). Because bromocriptine carries no obvious advantages and is the most expensive, this drug is the least preferred. Among the remaining three drugs, there is no clinical data favoring one over the others. Because pergolide is an ergot drug, it may have greater potential for side effects, although comparative studies are lacking.

The initial dosing principles are the same for all four drugs; each is started in very low dosage (subtherapeutic) and then slowly advanced. The pharmaceutical companies provide printed dosing escalation instructions for patients and such printed guides are advisable to avoid patient confusion.

CONCLUSION

Levodopa therapy remains the most efficacious treatment for PD, but motor fluctuations, dyskinesias, and levodopa-refractory symptoms eventually complicate the course. Early medication strategies have been proposed as means of reducing the subsequent development of these problems, but to date, none are supported by clinical evidence. Levodopa remains the most efficacious therapy for PD, but motor fluctuations and dyskinesias typically complicate the long-term course. Early treatment with a dopamine agonist has been proposed to reduce the subsequent frequency of these motor complications; however, it is unclear if that strategy would be just as effective if deferred until the time the motor complications actually develop.

REFERENCES

1. Olanow CW. Oxidation reactions in Parkinson's disease. *Neurology* 1990; 40(Suppl 3):32–37.
2. Fahn S, Cohen G. The oxidant stress hypothesis in Parkinson's disease: evidence supporting it. [Review]. *Ann Neurol* 1992; 32(6):804–812.
3. Dexter DT, Carter CJ, Wells FR, et al. Basal lipid peroxidation in substantia nigra is increased in Parkinson's disease. *J Neurochem* 1989; 52(2):381–389.
4. Dexter DT, Holley AE, Flitter WD, et al. Increased levels of lipid hydroperoxides in the parkinsonian substantia nigra: an HPLC and ESR study. *Mov Disord* 1994; 9:92–97.
5. Sanchez-Ramos J, Overvik E, LeWitt P, et al. A marker of oxyradical-mediated DNA damage (8-hydroxy-2'-deoxyguanosine) is increased in striatum of Parkinson's disease brain. *Mov Disord* 1993; 8:404.
6. Langston JW, Ballard P, Tetrud JW, et al. Chronic parkinsonism in humans due to a product of meperidine-analog synthesis. *Science* 1983; 219:979–980.
7. Snyder SH, D'Amato RJ. A neurotoxin relevant to the pathophysiology of Parkinson's disease. *Neurology* 1986; 36:250–258.
8. Fahn S. Levodopa-induced neurotoxicity: does it represent a problem for the treatment of Parkinson's disease? *CNS Drugs* 1997; 8:376–393.
9. Sweet RD, Mc Dowell FH. Five years' treatment of Parkinson's disease with levodopa: therapeutic results and survival of 100 patients. *Ann Intern Med* 1975; 83:456–463.
10. Diamond SG, Markham CH. Present mortality in Parkinson's disease: the ratio of observed to expected deaths with a method to calculate expected deaths. *J Neural Transm* 1976; 38:259–269.
11. Zumstein H, Siegfried J. Mortality among parkinson patients treated with l-dopa combined with a decarboxylase inhibitor. *Eur Neurol* 1976; 14:321–327.
12. Martilla RJ, Rinne UK, Siirtola T, et al. Mortality of patients with Parkinson's disease treated with levodopa. *J Neurol* 1977; 216:147–148.
13. Joseph C, Chassan JB, Koch ML. Levodopa in Parkinson's disease: a long-term appraisal of mortality. *Ann Neurol* 1978; 3:116–118.
14. Hoehn MM. Parkinsonism treated with levodopa: progression and mortality. *J Neural Transm* 1983; 19(Suppl 1):253–264.
15. Uitti RJ, Ahlskog JE, Maraganore DM, et al. Levodopa therapy and survival in idiopathic Parkinson's disease: Olmsted County Project. *Neurology* 1993; 43:1918–1926.
16. Przuntek H, Welzel D, Blumner E, et al. Bromocriptine lessens the incidence of mortality in L-dopa-treated parkinsonian patients: PRADO-study discontinued. *Eur J Clin Pharmacol* 1992; 43(4):357–363.
17. Ahlskog JE. Neuroprotective strategies in the treatment of Parkinson's disease: Clinical evidence. In: LeWitt P, Oertel W, (eds.). *Parkinson's Disease: The Treatment Options*. London: Martin Dunitz, 1998.
18. Yahr MD, Wolf A, Antunes J-L, et al. Autopsy findings in parkinsonism following treatment with levodopa. *Neurology* 1972; 22(Suppl):56–71.
19. Jellinger K. Overview of morphological changes in Parkinson's disease. *Adv Neurol* 1987; 45:1–18.
20. Markham CH, Diamond SG. Long-term follow-up of early dopa treatment in Parkinson's disease. *Ann Neurol* 1986; 19:365–372.
21. Olanow CW, Hauser R, Gauger L, et al. The effect of deprenyl and levodopa on the progression of Parkinson's disease. *Ann Neurol* 1995; 38:771–777.
22. Quinn N, Parkes D, Janota I, et al. Preservation of the substantia nigra and locus coeruleus in a patient

receiving levodopa (2 kg) plus decarboxylase inhibitor over a four-year period. *Mov Disord* 1986; 1:65–68.

23. Nygaard TG, Marsden CD, Fahn S. Dopa-responsive dystonia: long-term treatment response and prognosis. *Neurology* 1991; 41:174–181.

24. Rajput AH, Fenton ME, Dhand A. Is levodopa toxic to nondegenerating substantia nigra cells? clinical evidence. *Neurology* 1996; 46(Supplement):A371.

25. Riley D. Is levodopa toxic to human substantia nigra? *Mov Disord* 1998; 13:369–370.

26. Sahakian BJ, Carlson KR, De Girolami U, al. e. Functional and structural consequences of long-term dietary l-dopa treatment in mice. *Comm Psychopharmacol* 1980; 4:169–176.

27. Hefti F, Melamed E, Bhawan J, et al. Long-term administration of l-dopa does not damage dopaminergic neurons in the mouse. *Neurology* 1981; 31:1194–1195.

28. Cotzias GC, Miller ST, Tang LC, et al. Levodopa, fertility and longevity. *Science* 1977; 196:549–551.

29. Ahlskog JE, Uitti RJ, Low PA, et al. Levodopa and deprenyl treatment effects on peripheral indices of oxidant stress in Parkinson's disease. *Neurology* 1996; 46:796–801.

30. Mena MA, Casarejos MJ, Carazo A, et al. Glia conditioned medium protects fetal rat midbrain neurones in culture from L-DOPA toxicity. *Neuroreport* 1996; 7:441–445.

31. Mena MA, Casarejos MJ, Carazo A, et al. Glia protect fetal midbrain dopamine neurons in culture from L-DOPA toxicity through multiple mechanisms. *J Neural Transm* 1997; 104:317–328.

32. Mena MA, Davila V, Sulzer D. Neurotrophic effects of L-DOPA in postnatal midbrain dopamine neuron/cortical astrocyte cocultures. *J Neurochem* 1997; 69:1398–1408.

33. Parkinson Study Group. Effects of tocopherol and deprenyl on the progression of disability in early Parkinson's disease. *N Engl J Med* 1993; 328:176–183.

34. Parkinson Study Group. Impact of deprenyl and tocopherol treatment on Parkinson's disease in DATATOP subjects not requiring levodopa. *Ann Neurol* 1996; 39:29–36.

35. Parkinson Study Group. Impact of deprenyl and tocopherol treatment on Parkinson's disease in DATATOP patients requiring levodopa. *Ann Neurol* 1996; 39:37–45.

36. Brannan T, Yahr MD. Comparative study of selegiline plus l-dopa-carbidopa versus l-dopa-carbidopa alone in the treatment of Parkinson's disease. *Ann Neurol* 1995; 37:95–98.

37. Palhagen S, Heinonen EH, Hagglund J, et al. Seleglinie delays the onset of disability in de novo parkinsonian patients. *Neurology* 1998; 51:520–525.

38. Fowler JS, Volkow ND, Logan J, et al. Slow recovery of human brain MAO B after L-deprenyl (Selegeline) withdrawal. *Synapse* 1994; 18(2):86–93.

39. Lees AJ, on behalf of the Parkinson's Disease Research Group of the United Kingdom. Comparison of therapeutic effects and mortality data of levodopa and levodopa combined with selegiline in patients with early, mild Parkinson's disease. *BMJ* 1995; 311:1602–1607.

40. Olanow CW, Myllyla VV, Sotaniemi KA, et al. Effect of selegiline on mortality in patients with Parkinson's disease. A meta analysis. *Neurology* 1998; 51:825–830.

41. Olanow CW, Koller WC. An algorithm (decision tree) for the management of Parkinson's disease: treatment guidelines. *Neurology* 1998; 50(Suppl 3):S1–S57.

42. Felten DL, Felten SY, Fuller RW, et al. Chronic dietary pergolide preserves nigrostriatal neuronal integrity in aged Fischer 344 rats. *Neurobiol Aging* 1992; 13:339–351.

43. Ogawa N, Tanaka K, Asanuma M, et al. Bromocriptine protects mice against 6-hydroxydopamine and scavenges hydroxyl free radicals in vitro. *Brain Res* 1994; 657:207–213.

44. Hall ED, Andrus PK, Oostveen JA, et al. Neuroprotective effects of the dopamine D2/D3 agonist pramipexole against postischemic or amphetamine-induced degeneration of nigrostriatal neurons. *Brain Res* 1996; 742:80–88.

45. Sethy VH, Wu H, Oostveen JA, Hall ED. Neuroprotective effects of the dopamine agonist pramipexole and bromocriptine in 3-acetylpyridine-treated rats. *Brain Res* 1997; 754:181–186.

45a. Iida M, Miyazaki I, Tanaka K, Kabuto H, Iwata-Ichikawa E, Ogawa N. Dopamine D2 receptor-mediated antioxidant and neuroprotective effects of ropinirole, a dopamine agonist. *Brain Res* 1999; 838(1–2):51–9.

46. Carvey PM, Ling Z-D. The case for neuroprotection with dopamine agonists. *Clin Neuropharmacol* 1997; 20(Suppl. 1):S8–S21.

47. Carvey PM, Ling ZD. Attenuation of levodopa-induced toxicity in mesencephalic cultures by pramipexole. *J Neural Transm* 1997; 104:209–228.

48. Cassarino DS, Fall CP, Smith TS, et al. Pramipexole reduces reactive oxygen species production in vivo and in vitro and inhibits the mitochondrial permeability transition produced by the parkinsonian neurotoxin methylpyridinium ion. *J Neurochem* 1998; 71(1):295–301.

49. Rinne UK. Early combination of bromocriptine and levodopa in the treatment of Parkinson's disease: a 5-year follow up. *Neurology* 1987; 37:826–828.

50. Bergamasco B, Benna P, Scarzella L. Long-term bromocriptine treatment of de novo patients with Parkinson's disease. A seven-year follow-up. *Acta Neurol Scand* 1990; 81:383–387.

51. Nakanishi T, Iwata M, Goto I, et al. Nation-wide collaborative study on the long-term effects of bromocriptine in the treatment of Parkinson's disease: final report. *Eur Neurol* 1992; 32(Suppl 1):9–22.

52. Parkinson's Disease Research Group in the United Kingdom. Comparisons of therapeutic effects of levodopa, levodopa and selegiline, and bromocriptine

in patients with early, mild Parkinson's disease: three year interim report. *BMJ* 1993; 307:469–472.

53. Hely MA, Morris JGL, Reid WGJ, et al. The Sydney multicentre study of Parkinson's disease: a randomized, prospective five year study comparing low dose bromocriptine with low dose levodopa-carbidopa. *J Neurol Neurosurg Psychiatry* 1994; 57:903–910.

54. Mizuno Y, Kondo T, Narabayashi H. Pergolide in the treatment of Parkinson's disease. *Neurology* 1995; 45(Suppl 3):S13–S21.

55. Muenter MD, Tyce GM. L-dopa therapy of Parkinson's disease: plasma l-dopa concentration, therapeutic response, and side effects. *Mayo Clin Proc* 1971; 46:231–239.

56. Leenders KL, Palmer AJ, Quinn N, et al. Brain dopamine metabolism in patients with Parkinson's disease measured with positron emission tomography. *J Neurol Neurosurg Psychiatry* 1986; 49:853–860.

57. Papa SM, Engber TM, Kask AM, et al. Motor fluctuations in levodopa treated parkinsonian rats: relation to lesion extent and treatment duration. *Brain Res* 1994; 662:69–74.

58. Schneider JS. Levodopa-induced dyskinesias in parkinsonian monkeys: relationship to extent of nigrostriatal damage. *Pharmacol Biochem Behav* 1989; 34:193–196.

59. Ballard PA, Tetrud JW, Langston JW. Permanent human parkinsonism due to 1-methyl-4-phenyl-1,2,3,6-tetrahydropyridine (MPTP): seven cases. *Neurology* 1985; 35:949–956.

60. Chase TN. Levodopa therapy: consequences of the nonphysiologic replacement of dopamine. *Neurology* 1998; 50(Suppl 5):S17–25.

61. Chase TN. The significance of continuous dopaminergic stimulation in the treatment of Parkinson's disease. *Drugs* 1998; 55(Suppl 1):1–9.

62. Bedard PJ, DiPaolo T, Falardeau P, et al. Chronic treatment with l-dopa, but not bromocriptine induces dyskinesia in MPTP-parkinsonian monkeys. Correlation with [3H]spiperone binding. *Brain Res* 1986; 379:294–299.

63. Mouradian MM, Heuser JE, Baronti F, et al. Modification of central dopaminergic mechanisms by continuous levodopa therapy for advanced Parkinson's disease. *Ann Neurol* 1990; 27:18–23.

64. Baronti F, Mouradian MM, Davis TL, et al. Continuous lisuride effects on central dopaminergic mechanisms in Parkinson's disease. *Ann Neurol* 1992; 32:776–781.

65. Fahn S. Welcome news about levodopa, but uncertainty remains (Editorial). *Ann Neurol* 1998; 43:551–553.

66. Lesser RP, Fahn S, Snider SR, et al. Analysis of the clinical problems in parkinsonism and the complications of long-term levodopa therapy. *Neurology* 1979; 29:1253–1260.

67. DeJong GJ, Meerwaldt JD, Schmitz PIM. Factors that influence the occurrence of response variations in Parkinson's disease. *Ann Neurol* 1987; 22:4–7.

68. Cedarbaum JM, Gandy SE, Mc Dowell FH. "Early" initiation of levodopa treatment does not promote the development of motor response fluctuations, dyskinesias or dementia in Parkinson's disease. *Neurology* 1991; 41:622–629.

69. Blin J, Bonnet AM, Agid Y. Does levodopa aggravate Parkinson's disease? *Neurology* 1988; 38:1410–1416.

70. Roos RAC, Vredevoogd CB, van der Velde EA. Response fluctuations in Parkinson's disease. *Neurology* 1990; 40:1344–1346.

71. Caraceni T, Scigliano G, Musicco M. The occurrence of motor fluctuations in parkinsonian patients treated long-term with levodopa: role of early treatment and disease progression. *Neurology* 1991; 41:380–384.

72. Trabucchi M, Appollonio I, Battaini F, et al. Influence of treatment on the natural history of Parkinson's disease. In: Calne DB, ed. *Parkinsonism and Aging.* New York, N.Y.: Raven Press, 1989:239–254.

73. Bergmann KJ, Mendoza MR, Yahr MD. Parkinson's disease and long-term levodopa therapy. In: Yahr MD, Bergmann KJ, (eds.), *Advances in Neurology. Parkinson's Disease.* New York: Raven Press, 1986:463–467. vol 45).

74. Poewe WH, Lees AJ, Stern GM. Low-dose l-dopa therapy in Parkinson's disease: a 6-year follow-up study. *Neurology* 1986; 36:1528–1530.

75. Block G, Liss C, Reines S, et al. Comparison of immediate-release and controlled release carbidopa/levodopa in Parkinson's disease. *Eur Neurol* 1997; 37:23–27.

76. DuPont E, Andersen A, Boas J, et al. Sustained-release Madopar HBS compared with standard Madopar in the long-term treatment of de novo parkinsonian patients. *Acta Neurol Scand* 1996; 93:14–20.

77. Yeh KC, August TF, Bush DF, et al. Pharmacokinetics and bioavailability of Sinemet CR: a summary of human studies. *Neurology* 1989; 39(Suppl 2):25–38.

78. Bedard PJ, Mancilla BG, Blanchette P, et al. Levodopa-induced dyskinesia: facts and fancy. What does the MPTP monkey model tell us? *Can J Neurol Sci* 1992; 19:134–137.

79. Kurth MC, Adler CH. COMT inhibition: a new treatment strategy for Parkinson's disease. *Neurology* 1998; 50(Suppl 5):S3–S14.

80. Lupp A, Lucking CH, Koch R, et al. Inhibitory effects of the antiparkinson drugs memantine and amantadine on N-methyl-D-aspartate-evoked acetylcholine release in the rabbit caudate nucleus in vitro. *J Pharm Exp Ther* 1992; 263:717–724.

81. Stoof JC, Booij J, Drukarch B. Amantadine as N-methyl-D-aspartic acid receptor antagonist: new possibilities for therapeutic applications. *Clin Neurol Neurosurg* 1992; 94((Suppl)):S4–S6.

82. Kornhuber J, Weller M, Schoppmeyer K, et al. Amantadine and memantine are NMDA receptor antagonists with neuroprotective properties. [Review]. *J Neural Transmission.* 1994; 43:91–104.

83. Uitti RJ, Rajput AH, Ahlskog JE, et al. Amantadine treatment is an independent predictor of impro-

ved survival in parkinsonism. *Neurology* 1996; 46:1551–1556.

84. Rinne UK. Dopamine agonists as primary treatment in Parkinson's disease. In: Yahr MD, Bergmann KJ, (eds.). *Advances in Neurology*. New York, NY: Raven Press, 1986; 45:519–523.

85. Factor SA, Weiner WJ. Early combination therapy with bromocriptine and levodopa in Parkinson's disease. *Mov Disord* 1993; 8(No. 3):257–262.

86. Weiner WJ, Factor SA, Sanchez-Ramos JR, et al. Early combination therapy (bromocriptine and levodopa) does not prevent motor fluctuations in Parkinson's disease. *Neurology* 1993; 43:21–27.

87. Montastruc JL, Rascol L, Senard JM, et al. A randomized controlled study comparing bromocriptine to which levodopa was later added, with levodopa alone in previously untreated patients with Parkinson's disease: a five year follow up. *J Neurol Neurosurg Psychiatry* 1994; 57:1034–1038.

88. Przuntek H, Welzel D, Gerlach M, et al. Early institution of bromocriptine in Parkinson's disease inhibits the emergence of levodopa-associated motor side effects. Long term results of the PRADO study. *J Neural Transm* 1996; 103:699–715.

89. Gimenez-Roldan S, Tolosa E, Burguera JA, et al. Early combination of bromocriptine and levodopa in Parkinson's disease: a prospective randomized study of two parallel groups over a total follow-up period of 44 months including an initial 8-month double-blind stage. *Clin Neuropharmacol* 1997; 20:67–76.

90. Rascol O, Brooks D, Korczyn AD, et al. A five-year study of the incidence of dyskinesia in patients with early Parkinson's disease who were treated with ropinirole or levodopa. *N Engl J Med* 2000; 342:1484–1491.

91. Parkinson Study Group. A randomized controlled trial comparing the agonist pramipexole with levodopa as initial dopaminergic treatment for Parkinson's disease. *JAMA* 2000.

92. Quinn N. Young onset Parkinson's disease. *Mov Disord* 1987; 2:73–91.

93. Quinn NP. A case against early levodopa treatment of Parkinson's disease. *Clin Neuropharmacol* 1994; 17(suppl 3):S43–S49.

94. Nutt JG, Woodward WR, Hammerstad JP, et al. The "on-off" phenomenon in Parkinson's disease: Relation to levodopa absorption and transport. *N Engl J Med* 1884; 310:483–488.

45

Progress in Gene Therapy

M. Maral Mouradian, M.D.

National Institute of Neurological Disorders and Stroke, National Institutes of Health, Bethesda, Maryland

INTRODUCTION

Experience over the past three decades has demonstrated clearly that classical pharmacotherapy of Parkinson's disease (PD) is suboptimal because motor response fluctuations complicate the course of most patients with advanced disease (1). Furthermore, this approach provides only symptomatic relief and no current therapy has been definitively shown to retard the relentless loss of nigral dopaminergic neurons. Thus, the need to develop novel treatment strategies that would target the basic defect of PD in an effort to arrest or retard the degenerative process is well recognized. Although fetal nigral tissue implantation is promising, it is associated with a number of logistical and ethical issues that tend to limit the availability of this procedure to the large parkinsonian patient population (2). More practical and reproducible means for delivering therapeutic genes would allow larger scale systematic evaluation of efficacy. Advances in molecular biology and virology in recent years have enabled the technology of gene transfer to proceed forward. In fact, despite the disappointingly slow progress in initial clinical trials of gene therapy for other disorders, this novel therapeutic modality holds considerable potential for degenerative central nervous system (CNS) diseases.

Parkinson's disease is a particularly appropriate target for gene therapy because (1) the brain pathology is fully characterized and relatively well circumscribed largely within the nigrostriatal dopaminergic neurons; (2) animal models are available permitting preclinical testing in proof-of-principle experiments; and (3) several candidate genes known to favorably impact dopaminergic neurons in vitro and in vivo are cloned. In addition, the search for genetic mutations responsible for familial forms of PD has accelerated in recent years with several genes

or loci already identified (3–6). Thus, gene transfer could be envisioned to provide an adjunct to or a replacement for conventional pharmacotherapy in PD.

Although little doubt remains about the timeliness of gene-based therapy for PD, progress in gene delivery methods has lagged behind the conceptual development. This slow start is especially true for CNS disorders because of the inaccessibility of the brain and its structural and physiologic complexities. To date, clinical gene therapy has been attempted in only two CNS disorders, malignant brain tumors and Canavan disease (7,8). The current state of research in gene therapy for PD is typical of early development efforts for any novel therapeutic modality. Uncertainties about optimal gene transfer methodology have prompted testing a variety of available strategies. Thus, different combinations of delivery methods and candidate therapeutic genes have been tested in animal models of PD with various degrees of reported success (9–14).

The development of gene-based therapies for PD requires two primary considerations: (1) what gene should be targeted and (2) how to deliver that gene. Ideally, the development of a rational strategy for gene-based therapy first requires the identification of the defective gene and characterization of the normal gene product. Elucidation of the functional properties of a protein is essential before a feasible plan for gene delivery can be formulated. Finally, understanding the mechanism by which the mutation alters the phenotype is crucial, particularly knowing whether it results in loss of a normal function or gain of a toxic function. In case of the latter scenario, adding a normal copy of the gene would not eliminate the defective dominant mutant phenotype. Although the genes responsible for PD are being unraveled and their functions and pathogenic mechanisms are still not clear, current alternative gene-therapy approaches include either augmentation of dopaminergic neurotransmission or attempting to preserve residual nigral dopamine neurons by targeting compensatory or secondary molecular pathways. The latter can potentially be achieved by delivering neuroprotective or neurorestorative proteins, or by blocking toxic gene products. Thus, the goal of gene therapy for PD is not limited to replacement of a defective gene responsible for the basic disease process.

METHODS OF GENE TRANSFER TO THE BRAIN

Two main approaches to gene-based therapy are being pursued for PD (Figure 45-1). The first is the in vivo approach that involves direct introduction of a therapeutic gene into an appropriate brain region such as striatum or substantia nigra. The second is ex vivo approach that involves the introduction of a therapeutic gene into an appropriate cell type in culture, selection of appropriate clones, expansion to the necessary number of cells, followed by grafting the engineered cells into the brain.

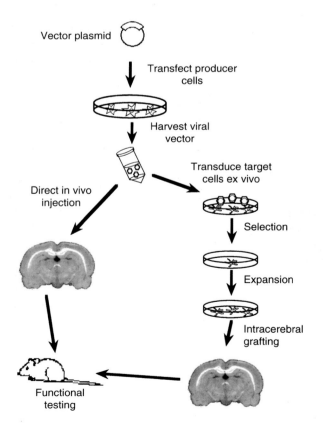

FIGURE 45-1. Schematic of procedures in the in vivo (left) and ex vivo (right) gene-transfer methods.

In vivo gene transfer can be achieved by viral vectors or by plasmids, but the former method remains the most efficient. In addition, viral vectors can be designed to accommodate one or more therapeutically relevant genes and can be sufficiently attenuated to prevent destructive infection in the brain. Plasmids, which can be used either as naked DNA or with cationic liposomes, result in shorter lived gene expression than viral vectors and, therefore, are generally not useful for a chronic disorder such as PD.

VIRAL VECTORS

Different viral vectors have been developed for somatic gene therapy (Table 45-1). In general, they are designed to be devoid of their cytopathogenic genes, which are replaced by the therapeutic gene(s). Many of these vectors have been used in experimental gene-transfer studies in animal models of PD. These vectors vary with respect to their physical and biologic characteristics as well as their tropism to the different cellular populations of the brain. Consequently, these properties dictate the suitability of each vector system for in vivo vs ex vivo gene-transfer methods.

Viral vectors that can be used for gene transfer to the brain should be neuronotropic such as those derived from herpes simplex virus type 1, adenovirus, adeno-associated virus or lentivirus. Although retroviruses generally require replicating cells for their life cycle, a lentiviral vector based on the human immunodeficiency virus 1, capable of infecting striatal and hippocampal neurons and expressing the transgene in adult rats, holds considerable promise (15).

Herpes Simplex Virus Type I

Herpes simplex virus type I (HSV-1) is a large neuronotropic virus that can infect a wide range of host cells and establishes latency indefinitely within neurons. HSV-1–based vectors have been used in a variety of experimental systems (16). Two different means of exploiting the HSV virus have been developed: (1) recombinant HSV-1 with various deletions that render the virus replication defective; and (2) HSV-1 amplicon based on plasmids containing the transgene with minimal HSV-1 sequences. Such a plasmid is transfected into a complementing cell line along with a helper virus for packaging. The term *amplicon* refers to the fact that multiple repeats of the plasmid are packaged allowing delivery of several copies of the transgene into a single cell, thus amplifying the signal.

Although HSV-1-based vectors were the first to introduce transgenes into postmitotic neurons

PROGRESS IN GENE THERAPY

509

Table 45-1 Viral Vectors for Gene Therapy

Virus	Integration in Host Genome	Target Cells	Advantages	Disadvantages
HSV-1	No	Neurons	Large insert size, latency	Cytotoxic
Adenovirus	No	Glia > Neurons	High titer, efficient	Immunogenic
AAV	Ch 19, some episomal	Neurons > Glia	Nonpathogenic	Low titer, needs helper virus
Retrovirus	Random integration	Dividing cells only	Most experience	For ex vivo gene transfer only
Lentivirus	Random integration	Dividing and nondividing, neurons	Low immune reaction	No packaging cell line, concerns about HIV virus

successfully, it has many disadvantages including the possibility of reversion from mutant to wild type HSV-1 resulting in lytic encephalitis. Because a high percentage of people have latent HSV-1 residing in the trigeminal ganglion, the theoretical possibility exists for a recombination event between latent HSV-1 and the engineered vector resulting in lytic infection or reactivation of latent HSV-1 in the CNS. A number of studies also reported cytotoxicity associated with several HSV-1 vectors. Part of the cytotoxicity could be due to the fact that these defective vectors require the presence of a helper virus to provide missing proteins needed to generate a virus stock. But recent attempts have been made to attenuate these risks. Newer generation vectors with multiple deletions to reduce the risk for neurovirulence and cytotoxicity (17–19) as well as an amplicon vector free of helper virus have been developed (20). Furthermore, the large genome of HSV-1, which expresses approximately 80 viral genes, also raises concerns about its safety as a gene delivery vector and highlights the need for detailed analysis of its biology. In addition to safety concerns, HSV-1–based vectors are limited by relatively low-infection efficiency and suboptimal long-term expression.

Adenovirus

Adenovirus is the common cold virus, which is considered a candidate for in vivo gene transfer in the brain because of its high titer virus stocks, efficient infection of postmitotic neuronal cells, and the relatively benign course of its infection (21,22). The adenoviral genome stays episomal, that is, nonintegrated in host chromosomal DNA, which makes it less than ideal for long-term expression of transgenes. The predominant cell type in the brain that is infected with adenovirus vector appears to be astrocytes (23). However, the main shortcoming of

adenoviral vectors is their tendency to elicit intense immune reaction from the host with inflammation and gliosis. Thus, current adenovirus vectors are useful for short-term experiments but do not appear to be practical for long-term treatment because of significant immunogenicity. Attempts are under way to develop vectors with reduced immunogenicity and toxicity.

AAV

AAV is a nonpathogenic parvovirus, which requires a helper virus such as adenovirus or HSV-1 for productive infection. It can infect both dividing and nondividing cells. AAV-derived vectors have several advantages including the fact that most of the wild-type viral genome is deleted and therefore have minimal deleterious consequences. AAV vectors can be obtained that are entirely free of helper viruses and that do not encode any viral proteins. This is a significant improvement over other viral vectors such as HSV-1 and adenovirus that retain the ability to synthesize viral proteins. Thus, the main advantage of AAV-based vectors is the apparent absence of significant cytotoxicity. In addition, AAV integrates into a specific site on chromosome 19, permitting increased DNA stability and longer expression time (24). Minor disadvantages include significantly lower viral titers than those obtained for adenovirus and small insert size which is generally not an issue for most currently known candidate therapeutic genes for PD. Largely due to their nonpathogenicity, AAV-based vectors are likely to be used initially in clinical applications for brain disorders.

Retroviruses

Retroviruses are RNA viruses that require dividing cells for their reverse transcription and integration into host chromosomal DNA. Disabled Moloney murine leukemia viruses have been widely used for ex vivo gene transfer for many years. Advantages include high infection rate and transgene expression as well as availability of packaging cell lines. In addition to relatively low viral titers, disadvantages include random integration in the host genome raising concerns about mutagenesis due to disruption of a tumor-suppressor gene or activation of an oncogene, although none has been observed to date. Homologous recombination of vector sequences with the retroviral genome in the packaging cell line could potentially generate wild type virus. However, current generations of packaging cells have minimal sequence overlap and helper virus genes are separated into separate plasmids. Finally, recombination of the retroviral vector with unsuspected dormant retroviral sequences in the host that lead to generation of a pathogenic virus is also a concern.

Lentiviruses

Lentiviruses unlike other retroviruses, have the ability to infect nondividing cells such as neurons. A vector based on the human immunodeficiency virus (HIV-1) has been shown to transduce nonproliferating adult rat brain neurons in vivo (15). Transgene expression is maintained for several months without appreciable decline and no obvious pathogenic changes or immune response has been detected. Because HIV-1 interferes with host cell division, development of packaging cell lines that can facilitate vector generation has been somewhat hampered.

CELL VEHICLES FOR EX VIVO GENE TRANSFER FOR PARKINSON'S DISEASE

Ex vivo engineering of cells with cDNAs encoding candidate therapeutic proteins is also being explored in Parkinson models. Several different cell types have been used in preclinical studies to assess their suitability for engineering in culture and subsequent transplantation into the brain to deliver secreted molecules (Table 45-2). Early studies that used cell lines including fibroblasts, Schwann cells, myoblasts, neuroblastoma, glioma, and neuroendocrine cells reported varying degrees of success and reproducibility (13,25,26). Not surprisingly, such cells were quickly abandoned for gene transfer applications because they generally either form large expanding tumors or are killed by host immune defense mechanisms.

The possibility of tumor formation as a result of grafting free floating cell lines is a major source of concern. This situation has stimulated the development

Table 45-2   Cell Types for Ex Vivo Gene therapy in Animal Models of Parkinson's Disease
Fibroblasts
Myoblasts
Astrocytes
Schwann cells
Transformed cell lines
CNS stem cells
Encapsulated cells

of polymer encapsulated cell technology using a semipermeable membrane that allows free exchange of nutrients, oxygen, and therapeutic gene products, while shielding the implanted cells from immune attack by the host. In addition, the physical barrier of the polymer device prevents uncontrolled cellular proliferation and mass formation. This approach has been tested in experimental animal models of PD to secrete dopamine (27) or GDNF (28–30) with variable degrees of success.

Another means of circumventing the limitations of grafted cell lines is the application of molecular techniques of conditional immortalization using nontransforming oncogenes such as the temperature sensitive allele of the SV 40 large tumor antigen. This manipulation allows cell growth at low permissive temperatures (around 33 °C) in culture but not at the body temperature of 37 °C. Immortalization of rat fetal mesencephalic neurons with this method has been tested in 6-OHDA lesioned rats demonstrating behavioral recovery without immune rejection or tumor formation (31). Delivery of the tyrosine hydroxylase (TH) cDNA using such cells increases levodopa production in rodent and nonhuman primate models of PD (32). Alternatively, the use of cell lines that differentiate into neurons under appropriate conditions has also been tried. For example, PC12 cells engineered with NGF under the control of the zinc-inducible metallothionein promoter differentiate into neurons when grafted in the rat striatum (33).

The idea of an autologous source of cells that are easily obtained from the patient and readily transduced by therapeutic genes in vitro has stimulated the use of primary skin fibroblasts as vehicles for gene transfer (34–36). However, survival of these cells in the brain is not reliably predictable. In addition, instead of integrating with host brain circuitry, they tend to displace the brain parenchyma by forming a globular clump of cells which itself can disrupt rotational behavior (35).

Astrocytes have also been tested because of their natural supportive role in brain, their efficient secretory mechanisms, their transducibility in vitro and their tendency to migrate from the graft site thus minimizing mass effect (37,38). Furthermore, astrocytes potentially represent autologous source of cell vehicles (39). Immature astrocytes from the rat brain transduced with the TH cDNA and transplanted in the striatum of 6-OHDA lesioned rats have been reported to survive and migrate. Although only few grafted cells expressed TH in vivo, some behavioral recovery was demonstrated (40). Astrocytes have also been used as cografts with embryonic ventral mesencephalic neuronal grafts that result in variable effects depending on the age of astrocytes and whether they expressed recombinant BDNF (41). An immortalized human fetal astrocyte cell line expressing TH injected in the striatum of 6-OHDA lesioned rats reportedly resulted in behavioral recovery but poor graft survival (42).

The ideal cell for CNS somatic gene therapy would be cells of CNS origin with many neuronal features such as storage mechanisms, secretory pathways, second messengers, and signal transduction pathways. Neural progenitor cells, which could potentially develop these characteristics, have been isolated from fetal and adult brains particularly from regions that undergo neurogenesis such as the subventricular zone, the olfactory system and the hippocampus (43). However, progenitor cells transplanted in the brain differentiate predominantly into the glial phenotype (43,44). Attempts to enhance the differentiation of these cells down the neuronal lineage would significantly improve the efficiency of this technology. Gene transfer with functional neuronal genes such as trophic factors might be necessary. This approach has the potential to produce universal donor cells with many of the desirable neuronal features. Among the different cell types tested experimentally, neural progenitors derived from embryonic mesencephalic cultures hold the best potential (45–49). Whether the mechanism(s) that kills nigral neurons in PD may also affect the survival of transplanted cells remains unknown at present and no evidence is available to address this issue.

CANDIDATE THERAPEUTIC GENES FOR PD

Two categories of candidate therapeutic genes are being considered for gene transfer studies in experimental parkinsonism. First, symptomatic molecules that relieve the phenotypic manifestations of the disorder, such as dopamine biosynthetic enzymes, without substantially influencing the underlying

---

Table 45.3 Categories of Candidate Therapeutic Genes for Parkinson's Disease

Symptomatic:
   Transmitter enzymes: TH, GTP-CH1, AADC
Restorative:
   Neurotrophic factors: GDNF, BDNF
   Anti-apoptotic molecules: *bcl-2*
   Free radical scavengers: Cu/Zn SOD

---

neurodegeneration. And second, restorative molecules that have the potential to retard the neurodegenerative process by one or more mechanisms (Table 45-3).

Symptomatic Gene Products

Because tyrosine hydroxylase (TH) is the rate-limiting enzyme in dopamine biosynthesis, attempts to deliver the cDNA encoding this protein have been a focus of intense investigational effort (11). One means of delivering the TH cDNA into the striatum is transplantation of a tissue that endogenously expresses tyrosine hydroxylase. The latter has been one of the rationales for transplantation of human fetal mesencephalic tissue. However, due to the limitations of this approach, a more readily available means of delivering the TH cDNA to the parkinsonian brain would be desirable. More recently, carotid body autotransplants were used in rodent and primate models of PD with favorable results (50–51). However, experience with this approach is limited and the ability to engraft an adequate number of cells with this approach in the human brain remains questionable.

Methods to deliver the TH cDNA in animal models of PD initially used cell lines such as AtT-20 and NIH3T3, but subsequently primary cells such as fibroblasts, myoblasts, astrocytes, and Schwann cells were used in ex vivo gene transfer studies (9,13,26,40). Immortalized cell lines generated from embryonic mesencephalic cultures have also been used for the delivery of TH into the striatum of Parkinson models (32). In addition, direct in vivo TH gene transfer has been tried with plasmid DNA using lipofectin (52–54). Several viral vectors have been used in proof-of-principle style experiments to deliver the TH cDNA in the rat 6-OHDA model of PD. An HSV-1-based amplicon vector expressing TH in the striatum of lesioned rats has resulted in behavioral recovery for a year (55). However, about 10 percent of the animals in this study died with evidence of HSV-1-mediated cytopathic effects presumably due to the presence of helper virus or the production of cytotoxic or immunogenic viral proteins. In addition, a diminution of TH expression was observed over time perhaps due to down regulation of the viral promoter in the vector. The TH cDNA has also been delivered using AAV to the rat striatum (56). Although most infected cells were neurons, transgene expression declined over four months and rotational recovery was reported for only two months. Similarly, adenovirus vector expressing TH results in functional recovery but only for a short time mainly due to the known short-lived expression of this vector (57). Interestingly, even TH expressed in glial cells under the influence of the GFAP promoter results in behavioral recovery in this model (54).

Another dopamine biosynthetic enzyme is aromatic amino acid decarboxylase (AADC), which converts levodopa to dopamine. But the importance of AADC in vivo is not clinically evident since levodopa is decarboxylated effectively in the brains of Parkinsonian patients despite loss of the majority of their dopamine neurons. Presumably, the required AADC function is provided by nondopaminergic cells such as glia, serotoninergic cells or vascular endothelial cells. The coadministration of two separate AAV vectors for TH and for AADC in the striatum of rats resulted in more efficient dopamine production and behavioral recovery than TH alone (58). Furthermore, in nonhuman primates that were rendered parkinsonian by MPTP administration, TH and AADC delivery in the striatum resulted in TH positive cells, biochemical, but no consistent behavioral, improvement (59). However, some reports also suggest a detrimental effect of AADC on dopamine production perhaps due to end product inhibition of TH (60). This effect might be cell type specific, perhaps seen in nonneuronal cells such as fibroblasts that do not have the ability to sequester dopamine into synaptic vesicles thus allowing it to interact with and inhibit cytoplasmic TH. To circumvent the problem of end product inhibition, constructs having a truncation of the N terminal regulatory domain of TH leaving only its catalytic domain have been developed (61).

TH is also critically dependent on the cofactor tetrahydrobiopterin (BH4) for its activity. The importance of BH4 has been shown in fibroblast cell lines which do not produce sufficient amounts of BH4 to permit production of levodopa in vitro or in vivo (62). Addition of BH4 to these cells is necessary for levodopa synthesis and behavioral recovery. So BH4 must either be supplemented exogenously or GTP cyclohydrolase (GTP-CH1), the rate-limiting enzyme in BH4 production from GTP, should be coexpressed. The expression of both TH and GTP-CH1 in fibroblasts grafted in denervated striata is reportedly required for detectable basal levodopa levels (35,36). Even in vivo microdialysis studies following gene transfer with AAV have

shown that TH alone is not enough for levodopa production and that GTH-CH1 is required in the absence of exogenous BH4 (63). So the role of GTH-CH1 appears to apply to both in vivo and ex vivo gene transfer.

Additional genes that alter the physiology of neurons have been tested in vivo and in vitro such as the catalytic domains of adenylate cyclase, protein kinase C (PKC) and calcium–calmodulin protein kinase II (9). Stereotaxic delivery of an HSV-1 vector in the nigra combined with cell specific expression using the TH promoter driving the expression of the constitutively active catalytic domain of PKCβII produced long-term changes in apomorphine induced rotational behavior in nonlesioned rats (64). Such genes can be used as adjuncts to other therapeutic genes to enhance the function of residual dopamine neurons.

Neurorestorative Genes

Because levodopa-associated motor response fluctuations arise in the context of severe neuronal loss in the substantia nigra, preservation of these dopaminergic neurons would be the optimal strategy for preventing the development of these complications and minimizing disease severity as well. Thus, the delivery of transgenes that enhance the survival of these cells should accomplish both objectives. Candidates at present include genes that encode neurotrophic or antiapoptotic factors or genes that reduce oxidative stress.

Because neurotrophic factors cannot cross the blood-brain barrier, and because of problems associated with intracerebroventricular delivery of proteins, gene-transfer approaches have been tried in animal models of PD. To date, two dopaminergic neurotrophic factors, namely GDNF and BDNF have been tested for this purpose (65,66). GDNF delivered in vivo with an adenoviral vector into the rat nigra (67) or striatum (68,69) protected against subsequent 6-OHDA lesions. A similar approach of delivering GDNF could also restore function even in rats with established 6-OHDA lesions (70). An adenovirus vector delivering GDNF is also effective in the mouse MPTP model (71). In addition, an AAV vector has been used to deliver the GDNF cDNA to the rat nigra resulting in functional recovery (72). Similarly, BDNF producing fibroblast implants in the striatum or nigra have been reported to protect against 6-OHDA and MPTP toxicity in experimental animals (73,74). Astrocytes have also been used to deliver BDNF yielding behavioral recovery although no improvement in TH immunoreactivity could be demonstrated leaving the mechanism of recovery unclear (37).

Other potential neuroprotective gene products such as the antiapoptotic molecule bcl-2 could be expressed in dopamine neurons to save them from demise. Transplantation of conditionally immortalized nigral cells that had been engineered with bcl-2 into the striatum of 6-OHDA lesioned rats has resulted in more behavioral recovery than control cell implants, but without differences in TH or GFAP immunoreactivity leaving the mechanism of recovery unclear (75). HSV-1 vector–mediated expression of bcl-2 has also been shown to prevent 6-OHDA–induced degeneration of neurons in the rat nigra (76). In addition, free radical scavenging enzymes such as Cu/Zn superoxide dismutase (SOD) protect dopamine neurons from MPTP and enhance survival of grafted neurons (77). Intrastriatal grafts of rat embryonic mesencephalic neurons with an adenovirus vector expressing Cu/Zn SOD result in more extensive functional recovery, more TH immunoreactivity and more cell survival (78). Furthermore, transplantation of cells from Cu/Zn SOD transgenic mice lead to longer survival and yield more extensive functional recovery than using cells from nontransgenic animals indicating improved graft survival (77).

COMPARISON OF IN VIVO AND EX VIVO GENE TRANSFER APPROACHES

Several advantages and disadvantages are unique to the ex vivo and in vivo gene transfer methods. Potential advantages of the in vivo method include the notion that host brain cells might be better equipped to express the desired functional protein because they may possess essential cofactors and biochemical pathways for posttranslational modifications as well as the ability to secrete the gene product. The ex vivo approach allows controlling the gene transfer process before implanting the engineered cells into the recipient's brain. The biochemical effects of the transgene can be characterized in vitro and toxicity of the virus can be screened. In addition, the ex vivo approach provides the possibility of either retrieving the graft especially with encapsulated cell implants or killing the cells in situ by inducing an incorporated suicide gene when the biologic effects are no longer wanted. However, there is generally more disturbance of the normal cytoarchitectural circuitry of the brain with implantation, except perhaps when neural progenitor cells are used. For the ex vivo method to generate sufficient protein expression, the graft might need to be large enough to result in a space occupying mass in the brain. Gene product delivery is limited by the process of diffusion through the brain parenchyma with the ex vivo approach and by both transfection efficiency as well as tissue diffusion with the in vivo approach. Although the generation of an immune response is not an issue with the implantation of autologous or encapsulated cells, it could be a significant problem with direct introduction of viral vectors into brain cells particularly with adenoviral vectors. Furthermore, the risk of helper virus is a frequent safety concern with the in vivo approach. Finally, the expression of functional intracellular survival genes, such as those that modulate apoptotic cascades, are achievable only with the direct introduction of transgenes into brain cells using the in vivo method.

Ideally, the requirements for in vivo gene-transfer methods include the achievement of long-term, cell-type specific, gene expression at therapeutic levels without causing cytotoxicity, insertional mutagenesis, immune reaction to viral antigens or the emergence of virulent viral particles. Unfortunately, none of the vectors used today in their present form fully satisfy all these criteria. Considerable improvements are still required to make these vectors safe and effective in a sustained manner. In addition to systematic efforts for improving the safety and efficacy profile of individual viral vector systems described, recent progress has included the generation of hybrid vectors such as HSV/AAV to combine essential features of each while eliminating undesirable genes (79). And the ex vivo approach requires that the cells be easily obtainable, readily cultured, capable of expressing the transgene, and able to undergo the selection process to enrich the transduced cell population. In addition, the cells should be nononcogenic, immunologically compatible with the recipient, and survive well in the brain. Such cells then could serve as biologic mini pumps at a localized site in the brain. Available evidence suggest that neural progenitor cells satisfy most if not all these requirements and are superior to other cell types tested to date.

FUTURE CONSIDERATIONS

The goal of therapeutic gene transfer is sustained transgene expression at therapeutic levels in a regulatable manner. The latter issue is largely ignored at present and only relatively simple gene delivery vectors are being tested at this initial stage. In addition, one of the main limitations of currently available gene-transfer methods is the inability to obtain prolonged sustained transgene expression in vivo. Although long-term expression can be readily obtained in vitro, transplantation of engineered cells in the brain is associated with rapid decline of expression. A major factor in loss of expression is promoter shutdown because of poorly understood mechanisms (80,81).

50. Leff SE, Rendahl KG, Spratt SK, et al. In vivo L-DOPA production by genetically modified primary rat

intrastriatal transplantation of carotid body cell aggregates. *Neuron* 1998; 20:197–206.

51. Luquin MR, Montoro RJ, Guillen J, et al. Recovery of chronic parkinsonian monkeys by autotransplants of carotid body cell aggregates into putamen. *Neuron* 1999; 22:743–750.

52. Cao L, Zheng Z-C, Zhao Y-C, et al. Gene therapy of Parkinson disease model rat by direct injection of plasmid DNA-lipofectin complex. *Hum Gene Ther* 1995; 6:1497–1501.

53. Imaoka T, date I, Ohmoto T, et al. Significant behavioral recovery in Parkinson's disease model by direct intracerebral gene transfer using continuous injection of a plasmid DNA-lipsome complex. *Hum Gene Ther* 1998; 9:1093–1102.

54. Segovia I, Vergara P, Brenner M. Astrocyte-specific expression of tyrosine hyrdoxylase after intracerebral gene transfer induces behavioral recovery in experimental Parkinsonism. *Gene Ther* 1998; 5:1650–1655.

55. During MJ, Naegele JR, O'Malley KL, et al. Long-term behavioral recovery in parkinsonian rats by an HSV vector expressing tyrosine hydroxylase. *Science* 1994; 266:1399–1403.

56. Kaplitt MG, Leone P, Samulski RJ, et al. Long-term gene expression and phenotypic correction using adeno-associated virus vectors in the mammalian brain. *Nat Genet* 1994; 8:148–154.

57. Horellou P, Mallet J. Gene therapy for Parkinson's disease. *Mol Neurobiol* 1997 15:241–256.

58. Fan DS, Ogawa M, Fujimoto KI, et al. Behavioral recovery in 6-hydroxydopamine-lesioned rats by cotransduction of striatum with tyrosine hydroxylase and aromatic L-amino acid decarboxylase genes using two separate adeno-associated virus vectors. *Hum Gene Ther* 1998; 9:2527–2535.

59. During MJ, Samulski RJ, Elsworth JD, et al. In vivo expression of therapeutic human genes for dopamine production in the caudates of MPTP-treated monkeys using an AAV vector. *Gene Ther* 1998; 5:820–827.

60. Wachtel SR, Bencsics C, Kang UJ. Role of aromatic L-amino acid decarboxylase for dopamine replacement by genetically modified fibroblasts in a rat model of Parkinson's disease. *J Neurochem* 1997; 69:2055–2063.

61. Moffat M, Harmon S, Haycock J, et al. L-dopa and dopamine-producing gene cassettes for gene therapy approaches to Parkinson's disease. *Exp Neurol* 1997; 144:69–73.

62. Uchida K, Tsuzaki N, Nagatsu T, et al. Tetrahydrobiopterin-dependent functional recovery in 6-hydroxydopamine-treated rats by intracerebral grafting of fibroblasts transfected with tyrosine hydroxylase cDNA. *Dev Neurosci* 1992; 14:173–180.

63. Mandel RJ, Rendahl KG, Spratt SK, et al. Characterization of intrastriatal recombinant adeno-associated virus-mediated gene transfer of human tyrosine hydroxylase and human GTP-cyclohydrolase I in a rat model of Parkinson's disease. *J Neurosci* 1998; 18:4271–4284.

64. Song S, Wang Y, Bak SY, et al. Modulation of rat rotational behavior by direct gene transfer of constitutively active protein kinase C into nigrostriatal neurons. *J Neurosci* 1998; 18:4119–4132.

65. Olson L. The coming of age of the GDNF family and its receptors: Gene delivery in a rat Parkinson model may have clinical implications. *Trends Neurol Sci* 1997; 20:277–279.

66. Bohn MC. A commentary on glial cell line-derived neurotrophic factor (GDNF). From a glial secreted molecule to gene therapy. *Biochem Pharmacol* 1999; 57:135–142.

67. Choi-Lundberg DL, Lin Q, Chang YN, et al. Dopaminergic neurons protected from degeneration by GDNF gene therapy. *Science* 1997; 275:838–841.

68. Bilang-Bleuel A, Revah F, Colin P, et al. Intrastriatal injection of an adenoviral vector expressing glial-cell-line-derived neurotrophic factor prevents dopaminergic neuron degeneration and behavioral impairment in a rat model of Parkinson's disease. *Proc Natl Acad Sci USA* 1997; 94:8818–8823.

69. Choi-Lundberg DL, Lin Q, Schallert T, Crippens D, et al. Behavioral and cellular protection of rat dopaminergic neurons by an adenoviral vector encoding glial cell line-derived neurotrophic factor. *Exp Neurol* 1998; 154:261–275.

70. Lapchak PA, Araujo DM, Hilt DC, et al. Adenoviral vector-mediated GDNF gene therapy in a rodent lesion model of late stage Parkinson's disease. *Brain Res* 1997; 777:153–160.

71. Kojima H, Abiru Y, Sakajiri K, et al. Adenovirus-mediated transduction with human glial cell line-derived neurotrophic factor gene prevents 1-methyl-4-phenyl-1,2,3,6-tetrahydropyridine-induced dopamine depletion in striatum of mouse brain. *Biochem Biophys Res Commun* 1997; 238:569–573.

72. Mandel RJ, Spratt SK, Snyder RO, et al. Midbrain injection of recombinant adeno-associated virus encoding rat glial cell line-derived neurotrophic factor protects nigral neurons in a progressive 6-hydroxydopamine-induced degeneration model of Parkinson's disease in rats. *Proc Natl Acad Sci USA* 1997; 94:14083–14088.

73. Frim DM, Uhler TA, Galpern WR, et al. Implanted fibroblasts genetically engineered to produce brain-derived neurotrophic factor prevent 1-methyl-4-phenylpyridinium toxicity to dopaminergic neurons in the rat. *Proc Natl Acad Sci USA* 1994; 91:5104–5108.

74. Levivier M, Przedborski S, Bencsics C, et al. Intrastriatal implantation of fibroblasts genetically engineered to produce brain-derived neurotrophic factor prevents degeneration of dopaminergic neurons in a rat model of Parkinson's disease. *J Neurosci* 1995; 15:7810–7820.

75. Anton R, Kordower JH, Kane DJ, et al. Neural transplantation of cells expressing the anti-apoptotic gene *bcl-2*. *Cell Transplant* 1995; 4:49–54.

76. Yamada M, Oligino T, Mata M, et al. Herpes simplex virus vector-mediated expression of Bcl-2 prevents 6-hydroxydopamine-induced degeneration of neurons in the substantia nigra in vivo. *Proc Natl Acad Sci USA* 1999; 96:4078–4083.

77. Nakao N, Frodl EM, Widner H, et al. Overexpressing Cu/Zn superoxide dismutase enhances survival of transplanted neurons in a rat model of Parkinson's disease. *Nature Med* 1995; 1:226–231.

78. Barkats M, Nakao N, Grasbon-Frodl EM, et al. Intrastriatal grafts of embryonic mesencephalic rat neurons genetically modified using an adenovirus encoding human Cu/Zn superoxide dismutase. *Neuroscience* 1997; 78:708–713.

79. Johnston KM, Jacoby D, Pechan PA, et al. HSV/AAV hybrid amplicon vectors extend transgene expression in human glioma cells. *Hum Gene Ther* 1997; 359–370.

80. Palmer TD, Rosman GJ, Osborne WR, et al. Genetically modified skin fibroblasts persist long after transplantation but gradually inactivate introduced genes. *Proc Natl Acad Sci USA* 1991; 88:1330–1334.

81. Qin L, Ding Y, Pahud DR, et al. Promoter attenuation in gene therapy: interferon-gamma and tumor necrosis factor-alpha inhibit transgene expression. *Hum Gene Ther* 1997; 8:2019–2029.

82. Song S, Wang Y, Bak SY, et al. An HSV-1 vector containing the rat tyrosine hydroxylase promoter enhances both long-term and cell type-specific expression in the midbrain. *J Neurochem* 1997; 68:1792–1803.

46

Tobacco Smoking, Nicotine, and Neuroprotection

Peter A. LeWitt, M.D.

Clinical Neuroscience Center, Southfield, Michigan

INTRODUCTION

Neither the distinctive signs and symptoms of Parkinson's disease (PD), nor its characteristic pattern of neuronal loss offer an explanation of how this disorder arises. Consequently, there has been considerable effort to unravel the cause(s) of PD from epidemiologic clues. Epidemiology has occasionally provided critical insights into the origins of medical disorders although such studies generally do not establish causality for any identified risk factor. For PD, which has been studied extensively in populations throughout the world, only a few associations have arisen from the analysis of environmental factors pertaining to occupation, diet, and other lifestyle exposures. One of the most robust findings from epidemiologic research, though perhaps the most puzzling, has been the discovery of an inverse (negative) association between PD and cigarette smoking[1]. A major influence of smoking at reducing the risk for PD has been validated. Whether derived from prospective studies, cross-sectional surveys of well-defined populations, or death certificate information, this inverse correlation generally has the same magnitude of effect. Coincidence does not prove causation, of course, but the circumstances of a strong association beg for explanation. Many details remain to be learned about why a history of smoking might lessen the risk for PD, and whether this information could be harnessed for therapeutic purposes. Because epidemiologic study of PD has yielded little else in the way of useful clues, the curious relationship between the occurrence of PD and a distinctive human behavior such as smoking offers a unique vantage point for further investigation into the pathogenesis of PD.

The preponderance of studies indicate that the risk for developing PD in a population of smokers is approximately half the risk for nonsmokers. Some investigations have further refined this observation by examining influences of age or the extent of smoking exposure on the risk for PD. Most evidence supports a conclusion that chronic smoking confers a neuroprotective action against the underlying disorder, rather than any artifactual action (such as a symptomatic action against parkinsonian signs and symptoms). Such a conclusion follows from guidelines for causality codified by Austin Hill in 1965 (1). In his classic monograph entitled *The Environment and Disease: Association or Causation?*, Hill proposed nine criteria by which causality might be inferred (e.g., supported, though not necessarily proven) by an association derived from an epidemiologic study:

1. if the *strength* of the association is especially large;
2. if the association is *consistently* found with different study designs or populations;
3. if the association has a high level of *specificity* (i.e., without *alternative explanations* for a presumed cause-and-effect relationship);
4. if a *reasonable chain of events* underlie the association (i.e., the temporal sequence of exposure and outcome is logical);
5. if the association provides for a *gradation of the biological effect* (i.e., a dose-response relationship, in further support of a cause-and-effect hypothesis);

---

[1] This habitual activity will hereafter be designated as "smoking" in this chapter. Burning tobacco can be inhaled from other smoking products, of course, and there can also be chronic use of noncombusted tobacco. However, the habitual use of tobacco is predominantly through cigarettes, and virtually all of the studies reviewed here deal with cigarette smoking (or, in a few instances, "cigarette equivalents" created from a conversion factor).

this relationship. The mean age of PD onset is greater in ever-smokers than in nonsmokers (110). Tzourio and colleagues (16) pointed out that previous case-control studies showing inverse relationships between smoking and PD were strongly over-represented by PD cases younger than 68 years. Failure to confirm the inverse association between smoking and PD occurred with study populations that tended to be older (17–20) than in studies finding reduced PD risk for smokers. The differential age effect was not found in all studies; Morens and colleagues (21) observed reduced incidence of PD in cigarette smokers at all ages over a span of 40 years. In older patients, occurrence of PD in first-order relatives is synergistic with not smoking in the risk for PD (109).

THE MAGNITUDE OF SMOKING'S EFFECTS AT REDUCING RISK FOR PARKINSON'S DISEASE

Smoking has been associated with a major reduction of risk for PD in several dozen studies that have appeared over almost four decades. The magnitude of this effect has clustered around a 50 percent reduction, although in a few studies even greater decrease of PD prevalence has been noted. For example, a prospective study by Morens and colleagues [21] (and providing follow-up on an earlier publication (15)), found the incidence of PD in 8,006 men was 94.2 per 10^5 person-years among nonsmokers but only 34.4 per 10^5 person-years for smokers.

CONSISTENCY AMONG STUDIES OF REDUCED RISK FOR PARKINSON'S DISEASE IN SMOKERS

Populations around the world have been investigated regarding the PD–smoking relationship. For the majority of these studies, the risk for PD has been assessed among groups in excess of 25 patients. A similar effect of smoking has been the consistent finding from most of these studies. No study has ever found smoking to be associated with increased risk for PD.

Not all studies have concluded that smoking confers a protective effect. Studies that did not find an association between smoking and PD include three case-control studies carried out in New York City (18), China (22), and a group of four European countries (23,16). Others that did not find significant associations were conducted in populations

from Hong Kong (24), Calgary (17), Rochester (Minnesota) (19,108), the United States (25), a rural community in Australia (102), and Spain (20). Several reports that did find reductions in the risk for PD nonetheless regarded these results as likely to be study artifacts rather than genuine phenomena (26–29,24). The report mentioned earlier by Tzourio and colleagues (16), one of the largest study populations examined to date, did not detect a protective effect from smoking for the entire group of 193 PD subjects matched to 535 controls. However, after the PD subjects were stratified by age, a strong reduction in risk for PD emerged for the younger PD cases. This study highlights the complexity of answering a deceptively simple question regarding the PD–smoking relationship.

Apart from the studies mentioned here, the rest of reports in Table 46-1 provide data for reduced risk for PD in association with smoking. The diversity of study designs and study populations argues against an artifactual basis for this conclusion.

SPECIFICITY OF CAUSE-AND-EFFECT RELATIONSHIP BETWEEN SMOKING AND REDUCED RISK FOR PARKINSON'S DISEASE

Several reports have considered alternatives to the conclusions that smoking imparts some manner of pharmacologic effect at reducing PD. Golbe and colleagues (30) regarded the association between PD and smoking as a possible epiphenomenon. They speculated that a particular personality trait (such as a pleasure-seeking or novelty-seeking factor) might be the actual link to the risk for PD, and that persons who are willing to smoke are biologically less at risk to develop PD. Paulson (31) has also hypothesized that factors conferring pleasure from smoking or nicotine addiction might be the same that lower the risk for PD. He speculated that the addictive habit of smoking might be due to high intrinsic brain levels of dopamine, which also could reduce the risk for developing PD. Despite the logic of these mechanisms, no evidence underlies this hypothesis. In the absence of alternative explanations, there seems to be reasonable specificity for the relationship between smoking and a reduced risk for PD.

THE CHAIN OF EVENTS UNDERLYING SMOKING AND THE RISK FOR PARKINSON'S DISEASE

Most cases of PD arise in the sixth decade, and only rarely does it start under the age of 40. Cigarette smoking generally begins by age 20, and so there are three to four decades after the start of the smoking habit and before the onset of PD. It is not known when the disease process actually begins in relation to the onset of signs and symptoms. However, the earlier start of exposure to smoking and a later age of PD onset are consistent with a logical sequence. One factor pertinent to the possible cause-and-effect relationship is whether smoking, in addition to lowering the risk for PD, might also increase the typical age of disease onset. This information has not been reported in most studies.

Morens and colleagues (14) considered the possibility that smoking might only appear to reduce the risk for PD because of smoking-related illnesses overshadowing the correct recognition of PD, a phenomenon termed *diagnostic displacement*. They regarded this possibility unlikely in prospective studies in which the ascertainment of patients was conducted by neurological specialists. They also rejected the concept of "selective mortality" as an alternative explanation. Several authors have argued that the inverse association between smoking and PD might be an artifact on the basis of smokers experiencing earlier mortality than nonsmokers (19,26,32). Riggs (33) has argued that the PD-smoking relationship is possibly only an "illusion of a neuroprotective effect." His argument and that of others has been that a differential survival bias might account for a lower incidence of PD among smokers. The hypothesis implies increased mortality among smokers destined to develop PD (and hence a cross-sectional study of all PD patients later in life will reveal more non-smokers). This hypothesis has been examined in several ways. Increased mortality for a PD-affected identical twin that smokes was not found (34) and in another analysis, a twin affected with PD was less likely to have smoked than his or her unaffected twin sibling (32). Another argument against differential survival bias has been that, since the difference in survival between smokers and nonsmokers increases with age, studies as to the risk for PD in smokers should show a greater effect in older than in younger individuals (35). However, contrary findings came from a case-controlled study of young- and old-onset PD (36). In another case-controlled study examining a patient population extending over 40-year age span, smoking was associated with a similar reduced incidence of PD at all ages (21).

Others have argued for the possibility that cigarette smokers might differ from fellow human beings in their personalities and other behavioral attributes that, in some way, are associated with avoiding a causative factor for PD. Alternatively, a "taste" for enjoying cigarettes or a biologic propensity for becoming addicted to nicotine might be an important correlate of a lower risk for PD (37). The possibility that certain personality traits might be associated with a lower risk for PD has not been examined in prospective studies. Most attempts to define a personality type at increased risk for PD, using, for example, populations of twins with one of them affected with PD, have been inconclusive at finding strong traits linked to either the occurrence or avoidance of PD.

Also untenable as an explanation for a faulty cause-and-effect assumption is the notion that PD's clinical features are suppressed by nicotine or some other byproduct of smoking. The reduced risk for PD has been found even among former smokers (38). A temporary improvement of Parkinsonian from smoking signs has been reported in young-onset PD patients (39), although similar experiences have not been observed by this author's PD patients who happen to smoke.

GRADATION OF BIOLOGIC EFFECT FROM SMOKING IN LOWERING THE RISK FOR PARKINSON'S DISEASE

Another criterion useful for inferring a causal relationship between smoking and reduction in risk for PD is whether there is a gradation of effect dependent on the duration or amount of smoking (or both). This concept of "dose-responsiveness" underlies most biologic effects of a pharmacologic nature. Although finding an outcome proportional to "dose" is not mandatory for inferring a biologic effect, the concept of a dose–response relationship is a useful argument in epidemiologic studies. The opportunity to gauge the possible gradation of smoking's anti-PD effect is fostered by observations that reduction of PD risk is only partial, and by the diversity in a population of cigarette users as to their smoking habits.

The "dose" of smoking can be conceived in several ways: as the duration of smoking, as the quantity of cigarettes smoked daily, or as the product of daily quantity and duration (i.e., a measure such as "pack-years"). The earliest studies to evaluate the "dose-response" question were those of Kahn (3) and Hammond (2), using death certificate information. A survey of 3,693 PD patients by a mailed questionnaire found no correlation between any measure of smoking and PD severity (30). A dose-response association has not appeared in all studies (including a case-controlled study (40,41)), but most reports supported a dose-related lowering of risk for PD (15,42–47). Several (but not all) have detected an intermediate lowering of PD risk among ex-smokers. For example, Checkoway and coworkers (100) found that the inverse relationship between

49. Vieregge P, Heberlein I. Nicotine consumption and Parkinson's disease – does the smoke clear up? *Mov Disord* 1995;10:359–360, and 1996; 11:613

50. Rowell PP, Laurence AC, Garner AC. Stimulation of (3H)-dopamine release by nicotine in rat nucleus accumbens. *J Neurochem* 1987; 49:1449–1454.

51. Fuxe K, Janson AM, Janson A, et al. Chronic nicotine treatment increases dopamine levels and reduces dopamine utilization in substantia nigra and surviving forebrain dopamine nerve terminal systems after a partial di-mesencephalic hemitransection. *Naunyn-Schmiedeberg's Arch Pharmacol* 1990; 341:171–181.

52. Gao ZG, Cui WY, Zhang HT, et al. Effects of nicotine on 1-methyl-4-phenyl-1,2,5,6-tetrahydropyridine-induced depression of striatal dopamine content and spontaneous locomotor activity in C57 black mice. *Pharmacol Res* 1998; 38:101–106.

53. Sershen H, Hashim A, Lajtha A. Behavioral and biochemical effects of nicotine in an MPTP-induced mouse model of Parkinson's disease. *Pharmacol Biochem Behav* 1987; 28:299–303.

54. Fagerström KO, Pomerleau O, Giordani B, et al. Nicotine may relieve symptoms of Parkinson's disease. *Psychopharmacology* 1994; 116:117–119.

55. Clemens P, Baron JA, Coffey D, et al. The short-term effect of nicotine chewing gum in patients with Parkinson's disease. *Psychopharmacology* 1995; 117:253–256.

56. Nishimura H, Tachibana H, Okuda B, et al. Transient worsening of Parkinson's disease after cigarette smoking. *Int Med* 1997; 36:651–653.

57. Nilsson A, Waller L, Rosengren A, et al. Cigarette smoking is associated with abnormal involuntary movements in the general male population – a study of men born in 1933. *Biol Psychiatr* 1997; 15;41:717–723.

58. Grenhoff J, Janson AM, Svensson TH, et al. Chronic continuous nicotine treatment causes decreased burst firing of nigral dopamine neurons in rats partially hemitransected at the meso-diencephalic junction. *Brain Res* 1991; 562:347–351.

59. Janson AM, Fuxe K, Goldstein M. Differential effects of acute and chronic nicotine treatment on MPTP (1-methyl-4-phenyl-1,2,3,6-tetrahydropyridine)-induced degeneration of nigrostriatal dopamine neurons in the black mouse. *Clin Invest* 1992; 70:232–238.

60. Janson AM, Moller A. Chronic nicotine treatment counteracts nigral cell loss induced by a partial mesodiencephalic hemisection: An analysis of the total number and mean volume of neurons and glia in substantia nigra of the male rat. *Neuroscience* 1993; 57:931–941.

61. Fung YK, Fiske LA, Lau YS. Chronic administration of nicotine fails to alter the MPTP-induced neurotoxicity in mice. *Gen Pharmacol* 1991; 22:669–672.

62. Wright SC, Zhong J, Zheng H, et al. Nicotine inhibition of apoptosis suggests a role in tumor promotion. *FASEB J* 1993; 7:1045–1051.

63. Baron JA. Beneficial effects of nicotine and cigarette smoking: The real, the possible, and the spurious. *Br Med Bull* 1996; 52:58–73.

64. McKenney J, Valeri CR, Mohandas N, et al. Decreased in vivo survival of hydrogen peroxide-damaged baboon red blood cells. *Blood* 1990; 76:206–211.

65. Calne DB, Langston JW. Aetiology of Parkinson's disease. *Lancet* 1983; 2:1457–1459.

66. Irwin I, Langston JW, DeLanney LE. 4-Phenylpyridine (4PP) and MPTP: The relationship between striatal MPP+ concentrations and neurotoxicity. *Life Sci* 1987; 40:731–740.

67. Soto-Otero R, Riguera-Vega R, Mendez-Alvarez E, et al. Interaction of 1,2,3,4-tetrahydroisoquinoline with some components of cigarette smoke: Potential implications for Parkinson's disease. *Biochem Biophys Res Com* 1996; 15; 222:607–611.

68. Balfour DJ, Fagerström KO. Pharmacology of nicotine and its therapeutic use in smoking cessation and neurodegenerative disorders. *Pharmacol Ther* 1996; 72:51–81.

69. Parkinson Study Group. DATATOP: A multicenter controlled clinical trial in early Parkinson's disease. *Arch Neurol* 1989; 46:1052–1060.

70. Parkinson Study Group. A controlled trial of lazabemide (Ro19-6327) in untreated Parkinson's disease. *Ann Neurol* 1993; 33:350–356.

71. Parkinson Study Group. Effects of tocopherol and deprenyl on the progression of disability in early Parkinson's disease. *N Engl J Med* 1993; 328:176–183.

72. Nelson LM, Longstreth WT, McGuire V, et al. Cigarette smoking and the risk of amyotrophic lateral sclerosis: A population-based case control study. *Neuroepidemiology* 1998; 17:210

73. Davis PH, Golbe LI, Duvoisin RC, et al. Risk factors for progressive supranuclear palsy. *Neurology* 1988; 38:1546–1552.

74. Graves AB, van Duijn CM, Chandra V, et al. Alcohol and nicotine consumption as risk factors for Alzheimer's disease: A collaborative re-analysis of case-controlled studies. *Int J Epidemiol* 1991; 20(suppl 2):S48–S57

75. Brenner D, Kukall WA, van Belle G, et al. Relationship between cigarette smoking and Alzheimer's disease in a population-based case-control study. *Neurology* 1993; 43:293–300.

76. van Duijn C, Hofman A. Relation between nicotine intake and Alzheimer's disease. *Br Med J* 1991; 302:1491–1494.

77. Calne DB, Eisen A, McGeer E, et al. Alzheimer's disease, Parkinson's disease, and motor-neurone disease: Abiotrophic interactions between ageing and environment? *Lancet* 1986; 2:1067–1070.

78. Ansari KA, Johnson A. Olfactory function in patients with Parkinson's disease. *J Chronic Dis* 1975; 28:493–497.

79. Baumann RJ, Johnson HD, McKean HE, et al. Cigarette smoking and Parkinson disease: 1. A comparison of cases with matched neighbors. *Neurology* 1980; 30:839–843.

80. Busenbark KL, Huber SJ, Greer G, et al. Olfactory function in essential tremor. *Neurology* 1992; 42:1631–1632.

81. Butterfield PG, Valanis BG, Spencer PS, et al. Environmental antecedents of young-onset Parkinson's disease. *Neurology* 1993; 43:1150–1158.

82. Cazzato G, Capus L, Monti F, et al. Abitudine al fumo e morbo di Parkinson. *Riv Neurol* 1985; 55:79–87.

83. Doll R, Peto R. Mortality in relation to smoking: 20 years' observations in British male doctors. *Br Med J* 1976; 2:1525–1536.

84. Duvoisin RC, Eldridge R, Williams A, et al. Twin study of Parkinson's disease. *Neurology* 1981; 31:77–80.

85. Granérus A-K, Mellström D, Himmelmann A, et al. Rökning och Parkinsons sjukdom. *Läkartidningen* 1987; 84:2025–2026.

86. Jiménez-Jiménez FJ, Mateo D, Giménez-Roldan S. Premorbid smoking, alcohol consumption, and coffee drinking habits in Parkinson's disease: A case-control study. *Mov Disord* 1992; 7:339–344.

87. Kessler II. Epidemiologic studies of Parkinson's disease. II. Smoking and Parkinson's disease: A hospital-based survey. *Am J Epidemiol* 1972; 95; 308–318.

88. Kessler II. Epidemiologic studies of Parkinson's disease. III. Smoking and Parkinson's disease: A community-based survey. *Am J Epidemiol* 1972; 96:242–254.

89. Martyn CN, Osmond C. Parkinson's disease and the environment in early life. *J Neurol Sci* 1995; 132:201–206.

90. Nefzger MD, Quadfasel FA, Karl VC. A retrospective study of smoking in Parkinson's disease. *Am J Epidemiol* 1968; 88:149–158.

91. Ngim CH, Devathasan G. Epidemiologic study on the association between body burden mercury level and idiopathic Parkinson's disease. *Neuroepidemiol* 1989; 8:128–141.

92. Smargiassi A, Mutti A, De Rosa A, et al. A case-control study of occupational and environmental risk factors for Parkinson's disease in the Emilia-Romagna region of Italy. *Neurotoxicology* 1998; 19:709–712.

93. Tanner CM, Koller WC, Gilley DC, et al. Cigarette smoking, alcohol drinking, and Parkinson's disease: Cross-cultural risk assessment. *Mov Disord* 1990; 5:11.

94. Wechsler LS, Checkoway H, Franklin GM, et al. A pilot study of occupational and environmental risk factors for Parkinson's disease. *Neurotoxicology* 12:387–392.

95. Wolf PA, Feldman RG, Saint-Hilaire M, et al. Precursors and natural history of Parkinson's disease: The Framingham study. *Neurology* 1991; 41(suppl 1):371.

96. Zuber M, Verdier-Taillefer M-H, Alperovitch A, et al. Smoking and Parkinson's disease: Differences according to age at disease onset. *Neuroepidemiology* 1991; 10:103–104.

97. Kondo K, Watanabe K. Lifestyles, risk factors, and inherited predispositions in Parkinson's disease. Preliminary report of a case-control study. *Adv Neurol* 1993; 60:346–351.

98. Hirayama Y. Epidemiological patterns of Parkinson's disease based on a cohort study. In: *Epidemiology of Intractable Diseases Research Committee.* Tokyo: Japan Ministry of Health and Welfare, 1985:219–227.

99. Maggio R, Riva M, Vaglini F, et al. Nicotine prevents experimental parkinsonism in rodents and induces striatal increase of neurotrophic factors. *J Neurochem* 1998; 71:2439–2446.

100. Checkoway H, Franklin GM, Costa-Mallen P, et al. A genetic polymorphism of MAO-B modifies the association of cigarette smoking and Parkinson's disease. *Neurology* 1998; 50:1458–1461.

101. Werneck AL, Alvarenga H. Genetic drugs and environmental factors in Parkinson's disease. A case-control study. *Arg Neuro-Psiguiatria* 1999; 57:347–355.

102. McCann SJ, LeCouteur DG, Green AC, et al. The epidemiology of Parkinson's disease in an Australian population. *Neuroepidemiology* 1998; 17:310–317.

103. Linert W, Bridge MH, Huber M, et al. In vitro and in vivo studies investigating possible antioxidant actions of nicotine: Relevance to Parkinson's and Alzheimer's disease. *Biochim Biophys Acta* 1999: 1454(2):143–152.

104. Ferger B, Spratt C, Earl CD, et al. Effects of nicotine on hydroxyl free radical formation in vitro and on MPTP-induced neurotoxicity in vivo. *Naunyn Schmiedebergs Arch Pharmacol* 1998; 358:351–359.

105. Soto-Otero R, Mendez-Alvarez E, Riguera-Vega R, et al. Studies on the interaction between 1,2,3,4-tetrahydro-beta-carboline and cigarette smoke: A potential mechanism of neuroprotection for Parkinson's disease. *Brain Res* 1998; 802:155–162.

106. Taylor CA, Saint-Hilaire MH, Cupples LA, et al. Environmental, medical, and family history risk factors for Parkinson's disease: A New England-based case control study. *Am J Med Genet* 1999; 88:742–749.

107. Chan DK, Woo J, Ho SC, et al. Genetic and environmental risk factors for Parkinson's disease in a Chinese population. *J Neurol Neurosurg Psychiatry* 1998; 65:781–784.

108. Benedetti MD, Bower JH, Maraganore DM, et al. *Neurology* 2000; 55:1350–1358.

109. Elbaz A, Manubens-Bertran JM, Baldereschi M, et al. Parkinson's disease, smoking, and family history. *J Neurol* 2000; 247:793–798.

110. Kuopio AM, Marttila RJ, Helenius H, Rinne UK. Environmental risk factors in Parkinson's disease. *Mov Disord* 1999; 14:928–939.

111. Preux PM, Condet A, Anglade C, et al. Parkinson's disease and environmental factors. Matched case-control study in the Limousin region of France. *Neuroepidemiololgy* 2000; 19:333–337.

47

Stereotactic Pallidotomy and Thalamotomy

Jung Y. Park, M.D., Andres M. Lozano, M.D., and Anthony E. Lang, M.D.
Toronto Western Hospital, Toronto, Ontario, Canada

INTRODUCTION

Surgical treatment of Parkinson's disease (PD) and other movement disorders has recently gained a level of importance that it had not previously achieved. This resurgence is mainly based on advances in understanding of the pathophysiology of the basal ganglia, in improvement of computer technology, and in elaboration of better imaging and stereotactic equipment that make neurosurgical procedures more accurate and safer. These developments and the need for treatment for those patients who derive insufficient benefit or experience complications of presently available pharmacotherapy have contributed to the reevalutaion of surgical procedures.

Generally, there are three main surgical approaches for PD: ablative surgery, deep brain stimulation (DBS), and "restorative" therapies, predominantly neural transplantation. These therapies are usually reserved for patients with advanced disease refractory to medications or who experience significant adverse effects most notably motor complications, such as fluctuations and dyskinesias. This chapter focuses on ablative surgery, specifically stereotactic pallidotomy and thalamotomy

HISTORICAL BACKGROUND

The first report of surgery for movement disorders was published more than a century ago and consisted of resection of premotor area to treat choreoathetosis (1). Surgical procedures for PD early in this century included lesioning the cerebral cortex or corticospinal system and replacing tremor with motor deficits (2–4). Meyers (5) first introduced surgical lesions directed at the basal ganglia. He found that sectioning of pallidofugal fibers could improve parkinsonism, particularly tremor, for the first time, without creating a pyramidal deficit. This pioneering work was followed by the development of more precise and safer methods using stereotactic guidance. Spiegel et al. (6) performed the first acknowledged stereotactic pallidotomy for movement disorders. Soon Leksell (7), Cooper (8), Guiot (9), and Narayabashi (10), developed their own instruments and surgical approaches to the globus pallidus and its output fibres. Because of the perceived variable and inconsistent results on tremor with pallidotomy as practiced at that time, Hassler introduced surgery of the ventrolateral (VL) nucleus of the thalamus (11). The procedure was based on a study of the anatomical connections between the pallidum and the thalamus. Beginning in the mid-to-late 1950s and reaching a peak in the 1960s, stereotactic neurosurgery, especially thalamotomy, became a prominent mode of therapy for PD. Microelectrode recording allowed the groups of Guiot (12) and Narabayashi (13,14) to define the ventral intermediate (VIM) nucleus of the thalamus as the best target to control the tremor in PD. But the VIM target was still disappointing for akinesia and rigidity. This provided a rationale for combining pallidotomy with thalamotomy, with the surgeon performing the second procedure as necessary depending upon the response to the initial lesion (15).

About a half century after the first discovery of dopamine by Guggenheim in 1913, levodopa treatment for PD was introduced in 1961 and was widely available by 1968. As it gained worldwide popularity the decline of stereotactic neurosurgery ensued, and the number of stereotactic procedures soon dramatically decreased (16).

Despite the striking benefits provided by levodopa, it quickly became evident that it too had shortcomings. As PD progresses, and with prolonged administration of levodopa, symptoms become refractory to the drug and disabling, abnormal, involuntary movements (dyskinesias), and "on-off" fluctuations appear. Because of these problems, stereotactic neurosurgery is being revisited and is more actively used. This new era was ushered in by advances in the understanding of basal ganglia pathophysiology (17,18) coincident with the work of Laitinen and coworkers (19,20), who reintroduced Leksell's pallidotomy and the development of better brain imaging and intraoperative electrophysiological techniques.

RATIONALE OF SURGERY

Pallidotomy

Together with the pars reticulata of the substantia nigra (SNr), the internal segment of the globus pallidus (GPi) constitutes the final output of the basal ganglia. As a result of the dopamine deficiency present in PD, the GABAergic output of the GPi is increased (21–26) Two main mechanisms are believed to contribute to this: (1) increased drive from the excitatory glutamatergic subthalamic nucleus (STN) via the indirect pathway from the striatum through the external segment of globus pallidus (GPe); and (2) decreased inhibition (dysinhibition) via a direct pathway from the motor striatum (25,27). Hyperactivitiy of the GPi is considered to be a hallmark of PD and is thought to exert an excessive inhibitory influence on the thalamus and downstream cortical motor system and on brainstem motor areas. This overinhibition of the cortical and brainstem motor systems is thought to be responsible for the disrupted and impoverished movement that characterizes PD. The surgical strategy is to make lesions selectively in the sensorimotor portions of the GPi so as to decrease the inhibitory influence of basal ganglia output thus releasing brainstem motor areas and normalizing thalamocortical activity. It is believed that lesions should be limited to the sensorimotor portions of the GPi as it is defined by the area populated by neurons that respond to movement. Lesions should spare the limbic and associative territories of the GPi to avoid unwanted complications and should avoid injury to the other adjacent territories including GPe, the optic tract, and the internal capsule.

VIM Thalamotomy

The VIM nucleus of the thalamus receives predominantly contralateral cerebellar inputs and projects it to the primary motor cortex, premotor, and supplementary motor cortical areas. Early investigations involving motor thalamus in PD patients revealed that many of its cells have a discharge pattern synchronized to the patient's tremor (28–30) These "tremor cells" were found in sites presumed to correspond to the Vim and Vop nuclei, that is the cerebellar and pallidal receiving areas respectively. Numerous studies (31–34) focused on the role of these ventral nuclear groups of the thalamus in the pathogenesis of tremor in PD. Moreover, intraoperative electrical stimulation in the regions where these tremor cells were recorded produced tremor arrest, whereas lesions at these same sites produced long-term tremor relief (35,36).

However, VIM lesions variably improve rigidity and have little effect on bradykinesia or the gait disturbances that are characteristic of PD. For this reason, the VIM target is of limited use in PD and should be restricted to a small group of patients, perhaps 5 percent, who have medication-resistant tremor-dominant PD and have shown over prolonged observation that their illness is unlikely to progress to akinesia, rigidity or gait disturbance.

INDICATIONS AND PATIENT SELECTION FOR SURGERY

Pallidotomy

Several recent trials (37–41) have documented significant benefits of pallidotomy including decrease in "off" periods, drug-induced dyskinesias, and improvement in activities of daily living, and functional independence.

The goal of pallidotomy is to improve the patient's most disabling symptoms on the most affected side of the body. Indications for GPi pallidotomy have been discussed in several recent articles (39,42–51). It is indicated for levodopa-induced dyskinesias, severe "on-off" fluctuations, rigidity, bradykinesia, "off" period dystonia, tremor, and gait disturbance, in that order of preference, as was rated in a multicenter survey (52). "Midline" symptoms persisting in the "on" periods (i.e., swallowing difficulty, hypophonic speech, postural instability, and freezing) are resistant and may even worsen with pallidotomy.

The ideal candidate for pallidotomy: (1) has asymmetric symptoms; (2) is young; (3) has bradykinetic idiopathic PD with symptoms responsive to levodopa, but continues to have significant motor impairment; (4) is cognitively intact; and (5) has reasonable expectations from surgery. Preoperative assessments include neurologic, neuroradiologic, and neuropsychologic evaluations to screen out secondary parkinsonism or "Parkinson-plus syndromes" and other problems that would contraindicate surgery. Patients who do not respond to levodopa for example, are unlikely to derive substantial benefits from pallidotomy. That is because most of them do not have idiopathic PD. Distinction between idiopathic PD and other causes of parkinsonism (e.g., multiple system atrophy (MSA), progressive supranuclear palsy (PSP), diffuse Lewy body disease, parkinsonism secondary to multifocal ischemic white matter disease) is important because preliminary evidence suggests that these disorders are much less likely to benefit from pallidotomy. Other contraindications for pallidotomy are dementia, severe depression, clinically significant medical disease that would increase the risk of developing pre- or postoperative complications (e.g., cardiac or pulmonary disease, diabetes mellitus, uncontrolled hypertension, coagulopathy).

MRI evidence of severe brain atrophy or multiple lacunar infarcts may also be relative contraindications. The presence of linear high signal in the posterolateral putamen (on T2 or proton MRI scans) sometimes combined with evidence of low signal on T2, indicative of iron dispostion, strongly suggests a diagnosis of MSA which is a definite contraindication (53). Patients with predominence of axial symptoms, postural instability, and severe contractures are generally not considered for pallidotomy (54). FDG-PET may also be used for patient selection, as patients who show lentiform hypometabolism should be excluded because this finding suggests the diagnosis of Parkinson's-plus syndromes, whereas IPD exhibits lentiform hypermetabolism and reduced striatal 18F-dopa uptake, particularly in the posterior putamen (55–57) Moreover, Eidelberg and his colleagues (58) reported that preoperative FDG/PET measurements of lentiform glucose metabolism showed significant correlation with clinical outcome following pallidotomy.

Age is not an absolute selection criterion, although some authors (37,39,43) suggest that younger patients derive more benefit than older patients, and there has even been a study showing a positive correlation of age with outcome (38). This also raises the controversial issue of when in the course of the illness, surgery is best performed. Surgery is generally reserved for patients who have reached a level of impairment that prevents them from carrying out important activities of daily living (e.g., work or self-care) despite (or because of, as in the case of dyskinesias) optimal medical therapy. Pallidotomy is not offered to end-stage, wheelchair-bound, or bedridden patients, based on the early experience of the limited benefits they derive and their often disabling associated features that are unresponsive to surgery (59).

Pre- and postoperative patients should be assessed according to the Core assessment program for intracerebral transplantation (CAPIT) protocol (60,61), which incorporates the UPDRS and Hoehn and Yahr staging scale. Recently, however, a new Core assessment program for surgical interventional therapies in PD (CAPSIT-PD) has been developed as a rating instrument, useful in evaluating surgical trials for PD (62). The cognitive and behavioral evaluation and more emphasis on quality of life, are included in this program. Thus it may provide a better tool in assessing various surgical trials for PD, in future.

A levodopa challenge test, a series of timed motor tasks, and a cognitive assessment of potential surgical candidates are also very important. Patients who score 25 or less out of 30 on the Folstein mini-mental status examination (63) are not considered to be good candidates. These patients may not be fully cooperative for the surgery, may be more prone to cognitive side effects with pallidal lesions, and because of their cognitive impairment, may derive less overall benefit associated with an improved motor status. However, this quick office screening test should not serve as the sole evaluation of cognitive function, whereas there are other neuropsychologic tests which can be included in the preoperative assessment (64–74).

Because the benefits of pallidotomy are predominantly unilateral, surgery is directed first toward the patient's worst side. When the disease is symmetrical, the dominant hemisphere is surgically treated. The efficacy and safety of bilateral pallidal lesions is still under active investigation. Although several recent reports (47,49,75,76) including over 100 bilateral pallidotomies show many "good" or "excellent" results with greater improvement than unilateral procedures, only one of these studies compared the outcome of these two procedures in a detailed quantified fashion using standard rating scales. There have also been a number of anecdotal reports of complications involving speech and cognitive function with bilateral procedures (47,77–79). Although some of these may be related to suboptimal placement of lesions, perhaps encroaching on the internal capsule or nonmotor portions of the GPi, it is prudent to proceed carefully and to rigorously assess both the benefits and the side effects of bilateral lesions.

By far the most striking effect of pallidotomy is the near complete (over 90%) (46) and sustained amelioration of drug-induced involuntary movements on the contralateral side (19,38–40,43,44,47,50,51,75, 78, 80–82). After pallidotomy, patients are better able to tolerate similar or even higher doses of medication than before surgery because of the striking diminution in contralateral and, to a lesser extent, ipsilateral dyskinesias. This translates into more dyskinesia-free "on" time and a striking improvement in their quality of life. The effects of pallidotomy on rigidity, tremor, and bradykinesia are also quite significant, with improvement in off-period scores, using validated rating scales, of 26 to 88 percent (20,37–40,43,46,83). There are many reports (38,41,43,51,75,84,85) demonstrating the improvements in axial features, but these are usually more modest, less predictable, and even less sustained than those for the other parkinsonian features (37,39,52,82). For this reason, patients whose primary disability is one or more of these are less suitable candidates for unilateral pallidotomy and should be considered for alternative surgical approaches, such as staged bilateral pallidotomy and other emerging surgical strategies, such as bilateral chronic electrical stimulation of the GPi or subthalamic nucleus (86–91).

In summary, unilateral pallidotomy is relatively safe and effective for patients with PD, with medically refractory bradykinesia, rigidity, and tremor, and those who experience significant drug-induced dyskinesia. The greatest and most consistent benefit from it is amelioration of dyskinesia. Other major advantages, compared to other surgical strategies such as deep brain stimulation, are it's wide availability, no implantation-related problems, and immediate benefit. The major drawbacks of pallidotomy are that it is irreversible and nonmodifiable. In this sense, a previous pallidotomy may preclude the full benefit of other therapeutic modalities in the future, and thus patients should be informed that they may be excluded from, or be ineligible for certain other medical and surgical therapeutic trials. Moreover, when a second procedure is contemplated on the opposite side, a series of complications and side effects are more common, than with a single unilateral procedure.

Thalamotomy

Thalamotomy directed to the Vim nucleus is indicated for asymmetric, severe, medically intractable tremor, especially when the tremor is not associated with significant disabilities from other features of PD. Vim thalamotomy is not effective for bradykinesia, micrographia, gait, and speech disturbances (92). There is evidence, however, that lesioning Vop, a pallidal receiving thalamic nucleus situated anterior to the Vim, can result in improvement of rigidity and dyskinesia through the possible mechanisms described earlier (93,94). It should be stressed that the majority of patients with PD eventually develop disabling symptoms other than tremor. Therefore, although thalamotomy may be an ideal therapeutic measure to treat the tremor, many patients will later require consideration of an additional procedure(s) for other disabilities. This is reflected in the slow decline in the number of thalamotomies being performed in patients with PD, in recent years. The same also applies to thalamic DBS (see Chapter 48). Thalamotomy on the second side is effective in ameliorating tremor but results in a high incidence of speech problems, and thus has largely been abandoned in favor of Vim-DBS and DBS of Gpi and STN, procedures that have the possibility of treating all major motor manifestations of PD.

Patient selection criteria for thalamotomy include: (1) tremor-dominant patients; (2) highly asymmetrical motor symptoms; (3) drug-resistance or intolerance; (4) lack of significant cognitive dysfunction; (5) disabilities because of tremor such that amelioration of tremor could result in an improvement in quality of life; (6) young age. Medical contraindications for thalamotomy are similar to pallidotomy (e.g., uncontrollable hypertension, diabetes mellitus, bleeding tendency, or cancer).

SURGICAL TECHNIQUES FOR PALLIDOTOMY AND THALAMOTOMY

The surgical procedures for pallidotomy and thalamotomy are described together because the basic techniques are similar. The detailed procedures are outlined in (95–98). Here, only a brief description of previously stereotactic pallidotomy and thalamotomy is presented. It is divided into three phases. First is stereotactic imaging; second, neuropsychologic mapping; and third, lesion making.

Imaging is used to obtain the location of the tentative surgical target in three-dimensional (3-D) stereotactic space. Currently, computed tomography (CT) and magnetic resonance imaging (MRI) are being used most commonly for this purpose. Initially, the stereotactic frame is applied to provide the terms of reference for the target in stereotactic space. This is done under local anesthesia. Generally, the patient is kept in an "off" state, the medications having been withheld for 12 hours overnight to accentuate the pathophysiological cellular activity in the basal ganglia and to allow direct observation of the effects of incremental lesions in either thalamus or pallidum. On the other hand, if the patient is extremely uncomfortable (e.g., because of painful off-period dystonia), it may be necessary to give some short acting anti-Parkinson medications first thing in the morning, perform the imaging with the patient "on" or partially "on," and then allow the medication to wear off before doing the physiological mapping. Target coordinates are chosen directly from the images or in relation to standard landmarks, such as the anterior and posterior commissures. The pallidal target usually corresponds

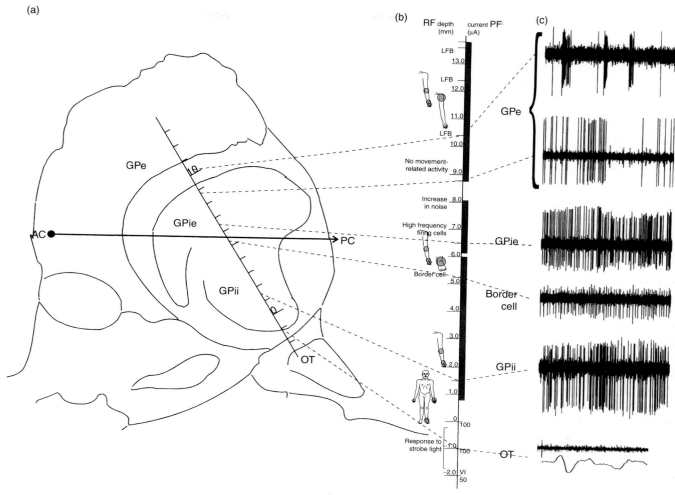

FIGURE 47-1. A, physiologic data obtained from one trajectory through the globus pallidus and optic tract (OP), plotted on the 20-mm sagittal map from the Schaltenbrand and Wahren stereotactic atlas. B, locations of neurons and their responses as well as intraoperative observations of the characteristics of recordings can be seen. Thick lines represent the cellular areas and thin lines represent the acellular (quiet) regions. Receptive fields (RFs) are shown to the left of the line along with the depth of the recordings along the trajectory. Projection fields (PFs), or the effects of microstimulation, are shown to the right of the line along with the current used. C, oscilloscope traces of representative examples of the neuronal types. GPe neurons have two distinct patterns of spontaneous firing: a low frequency discharge (10–20 Hz) punctuated by rapid bursts (so-called low frequency burst neurons) and an irregular pattern at a relatively slow frequency (30–60 Hz), also with intervening brief pauses (termed slow-frequency discharge-pause neurons). Neurons in GPi fire on the average at a higher frequency (82 ± 32 Hz, with ranges of 20–200 Hz) than that found in the GPe and normally lack audible pauses (termed high-frequency discharge neurons). Some of these neurons, termed "tremor cells," discharge in a rhythmic fashion in synchrony with peripheral tremor. Tremor cells tend to be found in the ventral half of the GP but have fond in some patients in the dorsal GPi as well. The white matter laminae which separate the GPe from GPi and GPi,e from GPi,i are flanked by "border cells" which often have wide spikes with a long after-potential. Border cells have the unique property of firing in a regular pattern at rates on the order of 20–40 Hz. The position of internal capsule is determined with microelctrodes, by its characteristic absence of somatodendritic action potentials, and the tetanization produced by stimulating corticospinal tract fibers. The somatotopic organization of the corticospinal system (face is medial, followed by the upper limb and leg most laterally) provides information on the laterality of the trajectory. For the TO (optic tract), a single-pass recording is shown above the multisweep potential responses to strobe light stimulation. LFB = low-frequency burst neurons; AC = anterior commissure; PC = posterior commissure. (Reprinted from Lozano A, Hutchison W, Kiss Z, et al. (95), with permission).

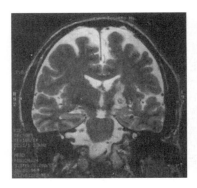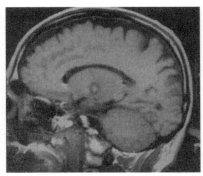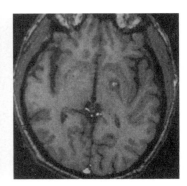

FIGURE 47-2. Postoperative MRI confirming the location of globus pallidus lesion in a patient with idiopathic Parkinson's disease in coronal (A) sagittal (B) and horizontal (C) planes. (Reprinted from Lozano A, Hutchison W, Kiss Z, et al. (95), with permission).

quite closely to the target initially described by Laitinen and coworkers (84) and is usually 2 to 3 mm anterior to the midcommissural point, 3 to 6 mm below the intercommissural (IC) line, and 20 to 21 mm from the midline. The thalamic target is usually 25 percent of AC-PC length, posterior to midcommissural point on the IC plane, and 13 to 17 mm from midline.

For the neurophysiologic mapping, a burr hole or twist drill opening just anterior to the coronal suture on the side opposite the worse Parkinsonian symptoms is made, so as to allow the introduction of a macroelectrode or canula to guide a microelectrode. There are currently two widely used techniques for physiologic mapping, microelectrode recording/stimulation and macroelectrode stimulation mapping. The macroelectrode technique allows mapping based on the interpretation of macrostimulation responses. It has the advantage of being rapid and requiring minimal equipment, but it does not allow the recording of neuronal activity. The microelectrode technique allows the acquisition of direct measures of cellular activity from individual neurons offering high level of physiologic resolution of nuclei based on the pattern of neuronal activity and the determination of their receptive fields. These advantages come at the price of extra time, extra equipment, and a high level of expertise required for the procedures.

The information required to place GPi lesions safely includes the identification of the optic tract, the internal capsule, and the sensorimotor GPi, defined as that part containing movement responsive neurons (Figure 47-1). For thalamotomy, important considerations in selecting the optimal target include: (1) lesions should be at least 2 to 3 mm anterior to the border of the tactile sensory relay thalamic nucleus, (2) lesions should be made in areas containing kinesthetic (movement-related) cells, (3) lesions should be placed in areas populated by tremor cells, (4) lesions should be made in areas where electrical stimulation produces

arrest of tremor, and (5) lesions should be made at the base of the thalamus to deafferent the entire dorsal ventral extent of VIM from incoming cerebellar fibres. Lesions are made by heating a 1-mm diameter probe whose last 2 or 3 mm is not insulated. The technique is to first make a test lesion at $60\,^\circ$C for 60s, followed by the formal lesioning by heating the electrode to $70\,^\circ$C, $80\,^\circ$C, up to $90\,^\circ$C for 60s. In the thalamus, 4-mm diameter lesions are made, whereas larger, 6-mm diameter lesions are usually made in the GPi. A spherical lesion that measures approximately 6-mm in height and 4 mm in diameter in the GPi is demonstrated on a T1-weighted MRI after surgery (Figure 47-2). Other groups make multiple smaller lesions on one or more electrode tracts. Some attempt to make the lesion depending on the somatotopic findings and the clinical distribution of signs and symptoms. On the other hand, there is no convincing evidence that the clinical outcome is any better using this approach than with the single larger lesion. Throughout lesion making, the patient's speech, vision, and motor function are tested. Although the optimal lesion size and location are yet to be determined, the lesion has to be sufficiently large enough to produce a longstanding clinical benefit, but small enough to avoid unwanted side effects. The benefits of pallidotomy and thalamotomy are seen immediately in the operating room.

CLINICAL RESULTS

Pallidotomy

Table 47-1 summarizes the contemporary reports of the effects of unilateral stereotactic pallidotomy in patients with PD as measured by standard rating scales. Striking improvements in motor functions have been obtained in patients in whom no further

Table 47-1   Summary of Published Results of Unilateral Pallidotomy for Parkinson's Disease as Measured by Standard Parkinson Rating Scale[a]

Authors	No. of patients	Mean F/U (mos)	Age Range (mean)	Total Scores; ADLs Changes Pre/Post(%)	Contralateral Change: "Off" Pre/Post(%)	Contralateral Change: "On" Pre/Post(%)	Ipsilateral Change	Effect on Midline/axial Symptoms	Effect on dyskinesia
J.K. Krauss et al.[b]	34	3	40–74 (59)	"off" motor: 29/25 (14) 7/34: no improvement	Tremor, bradykinesia (dexterity) significantly improved	NR	Marginal improvements in leg tremor, heel tapping	Arising from chair, gait and body bradykinesia significantly improved	NR
W.G. Ondo et al.[c]	36	6	40–75 (60)	"off" ADL: 31/18 (42)	UPDRS motor: 58/33 (43)	NR	NR	NR	NR
J.P. Sutton et al.[d]	5	2	60–75 (67.0)	ADL, total UPDRS, and S and E: no changes	No change	No change	No change	No change	Improved in 2, dystonia in 1
O. Kopyov et al.[e]	29	3	NR	ADL ("off" and "on"), motor H and Y and hours "off" per day significantly improved	NR	Tremor, bradykinesia, rigidity: significantly improved	"off" bradykinesia mostly unchanged, "on" improved	"Walking" (off vs on) significantly improved	Significantly improved (no direct scores)
I. Masterman et al.[f]	36	3–6	34–82 (65)	UPDRS improved 22%, motor "off" 24%, ADL 19%, S and E "off" 30%, and "on" 28%	UPDRS motor 24% improvement	UPDRS improved 29%	NR	Gait improved 30%, freezing 43%, dynamic balance improved	% time with dyskinesia improved 61%
Iacono et al.[g]	126	4.5	31–80 (62)	H and Y: 3.4/2.0 (41)	Tremor improved 65%, rigidity 70%	NR	NR	Posture, gait, and postural stability improved 50–57%	"all noted freedom from … dyskinesia"
M.S. Baron et al.[h]	15	12	38–71 (57.0)	Motor: 98.6/79.5 (19) ADL: 30.2/25.7 (15) S and E: 49/69	UPDRS motor: 33.4/46 (17) Tremor, rigidity, bradykinesia all significantly improved	NR	Some improvement at three months, not sustained at one yr	"off" gait, falling improved to one yr, postural stability not improved >3 mo; swallowing improved in 7–8 patients	Contra. dyskinesias markedly improved, ipsi. dyskinesias less affected

(continued)

Table 47-1 (Continued)

Authors	No. of patients	Mean F/U (mos)	Age Range (mean)	Total Scores; ADLs Changes Pre/Post(%)	Contralateral Change: "Off" Pre/Post(%)	Contralateral Change: "On" Pre/Post(%)	Ipsilateral Change	Effect on Midline/axial Symptoms	Effect on dyskinesia
I.L. Vitek et al.[i]	8	24	NR	UPDRS: 92/77 (16) S and E: 51/67	Motor: 51/42 (18)	NR	NR	NR	NR
M. Samuel et al.[j]	26	22 (3) 12(12)	40–72 (55.9)	"off" ADL: 32.5/26.5(16.9) "off" motor: 53.5/42.5(17.8) "on" no change	Motor: 16.5/12.0(27.3) Rigidity: 4/3(25) Tremor: 3/2 (33.3) Bradykinesia: 8.5/7.0(24)	No significant changes in motor, rigidity, tremor, bradykinesia	"off" ipsilateral motor NS, rigidity 22.2%, tremor and bradykinesia NS, timed tasks NS; "on" no change	"off" gait/postural stability marginal, timed walking 29.3% improvement	Significant improvements: 66.7% contralat. 50% axial, 45% ipsilateral
R. Scott et al.[k]	12	3	48–70 (56)	"off" motor: 78/57 (27) "off" ADL: 21/18 (14)	Unilateral motor 29% ADL 15% Bilateral motor 37% ADL 44%	Unilateral motor 27% ADL 28% Bilateral motor 47% ADL 30%	NR	NR	Unilateral: reduced by 73% Bilateral: reduced by 88%
R.J. Uitti et al.[l]	20	3	49–78 (66.5)	"off" UPDRS: 83/64 (23) "off" ADL: 21/17 (20)	Motor: 49/38 (22)	Motor: 27/20 (26)	No change in timed score	Severe gait disturbance preop in 6/11 were markedly improved	Goetz score (mean only 1.4 preop) not improved, Mayo dyskinesia score improved
P.R. Schuurman et al.[m]	15	18	17–74 (53)	"off" motor: 51.1/27.7 (47.8) "off" rigidity: 9.9/4.5 (54.5) "off" hypokinesia:19/11(42) "off" tremor: 4/0.8 (80) "off" H and Y: 3.7/2.9 (21.6) "off" S and E: 52.7/74 (40.4)	Rigidity: 5.1/1.5 (70.6) Hyperkinesia: 11.1/4.8 (57) Tremor: 2.3/0.1 (95.6)	NR	Rigidity: 3/2.1 (30) Hyperkinesia: 8.2/6.4 (22) Tremor: 1.6 (0.8 (50)	"off" posture 40%, gait 37.5%, balance 38.1% improvement	Peak-dose dyskinesias marked reduction and "off" time reduced
M. Dogali et al.[n]	18	12	42–79 (59.8)	"off" UPDRS improve by 65% "off" ADL: 18/8 (55) "on" scores also improved No significant change in Unoperated group	"off" motor: 35/13 (60) "off" CAPIT timed scores improved by 38.2%	Improved, numbers NR	"off" CAPIT timed scores improved by 38.2% "on" scores improved	"off" CAPIT walk scores improved by 45%, "on" scores improved	"resolution of … contralateral dyskinesias" – data NR

E. Fazzini et al.[o]	11	40	56–79 (61)	"off" ADL: 15/5 (66) ADL and motor scores remained significantly improved and did not change over 3 yrs of F/U	"off" motor: 32/8 (75) No decline in CAPIT improvements over the F/U period	NR	Some "minor" deterioration in CAPIT scores over the F/U	NR	"dyskinesias did not return on the operated side"
K.M. Shannon et al.[p]	26	6	NR (59.3)	"off" UPDRS motor: 15% improvement, ADL: no change "on": no change	"off" motor: 49/42 (15) 26% improvement in sum of tremor, rigidity and bradykinesia	No change	Not significant at 6 months	Short-lived improvement in "off" walking	Duration and severity(UPDRS) significantly improved at 6 months
C.A. Giller et al.[q]	55	2 wk	NR	"off" UPDRS, ADL: NR	"off" motor: 42/32 (24) significantly improved at 2 months (n = 35) in 71%; at 6 months (n = 27) 78%; at 12 months (n = 12) 75%	Improved but "less prominent"	NR	NR	70%, 89% reduction in total and contralateral scores
G. Linazasoro et al.[r]	27	12	NR	"off" UPDRS: 44.3%, 38.6% improvements at 1, 12 months Tremor: 90.9%, 96.8% improvements at 1, 12 months Rigidity: 71.7%, 54% improvements at 1, 12 months Bradykinesia: 69.4%, 52.3% improvements at 1, 12 months	NR	NR	NR	50.6%, 46.9% improvements of axial symptoms at 1, 12 months	100%, 95.8% improvements of dyskinesias at 1, 12 months

(continued)

Table 47-1 (*Continued*)

Authors	No. of patients	Mean F/U (mos)	Age Range (mean)	Total Scores; ADLs Changes Pre/Post(%)	Contralateral Change: "Off" Pre/Post(%)	Contralateral Change: "On" Pre/Post(%)	Ipsilateral Change	Effect on Midline/axial Symptoms	Effect on dyskinesia
F. Johansson et al.[s]	22	12	43–78 (63.8)	NR; no change in "off" occasions, "considerable" reduction in "on+" time	Maximum values of tremor and RAM of hands significantly improved Timed tests unchanged	NR	Not changed	Rising from chair, posture, and freezing not improved	12/13 with dyskinesias "completely vanished" at 4 mo, ipsi dyskinesia also improved
A.M. Lang et al.[t]	39	6–24	44–72 (58.8)	"off" UPDRS motor(28%), ADL(29%) significantly improved, sustained for 2 Years "on" ADL(30%) significantly improved, nil else and benefit not sustained >1 year	"off" bradykinesia and tapping significantly improved, sustained for two years for bradykinesia and rigidity	"on" tapping significantly improved but not sustained, nil else	"off" bradykinesia and tapping significantly improved, nil else, not sustained >3 months "on" tapping significant improvement, not sustained	"off" gait, postural stability, freezing and PIGD composite significantly improved, not sustained >3–6 months	Contralat. 83% reduction sustained with nonsignificant increase at two years Ipsi. 44% reduction lost between 1–2 years
A.M. Lozano et al.[u]	14	6	44–71 (58.9)	"off" UPDRS motor(30%), ADL(31%), akinesia(33%) significantly improved "on" no significant changes	"off" rigidity, tremor, akinesia significantly improved	Only tapping scores significantly improved	"off" akinesia significantly improved, nil else "on" only tapping scores significantly improved	"off" gait(15%),PIGD composite(23%) significantly improved "on" no changes	Contralateral: 92% reduction Ipsilateral : 32% reduction(NS)
A. Kishore et al.[v]	11	6–12	37–74 (61)	Significant improvement in "off" ADL; 24/18 (25) at 6 months 24/17 (29) at 12 months and motor UPDRS and "on" ADL(trend for motor)	"off" tremor(79%), Rigidity(55%), Bradykinesia(43%) and PPB(49%) significantly improved	"on" rigidity(38%) and PPB(20%) improvement	"off" tremor and bradykinesia significantly improved "on" PPB significantly improved	"off" gait and postural stability improved (not "on")	Contralateral: 76% improvement Ipsilateral: 41% improvement

A. Samii et al.[w]	20	24	37–74 (61)	No significant improvement in "off" ADL at 18 and 24 months but significantly worse than 3 months post-pallidotomy. No significant changes of UPDRS(IV-A,B) at 24 months. "on" ADL worsened by 75% compared with prepallidotomy	"off" tremor improvement (90%), but no significant PPB improvement	No "on" PPB score improvement at 24 months	No significant change of "off" PPB from prepallidotomy	No significant changes of "off" and "on", gait", and postural stability compared with prepallidotomy	Contralateral: 83% improvement Ipsilateral: no improvement

[a]Pre, preoperative; Post, postoperative; UPDRS, United Parkinson's Disease Rating Scale.

[b,c]See References 81, 40. UPDRS videos are rated blindly.

[d]See Reference 50. Microelectrode recording was not used during operation. Two patients H and Y five on and off after only four and five years of disease suggests possible alternative diagnosis such as multiple system atrophy. Three unilateral with two repeats, and two operated on bilaterally

[e]See Reference 115. UPDRS scores were determined blindly. "Improvement in onset in the single levodopa test".

[f]See Reference 99. Posturography, neuropsychologic and neuropsychiatric assessments were done.

[g]See Reference 71. Collaborated work with Kyushu University of Japan. 68 bilateral procedures with data lumped together with results from unilateral ones.

[h]See Reference 39. Young and nondemented patients had better responses; no significant changes in neuropsychologic or psychiatric evaluation.

[i]See Reference 160.

[j]See Reference 41. Significant correlation between magnitude of preop response to L-DOPA and total motor "off" improvement and between distance of most ventral point of lesion below AC-PC plane on MRI and improvement in contralateral bradykinesia.

[k]See Reference 47. Microelectrode recording was not used during operation. 8/20 bilateral procedures with separate results.

[l]See Reference 51. L lesions in R handed patients: mild decline in word generation(no other neuropsychologic changes); elderly patients responded as well as younger ones.

[m]See Reference 161. Four patients underwent staged bilateral procedure. Microelectrode recording or stimulation was not used during operation.

[n]See Reference 43. Eighteen operated patients compared to seven unoperated patients. Timed scores rated blindly from videos.

[o]See Reference 44. All patient were from M. Dogali et al. (43). Four had second procedures. F/U for two years in one, three years in five and four years in five.

[p]See Reference 48.

[q]See Reference 78. Review of 67 pallidotomies and 35 thalamotomies. Microelectrode recording was not used during operation. Report emphasized imaging technique. 49 unilateral, eight staged and three simultaneous bilateral procedures.

[r]See Reference 106. Seven patients had F/U up to 2–4 years and showed maintained effect on operated side but worsening of axial signs and the nonoperated side.

[s]See Reference 80. Two repeat operations. Not assessed at specific times related to medications (i.e., no true "off" and "on" assessments).

[t]See Reference 37. F/U in 39 at 6 months, 27 at one year, and 11 at two years. 44–52% of patients dependent in "off" state for ADL independent at six months and sustained to two years for feeding and dressing but reduced at one and two years for hygiene. Younger patients improved more than older patients.

[u]See Reference 46. Blinded investigators were used for all or part of the UPDRS score determination.

[v]See Reference 38. Microelectrode recording was not used during operation. F/U study up to one year (11 pts of 24 patients). Age correlated positively with improvement in "off" UPDRS motor scores.

[w]See Reference 116. Follow-up study on 20 of the original 24 patients reported by A. Kishore.[38]

Abbreviations:

ADL, Activities of Daily Living; Contra, contralateral; F/U, follow-up; H and Y, Hoehn and Yahr score; Ipsi, ipsilateral; NR, not reported; NS, not significant change; PIGD, postural instability/gait disorder composite score; PPB, purdue pegboard; RAM, rapid alternating movement; S and E, Schwab and England Scale improvement was obtainable with medical treatment. The improvements include: (1) marked amelioration of contralateral drug-induced dyskinesia, reaching to over 90 percent, (2) total UPDRS motor improvement (14–65%) and contralateral UPDRS motor improvements in the "off" state of approximately 32.2 percent (range 15–75%), at 6–12 months follow-up, including a substantial decrease in contralateral tremor score (about 33–97%), (3) at two-year evaluations, improvements in these scores over baseline remain significant, although quantitatively less than at one-year.

The motor improvements are most pronounced contralaterally. The benefit is primarily evident in the off-period. Measures of the activities of daily living (ADL) significantly improve in both the "on" and "off" phases with unilateral pallidotomy, ranging from 14 to 79 percent, and it can restore functional independence in certain patients with advanced and disabling disease. The improvement in "on" period ADL scores may be largely because of the reduction in peak-dose dyskinesias. Improvement of off-period bradykinesia ranges from 24 to 57 percent. In some patients this may be because of the fact that levodopa dose can be increased without producing dyskinesia but generally, the effect is seen without drug dosage changes. The improvements in rigidity scores range from 25 to 70 percent and improvements in axial symptoms (gait, posture, freezing, and falling) have been observed by many investigators, variably up to 57 percent (20,38,43,51,75,85,99), but in some studies these effects failed to reach statistical significance at longer evaluation times (39,46). Thus patients should be informed that significant improvement in axial symptomatology with unilateral pallidotomy is less predictable than that for other cardinal symptoms. Improvements in "off" period Parkinsonian features on the ipsilateral side to the pallidal lesion are seen (39,43,76,82), but these changes are not as striking or consistent, with the possible exception of a moderate reduction in bradykinesia. On the other hand, ipsilateral dyskinesias are consistently improved by up to 50 percent (37,38). However, the authors have found that this benefit is lost between one and two years following surgery.

A small number of studies evaluated performance on motor tasks aside from clinical rating scales. Jankovic et al. (100) demonstrated improvements in "off" period contralateral simple and complex reaction times and movement time. Bennett and coworkers (101) documented a reduction in the duration of movement and time spent in deceleration but at the "cost" of deterioration in movement patterning (reach to grasp, movements to objects of differing sizes). Pfann and colleagues (102) found no change in "on" period peak velocity or other mean "on" motor performance measures studied.

The effect of pallidotomy in response to levodopa has been evaluated beyond the simple assessment of "on" period clinical scores. Merello and coworkers (103) found a nonsignificant reduction (by 50%) in the latency to benefit from a single, oral dose of levodopa although the duration of effect was significantly prolonged bilaterally. Generally, the dose of dopaminergic medication remains the same postoperatively. However, this may vary because some patients are able to increase levodopa dosage because of improvement in dose-limiting dyskinesias, whereas others may reduce their daily drug intake because of improvement in off-periods. Studying responses to single oral doses and intravenous infusions of levodopa, Skalabrin and coworkers (104) found changes in motor benefit and dyskinesias that suggested that, pallidotomy significantly widens the therapeutic window of levodopa in PD.

The issue of bilateral pallidotomy is still controversial. Despite the beneficial effects described by some authors (20,49,75), most investigators have either avoided this approach or have given it up. This is primarily because of accompanying complications (e.g., speech deterioration, worsening of cognitive deficits) that are usually more frequent and more serious than with unilateral surgery. For this reason, the safety of bilateral pallidotomy needs further careful investigations. An alternative to bilateral lesioning is the use of DBS on the second side. This may be safer and equally or more effective. However, only one report of this approach has been published to date (86).

Data concerning the long-term effect of pallidotomy are limited, given that this is a newly reintroduced procedure, but it is generally agreed that improvements in Parkinsonism and drug-induced dyskinesias are maintained for at least two years (45,105). Although a study by Fazzini et al. (44) indicates its effects may be protracted up to four years, the data provided in this report are extremely difficult to accept. Linazasoro et al. (106) and Vitek et al. (53) have also reported prolonged benefit with respect to antidyskinetic effects. The preliminary evaluation of long-term effect has shown persistent significant improvements in off-period total motor scores, contralateral tremor, rigidity, and bradykinesia as well as contralateral dyskinesias.

The neuropsychologic effects of unilateral pallidotomy remain somewhat controversial. Although Baron and coworkers (39) and Soukup and coworkers (107) found no significant deterioration of cognitive abilities postoperatively, others have shown fairly consistent deficits in verbal phonemic or semantic fluencies, especially after left-side lesions (99,108–111). Scott and coworkers (47) and Perrine and coworkers (112) also reported a decline in verbal memory postoperatively in 3 of 12 (25%) and 5 of 28 (17.9%) patients, respectively. Stebbins and coworkers (113) reported that tasks assessing working memory capacity and other aspects of frontal executive functioning and visuoconstructional functions were performed poorly in 13 patients whose reports were studied 1 year after surgery. They found that performance on any task with strong working memory demands declined in the operated group, but not in an unoperated parkinsonian control group. Furthermore, frontal behavioral dyscontrol also has been observed, albeit rarely (44,48,81). Recently, a study of 42 unilateral pallidotomy patients evaluated in the "on"

state by Trépanier and coworkers (108) demonstrated that these behavioral changes interfered with patients' ability to function properly at work or in social settings. Lack of insight into these changes was noted in some patients, making behavioral management more difficult. However, these changes were outweighed by the positive clinical benefits obtained by the surgery.

Adverse effects and complications with pallidotomy are common. For many centers, these are new procedures requiring the acquisition of new technical, anatomical, physiological, and neurosurgical knowledge. The reports that have been reviewed in Table 47-2 represent the initial experience of several

Table 47-2 Published Complications of Unilateral Pallidotomy for Parkinson's Disease in Contemporary Series*

Death	0–7.7
Hemorrhage	0–15.4
Symptomatic	0–7.7
Cognitive (and/or behavioral change)	1.8–7.7
Persistent : Transient	5.0–7.7 : 1.8–2.5‡
Visual field deficits or scotoma	1.6–14
Persistent : Transient	1.6–8.0 : 0–14
Speech disturbance (or worsening)	1.8–27
Persistent : Transient	1.8–7.5 : 0.5–27
Hemiparesis	2.4–8.3
Persistent : Transient	0–3.8 : 1.8–8.2
Confusion	1.2–41.5
Persistent : Transient	0 : 1.2–41.5
Facial weakness	4.1–35.3
Persistent : Transient	5.0–12 : 2.2–30.3
Dysphagia	0–17.5
Persistent : Transient	0–15 : 3.8–12.5
Others:	
Frontal lobe syndrome	11.5% in 1 study (transient)
Hypersexuality	10.0% in 1 study (transient)
Psychosis	9.1% in 1 study (1/2 persistent)
Neglect of motor	8% in 1 study (persistent)
Reduced motivation	8% in 1 study (persistent)
Hallucination	8% in 1 study (transient)
Worsening of hand writing	5% in 2 studies (persistent)
Urinary incontinence	5% in 1 study (transient)
Infarct	3.9% in 4 studies (persistent)
(6 delayed capsular, 1 frontal venous, 1 hemorrhagic)	
Euphoria	2.9% in 1 study (transient)
Increased drooling	2.9% in 1 study (transient)
Worsening of dementia	2.9% in 2 studies (persistent)
Worsening of depression	2.5% in 1 study (persistent)
Infection	0.03–1.8% in 4 studies (all transient)
(1 scalp infection, 1 empyema, 1 abscess, 1 meningitis)	
Dyspraxia of foot	1.2% in 3 studies (transient)
Epileptic fit	1.1% in 5 studies (transient)

*Percent of cases based on data reported in the literature (20,37–41,43,44,46, 48,49,54,75,80,84,162–164).
‡Ranges of permanent and transient cases are based on only those specified.

groupswith variable past experience in functional neurosurgery. Overall, there is approximately a 10–15% incidence of persistent adverse effects with unilateral pallidotomy. Major complications of pallidotomy include visual field deficits and facial weakness related to thermolytic lesioning of adjacent structures (i.e., optic tract and capsular fibers of face). The most serious complication is intracerebral hemorrhage related to penetration of electrodes into arteries, arterioles, or veins. The incidence of cerebral hemorrhage ranges from 0% to 15% with mean of approximately 2%. The majority of these complications, however, are mild and well tolerated and appear to be far outweighed by the benefits of pallidotomy. The incidence of these complications appears to have substantially declined in recent years possibly because of increased awareness of the potential for these complications and modifications in surgical techniques to optimize the target and lesion.

Although concern has been expressed regarding a possible high incidence of complications associated with microelectrode techniques, careful review of the available literature indicates that there is little evidence to support this (39,43,46,80,114,115). Two year outcome data recently reported by one group who do not use microrecording showed less sustained benefit (116) than demonstrated in the author's own two year follow-up (45). Although the study populations may not be comparable, this difference could suggest differences in target selection based on the data made available with the microrecording technique.

Thalamotomy

Several reports suggest that up to 80% of patients achieve total abolition or marked reduction of contralateral tremor after unilateral thalamotomy for PD (Table 47-3) (32,36,94,97,117–127). It should be noted that thalamotomy is most effective in relieving appendicular tremor. Midline symptoms, such as head tremor and voice tremor, seem to respond less well and may progress relentlessly, and limit function in about 25% of patients (128–130). VanBuren et al. (129) found that impairment from the midline symptoms and speech deficits exceeded any gains from the reduced limb tremor, and their average patient functioned less well postthalamotomy. Therefore before making a final decision to proceed to operation, patients should be informed of what they can reasonably expect to avoid disappointment.

Published complications of unilateral thalamotomy for PD are listed in Table 47-4 (92,97,119,126–128, 130–134). The mortality rate is approximately 0.5% (range 0–5%), with intracranial hemorrhage being the major cause of death (incidence of intracranial

Table 47-3 Published Outcomes of Unilateral Thalamotomy for Tremor in Parkinson's Disease*	
Tremor	
Total abolition	45–93
Significant reduction	66–100

*Percentage of patients based on data reported in literature (32,36,94,97,117–127).

Table 47-4 Published Complications of Unilateral Thalamotomy for Parkinson's Disease*	
Death	0–5
Hemorrhage	1.5–6
Cognitive	
Persistent : Transient	0.8–14 : 1–43
Hemiparesis	
Persistent : Transient	0–9 : 0–26
Dysphasia	
Persistent : Transient	0–3 : 1.0–29
Dysarthria	
Persistent : Transient	0.8–11.2 : 1–43
Hand ataxia	
Persistent : Transient	1.3 : 5–61
Gait	
Persistent : Transient	1.2–6 : 1–30
Equinovarus deformity	
Persistent : Transient	3.5–5.3 : 2.7
Hyperkinesia	0.3–9
Numbness	
Persistent : Transient	0.5–3.3 : 1–20
Confusion	
Persistent : Transient	0–1 : 0–16
Blepharospasm	
Persistent : Transient	0–1 : 0–2
Hypertonia, transient	0–9
Seizure	0.5–8
Dyspagia/pseudobulbar symptoms	0.3–0.3
Infection	0.5–4
Dystonia, transient	0–3

*Percentage of patients based on data reported in the literature (92,97,119,126–128,130–134).

hematoma, 1.5–6%). Therefore, all patients should be screened for bleeding tendency, coagulopathy, and hypertension. Also, acetylsalicylic acid (ASA) or ASA containing products should be discontinued for at least one week before surgery. Hypertensive patients should have blood pressure strictly controlled before and during surgery. Special consideration should be given to those with significant cerebral atrophy because of the increased risk of subdural hematoma from traction injury to bridging veins. These steps should be taken for patients preparing for any surgical intervention. Other complications include dysarthria, cognitive difficulties, persistent hemiparesis or limb weakness, dystonia, unilateral auditory neglect, neglect of the contralateral extremities, arm dyspraxia, and "cerebellar" complications including limb ataxia and astasia. Side effects such as paresthesias or numbness with a predominant hand-mouth distribution may be seen often, but these usually subside spontaneously (92,97,119,126–128,130–134). Facial paresis also has been reported but is usually transient in the majority of cases. Memory and language dysfunctions following thalamotomy are probably more common than traditionally thought or recognized. They occur in about one third of patients and up to double this figure with bilateral thalamotomy. One half of these patients can be expected to recover to baseline within several months (135).

Although a blinded long-term follow-up study by Diederich et al. (118) showed significant persistent improvement of the tremor or amelioration of its rate of progression, other studies with follow-up periods up to 10 years indicated that as many as 48% of patients returned to their preoperative state and only 22 to 44% continued to show improvement from their preoperative baseline (117,121). Also as thalamotomy does not arrest general disease progression and has little effect on other parkinsonian symptoms, it is usually necessary to continue pharmacologic therapy.

Among patients who have undergone unilateral thalamotomy, many will eventually develop sufficiently disabling tremor on the other side so as to consider the contralateral surgery. Table 47-5 lists the outcome data for bilateral thalamotomy reported in the literature (32,121,132,133,136,137) Although its effect on abolishing tremor has been reported to be similar to that of the unilateral procedure (126), there has generally been significant reluctance to perform bilateral thalamotomy because of the high incidence of adverse effects. Most surgeons prefer bilateral or contralateral thalamic DBS over bilateral thalamotomy. Table 47-6 reviews the published complications of bilateral thalamotomy for PD (32,97,121,125,132,133,136,137).

Table 47-6 Published Complications of Bilateral Thalamotomy for Parkinson's Disease*

Death	0–4.3
Cognitive Dysphasia	1.8–34.8
Persistent : Transient	3.6 : 5.5
Hemiparesis	0.8–1.8
Dysphagia	3.6–5.4
Dysarthria	
Persistent : Transient	18–60 : 1.8–50
Gait disturbance	
Persistent : Transient	17.4 : 48
Equinovarus deformity	2.2
Hyperkinesis	5–7.2
Foot dystonia	0–1.8
Infection	0–3.6

*Percent of cases based on data reported in the literature (32,97,121,125,132,133,136,137).

Incidence of complications tends to be two to threefold higher than that for unilateral thalamotomy. The predominant complication is speech and language impairment, characterized by hypophonia, dysarthria, and dysphasia. Significant dysphagia and transient confusion may also be seen in up to 10% of cases. Cognitive dysfunction is also much more common and concerning following bilateral thalamotomy than after unilateral surgery.

CONCLUSION

Stereotactic pallidotomy results in unequivocal clinical benefits and has become an important treatment modality in patients with later stage PD who, despite optimal medical therapy, are disabled by levodopa-responsive off-period symptoms or levodopa-induced dyskinesias. The procedure is generally well tolerated, although side effects (mostly transient) are common. It is unclear whether patients who have undergone pallidotomy will respond to new treatment options, such as human fetal transplantation (138–141), xenotransplantation (142), infusion of trophic factors (143–149), implantation of encapsulated cells (140,150,151), or novel gene therapy (152–159). These future therapies may be beneficial, but it will require some time before they are applicable to patients. On the other hand, if DBS of GPi or STN is shown to be at least as safe and effective as pallidotomy, as suggested in some studies (87,88,91), it is reasonable to provide this nondestructive approach, especially to young patients, retaining the potential for

Table 47-5 Published Results on Bilateral Thalamotomy for Parkinson's Disease*

Tremor	
Complete abolition	33–100
Significant reduction	67–71

*Percentage of patients based on data reported in the literature (32,121,132,133,136,137).

unilateral pallidotomy for Parkinson's disease. *Ann Neurol* 1996; 39:450–459.

59. Lozano AM, Hutchison W. Pallidotomy: Indications and techniques. In: Germano IM (ed.). *Neurosurgical Treatment of Movement Disorders.* Park Ridge, Ill. : AANS Publications Committee, 1998:131–141.

60. Lang AE, Benabid AL, Koller WC, et al. The core assessment program for intracerebral transplantation [letter; comment] [see comments]. *Mov Disord* 1995; 10:527–528.

61. Langston JW, Winder H, Goetz CG. The core assessment program for intracerebral transplantation (CAPIT). *Mov Disord* 1992; 7:2–13.

62. Defer GL, Winder H, Marié RM, et al. Core assessment program for surgical interventional therapies in Parkinson's disease (CAPSIT-PD). *Mov. Disord* 1999; 14:572–584.

63. Folstein MF, Folstein SE, McHugh PR. "Mini-mental state." A practical method for trading the cognitive state of patients for the clinician. *J Psychiatr Res* 1975; 12:189–198.

64. Wechsler D. *WAIS-R: Manual.* New York: The Psychological Corporation, 1981.

65. Grace J, Malloy P. *Frontal lobe personality scale:* National Academy of Neuropsychology-Research Consortium, 1992.

66. Beck AT. *Depression Inventory: Manual.* San Antonio: The Psychological Corporation, 1987.

67. Delis DC, Kramer JH, Kaplan E. *California Verbal Learning Test: Adult version.* San Antonio: The Psychological Corporation, 1987.

68. Golden CJ. *Stroop color and word test.* Chicago: Stoelting, 1978.

69. Goodglass H, Kaplan E. *The Assessment of Aphasia and Related Disorders.* Philadelphia: Lea and Febiger, 1983.

70. Heaton RK. *Wisconsin Card Sorting Test: Manual.* Odessa, FL: Psychological Assessment Resources, 1981.

71. Hooper HE. *Hooper Visual Organization Test.* Los Angeles: Western Psychological Services, 1983.

72. Reitan RM, Wolfson D. *The Halstead-Reitan Neuropsychological Test Battery: Theory and Interpretation.* Tucson AZ: Neuropsychology Press, 1985.

73. Smith MC. Pathological findings subsequent to stereotactic lesions. *J Neurosurg* 1966; 35:443–445.

74. Grober E, Sliwinski M. Development and validation of a model for estimating premorbid verbal intelligence in the elderly. *J Clin Exp Neuropsychol* 1991; 13:933–949.

75. Iacono RP, Shima F, Lonser RR, The results, indications, and physiology of posteroventral pallidotomy for patients with Parkinson's disease [see comments]. *Neurosurgery* 1995; 36:1118–1125; discussion 1125–1127.

76. Laitinen LV, Hariz MI. Movement disorders. In: Yomans JR (ed.). *Neurological Surgery.* Philadelphia: WB Saunders Co., 1996:3575–3609.

77. Burchiel KJ, Favre J, Taha JM. *Risk of Speech Deterioration After Pallidotomy.* Congress of Neurological Surgeons Annual Meeting. Montreal, 1996.

78. Giller CA, Dewey RB, Ginsburg MI, et al. Stereotactic pallidotomy and thalamotomy using individual variations of anatomic landmarks for localization. *Neurosurgery* 1998; 42:56–62; discussion 62–65.

79. Lang AE. Medial pallidotomy. *Mov Disord* 1996; 11 [Suppl 1]:12.

80. Johansson F, Malm J, Nordh E, et al. Usefulness of pallidotomy in advanced Parkinson's disease. *J Neurol Neurosurg Psychiatry* 1997; 62:125–132.

81. Krauss JK, Desaloms JM, Lai EC, Microelectrode-guided posteroventral pallidotomy for treatment of Parkinson's disease: Postoperative magnetic resonance imaging analysis [see comments]. *J Neurosurg* 1997; 87:358–367.

82. Lozano AM, Lang AE, Galvez-Jimenez N. GPi pallidotomy improves motor function in patients with Parkinson's disease. *Lancet* 1995; 346:1383–1386.

83. Starr PA, Vitek JL, Bakay RAE. Pallidotomy: Clinical Results. In: Germano IM (ed.). *Neurosurgical Treatment of Movement Disorders.* Park Ridge, Ill: AANS Publications Committee, 1998:143–156.

84. Laitinen LV, Bergenheim AT, Hariz MI. Leksell's posteroventral pallidotomy in the treatment of Parkinson's disease [see comments]. *J Neurosurg* 1992; 76:53–61.

85. Roberts-Warrior D, Overby AS, Orr D, et al. Postural control in patients with Parkinson's disease after pallidotomy. *Ann Neurol* 1996; 40:534.

86. Galvez-Jimenez N, Lozano A, Tasker R, et al. Pallidal stimulation in Parkinson's disease patients with a prior unilateral pallidotomy [In Process Citation]. *Can J Neurol Sci* 1998; 25:300–305.

87. Kumar R, Lozano AM, Kim YJ, et al. Double-blind evaluation of subthalamic nucleus deep brain stimulation in advanced Parkinson's disease. *Neurology* 1998; 51:850–855.

88. Limousin P, Pollak P, Benazzouz A, et al. Bilateral subthalamic nucleus stimulation for severe Parkinson's disease. *Mov Disord* 1995; 10:672–674.

89. Limousin P, Pollak P, Benazzouz A, et al. Effect of parkinsonian signs and symptoms of bilateral subthalamic nucleus stimulation. *Lancet* 1995; 345:91–95.

90. Siegfried J, Lippitz B. Bilateral chronic electrostimulation of ventroposterolateral pallidum: A new therapeutic approach for alleviating all parkinsonian symptoms. *Neurosurgery* 1994; 35:1126–1129; discussion 1129–1130.

91. Bejjani B, Damier P, Arnulf I, et al. Pallidal stimulation for Parkinson's disease. Two targets? *Neurology* 1997; 49:1564–1549.

92. Tasker RR, Siqueira J, Hawrylyshyn P, et al. What happened to VIM thalamotomy for Parkinson's disease? *Appl Neurophysiol* 1983; 46:68–83.

93. Narabayashi H. Surgical treatment in the levodopa era. In: Stern G (ed.). *Parkinson's Disease.* London: Chapman and Hall, 1990:597–646.

94. Ohye C. Thalamotomy for Parkinson's disease and other types of tremor. In: Gildenberg PL, Tasker RR (eds.). *Textbook of Stereotactic and Functional Neurosurgery*. New York: McGraw-Hill, 1997:1167–1178.

95. Lozano A, Hutchison W, Kiss Z, et al. Methods for microelectrode-guided posteroventral pallidotomy [see comments]. *J Neurosurg* 1996; 84:194–202.

96. Lozano AM, Hutchison WD, Dostrovsky JO. Microelectrode monitoring of cortical and subcortical structures during stereotactic surgery. *Acta Neurochir Suppl* 1995; 64:30–34.

97. Tasker RR. Thalamotomy. *Neurosurg Clin N Am* 1990; 1:841–864.

98. Tasker RR, Lang AE, Lozano AM. Pallidal and thalamic surgery for Parkinson's disease. *Exp Neurol* 1997; 144:35–40.

99. Masterman D, DeSalles A, Baloh RW, et al. Motor, cognitive, and behavioral performance following unilateral ventroposterior pallidotomy for Parkinson's disease. *Arch Neurol* 1998; 55:1201–1208.

100. Jankovic J, Ben-Arie L, Schwartz K, et al. Movement and reaction times and fine coordination tasks following pallidotomy. *Mov Disord* 1999; 14:57–62.

101. Bennett KM, O'Sullivan JD, Peppard RF, et al. The effect of unilateral posteroventral pallidotomy on the kinematics of the reach to grasp movement. *J Neurol Neurosurg Psychiatry* 1998; 65:479–487.

102. Pfann KD, Penn RD, Shannon KM, et al. Pallidotomy and bradykinesia: Implications for basal ganglia function. *Neurology* 1998; 51:796–803.

103. Merello M, Nouzeilles MI, Cammarotta A, et al. Changes in the motor response to acute L-dopa challenge after unilateral microelectrode–guided posteroventral pallidotomy. *Clin Neuropharmacol* 1998; 21:135–138.

104. Skalabrin EJ, Laws ER Jr, Bennett JP Jr. Pallidotomy improves motor responses and widens the levodopa therapeutic window in Parkinson's disease [In Process Citation]. *Mov Disord* 1998; 13:775–781.

105. Vitek JL, Bakay RA, DeLong MR. Microelectrode-guided pallidotomy for medically intractable Parkinson's disease. *Adv Neurol* 1997; 74:183–198.

106. Linazasoro G, Guridi J, Vela L, et al. Stereotactic surgery in Parkinson's disease. *Neurologia* 1997; 12:343–353.

107. Soukup VM, Ingram F, Schiess MC, et al. Cognitive sequelae of unilateral posteroventral pallidotomy [see comments]. *Arch Neurol* 1997; 54:947–950.

108. Trepanier LL, Saint-Cyr JA, Lozano AM, et al. Neuropsychological consequences of posteroventral pallidotomy for the treatment of Parkinson's disease. *Neurology* 1998; 51:207–215.

109. Trepanier L, Saint-Cyr J, Lang A, et al. Hemisphere-specific cognitive and motor changes after unilateral posteroventral pallidotomy [letter; comment]. *Arch Neurol* 1998; 55:881–883.

110. Marsden CD, Olanow CW. The causes of Parkinson's disease are being unraveled and rational neuroprotective therapy is close to reality. *Ann Neurol* 1998; 44:S189–S196.

111. Rilling LM, Filoteo JV, Roberts JW, et al. Neuropsychological functioning in patients with Parkinson's disease pre- and post-pallidotomy. *Arch Clin Neuropsych* 1996; 11:442.

112. Perrine K, Dogali M, Fazzini E, et al. Cognitive functioning after pallidotomy for refractory Parkinson's disease [see comments]. *J Neurol Neurosurg Psychiatry* 1998; 65:150–154.

113. Stebbins GT, Goetz CG. Factor structure of the Unified Parkinson's disease rating scale: Motor examination section [in process citation]. *Mov Disord* 1998; 13:633–636.

114. Lozano AM, Lang AE. Pallidotomy for Parkinson's disease. *Neurosurg Clin N Am* 1998; 9:325–336.

115. Kopyov O, Jacques D, Duma C, et al. Microelectrode-guided posteroventral medial radiofrequency pallidotomy for Parkinson's disease. *J Neurosurg* 1997; 87:52–59.

116. Samii A, Trunbull IM, Kishore A, et al. Reassessment of unilateral pallidotomy in Parkinson's disease. A 2-year follow-up study. *Brain* 1999; 122:417–425.

117. Broggi G, Giorgi C, Servello D. Stereotactic neurosurgery in the treatment of tremor. *Acta Neurochir Suppl* 1987; 39:73–76.

118. Diederich N, Goetz CG, Stebbins GT, et al. Blinded evaluation confirms long-term asymmetric effect of unilateral thalamotomy or subthalamotomy on tremor in Parkinson's disease. *Neurology* 1992; 42:1311–1314.

119. Fox MW, Ahlskog JE, Kelly PJ. Stereotactic ventrolateralis thalamotomy for medically refractory tremor in post-levodopa era Parkinson's disease patients [see comments]. *J Neurosurg* 1991; 75:723–730.

120. Jankovic J, Cardoso F, Grossman RG, et al. Outcome after stereotactic thalamotomy for Parkinsonian, essential, and other types of tremor [see comments]. *Neurosurgery* 1995; 37:680–686; discussion 686–687.

121. Matsumoto K, Shichijo F, Fukami T. Long-term follow-up review of cases of Parkinson's disease after unilateral or bilateral thalamotomy. *J Neurosurg* 1984; 60:1033–1044.

122. Nagaseki Y, Shibazaki T, Hirai T, et al. [Long-term follow-up study of selective VIM-thalamotomy]. *No To Shinkei* 1985; 37:545–554.

123. Osenbach R, Burchiel K. Thalamotomy: Indications, techniques, and results. In: Germano IM (ed.). *Neurosurgical Treatment of Movement Disorders*. Park Ridge, IL: AANS Publications Committee, 1998:107–130.

124. Speelman JD, Bosch DA. Resurgence of functional neurosurgery for Parkinson's disease: A historical perspective. *Mov Disord* 1998; 13:582–588.

125. Tasker RR, DeCarvalho GC, Li CS, et al. Does thalamotomy alter the course of Parkinson's disease? *Adv Neurol* 1996; 69:563–583.

126. Tasker RR. The outcome of thalamotomy for tremor. In: Gildenberg PL, Tasker RR (eds.). *Textbook of Stereotactic and Functional Neurosurgery*. New York: McGraw-Hill, 1998:1179–1198.

127. Wester K, Hauglie-Hanssen E. Stereotaxic thalamotomy–experiences from the levodopa era. *J Neurol Neurosurg Psychiatry* 1990; 53:427–430.

128. Riechert T. Stereotaxic surgery for treatment of Parkinson's syndrome. *Progr Neurol Surg* 1973; 5:1–78.

129. Van Buren JM, Li CL, Shapiro DY, et al. A qualitative and quantitative evaluation of Parkinsonians three to six years following thalamotomy. *Confin Neurol* 1973; 35:202–235.

130. Van Manen J. Long-term results of stereotaxic operations for Parkinson's disease. *Psychiatry Neurol Neurochir* 1970; 73:365–374.

131. Tasker RR. Ablative therapy for movement disorders. Does thalamotomy alter the course of Parkinson's disease? *Neurosurg Clin N Am* 1998; 9:375–380.

132. Krayenbuhl H, Siegfried J. [Treatment of Parkinson's disease: L-dopa or stereotaxic technics?]. *Neurochirurgie* 1970; 16:71–76.

133. Kelly PJ, Gillingham FJ. The long-term results of stereotaxic surgery and L-dopa therapy in patients with Parkinson's disease. A 10-year follow-up study. *J Neurosurg* 1980; 53:332–337.

134. Ohye C. Stereotactic surgery in movement disorders: Choice of patient, localization with microelectrodes and long-term results. In: Tasker (ed.). *Neurosurgery: State of Art Reviews. Stereotactic Surgery*. Philadelphia, PA: Hanley and Belfus, 1987:193–208.

135. Rossitch EJ, Zeidman SM, Nashold BS. Evaluation of memory and language function pre- and postthalamotomy with an attempt to define those patients at risk for postoperative dysfunction. *Surg Neurol* 1988; 29:11–16.

136. Matsumoto K, Asano T, Baba T, et al. Long-term follow-up results of bilateral thalamotomy for parkinsonism. *Appl Neurophysiol* 1976; 39:257–260.

137. Smith MC. Stereotactic operations for Parkinson's disease – anatomical observations. *Mod Trends Neurol* 1967; 4:21–52.

138. Lindvall O. Update on fetal transplantation: The Swedish experience. *Mov Disord* 1998; 13:83–87.

139. Kordower JH, Freeman TB, Snow BJ, et al. Neuropathological evidence of graft survival and striatal reinnervation after the transplantation of fetal mesencephalic tissue in a patient with Parkinson's disease [see comments]. *N Engl J Med* 1995; 332:1118–1124.

140. Kordower JH, Liu YT, Winn S, et al. Encapsulated PC12 cell transplants into hemi-Parkinsonian monkeys: A behavioral, neuroanatomical, and neurochemical analysis. *Cell Transplant* 1995; 4:155–171.

141. Kordower JH, Freeman TB, Chen EY, et al. Fetal nigral grafts survive and mediate clinical benefit in a patient with Parkinson's disease. *Mov Disord* 1998; 13:383–393.

142. Galpern WR, Burns LH, Deacon TW, et al. Xenotransplantation of porcine fetal ventral mesencephalon in a rat model of Parkinson's disease: Functional recovery and graft morphology. *Exp Neurol* 1996; 140:1–13.

143. Gash DM, Zhang Z, Ovadia A, et al. Functional recovery in parkinsonian monkeys treated with GDNF. *Nature* 1996; 380:252–255.

144. Arenas E. GDNF, a multispecific neurotrophic factor with potential therapeutic applications in neurodegenerative disorders [news]. *Mol Psychiatry* 1996; 1:179–182.

145. Clarkson ED, Zawada WM, Freed CR. GDNF improves survival and reduces apoptosis in human embryonic dopaminergic neurons in vitro. *Cell Tissue Res* 1997; 289:207–210.

146. Date I, Ohmoto T. Neural transplantation and trophic factors in Parkinson's disease: Special reference to chromaffin cell grafting, NGF support from pretransected peripheral nerve, and encapsulated dopamine-secreting cell grafting. *Exp Neurol* 1996; 137:333–344.

147. Grondin R, Gash DM. Glial cell line-derived neurotrophic factor (GDNF): A drug candidate for the treatment of Parkinson's disease [In Process Citation]. *J Neurol* 1998; 245:35–42.

148. Lapchak PA, Jiao S, Collins F, et al. Glial cell line-derived neurotrophic factor: Distribution and pharmacology in the rat following a bolus intraventricular injection. *Brain Res* 1997; 747:92–102.

149. Sautter J, Meyer M, Spenger C, et al. Effects of combined BDNF and GDNF treatment on cultured dopaminergic midbrain neurons. *Neuroreport* 1998; 9:1093–1096.

150. Christenson L, Emerich DF, Sanberg PR. Encapsulated cell implantation for Parkinson's disease [letter]. *Mov Disord* 1992; 7:185–186.

151. Lindner MD, Emerich DF. Therapeutic potential of a polymer-encapsulated L-DOPA and dopamine-producing cell line in rodent and primate models of Parkinson's disease. *Cell Transplant* 1998; 7:165–174.

152. Barkats M, Bilang-Bleuel A, Buc-Caron MH, et al. Adenovirus in the brain: Recent advances of gene therapy for neurodegenerative diseases. *Prog Neurobiol* 1998; 55:333–341.

153. Bankiewicz KS, Bringas JR, McLaughlin W, Application of gene therapy for Parkinson's disease: Nonhuman primate experience. *Adv Pharmacol* 1998; 42:801–806.

154. Bowers WJ, Howard DF, Federoff HJ. Gene therapeutic strategies for neuroprotection: Implications for Parkinson's disease. *Exp Neurol* 1997; 144:58–68.

155. Cao L, Zheng ZC, Zhao YC, et al. Gene therapy of Parkinson's disease model rat by direct injection of plasmid DNA-lipofectin complex. *Hum Gene Ther* 1995; 6:1497–1501.

156. Horellou P, Mallet J. Gene therapy for Parkinson's disease. *Mol Neurobiol* 1997; 15:241–256.

157. Mouradian MM, Chase TN. Gene therapy for Parkinson's disease: An approach to the prevention or palliation of levodopa-associated motor complications. *Exp Neurol* 1997; 144:51–57.

158. Redmond DE Jr. Gene therapy approaches to Parkinson's disease: Preclinical to clinical trials, or what steps to take to get there from here? *Exp Neurol* 1997; 144:160–167.

159. Stern MB, Freese A. Parkinson's disease: The case for novel treatment strategies. *Exp Neurol* 1997; 144:2–3.

160. Vitek JL, Baron M, Bakay RA, et al. Pallidotomy for medically intractable Parkinson's disease: 2-year follow-up. *Ann Neurol* 1996(abstr); 40:488.

161. Schuurman PR, de Bie RM, Speelman JD, et al. Posteroventral pallidotomy in movement disorders. *Acta Neurochir Suppl* 1997; 68:14–17.

162. Vitek JL, Bakay RA, Hashimoto T, et al. Microelectrode-guided pallidotomy: Technical approach and its application in medically intractable Parkinson's disease. *J Neurosurg* 1998; 88:1027–1043.

163. Hariz MI, De Salles AA. The side-effects and complications of posteroventral pallidotomy. *Acta Neurochir Suppl* 1997; 68:42–48.

164. Lim JY, De Salles AA, Bronstein J, et al. Delayed internal capsule infarctions following radiofrequency pallidotomy. Report of three cases. *J Neurosurg* 1997; 87:955–960.

48

Thalamic Stimulation

William C. Koller, M.D., Ph.D.
University of Miami, Miami, Florida
and

Kelly Lyons, Ph.D., Rajesh Pahwa, M.D., and Steven Wilkinson SF, M.D.
University of Kansas Medical Center, Kansas City, Kansas

Stereotactic surgery was commonly used to treat tremor disorders 30 years ago (1,2). With advances in pharmacologic therapy, particularly with the advent of levodopa for Parkinson's disease (PD), these surgeries have been rarely performed during the past two decades. Currently, there is renewed interest in surgical therapies based on the recognition of the limitations of drug treatments, expanded understanding of the pathophysiologic mechanisms of PD, and technical advances in neuroimaging, electrophysiologic recording and stereotactic techniques. We will discuss the surgical approach of deep brain stimulation (DBS) of the thalamus for the treatment of tremor in PD.

CLINICAL BACKGROUND

Thalamotomies have been successfully performed for many years as a surgical treatment for tremor in PD (see Chapter 47). However, bilateral operations are usually not recommended because of the high prevalence of severe speech impairments. It has long been observed during the performance of thalamotomies that stimulation of the target site, usually the ventralis intermedius (VIM), has the same effect as its destruction, that is, there is an arrest of neuronal firing and amelioration of PD tremor. Benabid, Pollack, and colleagues have pioneered deep-brain or high-frequency stimulation for therapeutic use in PD over the last decade (3–5).

PATIENT SELECTION FOR DBS

Deep brain stimulation of the thalamus for PD is performed in patients who have severe and uncontrolled tremor of the upper extremity that causes significant disability. The tremor in study patients has typically been rated 3 or 4 on the UPDRS scale. The tremor also has to be refractory to pharmacologic therapy. In some studies, patients were chosen because it was thought that tremor was the main cause of disability. In general, candidates for this procedure need to be in good health and reasonable, surgical candidates. Dementia is a contraindication because cognition may be worsened with the procedure. Furthermore, a reduction in tremor, probably, will not change functional disability in a demented PD patient. Age, per se, is not a contraindication. The procedure has been successfully performed in patients older than 80 years of age. It should be stated that DBS of the VIM nucleus of the thalamus is only indicated for tremor of PD and not for the treatment of bradykinesia, rigidity, postural instability, dyskinesia or other complications of levodopa therapy.

SURGICAL PROCEDURE

On July 31, 1997, the U.S. Food and Drug Administration (FDA) approved the use of the Activa tremor control therapy which uses a DBS lead, the extension which connects the DBS lead to an Implantable pulse generator (IPG), and the Itrell II IPG, for the unilateral treatment of Parkinsonian tremor. The intracranial end of the DBS lead has four platinum–iridium contacts that are 1.5 mm in length, and separated by 1.5 mm. The DBS lead is connected to the IPG device by means of an the extension that is tunneled under the skin. The IPG is implanted subcutaneously in the subclavicular area. Any one of the stimulating contacts can be used for monopolar stimulation or any two or more can be used in combination for bipolar stimulation. Stimulation is usually initiated one day postoperatively and is programmed by using an external programming device. Adjustable parameters include pulse width, amplitude, stimulation frequency, and the choice of active contacts. The patient can turn the stimulator on or off using a hand-held magnet. The usual stimulation parameters are stimulation frequency of 135 to 185 hertz, pulse width of 60 to 120 microseconds and amplitude of 1 to 3 volts.

TEAM APPROACH

A team of neurologists, neurosurgeons, specialized nurses, neuropsychologists and electrophysiologists are needed to optimally perform DBS. DBS requires neurologic expertise to select patients that will benefit from the procedure. The neurosurgeon must have a high level of expertise in stereotactic techniques, stimulating and recording from the basal ganglia and the thalamus, and intra-operative programming of stimulation parameters to achieve maximum benefit. One member of the team must be familiar with programming the impulse generator and adjusting the stimulation parameters for optimal response. For some patients, programming the stimulator can be time-consuming. Continuing maintenance is needed and the battery in the impulse generator needs to be changed every three to five years. This procedure may be best suited for a university setting with special expertise in movement disorders and a multidisciplinary unit with advanced diagnostic facilities with imaging capabilities and ancillary medical services.

CLINICAL TRIALS

Clinical investigations of DBS of the thalamus in PD have demonstrated efficacy for reducing tremor (Table 48-1) (6–12). Two hundred and thirty four PD patients have been studied in these trials. Over 90% of patients were reported to have significant improvement. For the most part, unilateral stimulation was evaluated. The usual outcome variable was a clinical rating scale of tremor severity, for example 0–4, UPDRS. In some studies, the evaluator was blinded as to stimulation "on" or stimulation "off." Some patients had a "microthalamotomy" effect, a reduction of tremors after implantation of the electrode but before the stimulator was turned on. This is thought to be due to swelling at the electrode site. This effect usually lasts several weeks, but occasionally persists.

There is some disagreement as to what type of tremor responds best. Benabid (3) has suggested that rest tremor is better controlled than action tremor, distal tremor better than proximal, and upper extremity tremor better than lower limb tremor. However, it is clear that action tremor of the arms and legs may respond well to DBS of the thalamus (13). The amount of reduction of tremor varies from patient to patient. In one-third to one-half of patients, the tremor may be totally abolished. Total amelioration of tremor occurs infrequently with drug therapy. Several studies have reported long-term efficacy of thalamic DBS in PD tremor with follow-up of one year or more (9,10) As DBS does not halt the progression of PD, stimulation intensity might need to be increased over the period of implantation. In general, studies report the need to adjust stimulation parameters over time. Several studies have reported the effects of DBS

Investigation (yr)	No. Improved/ Total No. Patients	Persistent Morbidity
Blond et al. (1992) (6)	10/10	None
Speelman and Bosch (1995) (7)	5/5	Hemi-inattention
Alesch et al. (1995) (8)	18/23	Dysarthria, paresthesia, disequilibrium
Benabid et al. (1996) (9)	78/80	Dysarthria, paresthesia, dystonia of foot, disequilibrium
Koller et al. (1997) (10)	22/24	Paresthesia, dysarthria
Ondo et al (1998) (11)	18/19	Disequilibrium, paresthesia, dysarthria, diplopia
Limousin (1999) (12)	73/73	Dysarthria, disequilibrium, dystonia

Table 48-1   High-Frequency Thalamic Stimulation for Parkinson's Tremor

on patients who had a contralateral thalamotomy or bilateral stimulators (9,14). The effect of the DBS procedure is on the contralateral side of the body only and, as expected, tremor reduction on both sides occurred with bilateral procedures. Dysarthria may be more prominent with bilateral than unilateral procedures.

The effect of secondary outcome variables related to disability such as activities of daily living (ADL) and quality-of-life (QOL) measures, have been evaluated (9–12). Because Parkinson symptoms other than tremor are not affected by DBS of the VIM nucleus, there is often no change on these measures including UPDRS-ADL and the Schwab and England scale. However, the European multicenter trial did report a significant improvement in akinesia, rigidity, UPDRS-ADL and the Schwab and England scale (12). Patients in other trials often reported a subjective improvement in disability related to tremor. Subjective measures of global disability performed both by the patient and the physician often also show improvement.

Morbidity and mortality of DBS of the thalamus is low (6–12). The greatest risks are those directly related to the operation. Surgical complications have included intracerebral hemorrhage, subdural hematoma, seizures, and mental status changes. Asymptomatic intracerebral bleeds appear to be common. These hematomas most often quickly resolve. Seizures usually do not recur and postoperative mental confusion is usually short-lived. The precise prevalence of these adverse reactions is not clear. The training and experience of the neurosurgeon may be an important determinant of surgical complications.

Complications related to the device include wire erosion, lead fracture, infection of the IPG, malfunction of the IPG, electrical shocking, and lead migration. These events occur rarely. Side effects related to stimulation are reversible with stimulation reduction and are usually well tolerated. Transient paresthesias, lasting several seconds, are common. Other complications due to stimulation that may occur include dysarthria, disequilibrium, paresis, and gait disorders.

Neuropsychologic assessments of PD patients with unilateral DBS of the thalamus have been performed by Tröster and coworkers (15). The patients attained significantly high scores on word list recognition (discriminability) and delayed recall of prose passages after surgery than before surgery. In addition, there was a trend toward high scores on a visual confrontation naming test after surgery. Examination of individual patient data indicated that gains and losses in test scores exceeding two standard deviations, were rare. Changes of one standard deviation were also rare

and gains were more likely to occur than losses. The authors concluded that their observations supported the cognitive safety of unilateral DBS of the thalamus in PD.

THALAMOTOMY VS DBS OF THE THALAMUS

There have been no reported controlled, prospective, comparisons of chronic high-frequency stimulation of the VIM nucleus of the thalamus with thalamotomy. The impression of clinicians experienced with both procedures is that the effect on tremor is very comparable between ablative lesions and chronic stimulation, but that adverse effects are less in DBS because of the ability to adjust stimulation parameters. Tasker (16) reported a comparison between two series of patients, 19 with thalamic stimulation (16 PD patients, 3 with essential tremor) and 26 with thalamotomies (23 PD patients, 3 with essential tremor). Twelve (63%) of the stimulation patients and 17 (65%) of the thalamotomy recipients were observed for more than one year. Tasker found that control of tremor and the incidence of nonimplant-related complications (e.g., postoperative hemorrhage, dysarthria, ataxia) were the same. The recurrence of tremor was lower in the stimulation patients (5% vs. 15%), and 23% of the thalamotomies had to be repeated, though none of the implants were repeated. It was found that the amount of stimulating voltage needed to control tremor escalated with time, but this posed a problem for only one patient whose need eventually exceeded device capacity. Tasker concluded that stimulation was preferable because it was easier to obtain results.

MECHANISM OF ACTION

The precise mechanism of action of DBS is not known. The effect of neuronal destruction and high-frequency stimulation is similar. Benabid and coworkers (3) have suggested that tremor suppression could be the result of neuronal jamming, thus deactivating cyclic neuronal phenomenon. Dieber and coworkers (17) measured regional cerebral blood flow with positron emission tomography in six patients with PD who had thalamic stimulation. The suppression of tremor with thalamic stimulation was associated with decreasing activity in the cerebellum, indicating the importance of cerebellar deactivation in the mechanism of thalamic stimulation. Caparros-Lefebvre and coworkers (18) reported a patient with PD who died 43 months after the implantation of the stimulator. The extent of thalamic gliosis was very small. The stimulation site was in the medial inferior part of the VIM complex at the entrance of the cerebellothalamic fibers. They postulated that stimulation of the cerebellar afferent axons could be responsible for the clinical effect. It has also been postulated that DBS could have its effect by activation of inhibitory fibers (Hallett, personal communication).

ADVANTAGES AND DISADVANTAGES OF DEEP BRAIN STIMULATION

The main advantages of DBS are (1) its reversibility, there is no destruction of neuronal tissue; (2) adaptability, the ability to change stimulus parameters to either increase efficacy or to reduce adverse effects; (3) the ability to perform bilateral operations without causing permanent complications such as dysarthria. Drawbacks of DBS compared to an ablative procedure include: the cost of the system, the fact that a foreign material has been implanted, the future need to replace the battery, the possibility of equipment failure, and possible interaction with electromagnetic devices for example MRI. Infection can be problematic. If the IPG becomes infected, it must be removed to control the infection.

COSTS

The Activa tremor control system is manufactured by Medtronic, Inc. (Neurologic Division), Minneapolis, Minnesota. The device is made available to neurosurgeons for implantation in a hospital setting. Medtronic reports the cost of the Activa stimulator to be $9,000 to $10,000. The total cost of the procedure include cost of the device, charges of the neurosurgical team and hospital that can vary between $20,000 and $30,000. Reported hospital stays typically range from one to three days. Some centers first implant the stimulating lead and a day or two later implant the IPG. Additional costs may be incurred during follow-up care by repeated visits in the early postimplant period for stimulation parameter optimization.

REGULATORY STATUS

Under the PMA process, the FDA cleared the Activa thalamic stimulator for "unilateral thalamic

stimulation for the suppression of tremor in the upper extremity in patients who are diagnosed with essential tremor or parkinsonian tremor not adequately controlled by medications and where the tremor constitutes a significant functional disability." FDA approval of the Class II device was predicated on all physicians performing the implant being experienced in stereotactic and functional neurosurgery, and on the undertaking by Medtronic of postapproval studies. Medicare and most third party payers now reimburse for DBS of the thalamus in PD.

CONCLUSION

Deep brain stimulation of the VIM nucleus of the thalamus has both short-term and long-term efficacy in the treatment of the tremor of PD. In general, the procedure is safe and persistent morbidity is infrequent. The mechanism of action of DBS is not known. Functional disability in PD may not be significantly improved because DBS of the thalamus only reduces tremor and not other PD symptoms. Therefore, there is ongoing investigation of the effect of DBS on other brain targets, for example the globus pallidus and the subthalamus. DBS of these target sites may ameliorate many of the symptoms of PD (Chapter 49) (19,20)

REFERENCES

1. Cooper IS. Ligation of the anterior choroidal artery for involuntary movements of Parkinsonism. *Arch Neurol* 1956; 75:36–48.
2. Kelly PJ, Gillingham FJ. The long-terms results of stereotaxic surgery and L-dopa therapy in patients with Parkinson's disease: A 10-year follow-up study. *J Neurosurg* 1980; 53:332–337.
3. Benabid AL, Pollak P, Hoffman D, et al. Chronic high frequency thalamic stimulation in Parkinson's disease. In: Koller WC, Paulson GW (eds). *Therapy of Parkinson's Disease.* 2nd ed. New York: Marcel Dekker, 1994: 381–402.
4. Benabid AL, Pollak P, Gervason C, et al. Long-term suppression of tremor by chronic stimulation of the ventral intermediate thalamic nucleus. *Lancet* 1991; 337:403–406.
5. Benabid AL, Pollak P, Hommel M, et al. Treatment of Parkinson tremor by chronic stimulation of the ventral intermediate nucleus of the thalamus. *Rev Neurol (Paris)* 1989; 145:320–323.
6. Blond S, Caparros-Lefebvre D, Parker F, et al. Control of tremor and involuntary movement disorders by chronic stereotactic stimulation of the ventral

intermediate thalamic nucleus. *J Neurosurg* 1992; 77:62–68.

7. Speelman JD, Bosch DA. Continuous electric thalamus stimulation for the treatment of tremor resistant to pharmacotherapy. *Ned Tijdschr Geneeskd* 1995; 139:926–930.

8. Alesch F, Pinter MM, Helscher RJ, et al. Stimulation of the ventral intermediate thalamic nucleus in tremor dominated Parkinson's disease and essential tremor. *Acta Neurochir* 1995; 136:75–81.

9. Benabid AL, Pollak P, Gao D, et al. Chronic electrical stimulation of the ventralis intermedius nucleus of the thalamus as a treatment of movement disorders. *J Neurosurg* 1996; 84:203–214.

10. Koller W, Pahwa R, Busenbark K, et al. High-frequency unilateral thalamic stimulation in the treatment of essential and Parkinsonian tremor. *Ann Neurol* 1997; 42:292–299.

11. Ondo W, Jankovic J, Schwartz K, et al. Unilateral thalamic deep brain stimulation for refractory essential tremor and Parkinson's disease tremor. *Neurology* 1998; 51:1063–1069.

12. Limousin P, Speelman JD, Gielen F, et al. Multicenter European study of thalamic stimulation in parkinsonian and essential tremor. *J Neurol Neurosurg Psychiatry* 1999; 66:289–296.

13. Hubble JP, Busenbark KL, Wilkinson S, et al. Effects of thalamic deep brain stimulation based on tremor type and diagnosis. *Mov Disord* 1997; 12:337–341.

14. Pahwa R, Lyons KE, Wilkinson SB, et al. Bilateral thalamic stimulation for essential tremor. *Neurology* 1998; 50(Suppl 4):A19.

15. Tröster AK, Fields JA, Wilkinson SB, et al. Neuropsychological functioning before and after unilateral thalamic stimulating electrode implantation in Parkinson's disease. *Neurosurg Focus* 1997; 2(3):Article 9.

16. Tasker RR. Deep brain stimulation is preferable to thalamotomy for tremor suppression. *Surg Neurol* 1998; 49:145–153; discussion 153–154.

17. Dieber M-P, Pollak P, Passingham R, et al. Thalamic stimulation and suppression of parkinsonian tremor. *Brain* 1993; 116(Part 1):267–279.

18. Caparros-Lefebvre D, Ruchoux MM, Blond S, et al. Long-term thalamic stimulation in Parkinson's disease: Postmortem anatomoclinical study. *Neurology* 1994; 44:1856–1860.

19. Pahwa R, Wilkinson S, Smith D, et al. High-frequency stimulation of the globus pallidus for the treatment of Parkinson disease. *Neurology* 1997; 49:249–253.

20. Limousin P, Krack P, Pollak P, et al. Electrical stimulation of the subthalamic nucleus in advanced Parkinson's disease. *N Engl J Med* 1998; 339:1105–1111.

49

Pallidal and Subthalamic Stimulation

John P. Hammerstad, M.D.

Department of Neurology, Oregon Health Sciences University, Portland, Oregon

A BRIEF HISTORICAL ACCOUNT

Following the experience with thalamic stimulation for tremor in Parkinson's disease (PD), high-frequency deep-brain stimulation (DBS) of the globus pallidus interna (GPi) and subthalamic nucleus (STN) is rapidly gaining adherents. Initial results regarding the efficacy and safety of DBS in GPi or STN indicate it is as effective as lesions but is superior to pallidotomy because control of bilateral and midline symptoms can be achieved without the risk of complications commonly seen with bilateral lesions. In 1960 Hassler was the first to report the effects of stimulation of the pallidum (1). Low-frequency stimulation (4–8 per second) could evoke a tremor but higher frequencies (25–100 per second) reduced the intensity of tremor and in some cases completely arrested tremor and rigidity. Siegfried and Lippitz (2) in 1994 were the first to report the results of chronic bilateral high-frequency pallidal stimulation in three patients in whom all of the parkinsonian symptoms, including gait and speech, were improved.

Deep brain stimulation of the STN was a logical extension of ablation studies in monkeys. These studies confirmed the hypothesis that dopamine depletion in the striatum resulted in excessive excitation of the globus pallidus by the STN (3). Benabid and his colleagues demonstrated comparable remediation of experimental parkinsonism in animals with deep-brain stimulation of STN before they attempted the first human implantation (4,5). Since then, Benabid and coworkers in Grenoble, France, have concentrated their efforts on bilateral subthalamic nucleus stimulation in PD. Their experience suggests that STN stimulation is superior to pallidal stimulation in alleviating akinesia and rigidity, whereas both are equally efficacious in alleviating tremor, and pallidal stimulation is better for alleviating levodopa-induced dyskinesia (6).

TECHNIQUES

The equipment used for DBS of GPi and STN is the same as for thalamic stimulation. Target localization is performed with MRI imaging, sometimes in combination with positive contrast ventriculography (6). Electrophysiology is used to fine-tune the localization of the target. Macrostimulation is used to be certain the electrode tip is not too close to the internal capsule or optic tract when placement is in the GPi. Microelectrode recording of neural activity that is characteristic of the GPi (see Chapter 47) and STN is used to achieve the precise location (7–9). Further confirmation can be obtained by the neuronal response to intrasurgical systemic apomorphine administration (10). Implantation of the external leads in a programmable pulse generator is the same as for thalamic stimulation. Postoperative imaging with MR can be done safely to confirm the positioning of the electrodes (11,12).

Systematic programming of the stimulation parameters can be quite time consuming but the wide range of possibilities has a great advantage over lesioning because of the flexibility it provides in obtaining the best clinical results. The approach is to adopt a constant pulse width and stimulation frequency that depends on the target and the presence of tremor. Frequencies more than 100 hertz are the most effective with 120 to 130 hertz being most common. A frequency of 180 to 185 hertz is often necessary to control tremor, especially with stimulation of the GPi. Once the pulse width and rate of stimulation are chosen, monopolar stimulation of each of the four contacts is assessed, starting with an amplitude of one volt with stepwise increases from 0.1 to .5 volt until optimum improvement in parkinsonian signs or unwanted side effects are obtained. Voltages that are most effective in pallidal stimulation are higher than those required for optimum control with STN stimulation. If monopolar stimulation of one of the contacts produces insufficient alleviation of symptoms, bipolar stimulation combined with various contact combinations and polarities can then be explored.

RESULTS OF TREATMENT TRIALS: GPi STIMULATION

With one exception (13), DBS of GPi has been reported to be equally efficacious to lesioning in controlling all the symptoms of PD (2,14–22) (see Chapter 47). Only one direct comparison of posteroventral pallidotomy versus deep brain stimulation has been reported (23). A prospective series of 13 patients were randomized to receive either a unilateral thermal lesion or unilateral DBS. Comparable benefits were found with either and there were low rates of complications and side effects with both. Bilateral lesions versus DBS was not compared. The improvement in parkinsonian symptoms, especially akinesia, versus elimination of levodopa-induced dyskinesias (LID) may differ according to the sites stimulated within the GPi. Two groups have reported that monopolar stimulation of the more rostral contacts is best for alleviating akinesia but is less successful in controlling LID (14,18,24). Stimulation of the uppermost contact may even produce dyskinesia, whereas stimulation of the lowermost contact is best at eliminating LID but also may reduce the anti-akinetic effect of levodopa. The investigators have suggested that the best procedure is to determine which contact produces the best control of LID and then use the next higher contact to obtain the best compromise. Using apomorphine to study the dose response curve for dyskinesia, an examination of two patients found a different result, that is, the anti-parkinsonian and anti-LID effects could be obtained by stimulation of the same site (25). However, these studies are not necessarily comparable as the latter one used bipolar stimulation between the most upper and most lower contacts instead of monopolar stimulation. This may be the best strategy for some patients. Bipolar stimulation generates a longer and narrower current field, but often requires higher pulse widths and voltages, which results in higher energy consumption and shortened battery life.

RESULTS OF TREATMENT TRIALS: STIMULATION OF THE SUBTHALAMIC NUCLEUS

Benabid and his colleagues in Grenoble, France, pioneered bilateral stimulation of the subthalamic nucleus and have provided most of the published reports (17,26–33). In earlier studies in the MPTP monkey model of parkinsonism, it was shown that lesions of the subthalamic nucleus could reverse parkinsonian signs (3,34,35). These results supported the hypothesis that the excessive inhibitory output from the globus pallidus to the thalamus could be accounted for by excessive excitation of the globus pallidus by the subthalamic nucleus. Therefore, down-regulation of this excessive excitation by lesioning could restore a more normal output from the globus pallidus. A potential additional advantage is a reduction in excessive inhibitory output from the substantia nigra reticulata (Snr), which also receives innervation from the subthalamic nucleus and provides an inhibitory output to brain stem and spinal cord targets (36). Theoretically this may also improve midline symptoms such as speech and gait disorder (37). These symptoms may not be as effectively treated by pallidal stimulation alone. The Grenoble group also demonstrated that bilateral STN stimulation in the MPTP monkey could produce the same results as lesioning (4,5). They reported a beneficial effect on the first patient in 1994 (32) and recently reported the results of a long-term follow-up of 24 consecutive patients, 20 of whom had undergone bilateral stimulation of the subthalamic nucleus for at least one year (31). The patients' scores for activities of daily living and motor examination scores on the UPDRS off medication improved by 60%, including the subscores for limb akinesia, rigidity, tremor, and gait. The mean dose of dopaminergic drugs was reduced by half. The reduction in levodopa dose was thought to be the major factor in the alleviation of dyskinesia (38).

Comparable results and efficacy were obtained in the initial seven consecutive patients undergoing chronic STN DBS in Toronto (39). After 6 to 12 months of implantation, these patients underwent a two-day double-blind evaluation with stimulators on or off and with or without levodopa. In the medication "off" state, turning the stimulators on resulted in an improvement in the mean total UPDRS motor score by 58 percent with improvements in subscores ranging from 50 to 80 percent for akinesia, rigidity, tremor, gait, and postural stability. Levodopa-induced dyskinesias were reduced by 83 percent and total drug usage was decreased by 40 percent. They also found that the medication "off" state improved 17 percent without stimulation posing the question as to whether this was a lesion effect or a carry-over from chronic stimulation.

A study of seven patients with bilateral implants reported a marked improvement in five and moderate in the other two with a 41 percent improvement in UPDRS motor score off medication, on stimulation (40). The levodopa-equivalent daily dose of medication was reduced by 60%.

ADVERSE EFFECTS OF DEEP BRAIN STIMULATION

Surgical and Postoperative Morbidity

In the Toronto study of seven patients with STN stimulation (39) operative complications were common. The most serious was a cortical venous thrombosis resulting in infarction at the site of electrode insertion. Another patient developed a small thalamic lesion along one of the electrode tracks, which was associated with mild reduction of verbal memory. A third patient was noted by family members to have a mild personality change. A fourth, who had progressive cognitive decline before surgery, had an abrupt decline in most areas of cognition postoperatively. Despite these complications, the patients and their families felt that the motoric benefit outweighed any problems from the complications. A concern about inducing ballismus or chorea was not realized. Only two patients developed mild transient hemichorea during macroelectrode insertion.

The Grenoble group reported a lower rate of surgical morbidity (17,26,28–31). One patient had an intracerebral hematoma resulting in persistent severe paralysis and aphasia. Another had a lesion in the region of the upper thalamus and anterior limb of the internal capsule suggesting an infarction without any accompanying neurologic disability. One patient had a grand mal seizure after ventriculography. Three patients were confused for a few days after electrode implantation and one patient developed confusion and bradyphrenia for one month. This patient had an abnormal signal in the head of the left caudate nucleus and anterior limb of the internal capsule along the electrode trajectory. Among the postoperative complications in the Grenoble study of 20 patients (31), one developed a subcutaneous infection at the site of the extension lead. This was treated with antibiotics and the extension lead and pulse generator were removed for six months and then reimplanted. Eyelid opening apraxia was induced or worsened by the surgery in five patients. Hypophonia and postural instability worsened in one patient after three months. Transient postoperative confusion and hallucinations were more common, developing in eight of 20 patients. The effects lasted for a few days to two weeks with complete recovery.

The Grenoble group reported adverse events of GPi stimulation in only five patients (17). Four of them were confused for a few days after electrode implantation without any permanent adverse effects related to the surgical procedure. Postoperatively, two patients complained of a worsening of hypophonia, one had the "apraxia" of eyelid opening and another had a worsening of his "on"-period akinesia. Of 72 patients with either unilateral or bilateral implantation of electrodes in the GPi collected from eight other series (2,13,15,19–23) there was no operative mortality and minimal operative morbidity. A transient crural paresis was reported in one patient (23). A transient hemiparesis during surgery and an asymptomatic intracranial bleed occurred in another series (20). Several reports did not comment on any surgical or postoperative complications.

Complications of Stimulation

A variety of unwanted effects can occur during acute stimulation and they are usually alleviated by changing the contact stimulated or by lowering the voltage. The side effects include paresthesias, tonic contractions of the opposite side and dysarthria resulting from stimulation of the internal capsule. Nausea and unformed visual hallucinations are more common with GPi stimulation, diplopia, and feelings of panic or anxiety more common with STN stimulation. Dyskinesia can also be produced by either STN or GPi stimulation. In 18 of the 20 Grenoble STN patients, dyskinesias could be induced by increasing the stimulation voltage above the long-term level but adjustment to the subdyskinesia threshold eliminated the problem without loss of efficacy (28,31). One woman developed acute and reversible depression when the lowermost contact was stimulated (41). This contact was found to be in the substantia nigra reticulata, raising questions about the role of this nucleus in mood.

Neuropsychological Effects

A variety of studies have done preoperative and postoperative neuropsychological testing. Except for the occasional patient who has suffered hematoma or infarction along the needle tracks, no neuropsychological deficits have been found to be secondary to the procedure itself.

Other Concerns

One drawback of DBS that needs attention is the time and effort it takes to provide optimum programming. One of the challenges to improve the cost/benefit ratio of the procedure is to find a standard systematic approach that is most efficient in determining the optimum settings.

Hardware

Another challenge is to reduce the complications resulting from the hardware itself. The intracerebral electrodes have been reported to migrate, but this can be eliminated by a simple method of anchoring the electrode to the skull (42). There are occasional scalp erosions and subcutaneous infections from the extension leads, and seromas and subcutaneous infections can occur in the subcutaneous pocket into which the pulse generator is placed. The increased use of metal and magnetic detectors have also increased the likelihood of the pulse generators spontaneously turning off. Usually the patient is aware when this happens and can use a magnet to turn the generator back on. When there is uncertainty, a portable A.M. radio held next to the generator can be used to detect whether it is operating or not. The batteries have a finite life. Bipolar stimulation at higher frequencies and voltages will cause failure earlier, whereas monopolar stimulation at lower frequencies and voltages may prolong battery life for up to four to five years.

Long-Term Effects on Brain

The only information available on the effects of placement of the electrode and chronic stimulation of the brain comes from one autopsied patient who died after implantation of an electrode into the thalamus for control of tremor (43). Small areas of gliosis and spongiosis were observed in a 1 mm. perimeter around the track. There was an accumulation of lymphoid macrophages and giant cells 2 mm around the active tip of the electrode. The lymphoid cells appeared in front of the polyurethane sheath and were felt to be reactive T-lymphocytes. The volume of tissue that was affected was much smaller than the lesion from a microthalamotomy and a smaller volume than is estimated to be affected by the spread of the stimulation current.

OUTCOMES REMAINING TO BE ANSWERED

Mechanisms of Action

Because low-frequency stimulation produces facilitation and high-frequency stimulation of the GPi produces a result similar to lesioning, it has been proposed and assumed that high-frequency stimulation produces its effects by a depolarization block (6,44). However, in a study of nine patients with electrodes implanted in the GPi, Ashby, and coworkers (45) concluded that GPi stimulation may activate the corticospinal tract, even

when the stimuli are below the threshold for a visible muscle contraction, and that continuous stimulation may do so continuously. A study in MPTP monkeys showed that high-frequency stimulation of the internal globus pallidus restores the excessive firing to a more normal frequency approximating a normal firing rate (46). This raises the possibility that the effects are from activation of inhibitory GABA inputs from the GPe or a direct striatopallidal pathway. A similar result was obtained with subthalamic nucleus stimulation in the rat (47). At low-stimulation frequencies, there was an excitatory influence on the spontaneous activity of SNr cells. At higher stimulation frequencies, there was a substantial reduction in firing frequency. Thus, the net result of high-frequency stimulation of either GPi or STN may be to reduce the excessive inhibitory output and restore more normal activity in the thalamocortical circuit.

This hypothesis is supported by PET scan studies. GPi stimulation activates ipsilateral prefrontal cortical areas that show reduced activity in control patients (48). Another study compared six patients with STN and six with GPi stimulators (49). During effective STN stimulation, movement-related increases in cerebral blood flow were significantly higher in supplementary motor area, cingulate cortex and dorsal lateral prefrontal cortex (DLPFC). No significant change was observed in any of these areas during GPi stimulation. The difference between the effect of STN and GPi stimulation of movement-related activity was mainly localized to DLPFC. The greater activation of DLPFC with STN versus GPi stimulation may reflect the fact that STN projects to the cortex via both the GPi and SNr, whereas GPi projects by only one route. It has been suggested that this may account for a clinical impression that STN stimulation is more effective in improving Parkinsonian akinesia.

Choice of Targets

On the basis of their experience, Benabid and colleagues have proposed that STN stimulation is better at relieving Parkinsonian akinesia and tremor, whereas GPi stimulation may be better for controlling LID (6,26). This conclusion is based on a retrospective nonblinded comparison of GPi and STN stimulation in 13 young-onset patients (17). After six months of DBS, the "off" levodopa motor scores were improved by 39 percent in patients with GPi stimulation and 71% in the STN group. A similar, though less robust result, was reported by Kumar and coworkers (39), in 14 patients, eight with GPi (four unilateral, four bilateral) and six with STN (five bilateral, one unilateral) stimulation. Mean "off" levodopa motor score was improved by

27% after three months of GPi stimulation and 41% after one to six months of STN stimulation.

In a double-blind comparison of GPi versus STN stimulation, five patients were randomized to STN stimulation and four to GPi stimulation (50). All features of PD at both target sites improved from stimulation alone ("off" levodopa) with no significant difference between the target sites but a trend in favor of STN. Stimulation of both target sites markedly reduced dyskinesia. The main difference between the two groups was the requirement for levodopa which was substantially less in the STN group. The substantial reduction in the levodopa dose required by the STN patients could have accounted for an improvement in dyskinesia comparable to the GPi group whose levodopa doses did not change.

Both Bejjani and coworkers and Krack and coworkers (14,18), have reported that DBS of GPi may inhibit the anti-akinetic effect of levodopa. This appears to be related to the site stimulated within the GPi. Stimulation of the most inferior contact most reliably abolishes LID, but may also abolish the anti-akinetic effect of levodopa, whereas stimulation of the most dorsal contacts produce the best effect on akinesia but is less effective in counteracting LID. In the randomized blinded comparison by Hammerstadt and coworkers (50), bipolar stimulation of the intermediate contacts in GPi resulted in a positive interaction between stimulation and levodopa so that the combination was better than either alone.

A neurophysiologic study of upper limb akinesia in six patients with bilateral DBS of the GPi and six of the STN showed no significant differences between the two groups (51). In general, the effects of DBS at both target sites paralleled the effects of dopaminergic medication. Theoretically, STN stimulation may be more effective in improving posture and gait via its influence on SNr and its connections with motor centers in brainstem. However, the only systematic investigation of gait and posture was done in three patients with GPi stimulation (18,52). Comparison of stimulation in off and on conditions clearly showed improvement in all features measured when the stimulation was turned on.

Thus, the physiological and clinical evidence is mixed as to whether stimulation of one site is superior to the other or whether a particular feature responds better to stimulation at one site or the other. Nevertheless, the trend is in favor of subthalamic nucleus stimulation and some centers have concluded that STN stimulation is superior to GPi stimulation. Because of the difference in the effects of stimulation in dorsal and inferior portions of the GPi, it may take longer to achieve optimum programming with GPi stimulation. This fact alone favors STN, because programming time is the major factor in achieving optimum results.

Durability of Benefit

Most of the published results report response to stimulation over 6 to 12 months. A persistent good response has been noted during the second year of stimulation and beyond (21) in a small number of patients. However, a trend toward decreased efficacy was reported in six patients during the second year of GPi stimulation despite adjustments in stimulation parameters (15,18). In a report of chronic STN stimulation, five patients had a durable stable benefit after three years of stimulation (31). These results raise the possibility of a differential response to GPi and STN stimulation that is observable only in the long term.

Might Deep Brain Stimulation Be Neuroprotective?

Recent evidence from animal experiments would support the concept that excitotoxicity may play a role in the pathophysiology of PD (see Chapter 38). There is an excitatory input to the substantia nigra from the subthalamic nucleus (36). Animal experiments show a protective effect of lesioning the subthalamic nucleus in models of injury to the nigrostriatal tract (53,54). Any intervention that would reduce the excessive excitatory input from the subthalamic nucleus might not only ameliorate the symptoms of PD but reduce or abolish the excitotoxic contribution to the degenerative process (55). STN stimulation may have an advantage over GPi stimulation by more directly reducing the excitatory input to the substantia nigra. Long-term follow-up of DBS patients should provide valuable data to address this issue.

REFERENCES

1. Hassler R, Riechert T, Mundinger F, et al. Physiological observations in stereotatic operations in extrapyramidal motor disturbances. *Brain* 1960; 83:337–350.
2. Siegfried J, Lippitz B. Chronic electrical stimulation of the VL-VPL complex and of the pallidum in the treatment of movement disorders: Personal experience since 1982. *Stereotact Funct Neurosurg* 1994; 62(1–4):71–75.
3. Bergman H, Wichmann T, DeLong MR. Reversal of experimental parkinsonism by lesions of the subthalamic nucleus. *Science* 1990; 249:1436–1438.
4. Benazzouz A, Gross C, Feger J, et al. Reversal of rigidity and improvement in motor performance by subthalamic high-frequency stimulation in MPTP-treated monkeys. *Eur J Neurosci* 1993; 5(4):382–389.

5. Benazzouz A, Boraud T, Feger J, et al. Alleviation of experimental hemi-parkinsonism by high-frequency stimulation of the subthalamic nucleus in primates: a comparison with L-Dopa treatment. *Mov Disord* 1996; 11(6):627–632.

6. Benabid AL, Benazzouz A, Hoffmann D, et al. Long-term electrical inhibition of deep brain targets in movement disorders. *Mov Disord* 1998; 13(Suppl 3): 119–125.

7. Hutchison WD, Lozano AM, Davis KD, et al. Differential neuronal activity in segments of globus pallidus in Parkinson's disease patients. *Neuroreport* 1994; 5(12):1533–1537.

8. Hutchison WD, Lozano AM, Tasker RR, et al. Identification and characterization of neurons with tremor-frequency activity in human globus pallidus. *Exp Brain Res* 1997; 113(3):557–563.

9. Hutchison WD, Allan RJ, Opitz H, et al. Neurophysiological identification of the subthalamic nucleus in surgery for Parkinson's disease. *Ann Neurol* 1998; 44(4):622–628.

10. Hutchison WD, Levy R, Dostrovsky JO, et al. Effects of apomorphine on globus pallidus neurons in parkinsonian patients. *Ann Neurol* 1997; 42(5):767–775.

11. Kumar R, Chen R, Ashby P. Safety of transcranial magnetic stimulation in patients with implanted deep brain stimulators. *Mov Disord* 1999; 14(1):157–158.

12. Tronnier VM, Staubert A, Hahnel S, et al. Magnetic resonance imaging with implanted neurostimulators: an in vitro and in vivo study. *Neurosurgery* 1999; 44(1):118–125.

13. Tronnier VM, Fogel W, Kronenbuerger M, et al. Pallidal stimulation: an alternative to pallidotomy? *J Neurosurg* 1997; 87(5):700–705.

14. Bejjani BP, Damier P, Arnulf I, et al. Deep brain stimulation in Parkinson's disease: Opposite effects of stimulation in the pallidum. *Mov Disord* 1998; 13(6):969–970.

15. Ghika J, Villemure JG, Fankhauser H, et al. Efficiency and safety of bilateral contemporaneous pallidal stimulation (deep brain stimulation) in levodopa-responsive patients with Parkinson's disease with severe motor fluctuations: A 2-year follow-up review. *J Neurosurg* 1998; 89(5):713–718.

16. Iacono RP, Lonser RR, Maeda G, et al. Chronic anterior pallidal stimulation for Parkinson's disease. *Acta Neurochir* (Wien) 1995; 137(1–2):106–112.

17. Krack P, Pollak P, Limousin P, et al. Subthalamic nucleus or internal pallidal stimulation in young onset Parkinson's disease. *Brain* 1998; 121(Pt 3):451–457.

18. Krack P, Pollak P, Limousin P, et al. Opposite motor effects of pallidal stimulation in Parkinson's disease. *Ann Neurol* 1998; 43(2):180–192.

19. Kumar R, Lozano AM, Montgomery E, et al. Pallidotomy and deep brain stimulation of the pallidum and subthalamic nucleus in advanced Parkinson's disease. *Mov Disord* 1998; 13(Suppl 1):73–82.

20. Pahwa R, Wilkinson S, Smith D, et al. High-frequency stimulation of the globus pallidus for the treatment of Parkinson's disease. *Neurology* 1997; 49(1):249–253.

21. Siegfried J, Wellis G. Chronic electrostimulation of ventroposterolateral pallidum: Follow-up. *Acta Neurochir Suppl* (Wien) 1997; 68:11–13.

22. Volkmann J, Sturm V, Weiss P, et al. Bilateral high-frequency stimulation of the internal globus pallidus in advanced Parkinson's disease. *Ann Neurol* 1998; 44(6):953–961.

23. Merello M, Nouzeilles MI, Kuzis G, et al. Unilateral radiofrequency lesion versus electrostimulation of posteroventral pallidum: A prospective randomized comparison. *Mov Disord* 1999; 14:50–6.

24. Bejjani B, Damier P, Arnulf I, et al. Pallidal stimulation for Parkinson's disease. Two targets? *Neurology* 1997; 49(6):1564–1569.

25. Stanzione P, Mazzone P, Peppe A, et al. Antiparkinsonian and anti-levodopa-induced dyskinesia effects obtained by stimulating the same site within the GPi in PD [letter]. *Neurology* 1998; 51(6):1776–1777.

26. Krack P, Benazzouz A, Pollak P, et al. Treatment of tremor in Parkinson's disease by subthalamic nucleus stimulation. *Mov Disord* 1998; 13(6):907–914.

27. Krack P, Pollak P, Limousin P, et al. From off-period dystonia to peak-dose chorea. The clinical spectrum of varying subthalamic nucleus activity. *Brain* 1999; 122(Pt 6):1133–1146.

28. Limousin P, Pollak P, Benazzouz A, et al. Bilateral subthalamic nucleus stimulation for severe Parkinson's disease. *Mov Disord* 1995; 10(5):672–674.

29. Limousin P, Pollak P, Benazzouz A, et al. Effect of parkinsonian signs and symptoms of bilateral subthalamic nucleus stimulation. *Lancet* 1995; 345(8942): 91–95.

30. Limousin P, Pollak P, Hoffmann D, et al. Abnormal involuntary movements induced by subthalamic nucleus stimulation in parkinsonian patients. *Mov Disord* 1996; 11(3):231–235.

31. Limousin P, Krack P, Pollak P, et al. Electrical stimulation of the subthalamic nucleus in advanced Parkinson's disease. *N Engl J Med* 1998; 339(16):1105–1111.

32. Benabid AL, Pollak P, Gross C., et al. Acute and long-term effects of subthalamic nucleus stimulation in Parkinson's disease. *Stereotact Funct Neurosurg* 1994; 62:76–84.

33. Pollak P, Benabid AL, Limousin P, et al. Subthalamic nucleus stimulation alleviates akinesia and rigidity in parkinsonian patients. *Adv Neurol* 1996; 69:591–594.

34. Aziz T, Peggs D, Sambrook A, et al. Lesion of the subthalamic nucleus for the alleviation of 1-methyl-4-phenyl-1,2,3,6-tetra-hydropyridine (MPTP)-induced parkinsonism in the primate. *Mov Disord* 1991; 6:288–292.

35. Guridi J, Herrero MT, Luquin MR, et al. Subthalamotomy in parkinsonian monkeys: Behavioral and biochemical analysis. *Brain* 1996; 119:1717–1727.

36. Feger J, Hassani OK, Mouroux M. The subthalamic nucleus and its connections. New electrophysiological and pharmacological data. *Adv Neurol* 1997; 74:31–43.

37. Guridi J, Luquin MR, Herrero MT, et al. The subthalamic nucleus: A possible target for stereotaxic surgery in Parkinson's disease. *Mov Disord* 1993; 8(4):421–429.

38. Krack P, Limousin P, Benabid AL, et al. Chronic stimulation of subthalamic nucleus improves levodopa-induced dyskinesias in Parkinson's disease [letter]. *Lancet* 1997; 350(9092):1676.

39. Kumar R, Lozano AM, Kim YJ, et al. Double-blind evaluation of subthalamic nucleus deep brain stimulation in advanced Parkinson's disease. *Neurology* 1998; 51(3):850–855.

40. Moro E, Scerrati M, Romito LM, et al. Chronic subthalamic nucleus stimulation reduces medication requirements in Parkinson's disease. *Neurology* 1999; 53(1):85–90.

41. Bejjani BP, Damier P, Arnulf I, et al. Transient acute depression induced by high-frequency deep-brain stimulation. *N Engl J Med* 1999; 340(19):1476–1480.

42. Favre J, Taha JM, Steel T, et al. Anchoring of deep brain stimulation electrodes using a microplate. Technical note. *J Neurosurg* 1996; 85(6):1181–1183.

43. Caparros-Lefebvre D, Ruchoux MM, Blond S, et al. Long-term thalamic stimulation in Parkinson's disease: Postmortem anatomoclinical study. *Neurology* 1994; 44(10):1856–1860.

44. Starr PA, Vitek JL, Bakay RA. Deep brain stimulation for movement disorders. *Neurosurg Clin N Am* 1998; 9(2):381–402.

45. Ashby P, Strafella A, Dostrovsky JO, et al. Immediate motor effects of stimulation through electrodes implanted in the human globus pallidus. *Stereotact Funct Neurosurg* 1998; 70(1):1–18.

46. Boraud T, Bezard E, Bioulac B, et al. High frequency stimulation of the internal globus pallidus (GPi) simultaneously improves parkinsonian symptoms and reduces the ring frequency of GPi neurons in the MPTP-treated monkey. *Neurosci. Lett.* 1996; 215:17–20.

47. Benazzouz A, Piallat B, Pollak P, et al. Responses of substantia nigra pars reticulata and globus pallidus complex to high frequency stimulation of the subthalamic nucleus in rats: Electrophysiological data. *Neurosci Lett* 1995; 189:77–80.

48. Davis KD, Taub E, Houle S, et al. Globus pallidus stimulation activates the cortical motor system during alleviation of parkinsonian symptoms. *Nat Med* 1997; 3(6):671–674.

49. Limousin P, Greene J, Pollak P, et al. Changes in cerebral activity pattern due to subthalamic nucleus or internal pallidum stimulation in Parkinson's disease. *Ann Neurol* 1997; 42(3):283–291.

50. Burchiel KJ, Anderson VC, Favre J, Hammerstad JP. Comparison of pallidal and subthalamic nucleus deep brain stimulation for advanced Parkinson's disease: results of a randomized, blinded pilot study. *Neurosurgery* 1999; 45:1375–1384.

51. Brown RG, Limousin Dawsey P, Brown P, et al. Impact of deep-brain stimulation on upper limb akinesia in Parkinson's disease. *Ann Neurol* 1999; 45:473–488.

52. Grasso R, Peppe A, Stratta F, et al. Basal ganglia and gait control: Apomorphine administration and internal pallidum stimulation in Parkinson's disease. *Exp Brain Res* 1999; 126(2):139–148.

53. Piallat B, Benazzouz A, Benabid AL. Subthalamic nucleus lesion in rats prevents dopaminergic nigral neuron degeneration after striatal 6-OHDA injection: behavioral and immunohistochemical studies. *Eur J Neurosci* 1996; 8(7):1408–1414.

54. Piallat B, Benazzouz A, Benabid AL. Neuroprotective effect of chronic inactivation of the subthalamic nucleus in a rat model of Parkinson's disease. *J Neural Transm Suppl* 1999; 55:71–77.

55. Rodriguez MC, Obeso JA, Olanow CW. Subthalamic nucleus-mediated excitotoxicity in Parkinson's disease: a target for neuroprotection. *Ann Neurol* 1998; 44 (Suppl 1):S175–S188.

50

Neural Transplantation

J. Stephen Fink, M.D., Ph.D.

Boston University School of Medicine, Boston, Massachusetts

INTRODUCTION

Following the occurrence of neuronal injury, the adult mammalian central nervous system (CNS) has a limited capacity to generate new nerve cells. Although strategies are being considered to repair damaged neurons (1), this limited capacity of the CNS for self-repair remains the most fundamental obstacle in the treatment of neurodegenerative and other diseases of the CNS. Moreover, in the adult CNS, physical and trophic barriers limit reconstitution of new long-distance pathways. The complexity of the circuitry of the brain is an additional obstacle to the repair of damaged neuronal connections. Finally, the relative inaccessibility of the CNS (including the blood-brain barrier) limits, considerably, the range of therapeutics that might be available for treatment and repair of neurodegenerative disorders. For these reasons there is great interest in the possibility of using cell replacement to repair the damaged CNS. In this chapter the status of cell replacement therapy for the CNS is reviewed with particular reference to neurodegenerative diseases such as Parkinson's disease (PD).

HUMAN FETAL TRANSPLANTS IN PARKINSON'S DISEASE

The first demonstration that neuronal cells could be transplanted and that they could survive and repair motor deficits in the adult mammalian CNS was published in 1979 (2,3). Transplanted fetal rodent mesencephalic tissue, containing dopaminergic neurons, produced sufficient dopamine to ameliorate the motor deficits consequent to experimental damage to the nigrostriatal pathway. Over the subsequent decade, optimization of the fetal transplant procedure was accomplished, leading to the first reports in 1988 of human fetal transplantation in patients with PD (4,5).

Since the initial reports of human fetal transplantation, there have been more than 300 human fetal transplant procedures performed in PD patients. Although the outcome of only a small number of these transplanted patients have been reported in detail in the peer-reviewed literature (6–12), several conclusions can be made:

1. *Human fetal dopaminergic neurons are able to survive and grow when transplanted within species (allografts)*. The results of imaging with ^{18}F-DOPA position emission tomography (PET) and neuropathologic analysis of several autopsies have demonstrated that transplanted human fetal dopaminergic neurons are capable of differentiation and progressive fiber outgrowth that is accompanied by dopamine synthesis and release (6,10–15). Over 50 percent of the targeted putamen can be reinnervated by transplanted dopaminergic neurons (13,15). On the basis of studies on animals, it appears that this apparent functional and structural integration of transplanted fetal allograft tissue in humans is accomplished by the formation of reciprocal connections with host brain and regulated release of the neurotransmitter dopamine (16,17). As growth and differentiation of transplanted fetal neurons appear to be tightly regulated, the transplanted fetal cells appear to be responsive to intrinsic developmental programs and host epigenetic signals. The few isolated examples where overgrowth has occurred appear to be explained by deviation from standard dissection or surgical procedures (18,19).

2. *Long-term graft survival is possible.* In the longest reported case, graft survival has been demonstrated 10 years after transplantation (14). In this case, as in some other patients (6,11), striatal ^{18}F-DOPA PET signal was normalized by the graft. Using

sophisticated imaging techniques, regulated release of dopamine could also be demonstrated in this patient (14). Equally important is the observation that the grafted cells remained viable without loss of ^{18}F-DOPA PET signal, while the nontransplanted nigral dopamine cells continued to degenerate (6,10,11,14). This observation indicates that transplanted cells are apparently not susceptible, over the period of observation, to the ongoing degenerative process of PD.

3. *Sustained clinical improvement is possible, but the degree of improvement is variable.* In all reported studies, clinical improvement has been observed in many patients (6–12,14). This improvement can be quite substantial, such that some patients are able to stop anti-Parkinson medication. Some cases in which clinical improvement has been small have been given alternative diagnoses (i.e., multiple system atrophy) (6,11). Nonetheless, among patients with idiopathic PD, there has been a broad range of clinical improvement. It is important to acknowledge that all peer-reviewed reports of clinical outcomes after human fetal transplantation have been in open clinical trials, in which placebo effect and observer bias may influence clinical assessments (20). Additional results from human fetal transplants performed and assessed in controlled, blinded clinical trials will be required to accurately know the quantitative improvement in clinical status after transplantation. It appears, however, that human fetal transplants are able to alter the natural history of PD for some patients (6,14). Recently, the results of the first double-blind trial of human fetal transplants in PD were reported (21). Modest quantitative improvement was observed. Somewhat unexpectedly, there appeared to be an age-dependence to the degree of clinical improvement. Also, several patients developed spontaneous, disabling dyskinesias (off medication) more than one year after transplantation (21). Possible factors important to the variability in clinical response after human fetal transplantation within and among the transplantation centers include the number of surviving dopaminergic cells, surgical technique, regional placement of cells within the caudate and putamen, the preimplantation cell processing protocol, patient selection, and the type of immunosuppression (if any).

4. *Long-term immunosuppression may not be necessary for fetal allograft survival.* Allograft survival has been observed using immunosuppression protocols ranging from none to long-term regimens similar to those used for uncomplicated solid organ allografts (6–15). Robust graft survival has been observed with short-term, mild ("low-dose") cyclosporine, although at autopsy there was evidence of immune response at the site of surviving graft 18 months after transplantation and one year after immunosuppression had stopped (8,12,23). The significance of this observation for long-term graft viability is not known.

OTHER CELL SOURCES FOR PARKINSON'S DISEASE

Because of practical, ethical, and legal obstacles it is likely that use of human fetal cells for CNS transplantation will remain an experimental therapy. Although survival of fetal dopaminergic cells after transplantation has been improved severalfold by treatment with calcium channel antagonists, trophic factors, caspase inhibitors, or antioxidants (10,24), cell survival remains low (5–20%). Moreover, in current protocols it is necessary to acquire 3–4 acceptable fetuses over a two-day period to transplant one hemisphere in a PD patient. These technical considerations make human fetal neural tissue an impractical cell source for neural transplantation of PD and other neurodegenerative diseases.

There has, therefore, been great interest in finding an alternative cell source that could be used more routinely for transplantation in the CNS (Table 50-1). Adrenal medullulary tissue has the capacity to synthesize dopamine and was the first cell source to be used in transplantation protocols for PD. In autologous adrenal transplant protocols, poor cell survival, modest clinical benefit, and significant morbidity lead to the abandonment of this approach (25).

Xenogeneic Fetal Mammalian Tissue

Having seen the success of transplantation of human fetal mesencephalic cells in patients with PD, the use of xenogeneic fetal donor tissue has been considered. The main practical advantage of a xenogeneic source of tissue is, theoretically, the unlimited supply of transplantable fetal neural tissue that could be available. The pig has been considered the most desirable source species of whole organs (26,27). Pigs provide a large litter size, optimally staged embryonic porcine tissue, and the ability to reliably dissect the developing brain areas. Screening of animals for bacterial and viral

Table 50-1 Some Cell Sources for Transplantation in Parkinson's Disease

Cell	Source	Disease	Trials
Adrenal medulla	Autologous	PD	Yes
Human fetal	Human fetal brain	PD[1], HD[2]	Yes
Porcine fetal	Pig fetal brain	PD, HD	Yes
RPE cells[4]	Human	PD	Yes
hNT cells[3]	Human tumor	Stroke	Yes
Carotid body cells	Human	PD	No
Stem or progenitor cell	Human	PD, other	No

[1]Parkinson's disease,
[2]Huntington's disease
[3]Human teratocarcinoma-derived cells
[4]Retinal pigmented epithelial cells

diseases is possible as animals can be raised under controlled, quarantined conditions. Porcine tissue has been previously used in other medical applications such as heart valves, insulin replacement, pancreatic islet cell transplants, temporary skin for burn patients, and extracorporeal kidney and liver perfusion (28–31). On the basis of promising results of transplantation of porcine fetal cells in animal models of PD and Huntington's disease (HD) (32,33), pilot studies to assess the safety and efficacy of unilateral implantation of embryonic porcine cells into the striatum of patients with PD have been initiated (34,35).

In Phase 1 studies where porcine fetal neural cells were grafted unilaterally into 10 PD patients, clinical improvement of 19% was observed in the Unified Parkinson's Disease Rating Scale "off" state scores after 12 months. These patients received unilateral striatal transplantation of 12 million fetal porcine ventral mesencephalic cells. Several patients improved more than 30%. In a single autopsied PD patient, porcine fetal ventral mesencephalic cells were observed to survive seven months after transplantation (36), but the number of surviving porcine dopaminergic cells was small and not sufficient for reliable functional recovery. ^{18}F-DOPA PET scanning in this series of patients did not reveal increased dopamine synthesis capacity (34). Although the preliminary results from this Phase 1 trial are encouraging, particularly from the safety perspective, the open design of this trial cannot eliminate the possible influence of observer bias and placebo effect (20) in the efficacy results. Therefore the results of an ongoing, double blind trial, which employs an "imitation" surgery control, and a larger number of transplanted porcine fetal cells will be very informative.

In animal models of HD, transplanted embryonic striatal cells have been shown to integrate into the basal ganglia circuitry and to effect repair of some motor and cognitive deficits (33,37,38). Twelve HD patients

transplanted with fetal porcine cells derived from the lateral ganglionic eminence anlage of the striatum have shown a favorable safety profile in a Phase 1 trial (35). However, one year after unilateral striatal placement of up to 24 million fetal porcine striatal cells, there was slight worsening in total functional capacity score (35), consistent with the natural history of the disease (39).

The major challenges to the successful use of xenogeneic fetal neuronal cells in neurodegenerative diseases appear to be the management of the risk of xenotic infections (transmissions of pathogens outside the normal host range and in the setting of xenotransplantation) and minimizing immune-mediated rejection. When tissue is transplanted across species, there is a risk of transmission of infectious pathogens from the animal source (40). Two sets of porcine endogenous retrovirus (PERV), which are capable of replication in some human cells lines in vitro, have been identified (41–44). There was no evidence of PERV DNA in patient samples taken from 6 to 24 months after porcine fetal implantation in Phase 1 trials for PD or HD (34,35). Similar negative results for PERV transmission to humans have recently been observed in a large series of patients who have been exposed to living porcine tissue (45–47). These observations suggest that the propensity of PERV to establish a productive infection in humans, compared with other human pathogenic viruses, is low. Moreover, there is no known pathology of PERV in any species. However, risk of transmission of other porcine pathogens (known and unknown) from transplanted tissue remains a concern. This is particularly true because, in the absence of effective cryopreservation techniques for mammalian fetal neural tissue, current isolation protocols do not permit complete results of pathogen screening of fresh cells to be available before transplantation. Long-term monitoring of all patients receiving transplanted fetal porcine tissue will be necessary to accurately assess the risk of transmission of xenotic infections. Such protocols are, in effect, for those undergoing transplantation.

Although the requirements for immunosuppression for a xenograft placed in the CNS are clearly less than when the xenograft is placed outside the CNS, it is assumed that long-term immunosuppression is necessary for durable survival of CNS xenogeneic cell grafts. The identification of an optimal and tolerable immunosuppression regimen for CNS xenografts is, however, unresolved. Advances in modulation of host immune function (48), including transplantation on microcarrier beads (49), may permit long-term xenogeneic graft survival in the CNS with tolerable side effects from immunosuppression regimens. The use of xenogeneic fetal tissue remains a promising, but unproved, therapy for cellular repair in the nervous system.

Neural Stem Cells

Neural Stem Cell Biology

Neural stem cells have the potential to give rise to differentiated cell types of the mature brain in vivo (neuronal, astrocytes, and oligodendroglia), and to self-renew in an undifferentiated state (50,51). Differences among cells that are termed *embryonic stem cell*, *multipotent stem cell*, and *neural progenitors*, are based on their origin and the type of cells into which they have the capacity to develop (Figure 50-1). *Neural stem cells* are found within the CNS in vivo or have the capacity to develop into neural cell types.

The isolation of neural stem cells was first accomplished using rat brain (52). Cells were isolated from the ependymal and subependymal regions of the ventricular margin adjacent to the striatum and from the hippocampus. Once isolated, these cells are able to proliferate and respond to differentiation cues to form neurons (50,52). Multipotential neural stem cells have also been isolated from adult primate and human brain. In patients with laryngeal cancer who were administered bromodeoxyuridine (BrDU), postmortem analysis demonstrated that this mitotic marker was incorporated into neurons within the hippocampus (53), indicating that neurogenesis occurs in the adult human brain. Cells with proliferative capacity have also been identified in surgical biopsy specimens of adult human brain (54). The ependymal cell layer and the subependymal region (55–57) have been proposed as sites of origin of human neural stem cells that generate lineage-restricted precursor cells for neurons, astrocytes, and oligodendroglia.

These observations have several important implications for the neurobiology of CNS diseases. First, it raises the question of the role of neural stem cells in the

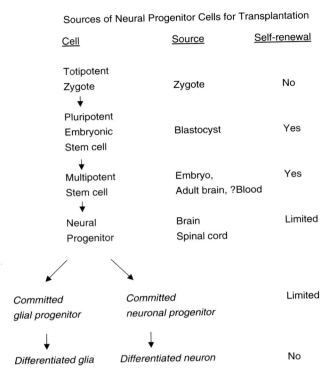

FIGURE 50-1. Possible sources of neural progenitor cells that may be used for transplantation and their presumptive developmental relationships. (adapted from Gage FH. Mammalian neural stem cells. *Science* 2000; 287:1433–1438) (50).

functioning of the adult CNS. Is neurogenesis in the adult a vestige of evolution from lower organisms or do neural stem cells function to contribute to plasticity of the adult CNS, perhaps in situations of injury or learning and memory? It has been demonstrated that the very small production of new neurons in the rodent hippocampus can be increased by mental activity, physical activity, and environmental enrichment (58–60). Second, the presence of neurogenesis in the CNS, which can be responsive to brain activity, raises the possibility that diffusible molecules might be identified that would induce neurogenesis in the mature mammalian CNS. Moreover, these inducers of neurogenesis might even be employed in a therapeutic context. The possible location of neural stem cells in the ependymal cell layer, directly adjacent to (CSF) in the ventricular system, might support this function of neural stem cells. It has been demonstrated that basic fibroblast growth factor (FGF-2) or brain-derived neurotrophic factor (BNDF) will increase in vivo neurogenesis in the CNS (61,62). Taken together, these observations of regulatable neurogenesis in the adult CNS raise the possibility that, for some diseases of the CNS, the identification of appropriate stimuli and molecules might be capable of harnessing the brain's capacity for intrinsic self-repair.

Neural Stem Cells for Transplantation

From the perspective of cellular therapy, the most important implication of the identification of neural stem cells is that, by combining ex vivo expansion and intracerebral delivery, these neural progenitors could be used as a renewable source of transplantable neural cells. It has been demonstrated by numerous laboratories that neural stem cells have the capacity to proliferate in vitro in an undifferentiated state and to retain some degree of ability to respond to differentiation signals. Fricker and coworkers (63) expanded human neural stem cells in culture and transplanted them into the uninjured rat brain. These cells migrated and integrated into several brain areas. These animal experiments suggest that transplanted human neural stem cells have the capacity to survive (across species) and to respond to local environmental cues by undergoing differentiation, migration, and integration into the host adult brain.

Neural stem cells can also be used as a source of glia. Two approaches have been demonstrated to have experimental utility in models of neurodegenerative disease. Duncan and coworkers (64) isolated neural stem cells, expanded them in vitro with mitogens, and induced these expanded cells to differentiate into oligodendroglia precursors. Snyder and colleagues (65) used an immortalized stem cell line derived from cerebellum. When these cells were transplanted into myelin-deficient rodents, there was evidence of migration and new myelin production. Taken together, these examples illustrate the potential for stem cells to serve as sources of neurons and glia in cell therapy paradigms.

There are several sources of neural progenitors (Figure 50-1) and several experimental approaches that have utilized expanded progenitor cells for the production of transplantable dopaminergic neurons. Dopaminergic neuron progenitors, obtained from cultures of fetal rat mesencephalon, were expanded with fibroblast growth factor. Mitogen withdrawal, prior to implantation, lead to modest dopaminergic differentiation (66). Progenitors have also been differentiated before implantation. In this approach, expanded lineage-restricted progenitors from rat mesencephalon were expanded (for months) in the presence of EGF in "neurospheres." Differentiation prior to transplantation was achieved using cytokines and undefined differentiation signals from membrane fragments from midbrain and conditioned medium from striatum (67). An "immortalized" neural stem cell, induced toward a dopaminergic neuron phenotype by transfection of a transcription factor (Nurr-1), underwent dopaminergic differentiation when exposed to the undefined differentiation factors contained in astrocyte-conditioned culture (68). After transplantation into the striatum of rodents, each approach yields survival and some degree of dopaminergic differentiation. However, survival of grafted neurons and, specifically, dopaminergic neurons was low, even when differentiation in vitro into neurons expressing some dopaminergic neuron phenotypes was efficient. This suggests that differentiation of these precursors did not achieve full dopaminergic phenotype, did not yield neurons with the ability to sustain differentiation or achieve critical synaptic connections required for survival, or that survival after transplantation of the differentiated DA cell was not complimented by other necessary neuronal or glial cell types.

Challenges of Neural Stem Cell Transplantation for Parkinson's Disease and Other Neurodegenerative Diseases

Parkinson's disease has advantages and disadvantages as a target disease for stem cell–based cellular therapy. It is a disease in which clinical symptoms are largely secondary to the loss of a single, chemically-defined neuronal phenotype. Thus it appears that replacement with only one differentiated cell type needs to be achieved. There are also excellent primate and rodent neurochemical models of nigrostriatal deficiency. Successful correction of motor deficits in these models by stem cell-derived dopaminergic cell transplants is likely to be highly predictive of clinical efficacy in PD patients.

However, the relative importance and effectiveness of region-specific signals in directing differentiation of transplanted progenitor cells is not fully understood, particularly when cells are placed outside the brain in areas where there is ongoing neurogenesis. This issue may be of particular importance in cellular repair strategies employing neural stem cells in PD. When transplanted into the hippocampus or subventricular zones (areas of neurogenesis), neuronal progenitor cells will migrate, and a small percentage will differentiate into neurons and glia, indicating the presence of local differentiation signals and the responsiveness of the progenitor cells to them (63,69,70). The likely target brain area for cell therapy in PD, the neostriatum, is not the normal site of dopaminergic cell generation, and it is not an area of active neurogenesis in the adult. Thus, if local (i.e., mesencephalic) signals are necessary to fully induce a stable dopaminergic phenotype, these differentiation signals may not be available if progenitor cells are implanted in the adult neostriatum. Region-specific differentiation signals in the adult brain may increase after injury and may direct differentiation of transplanted progenitors (71). However, it is not known if sufficient instructions will be present in the adult brain in certain neurodegenerative diseases such as PD to direct specification of transplanted progenitors into the desired dopaminergic phenotype.

The optimum stage of differentiation of the transplanted stem or precursor cell is also not known. Is it sufficient to transplant an uncommitted progenitor cell, or will it be more effective to "predifferentiate" the precursor cell toward a dopaminergic phenotype before transplantation? Finally, the process that regulates synaptogenesis and fiber outgrowth needs to be understood for stem cell-derived neurons. It appears that much is left to be learned about the process of stem cell differentiation, phenotype specification, integration, and establishment of synaptic connectivity before this source of transplantable dopaminergic neurons and other neural elements is ready for clinical application to PD and other neurodegenerative diseases.

Other Sources of Neuronal or Dopamine-Secreting Cells

A transformed cell line that generates large numbers of differentiated, postmitotic neurons has been used as a cell source for transplantation (Table 52-1). The NT2 line was established from a human teratocarcinoma. These cells are capable of differentiating into postmitotic neurons following treatment with retinoic acid. Following transplantation into rodent brain, a cell line (hNT, human teratocarcinoma-derived) derived from the original NT2 cell line displays features of a neuronal phenotype and integrates into host brain. Over the period of observation (one year) these transplanted hNT cells continue to survive and do not revert to the undifferentiated or neoplastic state. These cells have produced some recovery of function in animal models of stroke, although the mechanism of this recovery is not entirely understood (72). These cells are currently in clinical trials in patients with stroke (73). hNT cells also have the capacity to differentiate into cells that express tyrosine hydroxylase under certain treatment conditions (74), suggesting that they may be a source of transplantable dopaminergic neurons.

Neural cells for transplantation can be derived from other sources (Table 50-1). Rodent embryonic stem (ES) cells have been induced to differentiate into a population of cells enriched in oligodendroglia, which have been used as a cell source for transplantation in myelin-deficient animals (75). Marrow cells have also been reported to differentiate into cells of astrocytic lineage (76) and to repair motor deficits in a rat model of PD after genetic modification to produce dopamine (77). The ability of these cell sources to generate functional neurons and glia under controlled conditions need to be established before they can be

considered a useful source for transplantable neural cells.

The cell types discussed so far (embryonic, neural stem or progenitor and retinoic acid-treated transformed cell lines) have the capacity to differentiate into cells of neural lineage and integrate into the host brain. Cells that would be useful for the treatment of PD may not need to be "functional" neurons (i.e., capable of activity-dependent release of dopamine and synaptic connectivity). It is possible that cells that simply secrete dopamine, or synthesize dopamine from its precursor, may be sufficient to achieve functional benefit in PD. In addition to adrenal chromaffin cells, other cells in which DA secretion is the primary mechanism of benefit have been used in animal models of PD. Glomus cells from the carotid body (78) and nonneuronal cells that have been genetically engineered to produce high levels of dopamine or DOPA (79) can ameliorate motor deficits and reverse some of the neurochemical changes consequent to dopamine denervation in animal models of PD. To achieve maximum improvement of motor behavior in PD, it seems likely that other cellular functions subserved by dopaminergic neurons (reuptake and regulated release of dopamine) will be necessary characteristics of dopaminergic neurons derived from transplanted neural progenitors.

TRANSPLANTATION FOR OTHER NEURODEGENERATIVE DISEASES

The full promise of cellular therapy for CNS disorders is the potential to achieve *reconstruction* of neuronal circuitry of a damaged or diseased brain or spinal cord. Given the complexity of neuronal circuitry in the CNS, is cellular therapy likely to be able to achieve the necessary reconstruction to effect meaningful clinical improvement? The answer to this question may depend on the goal of the cellular replacement, which may be different for each target disease. For example, in PD, replacement of the dopamine synthetic capacity may be sufficient for, at least, partial recovery of function. However, maximum recovery of motor function in PD after transplantation may not entirely be due to restoration of DA synthesis, as there is a delay between the detectable increase in DOPA synthesis at the site of the graft as detected by ^{18}F-DOPA PET and recovery of motor cortex activation, suggesting that a process of synaptic maturation is required for full functional recovery (Lindvall O and Brooks DJ, *personal communication*).

Consideration of the goals of cellular therapy in HD serves as a useful paradigm for repair of neurologic disease that will require more complex reconstruction of neural pathways. In contrast to PD, in which some degree of recovery of motor function will result from an increase in dopamine synthetic capacity, recovery of function in HD is likely to require reinstatement of the cortico-striatal and the striatal outflow projections to pallidum and substantia nigra. The neurologic basis of the clinical symptoms is due, at least in part, to the disinhibition of efferent pallidal neuronal pathways. Animal models, which have used excitotoxic lesions to reproduce the cellular damage of HD, have been very useful in assessing the effects of cellular therapy. Fetal progenitor cells from the developing striatum engraft within the lesioned striatum and make connections with the efferent targets in the pallidum and receive synaptic inputs from the cortex. These connections are sufficient to improve lesion-induced motor and cognitive deficits in rodents and primates (33,37,38,80). Moreover, after transplantation, animals were able to learn motor tasks, suggesting that some degree of reinstatement of circuit complexity was achieved by the transplanted cells (81).

The challenge for establishment of reciprocal graft–host connections after transplantation in HD, from a spatial perspective, appears to be considerable. Efferent fibers from the graft will need to extend projections for considerable distances through adult (and, perhaps, diseased) brain to reach the output nuclei. Human fetal transplants in patients with HD are in progress and early results have demonstrated graft survival (82). Long-term, objective clinical improvement and evidence for establishment of reciprocal connections between host and graft remain to be determined. This evidence is awaited with great anticipation. Successful neuronal reconstruction by cellular transplants in HD will establish an important principal, which will serve to be the basis of cellular therapy in other neurologic diseases of the CNS such as stroke, brain trauma, and other neurologic diseases.

SUMMARY: PROSPECTS FOR NEW CELL SOURCES

The success of human fetal tissue transplants in PD has established as viable the principal of cell replacement therapy for diseases of the CNS. The lessons that have been learned from the use of fetal neural cells for transplantation will be instructive for the development of new cell therapies. Outcomes from the careful studies of human fetal transplants in PD and HD lead by the pioneering work of several groups will be the "gold standard" against which new cell sources will

initially be measured. Indeed, the accomplishments of human fetal transplants should not be minimized, and they include (1) attainment of approximate numbers of cells required for clinical efficacy in PD; (2) long-term cell survival; (3) apparent lack of need for long-term immunosuppression; (4) normalization or innervation of significant areas of the grafted striatum; (5) clinical benefit in PD sufficient in some cases to alter the natural progression of the disease; and (6) functional integration into the complex motor circuitry of the CNS (83). The attainment of these biologic outcomes, however, took time. It was nearly one decade between the first successful fetal graft in experimental animals and the first human clinical trials in PD and even longer before a protocol that led to clinically meaningful results was achieved. It is likely that the lessons learned from human fetal transplants, and the greater knowledge of cellular neurobiology, may accelerate these developmental timelines for new cell therapies.

The ability to isolate and maintain human neural stem cells in culture offers exciting possibilities for repair of neurodegenerative and other diseases of the nervous system. The challenge to reliably generate, from renewable neuronal precursor cells, mature neuronal elements capable of appropriate integration into the adult brain should not be underestimated. It is clear that additional knowledge must be gained about the identification of intrinsic and extrinsic signals that control neural differentiation, migration, and the development of synaptic connections in the setting of neural precursor cell transplantation. The rational maturation of cellular therapy using neural stem cells and other new cell sources as viable therapeutics for CNS disease will require the contributions of cell biologists and careful observations from clinical scientists.

REFERENCES

1. Olson L. Regeneration in the adult central nervous system: Experimental repair strategies. *Nat Med* 1997; 3:1329–1335.
2. Bjorklund A, Stenevi U. Reconstruction of the nigrostriatal pathway by intracerebral nigral transplants. *Brain Res* 1979; 177:555–560.
3. Perlow M, Freed W, Hoffer B, et al. Brain grafts reduce motor abnormalities produced by destruction of nigrostriatal dopamine system. *Neurosurgery* 1979; 204:643–647.
4. Lindvall O, Rehncrona S, Gustuvii B, et al. Embryonic dopamine-rich mesencephalic grafts in Parkinson's disease. *Lancet* 1988; 2:1483–1484.
5. Madrazo I, Leon V, Torres C, et al. Transplantation of embryonic substantia nigra and adrenal medulla to

the caudate nucleus in two patients with Parkinson's disease. *N Engl J Med* 1988; 318:51.

6. Lindvall O. Update on embryonic transplantation: The Swedish experience. *Mov Disord* 1998; 13:83–87.

7. Freed C, Breeze R, Rosenberg N, et al. Survival of implanted embryonic dopamine cells and neurologic improvement 12 to 46 months after transplantation for Parkinson's disease. *N Engl J Med* 1992; 237:1549–1555.

8. Hauser RA, Freeman TB, Snow BJ, et al. Long-term evaluation of bilateral embryonic nigral transplantation in Parkinson Disease. *Arch Neurol* 1999; 56:179–187.

9. Defer G, Geny C, Ricolfi F, et al. Long-term outcome of unilaterally transplanted parkinsonian patients: Clinical approach. *Brain* 1996; 119:41–50.

10. Brundin P, Pogarell O, Hagell P, et al. Bilateral caudate and putamen grafts of embryonic mesencephalic tissue treated with lazaroids in Parkinson's disease. *Brain* 2000; 123:1380–1390.

11. Wenning G, Odin P, Morish P, et al. Short- and long-term survival and function of unilateral intrastriatal dopaminergic grafts in Parkinson's disease. *Ann Neurol* 1997; 42:95–107.

12. Freeman T, Olanow C, Hauser R, et al. Bilateral embryonic nigral transplantation into the postcommissural putamen in Parkinson's disease. *Ann Neurol* 1995; 38:379–388.

13. Kordower J, Freeman T, Snow B, et al. Neuropathological evidence of graft survival and striatal reinnervation after the transplantation of embryonic mesencephalic tissue in a patient with Parkinson's disease. *N Engl J Med* 1995; 332:1118–1124.

14. Piccini P, Brooks DJ, Bjorklund A, et al. Dopamine release from nigral transplants visualized in vivo in a Parkinson's patient. *Nat Neurosci* 1999; 2:1137–1140.

15. Kordower J, Freeman TB, Chen EY, et al. Fetal grafts survive and mediate clinical benefit in a patient with Parkinson's disease. *Mov Disord* 1998: 13:383–393.

16. Fisher LJ, Young SJ, Tepper JM, et al. Electrophysiological characteristics of cells within mesencephalic suspension grafts. *Neuroscience* 1991; 40:109–122.

17. Doucet G, Murata Y, Brundin P, et al. Host afferents into intrastriatal transplants of fetal ventral mesencephalon. *Exp Neurol* 1989; 106:1–19.

18. Mamelak AN, Eggerding FA, Oh DS, et al. Fatal cyst formation after fetal mesencephalic allograft transplant for Parkinson's disease. *J Neurosurg* 1998; 89:592–598.

19. Folkerth RD, Durso R. Survival and proliferation of non-neural tissues, with obstruction of cerebral ventricles, in a parkinsonian patient treated with fetal allografts. *Neurology* 1996; 46:1219–1225.

20. Freeman TB, Vawter DE, Leaverton PE, et al. Use of placebo controlled surgery in controlled clinical trials of a cellular-based therapy for Parkinson's disease. *N Engl J Med* 1999; 341:988–992.

21. Freed CR, Greene PE, Breeze RE, et al. Transplantation of embryonic dopamine neurons for severe Parkinson's disease. *N Engl J Med* 2001; 344:710–719.

22. Watts RL, Raiser CD, Stover NO, et al. Stereotactic intrastriatal implantation of retinal pigmented epithelial cells attached to microcarriers in advanced Parkinson disease: A pilot study. *Neurology* 2001; 8(Suppl 3):A283.

23. Kordower J, Styren S, Clarke M, et al. Fetal grafting for Parkinson's disease: Expression of immune markers in patients with functional fetal nigral implants. *Cell Transplant* 1997; 6:213–219.

24. Brundin P, Karlsson J, Emgard M, et al. Improving the survival of grafted dopaminergic neurons: A review over current approach. *Cell Transplant* 2000; 9:179–195.

25. Goetz CG, Stebbin GT III, Klawans HL, et al. United Parkinson Foundation neurotransplantation registry on adrenal medullary transplants: Presurgical, and 1-year and 2-year follow up. *Neurology* 1991; 41:1719–1722.

26. Advisory group on the ethics of transplantation. *Animal Tissues into Humans*. Norwich, United Kingdom: Stationary Office, 1997:1–258.

27. Dunning J, White D, Wallwork J. The rationale for xenotransplantation as a solution to the donor organ shortage. *Pathol Biol* 1994; 42:231–235.

28. Breimer M, Bjorck E, Svalander C, et al. Extracorporeal connection of pig kidneys to humans: Clinical data and studies of platelet destruction. *Xenotransplantation* 1996; 3:328–339.

29. Chari R, Collins B, Magee J, et al. Treatment of hepatic failure with ex vivo pig-liver perfusion followed by liver transplantation. *N Engl J Med* 1994; 331:234–237.

30. Groth C, Korsgren O, Tibell A, et al. Transplantation of porcine embryonic pancreas to diabetic patients. *Lancet* 1994; 344:1402–1404.

31. Rydberg L, Bjorck S, Hallberg E, et al. Extracorporeal ("ex vivo") connection of pig kidneys to human II: The anti-pig antibody response. *Xenotransplantation* 1996; 3:340–353.

32. Galpern WR, Burns LH, Deacon TW, et al. Xenotransplantation of porcine embryonic ventral mesencephalon in a rat model of Parkinson's disease: Functional recovery and graft morphology. *Exp Neurol* 1996; 140:1–13.

33. Isacson O, Deacon TW, Pakzaban P, et al. Transplanted xenogeneic neural cells in neurodegenerative disease models exhibit remarkable axonal target specificity and distinct growth patterns of glial and axonal fibres. *Nat Med* 1995; 11:1189–1194.

34. Schumacher JM, Ellias SA, Palmer EP, et al. Transplantation of embryonic porcine mesencephalic tissue in patients with PD. *Neurology* 2000; 14:1042–1050.

35. Fink JS, Schumacher JM, Ellias SA, et al. Porcine xenografts in Parkinson's disease and Huntington's disease patients: Preliminary results. *Cell Transplant* 2000; 9:273–278.

36. Deacon T, Schumacher J, Dinsmore J, et al. Histological evidence of embryonic pig neural cell survival after transplantation into a patient with Parkinson's disease. *Nat Med* 1997; 3:350–353,34.

37. Kendall AL, Rayment FD, Torres EM, et al. Functional integration of striatal allografts in a primate model of Huntington's disease. *Nat Med* 1998; 4:727–729.

38. Palfi S, Conde F, Riche D, et al. Fetal striatal allografts reverse cognitive deficits in a primate model of Huntington's disease. *Nat Med* 1998; 4:963–966.

39. Quinn N, Brown R, Craufurd D, et al. Core assessment program for intracerebral transplantation in Huntington's disease (CAPIT-HD). *Mov Disord* 1996; 11:143–150.

40. Chapman L, Folks T, Salomon D, et al. Xenotransplantation and xenogenic infections. *N Engl J Med* 1995; 333:1498–1501.

41. Akiyoshi D, Denaro M, Zhu H, et al. Identification of a full-length cDNA for an endogenous retrovirus of miniature swine. *J Virol* 1998; 72:4503–4507.

42. LeTissier P, Stoye J, Yasuhiro Y, et al. Two sets of human-tropic pig retrovirus. *Nature* 1997; 389:681–682.

43. Patience C, Takeuchi Y, Weiss R. Infection of human cells by an endogenous retrovirus of pigs. *Nat Med* 1997; 3:282–286.

44. Wilson C, Wong S, Muller J, et al. Type C retrovirus released from porcine primary peripheral blood mononuclear cells infects human cells. *J Virol* 1998; 72:3082–3087.

45. Heneine W, Tibell A, Switzer WM, et al. No evidence of infection with porcine endogenous retrovirus in recipients of porcine islet-cell xenografts. *Lancet* 1998; 352:695–698.

46. Paradis K, Langford G, Long Z, et al. Search for cross-species transmission of porcine endogenous retrovirus in patients treated with living pig tissue. *Science* 1999; 285:1236–1241.

47. Patience C, Patton G, Takeuchi Y, et al. No evidence of pig DNA or retroviral infection in patients with short-term extracorporeal connection to pig kidneys. *Lancet* 1998; 352:699–701.

48. Auchincloss H Jr, Sachs DH. Xenogeneic transplantation. *Annu Rev Immunol* 1998; 16:433–470.

49. Saporta S, Borlongan C, Moore J, et al. Microcarrier enhances survival of human and rat fetal ventral mesencephalon cells implanted in the rat striatum. *Cell Transplant* 1997; 6:579–584.

50. Gage FH. Mammalian neural stem cells. *Science* 2000; 287:1433–1438.

51. Van der Kooy D, Weiss S. Why stem cells? *Science* 2000; 287:1439–1441.

52. Reynolds BA, Weiss S. Generation of neurons and astrocytes from isolated cells of the adult mammalian central nervous system. *Science* 1992; 255:1707–1710.

53. Eriksson PS, Perfilieva E, Bjork-Eriksson T, et al. Neurogenesis in the adult human hippocampus. *Nat Med* 1998; 4:1313–1317.

54. Kukekov VG, Laywell ED, Suslov O, et al. Multipotent stem or progenitor cells with similar properties arise from two different neurogenic regions of the adult human brain. *Exp Neurol* 1999; 156:333–344.

55. Johansson CB, Momma DL, Clarke DL, et al. Identification of a neural stem cell in the adult mammalian central nervous system. *Cell* 1999; 96:25–34.

56. Chiasson BJ, Tropepe V, Morsheas CM, et al. Adult mammalian forebrain ependymal and subependymal cells demonstrate proliferative potential, but only subependymal cells have neural stem cell characteristics. *J Neurosci* 1999; 19:4462–4471.

57. Doetsch F, Garcia-Verdugo JM, Alvarez-Buylla A. Regeneration of a germinal layer in the adult mammalian brain. *Proc Natl Acad Sci USA* 1999; 96:11619–11624.

58. Gould E, Beylin A, Tanapat P, et al. Learning enhances adult neurogenesis in the hippocampal formation. *Nat Neurosci* 1999; 2:260–265.

59. Van Praag H, Kempermann G, Gage FH. Running increases cell proliferation in the adult mouse dentate gyrus. *Nat Neurosci* 1999; 2:266–270.

60. Kempermann G, Kuhn HG, Gage FH. More hippocampal neurons in adult mice living in an enriched environment. *Nature* 1997; 386:493–495.

61. Wagner JP, Black IB, DiCicco-Bloom E. Stimulation of neonatal and adult brain neurogenesis by subcutaneous injection of basic fibroblast growth factor. *J Neurosci* 1999; 19:6006–6016.

62. Zigova T, Pencea V, Wiegand SJ, et al. Intraventricular administration of BDNF increase the number of newly generated neurons in the adult olfactory bulb. *Mol Cell Neurosci* 1998; 11:234–245.

63. Fricker RA, Carpenter MK, Winkler C, et al. Site-specific migration and neuronal differentiation of human neural progenitor cells after transplantation in the adult rat brain. *J Neurosci* 1999; 19:5990–6005.

64. Zhang S-C, Ge B, Duncan ID. Adult brain retains the potential to generate oligodendroglial progenitors with extensive myelination capacity. *Proc Natl Acad Sci USA* 1999; 96:4089–4094.

65. Yandava BD, Billiinghurst LL, Snyder EY. "Global" cell replacement is feasible via neural stem cell transplantation: Evidence from the dysmyelinated shiverer mouse brain. *Proc Natl Acad Sci USA* 1999; 96:7029–7034.

66. Struder L, Tabar V, McKay RDG. Transplantation of expanded mesencephalic precursors leads to recovery in Parkinsonian rats. *Nat Neurosci* 1998; 1:135–146.

67. Potter ED, Ling ZD, Carvey PM. Cytokine-induced conversion of mesencephalic-derived progenitor cells into dopamine neurons. *Cell Tissue Res* 1999; 296:235–246.

68. Wagner J, Akerud P, Castro DS, et al. Induction of a midbrain dopaminenergic phenotype in Nurr1-overexpressing neural stem cells by type 1 astrocytes. *Nat Biotech* 1999; 17:653–659.

69. Suhonen JO, Peterson DA, Ray J, et al. Differentiation of adult hippocampus-derived progenitors into olfactory neurons in vivo. *Nature* 1996; 383:624–627.

70. Gage FH, Coates PW, Palmer TD, et al. Survival and differentiation of adult neuronal progenitor cells

transplanted to the adult brain. *Proc Natl Acad Sci* 1995; 92:11879–11883.

71. Snyder EY, Yoon C, Flax JD, et al. Multipotent neural precursors can differentiate toward replacement of neurons undergoing targeted apoptotic degeneration in adult mouse neocortex. *Proc Natl Acad Sci USA* 1997; 94:11663–11668.

72. Saporta A, Borlongan CV, Sanberg PR. Neural transplantation of human neuroteratocarcinoma (hNT) neurons into ischemic rats. A qunatitative dose–response analysis of cell survival and behavioral recovery. *Neuroscience* 1999; 91:519–525.

73. Kondziolka D, Wechsler LR, Goldstein S, et al. Neuronal transplantation for stroke: Results of a Phase 1 study. *Neurology*, 2000; 54:A1.

74. Zigova T, Wiling AE, Tedesco EM, et al. Lithiuim chloride induces the expression of tyrosine hydroxylase in hNT neurons. *Exp Neurol* 1999; 157:251–258.

75. Brustle O, Jones KN, Learish RD, et al. Embryonic stem cell-derived glial precursors: A source of myelinating transplants. *Science* 1999; 285:754–756.

76. Kopen GC, Prockop DJ, Phinney G. Marrow stromal cells migrate throughout forebrain and cerebellum after injection into neonatal mouse brain. *Proc Natl Acad Sci USA* 1999; 96:10711–10716.

77. Schwarz EJ, Alexander GM, Prockop DJ, et al. Multipotential marrow stromal cells transduced to produce L-DOPA: Engraftment in a rat model of Parkinson disease. *Hum Gene Ther* 1999; 10:2539–2549.

78. Espejo EF, Montoro RJ, Armengol AJ, et al. Cellular and functional recovery of parkinsonian rats after intrastriatal transplantation of carotid body cell aggregates. *Neuron* 1998; 20:197–206.

79. Fisher LJ, Jinnah HA, Kale LC, et al. Survival and function of intrastriatally grafted primary fibroblasts genetically modified to produce l-DOPA. *Neuron* 1991; 371–380.

80. Dunnett SB. Functional repair of striatal systems by neural transplants: Evidence for circuit reconstruction. *Behav Brain Res* 1995; 66:133–142.

81. Brastad PJ, Watts C, Robbins TW, et al. Associative plasticity in striatal transplants. *Proc Natl Acad Sci USA* 1999; 96:10524–10529.

82. Hauser RA, Stoessl JA, Eichler SR, et al. Pilot evaluation of human fetal striatal transplantation for Huntington's disease. *Neurology* 2000; 54:A153.

83. Piccini P, Lindvall O, Bjorklund A, et al. Delayed recovery of movement-related cortical function in Parkinson's disease after striatal dopaminergic grafts. *Ann Neurol* 2000; 48:689–695.

51

Juvenile and Young-Onset Parkinsonism

Oscar S. Gershanik, M.D.

Centro Neurologico Hospital Francés, Buenos Aires, Argentina

INTRODUCTION

Parkinson's disease (PD) is a degenerative disorder of the central nervous system affecting approximately 1 in a 1,000 individuals with a predominant age of onset between 55 and 65 years of age (1). A small percentage of those affected (5–10%) have an age at onset below age 40 (2). This subgroup is generally referred to as early-onset parkinsonism, comprising, according to presently accepted criteria, those between the ages of 21 and 40 (young-onset cases, YOPD) and those below 21 (juvenile-onset cases, JP) (3). Interest in this age-related clinical subgroup of parkinsonian patients derives from several aspects : distinctive clinical features, a different natural history, peculiar response to medication, probable disease heterogeneity, and variable genetic background. From the time it was first recognized that PD could also affect younger individuals, there was a growing interest in this age segment, because it was thought that they could provide answers related to the genetics of the disease; the mechanisms underlying motor complications, both drug and disease-related; and the presence of cognitive decline, whether it is disease or age-related. This interest is reflected in the number of papers that have been published on the subject of early-onset parkinsonism.

However, review of past reports does not allow uniform conclusions for several reasons. Different publications use variable age limits to define the population under analysis, which makes a metanalysis almost impossible. Interpretation of findings in a comparable fashion is also difficult. Moreover, the precise nosologic placement of cases reported in earlier publications is quite difficult because of the lack of precise nosologic criteria to define the clinical boundaries, modern laboratory and imaging techniques and genetic markers at the time these cases were published, precluding a correct phenotypic–genotypic correlation.

Many of these limitations have been overcome in recent years because of the advances in molecular genetics, pharmacology, physiology, and clinical neuropsychology. At present clinical categories can be assigned to distinct disease entities accompanied by distinct genetic backgrounds, and this chapter reviews juvenile and young-onset parkinsonism in this new era.

HISTORICAL BACKGROUND

The occurrence of parkinsonism at an early age was first recognized in 1875, when Huchard, against prevailing knowledge, dared report a case of a child having clinical features strongly resembling PD, and, in fact, reported it as such (2). Although this report was soon discredited, it set in motion a search for additional cases of such early onset. Several isolated case reports followed that had in common not only their early age of onset but also the presence of strong familial aggregation. The first series of cases was that published by Willige (4) who commented on the clinical findings in 14 early-onset cases, the youngest of which had onset at age 18. Six of Willige's cases were familial, and although he believed his patients were in fact affected by PD, their early age of onset together with the presence of a positive family history prompted him to differentiate them from classical adult-onset PD. He even coined a new term, *paralysis agitans juvenilis familialis*, to underline the need for a more proper nosologic classification of PD cases according to age and family history.

From 1910 to the late 1950s there were several additional publications dealing with this peculiar disorder (5–7), including isolated cases, familial cases, small series, epidemiologic studies, and in some instances the inclusion of pathologic observations (2). What became evident was that no single disease could account for so much variation in clinical presentation and family background. New disorders were thus described, such as "primary atrophy of the globus pallidus" (5,6) and "pallidopyramidal disease" (7). In some cases the possibility of an encephalitic disease was entertained, without abandoning the idea that classical PD could start at a very early age, and that the presence of family aggregation could be the evidence of hereditary factors playing a role in the etiology of PD (2).

The introduction of levodopa to the treatment of PD in the later part of the 1960s shed new light on the issue of nosologic identity as this drug became the gold standard not only of treatment but also as a diagnostic tool. It became readily accepted that a positive response to levodopa was the hallmark of PD. The effects of levodopa helped, to some extent, in distinguishing cases of parkinsonism with a positive response to the drug from those in which no response could be elicited. However, a positive response to levodopa did not necessarily help in distinguishing classic Lewy body parkinsonism (PD) from other disorders presenting with parkinsonian features but corresponding to a different etiology. Such was the case with dopa-responsive dystonia, first reported by Segawa in the late 1960s (8), and selected cases of juvenile parkinsonism with marked response to levodopa, in whom postmortem examination revealed nigral cell loss without the presence of Lewy-body type inclusions (9,10).

Yokochi in 1979 (11) first drew attention to the high prevalence of "juvenile" and "young-onset" Parkinsonism in Japan in a comprehensive report including 40 patients with a mean age of onset of 26.1 ± 9.6 (range 6–39) collected from different hospitals. This investigator provided a detailed analysis of the clinical features, family history, and response to medication in these patients. According to Yokochi (11) and Yokochi and Narabayashi (12), "early-onset" parkinsonism cases accounted for almost 11% of all cases of parkinsonism seen in Japan and the frequency of a positive family history in these patients was substantially higher (42.5%) than previously reported for adult-onset cases. In addition, the clinical features of these cases differed somewhat from those usually seen in adult-onset patients. Gait disturbances and dystonic postures of the feet were particularly frequent in the younger patients, whereas tremor and autonomic disturbances were rarely present. A dramatic response to levodopa with rapid development of fluctuations and dyskinesias appeared to be the rule in these cases.

After Yokochi's publication and until now, there have been numerous reports originating in different regions of the world (3,13–25) providing detailed clinical descriptions of larger series of cases, allowing the comparative analysis of clinical presentation, pharmacologic response, development of complications, and natural history of the disease in contrast to adult-onset cases.

Perhaps the most important developments that have made a major impact in our present concept of early-onset parkinsonism are the findings of genetic markers for "dopa-responsive dystonia" and autosomal recessive "juvenile" or "young-onset parkinsonism" (26–28). Both these disorders, now precisely defined on the basis of their corresponding genetic mutations probably account for a large proportion of cases of parkinsonism of early onset. The possibility of making a correct diagnosis based on genetic analysis and not on artificially defined age limits or peculiar clinical manifestations exists now.

CLINICAL FEATURES

There is uniform agreement in the literature that regardless of underlying etiology, early-onset cases of parkinsonism have, in general, peculiar clinical features that differentiate them from late-onset cases. The earlier the age of onset, these differences tend to be more marked (2).

Distinguishing Clinical Features and Response to Medication

The majority of cases display predominantly rigid akinetic forms of the disease. Tremor is infrequently present although there is great variability among the different reported series. In most reports originating in Japan, tremor has been described as being predominantly of the postural type (12). Dystonia as a presenting feature, either alone and preceding the onset of parkinsonism, or at the same time has been frequently reported (2,29). Gait difficulties, on the contrary, are not often present at the onset of the disease. This is in contrast to older-onset patients who more commonly present with this complaint (24). In the youngest cases (juvenile parkinsonism), however, the presence of severe, lower limb or foot dystonia causes significant interference with gait. With a few exceptions, cognitive disturbances and autonomic symptoms have been reported to be less frequent than in older cases. In addition, diurnal fluctuations in symptomatology and marked sleep benefit may occur in early-onset cases, even before the introduction of levodopa (9,12,30).

The pattern of response to medication appears to be a very distinctive feature of early-onset parkinsonism.

Many published series have performed comparative studies between early-and late-onset cases specifically focusing on late complications of levodopa therapy in the two patient populations. Most investigators are in agreement that early-onset cases show a marked-to-dramatic response to levodopa, even in low doses, but the benefit obtained with the medication in significantly reducing the parkinsonian symptomatology is marred, early in the course of treatment, by the appearance of response fluctuations and sometimes severe dyskinesias (17,18,24;25).

Natural History and Progression

Few studies have addressed this issue and provided follow-up information in a systematic fashion. In Yokochi's original report (11), he concluded, based on a retrospective analysis of his cases, that parkinsonism of early onset (juvenile parkinsonism according to his nomenclature) tends to progress at a slower rate, and prognosis in these cases appears to be more benign.

This concept is applicable to PD in general, irrespective of specific age-group classifications. Goetz et al. (31) provided evidence that age at onset was the only contributory factor that helped distinguish the slowly from the rapidly progressing patients in a case-control study. Similarly, Diamond et al. (32), using a different approach, concluded that younger patients undergoing levodopa treatment had significantly lower disability scores from the onset of treatment than their older counterparts. This difference reached statistical significance after four years of treatment. At that time, the older-onset group had a 68% greater disability score. In addition, mortality ratios tended to be lower in the earlier-onset group confirming the more benign nature of the disease. In a prospective interventional study including a cohort of 800 "de novo" patients (from the DATATOP study), Jankovic and coworkers (33) analyzed the variable expression of PD within this group. Although early-onset cases had a similar degree of disability than the older cases when entering the study, these patients had, as a whole, a significantly longer estimated duration of symptoms. When comparing the course of the disease between different age groups, those with a benign course were significantly younger. Moreover, early-onset patients performed better than the older patients on a variety of neuropsychologic tests. Also those with late-onset disease were more occupationally disabled.

Recently, Schrag and coworkers (25) reviewed the natural history and mortality of a group of young-onset PD patients, a number of which were included in Quinn et al.'s original publication (3). After 10 years, 5% of patients were experiencing falls and 30% freezing, but all patients had developed levodopa-related fluctuations and dyskinesias. Cognitive function was fairly well preserved in the majority of patients after a median duration of disease of 18 years, more so in those who were less than 60 at the time of the second evaluation. Overall, mortality was twofold compared with the general population, which is comparable with the findings of Diamond and coworkers (32), who found a higher ratio for the older-onset group. The authors conclude that mortality in parkinsonism starting before the age of 40 is increased in comparison to the normal population and similar to that of the general PD population irrespective of age . Intellectual function and postural reflexes appear to remain well preserved despite a long history of the disease and the frequent occurrence of levodopa-related complications.

Along the same lines, Gomez Arévalo and coworkers (24) found that younger-onset patients (onset before age 40), irrespective of the duration of the disease, had a better response to levodopa and less involvement of postural stability and gait than those with a disease onset after 60. These authors speculated that the presence of a higher residual motor score, compounded by the presence of postural instability and gait disturbances, in older patients, was indicative of the involvement of nondopaminergic systems probably related to aging. This is in agreement with Blin and coworkers' (35) hypothesis on the mechanisms underlying a worsening of the response to levodopa with age.

DIAGNOSTIC CHALLENGES

When confronted with a patient presenting with an akinetic-rigid syndrome of early onset, the clinician should be particularly careful in diagnosing PD without the necessary imaging and laboratory workup, including a search for known genetic mutations. Moreover, it should be remembered that even the presence of a positive and sustained response to levodopa is not enough to warrant such a conclusion. Even after having ruled out the more frequent alternative diagnoses one cannot be entirely sure that what is diagnosed to be PD according to established criteria is in fact a definitive diagnosis. Based on recent findings, it is evident that the label idiopathic parkinsonism is not necessarily synonymous with PD (Lewy-body parkinsonism, sporadic or familial). Early-onset parkinsonism is in fact a heterogeneous category that includes a variety of idiopathic or primary disorders in addition to secondary or symptomatic ones.

Differential Diagnosis

Table 51-1 includes a list of known causes of early-onset parkinsonism (young-onset and juvenile-onset). Although many of the diseases listed in the table are rare or infrequent, they have been reported in the literature. However, they will not be dealt with separately as it would exceed the scope of this chapter.

Patients, whose parkinsonism begins around or under the age of 40, should be thoroughly evaluated. In addition to the usual criteria (both inclusionary and exclusionary) used in the diagnosis of PD, special attention has to be paid to the presence of clinical features that appear to be characteristic of some of the other disorders that usually present within this age range. Among these features, dystonia deserves a separate comment (27,10). The rate of occurrence of dystonia in parkinsonism increases with decreasing age. Thus, very early-onset cases (infancy or early adolescence) with predominant dystonia and mild parkinsonian features, sometimes associated with marked diurnal fluctuations in symptomatology (morning better than evening, rest-dependent improvement), should prompt a diagnosis of hereditary progressive dystonia or dopa-responsive dystonia (DRD) (8,10).

In older patients, with more marked Parkinsonian features, the presence of lower limb dystonia, brisk deep tendon reflexes and a history of consanguinity in their parents, or presence of affected siblings, autosomal recessive forms of parkinsonism (ARP) linked to chromosome 6 (PARK 2) should be considered (36,37,43). Although this last group also presents with diurnal fluctuations in disability, the response to levodopa is somewhat different. DRD cases show a dramatic response to very low doses of levodopa and rarely, if ever, develop long-term motor complications. On the contrary, ARP cases in spite of having an excellent response to the drug very early in the course of treatment develop motor fluctuations and dyskinesias. Dystonia may also be present as a prominent feature in cases of classic Lewy body PD of early onset (EOPD), and similar to what happens in ARP, early appearance of dyskinesias and response uctuations characterizes the pattern of response to levodopa in these cases (2).

Nonroutine metabolic studies (CSF biochemistry, fluorodopa PET (positron emission tomography) scanning, and dopamine transporter density measured with SPECT [single-photon-emission computed

Table 51-1 Differential Diagnosis of Young-Onset and Juvenile Parkinsonism	
Young-onset Parkinsonism (<40)	**Juvenile Parkinsonism (<21)**
Parkinson's disease (Lewy body) sporadic (15)	Dopa-responsive dystonia (DRD) (8)
Autosomal recessive parkinsonism (PARK 2) (43)	Autosomal recessive parkinsonism (ARP) (PARK 2) (43)
Parkinson's disease (Lewy body) familial (PARK 1) (41)	Juvenile parkinsonism/dystonia (Lewy bodies) (9,10)
Diffuse Lewy-body disease (62)	Rapid-onset dystonia-parkinsonism (63)
Rapid-onset dystonia-parkinsonism (63)	Postencephalitic parkinsonism (83)
X-linked dystonia parkinsonism (Lubag) (66)	Juvenile parkinsonism/dystonia (ARP) (Neuro brillary tangles) (44)
MPTP and other toxins (54)	Defects of the biosynthesis of DA (infantile forms of dystonia-parkinsonism) (67)
SCA 3 (Machado-Joseph's disease) (25)	Pallidopyramidal disease (7)
Postencephalitic parkinsonism (76,77)	Neuronal intranuclear hyaline inclusion disease (84)
Dominantly inherited early-onset parkinsonism (45)	Others: Wilson's disease, Huntington's disease, mitochondrial cytopathies, Niemann-Pick type C (81,82, personal observations)
Chromosome 17 linked-frontotemporal dementia and parkinsonism (78)	
Multiple system atrophy (79)	
Hemi-parkinsonism/hemiatrophy (80)	
Others: Wilson's disease, Huntington's disease, mitochondrial cytopathies, Prion's disease (81,82 personal observations)	

tomography]) may be helpful in distinguishing these cases. Furukawa et al. (27) reported their findings using these methods. They were able to separate patients with classic PD from early-onset parkinsonism with prominent dystonia and DRD on the basis of CSF levels of total biopterin, total neopterin, and fluorodopa PET scanning. CSF total biopterin levels were markedly reduced both in early-onset cases and DRD cases, whereas neopterin was reduced only in DRD. Fluorodopa PET scanning showed reduced striatal uptake both in PD and early-onset parkinsonism and was normal in DRD. Unfortunately, at the time these studies were performed, it was not possible to identify the genetic background of early-onset cases and it may well be that this group included both Lewy body parkinsonism and non-Lewy body ARP cases. More recently, Jeon and coworkers (38) measured the density of the dopamine transporter (DAT) by means of [123I]β-CIT SPECT in genetically confirmed cases of DRD and compared it with juvenile parkinsonism cases. DRD patients were shown to have normal levels of DAT, which corresponded with the absence of nigral cell loss found in postmortem studies in these cases (39), whereas in JP the levels of DAT were markedly decreased (Table 51-2). The presence of atypical features (excluding dystonia), and/or the lack of response to levodopa will be conducive to a more extensive search of alternative diagnosis (Table 51-1)

A comprehensive laboratory evaluation is mandatory and should include serum ceruloplasmin and urinary copper excretion. Wilson's disease, although infrequent, should be ruled out from the beginning as it is fatal if left untreated. The same is true for imaging techniques and electrophysiologic investigations that will be helpful in detecting structural damage or more extensive involvement of the central and peripheral nervous system. In selected patients, obtaining a biopsy specimen (muscle, peripheral nerve, bone marrow, brain) will be helpful in the diagnosis of early onset parkinsonism associated with more rare disorders (mitochondrial cytopathies, metabolic diseases, prion's disease).

At present, the possibility of detecting a specific genetic mutation has simplified the diagnostic process in a large number of cases of juvenile or young-onset parkinsonism. Mutations in the parkin gene (PARK 2) are diagnostic of ARP whereas those corresponding to GTP cyclohydrolase I will certify a diagnosis of DRD (26,28). However, genetic testing for these disorders is not available commercially at this time. There are numerous cases of parkinsonism with obvious familial incidence in which no specific mutation has been detected.

Table 51-2 Clinical, Biochemical, and Functional Differences Between Autosomal Recessive Parkinsonism (ARP), Early-Onset Parkinson's Disease (EOPD), and Dopa-Responsive Dystonia (DRD)

	ARP	EOPD	DRD
Heredity	AR	None	AD
Mean age at onset (yrs)	20s	30s	<10
Sleep benefit	+	−/+	++
Tremor	Fine, postural	Coarse, rest	Fine, postural
Dystonia	+	+	++
Effect of levodopa	+++	++	++++
Drug-induced dyskinesias	+++	++	−
Fluctuations	+++	++	−
CSF biopterin	↓↓	↓	↓
CSF neopterin	→	→	↓↓
Fluorodopa PET scanning	↓	↓	→
DAT/SPECT	↓	↓	→
Neuronal loss and gliosis in SN	Focal	Diffuse	None
Lewy bodies in SN	None	Diffuse	None
Depigmentation in SN	++	+	++
Neuronal loss in LC	+	++	−
Neurofibrillary tangles	+	−	−

AR: Autosomal recessive; AD: Autosomal dominant; DAT: Dopamine transporter

PATHOLOGY

The earliest autopsy reports of cases with parkinsonism of early onset will not be considered here because the pathologic concept of PD was not firmly established at the time these observations were made. They include the so-called "primary atrophies of the pallidal system" (5,6) and "pallidopyramidal disease" reported by Davison in 1947 (7).

Excluding those cases with a specific etiology, corresponding to degenerative, metabolic, toxic, or infectious disorders, the pathology of primary parkinsonism of early onset is, for the most part, restricted to the substantia nigra resulting in a syndrome of dopamine deficiency that can be subdivided into three main categories.

[1]　Lewy-body disease (familial or sporadic)
Patients with age of onset between 20 and 40 years have been reported as having pathology findings indistinguishable from classic late-onset PD. These include severe neuronal loss in the substantia nigra pars compacta (SNPC) Lewy bodies in some of the remaining neurons, extracellular melanin and melanin inside macrophages, together with marked gliosis. Mild-to-moderate cell loss, gliosis, and Lewy bodies in the locus ceruleus (LC), dorsal motor nucleus of the vagus, and substantia inominata are also seen (10,15,40). Pathologic features such as these have been found in sporadic cases of early onset and in autosomal dominant PD (PARK 1/alpha-synuclein mutation) in which early-onset cases have been documented (41).

[2]　Nigral cell loss without Lewy bodies
Autopsy reports of several cases of juvenile or young-onset parkinsonism with age of onset between 10 and 24 years have been published. In these cases the postmortem findings differed from classical Lewy-body parkinsonism. The neuropathologic features of these cases included marked depigmentation of the substantia nigra and locus ceruleus, neuronal loss with gliosis, and extraneuronal-free melanin in the ventrolateral and medial part of the intermediate group of the SNPC. The remaining neurons of the SNPC and those of the LC had smaller size and a reduced melanin content. Lewy bodies were not found anywhere in the central nervous system, even by ubiquitin immunostaining. In one of the cases the use of specific stains and immunohistochemical techniques revealed the presence of neurofibrillary tangles (NFT) in the SNPC, LC, red nucleus, posterior hypothalamus, and several cortical regions (42–44). All cases reported had a positive family history with an autosomal recessive mode of transmission (ARP). A few of them were later studied genetically and were found to carry mutations of the parkin gene (PARK 2) (44).
An exception to this is the case reported by Dwork and coworkers (45). This patient, whose symptoms started at age 28, died at age 46 after receiving an autologous adrenal transplantation, due to the occurrence of a glioblastoma multiform. Autopsy findings revealed severe neuronal loss in the SNPC and pars reticulata of the substantia nigra, and prominent gliosis was found in the pars reticulata. The remaining neurons in the SNPC were poorly pigmented, and no Lewy bodies or NFT were present in any of the regions studied. This case differed from the previous ARP cases discussed in that the hereditary mode of transmission was autosomal dominant (13 additional family members in three generations were affected, some with onset in early childhood). No genetic mutation has been detected in these cases.

[3]　Immature nigral cells with poor melanization
Only two patients with these neuropathologic features have been published and correspond to childhood-onset cases.
One was reported by Rajput in 1994 (39) and clinically fulfilled the criteria of DRD. In this case, the nigral cell population was normal except for reduced melanin content, especially in the ventral tier. Neurochemically, however, the levels of dopamine and tyrosine hydroxylase (TH) protein and the activity of TH were severely reduced in the striatum. In contrast, the substantia nigra showed normal levels of TH protein, normal TH immunoreactivity despite a substantial reduction of dopamine content.
The second case deserves separate comment as this patient was been reported and discussed in several publications, and the conclusions differ significantly from one another (46–48). This patient started at age six with gait disturbances and frequent falls, associated with inversion of the feet. She further developed generalized rigidity and limb dystonia before receiving levodopa. At age 24 a left-sided thalamotomy provided relief of both rigidity and dystonia on the

right side. After levodopa became available, the patient showed marked improvement but went on to develop left-sided involuntary movements that were subsequently relieved with a right-sided thalamotomy. From age 31 to 38 when she died with peritonitis, she functioned almost normally with small doses of levodopa and bromocriptine. The patient's younger brother was also affected, but he had milder dyskinesia on levodopa. Neuropathologic reports differ considerably: one of the publications emphasized a reduced number of neurons in the SNPC with numerous immature-appearing round cells, reduced melanin content comparable to that of a child 2 to 3 years old, and absence of microglial proliferation or fibrillary gliosis. By contrast, other authors found almost total nerve cell depletion and severe astrocytic gliosis in the ventrolateral part of the SNPC, presence of Lewy bodies, and reduced melanin content. These contradictory observations led to different interpretations of the pathogenetic mechanisms underlying this case, hypoplasia or dysgenesis vs. degenerative process. The question remains unresolved.

EPIDEMIOLOGY AND GENETICS

Despite the lack of a formal epidemiologic survey of early-onset parkinsonism, most reports agree that in western countries approximately 5 to 7 percent of patients with PD in referral populations develop their symptomatology before age 40 (2,49). The proportion is almost twice that in reports originating in Japan where confounding factors could be attributed to the inclusion of very early-onset cases (childhood or juvenile) probably corresponding to ARP and DRD (9,10,29).

Incidence and Etiology

The annual incidence of new cases of PD occurring between ages 35 and 39 is about 0.15 cases per 100,000 population, which is about 1/10 the incidence between ages 60 and 64, the age interval of peak occurrence of the disease (1,49). Although studied informally, it has been noticed that the mean age of patients being referred to specialized clinics has decreased. But, an analysis of the medical records of the population of Rochester, Minnesota, showed no difference in the distribution curves according to age of onset when comparing the years 1935 to 1966, 1945 to 1954, and 1967 to 1979, suggesting

that age of onset is not actually decreasing. It can be argued then, that this apparent decrease in the mean age of patients with PD seeking medical treatment is due to an improvement in public awareness, bringing patients to consultation sooner (1,49).

The prevailing hypotheses regarding etiology, propose that most cases of PD, including those of early onset, are the result of the combined interaction between genetically determined neuronal vulnerability and exogenous toxic factors (Chapter 27). Analysis of risk factors have yielded conflicting results with some studies finding an association between early onset and rural living and well-water consumption, others with occupational exposure to herbicides or pesticides, and finally some failing to find an association with either rural living or toxic exposure but with a positive family history of PD or head trauma (31,50–54).

Familial Aggregation

A higher incidence of familial cases has always been considered to be a distinctive feature of early-onset parkinsonism. In fact, studies of these cases have significantly contributed to the unravelling of the genetic background of PD and parkinsonism. It is evident, from an analysis of the different published series, that a higher incidence of familial aggregation is correlated with younger onset. Most of the reports originating in the western hemisphere failed to find any indication of a predominant hereditary component to this disorder, as the majority of cases were sporadic and only 1/5 of the cases had at least one affected relative. In contrast, Japanese publications report a significant number of familial cases among their early-onset parkinsonism patients. Ten out of 15 cases were familial in Yamamura's series (30); in the series of Yokochi and Narabayashi (12), 42.5% of patients with onset of parkinsonism between ages 6 and 39 had a first- or second-degree relative with PD; Ishikawa (36) found that 10 of 17 cases with a mean age at onset of 27.8 years had an affected sibling. The main differences between Western and Japanese cases are a younger onset (large number of patients with either childhood or juvenile onset) and an apparent autosomal recessive pattern of inheritance (9,10,29). This difference could be explained by the large number of ARP (PARK 2) cases found in Japan and perhaps the erroneous inclusion of DRD cases among them.

Genetic Aspects

A genetic contribution to the etiology of young-onset PD and juvenile parkinsonism is now well established.

This is based not only on the demonstration of familial aggregation of the disease found in several case-control studies, on the description of large multigenerational families with an autosomal dominant mode of transmission, or on families in which multiple siblings were affected (recessive), but also on the discovery of specific genetic mutations linked to the causation of the disease (55).

A gene locus has been mapped to the long arm of chromosome 4 (4q21-23) in a few families of Greek and Italian descent that manifested the disease in an autosomal dominant mode and were found to have typical Lewy body pathology at autopsy (41,56). These families carried a mutation in the alpha-synuclein gene. The mutation leads to an amino acid exchange in the alpha-synuclein protein (Ala53Thr) (57). Younger patients in these pedigrees fall within the range of young-onset PD (21–40 years).

Patients with an earlier age of onset, generally in the 20s and 30s, who have an autosomal recessive mode of transmission with a high degree of parental consanguinity have been found to correspond to a gene locus in the long arm of chromosome 6 (6q25.2-27) (28,37,58). The protein encoded by this gene has been denominated as *parkin*, and different mutations (single or multiple exon deletions or point mutations.) lead to a defect in the synthesis of this protein (28,59,60). The nature of this protein remains to be elucidated. The pathology in these cases differs from classic Lewy body parkinsonism in that there is a selective and severe degeneration of dopaminergic neurons in the SNPC but no Lewy bodies (44).

In addition, cases of DRD that present with prominent parkinsonian symptomatology at a very early age carry a gene abnormality on chromosome 14q that results in partial reduction of the GTP-cyclohydrolase I (GTP-CH I) activity in the nigrostriatal dopaminergic neurons (26,27,61). GTP-CH I is a crucial enzyme in the synthesis of tetrahydrobiopterin, a necessary cofactor for the synthesis of TH.

Furthermore, there are several reports of familial forms of either juvenile or young-onset parkinsonism in which genetic factors, as yet undiscovered, appear to play a role. Such is the case of the "Dominantly inherited, early-onset parkinsonism" reported by Dwork (90), the family reported by Ishikawa (45) with "Hereditary juvenile dystonia-parkinsonism" which also apparently has an autosomal dominant mode of transmission.

Atypical forms of early-onset parkinsonism have also been reported in which hereditary transmission is evident or genetic factors have been determined. The "pure" form of diffuse Lewy body disease may present initially with parkinsonian features of juvenile onset and the later development of dementia or psychosis. There appears to be a of familial incidence this disease (62). The cases of "rapid-onset dystonia parkinsonism" studied by Dobyns et al. (63) with onset between 14 and 45 years have been proposed as a distinct nosologic entity with an underlying genetic background as yet undiscovered. "Lubag" or X-linked dystonia parkinsonism is a disease that primarily affects Filipino men originating principally from the Panay Island. There have been two pathologically proven cases in non-Filipino men with juvenile onset (64,65). Linkage analysis has confirmed the mode of inheritance and localized the disease gene to the proximal long arm of the X-chromosome (66). The pathology of this disease characteristically involves a mosaic pattern of gliosis in the neostriatum (66). Infantile forms of dystonia-parkinsonism have also been reported and are most commonly caused by inborn errors of metabolism affecting the dopamine biosynthetic pathway (GTP-CH I deficiency, 6-pyruvoyltetrahydropterin synthase deficiency, dihydropteridine reductase deficiency, aromatic amino-acid decarboxylase deficiency, and TH deficiency) (67).

RESPONSE TO MEDICATIONS, THERAPEUTIC STRATEGIES

The peculiar pattern of response to medication that is characteristic of early-onset parkinsonism has been discussed. Table 51-3 provides a summarized review of all published reports in the literature in which an analysis of the response to levodopa has been made.

It is evident that younger patients respond to medication differently than older patients. Younger patients show a more complex pattern of pharmacologic response with more severe dyskinesias and a shorter duration of response to levodopa. However, the degree of improvement with levodopa therapy is qualitatively and quantitatively greater when compared with older patients. These differences are probably age-related and depend on central pharmacokinetics of pharmacodynamics of levodopa plus the involvement of nondopaminergic systems in older patients (24).

Whatever the reason underlying these differences, younger patients require a more cautious approach to medical treatment. Levodopa-sparing strategies are recommended in these cases, and de novo treatment with dopamine agonists is preferable as it has been demonstrated that their use may reduce the

Table 51-3 Response to Medication and Motor Complications in Young-Onset (YOPD) and Juvenile Parkinsonism (JP)

Author	No. of Cases	Degree of Response to Levodopa	Dyskinesias	Fluctuations	Latency
Yokochi and Narabayashi, 1981 (12)	Group 1 (10) Group 2 (22)	Dramatic Marked	+++ +++	No mention No mention	No mention No mention
Gershanik and Leist, 1986 (13)	13	Marked (low doses)	+++ (76%)	No mention	After 1 year (D)
Quinn et al. 1987 (3)	JP (4) YOPD (56)	Marked (80%) (group as a whole)	+++ (100%) (group as a whole)	+++ (96%) (group as a whole)	After 1 month (20%) (D) After 1 year (55%) (D) After 1 month (10%) (F) After 1 year (38%) (F) After 6 years (96%) (F) After years of treatment (D, F)
Ludin and Ludin, 1989 (16)	23	Not mentioned	+++ (16/23)	+++ (22/23)	
Askenasy et al. 1989 (84)	JP (3) YOPD (1)	Marked to dramatic (low doses)	No mention	+++	After 2 years (F)
Giovannini et al. 1991 (17)	60	Good (8.7%) at 6mo. Moderate (39.6%) at 6mo. Poor (51.7%) at 6mo.	++ (78%) (motor side effects considered as a whole)	++(78%) (motor side effects considered as a whole)	No mention
Bostanjopoulou et al. 1991 (20)	30 (<48y)	No mention	++(8/30)	++(8/30)	Evaluation at 6 years
Tsai and Lu, 1991 (19)	JP (8)	Dramatic	+++	No mention	(D, F)
Kostic et al. 1991 (18)	YOPD (17) 25	Dramatic No mention	+++ +++	No mention +++	After 4 years (83%)\(D) After 7 years (100%)\(D) After 2 years (48%)\(D)
Pantelatos and Fornadi, 1993 (22)	221	No mention	+++(>40%)	+++(>50%)	After 5 years (96%)\(D) After 2 years (40%)\(F) After 5 years (80%)\(F)
Muthane et al. 1994 (23)	JP (7) YOPD (16)	Excellent(28%), Good(72%) Good(22%), Poor (28%) Excellent(50%) Excellent (100%)	+++	+++	No mention After 6 months (33%)\(D) After 6 months (50%)\(D)
Gomez Arevalo et al. 1997 (24)	34	Excellent (100%)	+++	+++	After 5 years (82%)\(D) After 5 years (82%)\(F)
Schrag et al. 1998 (25)	JP (10) YOPD(139)	Excellent (81%) Good (15%) Poor (4%)	+++ ++(91%)	+++ ++(92%)	After 1 week (25%) (D/F) After 6 months (40%)\(D/F) After 5 years (91%)\(D/F) 100% at 10 years (D/F)

D: dyskinesias, F: fluctuations

incidence of levodopa-related motor complications in the long term. Whenever the use of levodopa becomes necessary it should be carefully introduced at the lowest dose necessary. It is advisable to maintain a stable therapeutic regime for as long as possible. Younger patients should receive psychologic support (psychotherapy, support groups) and be encouraged to engage regularly in physical activity and to preserve as much as possible an active life.

SPECIAL SITUATIONS AND NEEDS OF THE YOUNG PATIENT

Younger patients face special psychosocial problems and are often confronted with difficult situations in coping with a disease that has been traditionally attributed to advanced age. The issue of acceptance is paramount and the question "why me?" is frequently raised. The most valuable references on this topic are found in personal accounts on how to live with PD when young (68,69). People with PD at a young age are often reluctant to participate in support groups for the fear of facing the truth of what lies ahead for them. They feel conspicuous and out of place and do not share the same concerns with people of older age. The issues of family adjustment, marital and sexual life, concerns of being unable to continue being the provider for the family, although not unique to younger patients often have more impact.

Menstrual-Related Fluctuations and Pregnancy

Among the specific issues that have to be addressed in younger female patients are menstrual-induced alterations in symptoms and pregnancy. The menstrual cycle is associated with variations in disability and response to medication. Patients frequently complain that with each menstrual cycle there is a worsening of symptomatology and reduced response to levodopa for a few days before menstruation. This requires clarification and appropriate management (13,34,49,70,71).

Although pregnant women with PD do not experience excessive complications of gestation or parturition, there are reports that indicate that symptomatology tends to worsen during pregnancy and sometimes does not return to baseline after delivery. However, these reports did not find that activities of daily living or the ability to take care of the child appeared to be compromised significantly. Fortunately there has been no increased incidence of neonatal defects associated with the use of

levodopa or other anti-parkinsonian drugs, although no comprehensive studies on the subject have been performed (49,72–75).

Job-Related Demands

Finally, work place considerations for young Parkinsonian patients requires discussion. Parkinsonian patients are faced with a dilemma – they are confronted with a chronic, disabling disorder but they need to and want to continue living an active and productive life. The presence of conspicuous symptomatology often poses a risk of losing their jobs, especially if the symptoms are misinterpreted. Therefore they may require a more aggressive treatment strategy. A careful analysis of the risk–benefit ratio of any therapeutic intervention in these cases is mandatory and should be thoroughly discussed with the patient.

REFERENCES

1. Tanner CM, Hubble JP, Chan P. Epidemiology and genetics of Parkinson's disease. In: Watts RL, Koller WC (eds.). *Movement Disorders: Neurologic Principles and Practice*. New York: McGraw-Hill, 1997:137–152
2. Gershanik O. Early-onset parkinsonism. In: Jankovic J Tolosa E (eds.). *Parkinson's Disease and Movement Disorders*. 2nd. ed. Baltimore: Williams & Wilkins, 1993:235–252.
3. Quinn N, Critchley P, Marsden CD. Young onset parkinson's Disease. *Mov Disord*. 1987; 2:73–91.
4. Willige H. Uber paralysis agitans im jegendlichem alter. *Z Gesamte Neurol Psychiatry* 1910; 4:520–587.
5. Hunt JR. Progressive atrophy of the globus pallidus. *Brain* 1917; 40:58–148.
6. Van Bogaert L. Contribution clinique et anatomique a l'etude de la paralysie agitante juvenil primitive. *Rev Neurol* (France) 1930; 11:315–326.
7. Davison D. Pallido-pyramidal disease. *J Neuropathol Exp Neurol* 1947; 13:50–59.
8. Segawa M, Nomura Y, Kase M. Hereditary progressive dystonia with marked diurnal fluctuation: Clinico-pathophysiological identification in reference to juvenile Parkinson's disease. *Adv Neurol* 1985; 45:227–234.
9. Yokochi M, Narabayashi H, Iizuka R, et al. Juvenile parkinsonism. Some clinical, pharmacological, and neuropathological aspects. *Adv Neurol* 1984; 40:407–413.
10. Yokochi M. Familial juvenile parkinsonism. *Eur Neurol* 1997; 38(Suppl 1):29–33.
11. Yokochi M. Juvenile Parkinson's disease. Part 1: Clinical aspects. *Adv Neurol Sci* (Tokyo) 1979; 23:1048–1059.

12. Yokochi M, Narabayashi H. Clinical characteristics of juvenile parkinsonism. In: Rose FC, Capildeo R (eds.). *Research Progress in Parkinson's Disease*. Tunbridge Wells, England: Pitman, 1981:35–39.

13. Gershanik OS, Leist A. Juvenile onset Parkinson's disease. *Adv Neurol* 1986; 45:213–216.

14. Lima B, Neves G, Nora M. Juvenile parkinsonism: Clinical and metabolic characteristics. *J Neurol Neurosurg Psychiatry* 1987; 50:345–348.

15. Gibb WRG, Lees AJ. A comparison of clinical and pathological features of young- and old-onset Parkinson's disease. *Neurology* 1988; 38:1402–1406.

16. Ludin SM, Ludin HP. Is Parkinson's disease of early onset a separate disease entity? *J Neurol* 1989; 236(4):203–207.

17. Giovannini P, Piccolo I, Genitrini S, et al. Early-onset Parkinson's disease. *Mov Disord* 1991; 6(1):36–42.

18. Kostic V, Przedborski S, Flaster E, et al. Early development of levodopa-induced dyskinesias and response fluctuations in young-onset Parkinson's disease. *Neurology*. 1991; 41(2 (Pt 1)):202–205.

19. Tsai CH, Lu CS. Early onset parkinsonism in Chinese. *J Formos Med Assoc* 1991 Oct; 90(10):964–969.

20. Bostantjopoulou S, Logothetis J, Katsarou Z, et al. Clinical observations in early and late onset Parkinson's disease. *Funct Neurol* 1991; 6(2):145–149.

21. Ferreiro JL, Pugliese MI, Caride AE. Juvenile parkinsonism. 18 cases. *Medicina (B Aires)* 1991; 51(3):204–8.

22. Pantelatos A, Fornadi F. Clinical features and medical treatment of Parkinson's disease in patient groups selected in accordance with age at onset. *Adv Neurol* 1993; 60:690–697.

23. Muthane UB, Swamy HS, Satishchandra P, et al. Early onset Parkinson's disease: Are juvenile- and young-onset different? *Mov Disord* 1994; 9(5):539–544.

24. Gomez Arevalo G, Jorge R, Garcia S, et al. Clinical and pharmacological differences in early- versus late-onset Parkinson's disease. *Mov Disord* 1997; 12(3):277–284.

25. Schrag A, Ben-Shlomo Y, Brown R, et al. Young-onset Parkinson's disease revisited – clinical features, natural history, and mortality. *Mov Disord* 1998; 13(6):885–894.

26. Ichinose H, Ohye T, Takahashi E, et al. Hereditary progressive dystonia with marked diurnal fluctuation caused by mutations in the GTP cyclohydrolase I gene. *Nat Genet* 1994; 8:236–242.

27. Furukawa Y, Mizuno Y, Narabayashi H. Early-onset parkinsonism with dystonia. Clinical and biochemical differences from hereditary progressive dystonia or DOPA-responsive dystonia. *Adv Neurol* 1996; 69:327–337.

28. Kitada T, Asakawa S, Hattori N, et al. Mutations in the *parkin* gene cause autosomal recessive juvenile parkinsonism. *Nature* 1998; 392(6676):605–608.

29. Yokochi M. Nosological concept of juvenile parkinsonism with reference to the dopa-responsive syndrome. *Adv Neurol* 1993; 60:548–552.

30. Yamamura Y, Sobue I, Ando K, et al. Paralysis agitans of early onset with marked fluctuations of symptoms. *Neurology* 1973; 23:239–244.

31. Goetz CG, Tanner Cm, Stebbins GT, et al. Risk factors for progression in Parkinson's disease. *Neurology* 1988; 38:1841–1844.

32. Diamond SG, Markham CH, Hoehn MMM, et al. Effect of age at onset on progression and mortality in Parkinson's disease. *Neurology* 1989; 39:1187–1190.

33. Jankovic J, McDermott M, Carter J, et al. Variable expression of Parkinson's disease: A base-line analysis of the DATATOP cohort. The Parkinson Study Group. *Neurology* 1990; 40(10):1529–1534.

34. Quinn NP, Marsden CD. Menstrual-related fluctuations in Parkinson's disease. *Mov Disord* 1986; 1(1):85–87.

35. Blin J, Dubois B, Vidailhet M, et al. Does ageing aggravate parkinsonian disability? *J Neurol Neurosurg Psychiatry* 1991; 54:780–782.

36. Ishikawa A, Tsuji S. Clinical analysis of 17 patients in 12 Japanese families with autosomal-recessive type juvenile parkinsonism. *Neurology* 1996; 47(1):160–166.

37. Matsumine H, Yamamura Y, Kobayashi T, et al. Early onset parkinsonism with diurnal fluctuation maps to a locus for juvenile parkinsonism. *Neurology* 1998a; 50(5):1340–1345.

38. Jeon BS, Jeong JM, Park SS, et al. Dopamine transporter density measured by [123I]beta-CIT single-photon emission computed tomography is normal in dopa-responsive dystonia. *Ann Neurol* 1998; 43(6):792–800.

39. Rajput AH, Gibb WRG, Zhong XH, et al. Dopa-responsive dystonia; Pathological and biochemical observations in a case. *Ann Neurol* 1994; 35:396–402.

40. Gibb WR. Neuropathology in movement disorders. *J Neurol Neurosurg Psychiatry* 1989; Suppl:55–67.

41. Golbe LI, Di Iorio G, Bonavita V, et al. A large kindred with autosomal dominant Parkinson's disease. *Ann Neurol* 1990; 27(3):276–282.

42. Takahashi H, Ohama E, Suzuki S, et al. Familial juvenile parkinsonism: Clinical and pathologic study in a family. *Neurology* 1994; 44(3 Pt 1):437–41.

43. Ishikawa A, Takahashi H. Clinical and neuropathological aspects of autosomal recessive juvenile parkinsonism. *J Neurol* 1998; 245(11 Suppl 3):P4–p9.

44. Mori H, Kondo T, Yokochi M. Pathologic and biochemical studies of juvenile parkinsonism linked to chromosome 6q. *Neurology* 1998; 51(3):890–892.

45. Dwork AJ, Balmaceda C, Fazzini EA, et al. Dominantly inherited, early-onset parkinsonism: Neuropathology of a new form. *Neurology* 1993;43 (1):69–74.

46. Gibb WR, Narabayashi H, Yokochi M, et al. New pathologic observations in juvenile onset parkinsonism with dystonia. *Neurology* 1991; 41(6):820–822.

47. Mizutani Y, Yokochi M, Oyanagi S. Juvenile parkinsonism: A case with first clinical manifestation at the age of six years and with neuropathological findings

52

Is There a Familial Form of Parkinson's Disease?

Lawrence I. Golbe, M.D.

UMDNJ–Robert Wood Johnson Medical School, New Brunswick, New Jersey

The literature differentiates "familial Parkinson's disease (PD)" from "sporadic PD" or "idiopathic PD." About 10 percent of persons with PD have an affected parent or sibling, a figure two to four times that of controls (1–3). This chapter's title implies that PD occurring in such familial clusters differs from PD occurring sporadically. Most familial PD clusters comprise only two or three affected individuals. Such patients appear not to differ clinically from those with sporadic PD (4,5). This chapter reviews the evidence that familial clustering of PD is caused primarily by common genes rather than by common environmental exposures or by coincidence. Finally, the chapter discusses the clinical and molecular features of some large, well-studied family clusters of PD, not to catalog their highly varied clinical features but to point out what those families have taught us about PD.

HOW FAMILIAL IS PARKINSON'S DISEASE?

The lifetime incidence of PD among children of affected individuals is about 5 to 6 percent (6,7), whereas for the general population the figure is 2 percent (8). This datum is a more valid measure of family clustering than a raw prevalence statistic and answers a question frequently asked by patients and their families. For an asymptomatic individual who has both an affected parent and an affected sibling, the lifetime incidence of PD approaches 25 percent (6,7).

There are many pitfalls in quantifying family clustering in PD. First, not all patients with PD even claim to know whether PD was present in their relatives. Lazzarini and coworkers (6) found that only 20 percent of patients in our New Jersey clinic claimed enough knowledge of their first- and second-degree relatives to answer the question. Among that fraction of patients, the frequency of a family history of "probable" or "definite" PD on examination was 53 percent rather than the 22 percent for less well-informed patients.

Another difficulty is that families in which one member has PD may be more interested or proficient, and sometimes too proficient, than unaffected families in finding additional occurrences. Rajput and coworkers (9) have formally confirmed the presence of false positive family ascertainment bias in movement disorders. Uncritical acceptance of positive family allegations of PD in deceased individuals and failure to examine living individuals can exaggerate the genetic influence in a disease that usually starts late in life and has no readily available, objective diagnostic test.

One solution to the problems of false positive family reports is to measure the prevalence of the disease among asymptomatic relatives of the proband cases. One such approach was devised by Montgomery and coworkers (10), who administered sensitive tests of motor speed, olfaction, and mood to asymptomatic first-degree relatives of PD patients and controls. Abnormal results occurred in 22.5 percent of the relatives and 9 percent of controls (p < 0.05). Positron emission tomography (PET) in twins is a more sensitive test in asymptomatic relatives and will be discussed.

ARE FAMILIAL CLUSTERS GENETIC IN ORIGIN?

The hypothesis that familial clusters of PD may be explained by a common environmental exposure was examined by Uitti and coworkers (11) when they compared multiply affected families with families having only one affected member with regard to a history

591

of shared residence. They found shared residence to be actually less frequent for the familial than for the nonfamilial PD families. This failed to support an environmental cause of familial clustering. More studies are necessary to fully answer this important question.

If family clusters occurred randomly or for environmental reasons or as a result of multiple mutations (none predominant), then two affected relatives from a previous generation(s) are equally likely to both be on the father's side, to both be on the mother's side, and to be each from one side for a 2:1 unilateral–bilateral ratio. In fact the ratio for PD has repeatedly been observed to be far higher than 2:1 (6,12–15). This is the result predicted for an autosomal dominant trait, although in this case that trait has low penetrance. However, a strict Mendelian pattern as in Huntington's disease is the exception in familial PD, even when one accounts for the difference in onset age.

Two segregation analyses (16,17) (statistical analyses of the pattern of disease occurrence within families) supported a polygenic, non-Mendelian etiology, possibly with a nongenetic component rather than an autosomal dominant mechanism with low penetrance. Although a formal segregation analysis of the size needed to settle this issue has not been reported, one is under way. (D.M. Maraganore, personal communication)

The weight of opinion at this point is that an interplay of multiple genetic defects, probably with environmental exposure(s), is the etiology of most cases of PD, both familial and nonfamilial. The evidence for environmental risk factors is not reviewed here, but recent tests of combined genetic and environmental risk factor models have produced more robust results than either alone (18). So far, the strongest such interactions are those in which a hereditary insufficiency of detoxification mechanisms is combined with potential exposure to the corrresponding toxin (19,20).

CLINICALLY INAPPARENT PD

Lewy bodies (LB), the pathologic hallmark of degenerating neurons in PD, appear in the substantia nigra pars compacta in occasional autopsies of individuals dying with no clinical signs or symptoms of PD. This condition, known as incidental Lewy body disease (ILBD) has a prevalence among the autopsied population that increases from less than 1 percent during the fifth decade to 14 percent during the eighth (21,22). Neuronal degeneration accompanies the LBs, and it occurs in the same subregional distribution as in PD (23). ILBD also features early loss of reduced glutathione, one of the neurochemical defects characteristic of PD (24). Furthermore, LBs appear in

neurons of the cardiac plexus in patients whose brains show ILBD, as in PD (25). For all these reasons ILBD is thought to be the preclinical stage of PD.

Age adjustment of the ILBD autopsy data to the age structure of the living population suggests that 5 to 6 percent of individuals more than age 40 have ILBD, compared with 0.3 percent for clinically apparent PD. This suggests that there is a huge false negative rate inherent in clinical prevalence studies of PD and that if we include ILBD as part of the definition of PD, the frequency of a positive family history of PD may far exceed the 20 percent typically obtained in clinical surveys. However, the same "iceberg" phenomenon could as easily obscure clusters of PD of exogenous, toxic origin.

FLUORODOPA PET AND CLINICAL GENETICS

A standard technique for assessing the genetic contribution to disease etiology is to compare the concordance among monozygotic (MZ) twins with that among dizygotic (DZ) twins. A single-gene autosomal dominant model predicts MZ concordance to be twice DZ concordance. For an autosomal recessive trait, the ratio would be 4:1 and for a nongenetic trait, it would be unity. "Penetrance" of a genetic trait is the fraction of those carrying the gene defect who develop clinical disease.

Five published PD twin studies used purely clinical diagnosis. The four oldest and smallest of these (26–29) produced a total concordance rate of 5/82 (6.1%) MZ pairs and 3 of 66 (4.6%) DZ pairs – a result more compatible with a nongenetic etiology than with a single dominant or recessive mutation. The largest and most recent of the 5 clinically based twin studies is that of Tanner and coworkers (30). For those pairs in whom the first (or only) affected twin developed symptoms after age 50 there was no MZ–DZ concordance difference. This is again evidence against an important hereditary component in PD. However, in those few pairs in which PD first appeared before age 50, the MZ–DZ ratio was 6:1 suggesting a strong genetic etiologic component for younger onset patients.

The detection of preclinical PD is enhanced, at least in those few individuals of sufficient research interest to justify the cost, by ^{18}F-fluorodopa PET imaging of striatal dopamine terminals. PET can detect asymptomatic changes in healthy members of multiply affected sibships with PD (31–33).

In a recent landmark study, Piccini and coworkers (34) performed fluorodopa PET in clinically unaffected co-twins, finding the concordance at the initial evaluation to be 55 percent for MZ pairs and

18 percent for DZ pairs. After reevaluation with PET, an average of four years later, it was found that all 10 of the MZ co-twins had either developed clinical PD or showed a decline in striatal fluorodopa uptake far steeper than that in controls. Among the 10 DZ co-twins with follow-up evaluation, only two showed such a decline.

Even when Piccini and coworkers analyzed the subset of twins in which no other family member was alleged to have PD (i.e., instances of "sporadic" PD), the results were unchanged. This defuses criticism that the series was merely one of highly penetrant "familial PD," unrepresentative of PD. Furthermore, PD onset age among the proband twins of Piccini et al. averaged 57 years, which is nearly identical to the PD onset age in the community and suggests that the PET results were not driven by a large subgroup with atypically young-onset, familial PD. There is also the potential objection that many of the healthy co-twins who agreed to undergo PET scanning were concealing early symptoms of PD for which they sought evaluation. This bias could have raised the overall concordance rate, but unless it was far more frequent among MZ than DZ twins, it could not account for the large MZ–DZ concordance ratio discrepancy observed. Another potential objection is that the PET abnormality, reduced striatal uptake of labelled levodopa, is not necessarily diagnostic of PD. But the PET defect is too rare among control individuals to have influenced the result of the PD twin study.

The Piccini and coworkers twin study using PET strongly suggests that the previous twin studies, which were clinically based, simply failed to detect PD in its early, preclinical stages and that there exists a very strong genetic component to the etiology of PD. The significance of the twin data to the central hypothesis of this chapter is the notion that if we expand the definition of PD to include that which is undetectable except by serial PET, then all PD may be "familial." This may render moot the question of whether "familial" PD differs from "nonfamilial" PD in any medically interesting respect.

KNOWN PARKINSON'S DISEASE GENES OR LOCI

General Caveats

The discussion so far prompts the hypothesis that PD is an etiologically heterogeneous disease with genetic influences paramount but with varying degrees of penetrance. This, in turn, suggests that a variety of genetic defects, or combinations of defects, can produce PD. The simplest route to finding such a defect starts

with a family in which PD clusters in the manner of a classic Mendelian single-gene defect. If DNA is available from enough family members, typically about 10, depending on the proximity of the relationships, linkage analysis may permit identification of the general location of the disease gene. Then, sequencing of that region may reveal the precise defect.

For so many affected members to occur in one identifiable human family, the disease must be highly penetrant. This means that the illness must appear sufficiently early in life that its diagnosis will not be masked by mortality or by comorbid entities such as Alzheimer's disease, cerebrovascular disease, or arthritis. Clearly, PD occurring in so unusual a pattern is likely not to be caused by the same genetic defects that may cause "sporadic" PD, which becomes symptomatic at a mean age of nearly 60. Nevertheless, finding the genetic basis of such families can provide valuable clues to the pathogenesis of PD.

α-Synuclein Mutations

To date, two different single base-pair substitution mutations associated with PD have been found in the gene for α-synuclein, a small protein that is probably involved in axonal transport of synaptic vesicles (35). The first such mutation was found in 1997 (36,37) in an Italian-American family, the Contursi kindred, originating in the town of that name in the Campania region of south-central Italy (38,39). In affected members, typical LB's occur at autopsy (38). The same mutation was subsequently found in several Greek and Greek-American families that may be related to the Contursi kindred, given the frequent contact between southern Italy and Greece over the centuries (37,40). The other single base-pair substitution mutation in α-synuclein was found in a family from the Saxony-Anhalt region of Germany (41).

Clinical and Its Pathologic Aspects

The Contursi kindred includes 60 known affected individuals. The disease occurs in a very highly penetrant autosomal dominant fashion, and 40.1 percent of at-risk individuals (i.e., those with a sibling or parent with PD) became affected by age 50 (50 percent being full penetrance for a dominant trait). The frequency of rest tremor is slightly lower than in PD in the community, but the frequencies of dementia, depression, and other nonmotor features are typical for PD. Autopsy in one case showed typical LBs in the expected predominantly brainstem distribution (38) and in another case, a woman with prominent dementia and aphasia, there was wider distribution of LBs consistent with a diagnosis of dementia of the LB type. (L. Forno, personal communication) In both cases, the

LBs tended to occur in neuronal processes rather than in the predominantly perikaryal location typical of PD (L. Forno, W. Gibb, personal communications).

Although the motor aspects of PD in the Contursi kindred respond to levodopa in the usual fashion, the clinical course is collapsed to a mean survival of only 9.2 years. This compares to a mean survival of 20 to 25 years for PD of comparably young onset in the community. Furthermore, the mean PD symptom onset age in the Contursi kindred is only 45.6 years with a standard deviation of 13.48 and a range of 20 to 85 years. Although the mean onset age is about 15 years younger than that of PD in the community, the SD and range are typical.

In the German family, PD symptoms developed at ages 52, 55, and 60 in the three affected members. Two others, who were asymptomatic, showed objective signs of the disease at ages 50 and 33 (41). The onset age distribution therefore may be a bit older than in the Contursi kindred. Nevertheless, the range of clinical features appears similar to those of that family and of PD in the community. Opportunity for postmortem examination in the German family has not yet occurred.

Molecular Aspects

The primary pathogenetic mutation in the Contursi kindred was found by a linkage study to be a single base-pair substitution in the gene for α-synuclein, on chromosome 4q21 (36,37). The PD-1 or PARK-1 mutation, as the Contursi kindred's defect has been variously called, comprises a substitution of threonine for alanine at amino acid 53 (37).

Lewy bodies, abnormal intracellular aggregates whose causal role in the death of neurons in PD has long been debated, have now been found to stain heavily for α-synuclein in sporadic PD unassociated with mutations in the α-synuclein gene (42). The A53T amino acid substitution of the Contursi kindred and the A30P substitution of the German sibship (41) increase the normally high self-aggregation of the α-synuclein molecule (43). Furthermore, such aggregates in genetically engineered cultured cells expressing the mutant α-synuclein are associated with apoptotic neuronal death (44). In normal brain, α-synuclein appears to be expressed most heavily in pigmented neurons of the substantia nigra and other neurons in which LBs occur in PD (45).

Both α-synuclein mutations abolish the ability of that molecule to bind to vesicles being transported along the axon (46). It remains to be seen, however, whether this is the pathogenetic mechanism in PD, either in individuals with the known α-synuclein mutations or in others with PD. Another valuable pathogenetic clue is the identification of a novel protein, dubbed synphilin-1, which interacts with α-synuclein in neurons (47). Inducing cultured cells to produce both synphilin-1 and mutant α-synuclein produces intracellular protein aggregates similar to LBs. Synphilin-1 does not interact with normal α-synuclein or other proteins to produce such aggregates (47).

Neither of the two known α-synuclein mutations has been found in hundreds of patients with sporadic or familial PD outside the few original Italian, Greek, and German families in which they were described. However, one study found a dinucleotide repeat marker in the α-synuclein gene to differ markedly in frequency between familial and sporadic PD (48). Another found that the combination of the ε-4 allele of Apo E and a polymorphism in the promoter region of the α-synuclein gene was increased 12.8-fold in patients with PD relative to controls (49).

The prominence of α-synuclein in LBs reveals the role of that protein as central to the pathogenesis of all PD. Mutations in or near the α-synuclein gene, aside from their central role in a few rare families, may be a contributing factor in "sporadic" PD. Efforts are underway to further elucidate the role of normal α-synuclein and how genetic or acquired defects in that molecule can produce LBs and/or neuronal degeneration.

Ubiquitin Carboxy-Terminal Hydrolase L1 Mutation

In another German family with PD, but without autopsy confirmation, a specific mutation has been found in the gene for ubiquitin carboxy-terminal hydrolase L1(UCH-L1) (50), which codes for an enzyme involved in breakdown and disposal of damaged proteins. Attention was drawn to ubiquitin by the observation that LBs stain heavily for that protein (see Chapter 20).

A brother and sister whose PD began at ages 49 and 51 first experienced rest tremor that progressed to a typical parkinsonian picture of rigidity, bradykinesia, and postural instability with a good levodopa response. Their parents were deceased and allegedly unaffected, although two deceased paternal relatives were affected.

The mutation, a substitution of methionine for isoleucine at position 93, appears to reduce the catalytic activity of UCH-L1 by about half. The precise natural substrate for this protolytic enzyme is not known, but its involvement in some aspect of ubiquitin metabolism suggests that its insufficiency could allow damaged or superfluous proteins to accumulate and aggregate.

A subsequent study in 11 families with autosomal dominant-appearing PD has failed to reveal any carriers of this mutation, suggesting that it, like the α-synuclein mutations, is not a common etiologic factor in hereditary PD (51).

Parkin Mutations

The work of Mizuno and colleagues has revealed families with non-LB parkinsonism in whom the causative defect is a gene for a previously undescribed protein dubbed "parkin" (52,53). Its normal function is not yet known, but its sequence is, in part, similar to that of ubiquitin and it is expressed in the same neurons as α-synuclein [Penney, personal communication]. In the original Japanese families, in which the parkin mutation operated in recessive fashion, the typical PD onset age was in the late twenties (54), and the mutation was a deletion comprising most of the gene. However, since then, point substitutions or other modest alterations in the parkin gene have been found in patients with PD of midlife onset without familial clustering, both in Japan and in Western populations (55,56). The degree to which parkin mutations contribute to PD in the community has not been quantified, but the fact that LBs do not occur in the highly penetrant cases suggests that parkin mutations would have only an ancillary, although possibly frequent, contribution. The extent of this contribution is being elucidated by studies of non-Japanese populations (57–59) and could prove to be large.

Other Loci

Chromosomal locations, but not specific mutations, have to date been found on chromosome 2p in a northern European family with clinically typical PD ascertained by Wszolek and colleagues (60–63) and on chromosome 4p for another family of northern European origin, the "Iowa kindred," with PD and LBs but atypical for young onset and prominence of dementia (64,65).

CONCLUSIONS

Although patients from families with only two or three affected individuals have PD that is indiscernible from "sporadic" PD (4,5), it is clear that most of the large PD families, who are "large" by virtue of high gene penetrance do have clinically atypical disease. The most important atypical feature, relatively young onset, may result in part from a bias wherein younger onset PD is more likely not only to manifest during the human life span but also to be recognizable to family members. But being "atypical" does not place it outside the definition of PD. Furthermore, one may hypothesize

that many patients with nonfamilial PD have some atypical feature which, if shared by many members of a kindred, would prompt us to brand the family's PD "atypical."

Even correcting for these biases, highly penetrant PD tends toward atypicality in more than just its high penetrance. But we suspect that even nonfamilial PD is etiologically heterogenous. It should not be surprising to learn that PD, such as that in the Contursi kindred, etiologically different from all other PD by virtue of its unique mutation in α-synuclein, is also clinically or pathologically different. We would expect, similarly, that a single patient with nonfamilial PD that is clinically or pathologically atypical would also have a different etiology. The proof of this hypothesis awaits better understanding of the etiologies of PD.

It is also clear that much of what is called sporadic PD may actually be familial if we broaden the definition of PD to include preclinical dopaminergic dysfunction as detected by ^{18}F-dopa PET and other methods. If the recent PET study of Piccini et al. (34) is taken at face value (and it may be too early to do so), then indeed most sporadic PD may actually be familial PD, although with low penetrance. Other evidence, most prominently the ILBD data, has been presented supporting the view that familial clustering of PD is greater than that revealed by the routine family history in the clinic.

It is logical to conclude that there is no "familial form" of PD in the sense of a genetically determined PD different from an "idiopathic form" or "sporadic form." Present evidence supports the hypothesis that most PD is genetic but with variable penetrance. We now must learn the determinants of penetrance of PD genes. Understanding environmental exposures, ancillary genes, and stochastic factors could allow us to reduce the penetrance of PD genes to the point that the clinical manifestations of the disease no longer occur during the usual human life span.

REFERENCES

1. Elbaz A, Grigoletto F, Baldereschi M, et al. Familial aggregation of Parkinson's disease: A population-based case-control study in Europe. *Neurology* 1999; 52:1876–1882.

2. Marder K, Tang MX, Mejia H, et al. Risk of Parkinson's disease among first-degree relatives: A community-based study, *Neurology* 1996; 47: 155–160.

3. Payami H, Larsen K, Bernard S, et al. Increased risk of Parkinson's disease in parents and siblings of patients. *Ann Neurol* 1994; 36:659–661.

4. Röhl A, Friedrich H-J, Ulm G, et al. The relevance of clinical subtypes for disease course, family history, and epidemiological variables in Parkinson's disease. *Eur J Neurol* 1994; 1:65–72.

5. Hubble JP, Weeks CC, Nance M, et al. Parkinson's disease: Clinical features in sibships. *Neurology* 1999; 52(Suppl 2):A13.

6. Lazzarini AM, Myers RH, Zimmerman TR, et al. A clinical genetic study of Parkinson's disease: Evidence for dominant transmission. *Neurology* 1994; 44:499–506.

7. Bonifati V, Fabrizio E, Vanacore, et al. Familial Parkinson's disease: A clinical genetic analysis. *Can J Neurol Sci* 1995; 22:272–279.

8. Kurland LT. Epidemiology: Incidence, geographic distribution, and genetic considerations. In: Fields WS, (ed.). *Pathogenesis and Treatment of Parkinsonism.* Springfield, Ill.: Charles C. Thomas, 1958, 5–49.

9. Rajput AH, Fenton ME, George D, et al. Concordance of common movement disorders among familial cases. *Mov Disord* 1997; 12:747–751.

10. Montgomery EB Jr, Baker KB, Lyons K, et al. Abnormal performance on the PD test battery by asymptomatic first-degree relatives. *Neurology* 1999; 52:757–762.

11. Uitti RJ, Shinotoh H, Hayward M, et al. "Familial Parkinson's disease" – A case-control study of families. *Can J Neurol Sci* 1997; 24:127–132.

12. Campanella G, Idone M, De Michele G, et al. Paternal preponderance in familial Parkinson's disease. *Neurology* 1984; 34:1398–1400.

13. Young WI, Martin WE, Anderson VE. The distribution of ancestral secondary cases in Parkinson's disease. *Clin. Genet* 1977; 2:189–192.

14. Maraganore DM, Harding AE, Marsden CD. A clinical and genetic study of familial Parkinson's disease. Mov Disord 1990; 6:205–211.

15. De Michele G, Filla A, Volpe G, et al. Environmental and genetic risk factors in Parkinson's disease: A case-control study in southern Italy. *Mov Disord* 1996; 11:17–23.

16. Zareparsi S, Taylor TD, Harris EL, et al. Segregation analysis of Parkinson's disease. *Am J Med Gen* 1998; 80:410–417.

17. Martin WE, Young WI, Anderson VE. Parkinson's disease. A genetic study. Brain 1973; 96:495–506.

18. Golbe LI. Parkinson's disease: Nature meets nurture. *Lancet* 1998; 352:1328–1329.

19. Menegon A, Board PG, Blackburn AC, et al. Parkinson's disease, pesticides, and glutathione transferase polymorphisms. *Lancet* 1998; 352:1344–1346.

20. De Palma G, Mozzoni P, Mutti A, et al. Case-control study of interactions between genetic and environmental factors in Parkinson's disease. *Lancet* 1998; 352:1986–1987.

21. Forno LS. Concentric hyalin intraneuronal inclusions of Lewy type in the brains of elderly persons (50 incidental cases): Relationship to parkinsonism. *J Am Geriatr Soc* 1969; 17:557–575.

22. Gibb WRG, Lees AJ. The relevance of the Lewy body to the pathogenesis of idiopathic Parkinson's disease. *J Neurol Neurosurg Psychiatry* 1988; 349:704–706.

23. Fearnley JM, Lees AJ. Ageing and Parkinson's disease: Substantia nigra regional selectivity, *Brain* 1991; 114:2283–2301.

24. Dexter D, Sian J, Rose S, et al. Indices of oxidative stress and mitochondrial function in individuals with incidental Lewy body disease. *Ann Neurol* 1994; 35:38–44.

25. Iwanaga K, Wakabayaski K, Yoshimoto M, et al. Lewy body-type degeneration in cardiac plexus in Parkinson's and incidental Lewy body diseases. *Neurology* 1999; 52:1269–1271.

26. Ward CD, Duvoisin RC, Ince SE, et al. Parkinson's disease in 65 pairs of twins and in a set of quadruplets. *Neurology* 1983; 33:8815–824.

27. Marttila RJ, Kaprio J, Koskenvuo M, et al. Parkinson's disease in a nationwide twin cohort. *Neurology* 1988; 38:1217–1219.

28. Marsden CD. Parkinson's disease in twins. *J Neurol Neurosurg Psychiatry* 1987; 50:105–106.

29. Vieregge P, Schifke A, Kompf D. Parkinson's disease in twins. *Neurology* 1992; 42:1453–1461.

30. Tanner CM, Ottman R, Goldman SM, et al. Parkinson disease in twins: An etiologic study. *JAMA* 1999; 281:341–346.

31. Sawle GV, Wroe SJ, Lees AJ, et al. The identification of presymptomatic parkinsonism: Clinical and (18F)Dopa positron emission tomography studies in an Irish kindred, *Ann Neurol* 1992; 32:609–617.

32. Piccini P, Morrish PK, Turjanski N, et al. Dopaminergic function in familial Parkinson's disease: A clinical and ^{18}F-dopa positron emission tomography study. *Ann Neurol* 1997; 41:222–229.

33. Holthoff VA, Vieregge P, Kessler J, et al. Discordant twins with Parkinson's disease: Positron emission tomography and early signs of impaired cognitive circuits. *Ann Neurol* 1994; 36:176–182.

34. Piccini P, Burn DJ, Caravolo R, et al. The role of inheritance in sporadic Parkinson's disease: Evidence from a longitudinal study of dopaminergic function in twins. *Ann Neurol* 1999; 45:577–582.

35. Clayton DF, George JM. The synucleins: A family of proteins involved in synaptic function, plasticity, neurodegeneration, and disease. *TINS* 1998; 21:249–254.

36. Polymeropoulos MH, Higgins JJ, Golbe LI, et al. A gene for Parkinson's disease maps to 4q21-q23. *Science* 1996; 274:1197–1199.

37. Polymeropoulos MH, Lavedan C, Leroy E, et al. Mutation in α-synuclein identified in families with Parkinson's disease. *Science* 1997; 276:2045–2047.

38. Golbe LI, Di Iorio G, Bonavita V, et al. A large kindred with autosomal dominant Parkinson's disease. *Ann Neurol* 1990; 27:276–282.

39. Golbe LI, Di Iorio G, Sanges G, et al. Clinical genetic analysis of Parkinson's disease in the Contursi kindred. *Ann Neurol* 1996; 40:767–775.

40. Papadimitriou A, Veletza V, Hadjigeorgiou GM, et al. Mutated α-synuclein gene in two Greek kindreds with familial PD: Incomplete penetrance? *Neurology* 1999; 52:651–654.

41. Krüger R, Vieira-Saecker AMM, Kuhn W, et al. Increased susceptibility to sporadic Parkinson's disease by a certain combined α-synuclein/apolipoprotein E genotype. *Ann Neurol* 1999; 45:611–617.

42. Spillantini MG, Schmidt ML, Lee VM-Y, et al. α-synuclein in Lewy bodies. *Nature* 1997; 388:839–840.

43. El-Agnaf OMA, Jakes R, Curran MD, et al. Effects of the mutations Ala^{30} to Pro and Ala^{53} to Thr on the physical and morphologic properties of α-synuclein protein implicated in Parkinson's disease. *FEBS Lett* 1998; 440:67–70.

44. El-Agnaf OMA, Jakes R, Curran MD, et al. Aggregates from mutant and wild-type α-synuclein proteins and NAC peptide induce apoptotic cell death in human neuroblastoma cells by formation of -sheet and amyloid-like filaments. *FEBS Lett* 1998; 440:71–75.

45. Penney JB, Solano SM. α-Synuclein and parkin have restricted highly similar patterns of gene expression in human brain. *Neurology* 1999; 52(Suppl 2):A212.

46. Jensen PH, Nielsen MS, Jakes R, et al. Binding of α-synuclein to brain vesicles is abolished by familial Parkinson's disease mutation. *J Biol Chem* 1998; 273:26292–26294.

47. Engelender S, Kaminsky Z, Guo X, et al. Synphilin-1 associates with -synuclein and promotes the formation of cytosolic inclusions. *Nat Genet* 1999; 22:110–114.

48. Parsian A, Racette B, Zhang ZH, et al. Mutation, sequence analysis, and association studies of α-synuclein in Parkinson's disease, *Neurology* 1998; 51:1757–1759.

49. Krüger R, Kuhn W, Müller T, et al. Ala^{30}Pro mutation in the gene encoding alpha-synuclein in Parkinson's disease. *Nat Genet* 1998; 18:106–108.

50. Leroy E, Boyer R, Auburger G, et al. The ubiquitin pathway in Parkinson's disease. *Nature* 1998; 395:451–452.

51. Lincoln S, Vaughan J, Wood N, et al. Low frequency of pathogenic mutations in the ubiquitin carboxyterminal hydrolase gene in familial Parkinson's disease. *Neuroreport* 1999; 10:427–429.

52. Matsumine H, Saito M, Shimoda-Matsubayashi S, et al. Localization of a gene for autosomal recessive form of juvenile parkinsonism (AR-JP) linked to chromosome 6q25.2–27. *Am J Hum Genet* 1997; 60:588–596.

53. Kitada T, Asakawa S, Hattori N, et al. Mutations in the *parkin* gene cause autosomal recessive juvenile parkinsonism. *Nature* 1998; 392:605–608.

54. Lücking CB, Abbas N, Dürr A et al. Homozygous deletions in *parkin* gene in European and North African families with autosomal recessive juvenile parkinsonism. *Lancet* 1998; 352:1355–1356.

55. Ishikawa A, Tsuji S. Clinical analysis of 17 patients in 12 Japanese families with autosomal-recessive type juvenile parkinsonism. *Neurology* 1996; 47: 160–166.

56. Hattori N, Kitada T, Matsumine H, et al. Molecular genetic analysis of a novel *parkin* gene in Japanese families with autosomal recessive juvenile parkinsonism: Evidence for variable homozygous deletions in the *parkin* gene in affected individuals. *Ann Neurol* 1998; 44:935–941.

57. Jones AC, Yamamura Y, Almasy L, et al. Autosomal recessive juvenile parkinsonism maps to 6q25.2-q27 in four ethnic groups: Detailed genetic mapping of the linked region. *Am J Hum Genet* 1998; 63:80–87.

58. Tassin J, Dürr A, de Broucker T, et al. Chromosome 6-linked autosomal recessive early-onset parkinsonism: Linkage in European and Algerian families, extension of the clinical spectrum, and evidence of a small homozygous deletion in one family. *Am J Hum Genet* 1998; 63:88–94.

59. Lincoln S, Vaughan J, Wood N, et al. Homozygous deletions in *parkin* gene in European and North African families with autosomal recessive juvenile parkinsonism *Lancet* 1998; 352:1355–1356.

60. Wszolek ZK, Pfeiffer B, Fulgham JR, et al. Western Nebraska family (family D) with autosomal dominant parkinsonism. *Neurology* 1995; 45:502–505.

61. Wszolek ZK, Cordes M, Calne DB, et al. Hereditarer morbus parkinson: Bericht uber drie familien mit autosomal-dominantem erbgang, *Nervenarzt* 1993; 64:331–335.

62. Gasser T, Müller-Myhsok B, Wszolek ZK, et al. A susceptibility locus for Parkinson's disease maps to chromosome 2p13, *Nat Genet* 1998; 18: 262–265.

63. Denson MA, Wszolek ZK, Pfeiffer RF, et al. Familial parkinsonism, dementia, and Lewy body disease: Study of Family G. *Ann Neurol* 1997; 42:638–643.

64. Muenter MD, Howard FM, Okazaki H, et al. A familial Parkinson-dementia syndrome. *Neurology* 1986; 36(Suppl 1):115.

65. Farrer M, Gwinn-Hardy K, Muenter M, et al. A chromosome 4p haplotype segregating with Parkinson's disease and postural tremor. *Hum Mol Genet* 1999; 8:81–85.

53

Parkinson's Plus Syndromes

David Riley, M.D.

Mount Sinai Medical Center, Cleveland, Ohio

INTRODUCTION

Over the last few decades we have come to appreciate more clearly than ever that James Parkinson described a syndrome, not a disease, in his famous 1817 monograph. This syndrome has come to be known as *parkinsonism*. What we now call Parkinson's disease (PD) is a form of parkinsonism that, like other diseases, has characteristic clinical features, epidemiology, clinical course, prognosis, pathology, and treatment. The concept of "Parkinson's plus" diseases arises from the realization that there are a variety of diseases that mimic PD in some respects, but produce additional features that are not seen in PD (Table 53-1). Unfortunately, like PD, these diseases suffer from the same lack of knowledge regarding etiology, leading to an absence of curative measures. Furthermore, there is little in the way of symptomatic therapy available for these Parkinson's plus syndromes.

Parkinson's plus diseases share many of the symptoms and signs of PD, affect people of a similar age group and, at least at first, tend to develop in the same insidious, progressive fashion. Thus they are often mistaken for the more common and more familiar PD. Pathologic studies indicate that this is no small problem. Up to 25 percent of patients who are thought to have PD on a clinical basis, not just initially but up until death, have another disorder at autopsy (1,2). Our inability to identify these patients promptly after presentation means that first, the opportunity to study these other diseases is lost and second, inclusion of these patients confounds the results of studies of PD. Both PD and Parkinson's plus patients suffer as a result.

Parkinson's plus is a poor term to describe the major diseases discussed in this chapter. The implication of this phrase is that these diseases are similar to PD, only with some added features. This is certainly not the case. The Parkinsonism seen in so-called Parkinson's plus diseases differs in the frequency of individual features, their distribution, and their chronological occurrence in the course of the disease. For example, a resting tremor is a relatively rare finding in all Parkinson's plus diseases, whereas they cause disequilibrium and fall much earlier in their course. Because they usually lack the responsiveness to levodopa that characterizes PD, Quinn has suggested that *Parkinson's minus* might be a more appropriate designation for these diseases (3). In other words, PD is not a diagnosis of default that depends solely on the absence of other findings. There are both characteristic and relatively exclusionary clinical features for all of these diseases.

This chapter should be regarded as a fraction of the differential diagnosis of PD. The chief disorders under

Table 53-1 General Features of Parkinson's Plus Syndromes

Features in common with PD

Insidious onset in middle to late life
Progressive course measured in years
Akinesia and rigidity
Lack of diagnostic laboratory tests
Definitive diagnosis requires appropriate data from both clinical and pathologic sources
Lack of knowledge regarding etiology, prevention, and cure
Only symptomatic treatment is available

Features distinctive from PD

Description in the 1960s (except OPCA)
Poor recognition and understanding among lay public
Rest tremor unusual or rare
Frequent corticobulbar/corticospinal tract signs
Early postural instability
Frequent abnormal imaging studies
Poor response to anti-parkinsonian medication
More rapid progression, shorter life expectancy
Pathology involves many brain areas other than pigmented brainstem nuclei

consideration here are progressive supranuclear palsy (PSP), multiple system atrophy (MSA) and cortical-basal ganglionic degeneration (CBGD). Also reviewed briefly is frontotemporal dementia and parkinsonism linked to chromosome 17 (FTDP-17). Other secondary forms of parkinsonism will be found in Chapter 54.

PROGRESSIVE SUPRANUCLEAR PALSY

Progressive supranuclear palsy was first described in 1964 by three Canadian neurologists whose names have been honored in the eponym for this disease, the Steele-Richardson-Olszewski syndrome (4). Although in retrospect there were previous case reports, these authors merited this distinction by virtue of their thorough discussion of this entity.

Clinical Findings

Although the ocular motility disorder that Steele and colleagues chose to highlight remains the most distinctive feature of the clinical syndrome of PSP, strict reliance on this single physical sign leads to a lack of sensitivity, or at least a delay, in diagnosis. Most patients do not present with symptoms or signs related to their eyes. The most common initial feature of PSP is a disturbance of gait and a history of falling.

The parkinsonism of PSP differs from that of PD in the lack of resting tremor, the relative sparing of limb movement (except writing), the greater rigidity in the neck than the limbs, and the early development of freezing and marked micrographia. The speech disturbance also differs in the frequent presence of spastic dysarthria and dysphonia, although it shares the hypophonia and lack of modulation.

The distinctive supranuclear gaze palsy (SNGP) begins with slowing of vertical saccades, followed by a limitation of their range. Pursuit movements are affected later. Horizontal gaze eventually is impaired, but vertical gaze palsies precede and predominate. Other ocular motor findings include saccadic intrusions into fixation ("square-wave jerks"), loss of convergence, blepharospasm, and eyelid freezing, also known as apraxia of eyelid opening or closure.

Other clinical clues indicative of PSP include stuttering, palilalia, early dysphagia, personality changes, sleep disturbances, and dementia. One characteristic feature is a facial expression of perpetual astonishment, due to continuous frontalis contraction and a low blink rate. Another is extensor neck posturing, but this dystonia is to PSP as coprolalia is to Gilles de la Tourette syndrome. Both were features emphasized by

the original authors that have been overly stressed by subsequent authors and actually occur in fewer than 25 percent of cases. PSP patients may also manifest an action tremor, pseudobulbar palsy, hyperreflexia, and Babinski signs. Infrequent occurrences in PSP that lead to problems in diagnosis include an absence of ocular motor abnormalities, a resting tremor, hemidystonia, asymmetric apraxia, and urinary incontinence. Autonomic dysfunction is probably more common than generally appreciated, resulting in misdiagnosis of PSP as MSA. Patients who present with apraxia or aphasia also present a diagnostic challenge, as they run the risk of being mislabeled as having CBGD or Alzheimer's disease.

Symptoms invariably begin insidiously and progress gradually. Golbe and colleagues surveyed the clinical course of PSP and found that it took a mean of three years for patients to require gait assistance, eight years to become confined to a wheelchair or to bed, and 10 years to die (5). However, the duration of illness varies widely, from two to more than 15 years (6). The isolated triad of hypophonic stuttering speech, micrographia and freezing gait known as "pure akinesia" is a more benign form of PSP (7). Common causes of death include pulmonary and urinary tract infections, pulmonary emboli, head trauma, and complications of hip fractures.

Diagnostic criteria for clinical research in PSP were established at an international workshop in 1995 (8). These criteria were validated retrospectively with pathologically confirmed cases. The published report appended helpful descriptions of clinical and neuropsychological testing methods. Considered the most important clinical features in favor of the diagnosis of PSP were a vertical SNGP, slowing of vertical saccades, and prominent postural instability with falls within a year of onset (8).

Epidemiology and Genetics

Patients with PSP are uniformly older than those with PD. Cases beginning before age 40 are very rare. The mean age of onset is in the early seventh decade. Males outnumber females by as much as 2 : 1. Incidence rates in formal studies indicate that one can expect up to 11 new cases per million population per year (9), approximately one-fifth the incidence of PD. Moreover, the shorter life expectancy means that PSP patients make up a correspondingly lower proportion of patients in movement disorders clinics. No specific occupational or other environmental hazard is known.

Some families are known in which PSP is transmitted in an autosomal dominant fashion (10). Studies have detected a high frequency of the allele A0 of the tau gene on chromosome 17 in patients with PSP (11,12), but also in asymptomatic relatives of PSP patients. Tau is a family of microtubule-associated proteins that function to maintain neuronal structural integrity. Actual mutations of the tau gene have not been detected in familial PSP (13). One study discovered four identical sequence variants within the tau gene in 22 unrelated PSP patients (and not in 24 controls). It was concluded that this may represent a susceptibility haplotype. In other words, the presence of these variants may place a person at risk for PSP (13a). Another study demonstrated an alternative in tau mRNA isoform expression. There was an increase in the tau isoforms with four microtubule binding domains (as opposed to three) compared to Alzheimer's and controls in the vulnerable regions. It was thought that these may contribute to formation of neurofibrilliary tangles (NFTs) in this disorder (13b).

Investigations

There are no helpful indicators in common laboratory tests. Routine imaging studies may demonstrate atrophy of the midbrain (14), but usually too late in the course of the disease to be of diagnostic value. Formal neuropsychological testing indicates disproportionate impairment of frontal lobe function (15).

Pathology

There are no striking gross abnormalities in PSP. Minor changes include atrophy of the midbrain,

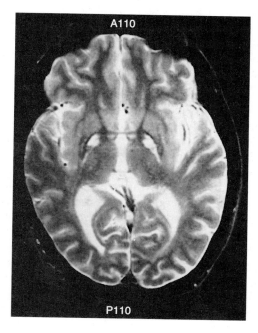

FIGURE 53-1.

milder cortical atrophy, pallor of the substantia nigra, and enlargement of the third ventricle and Sylvian aqueduct. Microscopically, the most consistent pathologic findings are in the basal ganglia, and particularly in the substantia nigra, subthalamic nucleus and internal globus pallidus. Other parts of the brainstem commonly affected in PSP include the superior colliculi, pretectal nuclei, periaqueductal gray matter, and pontine tegmentum. Involvement of the cerebral cortex is increasingly recognized (16,17). Aside from the neuronal loss and gliosis common in degenerative diseases, cytoplasmic inclusions known as neurofibrillary tangles (NFT) are found in surviving neurons. NFT are not specific to PSP, being also found in Alzheimer's disease, postencephalitic parkinsonism, dementia pugilistica and the parkinsonism-dementia complex of Guam. Ultrastructurally, the NFT of PSP are mainly composed of single straight filaments, in contrast to the paired helical filaments that predominate in Alzheimer's disease.

The major structural element of NFT in PSP appears to be abnormally phosphorylated tau, a protein normally associated with the microtubules responsible for axonal transport. Tau exists in multiple isoforms consisting of complete or partial translations of a single gene on chromosome 17. Its ability to promote formation of, and stabilize, microtubules is thought to derive from its state of phosphorylation. It is speculated that abnormal phosphorylation of tau interferes with microtubule function, impairs axonal transport and leads to tau aggregation as NFT. Tau-positive inclusions are also common in oligodendroglia in PSP, and may cause formation of "tufted" astrocytes. Thus abnormal tau modifications in both neurons and glia may be central to the pathophysiology of PSP. However, tau pathology is also seen in cortical-basal ganglionic degeneration (CBGD), Pick's disease and other degenerative diseases. In fact, the pattern of tau isoform accumulation in PSP is identical to that seen in CBGD, which suggests strong pathogenetic bonds between the two conditions (18).

Management

The treatment of PSP is difficult. There is no cure. Available medications provide no benefit in a majority of individuals (19), and when there are benefits they are usually modest (20). Nevertheless, there is opportunity to relieve many symptoms in a variety of ways (Table 53-2). The major goals of management are to identify the patient's major problems, decide which ones can be remedied, and treat them.

Most studies of medication for PSP have focused on the movement disorders. Medications are much less useful than in PD because of the multiplicity of

Table 53-2   Symptomatic Treatment of Parkinson's Plus Syndromes

Motor Problems	Available Treatments
Blepharospasm	Botulinum toxin, eye crutches, surgery
Disequilibrium, falls	Gait and safety training, canes, weighted walkers, hand rails, grab bars, low-heel nonstick shoes
Drooling	Conscious swallowing, drying medications, botulinum toxin
Dysarthria	Facial exercises, speech therapy, written communication, talking keyboard
Dysphagia	Head posturing, dietary changes, gastrostomy
Dystonia	Anticholinergics, clonazepam, botulinum toxin, surgery
Freezing of gait	Visual cues, rhythmic cues, arc (not pivot) turns
Hypophonia	Speech therapy (posture, breathing, swallowing, speaking), voice amplifiers
Micrographia	Change pen or wrist position, keyboard device
Myoclonus	Clonazepam, valproate
Oculomotor palsy	Prisms, pursuit (not saccade) movements, levodopa
Parkinsonism	Exercise, levodopa, dopamine agonists, amantadine, other medications, physical and occupational therapy
Tremor (action type)	Primidone, propranolol, methazolamide, gabapentin
Autonomic Problems	**Available Treatments**
Constipation	Increase fluids and fiber, exercise, bulk-forming agents, laxatives, suppositories, enemas
Postural hypotension	Eliminate causative drugs, increase salt and fluid intake, elevate head of bed, eat smaller meals, physical maneuvers, schedule afternoons for activity, midodrine, fludrocortisone, other medications, elastic stockings
Sexual dysfunction	Sildenafil, yohimbine, papaverine, vacuum pump, penile implant
Urinary incontinence/retention	Treat infection, oxybutinin, tolterodine, incontinence pads/diapers, catheterization
Other Problems	**Available Treatments**
Cognitive impairment	Simplify routines, reminders, donepezil, tacrine
Dental care	Avoid dry mouth, electric toothbrush
Depression	Psychotherapy, antidepressant medication
Hypersomnia	Treat insomnia, treat obstructive sleep apnea, stimulant medication
Insomnia	Treat depression, behavioral treatment, hypnotics
REM sleep behavior disorder	Clonazepam
Restless legs syndrome	Dopamine agonists, levodopa, clonazepam, gabapentin, opiates
Stridor	Tracheostomy

basal ganglia and other brain regions involved. In a retrospective review of treatment of 381 PSP patients, amitriptyline and other antidepressants, levodopa and dopamine agonists were somewhat useful (21). Perhaps not unexpectedly, in a disease that is complex and poorly understood, various medications appear to yield some benefit in some patients. Methysergide, a serotonin antagonist (in contrast with serotonergic antidepressants), initially showed success when used in some PSP patients; however, it has now been abandoned as ineffective. Similarly, anticholinergic drugs may occasionally improve motor symptoms, whereas the cholinergic agents donepezil and tacrine may help cognitive function. Amantadine is less effective than other anti-Parkinsonian drugs, but is worth trying. In the now-discarded category of noradrenergic agonists, idazoxan was somewhat effective for PSP but poorly tolerated, whereas efaroxan was better tolerated but ineffective. Zolpidem, a non-benzodiazepine hypnotic, was reported to help both motor symptoms and eye movements (22); these findings await confirmation. Limited studies of electroconvulsive therapy suggest it offers some benefit, but practical difficulties and posttreatment confusion limit its usefulness. The multifocal pathologic nature of PSP thwarts potential benefit from surgery.

Exercise programs are important for motor symptoms. Physical therapy and occupational therapy may be valuable for limitations of gait performance and motor independence. Hypophonia is best treated with breathing exercises, which may be taught by a speech therapist. Drooling patients need to be reminded to swallow consciously. The side effect of dry mouth caused by anticholinergic drugs such as atropine and glycopyrrolate can be exploited to relieve drooling. Botulinum toxin injections into the parotid and submandibular glands may also be helpful. Changing pens, stiffening the wrist, or typing may circumvent handwriting difficulties. Balance problems are poorly responsive to any intervention, although patients and families occasionally state they benefit from canes or walkers. Patients need frequent reminders to take precautionary measures against falls.

Dysarthria may be helped by facial exercises, but written or keyboard communication is often a necessary substitute. A formal swallowing evaluation is mandatory for dysphagia, which is best managed in early stages by a speech therapist who will advise patients and families regarding the mechanics of swallowing and possibly advantageous changes in dietary consistency. In later stages gastrostomy may be required. Dystonia is typically poorly responsive to medication (clonazepam, anticholinergics), but botulinum toxin may be very helpful, especially for blepharospasm. Management of nonmotor complications such as depression is similar to that of depressed patients without PSP.

MULTIPLE SYSTEM ATROPHY

From a tentative beginning three decades ago in the discussion of a single case report (23), the concept that striatonigral degeneration (SND), sporadic olivopontocerebellar atrophy (OPCA) and Shy-Drager syndrome (SDS) are variants of one and the same disease has taken firm hold. Multiple system atrophy (MSA) has emerged as the most difficult disease to distinguish from PD. The name not only describes the pathology but also helps keep in mind the various combinations of clinical manifestations encountered.

Clinical Findings

The clinical manifestations of MSA are often divided into motor and autonomic categories, the latter reflecting the autonomic nervous system involvement

emphasized in descriptions of SDS. The motor syndromes can be subdivided into basal ganglia (chiefly Parkinsonism) and cerebellar types, known as MSA-P and MSA-C, respectively, reflecting the presence of SND and OPCA. The most common presentation of MSA is Parkinsonism, but cerebellar or autonomic symptoms may predominate in the initial picture. These distinctions become arbitrary over time, because one sees all permutations of disease manifestations as it evolves. Ultimately, over 85 percent of MSA patients develop parkinsonism, about 75 percent have autonomic problems, and over 50 percent show evidence of cerebellar degeneration (24). Thus categorization as MSA-P or MSA-C is usually relevant only to the initial presentation, and sometimes the referral pattern through the health care system, until the time of diagnosis. From then on, one has to be prepared for a variety of potential developments. However, the concept of dividing MSA into clinical subtypes is also useful for research and management purposes (23A).

The parkinsonism of MSA tends to cause prominent akinesia, rigidity, and early postural instability, with tremor being uncommon. The tremor is more commonly an action type, not resting with low amplitude and high frequency. However, MSA mimics PD more closely than PSP in the prominence of limb involvement, often asymmetric, and the less-striking postural instability. Cerebellar findings in MSA include limb ataxia, a wide-based gait, dysarthric and scanning speech, and nystagmus. Dystonia is often quite prominent, with the most common manifestations being disproportionate antecollis and levodopa-induced action dystonia of facial muscles. Other motor signs (spasticity, hyperreflexia, Babinski signs) are attributable to corticospinal tract involvement. Common autonomic symptoms include orthostatic lightheadedness, syncope, urinary retention or incontinence, impotence (in males) or anorgasmia (in females), fecal incontinence, loss of sweating and paroxysmal bursts of excessive sweating. While many of these symptoms occur in PD, the diseases can be differentiated by the more profound autonomic "failure" of MSA. Other clinical features of MSA may include action myoclonus, respiratory stridor, dysphonia, Raynaud's phenomenon, pain, contractures, and REM sleep behavior disorder.

A consensus committee proposed formal criteria for the clinical diagnosis of MSA (25). The essential elements of diagnosis were felt to be a combination of autonomic dysfunction and either cerebellar ataxia or Parkinsonism poorly responsive to levodopa.

Epidemiology and Genetics

The mean age of onset of MSA is 54.2 years. This is slightly younger than that for PD and considerably younger than that for PSP. The youngest reported age of onset of MSA was 31 (26).

Current diagnostic criteria specify that the diagnosis of MSA should be restricted to patients with sporadic disease (25,27); thus, familial cases are not known. Although adherence to this diagnostic principle enhances the specificity of criteria for clinical research purposes, it closes off what has been a fruitful avenue of research for PD and PSP. In part, the reasons for adopting this position are historical. Authorities in this field have only recently managed to persuade medical orthodoxy to accept that sporadic OPCA occurring in the context of MSA is a different disease from the hereditary ataxias. It may be simply too soon to turn around and advance the argument that some cases of MSA are inherited, but still distinct from familial forms of ataxia. One can predict, however, that familial cases of MSA will eventually be discovered, as has occurred with nearly every other common degenerative neurologic disease. Identification of a biologic marker for MSA would naturally make this task much easier.

Investigations

There is no definitive test for MSA. What we have available is a "battery of nonspecific tests in which abnormal results help to sway the balance of diagnostic probability" (27). Two types of investigations are particularly useful in supporting a diagnosis of MSA. Formal autonomic testing can provide evidence of widespread autonomic dysfunction in a patient with a single autonomic symptom or sign, or it can detect dysautonomia in a patient with a pure parkinsonian or cerebellar syndrome. Some tests can be performed at the bedside including sweat test, cold pressor test, and evaluation of pupillary function. Others require availability of special technical abilities. A cardiovascular battery, including tilt table testing and measurement of cardiac responses to deep breathing and the Valsalva maneuver, and urodynamic testing are common tools for such clinical situations. Anal sphincter EMG may show denervation signifying degeneration of Onuf's nucleus.

Imaging studies can be diagnostically valuable. CT scans are relatively insensitive to changes in MSA, but may detect evidence of cerebellar, pontine, or putaminal atrophy. Far more helpful is MRI scanning, which is not only more sensitive to changes in structural appearance but also may show evidence of metabolic dysfunction. A variety of MRI abnormalities have been associated with MSA. Putaminal atrophy, a hyperintense putaminal rim, and infratentorial signal change (hyperintense middle cerebellar peduncles, transverse pontine fibers, and midline raphe) on T2-weighted or proton density images are thought to be highly sensitive findings in MSA (28). A combination of dorsolateral putaminal hypointensity with a lateral linear hyperintensity on T2-weighted studies may be particularly characteristic (29).

Supine plasma noradrenaline (NA) levels may distinguish MSA from pure autonomic failure (PAF) (3). Nerve conduction studies may disclose a mild sensorimotor polyneuropathy, although clinical evidence is much less common than upper motor neuron signs. Sleep studies in the majority of MSA patients demonstrate abnormalities consisting of REM sleep behavior disorder, obstructive sleep apnea, and periodic limb movements during sleep (30).

Pathology

The gross findings at autopsy can include atrophy and darkening of the putamina, and atrophy of the pons and cerebellum. Depigmentation of the substantia nigra may be present but is not universal. Microscopic examination reveals a distribution of degenerative changes (neuronal loss, gliosis) involving the putamen, substantia nigra, pontine nuclei, Purkinje cell layer of the cerebellum, inferior olives, locus ceruleus, and the intermediolateral columns of the spinal cord.

The hallmark of the pathology of MSA is the finding of oligodendroglial inclusions known as glial cytoplasmic inclusions (GCI) (31). These are found not only in the areas of greatest neuronal degeneration but also in the frontal cortex, globus pallidus, and cerebral and cerebellar white matter. Electron microscopy reveals GCI are composed of tubular filaments 20 to 30 nm in diameter. Immunostaining identifies α-synuclein as a major constituent of GCI.

Management

The management of MSA is more difficult than that of PD because of the greater resistance of its motor manifestations to treatment, and the wider assortment of problems usually encountered. Nevertheless, many of its symptoms are amenable to therapy (Table 53-2). Ten percent of MSA patients may show a dramatic response to levodopa comparable to that of patients with PD (27) especially in the early stages. Some patients may even develop motor fluctuations and dyskinesia. However, only a third of MSA patients show much response to levodopa at all, and then the response is almost always atypical in some way. If levodopa is unsuccessful or poorly tolerated, it is worth pursuing treatment with dopamine agonists or amantadine, because individual patients may respond better to one of these agents. The nonergot agents pramipexole and ropinirole may be preferable to older dopamine agonists because of their lesser tendency to provoke orthostatic hypotension, although this has not been proven in this patient group. There is no consistently effective treatment for most of the cerebellar manifestations, but isoniazid, clonazepam, or wrist weights occasionally dampen an ataxic tremor. Spasticity almost never reaches the point of requiring therapy.

Autonomic disturbances are the most amenable to treatment. A variety of measures treat orthostatic hypotension (32). A priority is to identify and reduce or eliminate medications that may be contributing to the problem. Nonpharmacologic measures include elevating the head of the bed, increasing salt and fluid intake, avoiding heat, and adopting certain body postures such as crossing the legs or squatting. Elastic stockings are effective but poorly tolerated because of the annoyance of constant pressure on the legs. Orthostatic hypotension is most pronounced upon getting up after prolonged recumbence, such as in the morning, and is best in the middle of the day. Slow, staged arising from bed is advised, and activities are best scheduled during afternoons. Smaller meals make lower demands on the circulatory system. The most effective medications for orthostatic hypotension are the peripheral alpha-adrenergic agonist midodrine and the mineralocorticoid fludrocortisone. Other effective medications include low-dose propranolol, desmopressin, phenylpropanolamine, yohimbine, and indomethacin (33).

Urinary incontinence may be related to detrusor hyperreflexia, which may respond to anticholinergics such as oxybutinin or tolterodine. Urinary retention usually can be managed by intermittent catheterization. Either of these problems may ultimately require indwelling catheterization. Consultation with a urologist to diagnose and treat these symptoms is highly recommended. Male sexual dysfunction may also be treated with a variety of pharmacologic and nonpharmacologic measures. Patients with Parkinsonism are frequently constipated. There are numerous measures to relieve this: increased fluid intake, exercise, a high-fiber diet, bulk-forming agents, laxatives, and others. Respiratory stridor demands a consultation with an otolaryngologist. Tracheostomy may be indicated.

CORTICAL-BASAL GANGLIONIC DEGENERATION

In 1968, a report entitled "Corticodentatonigral degeneration with neuronal achromasia" (34) described three cases of the disorder we now know as cortical-basal ganglionic degeneration (CBGD), often abbreviated as corticobasal degeneration. No further attention was paid to CBGD until 1985. Since then, however, CBGD has generated a level of study comparable to that of PSP and MSA, sufficient to warrant publication of a monograph on the subject (35).

Clinical Findings

The most striking aspect of the clinical picture of CBGD is the asymmetry with which it presents and progresses. It resembles PD more than any other type of degenerative Parkinsonism with regard to the asymmetry of initial findings. However, the addition of other motor findings such as dystonia, myoclonus, and apraxia result in CBGD being the least likely of the disorders in this chapter to be mistaken for PD. As is typical of degenerative diseases, CBGD develops insidiously and progresses gradually.

The clinical findings in CBGD can be divided into three categories: (1) movement disorders (usually reflecting dysfunction in the basal ganglia), (2) cerebral cortical signs, and (3) other findings. Of the movement disorders Parkinsonism is most prominent. The Parkinsonism in the limbs consists almost exclusively of akinesia and rigidity, with rest tremor being extremely rare. Other evidence of basal ganglia involvement includes dystonia of the involved limb, (usually fixed and often causing pronounced and/or painful deformities), postural instability, athetosis, and orofacial dyskinesias. Signs of cerebral cortical dysfunction consist of apraxia, cortical sensory loss, the alien limb phenomenon, dementia, and frontal lobe reflexes. Other manifestations include action tremor, focal reflex-action myoclonus, hyperreflexia, Babinski signs, and impaired ocular and eyelid motility.

The above description pertains to "classical" CBGD with a predominantly motor presentation. A variety of proposals for clinical diagnostic criteria have been published, the latest being that of Kumar and colleagues (36). The key concept in all these schemes is that patients must demonstrate a combination of signs pointing to both basal ganglia and cerebral cortical involvement. Recent pathologic series indicate that dementia may be the most common clinical syndrome associated with the pathologic picture of CBGD (37,37a). Unusual presentations include speech apraxia and progressive aphasia. It should also be noted that the "classical" CBGD picture described is not specific to CBGD and has been associated with a variety of other pathologic findings (38). Thus for a variety of reasons the definitive diagnosis of CBGD requires compatible findings in both clinical and pathologic domains.

Epidemiology and Genetics

CBGD is the least understood among Parkinson's plus disorders. Its relatively delayed rise to prominence has led to a lower profile among physicians in general and a high rate of false negative diagnoses. Nevertheless, it is likely that CBGD is somewhat less common than either PSP or MSA. The average patient with CBGD, as with PSP, is a little older than one with PD. No cases with onset under the age of 40 have been recognized. The mean life expectancy from onset is eight years (39). There are no known risk factors.

The status of hereditary CBGD is not clear. One report described two brothers with typical motor findings (40), but there has been no pathologic confirmation. Two families were reported where the pathology was characteristic of CBGD, but the clinical presentation consisted almost exclusively of cognitive and behavioral deterioration with only rare basal ganglia manifestations (41).

Investigations

The most helpful study is brain imaging, either computed tomography or magnetic resonance imaging (MRI). This will detect asymmetric atrophy of the cerebral cortex, greater on the side opposite that more clinically involved, in a little less than half of cases. Symmetric atrophy occurs in a like number. Signal hyperintensities on T2-weighted MRI in subcortical white matter may be found; these have been attributed to gliosis (42). A few patients will have normal scans (43). Other routine studies are normal. Positron emission tomography may demonstrate asymmetric striatal uptake of fluorolevodopa and reduction of cortical metabolism using fluorodeoxyglucose as a marker.

Pathology

The clinical findings and imaging studies presage the pathologic findings. The cerebral cortex and basal ganglia, particularly the substantia nigra, carry the burden of disease. Macroscopically, there is usually visible cerebral atrophy, often asymmetric, and predominating in the medial areas of the frontal and parietal lobes. Sectioning of the brain usually reveals pallor of the substantia nigra.

Microscopic abnormalities follow the same pattern. In the cerebral cortex, particularly the superior frontal, precentral and, postcentral gyri, are abundant swollen ("ballooned") poorly staining ("achromatic") neurons amid nonspecific degenerative changes. These abnormal neurons are the most characteristic pathologic finding of CBGD. They do not contain discrete inclusion bodies such as neurofibrillary tangles or Pick

bodies (although the latter are occasionally seen), but some surviving nonswollen cortical neurons do contain tau-positive inclusions. However, CBGD distinguishes itself from other tauopathies in that tau immunoreactivity predominates in cellular processes rather than in cell bodies, and these processes are mainly of glial origin. Tau-positive "astrocytic plaques" in CBGD (37) are distinct from the "tufted astrocytes" of the tauopathy seen in PSP (44). Oligodendroglial inclusions known as "coiled bodies" may be identified. In the substantia nigra, neuronal loss, depigmentation, extraneuronal melanin, and gliosis are found. Some residual nigral neurons contain inclusions known as "corticobasal bodies" that are morphologically similar to NFT. Tau-positive cell processes and glial abnormalities are abundant in the nigra. The putamen, caudate nucleus, globus pallidus and subthalamic nucleus usually show similar changes to a more modest degree. The tau that accumulates in CBGD contains the same isoforms as PSP.

Management

There is no specific treatment for CBGD, and therapy is currently symptomatic (Table 53-2). Parkinsonism in CBGD is particularly resistant to treatment, and rarely does medication provide any meaningful benefit. Somewhat more amenable to therapy are the myoclonus (with clonazepam or valproate) and dystonia (with botulinum toxin) (45), but treatment of CBGD is usually a dismal exercise in frustration for patients, families, and physicians.

FRONTOTEMPORAL DEMENTIA WITH PARKINSONISM

The term *frontotemporal dementia and parkinsonism linked to chromosome 17* (FTDP-17) has been coined to unify a group of hereditary disorders that share important clinical and pathologic features (46), as well as a genetic basis of mutations in the tau gene on the long arm of chromosome 17. FTDP-17 is included in this chapter because of the link to PSP and CBGD as fellow tauopathies. However, it is the obvious exception among these diseases in that there is a confirmatory diagnostic test, even though gene sequencing is not yet routine or widely available.

Although individual kindreds express seemingly distinctive clinical features, the presentation of FTDP-17 can be categorized as either dementia or Parkinsonism (47). If cognitive changes predominate, other manifestations including parkinsonism tend to occur late or not at all. In these patients behavioral abnormalities may be striking, including aggression, disinhibition, irritability, withdrawal, and paranoid actions. If an akinetic-rigid syndrome develops first, dementia soon follows and there are a greater variety of additional features such as amyotrophy, dystonia, spasticity, and ocular motor dysfunction. This broad division may reflect the presence of mutations in different regions of the tau gene (47). However, this is probably an oversimplification, in view of the clinical heterogeneity within families. For example, in one family with FTDP-17 the father developed a typical dementia whereas his son presented with a motor syndrome suggestive of CBGD (48).

The pathologic findings of FTDP-17 reflect the clinical features. The most consistent abnormality is atrophy, often with spongiform changes, of the cerebral cortex predominating in the frontal and temporal lobes. Depigmentation, neuronal loss, and gliosis in the substantia nigra are common. Degeneration of other basal ganglia including caudate nucleus, putamen, and subthalamic nucleus may be prominent (49). A variety of tau-positive neuronal and glial inclusions are present.

Recognition of FTDP-17 is a recent phenomenon and no general statements about management can be made.

CONCLUSION

Growing interest in Parkinson's plus diseases has resulted in the accumulation of an impressive body of information about PSP, MSA, and CBGD. Yet we are unable to make fundamental changes in the outlook for patients because the etiology and pathogenesis have eluded the grasp of research, and it appears that we remain a long way from developing definitive treatments. Fortunately, not only has frustration failed to set in, but efforts at untangling this mysterious area of neurology have intensified. Never has the degree of interest in these disorders been as great as it is at present.

Much of the recent scientific excitement surrounding Parkinson's plus diseases stems from the realization that mutations in the tau gene produce nervous system disease that is not far removed from PSP and CBGD. The potential that study of FTDP-17 holds for shedding light on the etiology and pathophysiology of PSP and CBGD is enormous. Furthermore, the discovery of FTDP-17 has accelerated a paradigm shift in the nosology of degenerative diseases, moving from clinicopathologic entities to clinicopathogenetic correlations. Unfortunately, this has reminded us that although genetic knowledge gives us crucial information regarding the identity or multiplicity of

hereditary conditions, it is insufficient to predict either clinical or pathologic effects on the nervous system. Production of seemingly disparate clinical syndromes from identical mutations is common to many genes other than that coding for tau (50). Clearly it is necessary to understand more than simply the genetic trigger to explain how members of the same family with the same mutations develop different clinicopathologic "entities".

Nevertheless, optimism that we are near to solving a major riddle of this complex puzzle is difficult to restrain. The identification of biologic markers for specific diseases, one of the most coveted among research goals, seems almost within our grasp. Perhaps the closest of these diseases to being understood is PSP, because of the number of well-documented affected families. The information we derive from them should enlighten us to a great degree about the pathogenesis and pathophysiology of PSP. However, there is no point in focusing on a single aspect of research and trying to predict the future. The most encouraging development in this field has been the increasing dedication of study of all the diseases covered in this chapter, and the tangible results obtained.

REFERENCES

1. Rajput AH, Rozdilsky B, Rajput A. Accuracy of clinical diagnosis in parkinsonism – a prospective study. *Can J Neurol Sci* 1991; 18:275–278.
2. Hughes AJ, Daniel SE, Kilford L, et al. Accuracy of clinical diagnosis of idiopathic Parkinson's disease: A clinico-pathological study of 100 cases. *J Neurol Neurosurg Psychiatry* 1992; 55:181–184.
3. Quinn N. Multiple system atrophy – the nature of the beast. *J Neurol Neurosurg Psychiatry* 1989; (suppl) 78–89.
4. Steele JC, Richardson JC, Olszewski J. Progressive supranuclear palsy. *Arch Neurol* 1964; 10:333–359.
5. Golbe LI, Davis PH, Schoenberg BS, et al. Prevalence and natural history of progressive supranuclear palsy. *Neurology* 1988; 38:1031–1034.
6. Litvan I, Mangone CA, McKee A, et al. Natural history of progressive supranuclear palsy and clinical predictors of survival: A clinicopathological study. *J Neurol Neurosurg Psychiatry* 1996; 61:615–620.
7. Riley DE, Fogt N, Leigh RJ. The syndrome of "pure akinesia" and its relationship to progressive supranuclear palsy. *Neurology* 1994; 44:1025–1029.
8. Litvan I, Agid Y, Calne D, et al. Clinical research criteria for the diagnosis of progressive supranuclear palsy (Steele-Richardson-Olszewski syndrome): Report of the NINDS-SPSP International Workshop. *Neurology* 1996; 47:1–9.

9. Bower JH, Maraganore DM, McDonnell SK, et al. Incidence of progressive supranuclear palsy and multiple system atrophy in Olmsted County, Minnesota, 1976 to 1990. *Neurology* 1997; 49:1284–1288.

10. Tetrud JW, Golbe LI, Forno LS, et al. Autopsy-proven progressive supranuclear palsy in two siblings. *Neurology* 1996; 46:931–934.

11. Bennett P, Bonifati V, Bonuccelli U, et al. Direct genetic evidence for involvement of tau in progressive supranuclear palsy. *Neurology* 1998; 51:982–985.

12. Morris HR, Janssen JC, Bandmann O, et al. The *tau* gene A0 polymorphism in progressive supranuclear palsy and related neurodegenerative diseases. *J Neurol Neurosurg Psychiatry* 1999; 66:665–667.

13. Hoenicka J, Perez M, Perez-Tur J, et al. The *tau* gene A0 allele and progressive supranuclear palsy. *Neurology* 1999; 53:1219–1225.

13a. Higgins JJ, Adler RL, Loveless JM. Mutational analysis of the tau gene in progressive supranuclear palsy. *Neurology* 1999; 53:1421–1424.

13b. Chambers CB, Lee JM, Trancoso JC et al. Over-expression of four-repeat tau mRNA isoforms in progressive supranuclear palsy but not in Alzheimer's disease. *Ann Neurol* 1999; 46:325–332.

14. Soliveri P, Monza D, Paridi D, et al. Cognitive and magnetic resonance imaging aspects of corticobasal degeneration and progressive supranuclear palsy. *Neurology* 1999; 53:502–507.

15. Litvan I, Mega M, Cummings JL, Fairbanks L. Neuropsychiatric aspects of progressive supranuclear palsy. *Neurology* 1996; 47:1184–1189.

16. Verny M, Duyckaerts C, Agid Y, et al. The significance of cortical pathology in progressive supranuclear palsy. *Brain* 1996; 119:1123–1136.

17. Bergeron C, Pollanen MS, Weyer L, et al. Cortical degeneration in progressive supranuclear palsy. A comparison with cortical-basal ganglionic degeneration. *J Neuropathol Exp Neurol* 1997; 56:726–734.

18. Sergeant N, Wattez A, Delacourte A. Neurofibrillary degeneration in progressive supranuclear palsy and corticobasal degeneration: Tau pathologies with exclusively "exon 10" isoforms. *J Neurochem* 1999; 72:1243–1249.

19. Nieforth KA, Golbe LI. Retrospective study of drug response in 87 patients with progressive supranuclear palsy. *Clin Neuropharmacol* 1993; 16:338–346.

20. Kompoliti K, Goetz CG, Litvan I, et al. Pharmacological therapy in progressive supranuclear palsy. *Arch Neurol* 1998; 55:1099–1102.

21. Litvan I, Chase TN. Traditional and experimental therapeutic approaches. In: Litvan I, Agid Y (eds.), *Progressive Supranuclear Palsy*. New York: Oxford, 1992; 254–269.

22. Daniele A, Moro E, Bentivoglio AR. Zolpidem in progressive supranuclear palsy. *N Engl J Med* 1999; 341:543–544.

23. Graham JG, Oppenheimer DR. Orthostatic hypotension and nicotine sensitivity in a case of multiple system atrophy. *J Neurol Neurosurg Psychiatry* 1969; 32:28–34.

23a. Shulman LM, Weiner WJ. Multiple system atroptty. In: Watts RL and Koller WC (eds.), *Movement Disorders*, New York: McGraw-Hill, 1947; 297–307.

24. Wenning GK, Tison F, Ben Shlomo Y, et al. Multiple system atrophy: A review of 203 pathologically proven cases. *Mov Disord* 1997; 12:133–147.

25. Gilman S, Low PA, Quinn N, et al. Consensus statement on the diagnosis of multiple system atrophy. *J Neurol Sci* 1999; 163:94–98.

26. Ben-Shlomo Y, Wenning GK, Tison F, et al. Survival of patients with pathologically proven multiple system atrophy: A meta-analysis. *Neurology* 1997; 48:384–393.

27. Quinn N. Multiple system atrophy. In: Marsden CD, Fahn S (eds.), *Movement Disorders 3*. Oxford: Butterworth-Heinemann, 1994; 262–281.

28. Schrag A, Kingsley D, Pharouros C, et al. Clinical usefulness of magnetic resonance imaging in multiple system atrophy. *J Neurol Neurosurg Psychiatry* 1998; 65:65–71.

29. Kraft E, Schwarz J, Trenkwalder C, et al. The combination of hypointense and hyperintense signal changes on T2-weighted magnetic resonance imaging sequences. *Arch Neurol* 1999; 56:225–228.

30. Plazzi G, Corsini R, Provini F, et al. REM sleep behavior disorders in multiple system atrophy. *Neurology* 1997; 48:1094–1097.

31. Lantos PL. The definition of multiple system atrophy: A review of recent developments. *J Neuropathol Exp Neurol* 1998; 57: 1099–1111.

32. Mathias CJ, Kimber JR. Treatment of postural hypotension. *J Neurol Neurosurg Psychiatry* 1998; 65:285–289.

33. Jordan J, Shannon JR, Biaggioni I, et al. Contrasting actions of pressor agents in severe autonomic failure. *Am J Med* 1998; 105:116–124.

34. Rebeiz JJ, Kolodny EH, Richardson EP. Corticodentatonigral degeneration with neuronal achromasia. *Arch Neurol* 1968; 18:20–33.

35. Litvan I, Goetz CG, Lang AE, Corticobasal degeneration and related disorders. *Adv Neurol* 2000; 82.

36. Kumar R, Bergeron C, Pollanen MS, et al. Cortical-basal ganglionic degeneration. In: Jankovic J, Tolosa E (eds.) *Parkinson's Disease and Movement Disorders*. 3rd ed. Baltimore: Williams & Wilkins, 1998; 297–316.

37. Feany MB, Dickson DW. Widespread cytoskeletal pathology characterizes corticobasal degeneration. *Am J Pathol* 1995; 146:1388–1396.

37a. Grimes DA, Lang AE, Bergeron CB. Dementia as the most common presentation of cortical-basal ganglionic degeneration. *Neurology* 1999; 53:1969–1974.

38. Boeve BF, Maraganore DM, Parisi JE, et al. Pathologic heterogeneity in clinically diagnosed corticobasal degeneration. *Neurology* 1999; 53:795–800.

39. Wenning GK, Litvan I, Jankovic J, et al. Natural history and survival of 14 patients with corticobasal degeneration confirmed at postmortem examination. *J Neurol Neurosurg Psychiatry* 1998; 64:184–189.

40. Verin M, Rancurel G, De Marco O, Edan G. First familial cases of corticobasal degeneration [abstract]. *Mov Disord* 1997; 12(suppl 1):55.

41. Brown J, Lantos PL, Roques P, Fidani L, Rossor MN. Familial dementia with swollen achromatic neurons and corticobasal inclusion bodies: A clinical and pathological study. *J Neurol Sci* 1996; 135;21–30.

42. Tokumaru AM, O'uchi T, Kuru Y, et al. Corticobasal degeneration: MR with histopathologic comparison. *Am J Neuroradiol* 1996; 17:1849–1852.

43. Ballan G, Tison F, Dousset V, et al. Study of cortical atrophy with magnetic resonance imaging in corticobasal degeneration. *Rev Neurol* 1998; 154:224–227.

44. Komori T, Arai N, Oda M, et al. Astrocytic plaques and tufts of abnormal fibers do not coexist in corticobasal degeneration and progressive supranuclear palsy. *Acta Neuropathol* 1998; 96:401–408.

45. Kompoliti K, Goetz CG, Boeve BF, et al. Clinical presentation and pharmacological therapy in corticobasal degeneration. *Arch Neurol* 1998; 55: 957–961.

46. Foster NL, Wilhelmsen K, Sima AA, et al. Frontotemporal dementia and parkinsonism linked to chromosome 17: A consensus conference. *Ann Neurol* 1997; 41:706–715.

47. Wszolek ZK, Markopoulou K. Molecular genetics of familial parkinsonism. *Parkinsonism Rel Disord* 1999; 5:145–155.

48. Bugiani O, Murrell JR, Giaccone G, et al. Frontotemporal dementia and corticobasal degeneration in a family with a P301S mutation in tau. *J Neuropathol Exp Neurol* 1999; 58:667–677.

49. Nasreddine ZS, Loginov M, Clark LN, et al. From genotype to phenotype: A clinical, pathological, and biochemical investigation of frontotemporal dementia and parkinsonism (FTDP-17) caused by the P301L tau mutation. *Ann Neurol* 1999; 45:704–715.

50. Bird T. Genotypes, phenotypes, and frontotemporal dementia. Take your pick. *Neurology* 1998; 50:1526–1527.

Table 54-1   A Classification of Parkinsonism

1. **Infections**
   Encephalitis lethargica and postencephalitic
     parkinsonism
   Other encephalitids
     Western equine encephalitis
     Japanese B encephalitis
     Cytomegalovirus
   Human immunodeficiency virus
   Creutzfeldt-Jakob's disease
   Fungal infections
   Mycoplasma pneumonia
   Tuberculosis
2. **Drug-Induced Parkinsonism (Table 54-2)**
3. **Toxin-Induced Parkinsonism**
   Manganese
   Carbon monoxide
   Cyanide
   Carbon disulfide
   Methyl alcohol
4. **Structural lesions**
   Hydrocephalus
   Brain tumors
   Intracranial hemorrhage
   Multiple Infarcts
5. **Miscellaneous**
   Posttraumatic parkinsonism
   Demyelinating disease
   Alcohol withdrawal
   Sjogren's syndrome
   Psychogenic parkinsonism

encephalitis (2,10,11). Parkinsonian features such as masked facies, tremors, rigidity, and gait impairment can be seen during the acute infection but usually resolve following recovery from the encephalitis. If Parkinsonian symptoms persist, neuroimaging may demonstrate lesions in the substantia nigra, thalamus, and basal ganglia (10).

Before the advent of levodopa, the treatment of PEP consisted of amphetamines and belladona. Levodopa was shown to be of benefit in a double-blind study (12). The response to levodopa in PEP is inconsistent and may wane after an excellent improvement. In a follow-up of 50 patients, a third continued to benefit, a third showed no response, and the others could not tolerate levodopa (13). OGC may respond to anticholinergics and levodopa. However, levodopa may worsen OGC in some patients.

Other Infectious Etiologies

Neurologic complications including parkinsonism may occur in patients with acquired immune deficiency syndrome (AIDS) (14). The Parkinsonian features may be caused by secondary AIDS-associated cerebral infections or primary cerebral HIV infection alone (14,15). In addition, AIDS patients are particularly sensitive to neuroleptics and may develop severe drug-induced Parkinsonism very quickly and on low doses. Some patients, including children with HIV–associated progressive encephalopathy and Parkinsonism, may respond to levodopa (16).

Other infectious processes may also rarely be associated with Parkinsonism. Adler and coworkers described a case of an intravenous drug user with subacute parkinsonism that was secondary to bilateral fungal striatal abscesses (17). Mycoplasma pneumonia may result in bradykinesia and chorea in some children (18). Parkinsonism associated with syphilis and cryptococcal and cysticercus infection has also been described (19–22).

DRUG-INDUCED PARKINSONISM

Drug-induced parkinsonism (DIP) is the most common cause of P and is often misdiagnosed as PD because their clinical features may be indistinguishable. Although several medications may be associated with P (Table 54-2), dopamine blocking agents (DBA) are the most common offending agents.

Dopamine Blocking Agents

Parkinsonism may be secondary to DBA such as neuroleptics (23,24) and metoclopromide (25). All classes of neuroleptics have been implicated. DIP may be indistinguishable on examination from PD and therefore may be unrecognized (24,25). The incidence of DIP is between 15% and 40% in patients receiving neuroleptics, and its prevalence increases with age (24). DIP tends to occur subacutely after drug exposure, but the duration from neuroleptic initiation to the onset of symptoms is variable, and in one series it was quite long and the mean exposure was 6.3 years (24).

All motor parkinsonian features may be seen in DIP and they include rigidity, bradykinesia, tremor, and a gait disturbance (24,26). Some authors suggest that symmetrical signs and the absence of tremor are typical of DIP (27); however, asymmetrical signs including asymmetrical tremor may be seen in 33 to 50 percent of patients (24,26). Rigidity is more common than tremor in DIP compared with idiopathic PD but tremor-dominant disorder may also be seen (24).

The exact pathophysiologic mechanism of DIP is not clear but it is probably related to a direct D2 dopamine receptor blockade. However, the majority of patients treated with neuroleptic medications will not develop

Table 54-2 Drugs Inducing Parkinsonism

Inhibitors of Dopamine Synthesis or Formation of a False Neurotransmitter
- Alpha methyl-paratyrosine
- Alpha methyldopa

Inhibitors of Presynaptic Dopamine Storage
- Reserpine
- Tetrabenazine

Blockade of Postsynaptic D2 Receptors:
- Neuroleptics

Trade Name	Generic Name
1. Phenothiazines	
Compazine	Prochlorperazine
Etrafon (Triavil)	Perphenazine and Amitriptyline
Mellaril	Thiordazine
Phenergan	Promethazine
Prolixin	Fluphenazine
Serentil	Mesoridazine
Stelazine	Trifluoperazine
Thorazine	Chlorpromazine
Torecan	Thiethylperazine
Trilafon	Perphenazine
2. Butyrophenones	
Haldol	Haloperidol
3. Thioxanthenes	
Navane	Thiothixene
4. Benzamides	
Reglan	Metoclopramide
5. Dihydroindolone	
Moban	Molindone
6. Dibenzoxazepine	
Loxitane	Loxapine
Miscellaneous D2 Blocking Agents	
Tetrabenazine	
Flunarizine	
Amoxapine	

DIP, suggesting that individual susceptibility to this complication exists. Risk factors include age, female gender, and higher potency DBA and possibly previous brain injury. There is some evidence that patients who develop DIP may have subclinical Lewy body PD that may be unmasked by DBA. This may be the reason why, in some patients, the parkinsonism fails to resolve following withdrawal of the DBA. In one clinicopathologic study of two patients with DIP, Lewy bodies were found at an autopsy, even though the symptoms and signs of parkinsonism had resolved after stopping the DBA (28). A PET study demonstrated similar findings. Patients with DIP with normal putamen ^{18}F-dopa uptake had improvement or resolution of their parkinsonism following neuroleptic withdrawal and so did patients with abnormal PET scans (29).

Treatment of DIP largely depends on the ability to withdraw the offending medication. If it is not possible to withdraw the neuroleptic medication, patients should be placed on the lowest dose possible or changed to an atypical agent such as clozapine, olanzapine, or quetiapine. Anticholinergics may be beneficial. Levodopa treatment has not been studied systematically and the concern is that levodopa may worsen any existing psychosis (24). Amantadine has been shown to be superior to anticholinergics in controlled studies (30).

Other Medications Associated with Parkinsonism

Dopamine depleting agents such as reserpine and tetrabenazine, may also produce DIP (31). These medications are currently used in the treatment of hyperkinetic movement disorders such as chorea and dystonia. Flunarizine and cinnarizine, calcium channel blockers that are chemically related to neuroleptics (currently unavailable in the United States), are also associated with parkinsonism. The parkinsonism may persist for long periods in some cases (32). Possible mechanisms include prevention of striatal cell activation by inhibiting calcium influx versus direct dopamine receptor antagonism (33). Other calcium channel blockers have also rarely been associated with parkinsonism and they include amlodipine, diltiazem, and verapamil (34–36). Lithium-induced parkinsonism is debatable (37). While the patients treated with lithium often have tremor and myoclonic jerks, typical parkinsonism appears to be rare. The symptoms resolve after the discontinuation of the drug.

A variety of other medications have been rarely associated with parkinsonism. These medications include chemotherapeutic agents (5-fluorouracil adriamycin), cardiac medications (amiodarone, alpha methyl dopa) histamine-2 (H2) antagonists (cimetidine), immunosuppressants (cyclosporin), antiepileptics (valproic acid), and antidepressants including serotonin-specific reuptake inhibitors (38–46).

TOXIN-INDUCED PARKINSONISM

Parkinsonism may be caused by a variety of toxins including carbon monoxide, 1-methyl-4-phenyl-1,2,5,6-tetrahydropyridine (MPTP), manganese, and cyanide. The onset of symptoms is usually subacute following the toxin exposure, and the course may be progressive. Historical clues can suggest possible toxin exposure leading to an appropriate diagnosis.

Carbon Monoxide

Carbon monoxide is a colorless, odorless, and nonirritating toxic gas. Sources of carbon monoxide that may lead to poisoning include natural gas, smoke inhalation, automobile exhaust, and methylene chloride in paint remover (47,48). The diagnosis of carbon monoxide exposure is usually suggested by the history and clinical suspicion. The diagnosis is confirmed by finding an elevated carboxyhemoglobin level in the blood (47).

Clinically, patients with carbon monoxide poisoning present with tachycardia, tachypnea, headache, nausea, syncope, seizures, or coma. The classic finding of cyanosis, cherry-red lips, and retinal hemorrhages rarely occurs (48). Delayed clinical presentations include neuropsychiatric symptoms such as cognitive and personality change, psychosis, dementia, and Parkinsonism (48,49). Although all features of Parkinsonism may be observed, rigidity, bradykinesia, and postural instability may be more common than tremor (49).

Carbon monoxide is easily absorbed from the lungs, and it competes with oxygen for binding to hemoglobin. The toxicity appears to result not only from hypoxia but also from direct cellular injury (48). The most common CT findings are symmetrical diffuse low-density lesions in the globus pallidus and cerebral white matter (47). Magnetic resonance imaging (MRI) changes may be dramatic with pallidal lesions being the dominant feature. The lesions represents necrosis.

In the acute setting the patient should be quickly removed from the source of carbon monoxide exposure and treated with 100% oxygen. A carboxyhemoglobin level should be checked; however, the level does not correlate well with clinical symptoms. Patients with respiratory compromise will need to be intubated for ventilatory assistance. The indications for hyperbaric oxygen therapy other than coma are debatable (48). The parkinsonism responds poorly to levodopa. The delayed clinical symptoms may resolve over time in some patients (49).

MPTP

MPTP (see Chapter 30) is a chemical by-product of 1-methyl-4-phenyl-4-propionoxy-piperidine (MPPP) synthesis and can contaminate MPPP manufactured in illicit drug operations. In fact, that is precisely what lead to the development of MPTP–induced parkinsonism. Irreversible parkinsonism associated with MPTP exposure was originally reported in a drug addict in 1979 (50) but was characterized more fully in 1983 (51).

Acute MPTP intoxication produces different symptoms than heroin such as severe burning at the injection site, dimming of vision during drug injection, and a different feeling of euphoria (52). Individuals exposed to MPTP may develop all the classic features of Parkinsonism subacutely with the onset of symptoms approximately two weeks following exposure (51). The most common clinical features include bradykinesia, rigidity, and postural instability. A rest tremor can occur but is much less common than in PD (52). The Parkinsonism becomes quite severe very quickly.

MPTP toxicity results in Parkinsonism by selectively damaging dopaminergic neurons in the substantia nigra. After intravenous injection, MPTP crosses the blood–brain barrier where it is converted to 1-methyl-4-phenyl-pyridine (MPP$^+$) by monoamine oxidase B in the glia. MPP$^+$ is taken up by dopamine-containing cells in the substantia nigra where it causes degeneration by inhibiting mitochondrial energy production (53). This selective destruction of nigrostriatal neurons lead to the development of animal models that have become an important research tool in PD (53).

Patients with MPTP-induced Parkinsonism respond to levodopa in a manner similar to PD. However, these patients developed levodopa-induced side effects including dyskinesia, fluctuations, and hallucinations very early (54).

Manganese

Manganese is used in the manufacturing of chlorine gas, dry cell batteries, paints, varnish, enamel, linoleum, and as an antiknock agent in gasoline. Manganese enters the body through the inhalation of dust particles or by ingestion (55).

The effects of chronic manganese intoxication were first described by Couper in 1837 (56). The clinical presentation is fairly stereotypical and includes bradykinesia, postural instability, and rigidity. The gait is characterized by extension of the spine, flexal elbows, and toe-walking (cock-walk). Tremor is less frequent and may have a flapping quality similar to Wilson's disease (56–57). A psychiatric prodrome of irritability, emotional instability, psychosis (locura manganica), and dystonia occur typically from manganese dust inhalation in miners; however, these features are not seen in industrial manganese intoxication (56).

The severity of clinical features of manganese intoxication do not correlate with tissue manganese levels (56,57). Pathologic studies have demonstrated degeneration in the internal segment of the pallidum, caudate nucleus, putamen, and rarely of the substantia nigra (55,56). Possible mechanisms of manganese toxicity include dopaminergic toxicity, free radical production, or 6-hydroxydopamine production (55). MRI scan generally shows metal deposition in the basal ganglia.

Treatment with chelating agents has proven ineffective possibly because of the fact that the tissue injury may occur even when tissue levels of manganese are not high (56,57). Removal of the manganese source may lead to stabilization or improvement. Levodopa may be beneficial in some patients; however, severely affected patients may not improve (55).

Carbon Disulfide

Carbon disulfide is a solvent that is used as a fumigant in the grain storage and rayon industry (58). Patients exposed to carbon disulfide may clinically exhibit cerebellar dysfunction, hearing loss, peripheral neuropathy, chorea and Parkinsonism. The Parkinsonian features include rest tremor, gait and postural instability, rigidity, and bradykinesia (58).

The exact mechanism by which carbon disulfide toxicity occurs is not known but may involve the binding of trace metals that interrupt enzymes activity (58). Brain MRI may reveal findings consistent with central demyelination (58).

Other Toxins

A variety of other toxic exposures have rarely been associated with parkinsonism. These include petroleum waste, hydrocarbons (n-hexane), diquat, paraquat, cyanide, and methanol (59–62).

STRUCTURAL LESIONS

Structural lesions that either directly or indirectly affect the basal ganglia may produce Parkinsonism. Lesions secondary to hypoxia, hydrocephalus, tumors, vascular disease (including strokes and vascular malformations), and demyelinating lesions have been associated with this syndrome.

Hydrocephalus

Hydrocephalus is rarely associated with parkinsonism (63). Patients may develop parkinsonian symptoms months or years after their initial presentation with hydrocephalus, or the parkinsonism may develop acutely because of shunt failure along with symptoms of increased intracranial pressure and resolution follows shunt revision (64). Clinically, patients may have tremor, rigidity, and bradykinesia. They can also have a characteristic gait disorder with shuffling, wide-based postural instability with normal arm swing. Patients often develop Parinaud's syndrome prior to the onset of parkinsonism (63).

Normal pressure hydrocephalus is a condition characterized by the triad of gait difficulty, mental status change, and urinary incontinence. Poor postural reflexes and flexed posture may be seen (65). This should be differentiated from dementia with atrophy and hydrocephalous exvacuo.

The hydrocephalus should be treated either by shunting or by shunt revision in the case of malfunction. If the parkinsonian symptoms do not respond to shunting, some patients will respond to dopaminergic therapy with a dopamine agonist or levodopa. Most patients will achieve adequate control of their symptoms, and some may eventually be weaned off their dopaminergic therapy (63).

The mechanism that leads to parkinsonism is not known. However, it is believed that pressure on the striatum from within plays a role.

Tumors

Tumors, appropriately placed, can be a rare cause of parkinsonism. The tumors associated with parkinsonism may occur in one of the several regions of the brain including the striatum, frontal lobe, temporal lobe, parietal lobe, thalamus or hypothalamus, substantia nigra, midbrain, and third ventricle (66,67). A variety of tumor types have been reported and they include glioma, meningioma, lymphoma, fibrosarcoma, and metastasis (66).

The pathologic mechanism leading to parkinsonism may be either the direct infiltration of tumor cells or indirect mass effect causing impaired metabolism of the striatum. Rarely does direct or indirect compression of the midbrain lead to parkinsonism (66).

Vascular Disease

The concept of vascular or arteriosclerotic parkinsonism was introduced by Critchley in 1929 (68) and has been a matter of debate for decades. The existence of this phenomenon now appears to be supported with both clinical and pathologic studies (69–71).

Vascular parkinsonism may have a variety of clinical presentations and may be acute or subacute in onset. The symptoms may include all the classic motor features of PD. Symptoms are usually bilateral but may be unilateral (72). The course may be stable from onset, may be progressive, or it may resolve spontaneously (73). A subgroup of patients may present with predominant lower extremity symptoms including a freezing gait disturbance with minimal upper extremity involvement, that is, lower body parkinsonism (74). The symptoms may occur as the result of multiple smalll vessel infarcts or a large single one (69,72). These patients have risk factors for stroke including hypertension and diabetes mellitus.

Vascular lesions may produce parkinsonian symptoms by interrupting the nigrostriatal pathway, direct involvement of the striatum, or the involvement of the globus pallidus externa, thereby decreasing the inhibitory input to the globus pallidus interna. This would lead to excessive inhibition of the thalamus by the globus pallidus interna thus producing parkinsonism (72).

Some patients with persistent symptoms may respond to levodopa, especially if the vascular lesion interrupts the nigrostriatal pathway. Cases secondary to direct striatal involvement may not respond (72).

Intracranial Hemorrhage

Intracranial hemorrhage may occur secondary to head trauma, arteriovenous or other vascular malformations, or aneurysm and may be subdural, epidural, intracerebral or subarachnoid in location. The first report of a chronic subdural hematoma-producing parkinsonism was by Samily in 1968 (66). This problem may also aggravate the symptoms already present in PD.

Clinically patients may exhibit any of the classic features of parkinsonism (75). Patients with hemorrhagic lesions may complain of headache or have other findings, such as altered mental status, suggestive of a diagnosis other than PD (66). Hemorrhagic lesions may cause parkinsonism by anatomically distorting the basal ganglia and midbrain structures. This may impact metabolic function of the involved neurons (75).

Surgical intervention such as draining a subdural hematoma or spontaneous resolution of the hemorrhage may result in improvement in the patient's symptoms (66,75). Levodopa may be useful in some cases with persistent symptoms (75).

Posthypoxic Parkinsonism

Anoxic brain injury from cardiac arrest or other event may result in Parkinsonism. Neuroimaging may reveal lesions in the striatum or the globus pallidus in these cases.

Demyelinating Disease or Multiple Sclerosis

There are a few cases reported in which parkinsonian symptoms emerged in patients with multiple sclerosis (MS). However, most are attributable to the coincidental occurrence of PD in patients with MS as a clear anatomic lesion correlating with the Parkinsonian features could not be identified (76). There is one case of a patient with MS who developed bilateral cogwheel rigidity and akinesia that was associated with a demyelinating lesion in the substantia nigra.

The patient's symptoms resolved with corticosteroid treatment (76).

Posttraumatic Parkinsonism

An isolated head injury usually does not lead to parkinsonism unless it is severe enough to cause loss of consciousness and significant brain damage, especially to the basal ganglia (77). However, multiple minor (subconcussive) head injuries may cause cumulative damage to the brain resulting in characteristic dysarthria, parkinsonism (all features) and dementia. This occurs in boxers who have had multiple knockouts (dementia pugilistic) (78). In this situation the severity of symptoms correlated with length of career, number of fights, and number of blows. The damage may be due to rotatory forces of the skull and brain in opposite directions and tearing of neurons. Despite cessation of fighting the encephalopathy usually progresses to very severe levels (78a). Radiologically, this is characterized by diffuse brain atrophy and a large cavum septum pellucidum. Pathologically, there are diffuse neurofibrillary tangles and neuronal loss. The parkinsonism may not respond to levodopa. Rarely, parkinsonism has been described following electrical injury (79).

Psychogenic Parkinsonism

Psychogenic parkinsonism is not common, whereas psychogenic tremor is seen often (80). This tremor is usually complex, (occurring at rest, with posture and action) and of variable frequency, direction, and muscle involvement. The bradykinesia takes the form of a deliberate slowness with no change in amptitude of movement and can be variable. These patients often have bizarre gait disorders, deliberate stiffness, and catastrophic response to shoulder pull without falling. Onset is usually abrupt and severe, secondary pain may be present and patients often have a history of psychiatric disease examination frequently reveals other psychogenic features, absence of a mask face, normal voice, and distractability of symptoms. Prolonged careful observation may be necessary to make this diagnosis. β-cit SPECT scanning may help in differentiating from PD since it is normal (80a). Early diagnosis, confrontation, and psychiatric therapy give the patient the best chance for recovery.

MISCELLANEOUS CAUSES OF SECONDARY PARKINSONISM

Parkinsonism may occur transiently during alcohol withdrawal (81). Metabolic causes include hypoparathyroidism with basal ganglia calcifications and hypothyroidism (82). There are a few reports of Sjögren's syndrome with associated parkinsonism. Whether Parkinsonism is related to Sjögren's syndrome directly or if the association is coincidental is not clear (83). Parkinsonian features have been reported in central pontine and extrapontine myelinolysis (84), following wasp sting (85) and in Behcet's disease (86).

REFERENCES

1. Blocq P, Marinesco G. Sur un cas tremblement Parkinsonien hémiplégique symptomatique d, une tumeur de pédoncule cérébral. *CR Cos Biol* (Paris) 1893; 45:105–111.

2. Duvoisin RC, Yahr MD. Encephalitis and parkinsonism. *Arch Neurol* 1965; 12:227–239.

3. Wilson SAK. Epidemic encephalitis in neurology. *Arnold London* 1940; 1:99–104.

4. Litvan I. Parkinsonism-dementia syndromes. In: Jankovic J, Tolosa E (eds.). *Parkinson's Disease and Movement Disorders*. Baltimore: Williams & Wilkins, 1998:827–828.

5. Oeckinghaus W. Encephalitis epidemica und Wilsonsches Krankleithild. *Dtsch Z Nervenkr* 1921; 72:294.

6. Calne DB, Lees AJ. Late progression of postencephalitic Parkinson's syndrome. *Can J Neurol Sci* 1988; 15:135–138.

7. Geddes JF, Hughes AJ, Lees AJ, et al. Pathological overlap in cases of parkinsonism associated with neurofibrillary tangles: A study of recent cases of postencephalitic Parkinsonism and comparison with progressive supranuclear palsy and Guamanian Parkinsonism–dementia complex. *Brain* 1993; 116:281–302.

8. Pramstaller PP, Lees AJ, Luxon LM. Possible clinical overlap between postencephalitic parkinsonism and progressive supranuclear palsy. *J Neurol Neurosurg Psychiatry* 1996; 60(5):589–590.

9. Litvan I, Agid Y, Jankovic J, et al. Accuracy of clinical criteria for the diagnosis of progressive supranuclear palsy (Steele-Richardson-Olszewski Syndrome). *Neurology* 1996; 46:922–930.

10. Shoji H, Watanabe M, Itoh S, et al. Japanese encephalitis and parkinsonism. *J Neurol* 1993; 240:59–60.

11. Solbrig MV, Nashef L. Acute parkinsonism is suspected herpes simplex encephalitis. *Mov Disord* 1993; 8(2):233–234.

12. Calne DB, Stern GM, Laurence DR, et al. L-dopa in postencephalitic parkinsonism. *Lancet* 1969; 12:744.

13. Hunter KR, Stern GM, Sharkey J. L-dopa in postencephalitic parkinsonism. *Lancet* 1970; 2:1366.

14. Nath A, Jankovic J, Pettigrew LC. Movement disorders and AIDS. *Neurology* 1987; 37:37–41.

15. Carrazana EJ, Rossitch E, Samuels MA. Parkinsonian symptoms in a patient with AIDS and cerebral toxoplasmosis. *J Neurol Neurosurg Psychiatry* 1989; 52:1445–1447.

16. Mintz M, Tardieu J, Hoyt L, et al. Levodopa therapy improves motor function in HIV-infected children with extrapyramidal syndromes. *Neurology* 1996; 47:1583–1585.

17. Adler CH, Stern MB, Brooks ML. Parkinsonism secondary to bilateral striatal fungal abscesses. *Mov Disord* 1989; 4(4):333–337.

18. Kim JS, Choi IS, Lee MC. Reversible parkinsonism and dystonia following probable *Mycoplasma pneumonia* infection. *Mov Disord* 1995; 10:510–512.

19. Neill KJ. An unusual case of syphilitic parkinsonism. *Br Med J* 1953; 2:320.

20. Milton WJ, Atlas SW, Lavi E, et al. Magnetic resonance imaging of Creutzfeldt-Jacob disease. *Ann Neurol* 1991; 29:438–440.

21. Wszolek Z, Monsour H, Smith P, et al. Cryptococcal meningoencephalitis with parkinsonian features. *Mov Disord* 1988; 3(3):271–273.

22. Verma A, Berger JR, Bowen BC, et al. Reversible parkinsonism syndrome complicating cysticercus midbrain encephalitis. *Mov Disord* 1995; 10(2): 215–219.

23. Lehmann HE, Hanrahan GE. Chlorpromazine: New inhibiting agent for psychomotor excitement and manic states. *Arch Neurol Psychiatry* 1954; 71:227.

24. Hardie RJ, Lees AJ. Neuroleptic-induced Parkinson's syndrome: Clinical features and results of treatment with levodopa. *J Neurol Neurosurg Psychiatry* 1988; 51:850–854.

25. Sethi KD, Patel B, Meador KJ. Metoclopramide-induced parkinsonism. *South Med J* 1989; 82: 1581–1582.

26. Sethi KD, Zamrini EY. Asymmetry in clinical features of drug-induced parkinsonism. *J Neuropsychiatry Clin Neurosci* 1990; 2(i):64–66.

27. Hausner RS. Neuroleptic-induced parkinsonism and Parkinson's disease: Differential diagnosis and treatment. *J Clin Psychiatry* 1983; 44:13–16.

28. Rajput AH, Rozdilsky B, Hornykiewicz O, et al. Reversible drug-induced parkinsonism: Clinicopathologic study of two cases. *Arch Neurol* 1982; 39:644–646.

29. Burn DJ, Brooks DJ. Nigral dysfunction in drug-induced parkinsonism: A ^{18}F-dopa PET study. *Neurology* 1993; 43:552–556.

30. Kelly JT, Zimmerman RL, Abuzzahab FS, et al. A double-blind study of amantidine hydrochloride versus benztropine mesylate in drug-induced parkinsonism. *Pharmacology* 1974; 12:65–73.

31. Jankovic J, Beach J. Long-term effects of tetrabenazine in hyperkinetic movement disorders. *Neurology* 1997; 48:358–362.

32. Marti-Masso JF, Poza JJ. Cinnarizine-induced parkinsonism: Ten years later. *Mov Disord* 1998; 13(3):453–456.

33. Micheli F, Pardal M, Gatto M, et al. Flunarizine and cinnarizine-induced extrapyramidal reactions. *Neurology* 1987; 37:881–884.

34. Sempere AP, Duarte J, Cabezas C, et al. Parkinsonism induced by amlodipine. *Mov Disord* 1995; 10(1):115–116.

35. Dick RS, Barold SS. Diltiazem-induced parkinsonism. *Am J Med* 1989; 87:95–96.

36. García-Albea E, Jiménez-Jiménez FJ, Ayuso-Peralta L, et al. Parkinsonism unmasked by verapamil. *Clin Neuropharmacol* 1993; 16(3):263–265.

37. Shopsin B, Gershon S. Cogwheel rigidity related to lithium maintenance. *Am J Psychiatry* 1975; 132:536–538.

38. Bergevin PR, Patwardhan VC, Weissman J, et al. Neurotoxicity of 5-fluorouracil. *Lancet* 1975; 1:410.

39. Boranic M, Raci F. A Parkinson-like syndrome as side effect of chemotherapy with vincristine and adriamycin in a child with acute leukaemia. *Biomedicine* 1979; 31:124–125.

40. Sechi GP, Demontis G, Rosati G. Relationship between Meige syndrome and alpha-methyldopa-induced parkinsonism. *Neurology* 1985; 35:1668–1669.

41. Dotti MT, Federico A. Amiodarone-induced parkinsonism: A case report and pathogenetic discussion. *Mov Disord* 1995; 10:233–234.

42. Handler CE, Besse CP, Wilson AO. Extrapyramidal and cerebellar syndrome with encephalopathy associated with cimetidine. *Postgrad Med J* 1982; 58:527–528.

43. Bird GLA, Meadows J, Goka J, et al. Cyclosporin-associated akinetic mutism and extrapyramidal syndrome after liver transplantation. *J Neurol Neursurg Psychiatry* 1990; 53:1068–1071.

44. Armon C, Shin C, Miller P, et al. Reversible parkinsonism and cognitive impairment with chronic valproate use. *Neurology* 1996; 47:626–635.

45. Di Rocco A, Brannan T, Prikhojan A, et al. Sertraline-induced extrapyramidal side effects may be related to interference with dopamine metabolism. *Mov Disord* 1997; 12(Suppl 1):66.

46. Albanese A, Rossi P, Altavista MC. Can trazodone induce parkinsonism? *Clin Neuropharmacol* 1988; 11(2):180–182.

47. Miura T, Mitomo M, Kawai R, et al. CT of the brain in acute carbon monoxide intoxication: Characteristic features and prognosis. *AJNR* 1985; 6:739–742.

48. Ernst A, Zibrak JD. Carbon monoxide poisoning. *NEJM* 1998; 339(22):1603–1608.

49. Min SK. A brain syndrome associated with delayed neuropsychiatric sequelae following acute carbon monoxide intoxication. *Acta Psychiatry Scand* 1986; 73:80–86.

50. Davis GC, Williams AC, Markey SP, et al. Chronic parkinsonism secondary to intravenous injection of meperidine analogs. *Psychiatry Res* 1979; 1: 249–254.

51. Langston JW, Ballard P, Tetrud JW, et al. Chronic parkinsonism in humans due to a product of meperidine-analog synthesis. *Science* 1983; 219: 979–980.

52. Tetrud JW, Langston JW, Irwin I, et al. Parkinsonism caused by petroleum waste ingestion. *Neurology* 1994; 44:1051–1054.

53. McCrodden JM, Tipton KF, Sullivan JP. The neurotoxicity of MPTP and the relevance to Parkinson's disease. *Pharmacol Toxicol* 1990; 67:8–13.

54. Tetrud JW, Langston JW, Garbe PL, et al. Mild parkinsonism in persons exposed to 1-methyl-4-phenyl-1,2,3,6-tetrahydropyridine (MPTP). *Neurology* 1989; 39:1483–1487.

55. Huang CC, Chu NS, Lu CS, et al. Chronic manganese intoxication. *Arch Neurol* 1989; 46:1104–1106.

56. Barbeau A. Manganese and extrapyramidal disorders. *Neurotoxicology* 1984; 5(1):13.

57. Mena I, Court J, Fuenzalida S, et al. Modification of chronic manganese poisoning: Treatment with L-dopa or 5-OH tryptophane. *NEJM* 1970; 282(1):5–10.

58. Peters HA, Levine RL, Matthews CG, et al. Extrapyramidal and other neurologic manifestations associated with carbon disulfide fumigant exposure. *Arch Neurol* 1988; 45:537–540.

59. Pezzoli G, Strada O, Silani V, et al. Clinical and pathological features in hydrocarbon-induced parkinsonism. *Ann Neurol* 1996; 40:922–925.

60. Sechi GP, Agnetti V, Piredda M, et al. Acute and persistent parkinsonism after use of diquat. *Neurology* 1992; 42:261–263.

61. Sanchez-Ramos JR, Hefti F, Weiner WJ. Paraquat and Parkinson's disease. *Neurology* 1987; 37:728.

62. Rosenow F, Herholz K, Lanfermann H, et al. Neurological sequelae of cyanide intoxication – the patterns of clinical, magnetic resonance imaging, and positron emission tomography findings. *Ann Neurol* 1995; 38:825–828.

63. Zeidler M, Dorman PJ, Ferguson IT, et al. Parkinsonism associated with obstructive hydrocephalus due to idiopathic aqueductal stenosis. *J Neurol Neurosurg Psychiatry* 1998; 64:657–659.

64. Keane JR. Tremor as the result of shunt obstruction: Four patients with cysticercosis and secondary parkinsonism: Report of four cases. *Neurosurgery* 1995; 37:520–522.

65. Krauss JK, Regel JP, Droste DW, et al. Movement disorders in adult hydrocephalus. *Mov Disord* 1997; 12:53–60.

66. Waters CH. Structural lesions and parkinsonism. In: Stern MB and Koller WC (eds.). *Parkinsonian Syndromes*. New York: Marcel Dekker, 1993:137–145.

67. Cicarelli G, Pellecchia MT, Maiuri F, et al. Brain stem cystic astrocytoma presenting with "pure" parkinsonism. *Mov Disord* 1999; 14(2):364–366.

68. Critchely M. Arteriosclerotic parkinsonism. *Brain* 1929; 52:23–83.

69. Murrow RW, Schweiger GD, Kepes JJ, et al. Parkinsonism due to a basal ganglia lacunar state: Clinicopathological correlation. *Neurology* 1990; 40:897–900.

70. Hughes AJ, Daniel SE, Kilford L, et al. Accuracy of clinical diagnosis of idiopathic Parkinson's disease: A clinico-pathological study of 100 cases. *J Neurol Neurosurg Psychiatry* 1992; 55:181–184.

71. Hurtig HI. Vascular parkinsonism In: Stern MB, Koller WC (eds.). *Parkinsonian Syndromes* New York: Marcel Dekker, 1993; 81–93.

72. Fénelon G, Houéto JL. Unilateral parkinsonism following a large infarct in the territory of the lenticulostriate arteries. *Mov Disord* 1997; 12(6):1086–1089.

73. Tolosa ES, Santamaría J. Parkinsonism and basal ganglia infarcts. *Neurology* 1984; 34:1516–1518.

74. FitzGerald PM, Jankovic J. Lower body parkinsonism: Evidence for vascular etiology. *Mov Disord* 1989; 4(3):249–260.

75. Turjanski N, Pentland B, Lees AD, et al. Parkinsonism associated with acute intracranial hematomas: A [18F] dopa positron-emission tomography study. *Mov Disord* 1997; 12(6):1035–1038.

76. Federlein J, Postert T, Allgeier A, et al. Remitting parkinsonism as a symptom of multiple sclerosis and the associated magnetic resonance imaging findings. *Mov Disord* 1997; 12(6):1090–1091.

77. Jankovic J: Posttraumatic movement disorders: Central and peripheral mechanisms. *Neurology* 1994; 44:2006–2014.

78. Koller WC, Wong, GF, Lang A. Posttraumatic movement disorders: A review. *Mov Disord* 1989; 4:20–36.

78a Factor SA. Posttraumatic parkinsonism. In: Stern MB, Koller WC (eds.). *Parkinsonian syndromes* New York, NY: Marcel Dekker, 1993:95–110.

79. Morris HR, Moriabadi NF, Lees AJ, et al. Parkinsonism following electrical injury to the hand *Mov Disord* 1998; 13(3):600–602.

80. Lang AE, Koller WC, Fahn S. Psychogenic parkinsonism. *Arch Neurol* 1995; 52:802–810.

80a. Factor SA, Seibyl J, Innis R, et al. Psychogenic Parkisonism: Confirmation of diagnosis with β-CIT SPECT scans. *Mov Disord* 1998; 13:860.

81. Shandling M, Carlen PL, Lang AE. Parkinsonism in alcohol withdrawl: A follow-up study. *Mov Disord* 1990; 5:36–39.

82. Sweeney PJ. Metabolic causes of parkinsonism. In: Stern MB, Koller WC (eds.). *Parkinsonian Syndromes*. New York: Marcel Dekker, 1993: 195–200.

83. Walker RH, Spiera H, Brin MF, et al. Parkinsonism associated with Sjogren's syndrome: Three cases and a review of the literature. *Mov Disord* 1999; 14(2):262–268.

84. Seiser A, Schwarz S, Aichinger-Steiner MM, et al. Parkinsonism and dystonia in central pontine and extrapontine myelinolysis. *J Neurol Neurosurg Psychiatry* 1998; 65(1):119–121.

85. Leopold NA, Bara-Jimenez W, Hallett M. Parkinsonism after a wasp sting. *Mov Disord* 1999; 14(1):122–127.

86. Bogdanova D, Milanov I, Georgiev D. Parkinsonian syndrome as a neurological manifestation of Behcet's disease. *Can J Neurol Sci* 1998; 25(1):82–85.

55

Quality of Life: Issues and Measurement

Mickie Welsh, R.N. DNSc.

University of Southern California, School of Medicine, Los Angeles, California

HISTORICAL PERSPECTIVE

At the turn of the century, infectious diseases posed the greatest threat to public health. Disease management was primarily of an episodic and curative focus. In the decades which followed, technologic advances and revolutionary discoveries reduced mortality and morbidity that resulted in longer life spans and greater numbers of individuals in all of the older age groups (1). Chronic cardiovascular, pulmonary, rheumatological, and neurological diseases replaced the life-threatening infections previously dominating the landscape. Early clinical trials of new technologies and therapeutics in oncology and cardiovascular diseases emphasized the impact that life-saving treatment choices and side effects presented to the patient living longer with a chronic illness. Increased longevity combined with the effects of both disease and treatment further heightened awareness to life-quality issues.

As many serious challenges to human health were met, medical practitioners began thinking about health as more than the absence of acute illness. With lengthening life spans, more individuals would be diagnosed with chronic and degenerative conditions, which could over time pose threats to functional ability, independence, and quality of life (QOL).

A growing array of medical and surgical therapies continues to enhance longevity with varying impact on quality of survival time. Today's health professionals are commonly faced with helping patients live full lives within disease boundaries. For many diseases that remain incurable, namely, Parkinson's disease (PD), maintaining or restoring quality of life is an important therapeutic goal. To do so, physicians must determine how a disease or a treatment affects the patient. The importance of recognizing and documenting the subjective impact of disease and the side effects of long-term medical therapy in illnesses such as PD is beginning to be fully appreciated (2). This appreciation follows the recognition that it is necessary to describe the overall results of diagnostic and treatment efforts in a way that makes sense to both patients and health professionals.

A transformation of thought and practice has occurred, where inclusion of concepts commonly subsumed under the term *quality of life* or *health related quality of life* (HRQOL) are considered for incorporation into clinical trials and clinical practice (3). Recent editorials in prominent neurological journals illustrate this shift in emphasis (2,4). This chapter provides an introduction and overview of quality-of-life concepts as they apply to PD clinical practice and research.

WHAT IS QUALITY OF LIFE?

Health-care applications of quality-of-life concepts are generally limited to those constructs that are most directly affected by health. Though no universal definition or conceptualization of HRQOL exists, five domains of quality of life are generally referred to by most authors: (1) physical status and functional abilities, (2) psychological status and well-being, (3) social interactions, (4) economic or vocational status and factors, and (5) religious or spiritual status (5).

Conceptual models of quality of life found in the literature illustrate the relationships of these somewhat abstract concepts and their functional manifestations in an illness situation. Ware conceptualized health-status concepts as a set of concentric circles with biologic functioning, central to human function, in the center surrounded by circles representing general well-being and behavioral functioning that contribute to the "wholeness" of the person (6). Biologic abnormalities can extend into an individuals behavioral and general well-being like a rock dropped into the center of a pond. Use of Ware's or other conceptual schema or models in clinical practice and research applications provide guidance for operationalizing outcomes, standardizing

Quality-of-life measurement applications include, but are not limited to, clinical settings, evaluation research, and clinical trials. In choosing HRQOL measures, trade-offs are most often necessary among competing goals of inquiry. The decision or problem being addressed, the objectives of measurement, and conceptual, methodologic and practical considerations all need to be weighed when designing quality-of-life studies (17). Different concepts of HRQOL apply differentially to the clinical decision or problem to be addressed. That is, no one single measure will be suitable for all applications. Selection criteria may include single or multiple indicators, general health-status measures or disease-specific measures.

As with all outcome variables, quality of life must be operationalized to be consistent with purpose and application. For research applications, conceptual and operational correspondence is necessary while selecting the appropriate instrument. In the clinical setting less rigor is required. The use of paradigms such as those of Ware (6) or Spilker (5) provides the investigator with a conceptual framework that helps to ensure methodological integrity. Additionally, for research applications, a conceptual framework provides a strategy for identifying the core variables and limiting design flaws. Such concerns are especially important when considering whether the instrument being considered for use in fact represents the intended concept or concepts. In Table 55-1, measures of physical status/ functional ability, psychological status, and social interactions suitable for use in PD clinical and research applications are illustrated.

METHODOLOGICAL CONSIDERATIONS

The strength of study findings is based upon choice of design, sampling decisions, and other means of controlling extraneous variables including the amount of control that exists within the indices of the conceptual variables. When the concept of control is applied to measurement, it refers to the ability of instruments to index the concepts with precision, accuracy and sensitivity (18). The more precise, accurate, and sensitive the instrument is, the more control exists within the study.

Adequate measurement properties are necessary conditions for any application of quality of life in research and evaluation. Measurement of health-related outcomes such as disability, handicap, and quality of life are increasingly recognized for their importance in evaluating therapeutic efficacy (19). In recent years considerable progress has been made in the area of psychometrics and outcomes measurement. Psychometrics is the science of using standardized tests or scales to measure one or more attributes of an individual or an object; in this case the attributes of health-related quality of life (6). Two necessary attributes for all measures are reliability and validity. A brief review of the necessary properties of instruments necessary for quality of life research indication follows.

Reliability

A measure which is reliable is one which produces results that are accurate, consistent, stable over time, and reproducible. Reliability is equal to the observed variance that is not random or fluctuating but is repeatable or true. When random error is low, reliability is high. The reliability coefficient is the portion of test variance that is true or nonrandom variance. This involves four different types of reliability (20).

Stability

The stability of a measure refers to the extent to which the same results are obtained over repeated administrations of the instrument. A commonly used method of assessing stability, test-retest reliability, confirms stability by computation of a correlation coefficient. A positive correlation provides support for how constant the measure's scores remain from one testing occasion to another.

Internal Consistency

An instrument is considered to be internally consistent or homogenous when all of its subparts measure the same characteristic (20). Commonly used estimates of internal consistency include the coefficient alpha (or Cronbach's alpha) and the Kuder Richardson (for instruments with dichotomous items). Each indicator, usually an item, is considered a separate but equal measure of the underlying concept.

Validity

Validity is an additional necessary instrument property. An indicator must be more than reliable if it is to provide an accurate representation of an abstract concept. It must also be valid (20). An instrument is considered valid when it measures what it is purported to measure. Like reliability, there are a number of different approaches to determining and establishing validity.

Content and face validity was once accepted as minimal criteria for validity. More substantial estimates of validity including construct and criterion validity are currently expected for publishable instruments. With abstract concepts such as quality of life, special attention should be applied to determining measurement accuracy and for confirming instrument appropriateness.

Construct Validity

Construct validity is concerned with the extent to which an instrument measures the concept or construct it was designed to measure (21). Variables used to establish construct validity, for example, may be directly concerned with the theoretical relationship of a variable to other variables. For example, decreasing motor function or disability is theoretically and practically linked to diminished quality of life.

Criterion Validity

Criterion validity is of a more practical issue than a scientific one because it is not concerned with understanding a process but merely with predicting it. In fact, criterion-related validity is often referred to as predictive validity (22). To have criterion-related validity, an item or scale is required only to have an empirical association with some other criterion or "gold standard." Criterion-related validity is often used in quality-of-life research applications where an external "gold standard" criterion exists but with a different theoretical basis. Such is the case in PD where the gold standard criterion is usually the UPDRS.

Sensitivity

For instruments to be used in prospective data collection, responsiveness or sensitivity is critical. The responsiveness of an instrument determines how small a variation in an attribute can be reliably detected and measured. Over time, responsiveness determines how discriminating an instrument's measurements will be in determining differences between individuals (23).

Practical Considerations

In the clinic, time and resources may be an over-riding consideration in the selection of instruments and the design of data collection methods. A valid, reliable and brief instrument may be the most suitable. Method of administration either by direct observation, face to face interview, telephone interview, self-administration or proxy respondents are options. Subject specific needs and potential bias must also be considered. Response burden (testing time, test difficulty) associated with extensive testing may affect outcome. Appropriateness for age group, culture and language should also be considered when selecting instruments. Practical considerations are especially important in diseases of aging, namely PD, where disease symptoms or timing of measurement may bias outcome measurement. For instance PD patients may respond differently when "on" or "off."

INTEGRATING QUALITY-OF-LIFE RESEARCH INTO PRACTICE

The ultimate goal of knowledge generation is improving practice through enhanced therapeutics, improving interventions and providing a better understanding of the disease process and its course. In order that this new knowledge is ultimately received and used by those who will benefit, a mechanism for dissemination and use needs to be employed. In many disciplines, integration, or use models exist for this purpose. Publication of study findings does not ensure that the knowledge reaches all that may use it or that the findings may be implemented to change or improve practice. Many of the studies which directly or indirectly address issues of quality of life involve pharmacologic interventions that are implemented into practice by physicians. Quality-of-life research presents a unique opportunity for studying how the myriad of services other than pharmacologic therapeutics provided by all health care professionals benefit the PD patient and their family. Many of the concepts and constructs in quality-of-life studies are of particular interest to the practice of nurses, occupational therapists, physical therapists, and social workers. Collaborative efforts with physicians, nurses, and other health care professionals must be expanded to explore the impact that nonpharmacologic interventions can have on quality of life in PD.

FUTURE APPLICATIONS

The rise in the number of individuals with chronic illnesses in our society has shifted the emphasis of disease management toward preservation of function and limitation of symptoms rather than on solely curative aspects of therapy. The focus of care and its outcomes broadened beyond survival and traditional biomedical measurements. Effects of disease and treatments on health status and quality of life increasingly receive attention by planners and providers of health care services. Noteworthy progress has been made both in the understanding of health status and quality of life and in the development of practical tools for measuring the most important aspects of these concepts (24).

Quality-of-life issues are now appreciated for their importance in the life of patients who struggle to live successfully with PD. Although scientists and scholars search for improved therapies and the eventual cure, patients and families live daily with the disabling changes that result from this disease. The progressive degenerative changes and the side effects of therapy often rob the patient and family of the life quality taken for granted by all of us. As health care professionals, we must actively expand our research and scholarly efforts to include these vital indicators of health on our daily practices.

REFERENCES

1. Read JL. The new era of quality of life assessment. In: Wallace SR, Rosser RM (eds),. *Quality of Life Assessment: Key Issues in the 1990s.* Dordrecht: Kluwer Academic Publishers, 1993:3–10.

2. Devinsky O. Outcomes research in neurology: Incorporating health-related quality of life. *Ann Neurol* 1995; 37:141.

3. Luce J, Dawson J. Quality of life. *Semin Oncol* 1995; 2:32–34.

4. Vickrey BG. Getting oriented to patient-oriented outcomes. *Neurology* 1999; 53:662–663.

5. Schipper H, Clinch JJ, Olweny CLM. Quality of life studies: Definitions and conceptual issues. In: Spilker B ed. *Quality of Life and Pharmacoeconomics in Clinical Trials.* Philadelphia: Lippincott, 1996:11–21.

6. Bungay KM, Ware JE. *Measuring and Monitoring Health-related Quality of Life.* Kalamazoo: The Upjohn Company, 1995.

7. Koller WC. Adverse effects of levodopa and other symptomatic therapies: impact on quality of life of the Parkinson's disease patient. In: Stern M (ed.). *Beyond the Decade of the Brain.* Tunbridge Wells: Tunbridge Wells, 1994:31–46.

8. Wallhagen MI, Brod M. Perceived control and well-being in Parkinson's disease. *WJ Nur Res* 1997; 19:11–31.

9. Shindler JS. Brown R, Welburn P, et al. Measuring quality of life of patients with Parkinson's disease. In: Wallace SR, Rosser RM (eds.), *Quality of Life*

10. Omnibus Reconciliation Act 1989. Public Law 101–239.

11. Chrischilles EA, Rubenstein LM, Voelker MD, et al. The health burdens of Parkinson's disease. *Mov Disord* 1998; 13:406–413.

12. Wasielewski PG, Koller WC. Quality of life and parkinson's disease: The CR FIRST Study. *J Neurol* 1998; 245(Suppl 1)S28–30.

13. Grandas F. Martinez-Martin P, Linazasoro G. Quality of life in patients with Parkinson's disease who transfer from standard levodopa to Sinemet CR: The STAR Study. The STAR Multicenter Study Group. *J Neurol* 1998; 245(Suppl)1:S31–33.

14. Fitzpatrick R, Peto V, Jenkinson C, et al. Health-related quality of life in Parkinson's disease: A study of outpatient clinic attenders. *Mov Disord* 1997; 12:916–922.

15. De Boer AGEM, Wijker W, Speelman JD, et al. Parkinson's disease Quality of life: Is it one construct? *Qual Life Res* 1998; 7:135–142.

16. Welsh M, McDermott M, Holloway R, et al. Development and testing of the PDQUALIF [abstract]. *Mov Disord* 1997; 12:836.

17. Patrick D, Erickson P. Assessing health-related quality of life for clinical decision-making. In: Walker SR, Rosser RM. *Quality of Life Assessment: Key Issues in the 1990s.* Dordrecht: Kluwer Academic Publishers, 1993.

18. Mishel M. Methodological studies: Instrument development. In: Brink PJ, Wood MJ (eds.). *Advanced Design in Nursing Research.* Newbury Park: Sage, 1989; 238–284.

19. Hobart JC, Lamping DL, Thompson AJ. Evaluating neurological outcome measures: The bare essentials. *J Neurol Neurosurg Psychiatry* 1997:136–139.

20. Carmines EG, Zeller RA. *Reliability and Validity Assessment.* Newbury Park: Sage, 1979.

21. Kirshner B, Guyatt G. A methodological framework for assessing health indices. *J Chron Dis* 1985; 38:27–36.

22. De Vellis RF. *Scale Development: Theory and Applications.* Newbury Park: Sage, 1991.

23. Guyatt GH, Bombardier C, Tugwell PX. Measuring disease-specific quality of life in clinical trials. *Can Med Assoc J* 1993; 134:869–895.

24. Deyo RA. Measuring functional outcomes in therapeutic trials for chronic disease. *Con Clin Trials* 1989; 5:223–240.

56

Family Caregiving

Julie H. Carter, R.N., M.N. ANP Patricia G. Archbold, R.N, D.N.Sc, F.A.A.N., Barbara J. Stewart, Ph.D.

Oregon Health Sciences University, Portland, Oregon

FAMILY CAREGIVING IN PARKINSON'S DISEASE

Caregiving is part of all relationships. It is the act of providing assistance to someone with whom one has a personal relationship. It is usually an extension of caring and a reciprocal act. In conditions of chronic progressive disease such as Parkinson's disease (PD), the act of caregiving is primarily from one person and reciprocal caregiving is diminished. In these situations, caregiving can become stressful and threaten the well-being of the caregiver and the care recipient with significant negative economic, social, and psychologic impacts.

DEMOGRAPHIC TRENDS IN FAMILY CAREGIVING FOR THE TWENTY-FIRST CENTURY

Growth of the Elderly Population

During the past century the United States experienced unprecedented growth in the part of the population that is 65 years of age and older. Indeed, the rate of growth for this subpopulation exceeded the rate of growth for the country as a whole – there was an 11-fold increase in elders between 1900 and 1994, compared with a threefold increase in the population younger than 65 years (1). A further dramatic increase in the actual numbers and relative percentage of elders is expected as the baby boomers enter old age between 2010 and 2030. The numbers of elderly are projected to grow from the current 35 million (12.8%) to 70 million (20%) (1).

It goes without saying that the elderly population is most at risk for functional loss and declines in health. The percentage of community-dwelling elders needing help with one or more activities of daily living (ADLs) (e.g., bathing and dressing) increases with age. Among those aged 65 to 74, only about 10% need help with such activities; but by age 85, about 50% need help (1). In 1990, 4.5 million elders needed assistance with one or more ADL.

IMPORTANT ROLE OF FAMILY CAREGIVING IN CHRONIC ILLNESS

The family is the "lynch pin" of the health and long-term care system for patients in this country. Families provide 80% to 90% of the care received by community-dwelling, chronically ill elders. Because families are the main providers of care and support to chronically ill persons, including persons with PD, the need for family care is undergoing unprecedented expansion as the number of persons with chronic illness increases. This can be expressed quantitatively as the parent-support ratio, or the number of persons 85 years old and over, divided by the number of persons 50 to 64 years old, times 100. In 1993 the parent-support ratio was 10; by 2050, it is projected to triple (1). Having living parents who are 85 and over will become commonplace in just over 50 years.

In 1996 a national phone survey of randomly selected English-speaking families was conducted to identify caregivers who provided unpaid assistance to a relative or friend aged 50 or older. Nearly one in four households contained at least one caregiver. Three quarters of these caregivers were providing care at the time of the phone survey and the remaining 24% had provided such care in the year preceding the survey (2). About half of the family caregivers who participated in the Caregiver Supplement of the National Long-term Care Survey had been providing unpaid assistance to an elder for one to four years; another quarter had been providing assistance for five years or more (3). Eighty percent of these caregivers provided unpaid assistance seven days a week and spent an average of four hours per day – more than a half-time job – on caregiving tasks (3). In a recent report of the economic burden of PD, Whetten-Goldstein and colleagues found that hidden costs of PD included the significant costs of uncompensated informal care (M = $5,386 per family per year) – costs that would be borne by the society if the family did not provide the care (4).

THE RISKS ASSOCIATED WITH FAMILY CAREGIVING

Not only are the number of potential caregivers not increasing as fast as the elders in our society but clinicians and researchers are also concerned that the strain of caregiving can bring with it health risks that threaten a caregiver's ability to continue in that role. In their 1995 review of the caregiving literature related to psychiatric and physical effects of dementia caregiving, Schulz and colleagues found that all studies reported elevated levels of depressive symptoms in caregivers (5). Studies that used clinician interviews reported high rates of clinical depression and anxiety. The authors of this chapter found a 27.1% prevalence rate of depressive symptoms in spouses of persons with late-stage PD, not quite as high as the 27.9% to 55% prevalence rates found with Alzheimer's disease (AD) caregivers (6).

Schulz and colleagues found that the evidence for physical health effects in AD caregivers was weaker and more equivocal than the psychiatric effects noted earlier, and it varied depending on the instrument used to measure of physical health (5). This area of inquiry is complex and developing rapidly. Statistically significant findings of interest to clinicians include: (1) caregivers who reported sleeping less than noncaregivers; (2) caregivers who experienced declines in cellular immunity over a 13-month period, and (3) caregivers who reported their self-rated health as worse than noncaregivers.

PREDICTORS OF CAREGIVER STRAIN

Most clinicians have had the experience of seeing patients with similar symptoms and dependencies, and yet, one family caregiver is coping well whereas another is visibly on the verge of burnout. Understanding this disparity may provide insight into how to help struggling families. A focus of many researchers has been to look at factors that predict strain and factors that reduce or buffer strain and, more complexly, the interaction between these two. Various models with theoretical underpinnings have been developed (7). A model offers a way to conceptualize this multifactorial problem. Rather than choosing a specific model, this chapter will synthesize the research on strain and the various factors that are linked to strain and organize them into three categories: (1) caregiver strain (i.e., perceived difficulty), (2) characteristics of the caregiver, and (3) the caregiving situation. Inherent in this thinking is that the greater the strain the greater the risk for negative outcomes such as decreased physical and emotional health of the caregiver, nursing home placement, and economic burden. Most caregiving research has been done in dementia. Research that is specific to PD will be mentioned.

CAREGIVER ROLE STRAIN

Caregiver strain is defined as the perceived difficulty in fulfilling the caregiving role. Strain can lead to negative outcomes that can prevent a family member from continuing in this role. Research in family caregiving has identified a number of variables that are associated with strain. Some of these predict higher strain and some attenuate strain. These factors will be reviewed in the next sections on caregiver characteristics and the caregiving situation. Understanding predictors of strain allows us to identify caregivers who are at risk for higher strain. It also holds the potential of developing interventions around factors that reduce strain.

In addition to understanding factors that are linked to strain, it is important to recognize that within the global concept of strain there are subtypes of strain. Archbold, Stewart, and colleagues identified nine subtypes of strain that include strain from worry, tension, frustration from communication, direct care, role conflict, mismatched expectations, economic burden, lack of personal resources, and feelings of being manipulated (8). As an example, if a clinician knows that frustration from communication is greater than the strain from lack of personal resources (e.g., exhaustion) they might refer them to a specialist in augmentative communication techniques rather than refer them for respite care.

In PD it has been shown that strain increases as the stage of disease progresses (6,9). By ferreting out types of strain, we can see that strain occurs at all stages of disease and accumulates with each advancing stage. In early-stage disease, when motor signs are minimal and before direct-care activities have started, worry emerges as an area of significant strain. In middle-stage disease, worry continues but now there is the addition of tension, frustration from communication problems, strain from direct care, and role conflict. By late-stage disease, significant levels of strain from lack of personal resources, economic burden, feelings of being manipulated, and mismatched expectations are added to the strain seen at earlier stages (6). As a clinician, having a general profile of the types of strain that a family member might be experiencing at different stages of disease is helpful in considering referral to appropriate resources.

CAREGIVER CHARACTERISTICS

The response to caregiving is directly influenced by characteristics of the caregiver. These include (1) age and gender, (2) economic status, (3) physical and emotional health, (4) whether the caregiver is a spouse or adult child, (5) ethnicity, (6) personality, (7) mutuality (i.e., positive quality of the relationship), and (8) preparedness (how prepared one feels for the caregiving role). Most of these variables cannot be influenced by interventions, but their relationship to caregiver burden is important to clinicians in identifying people at risk.

Age and Gender

Caregiver age has been inversely correlated with caregiver strain (5,10,11). It has been suggested that more strain in younger caregivers is because of the conflict of multiple role demands and economic burden.

In general, women caregivers report more negative, emotional, and physical responses to caregiving than do men (12,13). This may be because of a greater awareness by women of their emotions, differences in coping styles, differences in the amount and type of direct care tasks that women perform versus men, or differences in social support (13,14,15). Although most of the research examining gender differences has been done in dementia caregivers, the limited comparison of PD to AD would suggest that the findings are similar (16). The differences in strain between men and women have significance because the majority of caregivers are women.

Economic Status

The association of lower economic status and increased caregiver strain is more equivocal (10,11,17,18). A clear understanding of this relationship is difficult because better education is usually seen with better economic status. More education may result in better problem solving and coping skills, whereas more economic stability may allow for more paid support and respite opportunities (12).

Preexisting Health

The relationship of a family member's precaregiving physical and emotional health to caregiver outcomes has been difficult to study because most research is done after caregiving has begun. Poor health is a predictor of higher strain. It is understandable that poor physical and emotional health might limit the capacity to respond to the demands of caregiving and that caregiving might exacerbate underlying vulnerabilities (17–19). What is not clear is if this is reinforcing, with more strain producing worse health and worse health resulting in more strain. Longitudinal studies are needed to answer this question.

Relationship to Patient

The majority of caregivers are either spouses or adult children of the care recipient. Spouses compared with adult children experience more strain in the caregiver role (20). In spite of this, it should be considered that adult children have some unique characteristics that contribute to their strain and may limit side-by-side comparison to a spouse caregiver. Some of these are (1) a sense of filial responsibility, (2) employment demands, (3) conflict with other siblings regarding care of a parent, (4) responsibility to their own spouse and children, (5) prior relationship with parent, and (6) role reversals (21–24).

Ethnicity

A recent review of existing studies on ethnicity as a predictor of caregiving burden in dementia found that the majority of research compared Caucasian caregivers to African–American caregivers. Although there are many limitations in comparing these studies, the significant findings of interest are: (1) Caucasians reported higher levels of burden and depression than African–American caregivers, (2) African–American caregivers were more likely to be an adult child or friend, whereas Caucasian caregivers were more likely to be a spouse, (3) Caucasian caregivers identified support groups and health care professionals as a source of support whereas religion and prayer were identified for African-American caregivers, (4) a stronger belief regarding filial support as a reason for caregiving was held by African-American caregivers versus Caucasian caregivers (25).

who need relief from care activities. Obtaining respite can be difficult for families when it involves hiring a person or people to care for their loved one. The check list in Table 56-2 might be helpful to families.

Telephone and Computer Care

For over 15 years, telephone monitoring and support interventions have been successful in a wide range of health care situations including cardiac disease (45,46) and oncology (47,48). More recently, computer-based information and support interventions have been found effective for caregivers of persons with chronic illnesses, including AD (49). Telehealth technologies provide access to health advice and monitoring in the home for family-initiated questions or for provider-initiated monitoring. National Parkinson's organizations sponsor hotlines for people with PD and their families. These telephone intervention systems provide information and referral services, connecting persons with local and national PD resources. A list of hotlines is found in Table 56-3.

In-Home Interventions

A few studies have evaluated the effects of comprehensive, in-home interventions on elders and families – most involve extensive interdisciplinary in-home care along with telephone support (50–57). Each of these studies evaluated a new model of care for frail elders and their families. In each, an intervention that changed the nature of health-care delivery and the mix of health-care providers was evaluated. We will review two comprehensive in-home interventions as examples: PREP and the Comprehensive support program.

PREP was a comprehensive program of expanded in-home and telephone care for elders and their families referred for home health. PREP focused on three goals: increasing the skill and PReparedness of families for care, increasing Enrichment in family care, and

Table 56-2 Steps to Hire In-Home Respite Care
Hiring on Your Own
Create a job description
Conduct a search
Conduct interviews
Check references and public records for criminal history
Write an employee agreement
Set a work schedule
Talk with your insurance company
Talk with a tax accountant
Keep work records

Table 56-3 Parkinson's Disease Hotlines

National Parkinson Foundation, Inc.
1501 NW 9th Ave./Bob Hope Rd.
Miami, Florida 33136
USA
TEL: (305) 547-6666
FAX: (305) 243 4403
Web Site: www.parkinson.org

WE MOVE: Worldwide Education and Awareness For Movement Disorders.
A worldwide nonprofit organization that provides information, support, and educational materials to health care professionals and patients with movement disorders.
204 West 84th Street
New York, NY 10024
TEL: (212) 241-8567
FAX: (212) 987-7363

The American Parkinson's Disease Association
1250 Hylan Boulevard
Staten Island, New York 10305
USA
TEL: (800) 223-2732 / (718) 981-8001
FAX: (718) 981-4399
Web Site: www.apdaparkinson.com

Well Spouse Foundation
610 Lexington Avenue
Room 814
New York, NY 10022
TEL: (212) 644-1241
FAX: (212) 644-1338

(All the national organizations have free literature, a newsletter, and support group information.)

increasing Predictability in family care. PREP involved care planning and management, a PREP advice line (PAL) in which families could receive telephone advice about care when needed, and the Keep-in-touch (KIT) system through which nurses could monitor families. A pilot study of PREP found that mean levels of preparedness, enrichment, and predictability in PREP families were significantly higher than in control families ($P < 0.05$) and that PREP reduced mean health-care costs per family by $3,800 over a three-month period (50,58).

The Comprehensive support program of Mittelman and colleagues (1995,1996) was designed to treat the primary caregivers of persons with AD, over the course of the disease (54,55). The intervention included treatments to maximize formal and informal support for the caregivers and included individual and family counseling sessions directed at increasing the support of the primary caregiver by other family members.

In addition, the intervention included availability of a weekly support group and ad hoc consultation by project staff when needed by the caregiver. The intervention was designed to provide continuous support for the caregiver and family as long as it was needed. Over the period of a year, caregivers in the control group became more depressed; however, caregivers in the treatment group remained stable. After eight months of the intervention, treated caregivers were significantly less depressed than control-group caregivers.

Although comprehensive in-home interventions are not widely available, they hold great promise for persons with PD and their families. They provide highly individualized care to families, focus on developing family care skills, attend to long-term and acute problems, and monitor for transitions in health and care so that early intervention is possible.

Support Groups

Although support groups are the most available interventions for caregivers, there is great variability in the purpose and structure of these groups. Rigorous evaluation of support groups has been hampered by their enrollment practices – in general, caregivers self-select to join a support group when they are ready. Most evaluations of support groups in the literature depend on anecdotal comments from participants. Gonyea collected data from caregivers, some of whom had participated and others who had not participated in support groups, and examined the relationship between participation and caregiver well-being. Correlations between support group participation and three variables indicating well-being (objective burden, subjective burden, and morale) were small (ranging from 0.10 to 0.19) but statistically significant ($P < 0.05$). The strongest predictors of well-being in the multiple regression analyses, however, were caregiver and elder characteristics (59).

In some situations (e.g., people who are newly diagnosed with PD), support groups can be more frightening than comforting. In these cases, it may be desirable to refer the persons with PD and their families for peer support, typically to a person with a similar experience who is coping well. Such an approach is grounded in findings from Pillemer and Suitor, who highlighted the beneficial effects of interactions with people who have the same condition or experience (60).

CONCLUSION

For the estimated 1.5 million persons in the United States who have PD, family and friend caregivers are important mainstays in their everyday lives. These caregivers are also valuable resources for physicians, nurses, and other clinicians who provide health care to persons with PD. With the projected future increases in the elderly population, and the corresponding anticipated increases in the number of persons with PD, collaboration between family caregivers and health-care providers may be the key for improving the quality of care and quality of life of persons with PD. Such collaboration between families and providers may have the additional benefit of reducing caregiver strain and improving the satisfaction that families derive from caregiving. In the next century, we look forward to a growing number of creative interventions conducted by teams of clinicians and researchers to improve the health and well-being of persons with PD and of the families who care for them.

REFERENCES

1. Hobbs FB, Damon BL. United States Bureau of the Census. Current Population Reports, Special Studies, 65+ in the United States. Washington, D.C., United States Government Printing Office, 1996: 23–190.
2. National alliance for caregiving and the American association of retired persons. Family Caregiving in the United States: Findings from a National Survey. Bethesda, Md.: National alliance for caregiving and the American association of retired persons, 1997.
3. Stone R, Cafferata GL, Sangl J. Caregivers of the frail elderly: A national profile. The Gerontologist 1987; 27:616–626.
4. Whetten-Goldstein K, Sloan F, Kulas E, et al. The burden of Parkinson's disease on society, family, and the individual. JAGS 1997; 45:844–849.
5. Schulz R, OBrien AT, Bookwala J, et al. Psychiatric and physical morbidity effects of dementia caregiving: Prevalence, correlates, and causes. The Gerontologist 1995; 35:771–791.
6. Carter JH, Stewart BJ, Archbold PG, et al. Living with a person who has Parkinson's disease: The spouse's perspective by stage of disease. Mov Disord 1998; 13:20–28.
7. Pearlin LI, Mullan JT, Semple SJ, et al. Caregiving and the stress process: An overview of concepts and their measures. The Gerontologist 1990; 30(5):583–594.
8. Archbold PG, Stewart BJ, Greenlick MR, et al. Mutuality and preparedness as predictors of caregiver role strain. Res Nursing Health, 1990; 13:375–384.
9. Berry RA, Murphy JF. Well-being of caregivers of spouses with Parkinson's disease. Clin Nursing Res 1995; 4:373–386.
10. Montgomery RJV, Stull DE, Borgatta EF. Measurement and the analysis of burden. Res Aging 1985; 7(1):137–152.

a number of economic factors in her detailed analysis of the social and economic impact of PD. Among the findings in this study were that employment was substantially reduced among PD patients and that income from disability payments was increased compared with controls. There were also reductions in the ability to perform housework tasks and engage in leisure activities. More recent studies have attempted to arrive at a monetary figure for the annual cost of PD in the United States. These studies are made up of cost categories including direct costs such as formal medical services, home care and institutional care and medications, and indirect costs such as lost productivity and informal care provided by family members. These cost categories are summed to produce a cost per subject, and then the cost per subject is multiplied by an estimate of the prevalence of PD to arrive at an overall cost estimate. The components included in each study, variability in estimates of the cost of these components, and the estimate of the population prevalence of PD all contribute to differences between estimates.

The most detailed report on the economic impact of PD was prepared in 1998 for the Parkinson's Disease Foundation (PDF) (4). This study estimated the per-individual yearly cost of PD in 1997 at $24,041 ($24,425 in 1998). Based on a prevalence of one million affected individuals, the total economic burden was calculated at $24 billion. Direct medical costs contributed $8,872 or about one-third of the per-patient cost. These direct costs included physician visits and hospitalizations as well as use of allied medical professionals such as physical therapists, costs of assisted living, and nursing home costs. The estimate of drug costs of $2,137 used in this study may be an overestimate as the investigators used retail prices rather than wholesale costs. The remaining $15,169 per patient was made up by indirect costs including lost productivity in patients under 65 years of age and a fraction of patients between 65 and 74 years of age.

Few detailed reports of the costs associated with PD are published in the medical literature. In one study, Whetten-Goldstein and coworkers (11) interviewed 109 PD patients in central North Carolina. Measures in this study included direct medical costs, lost wages, and an estimate of the economic effect on family caregivers. The total costs per PD patient were estimated at $25,001 per year ($25,985 in 1998). Direct medical costs account for only $4,026 ($4,184 in 1998) of this cost, whereas lost wages of both patients and family caregivers comprise the remaining portion.

Rubenstein and coworkers (12) used data from the National Medical Expenditures Survey of 1987 to estimate the economic burden of PD. Out of a survey of 14,000 households, they identified 58 individuals with PD, of whom 43 had cost and health status estimates for an entire year. These individuals were compared to a control group matched for age, gender, race, urban-rural status, and presence of specific target conditions known to be highly associated with health resource use. People with PD were significantly more likely than controls to report lost productivity due to health problems, greater use of hospital visits, and longer duration of hospitalization for similar diagnoses. They were also more likely to visit physicians, use home health care services, and take significantly more prescription medications. Total direct medical expenditures in 1987 were $10,392 ($14,444 in 1998) per year for PD patients and $5,648 ($7,850 in 1998) more than that for controls. The authors commented that their estimates were somewhat imprecise because of their small sample. After adjusting for inflation, their estimate is also somewhat higher than the $4,026 estimate derived by Whetten-Goldstein and coworkers (11) and the $8,872 estimate used in the PDF study.

Dodel and coworkers (13) conducted a three-month prospective analysis of direct health care costs of PD including drug costs, hospitalization costs, office visits, diagnostic procedures, and nursing care among 20 PD patients in Germany. Informal care and lost productivity were not included in their estimate. Overall, these investigators found a three-month mean direct costs of 5,210 DM or $3,400 in 1995 ($3,639 in 1998). This annualized estimate ($14,556) is higher than those mentioned earlier and approximately 30 percent higher than an earlier estimate by the same investigators (14) based on review of medical records (i.e., retrospective) of 273 patients. Prospective measurements may lead to higher estimates of overall cost for several reasons. Prospective data collection may be more accurate as a result of more complete recall of resource use. However, prospective studies may also systematically inflate estimates because they tend to be made up of subjects who have recently come to medical attention. As a result the study sample may be biased toward patients with greater resource use. The ideal study would collect data on resource use prospectively from a sample of patients identified from a population of community dwelling individuals with PD. This information should also be validated by comparison with insurance claims.

INFLUENCE OF CLINICAL FEATURES ON RESOURCE USE

The study by Dodel and coworkers (13) also examined the impact of specific disease characteristics on resource use. These investigators found that patients with early disease (Hoehn and Yahr (H&Y) stage 1) were substantially less expensive than patients with advanced disease ($1,250 per year v5. $6,330 per year). They also found that patients experiencing motor fluctuations had substantially higher costs ($4,260) than those who did not have motor fluctuations ($1,960). This study is unique in that it is the only published report to express the impact of disease characteristics in monetary terms.

Several other studies have evaluated the effect of disease severity on resource use. Chrischilles and coworkers (15) conducted a detailed study of resource use in 193 patients with PD attending two university-based neurology clinics in Iowa. These investigators measured a number of economic factors including use of formal medical services, ancillary and community services, as well as durable medical equipment. Days out from work due to PD and premature retirement due to PD were recorded as measures of lost productivity. Caregiver burden was not assessed. There was a strong relationship between disease severity as measured by H&Y stage and use of resources. For example, three times as many patients with H&Y stage 3 disease reported use of emergency room services, compared with those with stage 1 or 1.5 (14.8% v. 40.7%) over a 12-month period of time.

We (unpublished data) conducted a survey of resource use of 428 patients attending a movement disorders clinic. Patients and caregivers completed a detailed questionnaire including items on disability for activities of daily living, use of direct medical services, drug use, and employment status. As in the study by Chrischilles and coworkers (15), a strong relationship between disease status and resource use was found. We also found that certain PD symptoms such as motor fluctuations, hallucinations, and confusion were strongly associated with resource use and negatively associated with employment. This is consistent with a previous study that showed that the presence of visual hallucinations was strongly associated with the need for nursing home placement (8). Our survey, although limited by lack of verification of patient self-report of resource use, suggests that nonmotor symptoms are an important factor associated with resource use in PD.

There are many other potential factors that may influence the costs associated with PD (Table 57-1). In other neurologic conditions, factors such as specialty of the treating physician and insurance type have been considered as additional determinants of health care costs (16,17). These factors are an area for future research in PD. Evaluation of these factors and population-based studies that use prospective and

Table 57-1 Determinants of Parkinson's Disease Cost

Patient-level factors:
  Disease severity
    Motor symptoms
    Nonmotor symptoms
  Patient age
  Employment status
  Co-morbidities
  Social factors
?Specialty of treating physician*
?Type of health insurance*
  Fee-for-service
  Capitated delivery system

*These factors have not been studied in PD but are important in other medical conditions.

verifiable methods to ascertain costs are needed to better characterize the economic burden of PD.

COST OF MEDICATIONS AND SURGERY FOR PARKINSON'S DISEASE

Spending on prescription drugs has grown much faster than spending for other types of health care goods and services (1). In the early 1990s (18), it was suggested that the introduction of new neurologic drugs including immuno-modulators for multiple sclerosis and triptans for migraine, among others, could result in increases in direct costs of over $6 billion per year. Drug treatment in PD is one of the largest contributors in the overall direct medical costs associated with this disorder (19). In 1997 two dopamine agonists (pramipexole and ropinirole) were approved for use in patients with PD, and in 1998 the catechol-O-methyltransferase inhibitor, tolcapone, was approved for use. These new medications have been shown to improve function for patients with PD. They are also relatively expensive. Table 57-2 shows the cost of commonly prescribed drugs used in PD. On the basis of average wholesale prices, it was found that a year of treatment with one of the new dopamine agonists is likely to cost approximately $2,000 (20). The cost of a year of treatment with tolcapone is likewise $2,000. These figures compare to a year of carbidopa/levodopa, which costs $600 based on six tablets per day (generic). Surgical therapies including pallidotomy and deep brain stimulation (DBS) have very high initial costs (21), but could be associated with long-term savings. Cost-effectiveness research can be used to assess the costs and health consequences of these new medical and surgical interventions and suggests that lost productivity and costs associated with informal care provided by family members account for the greatest part of the overall economic burden of PD. Direct medical costs become more important for patients with advanced disease who would have been unlikely to remain employed even without PD. These patients are also more likely to use expensive services such as ER visits, hospitalizations, home care, and nursing home care. The presence of specific PD symptoms such as motor fluctuations and nonmotor symptoms such as hallucinations are also associated with increasing resource use.

Cost-effectiveness research will provide new insights into the economics of PD and to the value of PD treatments. The economic toll of PD is of increasing importance as health care systems seek to contain costs while maintaining, or improving, quality of care. Because PD is highly disabling and expensive, it is likely that even modestly effective therapies are likely to be of good value. The burden of proof, however, depends on the careful conduct of cost-effectiveness analyses of PD-related technologies and the critical appraisal of the results. Only then can the medical community translate the knowledge learned from these studies into strategies for promoting improvements in the prevention and treatment of PD.

REFERENCES

1. Levit K, Cowan C, Braden B, et al. National health expenditures in 1997: More slow growth. *Health Affairs* 1998; 17:99–110.
2. Bodenheimer T. The movement for improved quality in health care. *New Engl J Med* 1999; 340:488–492.
3. Parkinson's Disease: Hope Through Research. Bethesda, MD: Office of Communication and Public Liaison, NINDS, 1994.
4. The Average Per-Patient Costs of Parkinson's Disease. New York: John Robbins Associates, 1998.
5. The Cost of Disorders of the Brain. Washington D.C.: National Foundation for Brain Research, 1992.
6. Schappert S. Office visits to neurologists: United States, 1991–1992. *Adv Data* 1995; 267:1–20.
7. Haupt B. An overview of home health and hospice care patients: 1996 national home and hospice care survey. *Adv Data* 1998; 297:1–36.
8. Goetz CG, Stebbins GT. Risk factors for nursing home placement in advanced Parkinson's disease. *Neurology* 1993; 43:2227–2229.
9. Mitchell SL, Kiely DK, Kiel DP, et al. The epidemiology, clinical characteristics, and natural history of older nursing home residents with a diagnosis of Parkinson's disease. *J Am Geriatr Soc* 1996; 44:394–399.
10. Singer E. Social costs of Parkinson's disease. *J Chron Dis* 1973; 26:243–254.
11. Whetten-Goldstein K, Sloan F, Kulas E, et al. The burden of Parkinson's disease on society, family, and the individual. *J Am Geriatr Soc* 1997; 45:844–849.
12. Rubenstein LM, Chrischilles EA, Voelker MD. The impact of Parkinson's Disease on health status, health expenditures and productivity. *Pharmacoeconomics* 1997; 12:486–497.
13. Dodel RC, Singer MS, Kohne-Volland R, et al. The economic impact of Parkinson's Disease. *Pharm Econ* 1998; 14:299–312.
14. Dodel RC, Eggert KM, Oertel WH. Costs of Parkinson's Disease – A preliminary retrospective survey, In: Stern MB (ed.). *Beyond the Decade of the Brain.* Kent, U.K. Wells Medical Limited, 1994:59–72.
15. Chrischilles EA, Rubenstein LM, Voelker MD et al. The health burdens of Parkinson's disease. *Mov Disord* 1998; 13:406–413.
16. Manone M, Kanter DS, Glynn RJ, et al. Variability in length of hospitalization for stroke: The role of managed care in an elderly population. *Arch Neurol* 1996; 53:875–880.
17. Mitchell JB, Ballard PA, Whisnant JP, et al. What role do neurologists play in determining the costs and outcomes of stroke patients? *Stroke* 1996; 27:1937–1943.
18. Gunderson CH. The impact of new pharmaceutical agents on the cost of neurologic care. *Neurology* 1995; 45:569–572.
19. Dodel RC, Eggert KM, Singer MS, et al. Costs of drug treatment in Parkinson's disease. *Mov Disord* 1998; 13:249–254.
20. Redbook. *1997 Drug Topics Red Book: Pharmacy's Fundamental Reference.* Montvale, N.J.: Medical Economic Company, 1998.
21. Siderowf A, Holloway R, Mushlin AI. Cost-effectiveness of pallidotomy and add-on medical therapy in advanced Parkinson's disease. *Ann Neurol* 1998; 44:517(Abstract).
22. Holloway RG. Cost-effectiveness analysis: What is it and how will it influence neurology. *Ann Neurol* 1996; 39:818–823.
23. Eisenberg JM. Clinical economics: A guide to the economic analysis of clinical practices. *JAMA* 1989; 262:2879–2886.
24. Hoerger TJ, Bala MV, Rowland C, et al. Cost-effectiveness of pramipexole in Parkinson's disease in the United States. *Pharmacoeconomics* 1998; 14:541–557.
25. Kurlan R, Clark S, Shoulson I, et al. Economic impact of protective therapy for early Parkinson's disease. *Ann Neurol* 1988; 24:153(Abstract).
26. Phelps CE, Mushlin AI. On the (near) equivalence of cost-effectiveness and cost–benefit analyses. *Int J Technol Assess Health Care* 1991; 7:12–21.
27. Drummond MF, O'Brien B, Stoddard Gl, et al. Cost-utility analysis. *Methods for the Economic Evaluation*

of Health Care Programmes. New York: Oxford University Press, 1997; 138–204.

28. Kaplan RM, Anderson JP. The general health policy model: An integrated approach, In: Spilker B (ed.). Quality of life and pharmacoeconomics in clinical trials, 2nd ed. Philadelphia: Lippincott-Raven, 1996:309–322.

29. Lee TT, Solomon NA, Heidenreich PA, et al. Cost-effectiveness of screening for carotid stenosis in asymptomatic patients. *Ann Intern Med* 1997; 126:337–346.

30. Weinstein MC, Siegel JE, Gold MR, Kamlet, MS, Russell LB. Recommendations of the panel on cost-effectiveness in health and medicine. *JAMA* 1996; 276:1253–1258.

58

Driving

Stewart A. Factor, D.O.

Parkinson's Disease and Movement Disorder Center of Albany Medical Center, Albany, New York
and

William J. Weiner, M.D.

University of Maryland School of Medicine, Baltimore, Maryland

INTRODUCTION

Driving is a complicated task that nearly all members of society now learn at a young age (15–20 yrs). It involves a variety of psychomotor activities including perception, information processing, judgement, decision making, sequential and simultaneous movements of limbs, reaction-time tasks, continuous tracking, and attentional tasks. These functions allow for appropriate judgement of distance and speed, application of control forces for braking and accelerating, and the negotiation of curves and hazards that may come up while driving. Over the years, driving ability becomes deeply ingrained with continuous practice so that loss of some function may not necessarily alter one's ability to drive in a noticeable way. Determining when a disease has progressed to the point of impairing driving can be difficult. Although assessment of the earlier noted parameters in elderly patients with and without neurodegenerative disease is complicated, there are other concerns that add to the complexity. They include the social and political ramifications. The reason driving is such an important social issue in North America is that the car provides a means to visit family, attend social and cultural events, shop, and visit health care providers. There is also a culturally engendered value where the car and a driver's license represent symbols of independence. If they are lost, so is independence. And alternative options are not always available. Some patients will not give up their license even if they do not use it. Pullen and coworkers (1) demonstrated in an in-patient study that 90 elderly patients who had given up driving on their own, years before the evaluation, maintained their driver's license. When interviewed, the elderly voiced the loss of the car as being a sign of becoming more dependent and requiring them to stay closer to home and having less social interactions. Many elderly patients are quite upset about the prospect of life without a car. "There is no public transportation in my area. I would be stranded in my apartment with no reliable means of getting to and from the store no less the doctor. I do not know what I would do." "Not driving means that I would have to move since I would become more dependent for the simplest activities. Moving means uprooting the whole range of social interactions and friends that I currently have. Not driving would be extremely disruptive (2)." The concerns of Parkinson's disease (PD) patients are quite similar. They also voice concerns regarding the increased reliance on other family members to take time to help them even when the family member freely volunteers to help out. They will go as far as trying to hide their illness from the motor vehicle bureau to maintain a license. Gimenez-Roldan and coworkers (3), on examining the issue of renewal of drivers licenses, found that at renewal time 63 percent of PD patients did not volunteer information on their disease for fear of losing their license.

We are faced with the issues of whether a PD patient should still drive on almost a daily basis. It is often broached by family members, spouses, or children, and the issue frequently causes a family rift. Attempts are made on both sides to get the treating neurologist to see their point of view. How can we deal with this issue in an educated manner? We hope to address this in this chapter. In doing so we will first discuss some important issues regarding the elderly, since most PD patients are elderly. Then we will discuss what is known about driving in PD. We will provide the treating neurologist with a plan to follow when dealing with this situation in practice.

DRIVING AND THE ELDERLY

Individuals over age 65 years make up between 13 and 17 percent of licensed drivers (4). In the traffic safety literature, there is an extensive field of study related to investigations of the elderly safe driver (2). Driving performance may be affected by several factors that relate to the physiologic changes of aging, disease processes, and the medications used to treat them. Although there has been criticism about the individual efforts to study aging drivers, suggesting that they are too focused on narrow measurable parameters not consistent with the overall everyday reality elderly drivers face, it is of more than passing interest to recognize studies that have examined sensory decrements, muscular degeneration, visual deficits, perception changes, attention problems, dichotic listening decrements, reaction times, psychomotor slowing, and glare impairment.

All of these studies lead to well-established facts concerning driving in the elderly. These facts may form the basis of public policy decisions because in North America the percentage of drivers over the age of fifty-five is expected to continue to increase into the next century. The major conclusions regarding the elderly healthy driver include: (1) Elderly drivers are under represented in accident statistics; (2) Studies based on actual miles driven in a year show that the elderly driver is the second-most accident prone group, second only to teenagers; (3) When the elderly are involved in automobile accidents, the most frequent problems include turning improperly, particularly to the left, failure to yield the right of way, starting up improperly in traffic, and ignoring traffic signals; (4) The elderly have a far better record with regard to alcohol-related motor vehicle accidents; (5) Physical fragility makes the elderly more prone to be a traffic fatality (5). Motor vehicle accidents are the leading cause of death by unintentional injury in the 65 to 74 age group and second for those who are 75 or older after falling (6); (6) Elderly people are poor judges of their own ability to drive, and this is especially true when health issues come into play (1).

Several studies examining characteristics of active elderly drivers are of interest. Although medical conditions and their associated morbidity, including visual and cognitive deficits, lead to driving cessation and decreased driving activity (7,8), many impaired patients continue to drive. In one study of outpatients seen in a geriatric clinic (9), drivers, as compared with nondrivers, were younger, more often male, and scored higher on a mental status exam. Even so, 40 percent of drivers were diagnosed with Alzheimer's disease and 26 percent were impaired with regard to activities of daily living. In another study of in-patients (1), 37 of 498 interviewed patients were active drivers and only five of these met the established medical criteria for safe driving. These findings underscore safety concerns related to the fact that unqualified people are on the road and the difficulty in determining whom of the elderly should not drive and how this decision can be established. Despite their decision to continue driving, there is evidence that the elderly compensate for increasing driving impairment. This includes (1) driving less at night, (2) avoiding unfamiliar roads, (3) avoiding rush hours, (4) avoiding poor weather conditions and (5) driving more slowly (5,7). However, they still drive frequently (5,7) but under familiar, safer surroundings. Despite this behavior and the fact that they receive fewer traffic violations, evidence indicates that while driving actively, their risk of involvement in a motor vehicle accident remains higher. Slower driving may lead to a more prolonged exposure to a high-risk situation (5). This may be the reason left turns appear to be so hazardous to the elderly.

Specific correlates that may lead to increased risk of motor vehicle accidents include that for drivers over the age of 64, and particularly over the age of seventy-four, the proportion of accidents occurring on poor road conditions at night is exaggerated (2). Also, data on the relative probability of accident responsibility by age in a large data set involving over 88,000 accidents clearly delineates that drivers over the age of seventy-five are more likely to be the cause of accidents (2).

What might explain the deterioration in driving seen in the elderly? Two broad areas are of particular concern in relation to the physiology of aging. The first is that visual disturbances are increasing problems for elderly drivers. Poor vision is the most common reason for cessation of driving. Sorting relevant information from a wide array of competing influences becomes increasingly difficult in the elderly. Recognition-response activities become harder, and when additional tasks are superimposed, for example, tuning on a car radio or speaking on a cellular phone, responsiveness becomes even more compromised. The second problem area is the decision-making process following extraction of pertinent information from the driving environment. Elderly drivers require more time to make such decisions. Elderly drivers are able to decide better to maintain the direction of the vehicle in a driving situation than to change directions on short notice. This is reflected by the increasing involvement of elderly drivers in motor vehicle accidents that occur at intersections. A test used to evaluate combined visual and cognitive changes is referred to as the "Useful field of view" (UFOV). This is a computer-administered test for visual attention. It is divided into three parts: (1) central vision and processing speed; (2) divided attention-recognizing objects both centrally and peripherally; and (3) selective attention, which utilizes distractors and forces the driver to focus on that object is of greater significance. The score leads to a measure of risk for motor vehicle accidents. This test has been used in studies (10) and in practice to evaluate driving ability in those who may be at risk.

Elderly drivers are also confronted with deterioration in information processing, depth judgement, and reaction speed. However, The degree and age when these difficulties in any given individual become significant is quite variable, and the exact relationship with these changes and accident risk are not entirely understood. Therefore, there is resistance to limiting driver licenses by a set age or even to determine a specific age of mandatory retesting.

Driving difficulties in the elderly may also relate to medical illnesses, functional disabilities, or the medications used to treat them. Several studies have examined these issues. Medical conditions frequently associated with motor vehicle accidents and ultimate driving cessation include cardiac disease, diabetes mellitus, Alzheimer's disease, Parkinson's disease, seizure disorders, stroke, and sleep apnea (4). One study (10) suggested that functional disabilities and nonspecific diagnoses or age predict at-fault motor vehicle accidents. In addition to visual difficulties measured by UFOV, falling was associated with increased crashes. The authors suggested that risk factors for crashes and falling were similar, but further study is needed. Falling with fractures was also associated with cessation of driving in women, perhaps due to osteoporosis (7). Another study found that foot abnormalities and decreased range of motion of the neck were important (4). In this study, association analyses demonstrated a strong predictive value of three factors – poor near vision (usually associated with poor distant vision as well), poor visual attention, and poor range of motion of the neck. These were retrospective studies, and one author felt that the results might lead to an office-based screening tool, but prospective evaluations would be needed to confirm their usefulness. Drug therapy (tricyclics, hypnotics, opiates) also play an important role in the occurrence of automotive crashes in the elderly, especially in males (11). The side effects of these drugs and resultant effect on driving ability may be enhanced due to advanced age, illness, or concomitant medication. Sims and coworkers (10) found that the use of beta-blockers was associated with fewer crashes. It may be that these drugs reduce anxiety and tremor therefore decreasing the risk of accidents. Many patients have more than one ailment or are on several drugs, so co-morbidity

issues are important, but proper studies have, as yet, not been completed.

It is clear that several concerns exist about the safe driving of elderly individuals. Further study is needed to sort out what factors result in the increased risk for crashes and how steps can be made to counsel drivers appropriately with regard to rescinding that privilege. One can see how the addition of a disease like PD with several motor and cognitive features could further complicate these issues. That is a concern we, as neurologists, must wrestle with often.

DRIVING IN PARKINSON'S DISEASE

Although it is known that PD is a common cause of driving cessation (12), in truth, the issue of driving has not been very well examined in this patient population. Patients with PD experience a number of abnormalities of function vital to driving safety. Motor function, visual perceptive activities, reaction time, attention maintenance, and information processing are all abnormal. Although the question of whether a PD patient should or should not drive is addressed frequently in movement disorder clinics, there is limited data that helps us to make an appropriate decision. The social issues delineated in the introduction make the decision to withdraw a patient's driving privileges more difficult. As one addresses this complicated topic, the main question that arises is what do we know about driving and PD? In the following paragraphs this information is reviewed.

Is Driving Impaired in PD?

Driving ability has been evaluated using simulators and driving tests with a series of computer-aided laboratory tests. Madeley et al. (13) used a simulator in which patients were evaluated for their ability to react with steering adjustments, respond to light changes, and utilize foot pedals. They examined 10 PD patients who were active drivers, four PD patients who had given up driving, and 10 age- and sex-matched controls. They found that the PD patients had impaired accuracy, driving reaction time, and light recognition, as they missed a number of light changes.

Lings and Dupont (14) also used a simulator ("mock car") to evaluate driving in 28 PD patients, 18 with a driver's license (five no longer driving) and 10 without (five gave it up and five never had one), and 109 controls. Controls were not age-matched and were, in fact, younger (median age 49) than the PD patients (median age 65). The duration of disease was 8.75 years and mean Hoehn and Yahr stage was 2.2. Twenty-one had mild motor fluctuations, 14 had mild dyskinesia, and none had on-off. The authors specified that patients were selected by their lack of major complicating problems. The simulator used measured the following items: grip strength, force applied by hand and foot, isometric force while turning the steering wheel, reaction time to audio and visual stimuli in hand and foot, choice reaction times, direction and speed of steering wheel turning, patterns of steering wheel movements, and erroneous reactions. Results demonstrated the following in PD patients: (1) reduced grip strength, (2) significantly reduced speed of movement, (3) significantly increased reaction times – the consequence of which was a prolonged reaction length, (4) increased frequency and more serious errors, mostly directional in nature (wrong turns). Sixty-one percent of PD patients compared with 32 percent of controls had one error, 21 percent PD and 6 percent controls had two or more errors. There were 57 percent of PD patients with directional errors, and 22 percent were seen in controls. Some patients completely failed to react to signals. When only licensed drivers were analyzed, similar results occurred.

Heikkila and coworkers (15) studied driving ability in PD patients using a 45-minute driving test and a series of computer-aided lab tests, including visual short-term memory, perceptual flexibility and decision making, vigilance, complex choice-reaction times, information-processing capacity reaction, and stress-tolerance test. They tested 20 men with PD stages I–III and 20 age-matched controls. The PD patients were regular drivers with no motor fluctuations. The driving test demonstrated an increase in risky faults that could lead to danger and infractions with the law. The patients had difficulty driving in traffic flow, difficulty turning left, as seen in the elderly, and greatest difficulty in urban conditions. Highway driving, surprisingly, was not impaired when compared with controls, perhaps because there is no need for a direction change. There was wide individual variation of driving ability in the PD group. The laboratory studies demonstrated more difficulties in the PD group with visual memory testing, choice-reaction time, and information-processing capacity. These findings were seen even in mild to moderate stages of disease, and they correlated with driving test difficulties, particularly the number of risky faults. The conclusions were that PD significantly influenced driving ability even in mild to moderate disease, although the milder patients were considered to be still competent.

These three studies indicate that, even in milder PD patients, driving impairment is detectable. Many of the patients tested were active drivers indicating, as seen

with the elderly in general, that some patients with substantial impairment remain behind the wheel.

Do PD Patients Have Insight into Their Driving Difficulties?

Dubinsky and coworkers (16) reported on the results of a retrospective survey of 150 PD patients and 100 controls with regard to driving ability. They found that 32 out of 150 (21 percent) stopped driving, 18 because they were concerned with their own safety and 10 because of safety concerns of the family. It was also noted that PD patients compensate for their difficulties by driving larger vehicles, driving under the speed limit and avoiding rush-hour traffic and hazardous weather conditions. Gimenez-Roldan and coworkers (17) used a semi-structured questionnaire in 166 PD patients and age-, sex-, social background-matched controls to assess this question. Of those PD patients, only 37 percent (62 patients) still had their driver's license; 19.2 percent (32 patients) were still active drivers. Only 40 percent of the patients were still driving after five years of disease. Eighty percent of exdrivers quit because of PD. 53 percent of active drivers were aware of difficulties with driving, including managing foot pedals and judging distances. These particular patients also made adjustments in their driving habits to compensate, including reducing speed and decreasing the number of hours behind the wheel. Thus these patients seem to have an awareness of their difficulties and limitations. In all likelihood, some continue to drive actively although they should not, and many know that they should not. The number of such patients is not known.

Do PD Patients Have Higher Incidences of Motor Vehicle Accidents or Moving Violations?

A review of the United Kingdom department of transportation records indicates that PD is not an important cause of motor vehicle accidents (18). Data from other countries suggest that fewer, not more, accidents than expected are due to PD because of the limitations and adjustments they place on themselves in driving. Dubinsky and coworkers (16) also found that PD patients did not have more frequent accidents; however, it was discovered that PD patients did experience more accidents per mile of driving.

Who Is the Best Judge for Driving Ability of PD Patients?

The patients usually believe they can judge. Family members try to leave it up to the neurologist. Despite their insight, patients themselves are not good judges of their own ability to drive, and in the report by Heikkila and coworkers (15), their own evaluation did not correlate with those of driving instructor. Neurologists tended to overestimate driving ability in PD patients in this study. This may relate to the apparent lack of correlation between severity of disease and driving inability. There is no correlation between Hoehn and Yahr stage, mini mental status exam, and levodopa dose with driving capability (15). This, however, is controversial. Madeley and coworkers (13) demonstrated a correlation between the results of simulator testing and the Webster severity scale but Lings and Dupont did not (14). However, Dubinsky and coworkers (16) demonstrated poor correlation between Northwestern University Parkinson's disease rating scale, Hoehn and Yahr scale, and Schwab and England scale with driving ability and number of motor vehicle accidents. However, they did show that there was some correlation between Hoehn and Yahr stage and motor vehicle accidents and that more occurred at Stage III. In an unpublished study by Weiner, patients with PD who were still driving were younger (66 vs. 74) and had a shorter duration of disease (5 vs. 8 years) compared with nondrivers. In addition, drivers had significantly lower total UPDRS scores and Schwab and England disability scores than nondrivers. It appears there is more to the driving difficulties of PD patients than motor disability as there is no consistent relationship. Finally, driving instructors using simulators or actual driving tests appear to be the best judges for driving ability in PD patients. There is no data on the ability of family members to judge.

What Clinical Features Particular to PD Impair Driving Ability?

Those that appear to have an impact on driving are motor symptomatology including dyskinesia, fluctuations, and tremor. As previously noted in nonparkinsonian elderly, correlation was observed between falling and motor vehicle accidents (7,10). This has not been studied in PD. The role of drug therapy is not clear (see Driving and "Sleep Attacks," p. 652). Aging may also play a role.

Cognitive difficulties such as dementia, hallucinations, and confusion occur in 20 to 30 percent of PD patients. The dementia has a progressive nature similar to Alzheimer's disease; in fact, some patients actually have Alzheimer's disease associated with their PD (see Chapters 15,16). The role of dementia in the driving difficulties of PD patients has not been studied. However, there is a substantive literature on Alzheimer's disease and, as a disease with purely cognitive deficits, the information gathered could provide some insight into the role of dementia on driving problems in PD. Although all Alzheimer patients eventually stop driving, several questions surround the issue, especially in the early years. During on-road tests, Alzheimer patients have demonstrated significant concern. One study of 19 patients with an average duration of disease of four years demonstrated a failure rate of >60 percent (19). Another demonstrated a 19 percent failure rate in "very mild" patients and a 41 percent rate in those considered "mild" compared with 3 percent in controls, indicating that driving impairment occurs very early in the course of disease (20). There is also an increased rate of motor vehicle accidents as demonstrated by simulator tests (21) and a questionnaire survey (22). The survey study demonstrated that the increased risk for crashes in the first 2 to 3 years of Alzheimer's disease is modest, and the yearly rate is lower than in young people up to the mid twenties. In addition, the accident rate is within the accepted risk for all registered drivers. However, the risk increases with duration of disease. There is marked variability in driving ability in the early years. Medical assessment and duration of disease do not correlate directly with the occurrence of unsafe driving practices. Drachman and coworkers (22) recommended the use of direct driving tests to decipher the individual's competence. There have been attempts to find parameters that will act as predictors to driving ability in the office setting. Those studied include tests of attention processing such as UFOV, Benton visual retention and digit span (23), and these seemed to be better than measures of dementia severity or other psychometric tests. A traffic sign naming test has also been used (24), but these need further study. It is clear that dementia alone can be a significant obstacle to safely guiding a motor vehicle. Consider the addition of those visual aspects associated with aging compounded with dementia and the motor features of PD and one can begin to realize the complexity of assessing driving in PD.

How Should Patients Be Evaluated for Driving Capability?

Road test under normal conditions, driving simulators and cognitive tests as described earlier (2–4) may all need to be used. None of these is sensitive enough when used alone. Certainly, medical evaluation is not sensitive as shown in one study (13), where only 30 percent of PD cases were detected and 10.8 percent had their license revoked. Many hospitals or rehabilitation centers have driving test programs as part of the occupational therapy programs. These programs not only assess driving ability but provide education, provide appropriate adaptive equipment, and train drivers to use it. They also teach compensatory techniques as needed. In one local program in upstate New York, the assessment is a two-step process. First is an initial screening phase in which a detailed review

Index

Note: Boldface numbers indicate illustrations; italic t indicates a table.

Speech and voice disorders (*Continued*)
  thyroarytenoid (TA) muscle weakness in, 76
  treatment for, 75
  tremor in, laryngeal, 76
  vidoestroboscopic examination in, 76
  voice onset time (VOT) assessment in, 77
  voice quality in (hoarseness, breathiness, etc.), 76
Sphygmograph to record tremors, 19, **20**
Spin trapping agents (*See also* Antioxidants), 306
Spinal cord, 189, 195, 203, 213, 220, 367
Spinocerebella ataxia, 32
Spondylotic myelopathy, 45
Sporadic olivopontocerebellar atrophy (OPCA), 603
Staging of disease in PD (*See also* Quantitative measures
    and ratings scales), 33, 37–38, 44–45, 51, 110–112
Start hesitation in gait disturbances, 59
Startle reflex, 247
Statistical parametric mapping (SPM) analysis, 251
Steele-Richardson-Olszewski syndrome (*See* Progressive
    supranuclear palsy)
Stem cells, neural, in transplantation, 570–572
Step-Seconds test, 414
Stereotactic pallidotomy (*See also* Neurosurgery;
    Pallidotomy), 27, 62–63, 485–486, 531
Stern, Matthew B., 481
Stewart, Barbara J., 627
Stiffness of muscles, 43
Striatum, 199, 235
Stress and PD, 274
Stress-activated protein kinase (SAPK), 293
Stria terminalis, 235
Striatofugal projections of basal ganglia, direct and indirect,
    212–213
Striatonigral degeneration (*See* Nigrostriatal degeneration)
Striatum (*See also* Basal ganglia), 3, 70, 71, 187–188, 195,
    196, 201–205, 211–216, 221, 235, 236, 238, 255, 292,
    330, 332, 340, 350, 427
Stride length in gait disturbances, 60
Stroke, 10, 46, 175–176, 266
Stroop Color-Word test for, 127
Structural lesions and parkinsonism, 615–617
Subdural hematoma, 175
Subnucleus compactus of PD brain, 184–185, **184**
Substance P, 71, 152, 175, 195, 204, 205, 233
Substantia nigra (SN), substantia nigra pars compacta
    (SNPC) (*See also* Basal ganglia), 190, **196**, 216, 235, 243,
    268, 273, 274, 281, 284, 285, 292, 332, 340, 344, 486,
    495, 611
  apoptosis and, 292
  basal ganglia and (*See* Basal ganglia)
  in cortical basal ganglionic degeneration (CBGD), 606
  dementia and, 127, 130–131
  dopamine receptors and, 236
  dopaminergic neuronal loss in, 41–42, 95, 109, 131, 200,
    215–216, 219
  excitatory amino acid receptor antagonists and, 423,
    427–430
  histopathology of PD and, 183–188, **184**, **185**
  intranigral selective vulnerability to MPTP in, 313–314

  MPTP-induced PD and, 300
  in multiple system atrophy (MSA), 604
  neurochemistry of PD and, 195, 200, 201, 205, 211
  neuronal damage and, 481
  nigrostriatal degeneration (*See* Nigrostriatal
    degeneration/loss)
  in progressive supranuclear palsy (PSP), 601
  sensory symptoms associated with, 70–71
  in young onset or juvenile PD, 582
Subthalamic nucleus (STN), 195, **196**, 211–217, 221, 301,
    344, 427–428, 450–451
  excitatory amino acid receptor antagonists and,
    430–431
  in gait disturbances, 63
  in progressive supranuclear palsy (PSP), 601
  stereotactic surgery for, 485
Subthalamic stimulation (*See also* Deep brain stimulation;
    Pallidal stimulation; Thalamic stimulation), 28, 559–565,
    559
Subtypes of dopamine receptors, 28
Super off states, 446
Superior colliculi, 195, 211, 213, 601
Superior temporal sulcus, **235**
Superoxides (*See also* Antioxidants), 281, 285, 307
Superoxide dismutase (SOD), 344, 429, 483, 488, 513
Supplementary motor area (SMA), 82, 212, 214, 220
Supplementary motor area (SMA)-associated loops, 60
Support groups, 635
Supranuclear gaze palsy (SNGP), 600
Surgical therapies (*See* Neurosurgery)
Surmontil (*See* Trimipramine)
Survey Assessment of Positive Symptoms (SAPS), 413
survival analysis in parkinsonism in, 35–36, **36**, **37**,
    346–347
Swallowing disorders (dysphagia), 9, 47, 75, 77–78,
    88–90, 459–460
  aspiration pneumonia and, 75
  behavioral modification vs., 78–79
  drug therapies for, 78
  gastrointestinal disorders and, 88
  incidence of, 75, 77
  Lee Silverman Voice Treatment (LSVT) in, 75, 82
  neurosurgical treatment of, 78
  oral phase dysfunction in, 78
  pallidotomy vs., 78
  pharyngeal phase dysfunction in, 78
  symptoms of, 75
  thalamotomy, bilateral, in treatment of, 78
  treatment for, 75, 82
  triggering of swallowing reflex in, 78
Sweating/flushing (*See also* Thermoregulation), 95,
    456–459, 603
Symmetrel (*See* Amantadine)
Sympathetic skin responses (SSRs), 96
Symptomatic parkinsonism, 611–619
Symptoms of PD, 6, 8, 14–15, 21–23, 32, 42–45, 110,
    202, 243, 244*t*, 295, 300, 437
  cardinal features of early PD, 41–56
  clinical presentation of, 110